# The Washington Manual™ of Medical Therapeutics

# The Washington Manual™ of Medical Therapeutics

31st Edition

Department of Medicine
Washington University
School of Medicine
St. Louis, Missouri

Gopa B. Green, M.D.
Ian S. Harris, M.D.
Grace A. Lin, M.D.
Kyle C. Moylan, M.D.
Editors

Robyn A. Schaiff, Pharm.D., B.C.P.S.
Associate Editor for
Pharmacotherapeutics

LIPPINCOTT WILLIAMS & WILKINS
A Wolters Kluwer Company
Philadelphia • Baltimore • New York • London
Buenos Aires • Hong Kong • Sydney • Tokyo

*Acquisitions Editor*: James Ryan
*Developmental Editor*: Erin McMullan
*Supervising Editor*: Michael Mallard
*Production Editors*: Erica Broennle Nelson and Lucinda Ewing, Silverchair Science + Communications
*Manufacturing Manager*: Colin Warnock
*Cover Designer*: Patricia Gast
*Compositor*: Silverchair Science + Communications
*Printer*: RR Donnelley Crawfordsville



Printed in the USA

ISBN 0781746388



10 9 8 7 6 5 4 3

**To our firm chiefs, Megan Wren, Gerald Medoff, and William Clutter, for their commitment to the education and well-being of the Medical House Staff at Barnes-Jewish Hospital**

# Contents

# Preface

This 31st edition of *The Washington Manual™ of Medical Therapeutics* is the first published since the appearance of the first edition of our companion text, *The Washington Manual™ of Ambulatory Therapeutics*. Since its inception in 1943 by the Department of Medicine at Washington University, *The Washington Manual™* has been used by house officers and medical students as a practical, portable reference for the care of hospitalized medical patients. As medicine has grown more complex, the *Manual* has necessarily grown in scope, encompassing topics relevant not only to inpatient medicine, but also to outpatient clinic and office practice. The development of *The Ambulatory Manual* has afforded us the opportunity to return to the original intent of this text and to focus our discussion on acute inpatient medicine.

In keeping with the tradition of the *Manual*, the authors are primarily junior faculty at Washington University—physicians who can recall what is practical and important when taking care of acutely ill patients in the middle of the night. The chapters have been somewhat reorganized to reflect our more keen focus on inpatient medicine. As always, the content has been extensively revised to ensure that it is consistent with current medical practice.

*The Washington Manual™* was originally produced as a small handbook designed for use by house officers within the Department of Medicine at Washington University. Over the past 60 years, it has grown to be not only the best-selling medical text in the world, but also a veritable institution of medical education, instantly familiar to generations of physicians around the globe. We are proud to be part of this tradition.

We are grateful for the assistance of the pharmacy staff at Barnes-Jewish Hospital, particularly that of Robyn Schaiff, our Associate Editor for Pharmacotherapeutics. We would also like to thank Katie Sharp and the editorial staff at Lippincott Williams & Wilkins for their assistance and Alison Whelan, an editor of the 27th edition of the *Manual*, for her support.

We have had the pleasure of serving as chief residents of the Shatz-Strauss, Karl-Flance, and Kipnis-Daughaday firms and of the Wohl Clinic of the Department of Medicine at Washington University, under the guidance of our firm chiefs Megan Wren, William Clutter, Gerald Medoff, and Jason Goldfeder, as well as Daniel Goodenberger, Chief of the Division of Medical Education, and Kenneth Polonsky, Chairman of Medicine.

We would especially like to thank our families Ashim, Bani, Doug, and Julia; Cliff, Mark, Lee, and Chris; George, Jean, Tammy, and Alice; and Lesli and Evan for their support.

G.B.G.
I.S.H.
G.A.L.
K.C.M.

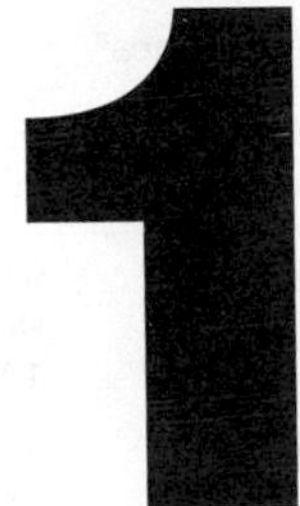

# Patient Care in Internal Medicine

Yoon Kang and
Michael E. Lazarus

## General Care of the Hospitalized Patient

Although a general approach to common problems can be outlined, **therapy must be individualized.** All diagnostic and therapeutic procedures should be explained carefully to the patient, including the potential risks, benefits, and alternatives. This explanation minimizes anxiety and provides the patient and the physician with appropriate expectations.

**I. Hospital orders**

**A. Admission orders** should be written promptly after evaluation of a patient. Each set of orders should bear the **date and time** of writing and the legible signature of the physician. Consideration should be given to including a **printed signature** and a **direct contact number** also. All orders should be clear, concise, organized, and legible.

**B.** To ensure that no important therapeutic measures are overlooked, the **content and organization** of admission orders should follow the outline below **(the mnemonic ADC VAAN DISML):**

1. **A**dmitting service and location and physician responsible for the patient
2. **D**iagnoses pertinent to nursing care
3. **C**ondition of the patient
4. **V**ital signs: type [temperature, heart rate (HR), respiratory rate, and BP], frequency, and parameters for notification of the physician (e.g., systolic BP <90, HR <60, respiratory rate <10, temperature >38.3°C) specified
5. **A**ctivity limitations
6. **A**llergies, sensitivities, and previous drug reactions
7. **N**ursing instructions (e.g., Foley catheter to gravity drainage, wound care, daily weights)
8. **D**iet
9. **I**V fluids, including composition and rate
10. **S**edatives, analgesics, and other prn medications
11. **M**edications, including dose, frequency, and route of administration
12. **L**aboratory tests and radiographic studies

**C. Orders should be re-evaluated frequently** and altered as patient status dictates. **When changing an order,** the old order must be specifically canceled before a new one is written.

**D. Venous thromboembolism (VTE) prophylaxis** should be considered for all hospitalized patients. **Risk factors** for VTE include advanced age, previous VTE, trauma, conditions associated with prolonged immobility (major surgery, stroke, paralysis), obesity, heart failure, malignancy, pregnancy, and coagulation factor deficiency. Commonly used **methods of prophylaxis** include heparin preparations (low-dose, unfractionated, and low-molecular-weight), oral anticoagulants, and intermittent pneumatic compression (*Chest* 119:132S–175S, 2001). **Method, timing, and duration of prophylaxis**

**Table 1-1.** Deep venous thrombosis anticoagulant prophylaxis guidelines[a]

| Drug | Abdominal surgery[b] | Total hip replacement[b] | Total knee replacement[b] | Medical conditions[c] |
|---|---|---|---|---|
| **Unfractionated heparin** | 5000 units SC q8–12h | — | — | 5000 units SC q8–12h |
| **Warfarin** | — | Start postop, target INR 2–3 | Start postop, target INR 2–3 | 1 mg PO qd for indwelling catheters |
| **Enoxaparin** | 40 mg SC qd, 1st dose 1–2 hr preop | 30 mg SC q12h, 1st dose 12–24 hr postop *or* 40 mg SC qd starting 12 hr preop | 30 mg SC qd, 1st dose 12–24 hr postop | 40 mg SC qd |
| **Dalteparin** | 2500 IU SC q24h, 1st dose 1–2 hr preop (moderate-risk patients) *or* 5000 IU SC q24h, 1st dose q8–12h preop (high-risk patients) | 2500 IU SC 2 hr preop and 6 hr postop then 5000 IU SC q24h (moderate-risk patients) *or* 5000 IU SC q8–12h preop, then q24h postop (high-risk patients) | — | — |
| **Fondaparinux** | — | 2.5 mg SC 6 hr postop, then 2.5 mg SC qd | 2.5. mg SC 6 hr postop, then 2.5 mg SC qd | — |

INR, international normalized ratio.
[a]Alternate dosing schedules may be appropriate based on specific risk profiles.
[b]Duration of postoperative prophylaxis is 7–10 days or until the patient is ambulatory.
[c]Major medical illness such as myocardial infarction, stroke, CHF, malignancy, pulmonary disease.
*Source:* Adapted from WH Geerts, et al. *Chest* 2001;119:132S–175S.

are based on the specific clinical setting and patient risk factors and are outlined in Table 1-1.

E. **Orders for medications to be taken prn** require careful consideration to avoid adverse drug interactions. The minimum dosing interval should be specified (e.g., q4h).

F. **Fall precautions** should be written for patients who have a history of falls or are at high risk of a fall (i.e., those with dementia, syncope, orthostatic hypotension). **Seizure precautions** should be considered for patients with a history of seizures or those at risk of seizing. Precautions include padded bed rails and an oral airway and tongue blade at the bedside. **Restraining orders** are written for patients who are at risk of injuring themselves or interfering with their treatment due to disruptive or dangerous behaviors. Restraining orders must be reviewed and renewed every 24 hours.

G. **Discharge planning** begins at the time of admission. Assessment of the patient's social situation and potential discharge needs should be made. **Early coordination** with nursing, social work, and case coordinators/managers facilitates efficient discharge and a complete postdischarge plan.

II. **Drug therapy**
   A. **Adverse drug reactions** occur frequently, and the rate increases in proportion to the number of drugs taken. Adverse reactions may be allergic, idiosyncratic, or dose-related magnification of known effects. Following the principles below may decrease the incidence of adverse drug reactions. Specific drug allergies are discussed in Chap. 10, Allergy and Immunology.
      1. **Record a careful history** of previous drug reactions, including the drug involved and the specific reaction, clearly on the chart.
      2. **Minimize number** of drugs used.
      3. **Consider drug interactions.** New medications should be added only after careful consideration of the current medical regimen. See Appendix C, Drug Interactions, for a list of commonly used medications and their interactions.
      4. **Consider the metabolism, route of excretion, and major adverse effects** associated with each drug used. Individualize dosages according to the patient's age, weight, and kidney and liver function. See Appendix E, Dosage Adjustments of Drugs in Renal Failure, for dose adjustments for commonly used medications.
      5. **Report unusual drug reactions** to the U.S. Food and Drug Administration. The MEDWATCH program provides an easy method for voluntary reporting of adverse drug reactions.
   B. **Prescriptions** should include the name of the patient, date, name of the drug, dosage, route of administration, amount dispensed, dosage schedule instructions, and signature of the physician. The number of refills should be limited, especially for patients who appear to be self-injurious. For **narcotics,** write out all numbers in parentheses [e.g., dispense 30 (thirty), refills 2 (two)].

III. **Pressure ulcers** typically occur within the first 2 weeks of hospitalization and can develop within 2–6 hours. Once they develop, pressure ulcers are difficult to heal and have been associated with increased mortality (AHCPR Publication 92-0652:15, 1994; *JAMA* 289:2; 2003).
   A. **Prevention** is the key to management of pressure ulcers. Prevention includes risk factor assessment, appropriate skin care, and interventions aimed at relieving or redistributing pressure. **Risk factors** for pressure ulcers include immobility, limited activity, incontinence, impaired nutritional status, and altered level of consciousness. **Patients at risk** include the elderly, patients with impairment of the microcirculatory system (i.e., diabetes, peripheral vascular disease), and orthopedic, spinal cord injury, and intensive care unit patients.
      1. **Skin care** includes daily inspection with particular attention to bony prominences, avoiding massage over bony prominences, and minimizing exposure to moisture from incontinence, perspiration, or wound drainage.
      2. **Interventions** include frequent repositioning (minimum of every 2 hours, or every 1 hour for wheelchair-bound patients), pillows or foam wedges between bony prominences, maintenance of the head of the bed at the lowest degree of elevation, and use of lifting devices when moving patients. Pressure-reducing devices (foam, dynamic air mattresses) and pressure-relieving devices (low-air-loss, air-fluidized beds) can also be used.
   B. **Treatment** begins with assessment of the ulcer for size, location, presence of necrotic and granulation tissue, and stage. The National Pressure Ulcer Task Force classifies ulcers as **stage I** (nonblanchable erythema; intact skin), **stage II** (extension through epidermis, shallow crater), **stage III** (full thickness without extension through fascia), and **stage IV** (full thickness with destruction of underlying tissue, muscle, and/or bone).
      1. **Initial interventions** include use of pressure-relieving devices, occlusive dressings, pain control, normal saline for cleansing, use of topical agents that promote wound healing [DuoDERM, silver sulfadiazine (Silvadene), bacitracin zinc, Neosporin, Polysporin], avoidance of agents that delay healing (antiseptic agents, such as Dakin's solution, hydrogen peroxide; wet-to-dry gauze), and removal of necrotic debris. **Adequate nutrition**

with particular attention to protein intake (1.25–1.50 g protein/kg/day) and vitamin C (500 mg PO qd) and zinc sulfate (220 mg PO qd) supplementation in the presence of deficiencies may also facilitate healing.

2. For clean pressure ulcers that continue to produce exudate or are not healing after 2–4 weeks of therapy, consider a 2-week trial of **topical antibiotic** (e.g., silver sulfadiazine, double antibiotic). **Surgical intervention** can be considered for nonhealing stage III or IV pressure ulcers, but rates of recurrence are relatively high. **Other adjunctive therapies** for nonhealing ulcers include electrical stimulation, radiant heat, and negative pressure therapy.

## Acute Inpatient Care

New or recurrent symptoms that require evaluation and management frequently develop in hospitalized patients. Evaluation should generally include a directed history, including a complete description of the symptom (i.e., palliating and precipitating factors, quality of the symptom, associated symptoms, and the course of the symptom, including acuity of onset, severity, duration, and previous episodes); physical examination; review of the medical problem list; review of medications with attention to recent medication discontinuation, addition, or dosage adjustment; and consideration of recent procedures. Further evaluation should be directed by the initial assessment, the acuity and severity of the complaint, and the diagnostic possibilities. An approach to selected common complaints is presented in this section.

I. **Chest pain** is a common complaint in the hospitalized patient, and the severity of chest discomfort and the gravity of its cause are not necessarily correlated. Chest pain should be evaluated to distinguish potentially life-threatening conditions, such as myocardial infarction (MI), aortic dissection, and pulmonary embolus, from less serious causes. **Initial history** should be taken in the context of the patient's other medical conditions, particularly previous cardiac or vascular history, cardiac risk factors, and factors that would predispose to a pulmonary embolus. Ideally, the **physical examination** is conducted during an episode of pain and includes vital signs with BP measured in both arms, a careful cardiopulmonary and abdominal examination, and inspection and palpation of the chest for possible trauma, herpes zoster rash, and reproducibility of the pain. **Assessment of oxygenation status, chest radiography, and ECG** are appropriate in most patients. **Management** of chest pain is guided by the diagnostic possibilities. If **cardiac ischemia** is a concern, initial therapy should include supplemental oxygen, chewed aspirin, and administration of nitroglycerin, 0.4 mg SL, or morphine sulfate, 1–2 mg IV, or both. Treatment of ischemic heart disease is discussed in Chap. 5, Ischemic Heart Disease. A combination of Maalox and diphenhydramine (30 ml of each in a 1:1 mix) can be administered if a **GI source** of chest pain is suspected. **Costochondritis** typically responds to nonsteroidal anti-inflammatory drug (NSAID) therapy.

II. **Dyspnea** is most often caused by a cardiopulmonary abnormality, such as CHF, cardiac ischemia, bronchospasm, pulmonary embolus, and/or infection, and must be promptly and carefully evaluated. **Initial evaluation** should include a review of the medical history for underlying pulmonary or cardiovascular disease, a directed history, and a detailed cardiopulmonary examination including vital signs with comparison of current findings to those documented earlier. **Assessment of oxygenation status and chest radiography** are useful in most patients. Other diagnostic and therapeutic measures should be directed by the findings in the initial evaluation and the severity of the suspected diagnoses.

III. **Acute hypertensive episodes** in the hospital are most often caused by inadequately treated essential hypertension. Evaluation and treatment decisions should consider baseline BP, presence of symptoms (e.g., chest pain or shortness of breath), and current and baseline antihypertensive medications. Hypertension associated with **withdrawal syndromes** (e.g., alcohol, cocaine, etc.) and **rebound hypertension** associated with sudden withdrawal of antihypertensive medications (i.e., clonidine, α-adrenergic antagonists) should be considered. These entities should be treated as discussed in Chap. 4, Hypertension. **Volume expansion** and **inadequate pain control** may exacerbate hypertension and should be recognized appropriately and treated.

**IV. Fever** accompanies many illnesses and is a valuable marker of disease activity. Because fever can cause increased tissue catabolism, increased oxygen consumption, dehydration, exacerbation of heart failure, delirium, and convulsions, the underlying cause of fever should be ascertained as quickly as possible. Infection is a primary concern; drug reaction, malignancy, VTE, vasculitis, and tissue infarction are other possibilities but are diagnoses of exclusion.

**A. Evaluation.** The differential diagnosis for fever is very broad, and the pace and complexity of the workup depend on the diagnostic considerations taken in the context of the clinical stability and immune status of the host.

1. **History** should include chronology of the fever and associated symptoms, medications, potential exposures, and a complete social and travel history. **Physical examination** should include **oral or rectal temperature** monitoring from a consistent site. In the hospitalized patient, special attention should be paid to any rash, new murmur, abnormal fluid accumulation, intravascular lines, and indwelling devices such as gastric tubes or Foley catheters. In the **neutropenic patient,** the skin, oral cavity, and perineal area should be examined carefully for breaches of mucosal integrity. See Chap. 20, Medical Management of Malignant Disease, for management of neutropenic fever.
2. **Diagnostic evaluation** generally includes chest radiography, CBC with differential, serum chemistries with liver function tests, urinalysis, and blood and urine cultures. Cultures of abnormal fluid collections, sputum, cerebrospinal fluid, and stool should be sent if clinically indicated.

**B. Treatment of fever** is indicated to prevent harmful sequelae and for patient discomfort. **Heat stroke and malignant hyperthermia** are medical emergencies that require prompt recognition and treatment (see Chap. 25, Medical Emergencies).

1. **Antipyretic drugs** can be given regularly until the underlying disease process has been controlled. Aspirin and acetaminophen are the drugs of choice (325–650 mg PO or per rectum q4h). **Aspirin should be avoided in adolescents** with possible viral infections because this combination has been associated with Reye's syndrome.
2. **Hypothermic (cooling) blankets** may be effective but require careful monitoring of rectal temperatures. Often, they produce excessive shivering and patient discomfort. The blanket should be discontinued when a patient's temperature falls below 39°C.
3. **Empiric antibiotics** should be considered in hemodynamically unstable patients in whom infection is a primary concern and in neutropenic and asplenic patients.

**V. Pain** is subjective, and therapy must be individualized. **Acute pain** usually requires only temporary therapy. For **chronic pain,** nonnarcotic preparations should be used when possible. Anticonvulsants and antidepressants are more useful than narcotics for **neuropathic pain.** If pain is refractory to conventional therapy, then nonpharmacologic modalities, such as nerve blocks, sympathectomy, and relaxation therapy, may be appropriate.

**A. Acetaminophen** has antipyretic and analgesic actions but does not have anti-inflammatory or antiplatelet properties.

1. **Preparations and dosage.** Acetaminophen, 325–1000 mg q4–6h (maximum dose, 4 g/day), is available in tablet, caplet, liquid, and rectal sup-

pository form. It should be avoided or used with caution at low doses in patients with liver disease.

2. **Adverse effects.** The principal advantage of acetaminophen is its lack of gastric toxicity. **Hepatic toxicity** may be serious, however, and acute overdose with 10–15 g can cause fatal hepatic necrosis (see Chap. 25, Medical Emergencies).

B. **Aspirin** has analgesic, antipyretic, and anti-inflammatory effects.

1. **Preparations and dosages.** Aspirin is given in a dosage of 325–1000 mg PO q4h prn (maximum dose, 3 g/day) for relief of pain. Rectal suppositories (300–600 mg q3–4h) may be irritating to the mucosa and have variable absorption. Enteric-coated tablets and nonacetylated salicylates may cause less injury to the gastric mucosa than buffered or plain aspirin. The nonacetylated salicylates also lack antiplatelet effects.

2. **Adverse effects.** Dose-related **side effects** include tinnitus, dizziness, and hearing loss. Dyspepsia and GI bleeding can develop and may be severe. Hypersensitivity reactions, including bronchospasm, laryngeal edema, and urticaria, are uncommon, but patients with asthma and nasal polyps are more susceptible. **Patients with allergic or bronchospastic reactions to aspirin should not be given NSAIDs.** Chronic excessive use can result in interstitial nephritis and papillary necrosis. Aspirin should be used with caution in patients with hepatic or renal disease.

3. **Antiplatelet effects.** These effects may last for up to 1 week after a single dose. **Aspirin should be avoided in patients with known bleeding disorders, in those who are receiving anticoagulant therapy, and during pregnancy.** Discontinuation of aspirin before elective surgery should be considered.

C. **NSAIDs** have analgesic, antipyretic, and anti-inflammatory properties mediated by inhibition of cyclooxygenase. All NSAIDs have similar efficacy and toxicities, with a side effect profile similar to that of the salicylates. **NSAIDs should be used with caution in patients with impaired renal or hepatic function** (see Chap. 23, Arthritis and Rheumatologic Diseases). **Ketorolac tromethamine** is an analgesic that can be given IM or IV and is often used postoperatively; however, parenteral therapy should not exceed 5 days. Nephrotoxicity is more pronounced with IM than with PO administration.

D. **Cyclooxygenase-2 (cox-2) inhibitors** act primarily on cox-2, which is an inducible form of cyclooxygenase and an important mediator of pain and inflammation. Cox-2 inhibitors have no significant effects on platelet aggregation or on the gastric mucosa. Currently available agents include **celecoxib, rofecoxib, and valdecoxib. Meloxicam** is also available but is less selective for cox-2. Cox-2 inhibitors should not be used in patients who have allergic or bronchospastic reactions to aspirin or other NSAIDs, and **celecoxib is contraindicated in patients with allergic-type reactions to sulfonamides.**

E. **Opioid analgesics** are pharmacologically similar to opium or morphine and are the drugs of choice when analgesia without antipyretic action is desired. Table 1-2 lists equianalgesic dosages.

1. **Preparations and dosages**

a. **Constant pain** requires continuous (around-the-clock) analgesia with supplementary (prn) doses for breakthrough pain. Medication dosages should be maintained at the lowest level that provides adequate analgesia. If frequent prn doses are required, the maintenance dose should be increased, or the dosing interval should be decreased.

b. **If adequate analgesia** cannot be achieved at the maximum recommended dose of one narcotic or if the side effects are intolerable, the patient should be changed to another preparation beginning at one-half the equianalgesic dose.

c. **Oral medications** should be used when possible. **Parenteral and transdermal administration** are useful in the setting of dysphagia, emesis, or decreased GI absorption. The lowest starting dose should

**Table 1-2.** Equianalgesic doses of opioid analgesics

| Drug | Onset (min) | Duration (hr) | IM/IV/SC (mg) | PO (mg) |
|---|---|---|---|---|
| Fentanyl | 7–8 | 1–2 | 0.1 | NA |
| Levorphanol | 30–90 | 6–8 | 2 | 4 |
| Hydromorphone | 15–30 | 4–5 | 1.5–2.0 | 7.5 |
| Methadone | 30–60 | 6–8 | 10 | 20 |
| Morphine | 15–30 | 4–6 | 10 | 60[a] |
| Oxycodone | 15–30 | 4–6 | NA | 30 |
| Meperidine | 10–45 | 2–4 | 75 | 300 |
| Codeine | 15–30 | 4–6 | 120 | 200 |

NA, not applicable.
*Note:* Equivalences are based on single-dose studies.
[a]An IM:PO ratio of 1:2–3.0 is used for repetitive dosing.

be given, with a gradual increase in the amount of drug administered until adequate analgesia is obtained.

d. **Continuous IV administration** provides steady blood levels and allows for rapid dose adjustment. Agents with short half-lives, such as morphine, should be used. **Patient-controlled analgesia** is often used to control pain in a postoperative or terminally ill patient. Advantages of patient-controlled analgesia include enhancement in pain relief, decrease in anxiety, and decrease in the total narcotic dose.

2. **Selected drugs**
   a. **Codeine** is usually given in combination with aspirin or acetaminophen. It is also an effective cough suppressant at a dosage of 10–15 mg PO q4–q6h.
   b. **Oxycodone and propoxyphene** are also usually prescribed orally in combination with aspirin or acetaminophen. Available tablets include oxycodone with acetaminophen (5 mg/325 mg PO q6h), oxycodone with aspirin (5 mg/325 mg PO q6h), and propoxyphene with acetaminophen (50 mg/325 mg or 100 mg/650 mg q6h).
   c. **Immediate and sustained-release morphine sulfate** preparations (immediate-release, 5–30 mg PO q2–8h; sustained-release, 15–120 mg PO q12h; or a rectal suppository) can be used. The liquid form can be useful in patients who have difficulty in swallowing pills. Larger doses of morphine may be necessary to control pain as tolerance develops.
   d. **Meperidine** (50–150 mg PO, SC, or IM q2–3h) causes less biliary spasm, urinary retention, and constipation than morphine but results in more respiratory depression and is a myocardial depressant. It is **contraindicated in patients who are taking monoamine oxidase inhibitors and in individuals with renal failure** (accumulation of active metabolites causes CNS excitement and seizures). Repetitive dosing is more likely to cause seizures; therefore, chronic administration is not recommended. Coadministration of **hydroxyzine** (25–100 mg IM q4–6h) may decrease nausea and potentiate the analgesic effect of meperidine.
   e. **Methadone** is very effective when administered orally and suppresses the symptoms of withdrawal from other opioids because of its extended half-life. Despite its long elimination half-life, its analgesic duration of action is much shorter.

f. **Hydromorphone** (2–4 mg PO q4–6h; 1–2 mg IM, IV, or SC q4–6h) is a potent morphine derivative. It can be given IV with caution. It is also available as a 3-mg rectal suppository.

g. **Fentanyl** is available in a transdermal patch with sustained release over 72 hours. Initial onset of action is delayed. Respiratory depression may occur more frequently with fentanyl.

h. **Mixed agonist-antagonist agents** (butorphanol, nalbuphine, oxymorphone, pentazocine) offer few advantages and produce more adverse effects than do the other agents.

3. **Precautions. Opioids are contraindicated** in acute disease states in which the pattern and degree of pain are important diagnostic signs (e.g., head injuries, abdominal pain). They may also increase intracranial pressure. **Opioids should be used with caution** in patients with hypothyroidism, Addison's disease, hypopituitarism, anemia, respiratory disease [e.g., chronic obstructive pulmonary disease (COPD), asthma, kyphoscoliosis, severe obesity], severe malnutrition, debilitation, or chronic cor pulmonale. The dosage should be adjusted for patients with impaired hepatic function. Drugs that potentiate the adverse effects of opioids include phenothiazines, antidepressants, benzodiazepines, and alcohol. **Tolerance** develops with chronic use and coincides with the development of physical dependence. **Physical dependence** is characterized by a withdrawal syndrome (anxiety, irritability, diaphoresis, tachycardia, GI distress, and temperature instability) when the drug is stopped abruptly. It may occur after only 2 weeks of therapy. Administration of an opioid antagonist may precipitate withdrawal after only 3 days of therapy. Withdrawal can be minimized by tapering the medication slowly over several days.

4. **Adverse and toxic effects.** Although individuals may tolerate some preparations better than others, at equianalgesic doses, few differences in side effects exist.

   a. **CNS effects** include sedation, euphoria, and pupillary constriction.

   b. **Respiratory depression** is dose related and is especially pronounced after IV administration.

   c. **Cardiovascular effects** include peripheral vasodilatation and hypotension, especially after IV administration.

   d. **GI effects** include constipation, nausea, and vomiting. Patients who are receiving opioid medications should be provided with stool softeners and laxatives. Nausea and vomiting can be limited by keeping the patient in a recumbent position. Benzodiazepines, dopamine antagonists (e.g., prochlorperazine, metoclopramide, etc.), and ondansetron can be used as antiemetics. Opioids may precipitate toxic megacolon in patients with inflammatory bowel disease.

   e. **Urinary retention** may be caused by increased bladder, ureter, and urethral sphincter tone.

   f. **Pruritus** occurs most commonly with spinal administration.

5. **Naloxone,** an opioid antagonist, should be readily available for administration in the case of accidental or intentional overdose. See Chap. 25, Medical Emergencies, for details of administration. Side effects include hyper- or hypotension, irritability, anxiety, restlessness, tremulousness, nausea, and vomiting. Naloxone can also precipitate seizure activity and cardiac arrhythmias.

F. **Tramadol** is similar to opioids but has less potential for addiction and abuse.

1. **Preparations and dosages.** Between 50 and 100 mg PO q4–6h can be used for acute pain. For elderly patients and those with renal or liver dysfunction, dosage reduction is recommended.

2. **Adverse effects.** Because CNS effects include sedation, concomitant use of alcohol, sedatives, or narcotics should be avoided. Nausea, dizziness, constipation, and headache also may occur. Respiratory depression

has not been described at prescribed dosages but may occur with overdose. **Tramadol should not be used in patients who are taking a monoamine oxidase inhibitor.**

G. **Anticonvulsants** (e.g., gabapentin, valproate) **and tricyclic antidepressants** (e.g., amitriptyline) are PO agents that can be used to treat neuropathic pain.

VI. **Mental status changes** have a broad differential diagnosis that includes neurologic (e.g., stroke, delirium), metabolic (e.g., hypoxemia, hypoglycemia), toxic (e.g., drug effects, alcohol withdrawal), and other etiologies. **Infection** (e.g., urinary tract infections, pneumonia, etc.) is a common cause of mental status changes in the elderly and patients with underlying neurologic disease. Management of specific disorders is discussed in Chap. 24, Neurologic Disorders.

A. **Medical history** should particularly focus on medications, underlying dementia, neurologic or psychiatric disorders, and a history of alcohol and drug use. Directed history should be obtained from the patient; family and nursing personnel may be able to provide additional details. **Physical examination** generally includes vital signs, a search for sites of infection, a complete cardiopulmonary examination, and a detailed neurologic examination including mental status evaluation.

B. In most patients **initial diagnostic evaluation** should include arterial oxygen saturation, blood glucose, serum electrolytes, creatinine, CBC, urinalysis, ECG, and chest radiograph. Other evaluation, including culture, toxicology screen, CT scan of the head, lumbar puncture, EEG, thyroid function tests, and syphilis serologies, should be directed by initial findings and diagnostic possibilities.

C. **Agitation and psychosis** may be features of a change in mental status. The neuroleptic haloperidol and the benzodiazepine lorazepam are commonly used in the **acute management** of these symptoms. In patients with **chronic agitation or psychosis,** the newer-generation neuroleptics (risperidone, olanzapine, quetiapine, clozapine) are preferred due to decreased incidence of extrapyramidal symptoms.

1. **Haloperidol** is the initial drug of choice for acute management of agitation and psychosis. The initial dose of 1–5 mg (0.25 mg in **elderly patients**) PO, IM, or IV can be repeated every 30–60 minutes until the desired effect is achieved. Sedation is usually achieved with 10–20 mg PO or IM. **IV infusions** (1–40 mg/hour) can also be used as an alternative to bolus injections. Compared with other antipsychotics with similar efficacy, haloperidol has fewer active metabolites and fewer anticholinergic, sedative, and hypotensive effects, although it may have more extrapyramidal side effects. In low dosages, haloperidol rarely causes hypotension, cardiovascular compromise, or excessive sedation.

   a. **Prolongation of the QT interval** with development of torsades de pointes may be seen with high-dose IV therapy. In patients who are receiving IV therapy, QTc and electrolytes (primarily potassium and magnesium) should be monitored. Use should be discontinued with prolongation of QTc greater than 450 msec or 25% above baseline.

   b. **Postural hypotension** may occasionally be acute and severe after IM administration. If significant hypotension occurs, administration of IV fluids with the patient in the Trendelenburg position are usually sufficient. If **vasopressors** are required, norepinephrine or phenylephrine should be used, as dopamine may exacerbate the psychotic state.

   c. **Neuroleptic malignant syndrome** is an infrequent, potentially lethal complication of antipsychotic drug therapy. Clinical manifestations include rigidity, akinesia, altered sensorium, fever, tachycardia, and alteration in BP. Severe muscle rigidity can cause rhabdomyolysis and acute renal failure. **Laboratory abnormalities** include elevations in creatine kinase, liver function tests, and white blood cell count (see Chap. 24, Neurologic Disorders).

2. **Lorazepam** is a benzodiazepine that is useful for agitation and psychosis in the setting of hepatic dysfunction and sedative or alcohol withdrawal,

**Table 1-3.** Characteristics of selected benzodiazepines

| Drug | Route | Usual dosage | Half-life (hr) |
|---|---|---|---|
| Alprazolam | PO | 0.75–4.0 mg/24 hr (in 3 doses) | 11–15 |
| Chlordiazepoxide | PO | 15–100 mg/24 hr (in divided doses) | 6–30 |
| Clorazepate | PO | 7.5–60.0 mg/24 hr (in 1–4 doses) | 30–100 |
| Diazepam | PO | 6–40 mg/24 hr (in 1–4 doses) | 20–50 |
| | IV | 2.5–20.0 mg (slow IV push) | 20–50 |
| Flurazepam | PO | 15–30 mg qhs | 50–100 |
| Lorazepam[a] | PO | 1–10 mg/24 hr (in 2–3 doses) | 10–20 |
| | IV or IM | 0.05 mg/kg (4 mg max) | 10–20 |
| Midazolam | IV | 0.01–0.05 mg/kg | 1–12 |
| | IM | 0.08 mg/kg | 1–12 |
| Oxazepam[a] | PO | 30–120 mg/24 hr (in 3–4 doses) | 5–10 |
| Prazepam | PO | 20–60 mg/24 hr (in 3–4 divided doses) | 36–70 |
| Temazepam[a] | PO | 15–30 mg qhs | 9–12 |
| Triazolam[a] | PO | 0.125–0.250 mg qhs | 2–3 |

qhs, every night at bedtime.
[a]Metabolites are inactive.

and in patients who are refractory to monotherapy with neuroleptics. The **initial dose** is 0.5–2.0 mg IV. The **key features** of lorazepam are its short duration of action and few active metabolites. The use of lorazepam, as with all benzodiazepines, is limited by excess sedation, respiratory depression, and the potential to precipitate agitation in the elderly and in patients with liver disease and low albumin.

**D. Sundown syndrome** refers to the appearance of worsening confusion in the evening and is associated with dementia, delirium, and unfamiliar environments. Behavioral interventions, such as increased lighting, maintenance of a familiar environment, and reorientation, should be attempted first; if these are ineffective, short-term antipsychotic therapy may be warranted.

**VII. Insomnia and anxiety** may be attributed to a variety of underlying medical or psychiatric disorders, and symptoms may be exacerbated by hospitalization. Possible causes of **insomnia** to consider include mood and anxiety disorders, substance abuse disorders, common medications (i.e., beta-blockers, steroids, bronchodilators, etc.), sleep apnea, hyperthyroidism, and nocturnal myoclonus. **Anxiety** may be seen in anxiety disorder, depression, substance abuse disorders, hyperthyroidism, and complex partial seizures.

**A. Selected medications for insomnia or anxiety, or both**

**1. Benzodiazepines** are frequently used in management of anxiety and insomnia. Table 1-3 provides a list of selected benzodiazepines and their dosages.

**a. Pharmacology.** Most benzodiazepines undergo oxidation to active metabolites in the liver. **Lorazepam, oxazepam, and temazepam** undergo glucuronidation to inactive metabolites; therefore, these agents may be particularly useful in the elderly and in those with liver disease. **Benzodiazepine toxicity** is increased by malnutrition, advanced age, hepatic disease, and concomitant use of alcohol, other CNS depressants, isoniazid, and cimetidine. Benzodiazepines with long half-lives may accumulate substantially, even with single daily dosing. This effect is a particular concern in the elderly, in whom the half-life may be increased twofold to fourfold.

b. **Relief of anxiety and insomnia** is achieved at the doses outlined in Table 1-3. Therapy should be started at the lowest recommended dosage with intermittent dosing schedules.

c. **Side effects** include drowsiness, dizziness, fatigue, psychomotor impairment, and anterograde amnesia. The elderly are more sensitive to these agents and may experience falls, paradoxical agitation, and delirium. **IV administration of diazepam and midazolam** can be associated with hypotension and respiratory or cardiac arrest. **Respiratory depression** can occur even with oral administration in patients with respiratory compromise.

d. **Tolerance** to benzodiazepines can develop. **Dependence** may develop after only 2–4 weeks of therapy. A **withdrawal syndrome** consisting of agitation, irritability, insomnia, tremor, palpitations, headache, GI distress, and perceptual disturbance begins 1–10 days after a rapid decrease in dosage or abrupt cessation of therapy and may last for several weeks. **Seizures and delirium** may also occur with sudden discontinuation of benzodiazepines. Although the severity and incidence of withdrawal symptoms appear to be related to dose and duration of treatment, withdrawal symptoms have been reported even after brief therapy at doses in the recommended range. Short-acting and intermediate-acting drugs should be decreased by 10–20% every 5 days, with a slower taper in the final few weeks; long-acting preparations can be tapered more quickly.

e. **Flumazenil,** a benzodiazepine antagonist, should be readily available in case of accidental or intentional overdose. See Chap. 25, Medical Emergencies, for details of administration. Common side effects include dizziness, nausea, and vomiting. **Flumazenil should not be used in patients with a known history of seizure disorder or if overdose with tricyclic antidepressants is suspected.**

2. **Trazodone** is an antidepressant that may be useful for the treatment of severe anxiety or insomnia. It is highly sedating, causes postural hypotension, and is associated with ventricular ectopy and priapism. No deaths or cardiovascular complications have been reported in patients taking trazodone alone. **A number of potential drug interactions can occur with trazodone** (see Appendix C, Drug Interactions).

3. **Zolpidem** is an imidazopyridine hypnotic agent that is useful for the treatment of insomnia. It has no withdrawal syndrome, rebound insomnia, or tolerance and, because of its rapid onset, is useful for initiating and for maintaining sleep. **Side effects** include headache, daytime somnolence, and GI upset. Zolpidem should be **avoided in patients with obstructive sleep apnea.** The starting dose is 5 mg PO every night at bedtime (qhs) for the elderly and 10 mg PO qhs for other patients, titrating up to 20 mg as needed. Doses should be reduced in cirrhosis.

4. **Zaleplon** is another nonbenzodiazepine hypnotic that is useful for insomnia. This agent has a half-life of approximately 1 hour and has no active metabolites. **Side effects** include drowsiness, dizziness, and impaired coordination. Zaleplon should be used with caution in those with compromised respiratory function. The starting dose is 5 mg PO qhs for the elderly or patients with hepatic dysfunction and 10–20 mg PO qhs for other patients.

5. **Over-the-counter antihistamines** can be used for insomnia and anxiety, particularly in patients with a history of drug dependence, but are only minimally effective in inducing sleep. Anticholinergic side effects limit the use of these agents.

VIII. **Depression.** Patients with a known history of depression or in whom depression is suspected should be evaluated for the presence of suicidal or homicidal ideations.

**Patients with active ideations or a plan of action, or both, should be monitored by a 1:1 sitter and undergo immediate psychiatric evaluation.** Psychiatric and medical conditions that may mimic or worsen depression, such as other mood disorders, substance abuse, and hypothyroidism, should be considered. **Psychiatric consultation** should be obtained for patients with psychotic features to determine the patient's capacity to make health care decisions.

**IX. Nausea/vomiting, diarrhea, and constipation** are discussed in Chap. 16, Gastrointestinal Diseases.

**X. Rash** may develop as a recurrence of a chronic skin condition, manifestation of a systemic illness, or a contact dermatitis or drug reaction. Stevens-Johnson drug reactions are discussed in Chap. 10, Allergy and Immunology.

## Perioperative Medicine

The major focus of the preoperative evaluation of patients about to undergo elective surgery is to identify those at increased risk for perioperative morbidity and mortality. The role of the medical consultant is to risk stratify patients, determine the need for further evaluation, and prescribe possible interventions to diminish or even eradicate risk.

**I. Preoperative cardiac evaluation.** Preoperative testing should be limited to circumstances in which the results will affect patient treatment and outcomes. Coronary artery disease is the most frequent cause of perioperative mortality and morbidity for noncardiac surgery.

**A. History.** Functional status is critical in assessing a patient's preoperative risk. Four metabolic equivalents (METs) is generally used as the standard to assess the adequacy of a patient's functional status related to cardiac risk for surgery (*Acta Anaesthesiol Scand* 34:144, 1990). Table 1-4 lists some activities equivalent to 4 METs of exercise. **Comorbid conditions** must be identified, especially diabetes, lung disease, heart disease, renal failure, immune status, hematologic diseases, and malignancy. The most widely used algorithm for the preoperative assessment of cardiac risk for noncardiac surgery was published in 1996 and updated in 2002 by the American Heart Association (AHA) (*J Am Coll Cardiol* 39:545, 2002) and uses the **following eight steps** (Fig. 1-1):

**Step 1: What is the urgency of the surgery?** If the surgery is emergent, the focus is perioperative medical management and surveillance.

**Step 2: Has the patient undergone coronary revascularization within the past 5 years?** If so, and the patient is asymptomatic, no further workup is needed.

**Step 3: Has the patient undergone a coronary evaluation within the last 2 years?** If so, and the patient remains asymptomatic, repeat testing is not indicated.

**Step 4: Does the patient have an unstable coronary syndrome or major clinical predictors?** In the setting of unstable coronary dis-

**Table 1-4.** Metabolic equivalents (METs) for certain activities

| METs | Representative activities |
|---|---|
| 4 or more | Walking at 4 mph on level ground, climbing stairs, climbing hills, riding a bicycle at 8 mph, golfing, bowling, throwing a baseball/football, carrying 25 lb (groceries from the store to the car), scrubbing the floor, raking leaves, mowing the lawn |
| >7 | Jogging at 5 mph on level ground, carrying 60-lb objects |

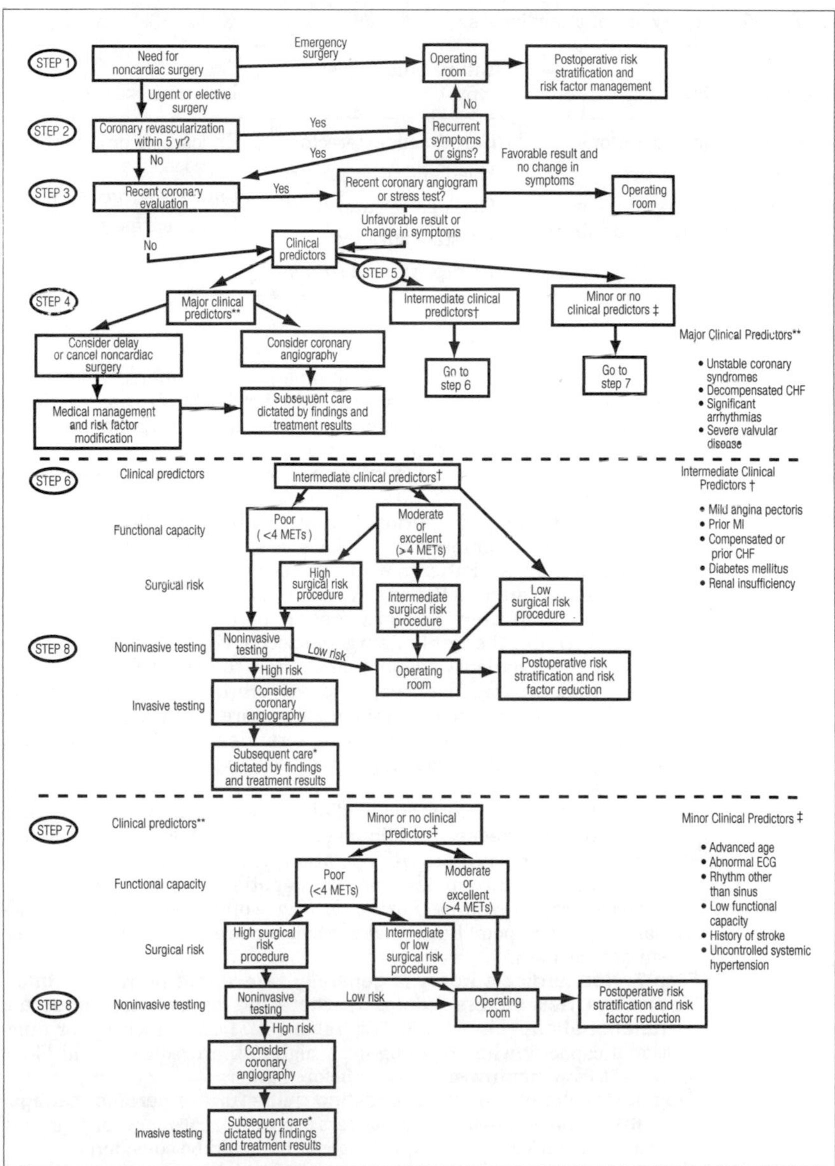


**Fig. 1-1.** Stepwise approach to preoperative cardiac assessment. *Subsequent care may include cancellation or delay in surgery, coronary revascularization followed by noncardiac surgery, or intensified care. METs, metabolic equivalents; MI, myocardial infarction. (From KA Eagle, BH Brundage, BR Chaitman, et al. Guidelines for perioperative cardiovascular evaluation for noncardiac surgery. Report of the American College of Cardiology/American Heart Association Task Force on Practice Guidelines. Committee on Perioperative Cardiovascular Evaluation for Noncardiac Surgery. *J Am Coll Cardiol* 39:545, 2002, with permission.)

**Table 1-5.** Surgery-specific cardiac risk

| High (risk >5%) | Intermediate (risk <5%) | Low (risk <1%) |
|---|---|---|
| Emergent major operations | Carotid endarterectomy | Endoscopic or superficial procedures |
| Major vascular surgery | Head and neck surgery | Cataract surgery |
| Anticipated prolonged procedures with large fluid shifts or blood loss | Orthopedic surgery | Breast surgery |
| | Prostate surgery | |
| | Intraperitoneal surgery | |

ease, decompensated CHF, symptomatic arrhythmias, high-grade atrioventricular block, or severe valvular heart disease, patients most often benefit from cardiac catheterization. Surgery may need to be delayed while medical therapy is optimized.

**Step 5: Does the patient have intermediate predictors of risk?** These include a history of prior MI, stable angina pectoris (Canadian class I or II), compensated or prior CHF, and diabetes mellitus. The most recent AHA recommendations have also included **renal insufficiency** in this list. Patients with intermediate predictors are considered through step 6. Patients without intermediate predictors are evaluated from step 7. Consideration of the functional capacity (Table 1-4) and the level of surgery-specific risk (Table 1-5) help to identify those patients who are most likely to benefit from noninvasive cardiac testing. The type of procedure is an important factor. Certain procedures (e.g., vascular) are more likely than others to result in prolonged perioperative alterations in HR and BP, fluid shifts, pain, bleeding, clotting tendencies, oxygenation, and neurohumoral activation.

**Step 6: Patients with intermediate clinical predictors of risk who have moderate to excellent functional capacity** (>4 METs) can generally undergo an intermediate-risk operation with little likelihood of perioperative cardiac complications. These patients should also tolerate low-risk procedures well. Further testing is often required for individuals who have poor functional capacity or are undergoing high-risk surgery, or both.

**Step 7: Noncardiac surgery is generally safe where no high or intermediate risk factors exist and where the patient has moderate functional capacity** (>4 METs; Table 1-4). Patients with poor functional capacity who are going for a high-risk procedure would likely benefit from noninvasive testing before surgery.

**Step 8: Results of noninvasive testing guide further cardiac management.** If the noninvasive cardiac test is positive, coronary angiography or maximization of medical management should be considered.

**B. Physical examination.** Vital signs are critical, with severe hypertension being a treatable but potentially dangerous preoperative condition. BP should be measured in both arms. A thorough physical examination is also necessary, including a funduscopic examination. On cardiac examination, the presence of a murmur may provide critical information on valvular disease or the need for endocarditis prophylaxis. An elevated jugular venous pressure, positive hepatojugular reflex, pulmonary crackles, or $S_3$ may indicate volume overload. Evidence of peripheral vascular disease should be sought, including carotid bruits, which may be the only clue to underlying atherosclerosis.

**C. Laboratory evaluation.** Adults age 50 and older should have a 12-lead ECG to evaluate for rhythms other than normal sinus and any evidence of old infarcts or ischemia. Any additional evaluation should be based on symptoms, comorbid conditions, and physical examination findings.

**D. Methods of assessing cardiac risk**

1. **Resting two-dimensional echocardiography.** A left ventricular (LV) ejection fraction of less than 35% and severe diastolic dysfunction both increase cardiac risk in noncardiac surgery. Knowledge of LV function is valuable for managing postoperative fluids.
2. **Exercise stress testing.** Evidence of myocardial ischemia on stress testing identifies patients with a sevenfold increased risk of untoward outcomes during noncardiac surgery. A gradient of increasing ischemic risk is seen in association with the degree of functional incapacity, symptoms of ischemia, and severity of ischemia (depth and rapidity of onset and the duration of ST-segment depression and evidence of hemodynamic or electrical instability during or after stress). This gradient also correlates with increasing likelihood of severe and multivessel coronary artery disease. In patients with **left bundle branch block,** exercise stress testing, even with nuclear imaging, is much less sensitive and specific than in those without left bundle branch block. Vasodilator (dipyridamole and adenosine)-based stress testing, however, has a high sensitivity and specificity in this situation.
3. **Pharmacologic stress testing**
   a. **Dipyridamole or adenosine thallium stress testing** has a high sensitivity and specificity for predicting perioperative cardiac events when used in patients with preexisting clinical predictors of risk such as angina, diabetes, and prior MI. Risk of perioperative ischemic events correlates well with the magnitude of ischemia that is present on the test (the presence of ECG evidence of ischemia and thallium or technetium redistribution after pharmacologic stress testing). The long-term risk of death or MI may be better predicted by the presence of reversible or fixed defects.
   b. **Dobutamine stress echocardiography** provides comparable information to thallium studies as well as an opportunity to evaluate LV and valvular function.
4. **Ambulatory ECG monitoring.** Detection of ischemia by preoperative 24- to 48-hour monitoring correlates with increased risk of early postoperative and late ischemic events. Higher-risk patients may have baseline ECG anomalies that preclude analysis.
5. **Coronary angiography.** Indications for preoperative angiography are the same as those in the nonoperative setting. Percutaneous transluminal coronary angioplasty (PTCA) or coronary artery bypass grafting surgery should be feasible options for patients who are sent for cardiac catheterization.

**E. Specific preoperative cardiovascular conditions**

1. **Hypertension.** Continuation of preoperative antihypertensive treatment throughout the perioperative period is critical, especially when the patient is receiving **beta-blockers or clonidine.** Withdrawal of these medications may result in tachycardia and rebound hypertension, respectively. Severe hypertension (BP >180/110) preoperatively often results in wider fluctuations in intraoperative BP and has been associated with an increased rate of perioperative cardiac events. **Cardioselective beta-blockers** have been shown to have a dramatic effect in reducing perioperative cardiovascular events (see sec. **E.7**). Evidence suggests that holding **angiotensin-converting enzyme inhibitors and angiotensin II–receptor blockers** on the day of surgery may reduce perioperative hypotension. This is believed to be due to the effect of this class of medication in blunting the compensatory activation of the

renin-angiotensin system perioperatively. In addition, all remedial causes of hypertension, such as pain, agitation, hypercarbia, hypoxia, hypervolemia, and bladder distention, should be excluded or treated. Many parenteral antihypertensive medications are available for patients who are unable to take medications orally. With the exception of beta-blockers and clonidine, it is not necessary for patients who are receiving chronic antihypertensive therapy to continue the same class of drug postoperatively (*JAMA* 287:2043, 2002). For management of postoperative hypertension, see Chap. 4, Hypertension.

2. **Valvular heart disease.** Symptomatic **stenotic lesions** such as mitral stenosis and aortic stenosis are associated with perioperative CHF and shock, and preoperative valvotomy or replacement is often needed. If surgery is emergent, elective valvular repair can be deferred to a later time. Symptomatic **regurgitant lesions** are generally better tolerated perioperatively and can be managed medically. Exceptions to this are those with regurgitant lesions with LV dysfunction, who may need surgical management preoperatively as these patients have reduced hemodynamic reserve.
3. **Myocardial heart disease.** Dilated cardiomyopathy and hypertrophic obstructive cardiomyopathy are both associated with a higher incidence of perioperative CHF. These patients should be managed by optimizing preoperative hemodynamic status and providing intensive postoperative medical treatment and surveillance.
4. **Arrhythmias and conduction anomalies.** When an arrhythmia is detected preoperatively, a thorough assessment for an underlying cause should be sought. The indications for preoperative arrhythmia management and pacemaker insertion are the same as in the nonoperative setting (see Chap. 7, Arrhythmias).
5. **Coronary artery bypass grafting.** Several observational studies have shown that patients with coronary artery disease who have undergone coronary artery bypass grafting are at lower cardiac risk when they undergo subsequent noncardiac surgery.
6. **Angioplasty.** No large randomized trials have compared perioperative cardiac outcome after noncardiac surgery for patients who had PTCA versus medical therapy. However, smaller observational studies have revealed that cardiac death is infrequent in patients who have PTCA before noncardiac surgery.
7. **Medical management.** Surgical stress can lead to release of large amounts of catecholamines that mediate arrhythmias and may predispose to coronary plaque rupture. **Perioperative beta-blockade** has been shown to reduce cardiac events. In high-risk patients (defined as having two or more of the following risk factors: age >65, hypertension, current smoking, cholesterol level >240 mg/dl, and diabetes) who are undergoing noncardiac surgery, **atenolol,** 5–10 mg IV 1 hour before surgery and immediately after surgery followed by 50–100 mg PO qd for 7 days postoperatively, produced a 15% absolute reduction compared to placebo in the combined end point of MI, unstable angina, CHF, myocardial revascularization, or death at 6 months. In addition, use of atenolol reduced mortality in these patients at 6 months and 2 years postsurgery (*N Engl J Med* 335:1713, 1996). The use of **bisoprolol** has produced dramatic results as well. When started 7 days preoperatively, titrated to a resting HR of 60 bpm, and continued for 30 days postoperatively, bisoprolol showed a 90% reduction in perioperative MI or death from cardiac events. The study was conducted in patients who had at least one cardiac risk factor (a history of CHF, prior MI, diabetes, angina pectoris, age >70, or poor functional status) and evidence of inducible myocardial ischemia on dobutamine echocardiography (*N Engl J Med* 341:1789, 1999). These landmark studies have resulted in the current American College of Cardiology/AHA guideline recommendations that

**patients who are at risk for perioperative myocardial events should be started on beta-blockers** days or weeks before elective surgery, with the dose titrated to achieve a resting HR of between 50 and 60 bpm.

**F. Intra- and postoperative period**

1. **Pulmonary artery catheters.** Current evidence suggests that the patients who are most likely to benefit from the use of pulmonary artery catheters are those with recent MI and associated CHF, those with severe coronary artery disease who are undergoing procedures that are routinely associated with hemodynamic stress, and patients with LV dysfunction, cardiomyopathy, or valvular disease who are undergoing high-risk operations.
2. **Continuous ECG monitoring.** Intra- and postoperative ST-segment changes are strong predictors of perioperative MI. Patients at high risk of cardiac complications should have continuous ECG monitoring perioperatively. Postoperative ischemia is a strong predictor of risk of long-term MI and cardiac death.
3. **Cardiac enzymes.** Routine postoperative assessment of cardiac enzymes should be discouraged. Enzymes should only be obtained in those patients who have clinical, ECG, or hemodynamic evidence of cardiovascular dysfunction.

**II. Preoperative pulmonary evaluation.** Clinically significant postoperative pulmonary complications are as common as postoperative cardiac complications. The most common complications include pneumonia, respiratory failure, bronchospasm, atelectasis, and exacerbation of underlying chronic lung disease (*N Engl J Med* 335:937, 1999).

**A. Modifiable patient-related risk factors**

1. Benefit from **smoking cessation** has been shown if patients stop smoking at least 8 weeks before surgery.
2. The incidence of complications in patients with **COPD** varies according to the severity of lung disease. Symptoms should be aggressively treated preoperatively. Bronchodilators, physical therapy, smoking cessation, and corticosteroids all reduce the risk of postoperative pulmonary complications. Although not all patients with COPD respond to **corticosteroid therapy,** a 2-week preoperative course is reasonable for symptomatic patients already receiving maximal bronchodilator therapy who are not at their best personal baseline level as determined by examination, chest x-ray, and spirometry. Patients with recent sputum changes may benefit from a preoperative course of **antibiotics.**
3. Before surgery, patients with **asthma** should be free of wheezing, with a peak expiratory flow rate greater than 80% of predicted or personal best level. See Chap. 10, Allergy and Immunology, for further management strategies.

**B. Procedure-related risk factors.** The surgical site is the most important predictor of pulmonary risk. Risk increases as the incision approaches the diaphragm. Upper abdominal and thoracic surgeries carry the greatest risk of postoperative pulmonary complications. Most studies have reported a lower risk of pulmonary complications for patients who undergo spinal or epidural anesthesia as compared to those who undergo general anesthesia. Regional anesthesia, such as an axillary block, carries even lower risk. The use of **pancuronium** should be avoided in patients with chronic pulmonary disease, as the risk of postoperative hypoventilation is higher due to neuromuscular blockade.

**C. Preoperative clinical evaluation with pulmonary function tests.** Routine preoperative use of pulmonary function tests remains controversial. Clinicians may reserve preoperative spirometry for patients who are to undergo thoracic or upper abdominal surgery and who have symptoms of cough, dyspnea, or exercise intolerance that remain unexplained after careful history and physical examination. Spirometry can be used for surveillance of lung volumes in patients with severe COPD or asthma in whom clinical assessment fails to elucidate the degree of airflow limitation.

**D. Arterial blood gas analysis.** Arterial blood gas analysis should not be used to identify patients for whom the risk of surgery would be prohibitive. It can be used to guide postoperative ventilatory management so that minute ventilations are directed to maintain preoperative levels of carbon dioxide retention.

**E. Reducing pulmonary risk postoperatively**

1. Postoperative use of **incentive spirometry** consistently reduces the relative risk of pulmonary complications by approximately 50% in repeated studies.
2. **Continuous positive airway pressure.** Clinicians should restrict the use of this modality to those patients who are unable to perform deep-breathing exercises or use an incentive spirometer.
3. The use of postoperative **epidural analgesia** is recommended in the setting of high-risk thoracic, abdominal, and major vascular surgery and has been shown to reduce the incidence of pulmonary complications.

**III. Hemostasis and transfusion issues in surgery**

**A. Strategies to reduce homologous blood exposure** include transfusing on a symptomatic basis only; correcting deficiencies in essential nutrients such as iron, folic acid, and vitamin $B_{12}$ preoperatively; pharmacologic stimulation of the bone marrow with recombinant erythropoietin; and avoidance of pharmacologic coagulopathies. Preoperative autologous blood donation can also be arranged. **Intraoperative measures** include normovolemic hemodilution for elective surgery, intraoperative blood salvage and autotransfusion, hypothermia, and positional blood pooling.

**B. General transfusion guidelines.** The patient's own blood is still the safest, but this strategy can usually only be used when the patient is not anemic and undergoing elective surgery with adequate time (3 weeks) available for blood donation. Arbitrary transfusion triggers (e.g., hemoglobin <10) are not supported by data and should not be used. Estimates of operative blood loss should be based on appropriately timed hematocrit measurements. **Erythropoietin,** 600 U/kg SC weekly starting 3 weeks before surgery (*Ann Thorac Surg* 54:101, 1992), has been approved for use perioperatively in mildly anemic patients (hemoglobin between 10 and 13) undergoing elective noncardiac surgery, but the clinical utility of this regimen has yet to be determined. The combination of erythropoietin with iron is indicated in patients with iron-deficiency anemia. Oral **iron supplementation** is sufficient in patients whose serum ferritin is greater than 100 ng/ml. For individuals whose ferritin level is less than 100 ng/ml, parenteral iron is indicated. Patients with **sickle cell anemia** require transfusion before surgery to reduce the percentage of hemoglobin S.

**IV. Surgery in the patient with liver disease.** The risk of perioperative morbidity or mortality is related to the extent of hepatic dysfunction. The **Child-Turcotte-Pugh score** (see Chap. 17, Liver Diseases, Table 17-5) has been shown to correlate with perioperative mortality in patients who are undergoing nonportacaval shunt surgery and in cirrhotic patients undergoing abdominal procedures. Patients with Child-Turcotte-Pugh class A, B, and C cirrhosis had mortalities of 10%, 31%, and 76%, respectively. The **serum albumin level, leukocytosis, and increased prothrombin time** are the most sensitive indicators of perioperative mortality independent of Child-Turcotte-Pugh score. Patients with acute symptomatic liver disease should have elective surgery postponed, if possible, until they have recovered. However, if surgery is emergent the following steps should be taken to optimize preoperative status.

**A. Coagulation status.** Vitamin K deficiency should be corrected by a single PO dose of 10 mg. Further coagulation anomalies may require fresh frozen plasma, given as needed. If the prothrombin time remains prolonged, cryoprecipitate can be used. Plasma exchange has been used for refractory coagulopathy. Prophylactic platelet transfusions can be considered for thrombocytopenia (platelet count <20,000).

**B. Renal and electrolyte abnormalities.** Careful attention should be paid to volume status. Nephrotoxic substances, such as NSAIDs and aminoglycosides, should be avoided. Patients with cirrhosis often have hypokalemia and alkalosis, and these conditions should be corrected preoperatively to minimize the risks of cardiac arrhythmias and to limit encephalopathy.

**C. Ascites.** Because the presence of ascites may influence respiratory mechanics and increase the risk of abdominal wound dehiscence, large-volume paracentesis is indicated preoperatively. Excessive use of saline solutions and medications containing sodium should be avoided. The use of albumin, blood products, or fresh frozen plasma may be useful for intravascular volume expansion and to slow reaccumulation of ascites. If hyponatremia occurs, free water restriction may be required (see Chap. 3, Fluid and Electrolyte Management).

**D. Encephalopathy.** Lactulose, 30 ml PO q6h, titrated to two to three soft bowel movements per day, should be started in patients with encephalopathy. Protein restriction has been recommended for individuals who respond poorly to lactulose but should be done cautiously, because excessive restriction may actually contribute to malnutrition. In addition, because encephalopathy may be worsened or precipitated by the use of sedatives, these should be avoided.

**E. Nutrition.** Malnutrition is common in patients with chronic liver disease and increases the risk of perioperative complications. Enteral nutrition (e.g., tube feeding) is helpful in improving Child class and reducing mortality in those with cirrhosis and malnutrition. A low-protein diet is advised only in patients with active encephalopathy.

**V. Perioperative diabetes management.** Patients with diabetes mellitus undergo surgical procedures at a higher rate than do nondiabetic persons (*Arch Intern Med* 159:2405, 1999). Major surgical operations require a period of fasting during which oral antidiabetic medications cannot be used. The stress of surgery itself results in metabolic perturbations that impair glucose regulation, and persistent hyperglycemia is a risk factor for postoperative sepsis. Elective surgery in patients with uncontrolled diabetes mellitus should preferably be scheduled after acceptable glycemic control has been achieved. If possible, the operation should be scheduled for early morning to minimize prolonged fasting.

**A. Patients managed with diet alone** may require no special intervention if diabetes is well controlled. Fasting and intraoperative blood glucose should be monitored. If fasting plasma glucose is 200 mg/dl or greater, small doses of SC short-acting insulin (regular or lispro) or IV infusion of insulin and 5% dextrose in water should be considered, depending on the duration and extent of surgery.

**B. Patients treated with oral antidiabetic agents. Short-acting sulfonylureas and other oral agents** should be withheld on the operative day. **Metformin and long-acting sulfonylureas** should be withheld 1 day before planned surgical procedures. Blood glucose should be monitored before and after surgery, and during surgery, for extensive procedures. Perioperative hyperglycemia (>200 mg/dl) can be managed with small SC doses of short-acting insulin (regular or lispro). Care must be taken to avoid hypoglycemia. For minor procedures, diabetes medications can be restarted once the patient starts eating. **Metformin therapy should be withheld for 48 hours postoperatively** and restarted after documentation of normal serum creatinine and absence of contrast-induced nephropathy. For extensive or stressful major procedures, hyperglycemia can be managed using an IV insulin infusion (see sec. **V.D**).

**C. Insulin-treated patients** can skip the morning dose of SC insulin on the day of surgery, depending on the nature of the operation. Patients treated with long-acting insulin can be switched to intermediate-acting forms 1–2 days before elective surgery. Close perioperative blood glucose monitoring is crucial to avoid extremes of glycemia.

**1. Patients undergoing minor surgery** of short duration require no special intervention if the fasting plasma glucose is 100–200 mg/dl. Glucose levels should be monitored q1h intraoperatively and immediately after surgery. Perioperative hyperglycemia can be managed with small SC doses of short-acting insulin (regular or lispro). The usual insulin treatment can be resumed once oral intake is established.

2. **Patients undergoing major surgery** should have preoperative measurement of blood glucose, serum electrolytes, and urine ketones. Ideally, metabolic and electrolyte abnormalities (e.g., hyponatremia, dyskalemia, acidosis) should be corrected before surgery. For patients treated with insulin, the most appropriate approach is IV insulin infusion (see sec. **V.D**). Another alternative is to give one-third to one-half of the total daily dose of insulin administered SC before surgery, depending on ambient glucose levels. Patients on insulin pumps can continue their usual basal rate of infusion.

**D. IV insulin infusion** is given for the management of diabetes in patients who are undergoing major procedures.

1. **Initial insulin infusion rate** can be estimated as one-half of the patient's total daily insulin dose divided by 24 hours expressed as units per hour. Regular insulin infusion from 0.5–1.0 U/hour is an appropriate starting dose for most patients with type 1 diabetes based on the degree of hyperglycemia; 5% dextrose in water (or 10% dextrose in water) at 100 ml/hour should also be started. An initial insulin infusion rate of 1–2 U/hour can be used in patients treated with oral antidiabetic agents who require perioperative insulin infusion.
2. **Maintenance infusion rates** for insulin and dextrose are determined using hourly blood glucose measurements; the goal is to maintain intraoperative plasma glucose in the 100- to 200-mg/dl range. In patients with persistent hyperglycemia, the insulin infusion rate should be increased by 25–50%. Conversely, if the blood glucose is less than 100 mg/dl or the decline of blood glucose is more than 100 mg/dl/hour, the insulin infusion should be stopped for 1 hour. The infusion can then be restarted at 25–50% of the initial rate.
3. **Potassium chloride,** 10 mEq, is added to each 500 ml dextrose to maintain normokalemia in patients with normal renal function.
4. **The duration of insulin and dextrose infusions** depends on the clinical status of the patient. The infusions should be continued postoperatively until oral intake is secure, after which the usual diabetes treatment can be resumed. It is prudent to give the first dose of SC insulin 30 minutes before disconnecting the IV route.

**VI. Perioperative corticosteroid management.** Surgery is one of the most potent activators of the hypothalamic-pituitary axis (HPA). The greatest cortisol and adrenocorticotropic hormone secretion occurs during reversal of anesthesia, extubation, and the immediate postoperative recovery period. Considerable variation is seen in the increased cortisol secretion among individuals undergoing surgery due to medication use, age, and associated illness. The adrenal gland produces 8–10 mg cortisol/day under normal conditions, 50 mg/day of cortisol during a minor surgical procedure, 75–100 mg/day during major procedures, and, rarely, in states of extreme stress and illness, up to 200 mg/day.

**A.** The following patients should be considered to have **functional suppression** of their HPA axis:

1. Any patient who has received more than 20 mg/day of prednisone or its equivalent for more than 3 weeks during the year preceding surgery
2. Any patient who has clinical Cushing's syndrome

**B.** In patients whose **HPA axis status is uncertain,** corticosteroids can be administered preoperatively or, time permitting, a cosyntropin stimulation test can be performed to assess HPA responsiveness.

**C. Guidelines for adrenal supplementation therapy** are based on extrapolation from small studies in the literature, expert opinion, and clinical experience.

1. Patients who receive 5 mg/day of prednisone or less should be given their normal daily replacement dose preoperatively.
2. Patients who are taking more than 5 mg/day should receive their normal daily dose in addition to supplementation therapy stratified according to the degree of surgical stress they are about to undergo (*JAMA* 287:236, 2002).
   a. **Minor surgical stress** (e.g., colonoscopy, cataract surgery): Administer 25 mg hydrocortisone or 5 mg methylprednisolone IV on the day of the procedure only.
   b. **Moderate surgical stress** (e.g., cholecystectomy, hemicolectomy): Administer 50–75 mg hydrocortisone or 10–15 mg methylprednisolone IV on the day of the procedure and taper quickly over 1 to 2 days to the usual dose.
   c. **Major surgical stress** (e.g., major cardiothoracic surgery, Whipple procedure): Administer 100–150 mg hydrocortisone or 20–30 mg methylprednisolone IV on the day of the procedure and taper to the usual dose over the next 1–2 days.
   d. **Critically ill patients undergoing emergent surgery** (e.g., sepsis, hypotension): Administer 50–100 mg hydrocortisone IV every 6–8 hours or 0.18 mg/kg/hour as a continuous infusion plus 50 mg/day of fludrocortisone until the shock has resolved. Then gradually taper the dose, monitoring vital signs and serum sodium closely.

**VII. Perioperative care of patients with kidney disease**

**A. Patients with end-stage renal disease (ESRD)** have estimated morbidity rates of 14–64% for cardiac and for noncardiac surgery (*Arch Intern Med* 154:1674, 1994). Causes include decreased abilities to concentrate urine, regulate fluid volume and sodium concentrations, handle acid loads, and excrete potassium and medications. **Hyperkalemia** is the most frequent complication, followed by infection, hemodynamic instability, bleeding, and arrhythmias.

**B. Strategies to reduce surgical risk in renal patients preoperatively**

1. A **potassium level** of less than 5.5 mmol/L is recommended to reduce the incidence of arrhythmias in the perioperative setting. This is achieved by giving polystyrene binding resins (30–60 g q6h either PO or via retention enema) or with preoperative hemodialysis in ESRD patients.
2. Although chronic **metabolic acidosis** has not been associated with elevated perioperative risk, some local anesthetics have reduced efficacy in acidotic patients. Preoperative metabolic acidosis should be corrected with sodium bicarbonate infusions.
3. Uremia-induced platelet dysfunction prolongs the bleeding time, and **all ESRD patients should undergo hemodialysis on the day before surgery.** The goal is to reduce the bleeding time to under 10–15 minutes. Other options for correcting bleeding times include
   a. **Desmopressin,** 0.3 μg/kg IV 1 hour before surgery
   b. **Cryoprecipitate,** 10 U over 30 minutes IV
   c. **Conjugated estrogens,** 0.6 mg/kg/day IV or PO for 5 days; some effect by 6 hours, peak effect at 7 days
4. **Anemia.** Patients with ESRD should have hematocrit levels greater than 26% before surgery (*Am J Surg* 134:765, 1977).
5. **Antibiotic prophylaxis.** Even for minor surgical procedures, prophylactic antibiotics using standard endocarditis protocols (see Table 13-1) are recommended for the first 6 months after the placement of synthetic vascular access grafts to prevent bacterial seeding before endothelialization.

**C. Postoperative renal insufficiency.** Common causes of postoperative renal insufficiency include acute tubular necrosis (a large percentage of which are accounted for by contrast-induced nephropathy) and hypoperfusion. The management of postoperative renal insufficiency involves early detection of worsening renal function, withdrawal of nephrotoxins (e.g., NSAIDs), prompt reversal of hypoperfusion, and correction of metabolic and electrolyte derangements. For further management, see Chap. 11, Renal Diseases.

**VIII. Common medication adjustments in the perioperative period**

**A. Aspirin** should be stopped at least 7 days before surgery. Stopping aspirin is especially important in the setting of neurosurgery, ophthalmologic surgery, and vascular procedures, where the risk of bleeding complications is highest. Aspirin is continued preferentially in many cardiac procedures. Postoperatively, aspirin should be restarted as soon as possible, when the risk of bleeding from surgery is diminished.

**B. NSAIDs.** Short-acting NSAIDs should be stopped 1 day before surgery, and longer-acting agents should be stopped 2–3 days in advance of any procedure to prevent antiplatelet effects. The newer cox-2 inhibitors have much less effect on platelet function than aspirin and nonselective NSAIDs. However, they have similar effects on renal prostaglandin synthesis as NSAIDs, and consequently use should be monitored closely in patients at risk for renal insufficiency.

**C. Lipid-lowering agents.** Niacin, fibric acid derivatives such as gemfibrozil, and the HMG (3-hydroxy-3-methyl-glutaryl)–coenzyme A reductase inhibitors (statins) may all cause myopathy or rhabdomyolysis, especially when used in combination. As a general precaution these agents should be discontinued the day before surgery and resumed when the patient is eating a full diet.

**D. Inhaled medications.** Inhaled β agonists, ipratropium, and corticosteroids should all be continued throughout the perioperative period.

**E. Thyroid medications.** Levothyroxine should be continued until the time of surgery on the patient's usual schedule. The drug has a half-life of 6–7 days and can be replaced IV at one half the oral dose if the patient remains NPO beyond this time. **Hyperthyroid patients** should continue taking their oral agents (i.e., propylthiouracil or methimazole) up to and including the day of surgery because control of the overactive gland is essential for safe surgery and recovery. Beta-blockers also can be used to control the effects of hyperthyroidism.

**F. Antiepileptics.** These agents should be continued in the perioperative period. If the patient is taking an agent that does not have an IV form and the surgery requires prolonged fasting, the patient can be converted to an antiepileptic with an IV form preoperatively.

**G. Antiparkinsonian medication.** Carbidopa/levodopa (Sinemet) should be continued in the perioperative period because worsening muscle rigidity complicates postoperative care. Sinemet interacts with many drugs used in anesthesia, which result in arrhythmias (see Appendix C, Drug Interactions).

**H. Benzodiazepines and opioid analgesics.** These medications, when used chronically, can lead to physiologic and psychological dependence. They should be continued in the perioperative period. IV and transdermal formulations exist for patients who are NPO. Due to tolerance issues dosage adjustments may be needed, especially with increased pain in the postoperative period.

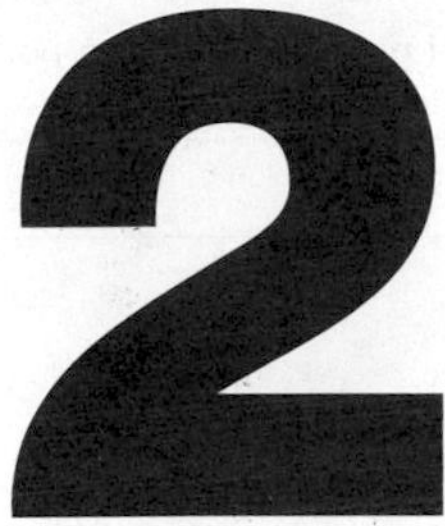

# Nutrition Support

Samuel Klein

An understanding of the fundamental aspects of clinical nutrition is important for the management of many hospitalized patients. Illness and injury can alter nutritional requirements and the ability to ingest, absorb, and process nutrients. The disruption in nutrient equilibrium can affect intermediary metabolism, organ function, body composition, and ultimately clinical outcome.

## I. Basic principles

**A. Energy stores.** Triglycerides present in adipose tissue are the body's major fuel reserve. During starvation, adipose tissue triglyceride becomes the major source of energy, and breakdown of body protein is decreased to conserve vital enzymatic, mechanical, and structural functions. The duration of survival during starvation depends largely on the amount of available body fat and lean tissue mass. Death from starvation is associated with body weight loss (loss of >35% of body weight), protein depletion (loss of >30% of body protein), fat depletion (loss of >70% of body fat stores), and body size [body mass index (BMI) of 13 kg/m$^2$ for men and 11 kg/m$^2$ for women] (see sec. **II.B.2**).

**B. Nutrient requirements**

1. **Energy.** Total daily energy expenditure (TEE) can be divided into resting energy expenditure (normally ~70% of TEE), thermic effect of food (normally ~10% of TEE), and energy expenditure of physical activity (normally ~20% of TEE). Malnutrition and hypocaloric feeding decrease resting energy expenditure to values 15–20% below those expected for actual body size, whereas metabolic stressors, such as inflammatory diseases or trauma, often increase energy requirements. However, it is rare for illnesses or injury to increase resting energy expenditure by more than 50% of preillness values. It is impossible to determine daily energy requirements precisely in hospitalized patients by using predictive equations because of the complexity of factors that affect metabolic rate. However, judicious use of predictive equations provides a reasonable estimate for most patients that should be modified as needed based on the patient's clinical course.

   a. **BMI approach.** A simple method for estimating total daily energy requirements in hospitalized patients based on BMI (see sec. **II.B.2**) is shown in Table 2-1. In general, energy requirements per kilogram of body weight are inversely related to BMI. The lower range within each category should be considered in insulin-resistant, critically ill patients—unless they are depleted in body fat—to decrease the risk of hyperglycemia and infection associated with overfeeding.

   b. The **Harris-Benedict equation** provides a reasonable estimate of resting energy expenditure (in kcal/day) in healthy adults:

$$\text{Men} = 66 + (13.7 \times W) + (5 \times H) - (6.8 \times A)$$

$$\text{Women} = 665 + (9.6 \times W) + (1.8 \times H) - (4.7 \times A)$$

   where W = adjusted body weight in kilograms, H = height in centimeters, and A = age in years. This equation takes into account the effect

**Table 2-1.** Estimated energy requirements for hospitalized patients based on body mass index (BMI)

| BMI ($kg/m^2$) | Energy requirements (kcal/kg/d) |
|---|---|
| <15 | 35–40 |
| 15–19 | 30–35 |
| 20–24 | 20–25 |
| 25–29 | 15–20 |
| ≥ 30 | <15 |

*Note:* These values are recommended for critically ill patients and all obese patients; add 20% of total calories in estimating energy requirements in non–critically ill patients.

of body size and lean tissue mass (which is influenced by gender and age) on energy requirements and can be used to estimate total daily energy needs in hospitalized patients. An **adjusted body weight** rather than actual body weight should be used in obese patients (BMI ≥ 30 $kg/m^2$) to avoid overfeeding. Adjusted body weight = ideal body weight + [(actual body weight − ideal body weight) × (0.25)]. **Ideal body weight** can be estimated based on height. For men, 106 lb is allotted for the first 5 ft, then 6 lb is added for each inch above 5 ft; for women, 100 lb is given for the first 5 ft, with 5 lb added for each additional inch. Providing total daily energy equal to the Harris-Benedict calculation should be considered in obese and critically ill patients. Providing total daily energy equal to the Harris-Benedict calculation plus an additional 20% is a reasonable goal for nonobese, non–critically ill patients who have increased metabolic demands. An additional 300–500 kcal should be added to Harris-Benedict estimates in patients who are underweight (BMI <18.5 $kg/m^2$).

2. **Protein.** Protein intake of 0.8 g/kg/day meets the requirements of 97% of the adult population. Individual protein requirements are affected by several factors, such as the amount of nonprotein calories provided, overall energy requirements, protein quality, and the patient's nutritional status. Inadequate amounts of any of the essential amino acids result in inefficient utilization. Table 2-2 lists approximate protein requirements during different clinical conditions.

**Table 2-2.** Recommended daily protein intake

| Clinical condition | Protein requirements (g/kg IBW/d)[a] |
|---|---|
| Normal | 0.8 |
| Metabolic "stress" (illness/injury) | 1.0–1.5 |
| Acute renal failure (undialyzed) | 0.8–1.0 |
| Hemodialysis | 1.2–1.4 |
| Peritoneal dialysis | 1.3–1.5 |

IBW, ideal body weight.
[a]Additional protein intake may be needed to compensate for excess protein loss in specific patient populations, such as those with burn injury, open wounds, and protein-losing enteropathy or nephropathy. Lower protein intake may be necessary in patients with chronic renal insufficiency who are not treated by dialysis and certain patients with hepatic encephalopathy.

3. **Essential fatty acids.** Most fatty acids can be synthesized by the liver, but humans lack the desaturase enzyme needed to produce the n-3 and n-6 fatty acid series. Therefore, linoleic acid should constitute at least 2% and linolenic acid at least 0.5% of the daily caloric intake to prevent the occurrence of essential fatty acid deficiency. The plasma pattern of increased triene-tetraene ratio (>0.4) can be used to detect essential fatty acid deficiency, even before the presence of clinical manifestations (dermatitis, coarse hair, alopecia, poor wound healing).
4. **Carbohydrate.** Certain tissues, such as bone marrow, erythrocytes, leukocytes, renal medulla, eye tissues, and peripheral nerves, cannot metabolize fatty acids and require glucose (~40 g/day) as a fuel, whereas other tissues, such as the brain, prefer glucose (~120 g/day) as a fuel.
5. **Major minerals.** Major minerals are important for ionic equilibrium, water balance, and normal cell function. The following are the daily recommended intakes (enteral and parenteral values, respectively): for sodium, 0.5–5.0 g and 60–150 mEq; for potassium, 2–5 g and 60–100 mEq; for magnesium, 300–400 mg and 8–24 mEq; for calcium, 800–1200 mg and 5–15 mEq; and for phosphorus, 800–1200 mg and 12–24 mEq.
6. **Micronutrients (trace elements and vitamins).** Trace elements and vitamins are essential constituents of enzyme complexes. The recommended dietary intake for trace elements, fat-soluble vitamins, and water-soluble vitamins (Table 2-3) is set at two standard deviations above the estimated mean so that it will cover the needs of 97% of the healthy population. Therefore, the recommended dietary intake exceeds the micronutrient requirements of most persons.
7. **Special considerations**
    a. **Mineral and vitamin supplementation in patients with severe malabsorption.** Patients who have an inadequate length of functional small bowel because of intestinal resection or intestinal disease require additional vitamins and minerals if they are not receiving parenteral nutrition. Table 2-4 provides guidelines for supplementation in these patients.
    b. **Patients with excessive GI tract losses** require additional fluids and electrolytes. An assessment of fluid losses through diarrhea, ostomy output, and fistula volume should be made to help determine fluid requirements. Knowledge of fluid losses is also useful in calculating intestinal mineral losses by multiplying the volume of fluid loss by an estimate of intestinal fluid electrolyte concentration (Table 2-5).

II. **Assessment of nutritional status.** The assessment of nutritional status can be divided into techniques that identify specific nutrient deficiencies and those used to assess protein-energy malnutrition. At present there is no gold standard for evaluating the nutritional status of hospitalized patients. The best overall approach involves a careful clinical evaluation, which includes a nutritional history and physical examination in conjunction with appropriate laboratory studies to evaluate further the abnormal findings obtained during clinical examination.

A. **Specific nutrient deficiencies.** A careful history and physical examination, routine blood tests, and selected laboratory tests can be used to diagnose specific macronutrient, major mineral, vitamin, and trace mineral deficiencies (Table 2-3).

B. **Protein-energy malnutrition.** Commonly used indicators of protein-energy malnutrition correlate with clinical outcome. However, all these indicators are influenced by illness or injury, making it difficult to separate the contribution of malnutrition from the severity of illness itself on outcome. The assessment techniques listed below can be used to determine subjectively

**Table 2-3.** Trace mineral, fat-soluble vitamin, and water-soluble vitamin requirements and assessment of deficiency

| Nutrient | Recommended daily enteral intake in normal adults | Recommended daily parenteral intake in normal adults | Symptoms or signs of deficiency | Laboratory evaluation |
|---|---|---|---|---|
| Chromium | 30–200 μg | 10–20 μg | Glucose intolerance, peripheral neuropathy, encephalopathy | Serum chromium |
| Copper | 2 mg | 0.3 mg | Anemia, neutropenia, osteoporosis, diarrhea | Serum copper, plasma ceruloplasmin |
| Iodine | 150 μg | 70–140 μg | Hypothyroidism, goiter | Urine iodine, thyroid-stimulating hormone |
| Iron | 10–15 mg | 1.0–1.5 mg | Microcytic hypochromic anemia | Serum iron and total iron-binding capacity, serum ferritin |
| Manganese | 1.5 mg | 0.2–0.8 mg | Hypercholesterolemia, dementia, dermatitis | Serum manganese |
| Selenium | 50–200 μg | 20–40 μg | Cardiomyopathy, muscle weakness | Serum selenium, blood glutathione peroxidase activity |
| Zinc | 15 mg | 2.5–4.0 mg | Growth retardation, delayed sexual maturation, hypogonadism, alopecia, acro-orificial skin lesion, diarrhea, mental status changes | Plasma zinc |
| Vitamin K (phylloquinone) | 50–100 μg | 100 μg | Easy bruising/bleeding | Prothrombin time |
| Vitamin A (retinol) | 5000 IU | 3300 IU | Night blindness, Bitot's spots, keratomalacia, follicular hyperkeratosis, xerosis | Serum retinol |
| Vitamin D (ergocalciferol) | 400 IU | 200 IU | Rickets, osteomalacia, osteoporosis, bone pain, muscle weakness, tetany | Serum 25-hydroxyvitamin D |

| | | | | |
|---|---|---|---|---|
| Vitamin E (alpha tocopherol) | 10–15 IU | 10 IU | Hemolysis, retinopathy, neuropathy, abnormal clotting | Serum tocopherol: total lipid (triglyceride and cholesterol) ratio |
| Vitamin $B_1$ (thiamine) | 1.0–1.5 mg | 3 mg | Beriberi, cardiac failure, Wernicke's encephalopathy, peripheral neuropathy, fatigue, ophthalmoplegia | RBC transketolase activity |
| Vitamin $B_2$ (riboflavin) | 1.1–1.8 mg | 3.6 mg | Cheilosis, sore tongue and mouth, eye irritation, seborrheic dermatitis | RBC glutathione reductase activity |
| Vitamin $B_3$ (niacin) | 12–20 mg | 40 mg | Pellagra (dermatitis, diarrhea, dementia), sore mouth and tongue | Urinary *N*-methyl-nicotinamide |
| Vitamin $B_5$ (pantothenic acid) | 5–10 mg | 10 mg | Fatigue, weakness, paresthesias, tenderness of heels and feet | Urinary pantothenic acid |
| Vitamin $B_6$ (pyridoxine) | 12 mg | 4 mg | Seborrheic dermatitis, cheilosis, glossitis, peripheral neuritis, convulsions, hypochromic anemia | Plasma pyridoxal phosphate |
| Vitamin $B_7$ (biotin) | 100–200 µg | 60 µg | Seborrheic dermatitis, alopecia, mental status change, seizures, myalgia, hyperesthesia | Plasma biotin |
| Vitamin $B_9$ (folic acid) | 400 µg | 400 µg | Megaloblastic anemia, glossitis, diarrhea | Serum folic acid, RBC folic acid |
| Vitamin $B_{12}$ (cobalamin) | 5 µg | 5 µg | Megaloblastic anemia, paresthesias, decreased vibratory or position sense, ataxia, mental status changes, diarrhea | Serum cobalamin, serum methylmalonic acid |
| Vitamin C (ascorbic acid) | 100 mg | 100 mg | Scurvy, petechia, purpura, gingival inflammation, and bleeding, weakness, depression | Plasma ascorbic acid, leukocyte ascorbic acid |

**Table 2-4.** Guidelines for vitamin and mineral supplementation in patients with severe malabsorption

| Supplement | Dose | Route |
|---|---|---|
| Prenatal multivitamin with minerals[a] | 1 tablet qd | PO |
| Vitamin D[a] | 50,000 U 2–3 times/wk | PO |
| Calcium[a] | 500 mg elemental calcium tid–qid | PO |
| Vitamin $B_{12}$[b] | 1 mg qd | PO |
| | 100–500 μg q1–2 mo | SC |
| Vitamin A[b] | 10,000–50,000 U qd | PO |
| Vitamin K[b] | 5 mg/d | PO |
| | 5–10 mg/wk | SC |
| Vitamin E[b] | 30 U/d | PO |
| Magnesium gluconate[b] | 108–169 mg elemental magnesium qid | PO |
| Magnesium sulfate[b] | 290 mg elemental magnesium 1–3 times/wk | IM/IV |
| Zinc gluconate or zinc sulfate[b] | 25 mg elemental zinc qd plus 100 mg elemental zinc/L intestinal output | PO |
| Ferrous sulfate[b] | 60 mg elemental iron tid | PO |
| Iron dextran[b] | Daily dose based on formula or table | IV |

[a]Recommended routinely for all patients.
[b]Recommended for patients with documented nutrient deficiency or malabsorption.

whether patients are well nourished, moderately malnourished, or severely malnourished (see sec. **IV.A**).

1. **History.** The patient and any appropriate family members should be interviewed to provide insight into the patient's current nutritional state and future ability to consume an adequate amount of nutrients. The nutritional history should evaluate the following:
   a. **Body weight.** The presence of mild (<5%), moderate (5–10%), or severe (>10%) unintentional body weight loss in the last 6 months should be established. In general, a 10% or greater unintentional loss in body weight in the last 6 months is associated with a poor clinical outcome (*Am J Med* 69:491, 1980).

**Table 2-5.** Electrolyte concentrations in gastrointestinal fluids

| Location | Na (mEq/L) | K (mEq/L) | Cl (mEq/L) | $HCO_3$ (mEq/L) |
|---|---|---|---|---|
| Stomach | 65 | 10 | 100 | — |
| Bile | 150 | 4 | 100 | 35 |
| Pancreas | 150 | 7 | 80 | 75 |
| Duodenum | 90 | 15 | 90 | 15 |
| Mid–small bowel | 140 | 6 | 100 | 20 |
| Terminal ileum | 140 | 8 | 60 | 70 |
| Rectum | 40 | 90 | 15 | 30 |

b. **Food intake.** A change in habitual diet pattern (number, size, and contents of meals) should be determined. If present, the reason for altered food intake (e.g., change in appetite, mental status or mood, ability to prepare meals, ability to chew or swallow, GI symptoms) should be investigated.
c. **Evidence of malabsorption**
d. **Specific nutrient deficiencies** (Table 2-3)
e. **Level of metabolic stress**
f. **Functional status** (e.g., bedridden, suboptimally active, change from baseline)

2. **Physical examination.** The physical examination corroborates and adds to the findings obtained by history and should include an assessment of the following:
a. **BMI,** which is defined as weight (in kilograms) divided by [height (meters)]$^2$ or weight (in pounds) times 704 divided by [height (inches)]$^2$. Patients can be classified by BMI as underweight (<18.5 kg/m$^2$), normal weight (18.5–24.9 kg/m$^2$), overweight (25.0–29.9 kg/m$^2$), class I obesity (30.0–34.9 kg/m$^2$), class II obesity (35.0–39.9 kg/m$^2$), or class III obesity (≥ 40.0 kg/m$^2$) (*Obes Res* 6[Suppl 2]:S53, 1998). Patients who are **extremely underweight** (BMI <14 kg/m$^2$) have a high risk of death and should be considered for admission to the hospital for nutritional support.
b. **Tissue depletion** (loss of body fat and skeletal muscle wasting)
c. **Muscle function** (strength testing of individual muscle groups)
d. **Fluid status** [signs and symptoms of either dehydration (hypotension, tachycardia, postural changes, mucosal xerosis, decreased axillary sweat, or dry skin) or excess body fluid (i.e., edema or ascites)]

3. **Laboratory studies** should be performed to determine specific nutrient deficiencies when clinically indicated (Table 2-3). The concentrations of several plasma proteins (e.g., albumin, prealbumin, retinol-binding protein, and transferrin) have been shown to correlate with clinical outcome. For example, a low serum albumin concentration is associated with an increased incidence of medical complications and death (*Crit Care Med* 10:305, 1982). However, illness or injury, not malnutrition, is responsible for hypoalbuminemia in sick patients (*Gastroenterology* 99:1845, 1990). Inflammation and injury decrease albumin synthesis, increase albumin degradation, and increase albumin transcapillary losses from the plasma compartment. In addition, certain GI, renal, and cardiac diseases can increase albumin losses through the GI tract and kidney, and albumin can be lost through surface tissues that have been damaged by wounds, burns, and peritonitis.

## III. Enteral nutrition

### A. General principles.
**A. General principles.** Whenever possible, oral/enteral rather than parenteral feeding should be used in patients who need nutritional support. Oral/enteral nutrition helps maintain the structural and functional integrity of the GI tract by preventing atrophy of the intestinal mucosa and pancreas, preserving mucosal digestive and pancreatic secretory enzyme activity, maintaining GI IgA secretion, and preventing cholelithiasis. In addition, oral/enteral nutrition is usually less expensive than parenteral nutrition. However, the intestinal tract cannot be used effectively in patients who have persistent nausea or vomiting, intolerable postprandial abdominal pain or diarrhea, mechanical obstruction, severe hypomotility, severe malabsorption, or high-output fistulas that do not permit feedings proximal or distal to the fistula.

### B. Types of feedings

1. **Hospital diets** include a regular diet and diets modified in either nutrient content (amount of fiber, fat, protein, or sodium) or consistency (liquid, pureed, soft). Food intake can often be increased by encouraging

patients to eat, providing assistance at mealtime, avoiding unpalatable diets, allowing some food to be supplied by relatives and friends, and limiting missed meals for medical tests and procedures.

2. **Defined liquid formulas** include monomeric formulas, oligomeric formulas, and polymeric formulas. Polymeric formulas are appropriate for most patients. **Elemental (monomeric) formulas** (e.g., Vivonex, Glutasorb) contain nitrogen in the form of free amino acids and small amounts of fat (<5% of total calories) and are hyperosmolar (550–650 mOsm/kg). These formulas are not palatable and require either tube feeding or mixing with other foods or flavorings for oral ingestion. Absorption of monomeric formulas is not clinically superior to that of oligomeric or polymeric formulas in patients with adequate pancreatic digestive function. **Semielemental (oligomeric) formulas** (e.g., Propeptide, Peptamen) contain hydrolyzed protein in the form of small peptides and sometimes free amino acids. **Polymeric formulas** contain nitrogen in the form of whole proteins and include blenderized food, milk-based, and lactose-free formulas. Milk-based formulas (e.g., Carnation Instant Breakfast) contain milk as a source of protein and fat and tend to be more palatable than other defined formula diets. Milk-based formulas can be problematic for some lactose-intolerant patients but are often tolerated when infused continuously because this approach decreases the rate of lactose delivered to the intestine. Lactose-free formulas (e.g., Osmolite, Ensure) are the most commonly used polymeric formulas in hospitalized patients. These formulas are available as standard iso-osmolar solutions, containing approximately 1 kcal/ml, 16% calories as protein, 55% calories as carbohydrate, and 30% calories as fat. Most patients can be fed with standard iso-osmolar lactose-free formulas. Predigested (elemental and semielemental) formulas are more expensive than standard formulas and do not usually provide additional clinical benefits, even in patients with limited digestive and absorptive function, such as those with pancreatic insufficiency treated with enzyme replacement and those with short-bowel syndrome. Other formulas are also available that have modified nutrient content, such as high-nitrogen (e.g., Promote, Perative) or high-calorie (e.g., Two Cal HN) formulas for patients who require fluid restriction, fiber-enriched formulas (e.g., Jevity) for individuals with constipation or loose stools or those receiving long-term enteral tube feeding, and reduced protein, fluid, phosphorus, potassium, and magnesium for patients with renal insufficiency (e.g., Nepro).
3. **Oral rehydration solutions.** Oral rehydration solutions stimulate sodium and water absorption by taking advantage of the sodium-glucose cotransporter present in the brush border of intestinal epithelium. Oral rehydration therapy can be useful in patients with severe GI fluid and mineral losses, such as those with short-bowel syndrome (*Clin Ther* 12[Suppl A]:129, 1990) and HIV infection (*Nutrition* 5:390, 1989). In patients with short-bowel syndrome, it is particularly important that the sodium concentration of the solution be between 90 and 120 mEq/L to avoid intestinal sodium secretion and negative sodium and water balance. The characteristics of several oral rehydration solutions are listed in Table 2-6.

C. **Enteral tube feeding.** Enteral tube feeding is useful in patients who have a functional GI tract but who cannot or will not ingest adequate nutrients. The type of tube-feeding approach selected (nasogastric, nasoduodenal, nasojejunal, gastrostomy, jejunostomy, pharyngostomy, and esophagostomy tubes) depends on physician experience, clinical prognosis, gut patency and motility, risk of aspirating gastric contents, patient preference, and anticipated duration of feeding.

1. **Short-term (<6 weeks) tube feeding** can be achieved by placement of a soft, small-bore nasogastric or nasoenteric feeding tube. These tubes

**Table 2-6.** Characteristics of selected oral rehydration solutions

| Product | Na (mEq/L) | K (mEq/L) | Cl (mEq/L) | Citrate (mEq/L) | kcal/L | CHO (g/L) | mOsm |
|---|---|---|---|---|---|---|---|
| Equalyte | 78 | 22 | 68 | 30 | 100 | 25 | 305 |
| CeraLyte 70 | 70 | 20 | 98 | 30 | 165 | 40 | 235 |
| CeraLyte 90 | 90 | 20 | 98 | 30 | 165 | 40 | 260 |
| Pedialyte | 45 | 20 | 35 | 30 | 100 | 20 | 300 |
| Rehydralyte | 74 | 19 | 64 | 30 | 100 | 25 | 305 |
| Gatorade | 20 | 3 | NA | NA | 210 | 45 | 330 |
| WHO[a] | 90 | 20 | 80 | 30 | 80 | 20 | 200 |
| Washington University[b] | 105 | 0 | 100 | 10 | 85 | 20 | 250 |

NA, not applicable; WHO, World Health Organization.
*Note:* Mix formulas with sugar-free flavorings as needed for palatability.
[a]WHO formula: Mix 3/4 tsp sodium chloride, 1/2 tsp sodium citrate, 1/4 tsp potassium chloride, and 4 tsp glucose (dextrose) in 1 L (4 1/4 cups) distilled water.
[b]Washington University formula: Mix 3/4 tsp sodium chloride, 1/2 tsp sodium citrate, and 3 tbsp + 1 tsp Polycose powder in 1 L (4 1/4 cups) distilled water.

are made of silicone or polyurethane and do not cause the tissue irritation and necrosis associated with larger polyvinyl chloride tubes. Because many patients are able to eat with the tube in place, tube feeding can be used to supplement oral intake. Although nasogastric feeding is usually the most appropriate route, orogastric feeding in patients with nasal injury or gross nasal deformity and nasoduodenal or nasojejunal feeding in patients with gastroparesis can also be used. Nasoduodenal and nasojejunal feeding tubes can be placed at the bedside with a success rate approaching 90% when inserted by experienced personnel (*Nutr Clin Pract* 16:258, 2001).

2. **Long-term (>6 weeks) tube feeding** usually requires a gastrostomy or jejunostomy tube that can be placed endoscopically, radiologically, or surgically, depending on the clinical situation and local expertise. **Percutaneous endoscopic gastrostomy** can be performed within 30 minutes and is successfully completed in more than 90% of attempts (*Am J Surg* 149:102, 1985). Gastrostomy tubes can be placed percutaneously without endoscopy by inserting the catheter directly into the stomach via a peel-away sheath introduced over a previously placed J-wire guide (*Am J Surg* 184:132, 1984). This approach permits tube placement in patients with an obstructing lesion of the esophagus or hypopharynx that prevents passage of an endoscope or gastrostomy tube. Jejunal tube placement can be achieved by threading a tube through an existing gastrostomy or by direct percutaneous endoscopic jejunostomy in patients with previous partial or total gastrectomy (*Gastrointest Endosc* 33:372, 1987). **Surgical gastrostomy and jejunostomy** can be performed by open and laparoscopic techniques and are particularly useful when endoscopic and radiologic approaches are technically impossible or cannot be performed safely because of prior abdominal surgeries or overlying bowel.
3. **Feeding schedules.** Patients who have feeding tubes in the stomach can often tolerate **intermittent bolus or gravity feedings,** in which the total amount of daily formula is divided into four to six equal portions. Bolus feedings are given by syringe as rapidly as tolerated, and gravity

feedings are infused over 30–60 minutes. The patient's upper body should be elevated by 30–45 degrees during and for at least 2 hours after feeding. Tubes should be flushed with water after each feeding. Intermittent feedings are useful for patients who cannot be positioned with continuous head-of-the-bed elevation or who require greater freedom from feeding. However, patients who experience nausea and early satiety with bolus gravity feedings may require continuous infusion at a slower rate. **Continuous feeding** can often be started at 20–30 ml/hour and advanced by 10 ml/hour every 6 hours until the feeding goal (see sec. **I.B**) is reached. Patients who have gastroparesis often tolerate gastric tube feedings when they are started at a slow rate (e.g., 10 ml/hour) and advanced by small increments (e.g., 10 ml/hour q8–12h). However, patients with severe gastroparesis require passage of the feeding tube tip past the ligament of Treitz. Continuous feeding should always be used when feeding directly into the duodenum or jejunum to avoid distention, abdominal pain, and dumping syndrome.

4. **Complications**
   a. **Mechanical complications. Nasogastric feeding tube misplacement** occurs more commonly in unconscious than in conscious patients. Intubation of the tracheobronchial tree has been reported in up to 15% of patients; intracranial placement can occur in patients with skull fractures. **Erosive tissue damage** can lead to nasopharyngeal erosions, pharyngitis, sinusitis, otitis media, pneumothorax, and GI tract perforation. **Tube occlusion** is often caused by inspissated feedings or pulverized medications given through small-diameter (<No. 10 French) tubes. Frequent flushing of the tube with 30–60 ml water and avoiding administration of pill fragments or "thick" medications help prevent occlusion. Techniques used to unclog tubes include the use of a small-volume syringe (10 ml) to flush warm water or pancreatic enzymes (Viokase dissolved in water) through the tube. Commercially made products can be obtained that either dissolve or mechanically remove the obstruction.
   b. **Hyperglycemia.** Management of blood glucose in tube-fed patients with diabetes can be challenging. Subcutaneously administered insulin can usually maintain good control. Intermediate-duration insulin can often be used safely once tube feedings reach 1000 kcal/day. Providing intermediate-duration insulin every 12 hours is appropriate for patients who are being given continuous (24 hours/day) feeding. A sliding-scale algorithm for regular insulin supplementation may be necessary to cover glucose excursions and should be designed to meet each patient's specific needs based on type of diabetes, tube-feeding regimen, and concurrent medical therapies.
   c. **Pulmonary aspiration.** The etiology of pulmonary aspiration can be difficult to determine in tube-fed patients because aspiration can occur from refluxed tube feedings or oropharyngeal secretions that are unrelated to feedings. Assessing the color of respiratory secretions after adding several drops of blue food coloring to the feeding formula has been used to aid in determining whether tube feedings are contributing to recovered secretions. However, several case reports suggest that food coloring can be absorbed by the GI tract in critically ill patients, which can lead to serious complications (i.e., refractory hypotension, metabolic acidosis) and death (*N Engl J Med* 343:1047, 2000). Therefore, if food coloring is added to enteral feedings, it should only be done for short periods of time and for valid indications. Prevention of reflux by decreasing gastric acid secretion, keeping the head of the bed elevated during feedings, checking gastric residuals, and avoiding gastric feeding in high-risk

patients (e.g., those with gastroparesis, gastric outlet obstruction, or frequent vomiting; dysphagia is not a contraindication for gastric tube feeding) is the best management approach.

d. **GI complications** include nausea, vomiting, abdominal pain, diarrhea, and intestinal ischemia/necrosis. Diarrhea is common in patients who receive tube feeding and occurs in up to 50% of critically ill patients. **Diarrhea** is often associated with antibiotic therapy (*JPEN J Parenter Enteral Nutr* 15:277, 1991) and the use of liquid medications that contain nonabsorbable carbohydrates, such as sorbitol (*Am J Med* 88:91, 1990). If diarrhea from tube feeding persists after proper evaluation of possible causes, a trial of antidiarrheal agents or fiber is justified.

## IV. Parenteral nutrition

**A. General principles.** Patients who are unable to consume "adequate" nutrients for a "prolonged" period of time by oral or enteral routes require parenteral nutritional therapy to prevent the adverse effects of malnutrition. However, the decision to use parenteral nutrition can be difficult because the precise definition of "adequate" and "prolonged" is not clear and depends on the patient's amount of body fat and lean tissue mass, the presence of preexisting medical illnesses, and the level of metabolic stress. In general, parenteral nutrition should be considered if energy intake has been, or is anticipated to be, inadequate (<50% of daily requirements) for more than 7 days and enteral feeding is not feasible. However, the efficacy of this approach has not been tested in clinical trials.

### B. Central parenteral nutrition (CPN)

1. **Catheters.** The infusion of hyperosmolar (usually >1500 mOsm/L) nutrient solutions requires a large-bore, high-flow vessel to minimize vessel irritation and damage. Percutaneous subclavian vein catheterization with advancement of the catheter tip to the junction of the superior vena cava and right atrium is the most commonly used technique for CPN access. The internal jugular, saphenous, and femoral veins are also used. Although these sites either decrease or eliminate the risk of pneumothorax, they are less desirable because of decreased patient comfort and difficulty in maintaining sterility. **Peripherally inserted central venous catheters,** which also eliminate the risk of pneumothorax, can be used to provide CPN in patients with adequate antecubital vein access.

2. **Macronutrient solutions**

   a. **Crystalline amino acid solutions,** containing 40–50% essential and 50–60% nonessential amino acids (usually with little or no glutamine, glutamate, aspartate, asparagine, tyrosine, and cysteine), are used to provide protein needs (Table 2-2). Infused amino acids are oxidized and should be included in the estimate of energy provided as part of the parenteral formulation. Some amino acid solutions have been modified for specific disease states, such as those enriched in branched-chain amino acids, advocated for use in patients who have hepatic encephalopathy, or those that contain mostly essential amino acids, advocated for patients with renal insufficiency.

   b. **Glucose (dextrose)** in IV solutions is hydrated; each gram of dextrose monohydrate provides 3.4 kcal. At least 150 g glucose/day is needed to maximize protein balance and provide energy to tissues that require and prefer glucose as a fuel (see sec. **I.B.4**).

   c. **Lipid emulsions** are available as a 10% (1.1 kcal/ml) or 20% (2.0 kcal/ml) solution and provide energy as well as a source of essential fatty acids. Emulsion particles are similar in size and structure to chylomicrons and are metabolized like nascent chylomicrons after acquiring apoproteins from contact with circulating endogenous high-density lipoprotein particles. Lipid emulsions are as effective as glucose in conserving body nitrogen economy once absolute tissue requirements for glucose are met. The optimal percentage of calories that should be infused as fat is not known, but 20–30% of total calories is reasonable for most patients. The **rate of infusion should not exceed 1.0 kcal/kg/hour** (0.11 g/kg/hour) because most complications associated with lipid infusions have been reported when providing more than this amount (*Curr Opin Gastroenterol* 7:306, 1991). A rate of 0.03–0.05 g/kg/hour is adequate for most patients who are receiving continuous CPN. Lipid emulsions should not be given to patients who have triglyceride concentrations of greater than 400 mg/dl. Moreover, patients at risk for **hypertriglyceridemia** should have serum triglyceride concentrations checked at least once during lipid emulsion infusion to ensure adequate clearance. Lipids may not be necessary in obese patients; underfeeding obese patients by the amount of lipid calories that would normally be given (e.g., 20–30% of calories) facilitates mobilization of endogenous fat stores for fuel and may improve insulin sensitivity and glucose control.

3. **Complications.** The incidence of most complications associated with the use of CPN is reduced with careful management and supervision, preferably by an experienced nutrition support team if available (*JAMA* 243:1906, 1980).

   a. **Mechanical complications,** such as pneumothorax, brachial plexus injury, subclavian and carotid artery puncture, hemothorax, thoracic duct injury, and chylothorax, may occur during central line insertion. Even when the subclavian vein is cannulated successfully, other mechanical complications can still occur. The catheter can be advanced upward into the internal jugular vein, or the tip can be sheared off completely if it is withdrawn back through an introducing needle. Air embolism can occur during insertion or whenever the connection between the catheter and IV tubing is disrupted.

   b. **Metabolic complications,** such as fluid overload, hypertriglyceridemia, hypercalcemia, hypoglycemia, hyperglycemia, and specific nutrient deficiencies, are usually caused by overzealous or inadequate nutrient administration. Blood glucose above 200 mg/dl should be avoided because it is associated with leukocyte and complement dysfunction and increases the risk of infection. Blood glucose goals for most patients are 100–200 mg/dl initially and 100–150 mg/dl when their conditions are stable. Blood glucose should be kept below 120 mg/dl in pregnant patients to avoid complications of gestational diabetes and large-for-gestational-age births.

      (1) **Management of patients with hyperglycemia or diabetes** (*Mayo Clin Proc* 71:587–594, 1996). If blood glucose is greater than 200 mg/dl or the patient has diabetes, consider obtaining better control of blood glucose before starting CPN. If CPN is started: (1) Limit dextrose to less than 200 g/day, (2) add 0.1 U of regular insulin for each gram of dextrose in CPN solution (e.g., 15 U for 150 g), (3) discontinue other sources of IV dextrose, and (4) order sliding-scale SC regular insulin with blood glucose monitoring by fingerstick every 4–6 hours or sliding-scale IV regular insulin infusion with blood glucose monitoring by fingerstick every 1–2 hours. If blood glucose remains greater than 200 mg/dl and the patient has been receiving SC insulin, add 50% of sliding-scale regular insulin given in the last 24 hours to the next day's CPN solution and double the amount of SC insulin sliding-scale dose for blood glucose values greater than 200 mg/dl. If the blood glucose remains greater than 200 mg/dl and the patient has been receiving IV insulin, add 50% of the IV insulin given in the last

24 hours to the next day's CPN solution and increase sliding-scale IV insulin by 50% for blood glucose values greater than 200 mg/dl. If the patient's blood glucose remains greater than 200 mg/dl, consider (1) discontinuing CPN until better glucose control can be established, (2) decreasing dextrose content in CPN, or (3) initiating insulin drip. Dextrose in CPN can be increased when blood glucose control (100–150 mg/dl) is achieved. The insulin-dextrose ratio in CPN formulation should be maintained while CPN dextrose content is changed.

c. **Thrombosis and pulmonary embolus.** Radiologically evident subclavian vein thrombosis occurs commonly (25–50% of patients), but clinically significant manifestations, such as upper extremity edema, superior vena cava syndrome, or pulmonary embolism, are rare. Patients with hypercoagulable conditions are at increased risk of catheter-induced central vein thrombosis. Prophylactic use of low-dose warfarin (1–2 mg/day), which rarely increases the international normalized ratio, should be considered in these patients, and the dose of warfarin should be increased to full therapeutic anticoagulation if central vein thrombosis or pulmonary embolism occurs. Fatal microvascular pulmonary emboli caused by nonvisible precipitate, containing calcium and phosphorus, in total nutrient admixtures underscore the importance of maintaining strict pharmacy standards regarding physical-chemical compatibility. Moreover, **inline filters** should be used with all parenteral nutrient solutions. The smallest pulmonary capillaries are 5 μm in diameter, and the size limit for visual detection of microprecipitates is 50–100 μm (*Clin Nutr* 10:114, 1995).

d. **Infectious complications.** Catheter-related sepsis is the most common life-threatening complication in patients who receive CPN and is most commonly caused by *Staphylococcus epidermidis* and *Staphylococcus aureus*. In immunocompromised patients (e.g., those with AIDS, immunosuppressive therapy, chemotherapy, absolute neutrophil count <200) and those with long-term (>2 weeks) CPN, *Enterococcus*, *Candida* species, *Escherichia coli*, *Pseudomonas*, *Klebsiella*, *Enterobacter*, *Acinetobacter*, *Proteus*, and *Xanthomonas* should be considered. The principles of evaluation and management of suspected catheter-related infection are outlined in Chap. 13, Treatment of Infectious Diseases.

Although antibiotics are often infused through the central line, the antibiotic lock technique has been used successfully to treat and prevent central catheter–related infections (*Nutrition* 14:466, 1998; *Antimicrob Agents Chemother* 43:2200, 1999). This technique involves injecting an antibiotic solution (e.g., vancomycin, 2 mg/ml) into the central catheter lumen and allowing the antibiotic to sit in the line for at least 12 hours. The catheter can be used to infuse fluids or parenteral nutritional solutions during the remaining 12 hours of the day. The catheter is periodically reinjected for a 14-day course. This approach is less expensive, delivers a higher antibiotic concentration into the catheter lumen, and has fewer side effects than systemic antibiotics.

e. **Hepatobiliary complications.** Hepatic abnormalities associated with CPN include biochemical (elevated serum aminotransferase and alkaline phosphatase) and histologic (steatosis, steatohepatitis, lipidosis and phospholipidosis, cholestasis, fibrosis, and cirrhosis) alterations [L Schiff, ER Schiff (eds). *Disease of the Liver* (7th ed). Philadelphia: JB Lippincott Co, 1993:1505–1516]. Although these abnormalities are usually benign and transient, more serious and progressive disease may develop in a small subset of patients, usually after 16 weeks of CPN therapy. The biliary complications associated with the use of CPN include acalculous cholecystitis, gallbladder sludge, and cholelithiasis and usually occur in patients who receive CPN for more than 3 weeks. Efforts to prevent hepatobiliary complications by providing a portion (20–40%) of calories as fat, cycling CPN so that the glucose infusion is stopped for at least 8–10 hours/day, encouraging enteral intake to stimulate gallbladder contraction and maintain mucosal integrity, and avoiding excessive calories should be routine in all patients who are receiving long-term CPN. If abnormal liver biochemistries or other evidence of liver damage occur, an evaluation for other possible causes of liver disease should be performed. Parenteral nutrition does not need to be discontinued, but the same principles used in preventing hepatic complications can be applied therapeutically. When cholestasis is present, copper and manganese should be deleted from the CPN formula to prevent accumulation in the liver and basal ganglia. A 4-week trial of metronidazole or ursodeoxycholic acid has been reported to be helpful in some patients.

f. **Metabolic bone disease** has been observed in patients receiving long-term (>3 months) CPN. The clinical manifestations of bone disease are seen in asymptomatic patients who have radiologic evidence of demineralization, those who have bone pain, and those who experience bone fracture (*Annu Rev Nutr* 11:93, 1991). Histologic examination has found osteomalacia or osteopenia, or both. The precise causes of metabolic bone disease are not known, but several mechanisms have been proposed, including aluminum toxicity, vitamin D toxicity, and negative calcium balance. Several therapeutic options should be considered in patients who have evidence of bone abnormalities: (1) Remove vitamin D from the CPN formulation, if the parathormone and 1,25-hydroxy vitamin D levels are low; (2) reduce protein to less than 1.5 g/kg/day because amino acids cause hypercalciuria; (3) maintain normal magnesium status because magnesium is necessary for normal parathormone action and renal conservation of calcium; (4) provide oral calcium supplements of 1–2 g/day; and (5) consider biophosphonate therapy to decrease bone resorption.

C. **Peripheral parenteral nutrition** is often considered to have limited usefulness because of the high risk of thrombophlebitis. However, appropriate adjustments in the management of peripheral parenteral nutrition can increase the life of a single infusion site to more than 10 days. The following guidelines are recommended: (1) Provide at least 50% of total energy as a lipid emulsion piggy-backed with the dextrose–amino acid solution, (2) add 500–1000 U heparin and 5 mg hydrocortisone/L (to decrease phlebitis), (3) place a fine-bore 22- or 23-gauge polyvinyl pyrrolidone-coated polyurethane catheter in as large a vein as possible in the proximal forearm using sterile technique, (4) place a 5-mg glycerol trinitrate ointment patch (or 1/4 in. of 2% nitroglycerin ointment) over the infusion site, (5) infuse the solution with a volumetric pump, (6) keep the total infused volume below 3500 ml/day, and (7) filter the solution with an inline 1.2-μm filter (*Nutrition* 10:49, 1994).

D. **Long-term home parenteral nutrition** is usually given through a tunneled catheter or an implantable subcutaneous port that is inserted in the subclavian vein and exits on the anterior chest. Nutrient formulations can be infused overnight to permit daytime activities. IV lipids may not be necessary in patients who are able to ingest and absorb adequate amounts of fat.

E. **Monitoring nutrition support** in the hospital is needed to ensure that nutritional therapy is safe and adequate. Adjustment of the nutrient formulation is often needed as medical therapy or clinical status changes. When nutrition support is initiated, other sources of glucose (e.g., peripheral IV dextrose infusions) should be stopped and the volume of other IV fluids adjusted to account for CPN. Vital signs should be checked every 8 hours. In certain patients, body weight, fluid intake, and fluid output should be followed daily. Serum electrolytes (including phosphorus) should be measured every 1 or 2 days after CPN is started until values are stable and then rechecked weekly. Serum glucose should be checked up to every 4–6 hours by fingerstick until blood glucose concentrations are stable and then rechecked weekly. If lipid emulsions are being given, serum triglycerides should be measured during lipid infusion in patients at risk for hypertriglyceridemia to demonstrate adequate clearance (triglyceride concentrations <400 mg/dl). Careful attention to the catheter and catheter site can help prevent catheter-related infections. Gauze dressings should be changed every 48–72 hours or when contaminated or wet, but transparent dressings can be changed weekly. Tubing that connects the parenteral solutions with the catheter should be changed every 24 hours. A 0.22-μm filter should be inserted between the IV tubing and the catheter when lipid-free CPN is infused and should be changed with the tubing. A 1.2-μm filter should be used when a total nutrient admixture containing a lipid emulsion is infused. When a single-lumen catheter is used to deliver CPN, the catheter should not be used to infuse other solutions or medications, with the exception of compatible antibiotics, and it should not be used to monitor central venous pressure. When a triple-lumen catheter is used, the distal port should be reserved solely for the administration of CPN.

**V. Refeeding the severely malnourished patient**

**A. Complications.** Initiating nutritional therapy in patients who are severely malnourished and have had minimal nutrient intake can have adverse clinical consequences known as the **refeeding syndrome,** which includes the following features.

1. **Hypophosphatemia, hypokalemia, and hypomagnesemia.** Rapid and marked decreases in these electrolytes occur during initial refeeding because of insulin-stimulated increases in cellular mineral uptake from extracellular fluid. For example, plasma phosphorus concentration can fall below 1 mg/dl and cause death within hours of initiating nutritional therapy if adequate phosphate is not given (*Am J Clin Nutr* 34:393, 1981).
2. **Fluid overload and CHF** are associated with decreased cardiac function and insulin-induced increased sodium and water reabsorption in conjunction with nutritional therapy containing water, glucose, and sodium.
3. **Cardiac arrhythmias.** Patients who are severely malnourished often have bradycardia. Sudden death from ventricular tachyarrhythmias can occur during the first week of refeeding in severely malnourished patients and may be associated with a prolonged QT interval (*Ann Intern Med* 102:49, 1985) or plasma electrolyte abnormalities.
4. **Glucose intolerance.** Starvation causes insulin resistance, so that refeeding with high-carbohydrate meals or large amounts of parenteral glucose can cause marked elevations in blood glucose concentration, glucosuria, dehydration, and hyperosmolar coma. In addition, carbohydrate refeeding in patients who are depleted in thiamine can precipitate Wernicke's encephalopathy.

**B. Clinical recommendations.** Careful evaluation of cardiovascular function and plasma electrolytes (history, physical examination, ECG, and blood tests) and correction of abnormal plasma electrolytes are important before initiation of feeding. Refeeding by the oral or enteral route involves the frequent or continuous administration of small amounts of food or an isotonic liquid formula. Parenteral supplementation or complete parenteral nutrition may be necessary if the intestine cannot tolerate feeding. During initial refeeding, fluid intake should be limited to approximately 800 ml/day plus insensible losses. However, adjustments in fluid and sodium intake are needed in patients who have evidence of fluid overload or dehydration. Changes in body weight provide a useful guide for evaluating the efficacy of fluid administration. Weight gain greater than 0.25 kg/day, or 1.5 kg/week, probably represents fluid accumulation in excess of tissue repletion. Initially, approximately 15 kcal/kg, containing approximately 100 g carbohydrate and 1.5 g protein/kg actual body weight, should be given daily. The rate at which the caloric intake can be increased depends on the severity of the malnutrition and the tolerance to feeding; however, in general, increases of 2–4 kcal/kg q24–48h are appropriate. Sodium should be restricted to approximately 60 mEq or 1.5 g/day, but liberal amounts of phosphorus, potassium, and magnesium should be given to patients who have normal renal function. All other nutrients should be given in amounts needed to meet the recommended dietary intake (Table 2-3). Body weight, fluid intake, urine output, and plasma glucose and electrolyte values should be monitored daily during early refeeding (first 3–7 days) so that nutritional therapy can be appropriately modified when necessary.

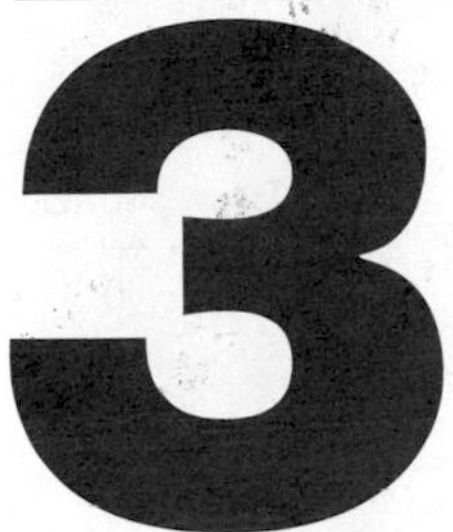

# Fluid and Electrolyte Management

Harry Giles and
Anitha Vijayan

## General Management of Fluids

**I. Maintenance therapy** can be provided enterally or intravenously for patients who are unable to take food or liquid by mouth. **This section assumes normal renal function and the absence of electrolyte or acid-base disturbances.**

**A. Minimum water requirements** for daily fluid balance can be approximated from the sum of the urine output necessary to excrete the daily solute load (500 ml/day) plus the insensible water losses from the skin and respiratory tract (500 ml/day), minus the amount of water produced from endogenous metabolism (250–350 ml/day). It is not uncommon to administer 2–3 L water per day to produce a urine volume greater than 1000–1500 ml/day, because there is no advantage to minimizing urine output. Weighing the patient daily is the best means of assessing net gain or loss of total body fluid, because GI, renal, and insensible fluid losses of patients are unpredictable. Table 3-1 lists commonly used IV fluid preparations.

**B.** The **electrolytes** that are usually administered during maintenance fluid therapy are $Na^+$ and $K^+$ salts. Requirements depend on minimum obligatory and ongoing losses. The kidneys are normally capable of compensating for wide fluctuations in dietary $Na^+$ intake—renal $Na^+$ excretion can fall to less than 5 mEq/day in the absence of $Na^+$ intake. It is customary to provide 50–150 mEq $Na^+$ daily (as NaCl). Generally, $K^+$ supplementation (20–60 mEq/day) is included if renal function is normal. Carbohydrate in the form of dextrose (100–150 g/day) is given to minimize protein catabolism and prevent ketoacidosis.

**C. A maintenance IV fluid regimen** can be provided by the administration of 2–3 L (90–125 ml/hour) 0.45% NaCl with 5% dextrose and 20 mEq/L KCl. Calcium, magnesium, phosphorus, vitamins, and protein replacement are necessary after 1 week of parenteral therapy (see Chap. 2, Nutritional Therapy). However, in very ill patients, this hypotonic solution can lead to severe hyponatremia (see Salt and Water, sec. **IV.A**).

**II. Replacement of abnormal water and electrolyte losses**

**A. Insensible water losses** from the skin and respiratory tract depend on respiratory rate, ambient temperature, humidity, and body temperature. Water losses increase by 100–150 ml/day for each degree of body temperature over 37°C. Fluid losses from sweating can vary enormously (100–2000 ml/hour) and depend on physical activity as well as body and ambient temperatures. Mechanical ventilation with humidified gases minimizes losses from the respiratory tract. Replacement of insensible water losses should be with 5% dextrose or hypotonic saline.

**B. Gastrointestinal losses** vary in composition and volume depending on their sources. Laboratory measurement of fluid composition can be performed to increase the accuracy of electrolyte replacement.

**Table 3-1.** Commonly used parenteral solutions

| IV solution | Osmolality (mOsm/kg) | [Glucose] (g/L) | $[Na^+]$ (mEq/L) | [Cl] (mEq/L) |
|---|---|---|---|---|
| $D_5W$ | 278 | 50 | 0 | 0 |
| $D_{10}W$ | 556 | 100 | 0 | 0 |
| $D_{50}W$ | 2778 | 500 | 0 | 0 |
| 0.45% NaCl[a] | 154 | —[b] | 77 | 77 |
| 0.9% NaCl[a] | 308 | —[b] | 154 | 154 |
| 3% NaCl | 1026 | — | 513 | 513 |
| Lactated Ringer's[c] | 274 | —[b] | 130 | 109 |

$D_5W$, 5% dextrose in water; $D_{10}W$, 10% dextrose in water; $D_{50}W$, 50% dextrose in water.
*Note:* One 50-ml ampule of 7.5% $NaHCO_3$ contains 44.6 mEq each of $Na^+$ and $HCO_3^-$. One 50-ml ampule of 8.4% $NaHCO_3$ contains 50 mEq each of $Na^+$ and $HCO_3^-$.
[a]NaCl 0.45% and 0.9% are half-normal and normal saline, respectively.
[b]Also available with 5% dextrose.
[c]Also contains 4 mEq/L $K^+$, 1.5 mEq/L $Ca^{2+}$, and 28 mEq/L lactate.

C. **Renal losses** of $Na^+$ may be significant, particularly in the setting of diuretic use, the recovery phase of acute tubular necrosis (ATN), postobstructive diuresis, interstitial renal disease, or mineralocorticoid deficiency. Kaliuresis may occur with the recovery phase of ATN, renal tubular acidosis (RTA), diuretic use, hyperaldosteronism, and catabolic states. If prolonged losses occur, measurement of the urine sodium and potassium may help guide replacement.

D. **Rapid internal fluid shifts** can occur with peritonitis, pancreatitis, portal vein thrombosis, extensive burns, severe nephrotic syndrome, ileus or intestinal obstruction, bacterial enteritis or colitis, crush injuries, and rhabdomyolysis, as well as during the postoperative period. Replacement of sequestered fluid with isotonic saline may be necessary in these situations.

## Salt and Water

I. **Total body water and $Na^+$.** Water comprises approximately 60% of body weight in men and 50% in women. Total body water is distributed in two major compartments: two-thirds intracellular fluid (ICF) and one-third extracellular fluid (ECF). The latter is further subdivided into intravascular and interstitial spaces in a ratio of 1:4. **Osmolality** is the solute or particle concentration of a fluid. Solutes that are restricted to the ECF ($Na^+$ and accompanying anions) or the ICF ($K^+$ salts and organic phosphate esters) determine the **effective osmolality or tonicity** of that compartment. Osmotic equilibrium occurs because water diffuses rapidly across cell membranes; this prevents differences in tonicity (ICF vs. ECF). The majority (85–90%) of total body $Na^+$ is extracellular. Water and $Na^+$ balance are regulated independently. Changes in $[Na^+]$ generally reflect disturbed water homeostasis and ICF volume, whereas alterations in $Na^+$ content are manifest as ECF volume contraction or expansion and imply abnormal $Na^+$ balance.

II. **ECF volume depletion**

A. **Manifestations.** Symptoms are usually nonspecific and secondary to electrolyte imbalances and tissue hypoperfusion. These include thirst, fatigue, weakness, muscle cramps, and postural dizziness. More severe degrees of volume contraction can lead to syncope and coma. Diminished skin turgor and dry mucous membranes are poor markers of decreased interstitial fluid. Signs of intravascular volume contraction include decreased jugular venous pressure, postural hypotension, and postural tachycardia. Mild degrees of volume depletion are often not clinically detectable. Weight loss can help estimate the magnitude of the volume deficit. Larger fluid losses often present as hypovolemic shock, heralded by hypotension, tachycardia, peripheral vasoconstriction, and hypoperfusion—cyanosis, cold and clammy extremities, oliguria, and altered mental status. A thorough history and physical examination are generally sufficient to determine the presence and cause of ECF volume contraction. Laboratory data confirm and support the clinical diagnosis. Measurement of the fractional excretion of $Na^+$ and BUN-creatinine ratio may provide additional diagnostic information (see Chap. 11, Renal Diseases). There may be a relative elevation in hematocrit (hemoconcentration) and plasma albumin concentration.

**B. Etiology.** ECF volume depletion reflects a deficit in total body $Na^+$ content as a result of renal or extrarenal losses that exceed $Na^+$ intake. Renal losses may be secondary to diuretics (pharmacologic or osmotic), interstitial renal disease ($Na^+$ wasting), or mineralocorticoid deficiency. Excessive renal losses of $Na^+$ and water may also occur during the diuretic phase of ATN and after the relief of bilateral urinary tract obstruction. Nonrenal causes of hypovolemia include fluid loss from the GI tract (vomiting, nasogastric suction, fistula drainage, diarrhea), skin and respiratory losses, third-space accumulations (burns, pancreatitis, peritonitis), and hemorrhage.

**C. Treatment.** The therapeutic goal is to restore normovolemia with fluid similar in composition to that which was lost, as well as to replace ongoing losses. Mild volume contraction can usually be corrected via the oral route. More severe cases of hypovolemia require IV therapy. Patients with significant hemorrhage, anemia, or third-spacing may require blood transfusion or colloid-containing solutions (albumin, dextran). Isotonic or normal saline (0.9% NaCl or 154 mEq/L $Na^+$) is the solution of choice in normonatremic and mildly hyponatremic individuals and should also be used initially in patients with hypotension or shock. Severe hyponatremia may require hypertonic saline (3.0% NaCl or 513 mEq/L $Na^+$, see sec. **IV.E.4**). Hypokalemia may be present initially or may ensue as a result of increased urinary $K^+$ excretion and should be corrected by adding appropriate amounts of KCl to replacement solutions. Finally, the appropriate management of hypovolemia must include correction of the underlying cause.

**III. ECF volume excess**

**A. Manifestations.** Because 75–80% of the ECF is extravascular, ECF volume excess results in expansion of the interstitial compartment, which presents as **edema.** Incipient edema may only be detected by the occurrence of weight gain. Overt edema is apparent only after 3–4 L fluid has accumulated. Clinical findings include dyspnea, tachypnea, tachycardia, pulmonary rales, elevated jugular venous pressure, hepatojugular reflux, presence of an $S_3$ gallop, and peripheral or presacral edema.

**B. Etiology.** ECF volume expansion is caused by salt intake in the presence of renal $Na^+$ retention. The latter may be caused by a primary renal disorder such as renal failure or the nephrotic syndrome. Alternatively, enhanced $Na^+$ reabsorption may be secondary to decreased effective circulating or arterial volume that results from heart failure or hypoalbuminemia (e.g., hepatic cirrhosis).

**C. Treatment** must address not only the ECF volume excess but also the underlying pathologic process. Treatment of the nephrotic syndrome and the volume overload associated with renal failure is discussed in Chap. 11, Renal Diseases. Treatment of heart failure and cirrhosis is discussed in Chaps. 6, Heart Failure, Cardiomyopathy, and Valvular Heart Disease, and 17, Liver Diseases, respectively.

**IV. Hyponatremia** is defined as a plasma [$Na^+$] of less than 135 mEq/L. In the absence of hyperglycemia, this usually reflects a hypo-osmolar state and an increased ICF volume. To maintain homeostasis and a normal plasma [$Na^+$], the ingestion of solute-free water must eventually lead to the loss of the same volume of electrolyte-free water. Three steps are required for the kidney to excrete a water load: (1) glomerular filtration and delivery of water (and electrolytes) to the diluting sites of the nephron, (2) active reabsorption of $Na^+$ and $Cl^-$ without water in the thick ascending limb of the loop of Henle, and (3) maintenance of a dilute urine due to impermeability of the collecting duct to water in the absence of vasopressin (antidiuretic hormone). Abnormalities of any of these steps can result in impaired free water excretion and eventual hyponatremia.

**A. Hyponatremia with a low plasma osmolality.** Most causes of hyponatremia are associated with a low plasma osmolality (high ICF volume). In general, hypotonic hyponatremia is caused either by a primary water gain or $Na^+$ loss. The ECF volume, reflecting total body $Na^+$ content, may be decreased, normal, or increased in hyponatremia.

1. **Hyponatremia associated with ECF volume depletion** may result from renal or nonrenal causes of net $Na^+$ loss (see sec. **II.B**). A decreased effective arterial volume stimulates thirst. It also stimulates vasopressin release from the posterior pituitary gland, which impairs the capacity to excrete a dilute urine. Hyponatremia develops as a consequence of electrolyte-free water retention. Furthermore, certain causes of hypovolemic hyponatremia (e.g., diuretics or vomiting) may be associated with a large $K^+$ deficit, resulting in transcellular ion exchange ($K^+$ exits and $Na^+$ enters cells), which contributes to hyponatremia.
2. **Hyponatremia associated with ECF volume excess** is usually a consequence of edematous states, such as CHF, hepatic cirrhosis, and the nephrotic syndrome. These disorders all have in common a decreased effective circulating volume, leading to increased thirst and vasopressin levels. The increase in total body $Na^+$ is exceeded by the rise in total body water. The degree of hyponatremia often correlates with the severity of the underlying condition and is therefore an important prognostic factor. Oliguric acute and chronic renal failure may be associated with hyponatremia if water intake exceeds the kidney's limited ability to excrete equivalent volumes.
3. **Hyponatremia associated with a normal ECF volume**
   a. **The syndrome of inappropriate antidiuretic hormone secretion (SIADH)** is the most common cause of normovolemic hyponatremia. This disorder is caused by the nonphysiologic release of vasopressin from the posterior pituitary or an ectopic source, resulting in impaired renal free water excretion. Common causes of SIADH include neuropsychiatric disorders, pulmonary diseases, and malignant tumors. SIADH is characterized by (1) hypo-osmotic hyponatremia, (2) an inappropriately concentrated urine (urine osmolality >100 mOsm/kg), (3) euvolemia, and (4) normal renal, adrenal, and thyroid function.
   b. **Glucocorticoid deficiency and hypothyroidism** may present with hyponatremia and should not be confused with SIADH. Although decreased mineralocorticoids may contribute to the hyponatremia of Addison's disease, it is the cortisol deficiency that leads to hypersecretion of vasopressin directly (cosecreted with corticotropin-releasing factor) and indirectly (secondary to volume depletion). The mechanisms by which hypothyroidism leads to hyponatremia include decreased cardiac output and glomerular filtration rate (GFR) and increased vasopressin secretion in response to hemodynamic stimuli.
   c. **Pharmacologic agents** may cause hyponatremia by one of at least three mechanisms: (1) stimulation of vasopressin release (e.g., nicotine, carbamazepine, tricyclic antidepressants, antipsychotic agents,

antineoplastic drugs, narcotics), (2) potentiation of antidiuretic action of vasopressin [e.g., chlorpropamide, methylxanthines, nonsteroidal anti-inflammatory drugs (NSAIDs)], or (3) vasopressin analogs [e.g., oxytocin, desmopressin acetate (DDAVP)].

d. **Physical and emotional stress** are often associated with vasopressin release, possibly secondary to nausea and/or hypotension associated with stress-induced vasovagal reactions.

e. **Acute hypoxia or hypercapnia** also stimulates vasopressin secretion.

f. **Psychogenic polydipsia** refers to a condition of compulsive water consumption that may overwhelm the normally large renal excretory capacity of 12 L/day. These patients often have psychiatric illnesses and may be taking medications, such as phenothiazines, that enhance the sensation of thirst by causing a dry mouth.

g. **Beer potomania** is similar to psychogenic polydipsia but with an associated lower renal excretory capacity of water. Urine can be maximally diluted to 50 mOsm/L. The low-solute and -protein diet seen with excessive beer intake may only result in the generation of 200–250 mOsm/day (600–900 mOsm/day is normal). Thus, only 4–5 L/day of urine can be generated. Beer drunk in excess of this capacity results in hyponatremia. A similar state, often referred to as the **tea-and-toast diet,** has been observed in malnourished elderly patients who maintain fluid intake without an adequate diet.

h. **Cerebral salt wasting** is a controversial and poorly understood syndrome that has been associated with neurosurgery and CNS trauma. It is purportedly distinguished from SIADH by a negative sodium balance and intravascular volume depletion after a CNS injury. The controversy centers on the tenet that the underlying hyponatremia is best treated with hydration and saline, and not with fluid restriction.

B. **Hyponatremia with a normal or high plasma osmolality**

1. **Pseudohyponatremia** is hyponatremia associated with a normal plasma osmolality. It occurs as a result of a decrease in the aqueous phase of plasma. Plasma is 93% water, with the remaining 7% consisting of plasma proteins and lipids. Because $Na^+$ ions are dissolved in plasma water, increasing the nonaqueous phase artificially lowers the [$Na^+$] measured per liter of plasma (except when $Na^+$-sensitive glass electrodes are used). The plasma osmolality and the [$Na^+$] measured per liter of plasma water remain normal.

2. **Hyponatremia associated with a hyperosmolar state** is usually caused by an increase in the concentration of a solute that is largely restricted to the ECF compartment. The resulting osmotic gradient causes water to shift from the ICF to the ECF, and hyponatremia ensues. Hypertonic hyponatremia is usually caused by hyperglycemia or, occasionally, IV administration of mannitol. Quantitatively, the plasma [$Na^+$] falls by 1.4 mEq/L for every 100 mg/dl rise in the plasma glucose concentration. Isotonic or slightly hypotonic hyponatremia can complicate transurethral resection of the prostate or bladder (*Br J Urol* 66:71, 1990).

C. **Manifestations.** The clinical features of **acute** hyponatremia are related to osmotic water shift leading to increased ICF volume, specifically cerebral edema. Therefore, the symptoms are primarily neurologic, and their severity is dependent on the rapidity of onset and absolute decrease in plasma [$Na^+$]. Patients may be asymptomatic or may complain of nausea and malaise. As the plasma [$Na^+$] falls, the symptoms progress to include headache, lethargy, confusion, and obtundation. Stupor, seizures, and coma do not usually occur unless the plasma [$Na^+$] falls acutely below 120 mEq/L. In **chronic** hyponatremia, adaptive mechanisms designed to defend cell volume occur and tend to minimize the increase in ICF volume and its symptoms.

D. **Diagnosis** (Fig. 3-1). The underlying cause of hyponatremia can often be ascertained from an accurate history and physical examination, including

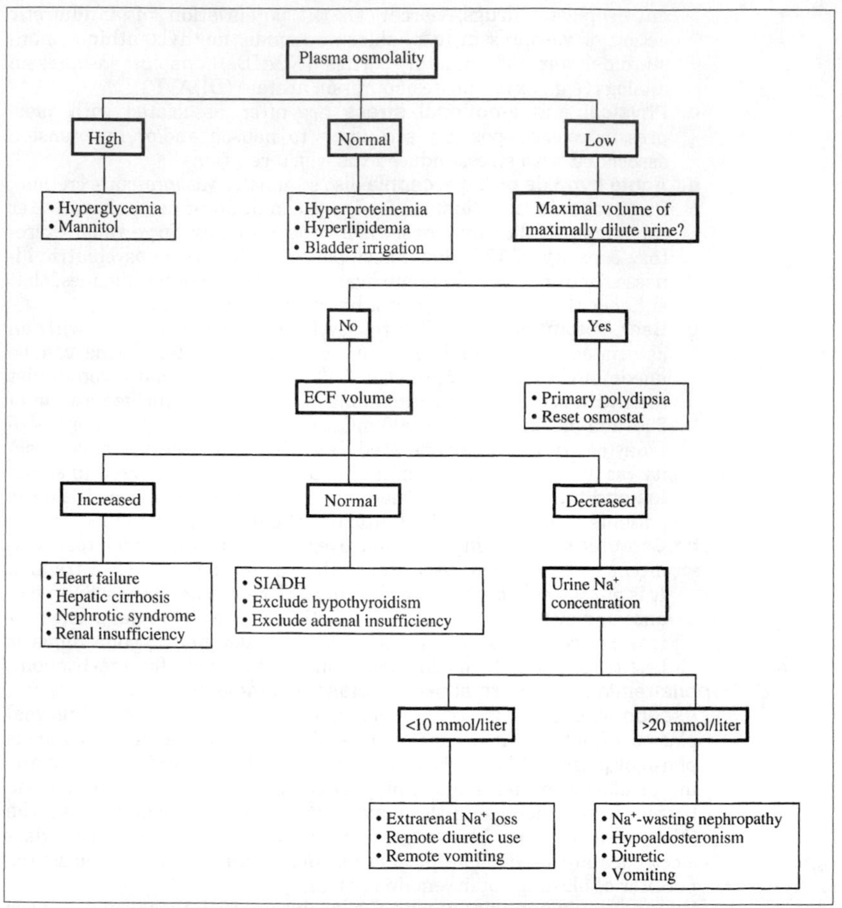


**Fig. 3-1.** Algorithm depicting clinical approach to hyponatremia. ECF, extracellular fluid; SIADH, syndrome of inappropriate antidiuretic hormone. [From GG Singer, BM Brenner. Fluid and electrolyte disturbances. In AS Fauci, et al. (eds). *Harrison's Principles of Internal Medicine* (15th ed). New York: McGraw-Hill, 2001, with permission.]

an assessment of ECF volume status and effective circulating arterial volume. Three laboratory findings often provide useful information and can narrow the differential diagnosis of hyponatremia: (1) the plasma osmolality, (2) the urine osmolality, and (3) the urine $[Na^+] + [Cl^-]$.

1. **Plasma osmolality.** Because ECF tonicity is determined primarily by the $[Na^+]$, most patients with hyponatremia have a decreased plasma osmolality. If the plasma osmolality is not low, pseudohyponatremia and hypertonic hyponatremia must be ruled out.
2. **Urine osmolality and volume.** The appropriate renal response to hypo-osmolality is to excrete the maximum volume of dilute urine, that is, urine osmolality and specific gravity of less than 100 mOsm/kg and 1.003, respectively. This occurs in patients with primary polydipsia. If this is not present, it suggests impaired free water excretion due to the action of vasopressin on the kidney. The secretion of vasopressin may be

a physiologic response to hemodynamic stimuli, or it may be inappropriate in the presence of hyponatremia and euvolemia. The maximal urine output is a function of the minimum urine osmolality achievable and the mandatory solute excretion. Metabolism of a normal diet generates 600–900 mOsm/day, and the minimum urine osmolality in humans is approximately 50 mOsm/kg. Therefore, the maximum daily urine output will be 12 L or more ($600 \div 50 = 12$). A solute excretion rate of greater than 900 mOsm/day is, by definition, an **osmotic diuresis.** A low-protein, low-salt diet may yield as few as 100 mOsm/day, which translates into a maximal urine output of 2 L/day at a minimum urine tonicity of 50 mOsm/kg (see sec. **IV.A.3.g**). Moreover, net $Na^+$ loss and ECF volume contraction lead to vasopressin release, further impairing free water excretion.

3. **Urine $Na^+$ concentrations.** Because $Na^+$ is the major ECF cation and is largely restricted to this compartment, ECF volume contraction represents a deficit in total body $Na^+$ content. Therefore, volume depletion in patients with normal underlying renal function results in enhanced tubule $Na^+$ reabsorption and a urine [$Na^+$] of less than 20 mEq/L. The finding of a urine [$Na^+$] of greater than 20 mEq/L in hypovolemic hyponatremia implies diuretic therapy, hypoaldosteronism, or occasionally, vomiting.

**E. Treatment.** The goals of therapy are threefold: (1) raise the plasma [$Na^+$] (lowering the ICF volume) by restricting water intake and promoting water loss, (2) replace the $Na^+$ and $K^+$ deficit(s), and (3) correct the underlying disorder. Mild asymptomatic hyponatremia is generally of little clinical significance and requires no treatment.

1. **ECF volume contraction.** Management of asymptomatic hyponatremia should include $Na^+$ repletion, generally in the form of saline that is isotonic to the patient, to avoid rapid changes in ICF volume.
2. **Edematous states.** Hyponatremia in CHF and cirrhosis tends to reflect the severity of the underlying disease and is usually asymptomatic. Treatment should include restriction of $Na^+$ and water intake, correction of hypokalemia, and promotion of water loss in excess of $Na^+$. The latter may require the use of loop diuretics with replacement of a proportion of the urinary $Na^+$ loss to ensure net free water excretion. Dietary water restriction should be less than the urine output. Correction of the $K^+$ deficit may raise the plasma [$Na^+$].
3. **The rate of correction of hyponatremia** depends on the absence or presence of neurologic dysfunction (*Lancet* 352:220, 1998). This, in turn, is related to the rapidity of onset and magnitude of the fall in plasma [$Na^+$]. The risks of correcting hyponatremia too rapidly are ECF volume excess and the development of osmotic demyelination or **central pontine myelinolysis.** This disorder, in its most overt form, is characterized by flaccid paralysis, dysarthria, and dysphagia. The diagnosis is occasionally suspected clinically and can be confirmed by appropriate neuroimaging studies (CT scan or MRI). In addition to rapid or overcorrection of hyponatremia, risk factors for osmotic demyelination include hypokalemia and malnutrition, especially secondary to alcoholism.
4. **Acute hyponatremia** tends to present with altered mental status or seizures, or both, and requires more rapid correction. Severe **symptomatic** hyponatremia should be treated with hypertonic saline, and the plasma [$Na^+$] should be raised only by 1–2 mEq/L/hour and by no more than 8 mEq/L during the first 24 hours. The quantity of $Na^+$ that is required to increase the plasma $Na^+$ concentration by a given amount can be estimated by multiplying the desired change in plasma [$Na^+$] by the total body water (e.g., 5 mEq/L $\times$ 30 L = 150 mEq = 300 ml 3% NaCl). In **asymptomatic** patients, the plasma [$Na^+$] should be raised by no more than 0.3 mEq/L/hr and equal to or less than 8 mEq/L over the first 24 hours.
5. Water restriction in primary polydipsia and IV saline therapy in ECF volume–contracted patients may also lead to overly rapid correction of

hyponatremia as a result of vasopressin suppression and a brisk water diuresis. This can be prevented by administration of water or use of a vasopressin analog to slow down the rate of free water excretion.

6. **The hyponatremia of SIADH** can be treated by limiting the intake of water or promoting its excretion, or both. The standard first-line therapy is water restriction. If this fails or if the patient is symptomatic, agents that enhance water excretion can be tried. Loop diuretics impair the ability to excrete concentrated urine and, when combined with $Na^+$ replacement in the form of salt tablets, can enhance free water excretion. In SIADH, the urine osmolality is relatively fixed. Therefore, the maximum urine output is a direct function of the solute excretion rate, which can be increased by dietary modification (high salt, high protein) or by administering urea, leading to increased urine output and water excretion. Drugs that interfere with the collecting tubule's ability to respond to vasopressin include lithium and demeclocycline. These agents are rarely used and should only be considered in severe hyponatremia that is unresponsive to more conservative measures.

V. **Hypernatremia** is defined as a plasma [$Na^+$] of greater than 145 mEq/L and represents a state of hyperosmolality. Maintenance of osmotic equilibrium in hypernatremia results in ICF volume contraction and cerebral cell shrinkage. Hypernatremia may be caused by a primary $Na^+$ gain or water deficit. The two components of an appropriate response to hypernatremia are increased water intake stimulated by thirst and the excretion of the minimum volume of maximally concentrated urine, reflecting vasopressin secretion in response to an osmotic stimulus.

A. **Impaired thirst.** The degree of hyperosmolality is typically mild unless the thirst mechanism is abnormal or access to water is limited. The latter occurs in infants, the physically handicapped, patients with impaired mental status, individuals in the postoperative state, and intubated patients in the ICU. Rarely, impaired thirst may be caused by **primary hypodipsia,** as a result of damage to the hypothalamic osmoreceptors that control thirst. Primary hypodipsia may be caused by a variety of pathologic changes, including granulomatous disease, vascular occlusion, and tumors.

B. **Hypernatremia due to water loss** accounts for the majority of cases of hypernatremia. Because water is distributed between the ICF and the ECF in a 2:1 ratio, a given amount of solute-free water loss results in the same percentage change but, quantitatively, a twofold greater absolute reduction in the ICF compartment than the ECF compartment.

1. **Nonrenal water loss** may be due to evaporation from the skin and respiratory tract (insensible losses) or loss from the GI tract. Insensible losses are increased with fever, exercise, heat exposure, severe burns, and in mechanically ventilated patients. Diarrhea is the most common GI cause of hypernatremia. Specifically, osmotic diarrheas (induced by lactulose, sorbitol, or malabsorption of carbohydrate) and viral gastroenteritides result in water loss exceeding that of $Na^+$ and $K^+$.

2. **Renal water loss** is the most common cause of hypernatremia and results from either osmotic diuresis or diabetes insipidus. The most frequent cause of an osmotic diuresis is hyperglycemia and glucosuria in poorly controlled diabetes mellitus. IV administration of mannitol and increased production of urea (high-protein diet) can also result in an osmotic diuresis. Hypernatremia secondary to nonosmotic urinary water loss is usually caused by (1) **central diabetes insipidus (CDI)** characterized by impaired vasopressin secretion or (2) **nephrogenic diabetes insipidus (NDI)** that results from resistance to the actions of vasopressin. The most common cause of CDI is destruction of the neurohypophysis as a result of trauma, neurosurgery, granulomatous disease, neoplasms, vascular accidents, or infection. In many cases, CDI is idiopathic and may occasionally be hereditary. NDI may either be inher-

ited or acquired. The latter can be further subdivided into disorders associated with renal medullary disease or with impaired vasopressin action. The causes of sporadic NDI are numerous and include drugs (especially lithium), hypercalcemia, hypokalemia, and conditions that impair medullary hypertonicity (e.g., papillary necrosis or osmotic diuresis).

**C. Hypernatremia due to $Na^+$ gain** occurs infrequently. This is most commonly seen in patients with diabetic ketoacidosis (DKA) and an osmotic diuresis (urine $[Na^+] \approx 50$ mEq/L) treated with isotonic saline. Inadvertent administration of hypertonic NaCl or $NaHCO_3$ or replacing sugar with salt in infant formula can also lead to hypernatremia.

**D. Transcellular water shift** from ECF to ICF occurs in rare circumstances (e.g., secondary to seizures or rhabdomyolysis). Hypernatremia is accompanied by ECF volume contraction with no change in body weight.

**E. Manifestations.** The major symptoms of hypernatremia are neurologic and include altered mental status, weakness, neuromuscular irritability, focal neurologic deficits, and occasionally coma or seizures. Patients may also complain of polyuria or thirst. For unknown reasons, patients with polydipsia from CDI tend to prefer ice-cold water. The signs and symptoms of volume depletion are often present in patients with a history of excessive sweating, diarrhea, or an osmotic diuresis. As with hyponatremia, the severity of the clinical manifestations is related to the acuity and magnitude of the rise in plasma $[Na^+]$. Chronic hypernatremia is generally less symptomatic as a result of adaptive mechanisms designed to defend cell volume.

**F. Diagnosis** (Fig. 3-2). A complete history and physical examination often provide clues as to the underlying cause of hypernatremia. The history should include a list of current and recent medications, and the physical examination is incomplete without a thorough mental status and neurologic assessment.

1. **Assessment of urine volume and osmolality** is essential in the evaluation of hyperosmolality. The appropriate renal response to hypernatremia is excretion of the minimum volume (500 ml/day) of maximally concentrated urine (urine osmolality > 800 mOsm/kg). These findings suggest extrarenal or remote renal water loss or administration of hypertonic $Na^+$ salt solutions. A primary $Na^+$ excess can be confirmed by the presence of ECF volume expansion and natriuresis (urine $[Na^+]$ usually >100 mEq/L). Many causes of hypernatremia are associated with polyuria and a submaximal urine osmolality. Calculation of the total daily solute excretion (24-hr urine volume × ruine osmolality) is helpful in determining the basis of the polyuria. To maintain a steady state, total solute excretion must equal solute production. As mentioned previously, a daily solute excretion in excess of 900 mOsm defines an osmotic diuresis (see sec. **IV.D.2**). This can be confirmed by measuring the urine glucose and urea.
2. **CDI and NDI** generally present with polyuria and hypotonic urine (urine osmolality <250 mOsm/kg). The degree of hypernatremia is usually mild unless the patient has an associated thirst abnormality. The clinical history, physical examination, and pertinent laboratory data can often rule out causes of acquired NDI. CDI and NDI can be distinguished by administering the vasopressin analog DDAVP (10 μg intranasally) after careful water restriction. The urine osmolality should increase by at least 50% in CDI and does not change in NDI. The diagnosis is sometimes difficult due to partial defects in vasopressin secretion and action.

**G. Treatment.** The therapeutic goals are (1) to stop ongoing water loss and (2) to correct the water deficit. The ECF volume should be restored in hypovolemic patients. The quantity of water required to correct the deficit can be calculated from the following equation:

$$\text{Water deficit} = \frac{(\text{plasma } [Na^+] - 140)}{140} \times \begin{array}{c}\text{total body water}\\ \text{(in liters)}\end{array}$$

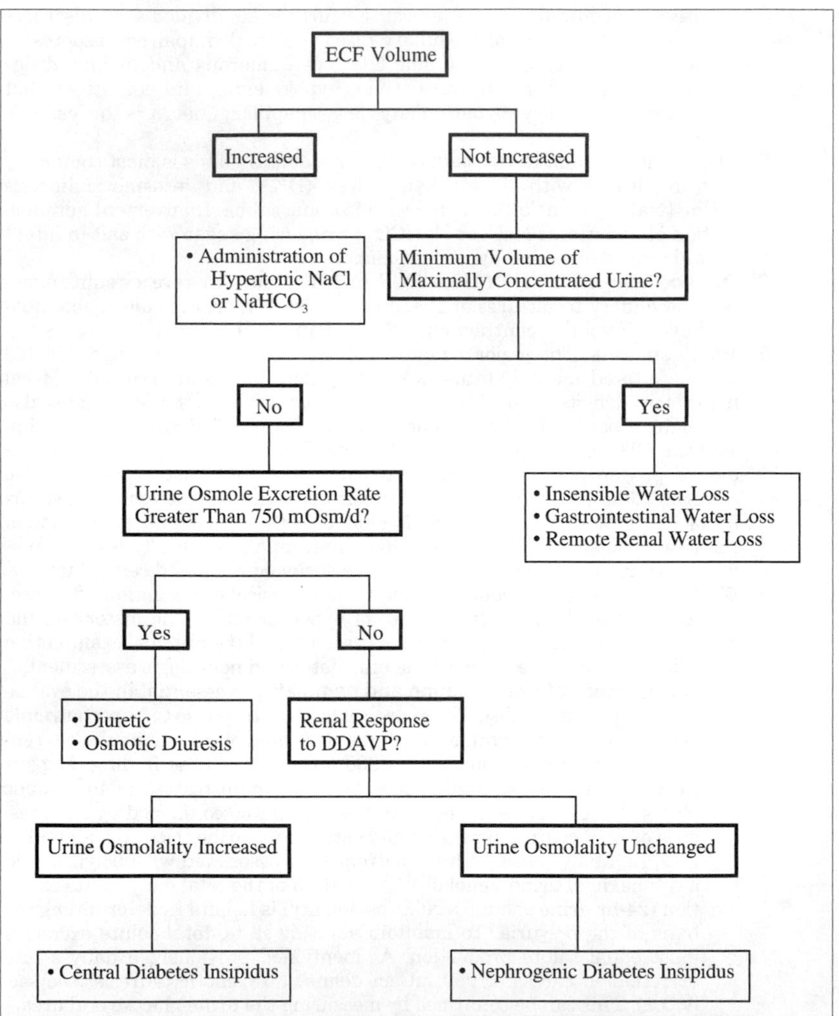


**Fig. 3-2.** Algorithm depicting clinical approach to hypernatremia. DDAVP, desmopressin acetate; ECF, extracellular fluid. [From GG Singer, BM Brenner. Fluid and electrolyte disturbances. In AS Fauci, et al. (eds). *Harrison's Principles of Internal Medicine* (15th ed). New York: McGraw-Hill, 2001, with permission.]

1. **The rate of correction.** As in hyponatremia, rapid correction of hypernatremia is potentially dangerous due to a rapid shift of water into brain cells, increasing the risk of seizures or permanent neurologic damage. Therefore, the water deficit should be corrected slowly over at least 48–72 hours. When calculating the rate of water replacement, ongoing losses should be taken into account, and the plasma [$Na^+$] should be lowered by 0.5 mEq/L/hour and by no more than 12 mEq/L over the first 24 hours. The safest route of administration of water is by mouth or via a nasogastric tube. Alternatively, half-isotonic or quarter-isotonic saline can be given IV.

2. **CDI.** The appropriate treatment of CDI consists of administering DDAVP intranasally.
3. **NDI.** The concentrating defect in NDI may be reversible by treating the underlying disorder or eliminating the offending drug. Symptomatic polyuria caused by NDI can be treated with a low-$Na^+$ diet and thiazide diuretics. This results in mild volume depletion, enhanced proximal reabsorption of salt and water, and decreased delivery to the site of action of vasopressin, the collecting duct. NSAIDs potentiate vasopressin action and thereby increase urine osmolality and decrease urine volume.

## Potassium

**Potassium** is the major intracellular cation. The normal plasma [$K^+$] is 3.5–5.0 mEq/L, whereas that inside cells is approximately 150 mEq/L. Therefore, the amount of $K^+$ in the ECF constitutes less than 2% of the total body $K^+$ content. The $Na^+$-$K^+$–adenosine triphosphatase pump actively transports $Na^+$ out of the cell and $K^+$ into the cell in a 3:2 ratio, and the passive outward diffusion of $K^+$ is quantitatively the most important factor that generates the resting membrane potential. The $K^+$ intake of individuals on an average Western diet is approximately 1 mEq/kg/day, 90% of which is absorbed by the GI tract. Maintenance of the steady state necessitates matching $K^+$ ingestion with excretion.

Renal excretion is the major route of elimination of excess $K^+$. Ninety percent of filtered $K^+$ is reabsorbed by the proximal convoluted tubule and loop of Henle. Net distal $K^+$ secretion or reabsorption occurs in the setting of $K^+$ excess or depletion, respectively. The principal cell is responsible for $K^+$ secretion in the distal convoluted tubule and cortical collecting duct (CCD). Virtually all regulation of renal $K^+$ excretion and total body $K^+$ balance occurs in the distal nephron. The driving force for $K^+$ secretion is a favorable electrochemical gradient across the luminal membrane of the principal cell. The generation of a lumen-negative transepithelial potential difference favors $K^+$ secretion and depends on the relative rates of reabsorption of $Na^+$ and its accompanying anion (primarily $Cl^-$). Equimolar reabsorption of $Na^+$ and $Cl^-$ at equivalent rates is electroneutral, whereas reabsorption of $Na^+$ in excess of $Cl^-$ is electrogenic.

Potassium secretion is regulated by two physiologic stimuli, aldosterone and hyperkalemia. Aldosterone is secreted in response to high renin and angiotensin II or hyperkalemia. The plasma [$K^+$], independent of aldosterone, can also directly affect $K^+$ secretion. In addition to the [$K^+$] in the lumen of the CCD, renal $K^+$ loss depends on the urine flow rate, a function of daily solute excretion. Because excretion is equal to the product of concentration and volume, increased distal flow rate can significantly enhance urinary $K^+$ output.

### I. Hypokalemia

**A. Manifestations.** The clinical features of $K^+$ depletion vary greatly, and their severity depends in part on the degree of hypokalemia. Symptoms seldom occur unless the plasma [$K^+$] is less than 3.0 mEq/L. Fatigue, myalgia, and muscular weakness (or cramps) of the lower extremities are common complaints. More severe hypokalemia may lead to progressive weakness, hypoventilation, and eventually complete paralysis. Profound $K^+$ depletion is associated with an increased risk of arrhythmias and also rhabdomyolysis. Smooth-muscle function may also be affected and manifest as paralytic ileus. The ECG changes of hypokalemia do not correlate well with the plasma [$K^+$]. Early changes include flattening or inversion of the T wave, a prominent U wave, ST-segment depression, and a prolonged QU interval. Severe $K^+$ depletion may result in a prolonged PR interval, decreased voltage and widening of the QRS complex, and an increased risk of ventricular arrhythmias. Hypokalemia may also enhance digitalis toxicity.

Hypokalemia is often associated with acid-base disturbances related to the underlying disorder. In addition, $K^+$ depletion results in enhanced proximal $HCO_3^-$ reabsorption, increased renal ammoniagenesis, and increased distal $H^+$ secretion. This contributes to the generation of metabolic alkalosis that is frequently present in hypokalemic patients. NDI can occur with $K^+$ depletion and is manifest as polydipsia and polyuria.

**B. Etiology.** Hypokalemia, defined as a plasma [$K^+$] of less than 3.5 mEq/L, may result from one or more of the following: decreased net intake, shift into cells, or increased net loss.

1. **Diminished intake** is seldom the sole cause of $K^+$ depletion because urinary excretion can be effectively decreased to less than 15 mEq/day. However, dietary $K^+$ restriction may exacerbate the hypokalemia secondary to increased GI or renal loss.
2. **Transcellular shift.** Movement of $K^+$ into cells may transiently decrease the plasma [$K^+$] without altering total body $K^+$ content. The magnitude of the change is relatively small, often less than 1 mEq/L, but may amplify the hypokalemia due to $K^+$ wasting. Metabolic alkalosis is always associated with hypokalemia as a result of $K^+$ redistribution as well as excessive renal $K^+$ loss. Insulin therapy for DKA may lead to hypokalemia. Furthermore, uncontrolled hyperglycemia often leads to $K^+$ depletion from an osmotic diuresis. Stress-induced catecholamine release and administration of $\beta_2$-adrenergic agonists directly induce cellular uptake of $K^+$, as well as promote insulin secretion by the pancreas. Anabolic states can potentially result in hypokalemia caused by a $K^+$ shift into cells. This may occur after rapid cell growth, seen in patients with pernicious anemia treated with vitamin $B_{12}$ or neutropenia treated with granulocyte-macrophage colony-stimulating factor. It can also be seen in patients receiving total parenteral nutrition and after treatment for DKA.
3. **Nonrenal $K^+$ loss.** Moderate to severe $K^+$ depletion is often associated with vomiting or nasogastric suction and is primarily due to increased renal $K^+$ excretion. Loss of gastric contents results in volume depletion and metabolic alkalosis, both of which promote kaliuresis. Hypovolemia stimulates aldosterone release, which augments $K^+$ secretion by the principal cells. In addition, bicarbonaturia enhances the electrochemical gradient favoring $K^+$ loss in the urine. Hypokalemia subsequent to increased GI loss can occur in patients with profuse diarrhea, villous adenomas, vasoactive intestinal polypeptide (VIP)omas, or laxative abuse. Excessive sweating that leads to hypovolemia may result in $K^+$ depletion from increased integumentary and renal $K^+$ losses (secondary to ECF volume contraction).
4. **Renal $K^+$ loss** accounts for most cases of chronic hypokalemia. This may be caused by factors that increase the $K^+$ concentration in the lumen of the CCD or augment distal flow rate. Diuretic use and abuse are common causes of $K^+$ depletion (*Kidney Int* 28:988, 1985). **Primary hyperaldosteronism** is caused by dysregulated aldosterone secretion by an adrenal adenoma, carcinoma, or adrenocortical hyperplasia. **Hyperreninemia** (and secondary hyperaldosteronism) is commonly seen in renovascular and malignant hypertension and can also occur secondary to decreased effective circulating volume. Renin-secreting tumors are a rare cause of hypokalemia. Enhanced distal nephron secretion of $K^+$ may result from increased production of nonaldosterone mineralocorticoids in congenital adrenal hyperplasia. The syndrome of apparent mineralocorticoid excess, due to 11 β-hydroxysteroid dehydrogenase deficiency or suppression, is associated with the ingestion of licorice, the use of chewing tobacco, and carbenoxolone. The presentation of Cushing's syndrome may include hypokalemia. Liddle's syndrome (pseudoaldosteronism) is a rare disorder that results from the constitutive activation of the renal epithe-

lial sodium channel and is associated with low renin and aldosterone and a hypokalemic metabolic alkalosis.

Hypokalemia can also be caused by increased distal delivery of $Na^+$ with a nonreabsorbable anion (without $Cl^-$), which enhances the electrochemical force that drives $K^+$ secretion. Typically, this is seen with vomiting, DKA, toluene abuse, and high doses of penicillin derivatives. Classic distal (type 1) RTA is associated with hypokalemia due to increased renal $K^+$ loss. Amphotericin B causes hypokalemia as a result of increased distal nephron permeability to $Na^+$ and $K^+$, and renal $K^+$ wasting.

**C. Diagnosis** (Fig. 3-3). In most cases, the etiology of $K^+$ depletion can be determined by a careful history. Diuretic and laxative abuse as well as surreptitious vomiting may be difficult to identify but should be excluded. After eliminating decreased intake and intracellular shift as potential causes of hypokalemia, examination of the renal response can help to clarify the source of $K^+$ loss. The appropriate response to $K^+$ depletion is to excrete less than 15 mEq/day $K^+$ in the urine. Hypokalemia with minimal renal $K^+$ excretion suggests that $K^+$ was lost via the skin or GI tract, or may be consistent with a remote history of vomiting or diuretic use. Renal $K^+$ wasting may be caused by factors that either increase the $[K^+]$ in the CCD or increase the distal flow rate. The ECF volume status, BP, and associated acid-base disorder may help to differentiate the causes of excessive renal $K^+$ loss.

**D. The transtubular $K^+$ concentration gradient (TTKG)** is a rapid and simple test designed to evaluate the driving force for net $K^+$ secretion (*Lancet* 352:135, 1998). The TTKG is the ratio of the $[K^+]$ in the lumen of the CCD ($[K^+]_{CCD}$) to that in peritubular capillaries or plasma ($[K^+]_P$). In general, reabsorption of $Na^+$ salts in the medullary collecting duct (MCD) has a small effect on the TTKG. Significant reabsorption or secretion of $K^+$ in the MCD seldom occurs, except in profound $K^+$ depletion or excess, respectively. When vasopressin is acting, the osmolality in the terminal CCD is the same as that of plasma, and the amount of water reabsorbed in the MCD can be calculated from the urine-plasma osmolality ratio ($Osm_U$-$Osm_P$). Therefore, the $K^+$ concentration in the lumen of the distal nephron can be estimated by dividing the urine $[K^+]$ ($[K^+]_U$) by the $Osm_U$-$Osm_P$ ratio:

$$[K^+]_{CCD} = [K^+]_U/(Osm_U/Osm_P)$$

The urine osmolality must exceed that of plasma to calculate the TTKG:

$$TTKG = [K^+]_{CCD}/[K^+]_P$$

Hypokalemia with a TTKG greater than 4 suggests renal $K^+$ loss due to increased distal $K^+$ secretion. Plasma renin and aldosterone levels are often helpful in differentiating the various causes of hyperaldosteronism. Bicarbonaturia and the presence of other nonreabsorbed anions also increase the TTKG and lead to renal $K^+$ wasting. Finally, hypomagnesemia may contribute to refractory hypokalemia and should be corrected if found.

**E. Treatment**

1. **The therapeutic goals** are to (1) prevent life-threatening complications (arrhythmias, respiratory failure, and hepatic encephalopathy), (2) correct the $K^+$ deficit, (3) minimize ongoing losses, and (4) treat the underlying cause.
2. **Oral therapy.** It is generally safer to correct hypokalemia via the oral route. The degree of $K^+$ depletion does not correlate well with the plasma $[K^+]$. A decrement of 1 mEq/L in the plasma $[K^+]$ may represent a total body $K^+$ deficit of 200–400 mEq. Furthermore, factors that promote $K^+$ shift out of cells may result in underestimation of the $K^+$ deficit. Therefore, the plasma $[K^+]$ should be monitored frequently when

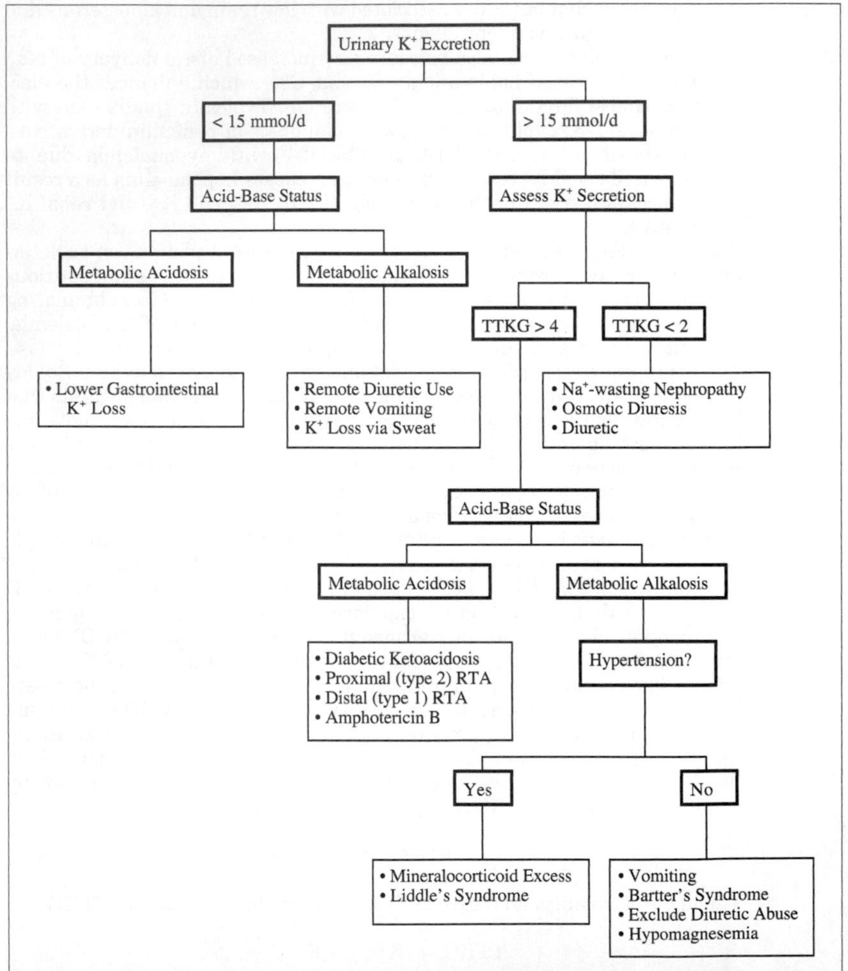


**Fig. 3-3.** Algorithm depicting clinical approach to hypokalemia. RTA, renal tubular acidosis; TTKG, transtubular $K^+$ concentration gradient. [From GG Singer, BM Brenner. Fluid and electrolyte disturbances. In AS Fauci, et al. (eds). *Harrison's Principles of Internal Medicine* (15th ed). New York: McGraw-Hill, 2001, with permission.]

assessing the response to treatment. KCl is usually the preparation of choice and promotes more rapid correction of hypokalemia and metabolic alkalosis than the other preparations. Potassium bicarbonate and citrate tend to alkalinize the patient and may be useful in correcting hypokalemia associated with chronic diarrhea or RTA.

3. **IV therapy.** Patients with severe hypokalemia or those who are unable to take anything by mouth require IV replacement therapy with KCl. The maximum concentration of administered $K^+$ should be no more than 40 mEq/L via a peripheral vein or 100 mEq/L via a central vein. The rate of infusion should not exceed 20 mEq/hour unless paralysis or malignant ventricular arrhythmias are present. Ideally, KCl should be

mixed in normal saline because dextrose solutions may initially exacerbate hypokalemia as a result of insulin-mediated movement of $K^+$ into cells. Rapid IV administration of $K^+$ should be used judiciously and requires close observation of the clinical manifestations of hypokalemia (ECG and neuromuscular examination).

## II. Hyperkalemia

**A. Manifestations.** The most serious effect of hyperkalemia is cardiac toxicity, which does not correlate well with the plasma [$K^+$]. The earliest ECG changes include increased T-wave amplitude, or peaked T waves. More severe degrees of hyperkalemia result in a prolonged PR interval and QRS duration, atrioventricular conduction delay, and loss of P waves. Progressive widening of the QRS complex and merging with the T wave produce a sine-wave pattern. The terminal event is usually ventricular fibrillation or asystole. Hyperkalemia causes partial depolarization of the cell membrane, which impairs membrane excitability and is manifest as weakness that may progress to flaccid paralysis and hypoventilation if the respiratory muscles are involved. Hyperkalemia also inhibits renal ammoniagenesis and reabsorption of $NH_4^+$ in the loop of Henle. Thus, net acid excretion is impaired and results in metabolic acidosis, which may further exacerbate the hyperkalemia because of $K^+$ movement out of cells.

**B. Etiology.** Hyperkalemia, defined as a plasma [$K^+$] of greater than 5.0 mEq/L, occurs primarily as a result of decreased renal loss, especially in chronic kidney disease.

1. **Increased $K^+$ intake** is rarely the sole cause of hyperkalemia. Iatrogenic hyperkalemia may result from overzealous parenteral $K^+$ replacement or in patients with renal insufficiency.
2. **Pseudohyperkalemia** represents an artificially elevated plasma [$K^+$] due to $K^+$ movement out of cells immediately before or following venipuncture. Contributing factors include repeated fist clenching, hemolysis, and marked leukocytosis or megakaryocytosis. Pseudohyperkalemia should be suspected in an otherwise asymptomatic patient with no obvious underlying cause.
3. **Transcellular shift.** Tumor lysis syndrome and rhabdomyolysis lead to $K^+$ release from cells. Metabolic acidoses, with the exception of those due to the accumulation of organic anions, can be associated with mild hyperkalemia resulting from intracellular buffering of $H^+$. Insulin deficiency and hypertonicity (e.g., hyperglycemia) promote $K^+$ shift from the ICF to the ECF. Exercise-induced hyperkalemia is due to release of $K^+$ from muscles, is usually rapidly reversible, and is often associated with rebound hypokalemia. Treatment with beta-blockers may contribute to the elevation in plasma [$K^+$] seen with other conditions. Hyperkalemic periodic paralysis is a rare cause of hyperkalemia. Depolarizing muscle relaxants such as succinylcholine can increase the plasma [$K^+$], especially in patients with massive trauma, burns, or neuromuscular disease.
4. **Decreased renal $K^+$ excretion** is virtually always associated with chronic hyperkalemia and is due to either impaired secretion or diminished distal solute delivery. Decreased $K^+$ secretion results from either impaired $Na^+$ reabsorption or increased $Cl^-$ reabsorption.
    a. **Impaired $Na^+$ reabsorption.** Decreased aldosterone synthesis may be due to primary adrenal insufficiency (Addison's disease) or congenital adrenal enzyme deficiency. Heparin inhibits the production of aldosterone and can lead to hyperkalemia in a subset of patients with underlying renal disease, diabetes mellitus, or those who are receiving $K^+$-sparing diuretics, angiotensin-converting enzyme (ACE) inhibitors, or NSAIDs. Pseudohypoaldosteronism is a rare disorder characterized by hyperkalemia, high renin and aldosterone levels, and hypertension. The kaliuretic response to aldosterone is also impaired by $K^+$-sparing diuretics. Spironolactone is a competi-

tive mineralocorticoid antagonist, whereas amiloride and triamterene block the apical $Na^+$ channel of the principal cell. Trimethoprim and pentamidine also impair $K^+$ secretion by blocking distal nephron $Na^+$ reabsorption. NSAIDs inhibit renin secretion and the synthesis of vasodilatory renal prostaglandins. The resultant decrease in GFR and $K^+$ secretion often manifests as hyperkalemia. ACE inhibitors block the conversion of angiotensin I to angiotensin II, resulting in impaired aldosterone release. Patients at increased risk for ACE inhibitor–induced hyperkalemia include those with diabetes mellitus, renal insufficiency, decreased effective circulating volume, bilateral renal artery stenosis, or concurrent use of $K^+$-sparing diuretics or NSAIDs. A similar effect may be seen with the use of angiotensin II receptor antagonists. Hyperkalemia frequently complicates acute oliguric renal failure due to increased $K^+$ release from cells and decreased excretion. In chronic renal insufficiency, adaptive mechanisms eventually fail to maintain $K^+$ balance when the GFR falls below 10–15 ml/minute or oliguria ensues.

b. **Increased $Cl^-$ reabsorption ($Cl^-$ shunt).** Hyperkalemia is commonly seen in mild renal insufficiency, diabetic nephropathy, or chronic tubulointerstitial disease. Patients frequently have an impaired kaliuretic response to exogenous mineralocorticoid administration, suggesting that enhanced distal $Cl^-$ reabsorption may account for many of the findings of hyporeninemic hypoaldosteronism. A similar mechanism may be partially responsible for the hyperkalemia associated with cyclosporine nephrotoxicity (*J Am Soc Nephrol* 2:1279, 1992). Hyperkalemic distal (type 4) RTA may be caused by either hypoaldosteronism or a $Cl^-$ shunt.

c. **Decreased distal flow rate** is seldom the only cause of impaired $K^+$ excretion but may significantly contribute to hyperkalemia in protein-malnourished (low urea excretion) and ECF volume–contracted (decreased distal NaCl delivery) patients.

C. **Diagnosis** (Fig. 3-4). With rare exceptions, chronic hyperkalemia is always caused by impaired $K^+$ excretion. If the etiology is not readily apparent and the patient is asymptomatic, pseudohyperkalemia should be excluded by drawing blood without fist clenching. Oliguric acute renal failure and severe chronic renal insufficiency should also be ruled out. The history should focus on medications that impair $K^+$ handling and potential sources of $K^+$ intake. Evaluation of the ECF compartment, effective circulating volume, and urine output are essential components of the physical examination. The appropriate renal response to hyperkalemia is the excretion of at least 200 mEq $K^+$ per day. In most cases, diminished renal $K^+$ loss is caused by impaired $K^+$ secretion, which can be revealed by finding a low TTKG (see sec. **I.C**). A TTKG of less than 10 implies a decreased driving force for $K^+$ secretion caused by either hypoaldosteronism or resistance to the renal effects of mineralocorticoid. This can be determined by evaluating the kaliuretic response after administration of mineralocorticoid [e.g., fludrocortisone (Florinef), 50–200 μg PO]. Primary adrenal insufficiency can be differentiated from hyporeninemic hypoaldosteronism by examining the renin-aldosterone axis. Renin and aldosterone levels should be measured in the supine and upright positions, after several days of $Na^+$ restriction ($Na^+$ intake <10 mEq/day) in combination with a loop diuretic to induce mild volume contraction. Aldosterone-resistant hyperkalemia can result from the various causes of impaired distal $Na^+$ reabsorption or, alternatively, from a $Cl^-$ shunt. The former leads to salt wasting, ECF volume contraction, and high renin and aldosterone levels. In contrast, enhanced distal $Cl^-$ reabsorption is associated with volume expansion and suppressed renin and aldosterone secretion.

D. **Treatment.** The approach to therapy depends on changes on the ECG and the degree of hyperkalemia.

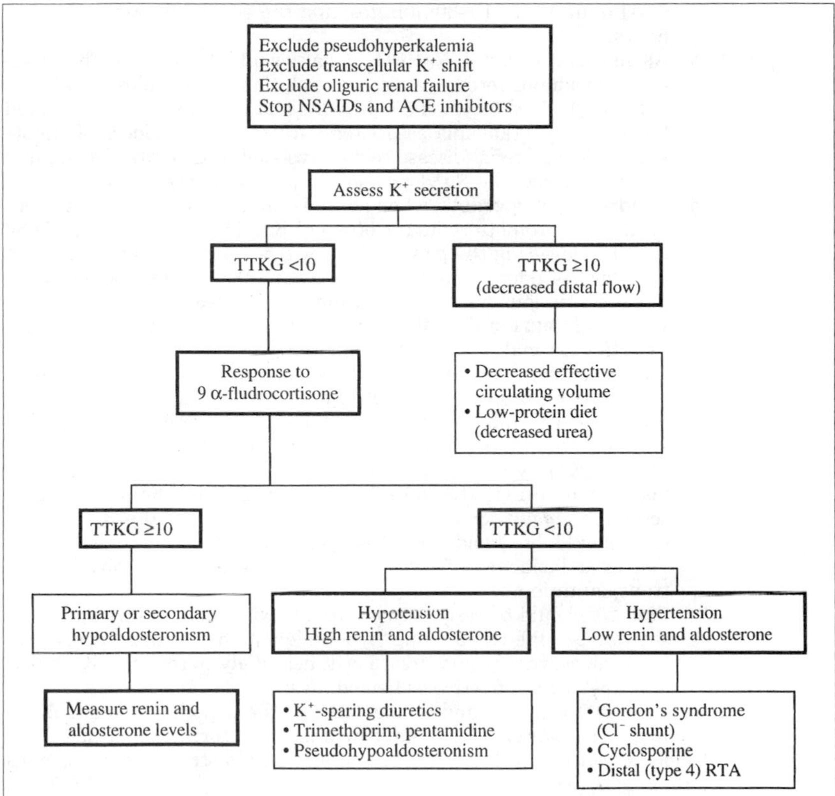


**Fig. 3-4.** Algorithm depicting clinical approach to hyperkalemia. ACE, angiotensin-converting enzyme; NSAIDs, nonsteroidal anti-inflammatory drugs; RTA, renal tubular acidosis; TTKG, transtubular $K^+$ concentration gradient. [From GG Singer, BM Brenner. Fluid and electrolyte disturbances. In AS Fauci, et al. (eds). *Harrison's Principles of Internal Medicine* (15th ed). New York: McGraw-Hill, 2001, with permission.]

1. **Acute therapy.** Severe hyperkalemia with ECG changes is a medical emergency and requires treatment directed at minimizing membrane depolarization over a few minutes, shifting $K^+$ into cells over the next 30–90 minutes, and longer-term objectives that promote $K^+$ loss. Exogenous $K^+$ intake and antikaliuretic drugs should be discontinued.
   a. **Administration of calcium gluconate** decreases membrane excitability. The usual dose is 10 ml of a 10% solution infused over 2–3 minutes. The effect begins within minutes but is short lived (30–60 minutes), and the dose can be repeated if no improvement in the ECG is seen after 5–10 minutes.
   b. **Insulin** causes $K^+$ to shift into cells and temporarily lowers the plasma [$K^+$]. Although **glucose** alone stimulates insulin release, a more rapid response generally occurs when exogenous insulin is administered (with glucose to prevent hypoglycemia). A commonly recommended combination is 10–20 units of regular insulin and 25–50 g glucose administered intravenously. Hyperglycemic patients should not be given glucose. If effective, the plasma [$K^+$] will fall by

0.5–1.5 mEq/L in 15–30 minutes, and the effect will last for several hours.

c. **Alkali therapy with IV $NaHCO_3$** can also shift $K^+$ into cells. This is safest when administered as an isotonic solution of 3 ampules of $NaHCO_3$ (134 mEq) added to 1 L of 5% dextrose and ideally should be reserved for severe hyperkalemia associated with metabolic acidosis. Patients with end-stage renal disease seldom respond to this intervention and may not tolerate the $Na^+$ load and resultant volume expansion.

d. **$\beta_2$-adrenergic agonists,** when administered parenterally or in nebulized form, promote cellular uptake of $K^+$. The onset of action is 30 minutes, lowering the plasma [$K^+$] by 0.5–1.5 mEq/L, and the effect lasts for 2–4 hours. Albuterol can be administered in a dose of 5–10 mg as continuous nebulized treatment over 30–60 minutes.

e. **Loop and thiazide diuretics,** often in combination, may enhance $K^+$ excretion if renal function is adequate.

f. **Cation exchange resins,** such as sodium polystyrene sulfonate (Kayexalate), promote the exchange of $Na^+$ for $K^+$ in the GI tract. When given by mouth, the usual dose is 25–50 g mixed with 100 ml 20% sorbitol to prevent constipation. This generally lowers the plasma [$K^+$] by 0.5–1.0 mEq/L within 1–2 hours and lasts for 4–6 hours. Sodium polystyrene sulfonate can also be administered as a retention enema consisting of 50 g resin in 150 ml tap water. Enemas should be avoided in postoperative patients because of the increased incidence of colonic necrosis, especially following renal transplantation.

g. **Dialysis** should be reserved for patients with renal failure and those with severe life-threatening hyperkalemia that is unresponsive to more conservative measures. Peritoneal dialysis removes $K^+$ but is only 15–20% as effective as hemodialysis.

2. **Chronic therapy.** The underlying cause of the hyperkalemia should be treated. This may involve dietary modification, correction of metabolic acidosis, cautious volume expansion, and administration of exogenous mineralocorticoid.

## Calcium

**Calcium** is essential for bone formation and neuromuscular function. Approximately 99% of body calcium is in bone; most of the remaining 1% is in the ECF. Nearly 50% of serum calcium is ionized (free), whereas the remainder is complexed, primarily to albumin. Changes in serum albumin, especially hypoalbuminemia, alter total serum calcium concentration without affecting the clinically relevant ionized calcium level. If serum albumin is abnormal, clinical decisions should be based on ionized calcium levels, which must lie within a narrow range (4.6–5.1 mg/dl) for normal neuromuscular function. **Calcium metabolism** is regulated by parathyroid hormone (PTH) and metabolites of vitamin D. PTH increases serum calcium by stimulating bone resorption, increasing renal calcium reabsorption, and promoting renal conversion of vitamin D to its active metabolite, calcitriol (1,25-dihydroxycholecalciferol; 1,25-dihydroxyvitamin $D_3$ [1,25$(OH)_2D_3$]). PTH also increases renal phosphate excretion. Serum calcium regulates PTH secretion by a negative feedback mechanism; hypocalcemia stimulates and hypercalcemia suppresses PTH release. Vitamin D is absorbed from food and synthesized in skin after exposure to sunlight. The liver converts it to 25-hydroxyvitamin $D_3$ [25$(OH)D_3$], which in turn is converted by the kidney to 1,25$(OH)_2D_3$. The latter metabolite increases serum calcium by promoting intestinal calcium absorption, and it plays a role in bone formation and resorption. It also enhances phosphate absorption by the intestine. Synthesis of 1,25(OH)$_2$D$_3$ is stimulated by PTH and hypophosphatemia and is inhibited by increased serum phosphorus.

I. **Hypercalcemia** is almost always caused by increased entry of calcium into the ECF (from bone resorption or intestinal absorption) and decreased renal calcium clearance. More than 90% of cases are due to primary hyperparathyroidism or malignancy.

A. **Primary hyperparathyroidism** causes most cases of hypercalcemia in ambulatory patients. It is a common disorder, especially in elderly women, in whom the annual incidence is approximately 2 in 1000. Nearly 85% of cases are due to an adenoma of a single gland, 15% to hyperplasia of all four glands, and 1% to parathyroid carcinoma. Most patients have asymptomatic hypercalcemia that is found incidentally. This disorder can cause symptoms of hypercalcemia (see sec. **I.D**), nephrolithiasis, osteopenia (primarily affecting cortical bone), or, rarely, osteitis fibrosa.

B. **Malignancy** is responsible for most cases of hypercalcemia among hospitalized patients, acting via two major mechanisms. In local **osteolytic hypercalcemia,** tumor cell products, such as cytokines, act locally to stimulate osteoclastic bone resorption. This form of malignant hypercalcemia occurs only with extensive bone involvement by tumor, most often due to breast carcinoma, myeloma, and lymphoma. In **humoral hypercalcemia of malignancy,** tumor products act systemically to stimulate bone resorption and, in many cases, to decrease calcium excretion. PTH-related peptide, which acts via PTH receptors but is not detected by PTH immunoassays, is an important mediator of this syndrome; tumor-derived growth factors may also play a role. Humoral hypercalcemia of malignancy is caused most often by squamous carcinoma of the lung, head and neck, or esophagus, or by renal, bladder, or ovarian carcinoma. Patients with malignant hypercalcemia almost always have advanced, clinically obvious disease.

C. **Other causes of hypercalcemia** (sarcoidosis, vitamin D toxicity, hyperthyroidism, lithium use, milk-alkali syndrome, and immobilization) are uncommon and are usually clinically evident. Thiazide diuretics cause persistent hypercalcemia in patients with increased bone turnover (e.g., mild primary hyperparathyroidism). 1,25(OH)$_2$D$_3$ levels are elevated in granulomatous disorders. **Familial hypocalciuric hypercalcemia** is a rare, autosomal-dominant disorder characterized by asymptomatic hypercalcemia from childhood and a family history of hypercalcemia.

D. **Clinical manifestations** generally are present only if serum calcium exceeds 12 mg/dl and tend to be more severe if hypercalcemia develops rapidly. Renal manifestations include polyuria and nephrolithiasis. GI symptoms include anorexia, nausea, vomiting, and constipation. Neurologic findings include weakness, fatigue, confusion, stupor, and coma. ECG manifestations include a shortened QT interval. Polyuria, nausea, and vomiting can cause marked dehydration, resulting in impaired calcium excretion and rapidly worsening hypercalcemia. If serum calcium rises above 13 mg/dl, renal failure and ectopic soft-tissue calcification may develop.

E. **Diagnosis of hypercalcemia** requires the distinction of primary hyperparathyroidism from other disorders. Increases in serum albumin can raise the total calcium level slightly without affecting ionized calcium concentration. Therefore, the serum ionized calcium should be measured to determine whether hypercalcemia actually is present.

1. **The history and physical examination** should focus on (1) the duration of hypercalcemia, (2) a history of renal stones, (3) clinical evidence of any of the unusual causes of hypercalcemia, and (4) symptoms and signs of malignancy (which almost always precede malignant hypercalcemia). If hypercalcemia has been present for more than 6 months without obvious cause, primary hyperparathyroidism is almost certainly the cause.

2. **The serum PTH level** should be measured. Assays measuring intact PTH should be used, as these are independent of renal function. Serum PTH levels are elevated in more than 90% of patients with primary hyperparathyroidism and invariably are suppressed in patients with hypercalcemia due to malignancy or other causes, except familial hypocalciuric hypercalcemia.
3. **Hypercalcemia** due to malignancy or uncommon causes is almost always evident from the history, physical examination, and routine laboratory tests; serum intact PTH levels are not elevated in these disorders. In a patient with chronic asymptomatic hypercalcemia, an elevated serum PTH, and no clinical evidence of malignancy, the diagnosis of primary hyperparathyroidism is secure. Some patients with the rare familial hypocalciuric hypercalcemia could present in this manner and can be distinguished by documenting low urinary calcium clearance. Malignancy or other causes should be sought if hypercalcemia is severe or develops rapidly and the serum PTH is not elevated.

F. **Acute management of hypercalcemia** includes measures that increase calcium excretion and decrease resorption of calcium from bone. The following regimen is warranted if severe symptoms are present or serum calcium is greater than 12 mg/dl. The goal is alleviation of symptoms rather than brisk normalization of serum calcium. The first step is replacement of ECF volume (see sec. **F.1**), followed by saline diuresis. An inhibitor of bone resorption should be given early; pamidronate is the drug of choice. Calcitonin can be used in patients with renal failure or can be added to a bisphosphonate to achieve rapid control of severe hypercalcemia. In patients with oliguric renal failure who cannot be treated with IV saline, hemodialysis with a low calcium dialysate lowers serum calcium temporarily.

1. **ECF volume restoration** with 0.9% saline constitutes initial therapy in severely hypercalcemic patients, who usually are volume depleted. The goal of this therapy is restoration of normal GFR. The initial infusion rate should be 300–500 ml/hour and should be reduced after the ECF volume deficit has been partially corrected. At least 3–4 L should be given in the first 24 hours, and a positive fluid balance of at least 2 L should be achieved.
2. **Saline diuresis** with 0.9% saline infusion (100–200 ml/hour) promotes calcium excretion after ECF volume is restored. Therapy should be monitored carefully, with frequent evaluation for evidence of heart failure. Serum electrolytes, calcium, and magnesium should be measured q6–12h. Adequate replacement of potassium and magnesium is essential. Furosemide, 20–40 mg IV bid–qid, adds little to the effect of saline diuresis and may prevent adequate restoration of ECF volume. It should not be given unless clinical evidence of heart failure develops. Thiazide diuretics must be avoided, as they impair calcium excretion.
3. **Pamidronate** is a bisphosphonate that inhibits bone resorption. A single dose of 60 mg in 500 ml 0.9% saline or 5% dextrose in water ($D_5W$) is infused over 2–4 hours; for severe hypercalcemia (>13.5 mg/dl), 90 mg in 1 L should be infused over 2–4 hours. Hypocalcemic response is seen within 2 days and peaks in nearly 7 days, and it may persist for 2 weeks or longer. Treatment can be repeated if hypercalcemia recurs. Side effects include hypocalcemia, hypomagnesemia, hypophosphatemia, and transient low-grade fever. **Zoledronate** is a newer, more potent bisphosphonate that is indicated for the treatment of hypercalcemia of malignancy. A single dose of 4 mg in 100 ml 0.9% saline or $D_5W$ is infused over a minimum of 15 minutes. Retreatment should not be considered for a minimum of 7 days. During treatment with bisphosphonates, renal dysfunction can occur from the precipitation of calcium bisphosphonate. Hydration should precede the use of bisphosphonates, and renal insufficiency is a relative contraindication to their use.

4. **Calcitonin** inhibits bone resorption and increases renal calcium excretion. Salmon calcitonin, 4–8 IU/kg IM or SC q6–12h, lowers serum calcium 1–2 mg/dl within several hours in 60–70% of patients. The hypocalcemic effect wanes after several days because of tachyphylaxis. Calcitonin is less potent than other inhibitors of bone resorption but has no serious toxicity, is safe in renal failure, and may have an analgesic effect in patients with skeletal metastases. It can be used early in the treatment of severe hypercalcemia to achieve a rapid response; concomitant use of a bisphosphonate ensures a prolonged effect. Side effects include flushing, nausea, and, rarely, allergic reactions.
5. **Glucocorticoids** lower serum calcium by inhibiting cytokine release, by direct cytolytic effects on some tumor cells, by inhibiting intestinal calcium absorption, and by increasing urinary calcium excretion. They are effective in hypercalcemia due to myeloma, other hematologic malignancies, sarcoidosis, and vitamin D intoxication. Other tumors rarely respond. The initial dose is prednisone, 20–50 mg PO bid, or its equivalent. Serum calcium may take 5–10 days to fall. After serum calcium stabilizes, the dose should be gradually reduced to the minimum needed to control symptoms of hypercalcemia. Toxicity (see Chap. 23, Arthritis and Rheumatologic Diseases) limits the usefulness of glucocorticoids for long-term therapy.
6. **Oral phosphate** inhibits calcium absorption and promotes calcium deposition in bone and soft tissue. It should be used only if the serum phosphorus level is lower than 3 mg/dl and renal function is normal, to minimize the risk of soft-tissue calcification. Doses of 0.5–1.0 g elemental phosphorus PO tid modestly lower serum calcium in some patients. Serum calcium, phosphorus, and creatinine should be monitored frequently, and the dose should be reduced if serum phosphorus exceeds 4.5 mg/dl or if the product of serum calcium and phosphorus (measured in mg/dl) exceeds 60. Side effects include diarrhea, nausea, and soft-tissue calcification. IV phosphate should never be used to treat hypercalcemia.
7. **Dialysis.** Hemodialysis using dialysate with low calcium and peritoneal dialysis are very effective means of treating hypercalcemia. This modality is particularly helpful for patients with CHF or renal insufficiency in whom hydration cannot be tolerated.

**G. Chronic management of hypercalcemia**

1. **For primary hyperparathyroidism,** parathyroidectomy is the only effective therapy. The natural history of asymptomatic hyperparathyroidism is not fully known, but in many patients the disorder has a benign course, with little change in clinical findings or serum calcium concentration for years. The possibility of progressive loss of bone mass and increased risk of fracture are the main concerns, but the likelihood of these outcomes appears to be low. Deterioration of renal function is possible but unlikely in the absence of nephrolithiasis. Currently, it is impossible to predict which patients will develop complications.
   a. **Indications for parathyroidectomy** include (1) symptoms caused by hypercalcemia, (2) nephrolithiasis, (3) reduced bone mass (more than 2 standard deviations below the mean for age), (4) serum calcium in excess of 12 mg/dl, (5) age younger than 50 years, and (6) unfeasibility of long-term follow-up (*N Engl J Med* 341:1249, 1999). Surgery is a reasonable choice in healthy patients even if they do not meet these criteria because it has a high success rate, with low morbidity and mortality. However, asymptomatic patients can be followed by assessing clinical status and serum calcium and creatinine levels at 6- to 12-month intervals. Bone mass at the hip should be assessed annually, using dual-energy absorptiometry. Surgery should be recommended if any of the aforementioned criteria develop or if progressive decline in bone mass or renal function occurs.

b. **Parathyroidectomy** performed by a surgeon experienced in the procedure has a success rate of 90–95%. Often a brief (1- to 2-day) period of mild, asymptomatic hypocalcemia ensues. In rare patients with overt bone disease, hypocalcemia may be severe and prolonged (the so-called **hungry bone syndrome**), requiring aggressive therapy with calcium and vitamin D. Other complications include permanent hypoparathyroidism and injury to the recurrent laryngeal nerve. Re-exploration is associated with a lower success rate and a greater risk of complications and should be performed at a referral center. Parathyroid localization procedures are not indicated before initial neck exploration but may be helpful before re-exploration.

c. **Medical therapy** has not been shown to affect the clinical outcome of primary hyperparathyroidism. However, in postmenopausal women, estrogen replacement therapy preserves bone mass with minimal effects on serum ionized calcium or PTH levels. In patients with symptomatic hypercalcemia who refuse or cannot tolerate surgery, physical activity should be encouraged, along with a diet that contains at least 2–3 L fluid and 8–10 g salt/day. Dietary calcium need not be restricted, and thiazide diuretics must not be used. Oral phosphate therapy may lower serum calcium but also raises serum PTH levels; its benefits do not clearly outweigh risks, and it should be used only if symptomatic hypercalcemia cannot be corrected surgically.

2. **Treatment of malignant hypercalcemia** may control symptoms until antineoplastic therapy takes effect, but it rarely succeeds for a long period of time unless the cancer responds to treatment. Because patients usually have extensive, unresectable disease, with a median survival of less than 3 months, the initial decision should be whether therapy is warranted. Treatment of hypercalcemia may palliate symptoms such as anorexia, nausea, and malaise. After acute management of hypercalcemia, physical activity and adequate fluid intake (at least 2–3 L/day) should be encouraged. Nausea should be treated, and a salt intake of 8–10 g/day is advisable; dietary calcium restriction is not beneficial. Repeated doses of IV pamidronate (see sec. **I.F.3**) can be given when hypercalcemia recurs. Plicamycin, an inhibitor of bone resorption, can be used as second-line therapy if pamidronate is ineffective, although its use is limited by hematologic, renal, and hepatic toxicity. Prednisone, 20–50 mg PO bid, usually controls hypercalcemia in multiple myeloma and other hematologic malignancies (see sec. **I.F.6**). Oral phosphate can be tried if the serum phosphorus level is low and renal function is normal.

3. **Hypercalcemia due to other disorders** should be treated with prednisone and a low-calcium diet (<400 mg/day). The effects of vitamin D itself may take up to 2 months to abate, but the toxicity of its metabolites is more short lived. Hypercalcemia due to sarcoidosis often responds to prednisone, and a dose of 10–20 mg/day may be sufficient for long-term control.

II. **Hypocalcemia** (low total serum calcium) is most commonly caused by hypoalbuminemia. If serum free (ionized) calcium is normal, no disorder of calcium metabolism is present. If ionized calcium cannot be measured, the total serum calcium can be corrected by adding 0.8 mg/dl for every 1 g/dl decrease of serum albumin below 4 g/dl, to determine whether true hypocalcemia is present. **Causes of low serum free calcium levels** include renal failure, hypoparathyroidism (either idiopathic or postsurgical), severe hypomagnesemia, hypermagnesemia, acute pancreatitis, rhabdomyolysis, tumor lysis syndrome, vitamin D deficiency, pseudohypoparathyroidism (PTH resistance), and, rarely, multiple citrated blood transfusions. A low serum free calcium level is common in critically ill patients, sometimes without evident cause. Drugs may cause hypocalcemia, including antineoplastic agents (cisplatin, cytosine arabinoside), antimicrobials (pentamidine, ketoconazole, foscarnet), and agents used to treat hypercalcemia (see sec. **I.F**).

**A. Clinical manifestations** vary with the degree and rate of onset. Chronic hypocalcemia may be asymptomatic. Alkalosis augments calcium binding to albumin and increases the severity of symptoms. Increased excitability of nerves and muscles causes paresthesias and tetany, including carpopedal spasms. **Trousseau's sign** is the development of carpal spasm when a BP cuff is inflated above systolic pressure for 3 minutes. **Chvostek's sign** refers to twitching of the facial muscles when the facial nerve is tapped anterior to the ear. The presence of these signs is known as **latent tetany.** Severe hypocalcemia may cause lethargy or confusion or, rarely, laryngospasm, seizures, or heart failure. The ECG may show a prolonged QT interval. Chronic hypocalcemia may cause cataracts and calcification of the basal ganglia.

**B.** The **history and physical examination** should focus on (1) previous neck surgery (as hypoparathyroidism may develop immediately or gradually over years), (2) disorders associated with idiopathic hypoparathyroidism (e.g., hypothyroidism, adrenal failure, candidiasis, vitiligo), (3) family history of hypocalcemia (which may be present in cases of familial hypocalcemia, hypoparathyroidism, or pseudohypoparathyroidism), (4) drugs that cause hypocalcemia or hypomagnesemia, (5) conditions that cause vitamin D deficiency, and (6) findings of pseudohypoparathyroidism (short stature, short metacarpals). **Laboratory studies** should include measurement of serum free calcium, phosphorus, magnesium, creatinine, and PTH. The serum phosphorus level is elevated in hypocalcemia resulting from most causes, although in hypocalcemia from vitamin D deficiency, it usually is low. Serum PTH is elevated in disorders other than hypoparathyroidism and magnesium deficiency.

**C. Acute management of symptomatic hypocalcemia** should be on an emergency basis with 2 g **calcium gluconate** (180 mg elemental calcium or 20 ml 10% calcium gluconate) IV over 10 minutes, followed by infusion of 6 g calcium gluconate in 500 ml $D_5W$ over 4–6 hours (10 ml 10% calcium gluconate = 1 g). Serum calcium should be measured q4–6h. The infusion rate should be adjusted to avoid recurrent symptomatic hypocalcemia and to maintain the serum calcium level at between 8 and 9 mg/dl. The underlying cause should be treated or long-term therapy started, and the IV infusion should be gradually tapered. Parenteral calcium is only necessary if the hypocalcemic patient is symptomatic or has a prolonged QT interval. **Hypomagnesemia,** if present, must be treated to correct hypocalcemia (see Magnesium, sec. **II.C**). In patients who take digoxin, the ECG should be monitored, as hypocalcemia potentiates digitalis toxicity. **Calcium and bicarbonate are not compatible IV admixtures.**

**D. Long-term management** of hypoparathyroidism and pseudohypoparathyroidism requires calcium supplements and vitamin D or its active metabolite to increase intestinal calcium absorption. Because PTH cannot limit urinary calcium excretion in these diseases, hypercalciuria and nephrolithiasis are potential side effects. The objective is to maintain serum calcium levels at slightly below the normal range (8.0–8.5 mg/dl), which usually prevents manifestations of hypocalcemia and minimizes hypercalciuria. While the dose of vitamin D is being titrated, serum calcium should be measured twice a week. When a maintenance dose is achieved, serum and 24-hour urinary calcium levels should be monitored every 3–6 months, because unexpected fluctuations may occur. If urine calcium exceeds 250 mg/24 hours, the dose of vitamin D should be reduced. If hypercalciuria develops at serum calcium levels of less than 8.5 mg/dl, hydrochlorothiazide (50 mg PO qd) can be used to reduce urinary calcium excretion.

1. **Oral calcium supplements. Calcium carbonate** (Os-Cal, 250 or 500 mg elemental calcium per tablet; Tums Calcium for Life Bone Health, 500

mg elemental calcium per tablet; or various generic formulations) is the least expensive compound. The initial dosage is 1–2 g elemental calcium PO tid during the transition from IV to oral therapy. For long-term therapy, the typical dosage is 0.5–1.0 g PO tid with meals. Calcium carbonate is well absorbed when taken with food, even in patients with achlorhydria. Side effects include dyspepsia and constipation.

2. **Vitamin D.** Dietary deficiency can be corrected by 400–1000 IU/day, but treatment of other hypocalcemic disorders requires much larger doses of vitamin D or use of an active metabolite. In patients with severe hyperphosphatemia, serum phosphorus should be lowered to less than 6.5 mg/dl with oral phosphate binders (see Phosphorus) before vitamin D is started. **Calcitriol** (0.25 or 0.5 μg/capsule) has a rapid onset of action. The initial dosage is 0.25 μg PO qd, and most patients are maintained on 0.5–2.0 μg PO qd. The dose can be increased at 2- to 4-week intervals. **Vitamin D** (50,000 IU or 1.25 mg/capsule) requires weeks to achieve full effect. The initial dosage is 50,000 IU PO qd, and usual maintenance dosages are 25,000–100,000 IU PO qd. The dose can be increased at 4- to 6-week intervals. Calcitriol is much more expensive than vitamin D, but its lower risk of toxicity makes it the best choice for most patients.

3. **Development of hypercalcemia.** In the event that hypercalcemia develops, vitamin D and calcium supplements should be stopped until serum calcium falls to a normal concentration; then both should be restarted at lower doses. Hypercalcemia due to calcitriol usually resolves within 1 week, and serum calcium should be monitored q24–48h. Hypercalcemia due to vitamin D may require more than 2 months to resolve. Symptomatic vitamin D–induced hypercalcemia should be treated with prednisone (see sec. **I.F.6**). In mild vitamin D toxicity, serum calcium can be monitored at weekly intervals until the level returns to normal.

## Phosphorus

**Phosphorus** is critical for bone formation and cellular energy metabolism. Approximately 85% of body phosphorus is in bone, and most of the remainder is within cells; only 1% is in the ECF. Thus, serum phosphorus levels may not reflect total body phosphorus stores. Phosphorus exists in the body as phosphate, but serum concentration is expressed as mass of phosphorus (1 mg/dl phosphorus = 0.32 mM phosphate). The normal range is 3.0–4.5 mg/dl, with somewhat higher values in children and postmenopausal women. Serum phosphorus is best measured in the fasting state, because there is diurnal variation, with a morning nadir. Carbohydrate ingestion and glucose infusion lower serum phosphorus, whereas a high-phosphate meal raises it. **Major regulatory factors** include PTH, which lowers serum phosphorus by increasing renal excretion; $1,25(OH)_2D_3$, which increases serum phosphorus by enhancing intestinal phosphate absorption; insulin, which lowers serum levels by shifting phosphate into cells; dietary phosphate intake; and renal function.

I. **Hyperphosphatemia** most often is caused by renal failure but also occurs in hypoparathyroidism, pseudohypoparathyroidism, rhabdomyolysis, tumor lysis syndrome, and metabolic and respiratory acidosis, and after excess phosphate administration. The latter is often seen when phospho-soda enemas (e.g., Fleet's) are given to patients with renal insufficiency, which can result in significant hypocalcemia.

A. **Clinical manifestations.** Symptoms and signs are those attributable to hypocalcemia (see Calcium, sec. **II.A**) and metastatic calcification of soft tissues, including blood vessels, cornea, skin, kidney, and periarticular tissue. Severe hyperphosphatemia may result in tissue ischemia or calciphylaxis. Chronic hyperphosphatemia contributes to renal osteodystrophy (see Chap. 11, Renal Diseases).

**B. Management**

1. **Dietary phosphate** should be restricted to 600–900 mg/day.
2. **Oral phosphate binders.** In patients with renal failure (see Chap. 11, Renal Diseases), **calcium carbonate** is given at an initial dosage of 0.5–1.0 g elemental **calcium PO tid with meals.** The dosage can be increased at intervals of 2–4 weeks to a maximum of 3 g tid. The goal of therapy is to maintain serum phosphorus levels between 4.5 and 6.0 mg/dl. Serum calcium and phosphorus levels should be measured frequently and the dose adjusted to keep the serum calcium level at less than 11 mg/dl and the calcium-phosphorus product at less than 60, to minimize the risk of ectopic calcification. **Sevelamer** is a phosphate binder that avoids the complications of hypermagnesemia, hypercalcemia, and aluminum toxicity. It is a nonabsorbable cationic polymer that binds phosphate through ion exchange and also lowers total cholesterol concentrations. Its major side effects are gastrointestinal complaints and worsening of metabolic acidosis. It is currently only approved for patients undergoing dialysis. **Aluminum hydroxide** and **aluminum carbonate** are no longer used in the dialysis population out of concern for their toxicity and because better alternatives are now available. **Calcium citrate** should not be used concurrently with aluminum gels because citrate increases aluminum absorption and can precipitate acute aluminum toxicity.
3. **Saline diuresis.** Acute hyperphosphatemia in patients who do not have renal failure is reduced by saline diuresis.
4. **Dialysis** is not very effective at removing phosphate due to the large intracellular stores. Extended or nocturnal hemodialysis is the only mode of dialysis that has been proven to lower phosphate levels.

**II. Hypophosphatemia** may be caused by impaired intestinal absorption, increased renal excretion, or redistribution of phosphate into cells. Causes of **severe hypophosphatemia** (<1 mg/dl) include alcohol abuse and withdrawal, respiratory alkalosis, malabsorption, oral phosphate binders, refeeding after malnutrition, hyperalimentation, severe burns, and DKA therapy; the presence of severe hypophosphatemia usually indicates total body phosphate depletion. **Moderate hypophosphatemia** (1.0–2.5 mg/dl) is common in hospitalized patients and may not indicate total body phosphate depletion. In addition, moderate hypophosphatemia may be caused by (1) infusion of glucose, (2) dietary vitamin D deficiency or malabsorption, and (3) increased renal phosphate loss due to hyperparathyroidism, the diuretic phase of ATN, renal transplantation, familial X-linked hypophosphatemia, Fanconi's syndrome, oncogenic osteomalacia, and ECF volume expansion.

**A. Clinical manifestations.** Signs and symptoms typically occur only if total body phosphate depletion is present and the serum phosphorus level is less than 1 mg/dl. Muscular abnormalities include weakness, rhabdomyolysis, impaired diaphragmatic function, respiratory failure, and heart failure. Neurologic abnormalities include paresthesias, dysarthria, confusion, stupor, seizures, and coma. Hemolysis, platelet dysfunction, and metabolic acidosis rarely occur. Chronic hypophosphatemia causes rickets in children and osteomalacia in adults.

**B. Diagnosis.** The cause is usually apparent, but, if not, measurement of urine phosphorus levels helps define the mechanism. Excretion of more than 100 mg/day during hypophosphatemia indicates excessive renal loss. Family history, serum calcium and PTH, and urine amino acids help distinguish among renal causes. Low serum 25(OH)$D_3$ suggests dietary vitamin D deficiency or malabsorption.

**C. Management**

1. **Moderate hypophosphatemia** (1.0–2.5 mg/dl) is usually asymptomatic and requires no therapy except correction of the underlying cause. Per-

sistent hypophosphatemia should be treated with oral phosphate supplements, 0.5–1.0 g elemental phosphorus PO bid–tid. Preparations include Neutra-Phos (250 mg elemental phosphorus and 7 mEq each sodium and potassium per capsule) and Neutra-Phos K (250 mg elemental phosphorus and 14 mEq potassium per capsule). The contents of capsules should be dissolved in water. Fleet Phospho-Soda (815 mg phosphorus and 33 mEq sodium per 5 ml) is an alternative oral agent. For patients who require long-term therapy, bulk powder is more economical; a 64-g bottle of Neutra-Phos dissolved in 1 gal water provides 250 mg elemental phosphorus per 75 ml. Serum phosphorus, calcium, and creatinine should be measured daily as the dose is adjusted. Side effects include diarrhea, which is often dose limiting, and nausea. Hypocalcemia and ectopic calcification are rare unless hyperphosphatemia occurs.

2. **Severe hypophosphatemia** (<1 mg/dl) may require IV phosphate therapy when associated with serious clinical manifestations. IV preparations include potassium phosphate (1.5 mEq potassium per mEq phosphate) and sodium phosphate (1.3 mEq sodium per mEq phosphate). An infusion of phosphate, 0.08–0.16 mEq/kg in 500 ml 0.45% saline, is given intravenously over 6 hours. If hypotension occurs, the infusion rate should be slowed. Further doses should be based on symptoms and on the serum calcium, phosphorus, and potassium levels, which should be measured q6h. IV infusion should be stopped when the serum phosphorus level is greater than 1.5 mg/dl or when oral therapy is possible. Because of the need to replenish intracellular stores, 24–36 hours of phosphate infusion may be required. Extreme care must be used to avoid hyperphosphatemia, which may cause hypocalcemia, ectopic soft-tissue calcification, renal failure, hypotension, and death. In renal failure, IV phosphate should be given only if absolutely necessary. Hypophosphatemic patients frequently also require correction of hypokalemia and hypomagnesemia. (Conversion factors for phosphate therapy are as follows: 1 mEq phosphate = 31 mg phosphorus, 1 mg phosphorus = 0.032 mEq phosphate.)

## Magnesium

**Magnesium** plays an important role in neuromuscular function. Approximately 60% of body magnesium is in bone, and most of the remainder is within cells. Only 1% is in the ECF, and serum magnesium levels often do not reflect total body magnesium content. Because clinical effects of magnesium disorders are determined primarily by tissue magnesium content, **serum magnesium levels** have limited diagnostic value. Normal serum concentrations are 1.3–2.2 mEq/L.

I. **Hypermagnesemia** occurs in renal failure, usually after therapy with magnesium-containing antacids or laxatives, and during treatment of preeclampsia with IV magnesium.

A. **Clinical manifestations.** Signs and symptoms are seen only if the serum magnesium level is greater than 4 mEq/L. Neuromuscular abnormalities usually include areflexia, lethargy, weakness, paralysis, and respiratory failure. Cardiac findings include hypotension; bradycardia; prolonged PR, QRS, and QT intervals; complete heart block; and asystole. Hypocalcemia may occur.

B. **Therapy.** Hypermagnesemia can be prevented by avoiding the use of magnesium preparations in renal failure. Asymptomatic hypermagnesemia requires only withdrawal of this therapy. Severe symptomatic hypermagnesemia should be treated with 10% calcium gluconate, 10–20 ml IV (1–2 g) over 10 minutes, to temporarily antagonize the effects of magnesium. Prompt supportive therapy is critical, including mechanical ventilation for respiratory failure and a temporary pacemaker for bradyarrhythmias. In severe renal failure, hemodialysis is required for definitive therapy. In the absence of severe renal failure, 0.9% saline with 2 g calcium gluconate per liter can be given at 150–200 ml/hour to promote magnesium excretion.

**II. Magnesium deficiency** may be caused by decreased intestinal absorption due to malnutrition, malabsorption, prolonged diarrhea, or nasogastric aspiration, or by increased renal excretion due to hypercalcemia, osmotic diuresis, and several drugs, including loop diuretics, aminoglycosides, amphotericin B, cisplatin, and cyclosporine. It often complicates alcoholism and alcohol withdrawal.

**A. Clinical manifestations.** Magnesium deficiency often causes hypokalemia and hypocalcemia, which contribute to the clinical picture. Neurologic abnormalities include lethargy, confusion, tremor, fasciculations, ataxia, nystagmus, tetany, and seizures. ECG abnormalities include prolonged PR and QT intervals. Atrial and ventricular arrhythmias may occur, especially in patients treated with digoxin.

**B. Diagnosis.** Magnesium deficiency should be suspected in the clinical situations described in sec. **II.A.** In these settings, hypomagnesemia is sufficient to establish the diagnosis of magnesium deficiency. However, routine measurement of serum magnesium without clinical suspicion of magnesium deficiency has little diagnostic value, and a normal serum level does not exclude total body magnesium deficiency. The etiology of hypomagnesemia usually is evident, but, if it is not, measurement of urine magnesium levels helps define the mechanism. Magnesium excretion of more than 2 mEq/day during hypomagnesemia indicates excessive renal loss.

**C. Therapy.** In patients with normal renal function, excess magnesium is readily excreted, and there is little risk of causing hypermagnesemia with recommended doses. However, magnesium must be given with extreme care in renal failure because of the risk of hypermagnesemia.

1. **Mild or chronic hypomagnesemia** can be treated with 240 mg elemental magnesium PO qd–bid. Magnesium oxide preparations include Mag-Ox 400 (240 mg elemental magnesium per 400-mg tablet) and Uro-Mag (84 mg elemental magnesium per 140-mg tablet). The major side effect is diarrhea.
2. **Severe symptomatic hypomagnesemia** can be treated with 1–2 g magnesium sulfate (4 mEq/ml) IV over 15 minutes, followed by an infusion of 6 g magnesium sulfate in 1 L or more IV fluid over 24 hours. Because of the need to replenish intracellular stores, the infusion should be continued for 3–7 days. Serum magnesium should be measured q24h and the infusion rate adjusted to maintain a serum magnesium level of less than 2.5 mEq/L. Tendon reflexes should be tested frequently, as hyporeflexia suggests hypermagnesemia. Reduced doses and more frequent monitoring must be used even in mild renal failure. (The conversion factors for magnesium therapy are as follows: 1 mmol = 24 mg elemental magnesium.)

## Acid-Base Disturbances

The normal ECF [$H^+$] is 40 nmol/L (pH 7.40) and is maintained within a narrow range. Perturbations in acid-base balance occur as a consequence of the gain or loss of $H^+$ or $HCO_3^-$. Individuals who consume a typical Western diet generate approximately 1 mEq/kg $H^+$ daily as a result of the metabolism of sulfur-containing (cysteine and methionine) and cationic (arginine and lysine) amino acids. To achieve $H^+$ balance, the dietary acid load must be excreted (and $HCO_3^-$ regenerated). Acid-base homeostasis is essential for normal cellular function and consists of three integral components: (1) chemical buffering by ECF ($HCO_3^-$) and ICF (proteins and organic and inorganic phosphates) buffers, (2) changes in alveolar ventilation to alter carbon dioxide tension ($PCO_2$), and (3) regulation of renal $H^+$ excretion to control ECF [$HCO_3^-$]. The latter is accomplished by proximal $HCO_3^-$ reabsorption and the generation of new $HCO_3^-$ as a result of titratable acid ($H_2PO_4^-$) and $NH_4^+$ excretion. The major adaptive response to an acid load is to stimulate ammoniagenesis and distal $H^+$ secretion, thereby increasing $NH_4^+$ excretion.

**I. Arterial blood gases (ABG).** Normal ABG values are pH, 7.40 ± 0.03 ([$H^+$] 40 ± 3 nmol/L); $PCO_2$, 40 ± 5 mm Hg; and [$HCO_3^-$], 24 ± 4 mEq/L. The relationship between these parameters is defined by the Henderson-Hasselbalch equation. For every 0.1 increase/decrease in pH, multiply/divide the [$H^+$] by 0.8 as follows:

| pH | 6.80 | 6.90 | 7.00 | 7.10 | 7.20 | 7.30 | 7.40 | 7.50 | 7.60 | 7.70 | 7.80 |
|---|---|---|---|---|---|---|---|---|---|---|---|
| [$H^+$] | 160 | 125 | 100 | 80 | 63 | 50 | 40 | 32 | 26 | 20 | 16 (nmol/L) |

Intermediate values can be estimated by interpolation.

**II. Primary acid-base disturbances.** The Henderson-Hasselbalch formula predicts that **acidemia** (high [$H^+$], low pH) can result from either a decreased [$HCO_3^-$] or an increased $PCO_2$. Likewise, **alkalemia** (low [$H^+$], high pH) is the consequence of an increased [$HCO_3^-$] or a decreased $PCO_2$. The compensatory responses (Table 3-2) tend to return the plasma [$H^+$] toward normal. A normal [$H^+$] implies either a mixed acid-base disorder or no acid-base disturbance.

**A. Metabolic acidosis** results from a primary decrease in plasma [$HCO_3^-$] due to either $HCO_3^-$ loss or the accumulation of acid. A compensatory fall in $PCO_2$ occurs as a result of alveolar hyperventilation.

**B. Metabolic alkalosis** is characterized by a primary increase in plasma [$HCO_3^-$] due to either $H^+$ loss or $HCO_3^-$ gain. The compensatory change is a rise in $PCO_2$ caused by decreased alveolar ventilation.

**C. Respiratory acidosis** is defined as a primary increase in $PCO_2$ (alveolar hypoventilation). The renal compensatory response is enhanced $H^+$ secretion. This occurs over 3–5 days and results in an increased plasma [$HCO_3^-$].

**Table 3-2.** Expected compensatory responses to primary acid-base disorders

| Disorder | Primary change | Compensatory response |
|---|---|---|
| Metabolic acidosis | ↓[$HCO_3^-$] | ↓$PCO_2$ by 1.0–1.3 mm Hg for every 1 mEq/L ↓[$HCO_3^-$] |
| | | $PCO_2$ should equal last two digits of pH × 100 |
| Metabolic alkalosis | ↑[$HCO_3^-$] | ↑$PCO_2$ 0.6–0.7 mm Hg for every 1 mEq/L ↑[$HCO_3^-$] |
| Respiratory acidosis | ↑$PCO_2$ | |
| Acute | | ↑[$HCO_3^-$] 1.0 mEq/L for every 10 mm Hg ↑$PCO_2$ |
| Chronic | | ↑[$HCO_3^-$] 3.0–3.5 mEq/L for every 10 mm Hg ↑$PCO_2$ |
| Respiratory alkalosis | ↓$PCO_2$ | |
| Acute | | ↓[$HCO_3^-$] 2.0 mEq/L for every 10 mm Hg ↓$PCO_2$ |
| Chronic | | ↓[$HCO_3^-$] 4.0–5.0 mEq/L for every 10 mm Hg ↓$PCO_2$ (pH usually in normal range) |

**D. Respiratory alkalosis** is manifest as hyperventilation that leads to a primary decrease in $PCO_2$. Chronically, a small compensatory decrease in renal $NH_4^+$ excretion occurs, leading to a fall in plasma $[HCO_3^-]$. The plasma pH is usually in the normal range.

## III. Diagnostic tests

**A. The plasma unmeasured anion gap (AG)** is the difference between the measured cations and the measured anions. Because the $[K^+]$ is usually unimportant quantitatively, it is often omitted from the calculation: $[Na^+] - ([Cl^-] + [HCO_3^-])$. The AG is normally 12 ± 2 mEq/L and is helpful in the differential diagnosis of metabolic acidosis. The normal AG is largely accounted for by anionic plasma proteins (i.e., albumin). A high AG generally signifies the overproduction of an organic acid or the presence of renal failure (see sec. **IV.B.1**). An increased AG may also be seen in metabolic alkalosis associated with ECF volume contraction. The causes of a low AG include hypoalbuminemia, halide ($Br^-$ or $I^-$) intoxication, severe hyperlipidemia, and some cases of multiple myeloma (cationic IgG paraprotein).

**B. The plasma osmolal gap** is the difference between the measured and the calculated plasma osmolality:

$$[Osm]_{meas} - [Osm]_{calc} = [Osm]_{meas} - (2\,[Na^+] + [glucose]/18 + [BUN]/2.8)$$

A high plasma osmolal gap reflects the presence of an unmeasured nonionized compound, usually an alcohol, such as methanol, ethanol, isopropanol, or ethylene glycol. This test is useful in distinguishing between the various causes of an increased AG metabolic acidosis (see sec. **IV.B.1**). Administration of IV mannitol or glycine is also detected as a high osmolal gap.

**C. The urine AG (UAG or urine net charge)** is useful when evaluating a normal AG metabolic acidosis (see sec. **IV.B.2**). The UAG is the difference between the major measured anions and cations:

$$[Na^+]_u + [K^+]_u - [Cl^-]_u$$

Because $NH_4^+$ is the major unmeasured urinary cation, a negative UAG reflects high $NH_4^+$ excretion. Conversely, a positive UAG signifies either low $NH_4^+$ excretion or the loss of $NH_4^+$ with a non-$Cl^-$ anion. If the latter is suspected, the **urine osmolal gap** (UOG) can help detect the presence of $NH_4^+$ in the urine.

**D. UOG** is the difference between the measured and the calculated urine osmolality:

$$[Osm]_{meas} - [Osm]_{estimated} = [Osm]_{meas} - 2([Na^+_{urine}] + [K^+_{urine}]) + [urea_{urine}]/2.8 + [glucose_{urine}]/18$$

The UOG is not affected by unmeasured anions (e.g., hippurate and β-hydroxybutyrate) and largely reflects the presence of $NH_4^+$ salts—the urine $[NH_4^+]$ is half the osmolal gap.

## IV. Metabolic acidosis

**A. Diagnosis.** After a thorough history and physical examination, the presence of metabolic acidosis is confirmed by finding a high $[H^+]$ and a low $[HCO_3^-]$. If the ventilatory compensation is inappropriate, a superimposed respiratory disorder is also present. In the absence of causes for a low AG (see sec. **III.A**), a normal AG metabolic acidosis suggests either loss of $HCO_3^-$ or gain of $H^+$ without a detectable accompanying plasma anion. The UAG and UOG should be determined to assess $NH_4^+$ excretion (see secs. **III.C** and **III.D**). Laboratory studies that are helpful in evaluating an increased AG metabolic acidosis include serum ketones (and β-hydroxybutyrate), lactate, creatinine, and a plasma osmolal gap (see sec. **III.B**). The ratio of the change in AG to the change in $[HCO_3^-]$ (Δ/Δ) is usually approximately 1:1. If the Δ/Δ is less than 1:1, a mixed normal and high AG metabolic acidosis should be suspected. Conversely, a Δ/Δ of greater than 1:1 suggests a concurrent metabolic alkalosis.

**B. Etiology and chronic treatment**

**1. Increased AG acidosis**

**a. Ketoacidosis** is due to relative insulin deficiency as a result of insulin-dependent diabetes mellitus, inhibition of insulin release, hypoglycemia, or liver disease. **DKA** is described in Chap. 21, Diabetes Mellitus and Related Disorders. **Alcoholic ketoacidosis** occurs when ethanol consumption is accompanied by impaired insulin release (β-adrenergic) and is usually due to vomiting, malnutrition, and ECF volume depletion. If enough ethanol remains in the blood, an osmolal gap, along with the increase in the AG, will be present. The osmolal gap should be equal to [ethanol] (in mg/dl)/4.6 unless there is an associated ingestion of another toxic alcohol. Because β-hydroxybutyrate initially predominates in the serum, the nitroprusside ketone reaction (Acetest), which detects acetoacetate and acetone, can underestimate the severity of the acidosis. Lactic acidosis may coexist, but lactate levels usually do not exceed 3 mEq/L. Serum glucose is typically normal or low. Treatment is directed at correction of ECF volume contraction. Thiamine should also be administered. The acidosis, unless severe, usually corrects with these measures. Hypokalemia, hypophosphatemia, and hypomagnesemia may occur, especially after 12–24 hours of therapy.

**b. Lactic acidosis** results from overproduction or decreased utilization of lactic acid. The former results from tissue hypoperfusion or impaired oxygenation, for example, cardiopulmonary arrest, shock, pulmonary edema, severe hypoxemia, carbon monoxide poisoning, or vascular insufficiency (mesenteric or limb ischemia). Hyperphosphatemia, hyperuricemia, and moderate hyperkalemia can accompany the acidosis. Conditions that cause a marked increase in the metabolic rate may also cause a lactic acidosis, for example, generalized seizures, anaerobic exercise, severe asthma, and hypothermic shivering. Other conditions associated with lactic acidosis include malignancy, diabetes mellitus, hypoglycemia, and D-lactate–producing bacteria in the short-bowel syndrome. Intoxication from cyanide, ethanol, methanol, propylene glycol, or salicylate should also be considered. Certain drugs (especially nucleoside reverse transcriptase inhibitors and metformin) have been shown to cause lactic acidosis. Of note, carnitine, thiamine, riboflavin, and coenzyme Q, which are involved in mitochondrial respiration, have all been used as therapies for drug-induced lactic acidosis. Their efficacy has not been established in randomized controlled trials.

**c. Renal failure** results in an AG acidosis when the GFR falls below 20–30 ml/minute (see Chap. 11, Renal Diseases). The AG is due to retained sulfate, phosphate, and organic anions. The AG does not account for the entire decrease in the serum $HCO_3^-$ because the acidosis is in part secondary to decreased $NH_4^+$ excretion.

**d. Intoxication** with methanol, ethylene glycol, and propylene glycol causes an increased AG metabolic acidosis along with an osmolal gap. Propylene glycol is used as a solvent in the IV formulations of drugs such as lorazepam, diazepam, and nitroglycerin. Paraldehyde may cause an increased AG acidosis, but without an osmolal gap. Salicylate intoxication usually results in respiratory alkalosis and metabolic acidosis. The metabolic acidosis may be due to increased lactate and ketoacid levels, as well as, to a minor degree, salicylic acid and its acid intermediates themselves. Diagnosis and treatment are described in Chap. 25, Medical Emergencies.

**2. Normal AG acidosis**

**a. Renal $HCO_3^-$ loss** or proximal (type 2) RTA is due to impaired proximal tubular $HCO_3^-$ reabsorption and ammoniagenesis. Proximal

RTA may be isolated or can occur in association with other transport defects (Fanconi's syndrome) such as glycosuria, aminoaciduria, hypouricemia, and hypophosphatemia. Causes include inherited disorders (cystinosis, galactosemia, Wilson's disease), toxins (heavy metals, outdated tetracycline, ifosfamide), multiple myeloma, autoimmune diseases (systemic lupus erythematosus, Sjögren's syndrome, chronic active hepatitis), amyloidosis, and acetazolamide. Bone disease (osteomalacia and osteopenia) is commonly associated with type 2 RTA. However, nephrocalcinosis seldom occurs. The diagnosis is made by administering $NaHCO_3$ intravenously and documenting bicarbonaturia as the plasma $[HCO_3^-]$ approaches normal: a urine pH of greater than 7.0 and a fractional excretion of $HCO_3^-$ greater than 15%. The fractional excretion of $HCO_3^-$ can be calculated using the following formula:

$$FE\ [HCO_3^-] = ([HCO_3^-]_{urine} \times [Cr]_{serum})/([HCO_3^-]_{serum} \times [Cr]_{urine})$$

Treatment should include attempts to correct the underlying cause. Large amounts of alkali (10–15 mEq/kg/day) are required. Citrate may cause fewer GI side effects than $HCO_3^-$. Administration of potassium salts minimizes the degree of hypokalemia associated with alkali therapy. Thiazide diuretics can be used to promote proximal tubule $HCO_3^-$ reabsorption by inducing mild ECF volume depletion.

b. **Enhanced $NH_4^+$ excretion** (negative UAG or high UOG, or both) indicates an appropriate renal response to metabolic acidosis and suggests two possible etiologies: GI $HCO_3^-$ loss or acid gain. The latter may result from the ingestion of HCl, $NH_4Cl$, lysine, arginine-HCl, or organic anions that are rapidly excreted in the urine (e.g., hippurate produced by patients who abuse toluene). GI loss of $HCO_3^-$ may be due to diarrhea, urinary diversion (ureterosigmoidostomy, long or obstructed ileal conduit), cholestyramine (especially in the presence of renal failure), or ingestion of calcium or magnesium chloride. GI losses may also be due to small-bowel, biliary, or pancreatic drainage or fistulas.

c. **Impaired $NH_4^+$ excretion** or distal RTA (positive UAG or UOG, $<100$ mOsm/kg) is associated with a heterogeneous group of disorders and results from either decreased $[NH_3]$ in the medullary interstitium (urine pH $<5.3$) or impaired distal $H^+$ secretion (urine pH $>5.8$). Historically, these conditions have been referred to as type 1 (distal or classic) and type 4 (hyperkalemic) RTA according to the plasma $[K^+]$. However, several unique mechanisms are implicated in the generation of a distal RTA that are not adequately addressed by the designations of types 1 and 4. Therefore, pathophysiologic classification allows a more rational approach to diagnosis and helps identify the possible etiologies. A low $[NH_3]$ in the renal medulla may be due to either decreased ammoniagenesis (usually associated with renal failure or hyperkalemia) or impaired medullary function due to various tubulointerstitial diseases (e.g., autoimmune diseases and hypergammaglobulinemia, nephrocalcinosis, analgesic use, chronic infection, or obstruction). Low distal $H^+$ secretion can result from (1) low $H^+$–adenosine triphosphatase pump activity (autoimmune or medullary interstitial diseases), (2) impaired voltage augmentation of $H^+$ secretion associated with hypoaldosteronism or mineralocorticoid resistance (see Potassium, sec. **II.B.4**), or (3) back-leak of $H^+$ due to increased membrane permeability (e.g., amphotericin B). **Treatment of distal RTA** should be directed at reversing the underlying disorder(s). Correction of the metabolic acidosis consists of $HCO_3^-$ replacement (usually 1–2 mEq/kg/day) with $NaHCO_3$ or sodium citrate. Hypokalemia should be corrected, and chronic potassium citrate replacement may be necessary for patients with nephrolithiasis or nephrocalcinosis. **Treatment of hyperkalemia** (see Potassium, sec. **II.D**) consists of dietary $K^+$ restriction (40–60 mEq/day) and possibly a loop diuretic. Chronic sodium polystyrene sulfonate therapy may also be necessary. Mineralocorticoid administration (fludrocortisone, 100–200 μg PO qd) should be considered in patients with primary adrenal insufficiency.

**C. Treatment with $NaHCO_3$** is appropriate for patients with a normal AG metabolic acidosis. Correcting severe acidemia to a pH of at least 7.20 decreases the risk of arrhythmias and enhances cardiac contractility. The plasma $[HCO_3^-]$ should be raised to approximately 5 mEq/L if the $PCO_2$ is less than 20 mm Hg. Calculation of the $HCO_3^-$ deficit $[0.5 \times \text{weight (kg)} \times (24 - [HCO_3^-])]$ assumes a volume of distribution of 50% of total body weight. The $HCO_3^-$ distribution space increases with the severity of the acidosis and may exceed 100% of total body weight in very severe metabolic acidosis. Rapid infusion of $NaHCO_3$ should only be considered for severe acidemia, and the tonicity of the $NaHCO_3$ administered depends on the patient's tonicity. Parenteral $NaHCO_3$ should always be prescribed with caution because of the potential adverse effects, including pulmonary edema, hypokalemia, and hypocalcemia.

## V. Metabolic alkalosis

**A. Etiology.** A primary increase in the plasma $[HCO_3^-]$ may be due to either $HCO_3^-$ gain ($H^+$ loss) or ECF volume contraction. To maintain electroneutrality, the addition of $HCO_3^-$ must be accompanied by either $Cl^-$ loss or $Na^+$ gain. In general, $Cl^-$ depletion results from either vomiting (or nasogastric suction, villous adenoma, or $Cl^-$-losing diarrhea) or diuretics (thiazide or loop). This leads to ECF volume contraction, $K^+$ depletion, ICF acidosis, and increased $NH_4^+$ excretion (new $HCO_3^-$ generation). Other causes of metabolic alkalosis that are associated with a decreased ECF volume include administration of nonreabsorbable anions (penicillin or carbenicillin), posthypercapnia, Bartter's syndrome, and $Mg^{2+}$ depletion. Exogenous administration of $NaHCO_3$, metabolism of organic anions (e.g., citrate, acetate, lactate, or ketoacid anions), or milk-alkali syndrome can result in metabolic alkalosis. Impaired renal $HCO_3^-$ excretion is required to maintain metabolic alkalosis. This occurs as a result of a decreased GFR and enhanced tubular $HCO_3^-$ reabsorption (due to effective circulating volume depletion, hypokalemia, and hyperaldosteronism). Metabolic alkalosis may also be associated with hypokalemia due to primary mineralocorticoid excess or secondary hyperaldosteronism (renal artery stenosis, malignant hypertension, renin-secreting tumor).

**B. Diagnosis** begins with a complete history, focusing on eating habits (vomiting) and drug use (diuretics). The physical examination should include an assessment of BP and ECF volume status. The two most common causes of metabolic alkalosis, vomiting and diuretic use, are both associated with ECF volume contraction. In contrast, patients with primary hyperreninemia or primary hyperaldosteronism tend to have a normal or expanded ECF compartment and are often hypertensive. Urine electrolytes are generally useful in identifying the etiology of metabolic alkalosis when the history is unrevealing. A low urine $[Cl^-]$ (<20 mEq/L) and decreased ECF volume suggest vomiting or remote diuretic use. Recent vomiting is associated with an alkaline urine (pH >7.0), a high TTKG (see Potassium, sec. **I.D**), and a urine $[Na^+]$ of greater than 20 mEq/L. The urine $[Na^+]$ and $[Cl^-]$ are both greater than 20 mEq/L after recent diuretic use. Without ECF volume contraction, the presence of hypertension, urine $[Na^+]$ and $[Cl^-]$ greater than 20 mEq/L, and a high TTKG is indicative of mineralocorticoid excess.

**C. Treatment** should be aimed at correcting the underlying disorder and replacing the deficits of NaCl and KCl. In the setting of ECF volume depletion, the latter is accomplished by giving isotonic NaCl. KCl should be administered to correct the $K^+$ deficit and intracellular acidosis. Metabolic alkalosis due to certain causes may be saline resistant, for example, edematous states, renal failure, mineralocorticoid excess, and severe $K^+$ or $Mg^{2+}$ depletion. These conditions are often associated with a normal or expanded ECF volume, and NaCl administration would be hazardous and ineffective. Hyperaldosteronism can be managed with a $K^+$-sparing diuretic (amiloride or spironolactone) with repletion of the $K^+$ and $Mg^{2+}$ deficits. Acetazolamide promotes bicarbonaturia, but renal $K^+$ loss is enhanced. Metabolic alkalosis associated with renal failure can be corrected with hemodialysis against a bath with a low [$HCO_3^-$]. Finally, severe alkalemia (pH >7.70) with ECF volume excess or renal failure, or both, can be treated with isotonic (150 mEq/L) HCl administered via a central vein (*Surgery* 75:194, 1974).

**VI. Respiratory acidosis**

**A. Diagnosis** is established by the detection of an increased [$H^+$] and an elevated $PCO_2$ on ABG. Hypercapnia almost always results from alveolar hypoventilation due to one of the following causes: (1) respiratory center depression (drugs, sleep apnea, obesity, CNS disease), (2) neuromuscular disorders (myasthenia gravis, Guillain-Barré syndrome, hypokalemia, myopathy), (3) upper airway obstruction, (4) pulmonary disease (chronic obstructive pulmonary disease, asthma, pulmonary edema, pneumothorax, pneumonia), or (5) mechanical hypoventilation. It is important to determine whether the change in [$H^+$] is appropriate for the change in $PCO_2$ to differentiate acute from chronic respiratory disturbances: For every mm Hg increase in $PCO_2$ from 40 mm Hg, the [$H^+$] should increase by 0.8 or 0.3 nmol/L in acute or chronic respiratory acidosis, respectively. The renal response occurs over several days, resulting in increased net acid excretion and an increased plasma [$HCO_3^-$] (Table 3-2).

**B. Treatment** is directed at correcting the underlying disorder and improving ventilation (see Chap. 9, Pulmonary Diseases). Administration of $NaHCO_3$ may exacerbate pulmonary edema, enhance hypercapnia, and lead to metabolic alkalosis. However, mechanically ventilated patients with severe status asthmaticus and acidosis (pH <7.15) may benefit from small doses of $NaHCO_3$ (44–88 mEq). Specifically, a higher plasma [$HCO_3^-$] allows the [$H^+$] to be controlled at a higher $PCO_2$ with a lower minute ventilation and peak airway pressures, thereby minimizing barotrauma.

**VII. Respiratory alkalosis**

**A. Diagnosis.** Respiratory alkalosis results from the temporary removal of carbon dioxide exceeding its generation, as a result of increased alveolar ventilation. The diagnosis is confirmed by finding a low [$H^+$] and a decreased [$PCO_3^-$] on ABG. Causes of respiratory alkalosis include (1) hypoxemia (pulmonary disease, anemia, heart failure, high altitude), (2) respiratory center stimulation [CNS disorders, liver failure, gram-negative sepsis, drugs (salicylates, progesterone, theophylline, catecholamines), pregnancy, psychogenic], (3) pulmonary disease (pneumonia, edema, emboli, interstitial fibrosis), and (4) mechanical hyperventilation. The compensatory renal response should be assessed (Table 3-2) and, if inappropriate, a mixed acid-base disturbance suspected.

**B. Treatment.** Treatment of respiratory alkalosis should focus on identifying and treating the underlying disease. In ICU patients this may involve changing the ventilator settings (see Chap. 8, Critical Care). Because alkalosis can lead to hypophosphatemia, hypokalemia, arrhythmias, and CNS disturbances, it needs to be corrected fairly promptly.

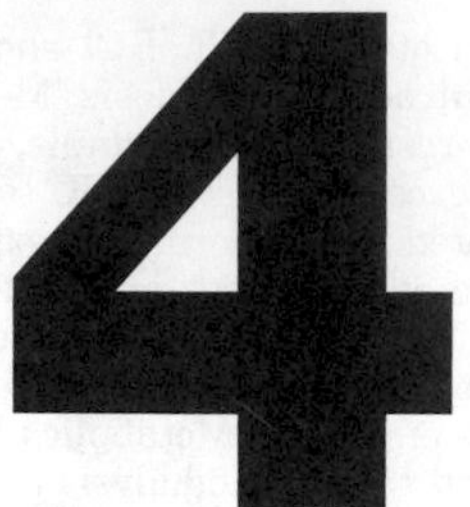

# Hypertension

Aubrey R. Morrison

## Definitions and Diagnostic Evaluation

**Hypertension** is defined as the presence of a BP elevation to a level that places patients at increased risk for target organ damage in several vascular beds, including the retina, brain, heart, kidneys, and large conduit arteries (Table 4-1). The public health burden of hypertension, characterized by a BP of greater than 140/90 mm Hg, is enormous, affecting an estimated 50 million Americans. Indeed, for individuals aged 55–65 years of age, the lifetime probability of development of hypertension is 90%. Of all hypertensive patients, 90% have essential hypertension; the remainder have hypertension secondary to causes such as renal parenchymal disease, renovascular disease, pheochromocytoma, Cushing's syndrome, primary hyperaldosteronism, coarctation of the aorta, and uncommon autosomal-dominant or -recessive diseases of the adrenal-renal axis that result in salt retention. Disease-associated morbidity and mortality, including atherosclerotic cardiovascular disease, stroke, heart failure (HF), and renal insufficiency, increase with higher levels of systolic and diastolic BP. Data derived from the Framingham study have shown that hypertensive patients have a fourfold increase in cerebrovascular accidents, as well as a sixfold increase in CHF, when compared to normotensive control subjects. Isolated systolic hypertension of the elderly is also associated with increased cardiovascular and cerebrovascular complications.

**I. Detection and classification.** BP measurements should be performed on multiple occasions under nonstressful circumstances (e.g., rest, sitting, empty bladder, comfortable temperature) to obtain an accurate assessment of BP in a given patient. Hypertension should not be diagnosed on the basis of one measurement alone, unless it is greater than 210/120 mm Hg or accompanied by target organ damage. Two or more abnormal readings should be obtained, preferably over a period of several weeks, before therapy is considered. Care should also be used to exclude pseudohypertension, which usually occurs in elderly individuals with stiff, noncompressible vessels. A palpable artery that persists after cuff inflation (Osler's sign) should alert the physician to this possibility. Home and ambulatory BP monitoring can be used to assess a patient's true average BP, which correlates better with target organ damage. Circumstances in which ambulatory BP monitoring might be of value include (1) suspected "white-coat hypertension" (increases in BP associated with the stress of physician office visits), (2) prehypertension (120–139 mm Hg systolic, 80–89 mm Hg diastolic), (3) evaluation of possible "drug resistance," and (4) episodic hypertension. Hypertension is present if a patient's average BP is greater than 140 mm Hg systolic or greater than 90 mm Hg diastolic (Table 4-2).

**II. Initial clinical evaluation.** BP elevation usually is discovered in asymptomatic individuals during screening. Optimal detection and evaluation of hypertension require accurate noninvasive BP measurement, which should be obtained in a

**Table 4-1.** Manifestations of target organ disease

| Organ system | Manifestations |
|---|---|
| Large vessels | Aneurysmal dilatation |
| | Accelerated atherosclerosis |
| | Aortic dissection |
| Cardiac | |
| Acute | Pulmonary edema, myocardial infarction |
| Chronic | Clinical or ECG evidence of CAD; LVH by ECG or echocardiogram |
| Cerebrovascular | |
| Acute | Intracerebral bleeding, coma, seizures, mental status changes, TIA, stroke |
| Chronic | TIA, stroke |
| Renal | |
| Acute | Hematuria, azotemia |
| Chronic | Serum creatinine >1.5 mg/dl, proteinuria >1+ on dipstick |
| Retinopathy | |
| Acute | Papilledema, hemorrhages |
| Chronic | Hemorrhages, exudates, arterial nicking |

CAD, coronary artery disease; LVH, left ventricular hypertrophy; TIA, transient ischemic attack.

seated patient with the arm level with the heart. A calibrated, appropriately fitting BP cuff should be used because falsely high readings can be obtained if the cuff is too small. Two readings should be taken, separated by 2 minutes. Systolic BP should be noted with the appearance of Korotkoff sounds (phase I) and diastolic BP with the disappearance of sounds (phase V). In certain patients,

**Table 4-2.** Classification of blood pressure for adults aged 18 years and older[a]

| Category | Systolic pressure (mm Hg) | Diastolic pressure (mm Hg) |
|---|---|---|
| Normal[b] | <120 | <80 |
| Prehypertension | 120–139 | 80–89 |
| Hypertension[c] | | |
| Stage 1 | 140–159 | 90–99 |
| Stage 2 | >160 | >100 |

[a]Not taking antihypertensive drugs and not acutely ill. When systolic and diastolic pressures fall into different categories, the higher category should be selected to classify the individual's BP status. Isolated systolic hypertension is defined as a systolic BP of 140 mm Hg or more and a diastolic BP of less than 90 mm Hg and staged appropriately (e.g., 170/85 mm Hg is defined as stage 2 isolated systolic hypertension). In addition to classifying stages of hypertension on the basis of average BP levels, the clinician should specify the presence or absence of target organ disease and additional risk factors. This specificity is important for risk classification and management.
[b]Optimal BP with respect to cardiovascular risk is less than 120 mm Hg systolic and less than 80 mm Hg diastolic. However, unusually low readings should be evaluated for clinical significance.
[c]Based on the average of two or more readings taken at each of two or more visits after an initial screening.
*Source:* Seventh Report of the Joint National Committee on Detection, Evaluation, and Treatment of High Blood Pressure. *JAMA* 289:2560, 2003, with permission.

the Korotkoff sounds do not disappear but are present to 0 mm Hg. In this case, the initial muffling of Korotkoff sounds (phase IV) should be taken as the diastolic BP (*Hypertension* 11:211A, 1988). One should be careful to avoid spuriously low BP readings due to an auscultatory gap, which is caused by the disappearance and reappearance of Korotkoff sounds in hypertensive patients and may account for up to a 25–mm Hg gap between true and measured BP. Hypertension should be confirmed in both arms, and the higher reading should be used. The history should seek to discover secondary causes of hypertension and note the presence of medications that can affect BP (e.g., decongestants, oral contraceptives, appetite suppressants, nonsteroidal anti-inflammatory agents, exogenous thyroid hormone, recent alcohol consumption, and illicit stimulants such as cocaine). A diagnosis of secondary hypertension should be considered in the following situations: (1) age at onset younger than 30 or older than 60 years, (2) hypertension that is difficult to control after therapy has been initiated, (3) stable hypertension that becomes difficult to control, (4) clinical occurrence of a hypertensive crisis (see Therapeutic Considerations, sec. **I.D**), and (5) the presence of signs or symptoms of a secondary cause such as hypokalemia or metabolic alkalosis that is not explained by diuretic therapy. In patients who present with significant hypertension at a young age, a careful family history may give clues to forms of hypertension that follow simple mendelian inheritance. The physical examination should include investigation for target organ damage or a secondary cause of hypertension by noting the presence of carotid bruits, an $S_3$ or $S_4$, cardiac murmurs, neurologic deficits, elevated jugular venous pressure, rales, retinopathy, unequal pulses, enlarged or small kidneys, cushingoid features, and abdominal bruits.

**III. Laboratory evaluation.** All newly diagnosed hypertensive patients should have a laboratory assessment, which may include a urinalysis, hematocrit, plasma glucose, serum potassium, serum creatinine, calcium, uric acid, chest radiography, and ECG. Fasting serum cholesterol and triglyceride levels should be obtained to screen for hyperlipidemia. This battery of tests helps to identify patients with possible target organ damage and provides a baseline for assessing adverse effects of therapy. Assessment of cardiac function or detection of left ventricular hypertrophy (LVH) by echocardiography may be of value for certain patients.

## Therapeutic Considerations

**I. General considerations and goals.** The goal of treatment for hypertension is to prevent long-term sequelae (i.e., target organ damage). Barring an overt need for immediate pharmacologic therapy, most patients should be given the opportunity to achieve a reduction in BP over an interval of 3–6 months by applying nonpharmacologic modifications. The primary goal is to reduce BP to less than 140/90 mm Hg while concurrently controlling other modifiable cardiovascular risk factors. As isolated systolic hypertension is also associated with increased cerebrovascular and cardiac events, the therapeutic goal in this subset of patients should be to lower BP to less than 140 mm Hg systolic. Treatment should be more aggressive, with a goal BP of <130/80 in patients with chronic kidney disease or diabetes. Discretion is warranted in prescribing medication to lower BP that may affect cardiovascular risk adversely in other ways (e.g., glucose control, lipid metabolism, uric acid levels). In the absence of hypertensive crisis (see sec. **I.D**), BP should be reduced gradually to avoid end-organ (e.g., cerebral) ischemia. Patient education is an essential component of the treatment plan and promotes patient compliance. Physicians should emphasize that (1) lifelong treatment usually is required, (2) symptoms are an unreliable gauge of severity of hypertension, and (3) prognosis improves with proper management. Cultural and other individual differences among patients must be considered in planning a therapeutic regimen. Although classification of adult BP is somewhat arbitrary, it may nevertheless be useful in making clinical decisions (Table 4-2).

**A. Normal BP** is defined as <120/<80; pharmacologic intervention is not indicated.

**B. Prehypertension** is defined as a BP of 120–139/80–89. In these patients with no more than one cardiovascular risk factor, excluding diabetes mellitus, and no target organ damage, BP can be followed for up to 6 months with nonpharmacologic therapy. If treatment is ineffective or the patient has evidence of end-organ damage or diabetes, or both, pharmacologic therapy should be initiated. Lifestyle modifications should be encouraged.

**C. In stages 1** (140–159/90–99) **and 2** (>160/>100) **hypertension,** pharmacologic therapy should be initiated in addition to lifestyle modification. Patients with BP levels greater than 180/110 mm Hg often require more than one medication and frequent intervals of follow-up before adequate control is achieved. Patients with an average BP of 200/120 or greater require immediate therapy and, if symptomatic end-organ damage is present, hospitalization.

**D. Hypertensive crisis** includes hypertensive emergencies and urgencies (see Special Considerations, sec. **III**). It usually develops in patients with a previous history of elevated BP but may arise in those who were previously normotensive. The severity of a hypertensive crisis correlates not only with the absolute level of BP elevation but also with the rapidity of development, because autoregulatory mechanisms have not had sufficient time to adapt.

1. **Hypertensive urgencies** are defined as a substantial increase in BP, usually with a diastolic BP of greater than 120–130 mm Hg, and occur in approximately 1% of hypertensive patients. Hypertensive urgencies (i.e., upper levels of stage 2 hypertension, hypertension with optic disk edema, progressive end-organ complications rather than damage, and severe perioperative hypertension) warrant BP reduction within several hours (*Arch Intern Med* 157:2412, 1997).
2. **Hypertensive emergencies** include **accelerated hypertension,** defined as a systolic BP typically exceeding 210 and diastolic BP greater than 130 presenting with headaches, blurred vision, or focal neurologic symptoms, and **malignant hypertension,** which requires the presence of papilledema. Hypertensive emergencies require immediate BP reduction by 20–25% (see Special Considerations, sec. **III**) to prevent or minimize end-organ damage [i.e., hypertensive encephalopathy, intracranial hemorrhage, unstable angina pectoris, acute myocardial infarction (MI), acute left ventricular failure with pulmonary edema, dissecting aortic aneurysm, progressive renal failure, or eclampsia].

**E. Isolated systolic hypertension.** Isolated systolic hypertension—defined as a systolic BP greater than 140 mm Hg—occurs frequently in the elderly (beginning after the fifth decade and increasing with age). Nonpharmacologic therapy should be attempted initially. If it fails, medication should be used to lower systolic BP to less than 140 mm Hg. Patient tolerance of antihypertensive therapy should be assessed frequently.

**II. Nonpharmacologic therapy.** Lifestyle modifications should be encouraged in all hypertensive patients regardless of whether they require medication. These changes may have beneficial effects on other cardiovascular risk factors. Some of these lifestyle modifications include cessation of smoking, reduction in body weight if the patient is overweight, judicious consumption of alcohol, and adequate nutritional intake of minerals and vitamins.

**III. Pharmacologic therapy**

**A. Diuretics** (Table 4-3) are effective agents in the therapy of hypertension, and data have accumulated to demonstrate their safety and benefit in reducing the incidence of stroke and cardiovascular events. Chlorthalidone, a thiazide diuretic, may be more effective than α-adrenergic antagonists

**Table 4-3.** Commonly used antihypertensive agents by functional class

| Drugs by class | Properties | Initial dose | Usual dosage range (mg) |
|---|---|---|---|
| **β-Adrenergic antagonists** | | | |
| Atenolol[a,b] | Selective | 50 mg PO qd | 25–100 |
| Betaxolol | Selective | 10 mg PO qd | 5–40 |
| Bisoprolol[a] | Selective | 5 mg PO qd | 2.5–20 |
| Metoprolol | Selective | 50 mg PO bid | 50–450 |
| Metoprolol XL | Selective | 50–100 mg PO qd | 50–400 |
| Nadolol[a] | Nonselective | 40 mg PO qd | 20–240 |
| Propranolol[b] | Nonselective | 40 mg PO bid | 40–240 |
| Propranolol LA | Nonselective | 80 mg PO qd | 60–240 |
| Timolol[b] | Nonselective | 10 mg PO bid | 20–40 |
| Carteolol[a] | ISA | 2.5 mg PO qd | 2.5–10 |
| Penbutolol | ISA | 20 mg PO qd | 20–80 |
| Pindolol | ISA | 5 mg PO qd | 10–60 |
| Labetalol | α- and β-antagonist properties | 100 mg PO bid | 200–1200 |
| Carvedilol | α- and β-antagonist properties | 6.25 mg PO bid | 12.5–50 |
| Acebutolol[a] | ISA, selective | 200 mg PO bid, 400 mg PO qd | 200–1200 |
| **Calcium channel antagonists** | | | |
| Amlodipine | DHP | 5 mg PO qd | 2.5–10 |
| Diltiazem | — | 30 mg PO qid | 90–360 |
| Diltiazem SR | — | 60–120 mg PO bid | 120–360 |
| Diltiazem CD | — | 180 mg PO bid | 180–360 |
| Diltiazem XR | — | 80 mg qd | 180–480 |
| Isradipine | DHP | 2.5 mg PO bid | 2.5–10 |
| Nicardipine[b] | DHP | 20 mg PO tid | 60–120 |
| Nicardipine SR | DHP | 30 mg PO bid | 60–120 |
| Nifedipine | DHP | 10 mg PO tid | 30–120 |
| Nifedipine XL (or CC) | DHP | 30 mg PO qd | 30–90 |
| Nisoldipine | DHP | 20 mg PO qd | 20–40 |
| Verapamil[b] | — | 80 mg PO tid | 80–480 |
| Verapamil COER | — | 80 mg PO qd | 180–480 |
| Verapamil SR | — | 120–140 mg PO qd | 120–480 |
| **Angiotensin-converting enzyme inhibitors** | | | |
| Benazepril[a] | — | 10 mg PO bid | 10–40 |
| Captopril[a] | — | 25 mg PO bid–tid | 50–450 |
| Enalapril[a] | — | 5 mg PO qd | 2.5–40 |
| Fosinopril | — | 10 mg PO qd | 10–40 |
| Lisinopril[a] | — | 10 mg PO qd | 5–40 |

*(continued)*

**Table 4-3.** Continued

| Drugs by class | Properties | Initial dose | Usual dosage range (mg) |
|---|---|---|---|
| Moexipril | — | 7.5 mg PO qd | 7.5–30 |
| Quinapril[a] | — | 10 mg PO qd | 5–80 |
| Ramipril[a] | — | 2.5 mg PO qd | 1.25–20 |
| Trandolapril | — | 1–2 mg PO qd | 1–4 |
| **Angiotensin II receptor blocker** | | | |
| Candesartan | — | 8 mg PO qd | 8–32 |
| Irbesartan | — | 150 mg PO qd | 150–300 |
| Losartan | — | 25 mg PO qd | 25–100 |
| Telmisartan | — | 20 mg PO qd | 20–80 |
| Valsartan | — | 80 mg PO qd | 80–320 |
| **Diuretics** | | | |
| Bendroflumethiazide | Thiazide diuretic | 5 mg PO qd | 2.5–15 |
| Benzthiazide | Thiazide diuretic | 25 mg PO bid | 50–100 |
| Chlorothiazide | Thiazide diuretic | 500 mg PO qd (or IV) | 125–1000 |
| Chlorthalidone | Thiazide diuretic | 25 mg PO qd | 12.5–50 |
| Hydrochlorothiazide | Thiazide diuretic | 25 mg PO qd | 12.5–50 |
| Hydroflumethiazide | Thiazide diuretic | 50 mg PO qd | 50–100 |
| Indapamide | Thiazide diuretic | 1.25 mg PO qd | 2.5–5.0 |
| Methyclothiazide | Thiazide diuretic | 2.5 mg PO qd | 2.5–5.0 |
| Metolazone | Thiazide diuretic | 2.5 mg PO qd | 1.25–5 |
| Polythiazide | Thiazide diuretic | 2.0 mg PO qd | 1–4 |
| Quinethazone | Thiazide diuretic | 50 mg PO qd | 25–100 |
| Trichlormethiazide | Thiazide diuretic | 2.0 mg PO qd | 1–4 |
| Bumetanide | Loop diuretic | 0.5 mg PO qd (or IV) | 0.5–5 |
| Ethacrynic acid | Loop diuretic | 50 mg PO qd (or IV) | 25–100 |
| Furosemide | Loop diuretic | 20 mg PO qd (or IV) | 20–320 |
| Torsemide | Loop diuretic | 5 mg PO qd (or IV) | 5–10 |
| Amiloride | Potassium-sparing diuretic | 5 mg PO qd | 5–10 |
| Triamterene | Potassium-sparing diuretic | 50 mg PO bid | 50–200 |
| Eplerenone | Aldosterone antagonist | 25 mg PO qd | 25–100 |
| Spironolactone | Aldosterone antagonist | 50 mg PO qd | 25–100 |
| **α-Adrenergic antagonists** | | | |
| Doxazosin | — | 1 mg PO qd | 1–16 |
| Prazosin | — | 1 mg PO bid–tid | 1–20 |
| Terazosin | — | 1 mg PO qhs | 1–20 |

(*continued*)

**Table 4-3.** Continued

| Drugs by class | Properties | Initial dose | Usual dosage range (mg) |
|---|---|---|---|
| **Centrally acting adrenergic agents** | | | |
| Clonidine[b] | — | 0.1 mg PO bid | 0.1–1.2 |
| Clonidine patch | — | TTS 1/wk (equivalent to 0.1 mg/d release) | 0.1–0.3 |
| Guanfacine | — | 1 mg PO qd | 1–3 |
| Guanabenz | — | 4 mg PO bid | 4–64 |
| Methyldopa[b] | — | 250 mg PO bid–tid | 250–2000 |
| **Direct-acting vasodilators** | | | |
| Hydralazine | — | 10 mg PO qid | 50–300 |
| Minoxidil | — | 5 mg PO qd | 2.5–100 |
| **Miscellaneous** | | | |
| Reserpine[b] | — | 0.5 mg PO qd | 0.01–0.25 |

DHP, dihydropyridine; ISA, intrinsic sympathomimetic activity; TTS, transdermal therapeutic system.
[a]Adjusted in renal failure.
[b]Available in generic form.

(doxazosin) in the treatment of hypertension and may also lessen the risk of cardiovascular disease and stroke in patients with hypertension and at least one risk factor for coronary heart disease [Antihypertensive and Lipid Lowering Treatment to Prevent Heart Attack Trial (ALLHAT). *JAMA* 283:1967, 2000]. The effectiveness of thiazide-like diuretics in the management of hypertension has been reinforced as updated results of the ALLHAT trial have been released (*JAMA* 288:2981,2002). These relatively inexpensive agents were shown to be effective for BP control and reduction in end points such as fatal and nonfatal MI.

1. **The mechanism of action** is to initiate a natriuresis and subsequently to decrease intravascular volume. Diuretics may initially cause an increase in peripheral resistance and a decrease in cardiac output, but, with chronic administration, these parameters return to normal. Diuretics may also produce mild vasodilation by inhibiting sodium entry into vascular smooth-muscle cells. Indapamide in particular has a pronounced vasodilating effect.
2. **Several classes of diuretics** are available, generally categorized by their site of action in the kidney. Thiazide and thiazide-like diuretics (e.g., hydrochlorothiazide, chlorthalidone) block sodium reabsorption predominantly in the distal convoluted tubule by inhibition of the thiazide-sensitive Na/Cl cotransporter. Loop diuretics (e.g., furosemide, bumetanide, ethacrynic acid, and torsemide) block sodium reabsorption in the thick ascending loop of Henle through inhibition of the Na/K/2Cl cotransporter and are the most effective agents in patients with renal insufficiency (creatinine >2.5 mg/dl). Spironolactone, a potassium-sparing agent, acts by competitively inhibiting the actions of aldosterone on the kidney. Triamterene and amiloride are potassium-sparing drugs that inhibit the epithelial $Na^+$ channel in the distal nephron to inhibit reabsorption of $Na^+$ and secretion of potassium ions. Potassium-sparing diuretics are weak agents when used alone; thus, they are often combined with a thiazide for added potency. Aldosterone antagonists may

have an additional benefit in improving myocardial function in HF; this effect may be independent of its effect on renal transport mechanisms.

3. **Side effects** of diuretics vary by class. Thiazide diuretics can produce weakness, muscle cramps, and impotence. Metabolic side effects include hypokalemia, hypomagnesemia, hyperlipidemia (with increases in low-density lipoproteins and triglyceride levels), hypercalcemia, hyperglycemia, hyperuricemia, hyponatremia, and, rarely, azotemia. Thiazide-induced pancreatitis also has been reported. Metabolic side effects may be limited when thiazides are used in low doses (e.g., hydrochlorothiazide, 12.5–25.0 mg/day). Loop diuretics can cause electrolyte abnormalities, such as hypomagnesemia, hypocalcemia, and hypokalemia, and also can produce irreversible ototoxicity (usually dose related and more common with parenteral therapy). Spironolactone can produce hyperkalemia; gynecomastia may occur in men, and breast tenderness has been noted in women. Triamterene (usually in combination with hydrochlorothiazide) can cause renal tubular damage and renal calculi. Unlike thiazides, potassium-sparing and loop diuretics do not cause adverse lipid effects.

**B. Sympatholytic agents**

1. **β-Adrenergic antagonists** (Table 4-3) are effective antihypertensive agents and are part of medical regimens that have been proven to decrease the incidence of stroke, MI, and HF.
   a. The **mechanism of action** of β-adrenergic antagonists is competitive inhibition of the effects of catecholamines at β-adrenergic receptors, which decreases heart rate and cardiac output. These agents also decrease plasma renin and cause a resetting of baroreceptors to accept a lower level of BP. β-Adrenergic antagonists cause release of vasodilatory prostaglandins, decrease plasma volume, and also may have a CNS-mediated antihypertensive effect.
   b. **Classes of β-adrenergic antagonists** can be subdivided into those that are cardioselective, with primarily $\beta_1$-blocking effects, and those that are nonselective, with $\beta_1$- and $\beta_2$-blocking effects. At low doses, the cardioselective agents can be given with caution to patients with mild chronic obstructive pulmonary disease, diabetes mellitus, or peripheral vascular disease. At higher doses, these agents lose their $\beta_1$ selectivity and may cause unwanted effects in these patients. β-Adrenergic antagonists also can be categorized according to the presence or absence of partial agonist or intrinsic sympathomimetic activity (ISA). β-Adrenergic antagonists with ISA cause less bradycardia than do those without it.
   c. **Side effects** include high-degree atrioventricular block, HF, Raynaud's phenomenon, and impotence. Lipophilic β-adrenergic antagonists, such as propranolol, have a higher incidence of CNS side effects, such as insomnia and depression, than do the more hydrophilic agents. Propranolol also can cause nasal congestion. β-Adrenergic antagonists can cause adverse effects on the lipid profile; increased triglyceride and decreased high-density lipoprotein (HDL) levels occur mainly with nonselective β-adrenergic antagonists but generally do not occur when β-adrenergic antagonists with ISA are used. Pindolol, a selective β-adrenergic antagonist with ISA, may actually increase HDL and nominally increase triglycerides. Because β-receptor density is increased with chronic antagonism, abrupt withdrawal of these agents can precipitate angina pectoris, increases in BP, and other effects attributable to an increase in adrenergic tone (*Br Heart J* 45:637, 1981).
2. **Selective α-adrenergic antagonists,** such as prazosin, terazosin, and doxazosin, have replaced nonselective α-adrenergic antagonists, such as phenoxybenzamine (Table 4-3), in the treatment of essential hypertension.

However, based on the ALLHAT trial, they appear to be less efficacious than diuretics, calcium channel blockers, and angiotensin-converting enzyme (ACE) inhibitors in reducing primary end points of cardiovascular disease when used as monotherapy (*JAMA* 288:2981, 2002).

a. The **mechanism of action** of selective $\alpha_1$-adrenergic antagonists is to block postsynaptic $\alpha$-receptors, producing arterial and venous vasodilation.

b. **Side effects** of these agents include a "first-dose effect," which results from a greater decrease in BP with the first dose than with subsequent doses. Selective $\alpha_1$-adrenergic antagonists can cause syncope, orthostatic hypotension, dizziness, headache, and drowsiness. In most cases, side effects are self-limited and do not recur with continued therapy. Selective $\alpha_1$-adrenergic antagonists may improve lipid profiles by decreasing total cholesterol and triglyceride levels and increasing HDL levels. Additionally, these agents can improve the negative effects on lipids induced by thiazide diuretics and $\beta$-adrenergic antagonists (*Am Heart J* 121:1307, 1991). However, doxazosin specifically may be less effective in lowering systolic BP than thiazide diuretics and may additionally be associated with a higher risk of cardiovascular disease, particularly HF, and stroke in patients with hypertension and at least one additional risk factor for coronary heart disease (ALLHAT, *JAMA* 283:1967, 2000).

3. **Agents with mixed properties** (labetalol, carvedilol) have $\alpha$- and $\beta$-adrenergic antagonist actions (Table 4-3). In addition, carvedilol may have antioxidant properties. These agents are effective in white and in black hypertensive patients.

a. The **mechanism of action** of these drugs is to antagonize the effects of catecholamines at $\beta$-receptors and peripheral $\alpha_1$-receptors. The effects of labetalol on $\alpha$-receptors decrease with chronic administration and are essentially gone within a few months.

b. **Side effects** of labetalol include hepatocellular damage, postural hypotension, a positive antinuclear antibody test (ANA), a lupus-like syndrome, tremors, and potential hypotension in the setting of halothane anesthesia. Labetalol has negligible effects on lipids. Carvedilol appears to have a similar side effect profile to other $\beta$-adrenergic antagonists. Rarely, reflex tachycardia may occur because of the initial vasodilatory effect of labetalol and carvedilol.

4. **Centrally acting adrenergic agents** (Table 4-3) are potent antihypertensive agents. In addition to its oral dosage forms, clonidine is available as a transdermal patch that is applied weekly.

a. The **mechanism of action** of centrally acting adrenergic agents is to stimulate the presynaptic $\alpha_2$-adrenergic receptors in the CNS. This stimulation leads to a decrease in peripheral sympathetic tone, which reduces systemic vascular resistance. Also, it causes a modest decrease in cardiac output and heart rate. Renal blood flow is not compromised by centrally acting adrenergic agents, but fluid retention may occur.

b. **Side effects** may include bradycardia, drowsiness, dry mouth, orthostatic hypotension, galactorrhea, and sexual dysfunction. Transdermal clonidine causes a rash in up to 20% of patients. These agents can precipitate HF in patients with decreased left ventricular function, and abrupt cessation can precipitate an acute withdrawal syndrome (AWS) of elevated BP, tachycardia, and diaphoresis (see Special Considerations, sec. **II**). Methyldopa produces a positive direct antibody (Coombs') test in up to 25% of patients, but significant hemolytic anemia is much less common. If a hemolytic anemia develops secondary to methyldopa, the drug should be withdrawn. Severe cases of hemolytic anemia may require treatment with glucocorticoids. Methyldopa also causes positive ANA test results in approximately 10% of patients and can cause an inflammatory reaction in the liver that is indistinguishable from viral hepatitis; fatal hepatitis has been reported. Guanabenz and guanfacine decrease total cholesterol levels, and guanfacine also can decrease serum triglyceride levels.

5. **Other sympatholytics** (reserpine, guanethidine, guanadrel). These agents (Table 4-3) were among the first effective antihypertensive agents available. Currently, these drugs are not regarded as first- or second-line therapy because of their significant side effects.
   a. The **mechanism of action** of these agents is to inhibit the release of norepinephrine from peripheral neurons. Reserpine, which is more lipophilic than are other drugs in this class, also affects the CNS. Reserpine depletes biogenic amines from being packaged into storage vesicles within neurons, thereby allowing norepinephrine to be degraded by cytoplasmic monoamine oxidase. Guanethidine and guanadrel directly inhibit the release of norepinephrine from peripheral nerve terminals.
   b. **Side effects** of reserpine include severe depression in approximately 2% of patients. Sedation and nasal stuffiness also are potential side effects. Guanethidine can cause severe postural hypotension by effecting a decrease in cardiac output, a decrease in peripheral resistance, and venous pooling in the extremities. Patients who are receiving guanethidine with orthostatic hypotension should be cautioned to arise slowly and to wear support hose. Guanethidine also can cause ejaculatory failure and diarrhea.

C. **Calcium channel antagonists** (Table 4-3) are effective agents in the treatment of hypertension. Generally, they have no significant CNS side effects and can be used to treat diseases, such as angina pectoris, that can coexist with hypertension. Concern has arisen that the use of short-acting dihydropyridine calcium channel antagonists may increase the number of ischemic cardiac events (*JAMA* 274:620, 1995); however, long-acting agents are safe in the management of hypertension (*Am J Cardiol* 77:81, 1996).

1. The **mechanism of action** is to cause arteriolar vasodilation by selective blockade of the slow inward calcium channels in vascular smooth-muscle cells. These agents also cause an initial natriuresis, which may dissipate with time.
2. **Classes of calcium channel antagonists** include diphenylalkylamines (e.g., verapamil), benzothiazepines (e.g., diltiazem), and dihydropyridines (e.g., nifedipine). The dihydropyridines include many newer second-generation drugs (e.g., amlodipine, felodipine, isradipine, and nicardipine), which are more vasoselective and have longer plasma half-lives than nifedipine. Verapamil and diltiazem have negative cardiac inotropic and chronotropic effects. Nifedipine also has negative inotropic effect, but, in clinical use, it is much less pronounced than that of verapamil or diltiazem because of peripheral vasodilatation and reflex tachycardia. Less negative inotropic effects have been observed with the second-generation dihydropyridines. All calcium channel antagonists are metabolized in the liver; thus, in patients with cirrhosis, the dosing interval should be adjusted accordingly. Some of these drugs also inhibit the metabolism of other hepatically cleared medications (e.g., cyclosporine; see Appendix C, Drug Interactions). Verapamil and diltiazem should be used with caution in patients with cardiac conduction abnormalities and can cause or worsen HF in patients with decreased left ventricular function.
3. **Side effects** of verapamil include constipation, nausea, headache, and orthostatic hypotension. Diltiazem can cause nausea, headache, and rash. Dihydropyridines can cause lower extremity edema, flushing, headache, and rash. Calcium channel antagonists have no significant effects on glucose tolerance, electrolytes, or lipid profiles. In general, calcium channel

antagonists should not be initiated in patients immediately after MI because of increased mortality in all but the most stable patients without evidence of HF (see Chap. 5, Ischemic Heart Disease). Additionally, in patients with hypertension and non–insulin-dependent diabetes mellitus, nisoldipine may be associated with a higher incidence of fatal and nonfatal MIs [Appropriate Blood Pressure Control in Diabetes (ABCD) trial, *N Engl J Med* 338:645, 1998], although amlodipine appears to be safe and effective in this population.

D. **Inhibitors of the renin-angiotensin system** (Table 4-3) are effective antihypertensive agents in a broad array of patients.

1. **ACE inhibitors** may have beneficial effects in patients with concomitant HF or kidney disease. One study has also suggested that ACE inhibitors (ramipril) may significantly reduce the rate of death, MI, and stroke in patients without HF or low ejection fraction (*N Engl J Med* 342:145, 2000). Additionally, they can reduce hypokalemia, hypercholesterolemia, hyperglycemia, and hyperuricemia caused by diuretic therapy and are particularly effective in states of hypertension associated with a high renin state (e.g., scleroderma renal crisis) (*Med Clin North Am* 71:979, 1987). Fosinopril is unique in that 50% of the drug is eliminated by the liver under normal conditions, but this percentage increases in the presence of renal insufficiency.

   a. **Mechanism of action.** ACE inhibitors block the production of angiotensin II, a vasoconstrictor, by inhibiting ACE competitively, thereby leading to arterial and venous vasodilation and to natriuresis. Furthermore, ACE inhibitors, by inhibiting the formation of angiotensin II, reduce aldosterone secretion, thus producing a mild natriuresis and a decrease in $K^+$ secretion. Additionally, ACE inhibitors increase levels of vasodilating bradykinins. Some agents (i.e., captopril) directly stimulate production of renal and endothelial vasodilatory prostaglandins. Despite these vasodilating effects, ACE inhibitors do not cause significant reflex tachycardia, perhaps owing to a resetting of the baroreceptor reflex.

   b. **Side effects** associated with the use of ACE inhibitors are infrequent. They can cause a dry cough (up to 20% of patients), angioneurotic edema, and hypotension, but they do not cause levels of lipids, glucose, or uric acid to increase. ACE inhibitors that contain a sulfhydryl group (e.g., captopril) may cause taste disturbance, leukopenia, and a glomerulopathy with proteinuria. Because ACE inhibitors cause preferential vasodilation of the efferent arteriole in the kidney, worsening of renal function may occur in patients who have decreased renal perfusion or who have preexisting severe renal insufficiency. ACE inhibitors can cause hyperkalemia and should be used with caution in patients with a decreased glomerular filtration rate who are taking potassium supplements or who are receiving potassium-sparing diuretics.

2. **Angiotensin-receptor blockers (ARBs)** are a class of antihypertensive drugs that are effective in diverse patient populations (*N Engl J Med* 334:1649, 1996). Several of these agents are now approved for the management of mild to moderate hypertension (Table 4-3). Additionally, ARBs may be useful alternatives in patients with HF who are unable to tolerate ACE inhibitors [*Lancet* 355:1582, 2000; *N Engl J Med* 354:1667, 2001; *Lancet* 362(9386):772, 2003].

   a. **The main mechanisms of action** of these drugs are to antagonize the vasoconstrictor effects on smooth muscle and the secretory effects on the zona glomerulosa of angiotensin II at the angiotensin II type 1 receptor. These actions result in decreased peripheral vascular resistance.

   b. **Side effects** of ARBs occur rarely but include angioedema, allergic reaction, and rash. ARBs cause cough much less frequently than

ACE inhibitors; the side effect profile is otherwise similar to that of the ACE inhibitors. Losartan specifically is uricosuric. These agents do not appear to affect lipids.

**E. Direct-acting vasodilators** are potent antihypertensive agents (Table 4-3) now reserved for refractory hypertension or specific circumstances, such as the use of hydralazine in pregnancy. Hydralazine in combination with nitrates is useful in treating patients with hypertension and HF (see Chap. 6, Heart Failure, Cardiomyopathy, and Valvular Heart Disease).

1. **The mechanism of action** of these agents (e.g., minoxidil and hydralazine) is to produce direct arterial vasodilation. Minoxidil hyperpolarizes and relaxes smooth muscle by stimulating an adenosine triphosphate–dependent $K^+$ channel. The mechanism of action of hydralazine is unknown. Although these drugs lower BP when used alone, their sustained antihypertensive action is limited because of reflex sodium and fluid retention and sympathetic hyperactivity producing tachycardia. Often, concomitant diuretic or β-adrenergic antagonist use is required to ameliorate these unwanted effects. These agents should be used with caution or avoided in patients with ischemic heart disease because of the reflex sympathetic hyperactivity that they induce.
2. **Side effects** of hydralazine therapy may include headache, nausea, emesis, tachycardia, and postural hypotension. Asymptomatic patients may have a positive ANA test result, and a hydralazine-induced systemic lupus–like syndrome may develop in approximately 10% of patients. Patients who may be at increased risk for this latter complication include (1) those treated with excessive doses (e.g., >400 mg/day), (2) those with impaired renal or cardiac function, and (3) those with the slow acetylation phenotype. Hydralazine should be discontinued if clinical evidence of a lupus-like syndrome develops and a positive ANA test result is present. The syndrome usually resolves with discontinuation of the drug, leaving no adverse long-term effects. Side effects of minoxidil include weight gain, hypertrichosis, hirsutism, ECG abnormalities, and pericardial effusions.

**F. Parenteral antihypertensive agents** are indicated for the immediate reduction of BP in patients with hypertensive emergencies. Judicious administration of these agents (Table 4-4) may also be appropriate in patients with hypertension complicated by HF or MI. These drugs are also indicated for individuals who have perioperative hypertensive urgency or are in need of emergency surgery. If possible, an accurate baseline BP should be determined before the initiation of therapy. In the setting of hypertensive emergency, the patient should be admitted to an ICU for close monitoring, and an intra-arterial monitor should be used when available. Although parenteral agents are indicated as a first line in hypertensive emergencies, oral agents may also be effective in this group (see sec. **III.G**); the choice of drug and route of administration must be individualized. If parenteral agents are used initially, oral medications should be administered shortly thereafter to facilitate rapid weaning from parenteral therapy.

1. **Sodium nitroprusside,** a direct-acting arterial and venous vasodilator, is the drug of choice for most hypertensive emergencies (Table 4-4). It reduces BP rapidly and is easily titratable, and its action is short lived when discontinued. Patients should be monitored very closely to avoid an exaggerated hypotensive response. Therapy for more than 48–72 hours with a high cumulative dose or renal insufficiency may cause accumulation of thiocyanate, a toxic metabolite. Thiocyanate toxicity may cause paresthesias, tinnitus, blurred vision, delirium, or seizures. Serum thiocyanate levels should be kept at less than 10 mg/dl. Patients on high doses (>2–3 mg/kg/minute) or those with renal dysfunction should have serum levels of thiocyanate drawn after 48–72 hours of therapy. In patients with normal renal function or those receiving lower doses, levels can be drawn after 5–7 days. Hepatic dysfunction may

**Table 4-4.** IV antihypertensive drug preparations

| Drug | Adminis-tration | Onset | Duration of action | Dosage | Adverse effects and comments |
|---|---|---|---|---|---|
| Sodium nitroprusside | IV infusion | Immediate | 2–3 min | 0.5–10 μg/kg/min (initial dose, 0.25 μg/kg/min for eclampsia and renal insufficiency) | Hypotension, nausea, vomiting, apprehension. Risk of thiocyanate and cyanide toxicity increased in renal and hepatic insufficiency, respectively; levels should be monitored. Must shield from light. |
| Diazoxide | IV bolus | 15 min | 6–12 hr | 50–100 mg q5–10min, up to 600 mg | Hypotension, tachycardia, nausea, vomiting, fluid retention, hyperglycemia; may exacerbate myocardial ischemia, heart failure, or aortic dissection. |
| Labetalol | IV bolus | 5–10 min | 3–6 hr | 20–80 mg q5–10min, up to 300 mg | Hypotension, heart block, heart failure, bronchospasm, nausea, vomiting, scalp tingling, paradoxical pressor response; may not be effective in patients receiving α or β antagonists. |
| | IV infusion | | | 0.5–2 mg/min | |
| Nitroglycerin | IV infusion | 1–2 min | 3–5 min | 5–250 μg/min | Headache, nausea, vomiting; tolerance may develop with prolonged use. |
| Esmolol | IV bolus | 1–5 min | 10 min | 500 μg/kg/min for first 1 min | Hypotension, heart block, heart failure, bronchospasm. |
| | IV infusion | | | 50–300 μg/kg/min | |

| | | | | | |
|---|---|---|---|---|---|
| Phentolamine | IV bolus | 1–2 min | 3–10 min | 5–10 mg q5–15min | Hypotension, tachycardia, headache, angina, paradoxical pressor response. |
| Hydralazine (for treatment of eclampsia) | IV bolus | 10–20 min | 3–6 hr | 10–20 mg q20min (if no effect after 20 mg, try another agent) | Hypotension, fetal distress, tachycardia, headache, nausea, vomiting, local thrombophlebitis; infusion site should be changed after 12 hr. |
| Methyldopate (for treatment of eclampsia) | IV bolus | 30–60 min | 10–16 hr | 250–500 mg | Hypotension. |
| Nicardipine | IV infusion | 1–5 min | 3–6 hr | 5 mg/hr, increased by 1.0–2.5 mg/hr q15min, up to 15 mg/hr | Hypotension, headache, tachycardia, nausea, vomiting. |
| Enalaprilat | IV bolus | 5–15 min | 1–6 hr | 0.625–5 mg q6h | Hypotension. |

*Source:* DA Calhoun, S Oparil. Treatment of hypertensive crisis. *N Engl J Med* 323:1177, 1990, with permission.

result in accumulation of cyanide, which can cause metabolic acidosis, dyspnea, vomiting, dizziness, ataxia, and syncope. Hemodialysis should be considered for thiocyanate poisoning. Nitrites and thiosulfate can be administered intravenously for cyanide poisoning.

2. **Nitroglycerin** given as a continuous IV infusion (Table 4-4) may be appropriate in situations in which sodium nitroprusside is relatively contraindicated, such as in patients with severe coronary insufficiency or advanced renal or hepatic disease. It is the preferred agent for patients with moderate hypertension in the setting of acute coronary ischemia or after coronary artery bypass surgery because of its more favorable effects on pulmonary gas exchange and collateral coronary blood flow. In patients with severely elevated BP, sodium nitroprusside remains the agent of choice. Nitroglycerin reduces preload more than afterload and should be used with caution or avoided in patients who have inferior MI with right ventricular infarction and are dependent on preload to maintain cardiac output.
3. **Labetalol** can be administered parenterally (Table 4-4) in hypertensive crisis, even in patients in the early phase of an acute MI, and is the drug of choice in hypertensive emergencies that occur during pregnancy. When given intravenously, the β-adrenergic antagonist effect is greater than is the α-adrenergic antagonist effect. Nevertheless, symptomatic postural hypotension may occur with IV use; thus, patients should be treated in a supine position. Labetalol may be particularly beneficial during adrenergic excess (e.g., clonidine withdrawal, pheochromocytoma, postcoronary bypass grafting). As the half-life of labetalol is 5–8 hours, intermittent IV bolus dosing may be preferable to IV infusion. IV infusion can be discontinued before oral labetalol is begun. When the supine diastolic BP begins to rise, oral dosing can be initiated at 200 mg PO, followed in 6–12 hours by 200–400 mg PO, depending on the BP response.
4. **Esmolol** is a parenteral, short-acting, cardioselective β-adrenergic antagonist (Table 4-4) that can be used in the treatment of hypertensive emergencies in patients in whom beta-blocker intolerance is a concern. Esmolol is also useful for the treatment of aortic dissection. β-Adrenergic antagonists may be ineffective when used as monotherapy in the treatment of severe hypertension and frequently are combined with other agents (e.g., with sodium nitroprusside in the treatment of aortic dissection).
5. **Nicardipine** is an effective IV calcium antagonist preparation (Table 4-4) approved for use in postoperative hypertension. Side effects include headache, flushing, reflex tachycardia, and venous irritation. Nicardipine should be administered via a central venous line. If it is given peripherally, the IV site should be changed q12h. Fifty percent of the peak effect is seen within the first 30 minutes, but the full peak effect is not achieved until after 48 hours of administration.
6. **Enalaprilat** is the active de-esterified form of enalapril (Table 4-4) that results from hepatic conversion after an oral dose. Enalaprilat (as well as other ACE inhibitors) has been used effectively in cases of severe and malignant hypertension. However, variable and unpredictable results also have been reported. ACE inhibition can cause rapid BP reduction in hypertensive patients with high renin states, such as renovascular hypertension, concomitant use of vasodilators, and scleroderma renal crisis, but should be used cautiously to avoid precipitating hypotension. Therapy can be changed to an oral preparation when IV therapy is no longer necessary.
7. **Diazoxide and hydralazine** now are used rarely in hypertensive crises and offer little or no advantage to the agents discussed in sec. **III.F.1–6.** It should be noted, however, that hydralazine is a useful agent in preg-

nancy-related hypertensive emergencies because of its established safety profile.

G. **Oral loading of antihypertensive agents** has been used successfully in patients with hypertensive crisis when urgent but not immediate reduction of BP is indicated.

1. **Oral clonidine loading** is achieved by using an initial dose of 0.2 mg PO followed by 0.1 mg PO q1h to a total dose of 0.7 mg or a reduction in diastolic pressure of 20 mm Hg or more. BP should be checked at 15-minute intervals over the first hour, 30-minute intervals over the second hour, and then hourly. After 6 hours, a diuretic can be added, and an 8-hour clonidine dosing interval can be begun. Sedative side effects are significant.

2. **Sublingual nifedipine** has an onset of action within 30 minutes but can produce wide fluctuations and excessive reductions in BP. **Because of the potential for adverse cardiovascular events (stroke/MI), sublingual nifedipine should be avoided in the acute management of elevated BP** (*Ann Intern Med* 107:185, 1987). Side effects include facial flushing and postural hypotension.

IV. **Individual patient considerations.** A vast array of effective antihypertensive agents is available. Logical therapeutic choices require consideration of a patient's pathogenic derangement of renin secretion, sympathetic tone, and renal sodium excretion and the attendant changes in cardiac output, peripheral vascular resistance, and volume status.

A. **The elderly hypertensive patient** (>60 years) generally is characterized by increased vascular resistance, decreased plasma renin activity, and greater LVH than in younger patients. Often, elderly hypertensive patients have coexisting medical problems that must be considered in initiating antihypertensive therapy. Drug doses should be increased slowly to avoid adverse effects and hypotension. Diuretics as initial therapy have been shown to decrease the incidence of stroke, fatal MI, and overall mortality in this age group [*JAMA* 283:1967, 2000; Systolic Hypertension in the Elderly Program (SHEP), *JAMA* 265:3255, 1991; *Lancet* 1:1349, 1985]. Calcium channel antagonists decrease vascular resistance, have no adverse effects on lipid levels, and also are good choices for elderly patients. Even though elderly patients tend to have low plasma renin activity, ACE inhibitors and ARBs may be effective agents in this population (*N Engl J Med* 328:914, 1993). Long-term studies have documented the safety and efficacy of β-adrenergic antagonists, especially after acute MI; however, they may increase peripheral resistance, decrease cardiac output, and decrease HDL cholesterol. Agents that produce postural hypotension (i.e., prazosin, guanethidine, guanadrel) should be avoided. Central α-adrenergic agents generally are effective in elderly patients but commonly cause sedation. In elderly patients with isolated systolic hypertension, the same approach to initiating therapy should be used, but smaller doses should be given, and adjustments should be made less frequently.

B. **Black hypertensive patients** generally have a lower plasma renin level, higher plasma volume, and higher vascular resistance than do white patients. Thus, black patients respond well to diuretics, alone or in combination with calcium channel antagonists. ACE inhibitors, ARBs, and labetalol (an α- and β-adrenergic antagonist) are also effective agents in this population.

C. **The obese hypertensive patient** is characterized by more modest elevations in vascular resistance, higher cardiac output, expanded intravascular volume, and lower plasma renin activity at any given level of arterial pressure. Weight reduction is the primary goal of therapy and is effective in reducing BP and causing regression of LVH. Weight reduction should be part of any therapeutic regimen.

D. **The diabetic patient** with nephropathy may have significant proteinuria and renal insufficiency, which can complicate management (see Chap. 11, Renal

Diseases). Control of BP is the most important intervention shown to slow loss of renal function. ACE inhibitors should be used as first-line therapy, as they have been shown to decrease proteinuria and to slow progressive loss of renal function independent of their antihypertensive effects (*N Engl J Med* 329:1456, 1993). ACE inhibitors also may be beneficial in reducing the rates of death, MI, and stroke in diabetics who have cardiovascular risk factors but lack left ventricular dysfunction (*N Engl J Med* 342:145, 2000). Furthermore, patients receiving ACE inhibitors may have a lower incidence of MI than those receiving the dihydropyridine class of calcium channel antagonists (ABCD, *N Engl J Med* 338:645, 1998), although this observation was not evident in the ALLHAT trial. Hyperkalemia is a common side effect in diabetic patients treated with ACE inhibitors, especially in those with moderate to severe impairment of their glomerular filtration rate. ARBs also are effective antihypertensive agents and have been shown to slow the rate of progression to end-stage renal disease, thus supporting a renal protective effect [Reduction of Endpoints in Non–Insulin-Dependent Diabetes Mellitus with the Angiotensin II Antagonist Losartan (RENAAL) and irbesartan trials].

**E. The hypertensive patient with chronic renal insufficiency** has hypertension that usually is partially volume dependent. Retention of sodium and water exacerbates the existing hypertensive state, and diuretics are important in the management of this problem. With a serum creatinine greater than 2.5 mg/dl, loop diuretics are the most effective class. BP control in this patient group decreases progression to end-stage renal disease (*N Engl J Med* 334:13, 1996). Increasing evidence has shown that ACE inhibitors can slow the rate of deterioration of renal function in diverse primary renal diseases and are worth considering as part of the therapeutic regimen in this clinical setting.

**F. The hypertensive patient with LVH** is at increased risk for sudden death, MI, and all-cause mortality. Although there is no direct evidence, regression of LVH could be expected to reduce the risk for subsequent complications. Sodium restriction, weight loss, and all drugs except direct-acting vasodilators can decrease left ventricular mass and wall thickness. ACE inhibitors appear to have the greatest effect on regression (*JAMA* 275:1507, 1996).

**G. The hypertensive patient with coronary artery disease** is at increased risk for unstable angina and MI. β-Adrenergic antagonists can be used as first-line agents in these patients, as they can decrease cardiac mortality and subsequent reinfarction in the setting of acute MI and can decrease progression to MI in those who present with unstable angina. β-Adrenergic antagonists also have a role in secondary prevention of cardiac events and in increasing long-term survival after MI (*Arch Intern Med* 156:1267, 1996). Care should be exercised in those with cardiac conduction system disease. Calcium channel antagonists should be used with caution in the setting of acute MI, as studies have shown conflicting results from their use. ACE inhibitors are also useful in patients with coronary artery disease and decrease mortality in individuals who present with acute MI, especially those with left ventricular dysfunction, and more recently have been shown to decrease mortality in patients without left ventricular dysfunction (*N Engl J Med* 342:145, 2000).

**H. The hypertensive patient with HF** is at risk for progressive left ventricular dilatation and sudden death. In this population, ACE inhibitors decrease mortality (*N Engl J Med* 327:685, 1992), and in the setting of acute MI, they decrease the risk of recurrent MI, hospitalization for HF, and mortality (*N Engl J Med* 327:669, 1992; *Lancet* 345:669, 1995). ARBs have similar beneficial effects, and they appear to be an effective alternative in patients who are unable to tolerate an ACE inhibitor (*Lancet* 355:1582, 2000; *N Engl J Med* 345:1667, 2001; *Lancet* 362(9386:772, 2003). Nitrates and hydralazine also decrease mortality in patients with HF irrespective of hypertension, but hydralazine can cause reflex tachycardia and worsening ischemia in patients with unstable coronary syndromes and should be used with caution. Calcium channel antagonists should generally be avoided in patients in whom negative inotropic effects would affect their status adversely.

V. **Initial drug therapy.** Data from the ALLHAT trial have shown decreased cardiovascular and cerebrovascular morbidity and mortality with the use of thiazide diuretics; thus, this class of drugs is favored as first-line agents in the absence of a contraindication to their use or if characteristics of a patient's profile (concomitant disease, age, race) mandate institution of a different agent. Calcium channel antagonists and ACE inhibitors have been shown to decrease BP to degrees similar to those observed with diuretics and β-adrenergic antagonists and also are reasonable initial agents because of their low side effect profile; however, it may be justifiable to choose agents that are off-patent to allow for cost containment. Initial drug choice may be affected by coexistent factors, such as age, race, angina, HF, renal insufficiency, LVH, obesity, hyperlipidemia, gout, and bronchospasm. Cost and drug interactions also should be considered. The BP response usually is consistent within a given class of agents; therefore, if a drug fails to control BP, another agent from the same class is unlikely to be effective. At times, however, a change within drug class may be useful in reducing adverse effects. The lowest possible effective dosage should be used to control BP, adjusted every 1–3 months as needed. The majority of patients with stage 1 hypertension can attain adequate BP control with single-drug therapy.

VI. **Additional therapy.** When a second drug is needed, it can generally be chosen from among the other first-line agents. A diuretic should be added first, as doing so may enhance effectiveness of the first drug, yielding more than a simple additive effect. Several combination preparations of first-line agents are available.

VII. **Adjustments of a therapeutic regimen.** In considering a modification of therapy because of inadequate response to the current regimen, the physician should investigate other possible contributing factors. Poor patient compliance, use of antagonistic drugs (i.e., sympathomimetics, antidepressants, steroids, nonsteroidal anti-inflammatory drugs, cyclosporine, caffeine, thyroid hormones, cocaine, erythropoietin), inappropriately high sodium intake, or increased alcohol consumption should be considered before antihypertensive drug therapy is modified. Unacceptable side effects from a particular agent may contribute to poor patient compliance. Excessive fluid retention should be evaluated and treated. Secondary causes of hypertension must be considered when a previously effective regimen becomes inadequate and other confounding factors are absent.

## Special Considerations

I. **Hypertension associated with withdrawal syndromes.** Hypertension may be part of several important syndromes of withdrawal from drugs, including alcohol, cocaine, and opioid analgesics. Rebound increases in BP also may be seen in patients who abruptly discontinue antihypertensive therapy.

A. **Cocaine and other sympathomimetic drugs** (e.g., amphetamines, phencyclidine hydrochloride) can produce hypertension in the setting of acute intoxication and when the agents are discontinued abruptly after chronic use. Hypertension often is complicated by other end-organ insults, such as ischemic heart disease, stroke, and seizures. Phentolamine is effective in acute management, and sodium nitroprusside or nitroglycerin can be used as an alternative (Table 4-3). β-Adrenergic antagonists should be avoided due to the risk of unopposed α-adrenergic activity, which can exacerbate hypertension.

**B. Monoamine oxidase inhibitors** used in association with certain drugs or foods can produce a catecholamine excess state and accelerated hypertension. Interactions are common with tricyclic antidepressants, meperidine, methyldopa, levodopa, sympathomimetic agents, and antihistamines. Tyramine-containing foods that can lead to this syndrome include certain cheeses, red wine, beer, chocolate, chicken liver, processed meat, herring, broad beans, canned figs, and yeast. Nitroprusside, labetalol, and phentolamine have been used effectively in the treatment of accelerated hypertension associated with monoamine oxidase inhibitor use (Table 4-4).

**II. Withdrawal syndrome associated with discontinuation of antihypertensive therapy.** In substituting therapy in patients with moderate to severe hypertension, it is reasonable to increase doses of the new medication in small increments while tapering the previous medication to avoid excessive BP fluctuations. On occasion, an AWS develops, usually within the first 24–72 hours. Occasionally, BP rises to levels that are much greater than those of baseline values. The most severe complications of AWS include encephalopathy, stroke, MI, and sudden death. The AWS is associated most commonly with centrally acting adrenergic agents (particularly clonidine) and β-adrenergic antagonists but has been reported with other agents as well, including diuretics. Rarely should BP medications be withdrawn, but, in discontinuing therapy, these drugs should be tapered over several days to weeks unless other medications are used to substitute in the interim. Discontinuation of antihypertensive medications should be done with caution in patients with preexisting cerebrovascular or cardiac disease. Management of AWS by reinstitution of the previously administered drug generally is effective. Sodium nitroprusside (Table 4-3) is the treatment of choice when parenteral administration of an antihypertensive agent is required or when the identity of the previously administered agent is unknown. In the AWS caused by clonidine, β-adrenergic antagonists should not be used because unopposed α-adrenergic activity will be augmented and may exacerbate hypertension. However, labetalol (Table 4-3) may be useful in this situation.

**III. Hypertensive crisis** (see Therapeutic Considerations, sec. **I.D**). In hypertensive emergency, control of acute or ongoing end-organ damage is more important than the absolute level of BP. BP control with a rapidly acting parenteral agent should be accomplished as soon as possible (within 1 hour) to reduce the chance of permanent organ dysfunction and death. A reasonable goal is a 20–25% reduction of mean arterial pressure or a reduction of the diastolic pressure to 100–110 mm Hg over a period of minutes to hours. A precipitous fall in BP may occur in patients who are elderly, volume depleted, or receiving other antihypertensive agents, and caution should be used to avoid cerebral hypoperfusion. BP control in hypertensive urgencies can be accomplished more slowly. The initial goal of therapy in urgency should be to achieve a diastolic BP of 100–110 mm Hg. Excessive or rapid decreases in BP should be avoided to minimize the risk of cerebral hypoperfusion or coronary insufficiency. Normal BP can be attained gradually over several days as tolerated by the individual patient.

**IV. Aortic dissection.** Acute, proximal aortic dissection (type A) is a surgical emergency, whereas uncomplicated, distal dissection (type B) can be treated successfully with medical therapy alone. All patients, including those treated surgically, require acute and chronic antihypertensive therapy to provide initial stabilization and to prevent complications (e.g., aortic rupture, continued dissection). Medical therapy of chronic stable aortic dissection should seek to maintain systolic BP at or below 130–140 mm Hg if tolerated. Antihypertensive agents with negative inotropic properties, including calcium channel antagonists, β-adrenergic antagonists, methyldopa, clonidine, and reserpine, are preferred for management in the postacute phase.

**A. Sodium nitroprusside** is considered the initial drug of choice because of the predictability of response and absence of tachyphylaxis. The dose should be titrated to achieve a systolic BP of 100–120 mm Hg or the lowest possible BP that permits adequate organ perfusion. Nitroprusside alone causes an increase in left ventricular contractility and subsequent arterial shearing forces, which contribute to ongoing intimal dissection. Thus, when using sodium nitroprusside, adequate simultaneous **β-adrenergic antagonist therapy is essential,** regardless of whether systolic hypertension is present. Traditionally, propranolol has been recommended. **Esmolol,** a cardioselective IV β-adrenergic antagonist with a very short duration of action, may be preferable, especially in patients with relative contraindications to β antagonists. If esmolol is tolerated, a longer-acting β-adrenergic antagonist should be used.

**B. IV labetalol** has been used successfully as a single agent in the treatment of acute aortic dissection (*JAMA* 258:78, 1987). Labetalol produces a dose-related decrease in BP and lowers contractility. It has the advantage of allowing for oral administration after the acute stage of dissection has been managed successfully.

**C. Trimethaphan camsylate,** a ganglionic blocking agent, can be used as a single IV agent if sodium nitroprusside or β-adrenergic antagonists cannot be tolerated. Unlike sodium nitroprusside, trimethaphan reduces left ventricular contractility. Because trimethaphan is associated with rapid tachyphylaxis and sympathoplegia (e.g., orthostatic hypotension, blurred vision, and urinary retention), other drugs are preferable.

**V. Pregnancy and hypertension.** Hypertension in the setting of pregnancy is a special situation because of the potential for maternal and fetal morbidity and mortality associated with elevated BP and the clinical syndromes of preeclampsia and eclampsia. The possibility of teratogenic or other adverse effects of antihypertensive medications on fetal development also should be considered.

**A. Classification of hypertension** during pregnancy has been proposed by the American College of Obstetrics and Gynecology (*N Engl J Med* 335:257, 1996).

1. **Preeclampsia or eclampsia.** Preeclampsia is a condition defined by pregnancy, hypertension, proteinuria, generalized edema, and, occasionally, coagulation and liver function abnormalities after 20 weeks' gestation. Eclampsia encompasses those physical signs in addition to generalized seizures.
2. **Chronic hypertension.** This disorder is defined by a BP greater than 140/90 mm Hg before the twentieth week of pregnancy.
3. **Chronic hypertension with superimposed preeclampsia or eclampsia.**
4. **Transient hypertension.** This condition results in increases in BP without associated proteinuria or CNS manifestations. BP returns to normal within 10 days of delivery.

**B. Therapy.** Treatment of hypertension in pregnancy should begin if the diastolic BP is greater than 100 mm Hg. Nonpharmacologic therapy, such as weight reduction and vigorous exercise, is not recommended during pregnancy. Alcohol and tobacco use should be discouraged strongly. Pharmacologic intervention with methyldopa is recommended as first-line therapy because of its proven safety. Hydralazine and labetalol are also safe and can be used as alternative agents; both can be used parenterally. Other antihypertensives have theoretical disadvantages, but none except the ACE inhibitors has been proven to increase fetal morbidity or mortality. If a patient is suspected of having preeclampsia or eclampsia, urgent referral to an obstetrician who specializes in high-risk pregnancy is recommended.

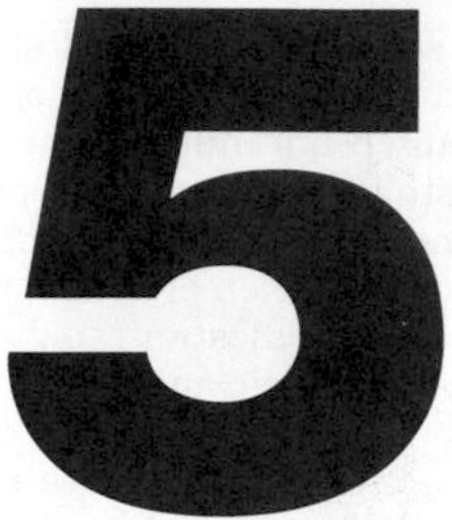

# Ischemic Heart Disease

David Schwartz and
Anne Carol Goldberg

**Coronary artery disease** (CAD) is the leading cause of morbidity and mortality in Western society. The manifestations of CAD include stable angina, acute coronary syndromes (ACS), congestive heart failure, sudden cardiac death, and silent ischemia. Stable angina most often results from fixed coronary lesions that produce a mismatch of myocardial supply and demand with increasing cardiac workload. ACS encompass a spectrum of clinical conditions from unstable angina to ST-elevation myocardial infarction (MI). The acute event usually represents rupture of a vulnerable atherosclerotic plaque, exposing a thrombogenic surface within the vessel. Platelet aggregation of varying degrees ensues, limiting blood flow to the myocardium distal to the lesion. The resulting myocardial oxygen supply-demand mismatch can result in tissue ischemia (unstable angina) or necrosis (MI). Other clinical conditions may also lead to a supply-demand mismatch, including aortic stenosis, thyrotoxicosis, and profound anemia. The presence of ischemic heart disease can predispose patients to additional problems, including heart failure, cardiac arrhythmias, and sudden cardiac death.

I. **Risk factors.** Epidemiologic studies have identified several major risk factors associated with an increased risk of cardiovascular disease including atherosclerotic CAD. Cigarette smoking, hypertension, hypercholesterolemia, and diabetes mellitus all confer an increased risk of cardiovascular disease as well as an increase in cardiac morbidity and mortality. In addition, advanced age, male gender (or postmenopausal state in women), a family history of premature coronary disease (first-degree male relatives <55 years old or female relatives <65 years old), physical inactivity, obesity, and chronic inflammation (reflected by elevated C-reactive protein levels) are associated with an increased incidence of CAD.

II. **Differential diagnosis.** The presenting symptoms for ischemic heart disease can be quite variable. Silent ischemia can be manifest as labile ST-segment depression on an ambulatory ECG or during exercise testing. Classic angina is often described as a retrosternal pressure or "heartburn" that may radiate to the neck, jaw, and/or shoulders. The patient may also experience associated symptoms of dyspnea, nausea, or diaphoresis. The predictive value of anginal symptoms representing underlying coronary atherosclerosis depends on the patient's prior probability of disease and can range from as low as 5% to almost 90%. These anginal symptoms are not specific for ischemic heart disease. As additional findings from the patient's clinical history and physical examination warrant, **nonischemic causes of chest pain** should also be considered. Cardiovascular-related symptoms that are not due to atherosclerotic disease of the epicardial vessels may be due to aortic dissection, coronary spasm, or pericarditis. **Syndrome X** refers to ischemic chest pain in the presence of normal coronary arteries. The etiology of the ischemia is not fully understood but may represent microvascular disease in the heart. Compared with patients with classic coronary disease, those with syndrome X have a good prognosis (*J Am Coll Cardiol* 17:491, 1991).

**Noncardiac causes of angina-like symptoms** include esophageal disease (gastroesophageal reflux and motility disorders), biliary colic, musculoskeletal pain, and cervical radiculitis. Pulmonary disease should also be considered,

**Table 5-1.** Selected differential diagnosis of myocardial infarction

| Diagnosis | ECG findings | Diagnostic evaluation |
|---|---|---|
| Pericarditis | PR depression, diffuse or focal ST elevation | Echocardiography |
| Myocarditis | ST elevation, Q waves | Cardiac enzymes (e.g., troponin) |
| Acute aortic dissection | ST elevation or depression, nonspecific ST- and T-wave changes | Transesophageal echocardiography, chest CT, MRI, or aortography |
| Pneumothorax | New poor R-wave progression in precordial leads, acute QRS-axis shift | Chest radiography |
| Pulmonary embolism | Inferior ST elevation, ST shifts in leads $V_1$–$V_3$ | Ventilation-perfusion scan, D-dimer, or spiral CT scan |
| Acute cholecystitis | Inferior ST elevation | Gallbladder ultrasound or radioisotope scan |

including pulmonary embolism, severe pulmonary hypertension, or pneumonia (Table 5-1).

This list is not all-inclusive. The need to pursue a workup of nonischemic causes of angina should be individualized to each patient depending on the patient's physical examination, clinical course, and results of laboratory studies and diagnostic testing.

**III. Primary prevention.** In contrast to genetic factors that are not modifiable, the majority of environmental factors associated with an increased risk in cardiovascular disease can be altered, with a corresponding benefit in terms of morbidity and mortality. Institution of lifestyle changes that lower rates of smoking, promote physical activity, and lower trends in obesity all have a positive impact on chronic medical conditions, including hypertension, diabetes, and hyperlipidemic syndromes, each of which contributes to increased cardiovascular risk. Prevention or treatment of these diseases lowers the rate of cardiovascular events. Risk factor screening in adults should begin at age 20 years and be re-evaluated every 5 years, or sooner if changes in clinical status warrant (*Circulation* 106:388, 2002).

**A. Cigarette smoking** increases the risk of CAD and has a synergistic effect with other risk factors. Environmental exposure to smoke (second-hand smoke) may also increase the risk of heart disease. Successful smoking cessation restores the risk of CAD to that of a nonsmoker within approximately 3 years (*J Clin Epidemiol* 44:1247, 1991).

**B. Hypertension,** systolic as well as diastolic, is associated with increased cardiovascular risk. Lifestyle modification and pharmacologic therapy (if needed) should be used to achieve a goal of less than 140/90 mm Hg. More stringent control (<130/80 mm Hg) is appropriate if comorbid disease, including renal insufficiency, diabetes, or heart failure, is present (see Chap. 4, Hypertension).

**C. Diabetes mellitus** and the prediabetic condition of impaired glucose tolerance are strongly associated with premature CAD. Appropriate dietary modifications and hypoglycemic therapy should be instituted, with a goal of normal fasting plasma glucose (<110 mg/dl) and near-normal hemoglobin $A1_c$ of less than 7.0%.

**D. Hyperlipidemia** significantly increases the risk of developing CAD. Current guidelines identify low-density lipoprotein (LDL) levels as the primary value to guide therapy. The LDL goal is dependent on the patient's risk category.

For patients with zero to one major risk factors [cigarette use, hypertension, high-density lipoprotein (HDL) <40 mg/dl, family history of premature coronary heart disease (CHD), or age (>45 years for men, >55 years for women)], the LDL goal for primary prevention is less than 160 mg/dl. If multiple risk factors are present, the LDL goal is less than 130 mg/dl. Finally, if CHD risk equivalents (diabetes or other forms of atherosclerotic disease) are present, the recommended LDL goal is less than 100 mg/dl. Primary prevention of lipid abnormalities can reduce cardiac events by up to 60%. Elevated triglyceride levels may also be an independent risk factor for CHD. Values over 200 mg/dl warrant intervention (see Hyperlipidemia in Patients with Ischemic Heart Disease).

E. **Obesity** increases the risk of CAD and is associated with additional cardiac risk factors, including hypertension, diabetes, and lipid abnormalities. The weight goal is a body mass index of less than 25 kg/m$^2$.

F. **Physical activity** for at least 30 minutes/day is recommended. Activity should be of moderate intensity. If the patient has coexisting medical conditions or is middle aged or older and sedentary, consultation with a physician is appropriate before an exercise program is initiated.

G. The role of **hormone replacement therapy** (HRT) in primary prevention has not been clearly defined but may be associated with increased cardiovascular events. The benefits of folate supplementation in primary prevention are unknown.

H. **Aspirin** use should be considered in persons at higher risk of cardiovascular events (>10% risk of stroke or MI over 10 years), providing that the patient is not aspirin intolerant. Low-dose aspirin (75–160 mg/day) is as effective as higher doses at lowering cardiovascular risk (*N Engl J Med* 318:262, 1988).

## IV. Diagnostic testing

A. **History and physical examination.** A careful history and physical examination are usually sufficient to provide information to establish an appropriate pretest probability of coronary disease. Angina is typically described as a chest discomfort or heaviness that may radiate to the neck, jaw, or arm(s). Symptoms may be associated with dyspnea, diaphoresis, nausea, vomiting, dizziness, or palpitations. The patient's complaints may also be atypical in nature, such as epigastric discomfort. Women and diabetic patients are more likely than nondiabetic men to experience atypical symptoms. The patient's clinical presentation, along with the physician's level of suspicion for disease, dictates the appropriate testing that should be pursued. The patient should be questioned for the presence of known cardiac risk factors, including age, tobacco use, family history, and the presence of comorbid diseases, such as previously diagnosed coronary disease, diabetes, hypertension, and hypercholesterolemia. The clinical examination should evaluate for the presence or absence of heart failure (e.g., pulmonary rales, peripheral edema) or cardiac dysfunction (e.g., abnormal heart sounds, murmurs, or cardiac impulse).

B. **Noninvasive testing**

1. **Electrocardiogram.** A baseline ECG should be recorded in all patients with suspected CAD. A normal tracing does not exclude the presence of disease, and an abnormal ECG does not indicate with certainty the presence of disease. Findings of significant Q waves or ST-T–wave abnormalities are consistent with (but not diagnostic of) underlying CAD. In addition to the baseline tracing, an ECG should be obtained if the patient is having anginal symptoms to assess for labile changes consistent with underlying ischemic disease.
2. **Exercise stress testing.** Patients can be exercised on a treadmill following a prescribed protocol. The Bruce protocol is most commonly used, consisting of 3-minute stages of increasing treadmill speed and incline. The patient is monitored for an appropriate physiologic response to exercise with BP and heart rate measurements during the walk and into the

recovery period. The patient should be questioned for the presence of anginal symptoms. Finally, the patient's ECG is monitored throughout the study to evaluate for ischemic changes. The study can be done either as a screening tool (i.e., to determine if CAD is present) or to assess the degree of ischemia in patients with known disease. Patients with active anginal symptoms or evidence of ongoing ischemia should not be studied. In properly selected patients the exercise stress test has a sensitivity and specificity of 70–80% to detect disease if the patient has a normal resting ECG and a target heart rate of 85% of the maximum heart rate for age is achieved. The sensitivity and specificity of the test are increased if it is performed in conjunction with an imaging modality such as a nuclear imaging or an echocardiographic study. Prognostic information can be quantified by the Duke treadmill score, which incorporates the duration of exercise on the Bruce protocol, maximal ST-segment deviation on the ECG, and anginal symptoms (Duke score = minutes exercise – [5 × mm ST-segment deviation] – [4 × anginal score]). Scores of ($>^{+}5$), ($^{-}10$–$^{+}4$) and ($<^{-}11$) are associated with low, moderate, and high risks, respectively, of subsequent cardiovascular events. A positive study is present if new ST-segment depressions (>1 mm in multiple leads), a hypotensive response, new heart failure, or sustained ventricular arrhythmias develop. In contrast, the ability to complete 12 minutes of a standard Bruce protocol, even in patients with known CAD, is associated with an excellent prognosis with medical therapy alone.

An abnormal baseline ECG is associated with increased false-positive ECG test results. If the patient has a left bundle branch block or significant ST-segment abnormalities on the baseline ECG, the stress test should be performed with either nuclear or echocardiographic imaging if patients are at intermediate or high risk by clinical assessment.

3. **Pharmacologic stress testing.** In patients who are unable to exercise or who have a significantly abnormal ECG (e.g., left bundle branch block, significant ST-T–wave changes, etc.), myocardial stress can be induced pharmacologically. Infusions of adenosine or dipyridamole can be used in conjunction with nuclear imaging to assess for ischemia. Dobutamine can be used with nuclear or echocardiographic imaging.
4. **Nuclear imaging.** The radioactive tracers thallium-201 and technetium-99m are commonly used in conjunction with exercise or pharmacologic stress testing. The tracers permit evaluation of myocardial perfusion, which can be used to assess the presence of myocardial ischemia, infarction, or viability. Although false-positive and -negative studies occur, the addition of nuclear imaging to an exercise stress test increases the sensitivity and specificity of the study to approximately 80–90% in properly selected patients (*Circulation* 83:363, 1991).
5. **Echocardiographic imaging.** Exercise or dobutamine stress testing can be performed with echocardiography to aid in the diagnosis of CAD. As with nuclear imaging, echocardiography adds to the sensitivity and specificity of the test.
6. **Electron beam computed tomography (EBCT).** Coronary calcification is often present in the advanced stages of atherosclerotic lesion formation. EBCT has a high sensitivity but a much lower specificity for the detection of functionally significant CAD. The overall predictive accuracy is approximately 70% in typical CAD patients, which is roughly equivalent to or less than that of alternate noninvasive testing procedures. Current data do not clearly define which asymptomatic people may benefit from EBCT. Given this fact and the potential for unnecessary additional testing in patients with false-positive results, current American Heart Association/American College of Cardiology guidelines do not recommend EBCT for diagnosing obstructive CAD.

7. **Magnetic resonance.** The proximal portions of the coronary vasculature can be examined by MRI. However, the procedure has significant technical limitations at this time, precluding its use in the diagnosis and management of CAD.

**C. Invasive testing**

1. **Coronary angiography.** The "gold standard" for evaluating the coronary anatomy is selective angiography of the left and right coronary arterial systems. The presence and severity of atherosclerotic lesions can be directly identified. The rate of coronary flow down the epicardial vessels may be of prognostic value in patients who present with acute ischemic syndromes or after percutaneous revascularization. Coronary angiography may also be of benefit in defining aberrant anatomy or vasospasm. In selected patients, more definitive assessment of the coronary vasculature can be obtained at the time of the cardiac catheterization using **intravascular ultrasound** to assess plaque burden or a Doppler flow probe to determine the functional significance of a coronary lesion by measuring fractional flow reserve across the stenosis.
2. **Left ventricular (LV) catheterization.** An assessment of LV function can be made at the time of cardiac catheterization. LV filling pressure and the gradient across the aortic valve can be measured. In addition, the presence of regional wall motion abnormalities can be evaluated by contrast ventriculography.
3. **Pulmonary arterial catheterization.** Invasive hemodynamic monitoring is generally not necessary in patients with a clinically uncomplicated MI. In contrast, in patients with MI complicated by refractory hypotension, progressive renal dysfunction, or congestive heart failure, measurement of cardiac filling pressures, pulmonary arterial pressures, and cardiac function (cardiac output) with a pulmonary arterial catheter may aid in establishing a diagnosis and guide the therapeutic intervention. For a complete discussion of hemodynamic monitoring, see sec. **VIII.H.**
4. **Esophageal Doppler monitoring (EDM).** Minimally invasive monitoring devices are available to estimate cardiac output in the intensive care unit setting. Among these devices is EDM, which uses Doppler technique to measure blood flow in the aorta. Cardiac output is calculated as a product of blood flow × cross-sectional area of the aorta × heart rate. In selected patients, EDM may yield data that are beneficial in clinical management, with results correlating well with the "gold standard" of pulmonary arterial catheterization. Extensive experience with this technique in patients with ischemic heart disease is lacking.

**V. Risk assessment in asymptomatic patients.** A patient's risk profile can be established by means of a careful cardiac history, physical examination, and ECG. In symptomatic patients, further testing is clearly warranted to determine whether the symptoms are cardiac in origin and to guide management decisions in patients with ischemic heart disease as the source of their symptoms. The decision on noninvasive versus invasive testing should be individualized to the patient.

In asymptomatic patients, the decision must also be focused on the patients' particular circumstances. The asymptomatic patient population includes a wide spectrum of individuals, from those with no known CAD and no risk factors to those with known disease and a history of MI, heart failure, or prior revascularization. The decision to test this patient population should balance the risks of the procedure and possible consequences of a false-positive test with the benefit of identifying silent ischemia and providing an intervention before a cardiac event occurs.

**A. Patients without known coronary disease.** In general, a "screening" exercise test is not warranted in asymptomatic patients at low risk for CAD. Patients can be considered for testing if they are at intermediate risk for CAD and (1) their occupation is such that impairment might have an impact on public safety (e.g., airline pilot), or (2) they plan to begin a vigorous exercise program. Asymptomatic patients at high risk for CAD due to other diseases, such as diabetes, can also be considered for testing.

**B. Patients with known coronary disease.** Stress testing after MI provides useful prognostic information in patients who remain symptom free after their infarction and have not undergone coronary angiography. A submaximal study performed 4–7 days after acute MI or a maximal exercise stress test 4–6 weeks after MI aids in determining the patient's ischemic burden, which, if present, should prompt consideration for cardiac catheterization to define the coronary anatomy. A stress test after acute MI, either with or without revascularization, helps guide recommendations for a cardiac rehabilitation program. Risk assessment may be appropriate in asymptomatic patients with known disease who are scheduled to undergo elective surgical procedure (see Chap. 1, Patient Care in Internal Medicine, the section Perioperative Medicine, Fig. 1-1).

The routine use of stress testing in asymptomatic patients after percutaneous or surgical revascularization remains controversial. If testing is done, it should be performed in conjunction with an imaging modality (nuclear or echocardiographic) to increase the sensitivity of the test and to localize area(s) of ischemia that may exist.

In the Coronary Artery Surgery Study Registry, patients with left main disease who underwent coronary artery bypass grafting (CABG) had a better outcome than patients treated with medical therapy (*Circulation* 79:1171, 1989). This study was not a randomized trial and was performed before the current percutaneous coronary intervention (PCI) era. In the Asymptomatic Cardiac Ischemia Pilot study, patients who were either free of angina or had well-controlled symptoms and were revascularized had a lower cardiac event rate than those who were randomized to medical management. The degree to which the results of these trials can be applied to minimally symptomatic or truly asymptomatic patients is uncertain.

**VI. Stable coronary syndrome.** Chronic stable angina is the manifestation of ischemic heart disease in approximately half of patients with CAD. The angina is most commonly due to a mismatch between myocardial oxygen supply and demand. A fixed stenosis of an epicardial coronary artery, usually greater than 70% of the original luminal diameter of the vessel, is sufficient to limit blood flow distal to the lesion. When myocardial workload (oxygen demand) exceeds the capacity of myocardial blood supply (oxygen delivery), angina may ensue. In addition to coronary atherosclerotic lesions, myocardial supply-demand mismatch may result from disease of the coronary microvasculature (syndrome X), hypertrophic heart disease, coronary spasm (Prinzmetal's angina), uncontrolled hypertension, or valvular heart disease (e.g., aortic stenosis). Clearly, the approach to diagnosis and treatment depends on the suspected or known underlying pathology.

**A. Diagnosis.** A detailed review of the patient's symptoms and focused physical examination are often helpful at directing further diagnostic testing. Classic angina is described as chest discomfort (heaviness or pressure) that may radiate to the jaw, shoulder, back, or arm(s). The symptoms are usually provoked by exertion or emotional stress and relieved by rest or nitroglycerin. Associated symptoms include dyspnea, diaphoresis, nausea, vomiting, or palpitations. The angina may also be atypical in nature. For example, women (more than men) may complain of epigastric discomfort that otherwise presents like typical angina. Diabetic patients may experience anginal equivalent symptoms (e.g., epigastric distress) that are suspicious for underlying ischemia.

Patients with typical angina often have CAD of one or more epicardial arteries. Cardiac risk factors, including smoking, diabetes, hypertension, and family history, should be reviewed. A history of peripheral or cerebrovascular disease increases the likelihood that CAD will be present. Patients can be characterized as being at low, intermediate, or high probability of significant CAD based on their symptoms and cardiac risk profile.

Patients with noncardiac chest pain are usually at low risk for ischemic heart disease.

The initial evaluation of a patient with suspected stable angina should include laboratory testing for (1) hemoglobin, (2) fasting glucose, and (3) fasting lipid profile. Recent data suggest that C-reactive protein level is also of benefit in determining a patient's cardiovascular risk. A rest ECG should be obtained when the patient is pain free and during an episode of chest pain, if possible. A rest ECG will be normal in fewer than 50% of patients with chronic stable angina, and a normal rest ECG does not exclude the presence of significant CAD. Evidence of LV hypertrophy, ischemic ST-T–wave changes, or Q waves increases the likelihood that chest discomfort is cardiac in origin. Although a chest x-ray is often normal in patients with stable angina, one can be obtained if the patient exhibits signs or symptoms of CHF, valvular heart disease, or pericardial disease.

**B. Noninvasive testing.** Patients with an intermediate or high pretest probability of CAD should be evaluated with a noninvasive stress test. Exercise testing is the preferred technique and can be used to establish a diagnosis of CAD or to assess functional capacity and prognosis in patients with known disease. The exercise test can be performed without an accompanying imaging modality if the patient's baseline ECG is normal or near normal. If the patient's ECG demonstrates (1) left bundle branch block, (2) 1 mm or greater ST depression at rest, (3) ventricular paced complexes, or (4) preexcitation syndrome, or if the patient is unable to exercise and has a pharmacologic stress test, then either nuclear or echocardiographic imaging is warranted. An imaging modality is also recommended in patients in whom an exercise test is nondiagnostic or positive (if they do not proceed directly to cardiac catheterization) or if the test is to evaluate for restenosis after a previous coronary revascularization. Noninvasive diagnostic testing is most useful when the pretest probability of CAD is intermediate. An echocardiogram should be obtained if the patient's clinical history or physical examination is suggestive of aortic stenosis or hypertrophic cardiomyopathy. The utility of EBCT in patient management is unclear at the present time.

**C. Invasive testing.** Coronary angiography is considered the "gold standard" technique for diagnosing CAD. As with noninvasive testing, angiography can be used to establish a diagnosis or to characterize the degree of atherosclerosis in patients with known disease. Coronary angiography should be performed in patients with known or suspected angina who have survived sudden cardiac death. Invasive testing should be considered, as well, for patients with a high pretest probability of left main or three-vessel CAD or for those whose occupation requires a definitive diagnosis. Angiography can also be considered for patients if a recent stress test is nondiagnostic and for individuals who are unable to undergo noninvasive testing. In selected patients with recurrent hospitalizations for chest pain or those with an overriding desire for a definite diagnosis and an intermediate or high pretest probability of CAD, invasive testing can be used to document the presence or extent of disease and facilitate long-term management. Coronary angiography may also be useful in patients with angina who are suspected of having a nonatherosclerotic cause of ischemia (e.g., coronary anomaly, coronary dissection, radiation vasculopathy).

**D. Risk assessment.** Risk assessment of patients with stable angina should be used to help guide decisions on referral for noninvasive or invasive cardiac testing in patients with an intermediate or high probability of CAD. The Duke treadmill score provides useful information on survival. Patients in the low-risk group (Duke score $\geq {}^{+}5$) have an annual mortality of 0.25%. Those in the moderate-risk group (Duke score ${}^{-}10$–${}^{+}4$) have a mortality of 1.25% per year, and those in the high-risk group (Duke score $< {}^{-}10$) have an annual mortality exceeding 5%. Patients at low risk can often be managed medically. Those at high risk should be referred for coronary angiography.

Management of a patient at intermediate risk should be individualized, taking into account the patient's clinical history, lifestyle, and comorbid conditions.

The probability of a patient having severe (three-vessel or left main) CAD can be estimated by review of the clinical history, physical examination, and demographic characteristics. Independent predictors of severe CAD include age (>65), diabetes, evidence of a prior MI by history and ECG, complaints of typical angina, and male sex. Absence of all of these predictors is associated with a probability of severe disease ranging from less than 5% (30-year-old patient) to 20% (80-year-old patient). The probability of disease increases with an increasing number of predictors. With all five predictors present, the probability of severe disease ranges from 40–80%, depending on the age of the patient.

In clinically stable patients, once risk is assessed and a plan for management enacted (invasive testing or medical management), there is no need for routine reassessment. If the patient experiences a significant worsening of symptoms or a change in therapy is contemplated, repeat testing may be warranted.

**E. Treatment.** The major purposes of treatment of patients with stable angina are to prevent MI and death and to reduce or relieve symptoms, leading to an improved quality of life. One approach to guide the treatment of patients with ischemic heart disease is the ABCDE mnemonic. Medical therapy and lifestyle modification are important factors to consider.

**1. Aspirin and antianginal therapy.** Aspirin use in patients with stable angina has been shown to reduce cardiovascular events by 33%. In asymptomatic patients in the Physician's Health Study, aspirin (325 mg, every other day) decreased the incidence of MI. Clopidogrel (75 mg/day) can be used in patients who are allergic or intolerant of aspirin.

A number of medications have antianginal properties. Beta-blockers are a key first choice of therapy (Table 5-2). Calcium channel blockers can be used in lieu of a beta-blocker if beta-blockers are contraindicated or not tolerated due to significant adverse effects. Calcium antagonists can also be used in conjunction with beta-blockers if the latter are not fully effective at relieving anginal symptoms (Table 5-3). Long-acting dihydropyridines and nondihydropyridine agents can be used. Use of short-acting dihydropyridines (e.g., nifedipine) should be avoided due to the potential to enhance the risk of adverse cardiac events.

**Table 5-2.** Beta-blockers commonly used for ischemic heart disease

| Drug | β-Receptor selectivity | Usual dosage |
|---|---|---|
| Propranolol | None | 20–80 mg bid |
| Metoprolol | $\beta_1$ | 50–200 mg bid |
| Atenolol | $\beta_1$ | 50–200 mg qd |
| Nadolol | None | 40–80 mg qd |
| Timolol | None | 10–30 mg bid |
| Acebutolol | $\beta_1$ | 200–600 mg bid |
| Bisoprolol | $\beta_1$ | 10–20 mg/d |
| Esmolol (IV) | $\beta_1$ | 50–300 μg/kg$^{-1}$min$^{-1}$ |
| Labetalol | None (combined alpha-/beta-blocker) | 200–600 mg bid |
| Pindolol | None | 2.5–7.5 mg tid |

**Table 5-3.** Calcium channel blockers commonly used for ischemic heart disease

| Drug | Duration of action | Usual dosage |
|---|---|---|
| Dihydropyridines | | |
| Nifedipine | | |
| Slow release | Long | 30–180 mg/d |
| Amlodipine | Long | 5–10 mg/d |
| Felodipine (SR) | Long | 5–10 mg/d |
| Isradipine (SR) | Medium | 2.5–10 mg/d |
| Nicardipine | Short | 20–40 mg tid |
| Other | | |
| Diltiazem | | |
| Immediate release | Short | 30–80 mg qid |
| Slow release | Long | 120–360 mg/d |
| Verapamil | | |
| Immediate release | Short | 80–160 mg tid |
| Slow release | Long | 120–480 mg/d |

Nitrates, either long-acting formulations for chronic use or sublingual preparations for acute anginal symptoms, can be used as adjuncts to baseline therapy with beta-blockers or calcium antagonists, or both (Table 5-4). The patient should take the medication while seated because of possible side effects of hypotension. Sublingual preparations should be used at the first indication of angina or prophylactically before engaging in activities that are known to precipitate angina. Patients should seek prompt medical attention if angina occurs at rest or fails to respond to the third sublingual dose.

2. **β-Adrenergic antagonists and BP control.** All beta-blockers appear to be effective in controlling angina by decreasing heart rate and BP. The dosage can be adjusted to result in a resting heart rate of 50–60 beats/minute. In patients with persistent angina, a target heart rate of less than 50 beats/minute is warranted providing that no symptoms are associated with the bradycardia and that heart block does not develop. If stress testing is performed as part of the evaluation, beta-blocker therapy in patients with known heart disease should limit the heart rate response with exercise to less than 75% of the heart rate associated with the onset of ischemia. Use of beta-blockers is contraindicated in patients with severe bronchospasm, significant atrioventricular (AV) block, marked resting bradycardia, or poorly compensated heart failure. If additional BP control is necessary after incorporation of beta-blocker and calcium antagonist therapy, supplemental agents can be used, as outlined in Chap. 4, Hypertension.
3. **Cholesterol-lowering agents** and **cigarette-smoking cessation.** When used for primary or secondary prevention, use of lipid-lowering agents in patients with elevated baseline total cholesterol levels was associated with a significant reduction in fatal and nonfatal MI and the need for revascularization. Lovastatin, pravastatin, and simvastatin, as well as gemfibrozil, reduced cardiovascular events by 22–37% (*N Engl J Med* 335:1107, 1996; see Hyperlipidemia in Patients with Ischemic Heart Disease, sec. **IV**).

**Table 5-4.** Nitrate preparations commonly used for ischemic heart disease

| Preparation | Dosage | Onset (min) | Duration |
|---|---|---|---|
| Sublingual nitroglycerin | 0.3–0.6 mg prn | 2–5 | 10–30 min |
| Aerosol nitroglycerin | 0.4 mg prn | 2–5 | 10–30 min |
| Oral isosorbide dinitrate | 5–40 mg tid | 30–60 | 4–6 hr |
| Oral isosorbide mononitrate | 10–20 mg bid | 30–60 | 6–8 hr |
| Oral isosorbide mononitrate SR | 30–120 mg qd | 30–60 | 12–18 hr |
| 2% Nitroglycerin ointment | 0.5–2.0 in. tid | 20–60 | 3–8 hr |
| Transdermal nitroglycerin patches | 5–15 mg qd | >60 | 12 hr |
| Intravenous nitroglycerin | 10–200 μg/min | <2 | During infusion |

Successful smoking cessation is associated with a 4–47% decrease in cardiac event rate in patients without a previous cardiovascular history. Bupropion (150 mg bid) for 7 weeks to 1 year or nicotine preparations along with support group participation dramatically increases success rates.

4. **Diabetes and diet.** Although no direct data are available to demonstrate the benefit of tight glucose control and weight reduction on cardiac events, current recommendations favor aggressive treatment of these two conditions. Effective treatment of both conditions leads to a more favorable profile of other known cardiac risk factors, including hypertension and lipid abnormalities.
5. **Exercise and education.** Patients who participate in exercise training have a statistically significant increase in exercise tolerance compared with a "no-exercise" control group of patients. No clear evidence has shown that exercise reduces the risk of subsequent cardiac events. Referral to a cardiac rehabilitation program may be appropriate to define the level of exercise that can safely keep the patient under the threshold of an ischemia. As with diet control, exercise yields additional benefit by means of its favorable effects on other cardiac risk factors including hypertension and hyperlipidemia. Education of the cardiac patient serves multiple purposes, including allaying the patients' natural fears and anxieties regarding their disease, improving their medical compliance, and informing them of pertinent signs or symptoms that should prompt elective, urgent, or emergent evaluation.

F. **Revascularization.** Medical therapy with at least two, and preferably three, classes of antianginal agents should be attempted before treatment is considered a failure. Patients who are refractory to medical therapy should be assessed with coronary angiography, if the anatomy has not already been defined. Revascularization with PCI or CABG should be considered, as the clinical history and anatomy dictate and may be associated with lower rates of death, nonfatal MI, or recurrent hospitalization (*Circulation* 95:2037, 1997). CABG is optimal for patients at high risk for cardiac mortality, including those with (1) left main disease, (2) two-vessel or three-vessel disease involving the proximal left anterior descending artery and LV dysfunction, and (3) diabetes and multivessel coronary disease. The risk of surgery includes a 1–3% mortality, a 5–10% incidence of perioperative MI, a small risk of perioperative stroke or cognitive dysfunction, and a 10–20% risk of vein graft failure in the first year. Approximately 75% of patients remain free of recurrent angina or adverse cardiac events at 5 years of follow-up. The use of internal mammary artery grafts is associated with 90% graft patency at 10 years, compared with 40–50% for saphenous vein grafts. The long-term patency of radial artery grafts is currently under review. After 10 years of follow-up, 50% of patients develop recurrent angina or other adverse cardiac events related to late vein graft failure or progression of native CAD.

Current percutaneous techniques include balloon angioplasty, atherectomy devices, and intracoronary stenting. In appropriately selected cases, a clinical success rate of greater than 90% can be expected. The risks of elective PCI include a less than 1% mortality, a 2–5% rate of nonfatal MI, and a less than 1% need for emergent CABG for an unsuccessful procedure. The rate of coronary restenosis is related to the revascularization technique used; the nature of the lesion; and the presence of comorbid risks, such as diabetes and continued tobacco abuse. Use of recently developed sirolimus-eluting stents has been demonstrated to be associated with significantly lower rates of restenosis and failure at 9 months compared to standard stents (*N Engl J Med* 349:1315, 2003). All patients who receive coronary stents should be given aspirin indefinitely and additional antiplatelet therapy (clopidogrel, 300-mg load, then 75 mg/day) for a minimum of 1 month.

**G. Alternate therapies** are available for patients with chronic stable angina who are refractory to medical management and who are not candidates for percutaneous or surgical revascularization. Transmyocardial laser revascularization has been delivered by percutaneous technique [YAG (yttrium-aluminum-garnet) laser] and by epicardial surgical techniques ($CO_2$ or YAG laser). The percutaneous approach has not been approved by the U.S. Food and Drug Administration and should therefore be considered experimental therapy. The goal in either approach is to create a series of transmural endomyocardial channels. Surgical transmyocardial laser revascularization has been shown to improve symptoms in patients with stable angina, although the mechanism that is responsible is controversial. The data on whether exercise capacity is improved are conflicting, and no benefit has been demonstrated in terms of increasing myocardial perfusion.

Enhanced external counterpulsation is a nonpharmacologic technique for which 35 hours/week of treatment in patients with chronic stable angina and a positive stress test was shown to decrease the frequency of angina and increase the time to exercise-induced ischemia [*J Am Coll Cardiol* 37(1):93, 2001]. The treatment improved anginal symptoms in approximately 75–80% of patients; however, additional clinical trial data are required before enhanced external counterpulsation can be definitively recommended.

Spinal cord stimulation is another nonpharmacologic technique that was proposed to provide analgesia for patients with refractory symptoms. Preliminary data in multiple small clinical trials suggest that a stimulating electrode in the C-7 to T-1 epidural space results in improved anginal symptoms. Additional data are necessary to define the intermediate- and long-term benefit of these devices.

**H. Patient follow-up** is discussed in detail in sec. **X.** Minor changes in the patient's anginal complaints can be treated with titration or adjustment of the antianginal regimen. If the patient has a significant change in anginal complaints (frequency, severity, or time to onset with activity), a reassessment with a stress test (likely in conjunction with an imaging modality) or a cardiac catheterization is warranted. If the anatomy is amenable to revascularization (either percutaneous or surgical), this approach should be considered.

**VII. Acute coronary syndromes (unstable angina and non–ST-elevation myocardial infarction).** ACS is a spectrum of disease characterized by either (1) new-onset angina, (2) angina at rest, or (3) progression of angina of increasing frequency or severity or in response to lower levels of exertion. ACS may present in patients with a history of angina or may occur in individuals without previously recognized coronary disease. ACS most often represents acute atherosclerotic plaque rupture with exposure of a thrombogenic subendothelial matrix.

Thrombus formation, which may be episodic in nature, is the mechanism underlying the compromise in coronary blood flow. Prevention of thrombus, restoration of coronary flow, and reduction in myocardial oxygen demand are the primary goals of therapy.

**Unstable angina** may be due to causes other than plaque rupture. It may be a result of dynamic obstruction of the coronary artery (vasospasm, Prinzmetal's angina); a progressive mechanical obstruction of the coronary artery (advancing atherosclerotic disease or restenosis after percutaneous intervention); cardiac inflammation or infection, or both; or some secondary factor extrinsic to the coronary vasculature that results in a myocardial supply-demand mismatch, such as aortic stenosis, severe anemia, hypoxemia, or marked hypertension and cardiac hypertrophy. The approach to the most common etiology of unstable angina, that is, a disrupted atherosclerotic plaque, is discussed in sec. **VIIA–C,** but noncoronary causes to explain the development of symptoms should be considered. The causes of unstable angina are not mutually exclusive. Evaluation and management should be individualized to the patient's clinical presentation.

The diagnosis of unstable angina confers a 10–20% risk of progression to acute MI in the untreated patient. Medical treatment reduces the risk of progression to MI to 5–7%. Patients at highest risk for progression include those with rest angina, those with associated labile ischemic ECG changes (ST-segment deviations or T-wave inversions), and those with continued symptoms despite initiation of medical therapy. The presence of severe underlying coronary disease is suggested in patients with clinical evidence of LV dysfunction, congestive heart failure, or transient ischemic ECG changes.

**A. Diagnosis.** Individuals who present with ACS represent a spectrum of patients, from those with unstable angina to those with non–ST-segment elevation myocardial infarction (NSTEMI). These patients can be difficult to distinguish from one another solely on the basis of clinical symptoms and ECG findings. Approximately three-fourths of patients with ACS have an abnormal ECG, more often seen as labile ST-segment depression or T-wave inversions, or less frequently transient ST-segment elevations. NSTEMI is defined by an elevation of cardiac isoenzymes [creatine kinase MB (CK-MB) or troponin] and the absence of persistent ST-segment elevation. In patients with ACS, approximately 60% have unstable angina and 40% are diagnosed with MI. Of the patients with MI, two-thirds have NSTEMI and the remaining one-third present with acute ST-segment elevation MI.

**B. Immediate assessment.** Initial medical management of ACS includes presentation to a hospital for clinical evaluation (history and physical examination), 12-lead ECG recording, and measurement of cardiac-specific marker (troponin or CK-MB). In patients with ACS, the risk of subsequent cardiac death is directly proportional to the increase in cardiac-specific troponin, even if CK-MB levels are not elevated. Troponin T or I levels increase 3–12 hours after the onset of MI and peak at 24–48 hours, then return to baseline over 5–14 days. C-reactive protein levels may aid in initial risk assessment in ACS patients. Patients with levels greater than 3 mg/L represent a high-risk group. The goal is to determine if the patient's symptoms are ischemia related and attempt to stratify the patient according to the level of risk. If the symptoms are ischemia related, treatment is directed at relieving ischemic symptoms with medications that target coronary thrombosis and the mismatch in supply and demand of myocardial oxygenation.

**C. Risk profile.** The clinical history and examination, along with the ECG and laboratory test results, can be used to determine the patient's short-term risk of death or non-fatal MI. Patients can be classified as low, intermediate, or high risk on the basis of their clinical profile. Several authors have devised risk-scoring systems. Antman et al. (*JAMA* 284:835, 2000) developed a seven-point Thrombolysis in Myocardial Infarction (TIMI) Risk Score, with risks including (1) age greater than 65 years, (2) three or more

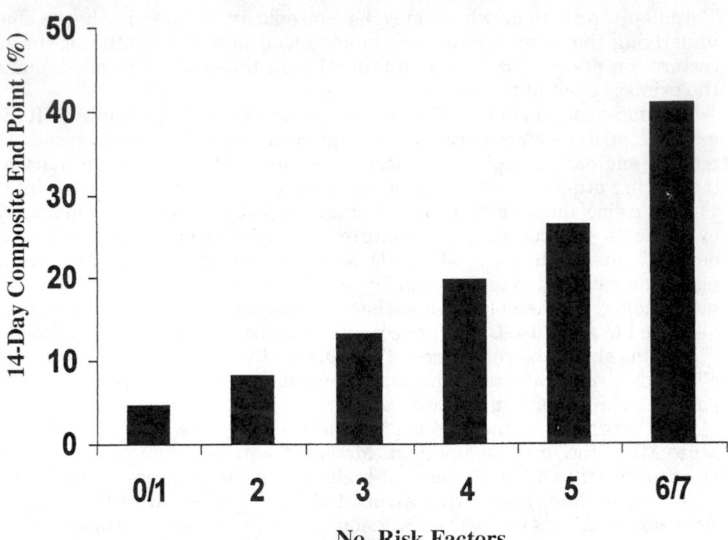


**Fig. 5-1.** Effect of Thrombolysis in Myocardial Infarction (TIMI) Risk Score on cardiovascular events. Rate of death, myocardial infarction, or urgent revascularization after presentation with acute coronary syndromes. TIMI risk factors include (1) age >65 years, (2) three coronary artery disease (CAD) risk factors, (3) known CAD, (4) ST-segment deviation, (5) severe angina, (6) acetylsalicylic acid (ASA) use in the past, and (7) positive cardiac enzyme. (Adapted with permission from EM Antman, M Cohen, PJ Bernink, et al. The TIMI Risk Score for unstable angina/non-ST elevation MI: a method for prognostication and therapeutic decision making. *JAMA* 284:835–842, 2000. Copyrighted 2000, American Medical Association.)

coronary risk factors, (3) angiographically documented prior CAD, (4) more than two anginal episodes within 24 hours, (5) ST-segment deviation on ECG, (6) aspirin use within 7 days, and (7) elevated cardiac enzymes. The risk of experiencing an adverse outcome [death, (re)infarction, severe ischemia requiring revascularization] was directly proportional to the risk score (*JAMA* 284:835, 2000) (Fig. 5-1). The choice of clinical testing and pharmacologic treatment, and the timing of possible invasive therapy, can be guided, in part, by the severity of the patient's risk. The higher the risk, the more aggressive the approach to care should be (Table 5-5).

1. **Low-risk** patients may be initially observed in a facility with cardiac monitoring (chest pain or observation unit). If the patient remains pain free and a subsequent ECG cardiac marker at 6–12 hours is normal, a stress test to provoke ischemia can be performed. Low-risk patients with a negative stress test can be managed as outpatients. If the stress test is positive, the course of management with medication and invasive testing should be individualized according to the patient's clinical status and the severity of the ischemic burden.
2. **Intermediate- and high-risk** patients should be admitted to the hospital for observation and management. The choice between admission to the intensive care unit or a high-risk cardiac ward depends on the patient's clinical course. If the patient is rendered pain free with pharmacotherapy, he or she does not necessarily need ICU monitoring and the decision to proceed with noninvasive versus invasive testing must be made (discussed in sec. **VII.E**). (Recent studies suggest that intermediate-risk

**Table 5-5.** Risk assessment in patients presenting with acute coronary syndrome

| Feature | High risk (at least 1 of the following) | Intermediate risk (no high-risk features, but at least 1 of the following) | Low risk (no high- or intermediate-risk features but may have any of the following) |
|---|---|---|---|
| Clinical history | — | Prior MI, peripheral or cerebrovascular disease, CABG, or prior aspirin use | — |
| Characteristic of pain | Prolonged ongoing (>30 min) rest pain | Prolonged (>20 min) rest angina, now resolved, with moderate or high likelihood of CAD; rest angina (<20 min) or relieved with rest or SL-TNG | New-onset or progressive angina in the past 2 wk with moderate or high likelihood of CAD |
| Clinical findings | Pulmonary edema; new or worsening MR murmur; $S_3$, or new or worsening rales; hypotension, bradycardia, or tachycardia; age >75 yr | Age >70 yr | — |
| ECG | Angina at rest with transient ST changes >0.05 mV; new (or presumed new) bundle branch block; sustained ventricular tachycardia | T-wave inversions >0.02 mV; pathologic Q waves | Normal or unchanged ECG during an episode of angina |
| Biochemical cardiac markers | Elevated (troponin or CK-MB) | Borderline elevated (troponin or CK-MB) | Normal |

ACS, acute coronary syndrome; CABG, coronary artery bypass graft; CAD, coronary artery disease; CK-MB, creatine kinase MB; SL-TNG, sublingual nitroglycerin.
*Source:* Adapted with permission from E Braunwald, EM Antman, JW Beasley, et al. ACC/AHA guidelines for the management of patients with unstable angina and non–ST-segment elevation myocardial infarction: executive summary and recommendations. A report of the American College of Cardiology/American Heart Association task force on practice guidelines (committee on the management of patients with unstable angina). *Circulation* 102:1193, 2000.

patients can be safely managed in the same fashion as low-risk patients; however, additional data are necessary to address this question more clearly.) In general, the higher risk the patient, the greater the likelihood of significant coronary disease. Patients with ongoing symptoms should be admitted to the ICU for more aggressive intervention. They should be treated with anti-ischemic therapies and, if necessary, urgent cardiac catheterization with the goal of reperfusion of the culprit coronary lesion(s). An intra-aortic balloon pump can be used in appropriate individuals to stabilize the patient clinically before revascularization with PCI or CABG. Thrombolytic therapy is not indicated in unstable angina or non–ST-elevation MI (TIMI IIIB trial, *Circulation* 89:1545, 1994).

**D. Pharmacotherapy.** The goal of treatment is to provide relief of ischemia and prevent serious adverse outcomes (death or MI). The approach should be threefold, including anti-ischemia, antiplatelet, and anticoagulant (antithrombotic) therapies. As with patients who present with ST-elevation MI, those with an unstable ACS should be restricted to bed rest and provided supplemental oxygen and adequate morphine (for control of pain and anxiety), as tolerated.

1. **Antiplatelet therapy.** All patients should receive aspirin unless a contraindication exists. **Aspirin** reduces subsequent MI and cardiac death in patients with unstable angina. Although doses as low as 75 mg/day have been used, the current American Heart Association/American College of Cardiology recommendation is 160–325 mg/day starting at the time of presentation and continued indefinitely. **Clopidogrel** (75 mg/day) can be used in patients who are intolerant or allergic to aspirin. Additional data suggest that clopidogrel (300-mg loading dose, then 75 mg/day) decreases the composite end point of cardiovascular death, MI, or stroke from 11.5% to 9.3% (*N Engl J Med* 345:494, 2002). This effect was seen at the expense of increased bleeding and delays or complications with CABG if urgent surgical intervention was required. The optimal time to initiate clopidogrel therapy should factor in the risk of surgical disease. A minimum of 1 month of therapy should be given if medical or percutaneous treatment is expected and can be continued for up to 9 months. The use of a **glycoprotein (GP) IIb/IIIa antagonist** (e.g., abciximab, eptifibatide, or tirofiban) should also be considered for high-risk patients (*Circulation* 100:2045, 1999) (Table 5-6). If early catheterization and PCI are planned, any of the agents can be used. If the plan for management does not involve an early invasive strategy, one of the small-molecule GP IIb/IIIa antagonists (eptifibatide or tirofiban) should be used. GP IIb/IIIa antagonists should be used in conjunction with therapeutically dosed heparin, either unfractionated heparin (UFH) or enoxaparin.
2. **Anticoagulant therapy** is a key component of the antithrombotic management of patients with ACS. Treatment with heparin has been shown to reduce the early rate of death or MI by up to 60%. **Enoxaparin** [low-molecular-weight heparin (LMWH), 1 mg/kg bid subcutaneously] or intravenous **UFH** (loading dose of 60 U/kg followed by a maintenance infusion of 12 U/kg/hour with a maximum of 5000 units and 1000 U/hour, respectively) can be used. The activated partial thromboplastin time (aPTT) should be adjusted to maintain a value of 1.5–2.0 times control (50–70 seconds) for UFH therapy. Randomized trials demonstrated a moderate benefit of LMWH over UFH (*N Engl J Med* 337:447, 1997). In addition, LMWH is easier to dose and does not require monitoring for clinical effect. To date, however, there has been greater experience with the use of UFH in patients who proceed to cardiac catheterization. Thus far, enoxaparin is the only LMWH that has been shown to confer greater cardiac benefit than UFH in the ACS patient. Trials with dalteparin and nadroparin have yielded neutral or unfavorable trends. **Heparin-induced thrombocytopenia** develops in approximately 1–3% of patients receiving heparin. Platelet counts usually drop after 5–7 days of therapy. If this occurs, the heparin should be discontinued, and if additional anticoagulation is needed, **lepirudin** can be used and is administered as a 0.4-mg/kg bolus IV (maximum, 44 mg) and then continuously infused at 0.15 mg/kg/hour. A dose reduction is required in renal impairment. (Refer to Chap. 11, Renal Diseases, for further details.)

**Table 5-6.** Platelet glycoprotein IIb/IIIa receptor inhibitors in acute coronary syndromes

| | Abciximab | Eptifibatide | Tirofiban |
|---|---|---|---|
| Drug type | Monoclonal antibody | Cyclic heptapeptide | Nonpeptide small molecule |
| Dosage | 0.25-mg/kg IV bolus, then 0.125 μg/kg/min (max 10 μg/min) × 12 hr (for ACS and planned PCI) | 180-μg/kg bolus, then 2 μg/kg/min × 24–48 hr | 0.4 μg/kg/min for 30 min, then 0.1 μg/kg/min × 24–48 hr |
| Metabolism/excretion | Cellular catabolism | Renal excretion (dosage should be adjusted for patients with a serum creatinine >2.0) | Renal excretion (dosage should be adjusted for patients with a serum creatinine clearance <30 ml/min) |
| Recovery of platelet inhibition | 48–96 hr | 4–6 hr | 4–6 hr |
| Reversibility | Platelet transfusion | None | None |

ACS, acute coronary syndrome; PCI, percutaneous coronary intervention.
*Note:* Contraindications to glycoprotein IIb/IIIa receptor inhibition include a history of bleeding diathesis or active bleeding within the previous 30 days (2 years for abciximab), major surgery within the previous 6 weeks, a history of stroke, severe hypertension, platelet count less than 100,000, or international normalized ratio greater than 1.2. All patients should be monitored for thrombocytopenia every 6–8 hours while receiving a glycoprotein IIb/IIIa inhibitor. All patients should receive weight-adjusted heparin therapy [unfractionated or low molecular weight (enoxaparin)].

3. **Nitroglycerin** reduces myocardial oxygen demand while enhancing myocardial oxygen delivery. The choice of preparation depends on the acuity of the patient's symptoms. **Nitroglycerin use is contraindicated in the presence of hypotension or if the patient has used sildenafil (Viagra) within the previous 24 hours.** Treatment can be initiated at the time of presentation with sublingual nitroglycerin (spray or tablets, 0.4 mg every 5 minutes for a total of 3 doses). If the patient is clinically stable, topical or oral preparations can be used (Table 5-4). Less stable patients, or those who require additional agents to control significant hypertension, should be treated with intravenous nitroglycerin (10 μg/minute, titrated up by 10–20 μg/minute every 3–5 minutes until pain relief, hypertension control, or both are achieved). Significant antianginal effects are not seen above 200 μg/minute, but doses of up to 400 μg/minute can be used, if necessary, for BP control.
4. **β-Adrenergic blockers** should be started early in the absence of contraindications. In high-risk patients, intravenous, followed by oral, preparations can be used (Table 5-2). Treatment with only an oral preparation is acceptable in intermediate- and low-risk patients. The initial choice of agents includes metoprolol, atenolol, and propranolol. Esmolol can be used if a short-acting agent is required. After the patient has stabilized and proved an ability to tolerate beta-blocker therapy, conversion to a long-acting agent can be considered.
5. **Calcium antagonists** vary in the degree to which they produce decreased myocardial contractility, peripheral vasodilation, AV block, and a slowing of sinus node activity. Nifedipine, diltiazem, verapamil,

and amlodipine appear to have similar coronary dilatory properties. Calcium antagonists can be used to control ongoing or recurrent ischemia if patients are either intolerant of or inadequately managed by beta-blocker therapy. **Short-acting nifedipine preparations must be avoided** in the absence of adequate concurrent beta-blockade because of increased adverse outcomes with this medication. Verapamil and diltiazem should be avoided in patients with evidence of severe LV dysfunction or pulmonary congestion (Table 5-3).

6. **Angiotensin-converting enzyme (ACE) inhibitors** are effective antihypertensive agents. Ischemia relief may be facilitated by this mechanism if hypotension or concerns of renal dysfunction do not preclude the use of these agents. In addition, ACE inhibitors have been shown to reduce mortality in patients with MI and LV systolic dysfunction, particularly the diabetic population. These agents may also have mortality benefit in high-risk patients with normal systolic function.

**E. Early conservative versus invasive strategies.** Two different strategies have evolved for patients with ACS. In the **early conservative strategy,** the patient is treated with medical therapy at maximally tolerated doses and coronary angiography is reserved for patients with evidence of recurrent ischemia or a strongly positive stress test, despite medical therapy. In the **early invasive strategy,** patients are routinely recommended for coronary angiography and subsequent revascularization, as warranted.

Although the choice should always be individualized to a particular patient, in general an early conservative approach can be used for low-risk patients and selected intermediate-risk patients without adverse effects on clinical outcomes. **High-risk patients** include those with recurrent ischemia on medical therapy, evidence of congestive heart failure, LV dysfunction, sustained ventricular tachycardia (VT), or prior coronary revascularization (PCI within 6 months or CABG). These patients are best assessed with an early invasive approach. Angiography in these individuals defines the anatomy and directs the choice of revascularization options, if appropriate. An early invasive strategy is also warranted in low- or intermediate-risk patients with repeated ACS presentations despite therapy. Catheterization of these patients provides a convenient approach to distinguish between those with no significant coronary disease and those with anatomy that is amenable to revascularization.

**F. Coronary revascularization.** In general, the indications for PCI and CABG in patients with ACS are similar to those for individuals with stable angina. Patients who are optimally treated with CABG include those with (1) significant left main CAD, (2) three-vessel disease and abnormal LV function (ejection fraction <50%), (3) two-vessel disease with a significant proximal left anterior descending artery stenosis and abnormal LV function by ischemia on noninvasive testing, or (4) diabetes and multivessel disease. The remaining patients with coronary disease requiring revascularization can be treated with CABG or PCI. Patients who are treated with CABG tend to have a lower incidence of angina and less need for subsequent revascularization, but there is no difference in the rates of cardiac death or MI between the two treatment strategies.

**G. Hospital discharge.** The highest rate of progression to MI or development of recurrent MI is in the first 2 months after presentation with the index episode. Beyond that time point, most patients have a clinical course similar to those with chronic stable angina. It is incumbent on the entire hospital staff (physicians, nurses, dietitians, pharmacists, and rehabilitation specialists) to prepare the patient for hospital discharge. The patient should be discharged on a medical regimen, as tolerated, to take advantage of proven methods of secondary prevention (see sec. **IX–X**). The patient should also be provided a sublingual or spray formulation of nitroglycerin and instructed on its appropriate use. Risk factor modification should be addressed, including smoking cessation, weight loss, exercise, and control of hypertension, diabetes, and hyperlipidemia, as warranted. Arrangements for follow-up care should also be established before hospital discharge.

**VIII. Acute (ST-elevation) myocardial infarction.** ST-elevation MI most commonly results from an atherosclerotic plaque rupture and the subsequent formation of an occlusive coronary thrombus. Over the past four decades, there has been a dramatic improvement in short-term mortality to the current rate of 6–10%. Almost half of the deaths associated with an acute MI occur within the first hour of symptoms, often before presentation to the hospital for medical attention. Mortality in these patients is most often due to ventricular fibrillation.

**A. Diagnosis.** The diagnosis of acute MI requires at least two of the following criteria: (1) chest discomfort or an anginal equivalent, (2) ECG changes consistent with ischemia or infarction, or (3) elevated cardiac-specific enzymes. Because the morbidity and mortality associated with an acute MI are proportional to the time to treatment, the goal should be rapid evaluation and therapy.

**B. Initial therapy.** Before presentation to the hospital, patients and the general public should be educated and informed of the signs and symptoms consistent with an acute MI that should lead them to seek urgent medical care. Availability of "911" access and emergency medical services facilitate delivery of patients to emergency medical care. Once in the emergency department, care using an **acute MI protocol** should yield a targeted clinical examination and a 12-lead ECG within 10 minutes and an initial triage management plan shortly thereafter. In patients with an inferior MI, right-sided chest leads should be recorded to detect right ventricular involvement. ST elevation of 1 mm or more in lead $V_4R$ is most suggestive of a right ventricular MI. Repeat 12-lead ECG tracings should be performed, either to monitor the response to therapy or if the initial ECG does not demonstrate ischemic changes and the patient has ongoing chest pain.

**Routine initial care of a suspected MI patient** includes supplemental oxygen for at least the first 2–3 hours after presentation. More prolonged oxygen treatment is appropriate for patients with pulmonary congestion, $SaO_2$ (arterial oxygen saturation) of less than 90%, or other clinical complications. Adequate intravenous access should be obtained and the patient placed on continuous ECG monitoring. As with patients with ACS, blood samples should be sent for cardiac enzyme levels, CBC, and electrolytes (including magnesium).

1. **Coronary care unit (CCU)** use was the first major advance in the modern era of treatment of patients with acute MI. The majority of patients benefit from the specialized training of the nursing and support staff in the CCU. The ability to intervene acutely in the event of lethal arrhythmias has led to a dramatic reduction in in-hospital mortality of patients with acute MI. The CCU environment also offers the opportunity of hemodynamic monitoring and ventilator, pressor, and inotropic support. Although there may be a subset of patients with an uncomplicated MI who can safely be triaged initially to an intermediate level of care, most patients with acute MI should be observed for at least the first 12–24 hours in the CCU.
2. **Aspirin** (160–325 mg) should be given on presentation (preferably chewed to facilitate absorption) and then continued indefinitely on a daily basis (81–325 mg). **Clopidogrel** (75 mg/day) can be substituted in patients with a true aspirin allergy. Treatment with a **GP IIb/IIIa inhibitor** is not indicated in the setting of an ST-elevation MI unless it is used as adjunctive therapy to PCI.
3. **Nitroglycerin** is appropriate for all patients with acute MI for the first 24–48 hours unless hypotension (systolic BP <90 mm Hg) precludes its use. Initial treatment should be with sublingual nitroglycerin (0.4 mg) followed by intravenous nitroglycerin at 10 μg/minute. The dose should be titrated upward for relief of ischemic pain. BP and heart rate should

be carefully monitored for hypotension and excessive bradycardia or tachycardia (heart rate <50 beats/minute or >120 beats/minute).

4. **Atropine** (0.5 mg IV) can be used to treat sinus bradycardia in symptomatic patients or if the bradycardia is associated with a low cardiac output, peripheral hypoperfusion, or AV block at or above the level of the AV node.
5. **Beta-blocker therapy** reduces myocardial ischemia and may limit infarct size. Therapy can be initiated with IV metoprolol (5 mg), which can be repeated every 5 minutes × 3 doses. Patients who tolerate beta-blocker therapy can then be started on an oral agent (metoprolol, 25–50 mg q6–12h) and then converted to maintenance therapy with bid dosing (25–100 mg) as heart rate and BP permit. Alternatively, atenolol (50–100 mg/day) can be used for maintenance therapy.

   These agents should be used with extreme caution or possibly avoided in patients (1) in clinical heart failure, (2) with a heart rate of less than 60 beats/minute, (3) who are hypotensive with a systolic BP of less than 90 mm Hg, (4) with marked first-degree (PR interval >250 msec) or advanced heart block, or (5) with significant bronchospastic lung disease. Although no data have demonstrated the mortality benefit of esmolol, its short half-life (9 minutes) makes this agent useful in patients at high risk for beta-blocker therapy. If treatment with esmolol is successful, continued therapy with an oral agent is also likely to be tolerated.
6. **Anticoagulation** should be started in all patients except those who are receiving nonselective fibrinolytic therapy (streptokinase) or those with a contraindication to heparin therapy. The choice of anticoagulant depends, in part, on the course of treatment chosen for the patient (see below). **UFH** is used in patients who are undergoing reperfusion with alteplase (rt-PA) or one of the other selective thrombolytic agents. A heparin bolus of 60 units/kg is followed by a maintenance infusion of 12 units/kg/hour, with a maximum of 5000 units and 1000 units/hour, respectively. The aPTT should be adjusted to maintain a value of 1.5–2.0 times control (50–70 seconds). Heparin should be continued for 48 hours, at which time a decision on continued anticoagulation therapy should be individualized to the patient's clinical needs. If streptokinase is used, heparin therapy can be initiated 6 hours after administration of the thrombolytic agent and given as previously outlined. Intravenous UFH (dosed as outlined above) or subcutaneous LMWH (enoxaparin, 1 mg/kg bid) can be used in patients who were initially committed to medical therapy or percutaneous revascularization.
7. **Morphine sulfate** or comparable analgesics should be used for adequate pain control. Morphine induces modest arterial and venous dilation, resulting in reduced myocardial oxygen demands from its effects on afterload and preload, respectively. Doses of 2–4 mg can be given at intervals of 5–15 minutes until the pain is relieved or side effects (hypotension, respiratory depression, vomiting) develop.
8. **Glucose-insulin-potassium (GIK)** therapy shows promise as a low-cost pharmacologic intervention in patients with acute MI, particularly those without evidence of clinical heart failure. Treatment with high-dose (25% glucose; 50 IU/L insulin; 80 mmol/L KCl) GIK at 1.5 ml/kg/hour resulted in a 30% relative risk reduction in death in a recent clinical trial of diabetic patients. A larger randomized clinical trial is in progress to determine the role of GIK therapy in the nondiabetic patient.
9. **Intra-aortic balloon counterpulsation** should be considered in patients who are experiencing cardiogenic shock or hemodynamic instability. A balloon pump can be used as a stabilizing measure before cardiac catheterization and presumed revascularization. It may also be of use in patients who have experienced a mechanical complication of MI, such as

**Table 5-7.** Doses of thrombolytic agents for myocardial infarction

**Agents with fibrin specificity**

Alteplase (rt-PA): IV bolus of 15 mg, followed by 0.75 mg/kg (up to 50 mg) by IV infusion over 30 min, then 0.5 mg/kg (up to 35 mg) by IV infusion over 60 min; maximum dose: 100 mg IV over 90 min

Reteplase (r-PA): IV bolus of 10 mg over 2 min, followed by another IV bolus of 10 units after 30 min

Tenecteplase (TNK-tPA): IV bolus of 0.5 mg/kg; ≤60 kg = 30 mg; 61–70 kg = 35 mg; 71–80 kg = 40 mg; 81–90 kg = 45 mg; ≥90 kg = 50 mg

**Agents without fibrin specificity**

Streptokinase (SK): IV infusion of 1.5 million units over 60 min

a VSD or acute mitral regurgitation due to papillary muscle rupture, before definitive surgical repair.

10. **Magnesium** and **calcium antagonist** therapy is not currently recommended in the setting of acute MI.

C. **Early therapy.** Once the patient with acute MI has been started on the appropriate initial medical therapy, the next urgent decision is the choice of reperfusion therapy. Approximately 90% of patients with an acute MI and ST-segment elevation have a thrombotic occlusion of the infarct-related coronary artery. Early restoration of flow down the vessel limits infarct size, preserves LV function, and reduces mortality.

The American College of Cardiology/American Heart Association publishes guidelines with periodic updates outlining the management of patients with acute MI. The choice of therapy is influenced by the duration of symptoms, the anatomic localization of the infarct, the presence of comorbid illnesses, and the rapid availability of a cardiac catheterization laboratory with qualified staff. Unless spontaneous resolution of the infarction occurs (as determined by dissipation of angina and normalization of the ischemic changes on the ECG), the choices of reperfusion strategies include (1) thrombolytic therapy, (2) primary PCI, or (3) emergent CABG.

1. **Thrombolytic therapy** (Table 5-7) offers the advantages of availability and rapid administration. The primary disadvantage of thrombolytic therapy is the risk of intracranial hemorrhage (0.7–0.9%) and the uncertainty of whether normal coronary flow has been restored to the infarct-related artery. When assessed at 90 minutes, thrombolysis induces clot lysis in 60–90% of patients but restores normal flow in only 30–60%. Normal flow in the infarct-related artery is directly related to improved LV function and survival.

   Thrombolytic therapy should be considered in patients with ST-segment elevation in two or more contiguous ECG leads. It is most effective if given within 12 hours of the onset of symptoms but can be administered for up to, but not beyond, 24 hours. Thrombolytic therapy is not indicated if the symptoms have resolved or for patients with ST-segment depression on the presenting ECG.

   Contraindications to thrombolytic therapy may be relative or absolute (Table 5-8). The risk of intracranial hemorrhage is increased twofold in the elderly (>75 years old), in those who weigh less than 70 kg, and in those with severe hypertension. In patients with a relative contraindication to thrombolytic therapy, the decision to treat should be individualized, assessing the risk of bleeding with the risk of MI complications. Primary PCI is an alternative to thrombolytic therapy.

   **Heparin** is used as adjunctive therapy for all of the selective fibrinolytic agents. See sec. **VIII.B.6.**

**Table 5-8.** Contraindications to thrombolytic therapy

| Absolute contraindications | |
|---|---|
| Active bleeding | Active inflammatory bowel disease |
| Defective hemostasis | Active cavitary lung disease |
| Recent major trauma | Pregnancy |
| Surgical procedure <10 d | **Relative contraindications** |
| Invasive procedure <10 d | Systolic BP >180 mm Hg |
| Neurosurgical procedure <2 mo | Diastolic BP >110 mm Hg |
| GI/genitourinary bleeding <6 mo | Bacterial endocarditis |
| Prolonged CPR >10 min | Hemorrhagic diabetic retinopathy |
| Stroke/transient ischemic attack (TIA) <12 mo | History of intraocular bleeding |
| History of CNS tumor, aneurysm, or arteriovenous malformation | Stroke or TIA ≥12 mo ago |
| Acute pericarditis | Brief CPR <10 min |
| Suspected aortic dissection | Chronic warfarin therapy |
| Active peptic ulcer disease | Severe renal or liver disease |
| | Severe menstrual bleeding |

a. **Recombinant tissue-plasminogen activator** (rt-PA) is more clot selective than streptokinase and does not cause allergic reactions or hypotension. rt-PA is administered as an IV bolus of 15 mg followed by an IV infusion of 0.75 mg/kg (up to 50 mg) over 30 minutes, then 0.5 mg/kg (up to 35 mg) by IV infusion over 60 minutes. Thus, patients with a body weight of 70 kg or more receive a maximum dose of 100 mg over 90 minutes. Concomitant use of IV heparin reduces the risk of subsequent coronary occlusion.

b. **Reteplase** (r-PA) has reduced fibrin specificity but a longer half-life than does rt-PA, permitting bolus administration. r-PA resulted in a similar decrease in mortality when compared to streptokinase and rt-PA in randomized trials. The initial dose is 10 units by IV bolus, with a second 10-unit bolus administered 30 minutes later. Guidelines for heparin administration are the same as for rt-PA.

c. **Tenecteplase** (TNK-tPA) is a genetically engineered variant of rt-PA with slower plasma clearance, better fibrin specificity, and high resistance to plasminogen-activator inhibitor-1, allowing single-bolus administration. When compared to rt-PA, TNK-tPA had a similar decrease in mortality in randomized trials. However, the incidence of mild to moderate bleeding was less in patients who received TNK-tPA. Dosing is approximately 0.5 mg/kg IV, with minimum and maximum doses of 30 and 50 mg, respectively. Guidelines for heparin administration are the same as those for rt-PA.

d. **Streptokinase** is a nonselective agent that induces a generalized fibrinolytic state characterized by extensive fibrinogen degradation. It is administered as an IV infusion of 1.5 million units over 60 minutes. Allergic reactions (skin rashes and fever) may be seen in 1–2% of patients. Hypotension occurs in 10% of patients and usually responds to volume expansion. Allergic reactions and severe hypotension are treated as anaphylactic reactions, with IV antihistamines and steroids. Because of the development of antibodies, patients who were previously treated with streptokinase should be given an alternate thrombolytic agent if such treatment is warranted.

The choice of thrombolytic agent is guided by considerations of cost, efficacy, and ease of administration. rt-PA, r-PA, and TNK-tPA are more expensive than streptokinase. Compared with streptokinase, rt-PA is associated with a slightly greater risk of intracranial hemorrhage but offers the net clinical benefit of an additional ten lives saved per 1000 patients treated.

The therapeutic efficacy of thrombolytic treatment can be monitored by clinical response (resolution of chest pain) and improvement in ST-segment elevation on the ECG. In patients who demonstrate a 50% or greater reduction in ST-segment elevation and relief of chest pain, there is an 80–90% chance that TIMI 2 flow has been restored in the infarct-related artery. However, fewer than half of the patients demonstrate successful reperfusion. Individuals with persistent angina or persistent ischemic changes on the ECG (<50% reduction in ST-segment elevation) at 60–90 minutes after the initiation of fibrinolytic therapy should be considered for urgent coronary angiography and rescue PCI.

Bleeding complications are the most common adverse effect of thrombolytic therapy. Careful monitoring of the patient should be performed along with daily monitoring of the hematocrit and platelet count. Routine monitoring of fibrinogen and fibrin degradation products is not necessary. Venipuncture should be limited and arterial puncture avoided in patients treated with thrombolytic therapy for 24 hours after the initiation of treatment. Major bleeding complications that require blood transfusion occur in approximately 10% of patients. Intracranial hemorrhage is the most dreaded complication and generally results in death or permanent disability. In patients who experience a sudden change in neurologic status, anticoagulant and thrombolytic therapies should be terminated and evaluation with an urgent head CT scan should be undertaken. In patients who hemorrhage, fresh frozen plasma can be given to reverse the lytic state. Cryoprecipitate can also be used to replenish fibrinogen and factor VIII levels. Because platelet dysfunction often accompanies the lytic state, platelet transfusions may be useful in patients with markedly prolonged bleeding times.

2. **Primary PCI** is an alternative to thrombolytic therapy in patients with acute MI and ST-segment elevation or new (or presumed new) LBBB. Primary PCI results in mechanical reperfusion of a thrombosed coronary vessel with normal arterial flow (TIMI 3) in greater than 95% of patients with ST-segment elevation MI. Other advantages of primary PCI are immediate assessment of LV function and identification of other diseased vessels. Primary PCI should be considered when a catheterization facility with experienced staff can anticipate providing a "door-to-balloon time" of less than 90 minutes. Treatment is optimal when the angioplasty is performed within 12 hours of symptom onset but is effective beyond that point if symptoms persist. PCI should be considered in patients with contraindications to thrombolytic therapy or those in whom cardiogenic shock develops within 36 hours of presentation with acute MI. If the patient has multivessel coronary disease, the decision on revascularization of the noninfarct-related arteries can be made after he or she has been stabilized. In general, the approach to this question can be similar to that of patients with stable coronary disease. The functional significance of the lesion can be assessed by noninvasive testing and the vessel treated, if appropriate. Alternatively, the lesion can be treated empirically (without a prior noninvasive evaluation) if this is warranted in the judgment of the interventional cardiologist.

   **The choice of therapy** between thrombolysis and PCI should almost be considered of secondary importance to the imperative of the overall goal of achieving reperfusion in a timely fashion with pharmacologic or mechanical intervention. The morbidity and mortality associated with an acute MI is linearly related to the time to treatment. In general, primary PCI has been shown to result in improved outcomes compared with thrombolytic therapy, regardless of the anatomic distribution of the infarction or the age of the patient. Preliminary data indicate that the added benefit of PCI is also present in patients who can be transferred emergently from a community hospital to a tertiary care center with catheterization facilities. The utility of "facilitated PCI," a strategy of reduced dose of thrombolytic agent combined with PCI, remains to be determined.

3. **Emergency CABG** is a high-risk procedure that should be considered only if the patient has refractory ischemia or cardiogenic shock and the coronary vasculature is not amenable to PCI, or the procedure has failed. Emergency surgery should also be considered for patients with acute mechanical complications of MI, including papillary muscle rupture, VSD, ventricular aneurysm formation in the setting of intractable ventricular arrhythmias or pump failure, or ventricular free wall rupture.

**D. Intermediate care**

1. **Bed rest** is appropriate for the first 24 hours after presentation with an acute MI. Bedside commode privileges are acceptable in hemodynamically stable patients if they are free of anginal symptoms. Patients should be cautioned to avoid the Valsalva maneuver, which may predispose to ventricular arrhythmias. After 24 hours, clinically stable patients can progressively advance their activity with sitting, assisted bathing, standing, and finally walking, as tolerated. Pain relief and treatment of anxiety should be provided, as required.
2. **Hemodynamic monitoring** may be useful to assess ambiguous clinical data or to optimize medical therapy (see sec. **VIII.H**).
3. **Cardiac pacing** may be required in the setting of an acute MI. The rhythm disturbance may be transient in nature, in which case temporary pacing is sufficient until a stable rhythm returns. In some patients, the arrhythmia persists beyond the acute time period of the MI, and permanent pacing is required (see Chap. 7, Arrhythmias). Transcutaneous patches can be used if the need for pacing is anticipated but not required. Because use of the transcutaneous system is associated with significant pain, patients at high risk or who have proven to have a need for pacing should receive a temporary transvenous pacemaker.

**E. Secondary prevention measures** have been shown to reduce the morbidity and mortality after an acute MI (see sec. **IX**).

1. **Aspirin,** initially started at the time of presentation, should be continued indefinitely. The minimum daily dose is 81 mg. Clopidogrel (75 mg/day) can be used in aspirin-allergic patients.
2. **Beta-blockers** confer a 23% mortality benefit in the first 30 days after an acute MI. Treatment should begin as soon as possible (preferably within the first 24 hours) and continue indefinitely. **Calcium channel blockers** (other than short-acting nifedipine) can be used in patients with normal ventricular function and no evidence of heart failure or AV block if beta-blocker therapy is contraindicated or ineffective for relief of ongoing ischemia or for arrhythmia management. **Diltiazem should not be used in patients with ventricular dysfunction** because it has been shown to increase mortality in this patient population.
3. **ACE inhibitors** provide a reduction in short-term mortality when initiated within the first 24 hours of an acute MI. Benefit is seen in all groups of patients but is greatest in high-risk patients, including those with anterior infarctions and heart failure. Therapy can be initiated with captopril, ramipril, trandolapril, or enalapril and titrated as BP permits. ACE inhibitors should be used with caution in patients with

renal insufficiency and are contraindicated in individuals with hypotension. **IV enalaprilat should be avoided** as the initial therapeutic agent because of the possible increased mortality if BP is reduced excessively. Patients with heart failure or asymptomatic LV dysfunction (ejection fraction <40%) should receive ACE inhibitors indefinitely.

4. **Anticoagulant therapy** should be given on initial presentation, either as an adjunct to thrombolytic therapy or in association with cardiac catheterization. IV heparin should be continued for 48 hours. The role of LMWH (enoxaparin) in this setting has not been defined. Beyond 48 hours, the use of anticoagulant therapy should be customized to the patient's needs. If the patient is not ambulatory, prophylactic dosing to prevent deep venous thrombosis is appropriate (see Chap. 1, Patient Care in Internal Medicine).

   Warfarin should be used, absent contraindications, in patients with atrial fibrillation, a large anterior MI, or a documented LV thrombus. Heparin can be used until a therapeutic international normalized ratio (INR) of 2–3 is achieved. **Chronic anticoagulation** is appropriate for patients with LV dysfunction and a documented embolic event. Long-term use should also be considered in patients with severe LV dysfunction. In patients with an extensive anterior wall motion abnormality or a documented LV thrombus, warfarin can be used as prophylaxis against an embolic event and then discontinued after 3–6 months unless other indications warrant its continued use.

5. **Lipid assessment and management** are warranted in all cardiac patients. Details are discussed in Hyperlipidemia in Patients with Ischemic Heart Disease.

**F. Risk assessment.** In patients who present with an acute ST-segment MI, some undergo cardiac catheterization and PCI of the infarct-related artery, if appropriate. The remaining patients are treated with medical therapy alone, including the possible use of a thrombolytic agent. If this latter group of patients experiences any complications associated with the MI, including recurrent angina/ischemia, heart failure, a significant ventricular arrhythmia in the absence of ongoing ischemia, or a mechanical complication of the MI, it is appropriate to proceed directly to cardiac catheterization to assess the coronary anatomy and offer a revascularization strategy as the anatomy dictates.

On the other hand, for the patient treated medically who has an uncomplicated post-MI course, two possible strategies can be considered. One course to follow is a noninvasive (stress test) evaluation to determine prognosis or functional capacity. The stress test can be a submaximal study performed 4–6 days after the MI or a symptom-limited study at 10–14 days. The stress test can also be performed early after hospital discharge (2–3 weeks) or late after discharge (3–6 weeks) if the initial postinfarction stress test was submaximal. With any of the approaches, a diagnostic cardiac catheterization should be performed only if a significant ischemic burden is identified.

The alternate approach to the patient who was successfully managed medically at the time of initial presentation is to proceed directly to catheterization without prior noninvasive assessment. At the time of catheterization, decisions on revascularization should be made based on the patient's anatomy, ventricular function, and clinical status. Which patients are optimally treated with the "conservative" versus the "early invasive" approach to patient management has not yet been clearly defined.

**G. Complications of MI.** ST-elevation and non–ST-elevation MI are most commonly due to rupture of a vulnerable plaque and subsequent thrombus formation with compromise of coronary flow distal to the lesion. Myocardial damage predisposes the patient to several potential adverse consequences or complications that should be considered if the patient presents after the original event with new clinical signs or symptoms.

1. **Recurrent chest pain.** Recurrent pain may be due to ischemia in the territory of the original infarction. The ischemia may result from incomplete revascularization, either by natural or pharmacologic fibrinolytic activity or by early restenosis at the site of a percutaneous intervention. Additional causes of chest pain to be considered include pericarditis, pulmonary embolism, and cardiac rupture. Evaluation of the patient should include a careful clinical examination for new murmurs or friction rubs. An ECG should be examined for evidence of ischemic changes or findings consistent with pericarditis. Cardiac enzymes may help to establish whether additional myocardial damage has occurred. Echocardiography or (repeat) angiography may also be indicated.
   a. **Recurrent ischemia.** Ischemia recurs in 20–30% of patients after MI, with or without recent fibrinolytic therapy, and up to 10% of patients in the early time period after percutaneous revascularization. Patients with signs or symptoms of recurrent ischemia should continue on heparin, nitrate, and β-adrenergic antagonist therapy. If the ischemia is refractory to medical treatment, (repeat) angiography should be considered along with (repeat) dilation of the coronary lesion and stabilization with an intra-aortic balloon pump.
   b. **Recurrent infarction.** Extension or recurrence of infarction occurs in up to 20% of patients after MI and is usually heralded by recurrent anginal symptoms. Patients with recurrent chest pain should be evaluated for new ischemic ECG changes or a significant rise in cardiac enzyme levels. Patients with recurrent ST elevation after fibrinolytic therapy should be considered for rescue angioplasty. If revascularization is not available on-site, or in a timely fashion with hospital transfer, patients can be treated 24 hours after the initial fibrinolytic therapy with additional doses of rt-PA or r-PA. Because reinfarction increases the probability of death, heart failure, arrhythmias, and cardiac rupture, these patients should be monitored in-hospital for an extended period of time.
   c. **Acute pericarditis.** Postinfarction pericarditis occurs in approximately 15–20% of patients with large MIs. Pericarditic pain is often pleuritic in nature and may be relieved in the upright position. A friction rub may be noted on clinical examination.
   d. **Dressler's syndrome.** The post-MI syndrome is characterized by malaise, fever, pericardial pain, leukocytosis, elevated sedimentation rate, and often a pericardial effusion occurring between the first and tenth week after acute MI. Symptoms may be mistaken for recurrent ischemia. The ECG may show diffuse ST-segment elevation. Dressler's syndrome is thought to be an autoimmune process. Treatment is directed at pain management using nonsteroidal anti-inflammatory drugs (NSAIDs) such as aspirin (650 mg PO qid) or indomethacin (25–50 mg qid). Glucocorticoids (prednisone, 1 mg/kg qd) may be useful if symptoms are severe and refractory to initial therapy. Steroid use should be deferred until at least 4 weeks after acute MI due to their adverse impact on infarct healing and risk of ventricular rupture.
2. **Arrhythmias.** Cardiac rhythm abnormalities are common in patients with acute MI. Multiple factors may contribute to the rhythm disturbances, including conduction system disease (sinus bradycardia and AV block), increased sympathetic stimulation (sinus tachycardia, atrial fibrillation/flutter, paroxysmal sustained VT), and electrical instability (VT, ventricular fibrillation, accelerated idioventricular rhythm). Arrhythmias that result in hemodynamic compromise require prompt, aggressive intervention. If the arrhythmia precipitates refractory angina or heart failure, urgent therapy is also warranted. For all rhythm disturbances,

even those that are not life-threatening, exacerbating conditions should be addressed, including electrolyte imbalances, hypoxia, acidosis, and adverse drug effects.

3. **Intraventricular conduction disturbances.** One or more of the three fascicles of the His-Purkinje system may be affected in patients who present with acute MI. The left anterior fascicle is most commonly affected because of isolated coronary blood supply, compared with the left posterior and right fascicles, which receive dual coronary supply. Bifascicular or trifascicular block is associated with a high incidence of progression to complete heart block and other rhythm disturbances.
4. **Bradycardia and heart block**
   a. **Sinus bradycardia.** Sinus bradycardia is common in patients with acute MI, particularly that involving the right coronary artery. In the absence of hypotension or significant ventricular ectopy, observation alone is indicated. If treatment is necessary, atropine (0.3–0.6 mg IV every 3–10 minutes; dose not to exceed 2 mg) can be used to achieve a rate of 60 beats/minute. Temporary pacing may be required for more prolonged or refractory periods of bradycardia.
   b. **First-degree AV block.** First-degree AV block usually does not require specific treatment. The conduction disturbance may be due to use of digoxin or other agents that slow AV conduction. Beta-blocker therapy is contraindicated only if marked PR-interval prolongation or hemodynamic compromise from the loss of AV synchrony is noted.
   c. **Second-degree AV block.** Wenckebach (Mobitz I) second-degree AV block occurs more often with inferior than anterior MI. The block is usually within the His bundle and does not require treatment unless symptomatic bradycardia is present. Mobitz II second-degree AV block originates below the His bundle and is more commonly associated with anterior infarctions. Because of the significant risk of progression to complete heart block, Mobitz II block should be treated with temporary pacing, regardless of the patient's symptoms.
   d. **Third-degree AV block.** Complete dissociation of atrial and ventricular rhythms may develop in up to 15% of patients with MI. Mortality in these individuals may approach 15% (or higher if right ventricular infarction is present). In patients with anterior MI, third-degree heart block often occurs 12–24 hours after initial presentation and may appear suddenly. Temporary pacing is recommended because of the risk of progression to ventricular asystole.
5. **Asystole.** Complete loss of ventricular complexes may occur abruptly in patients with high-grade AV block or complex fascicular blocks. Temporary transvenous pacing is warranted in these patients.
6. **Indications for pacing.** Conduction system disease at risk for progression to complete heart block or significant symptomatic bradycardia can be effectively treated with cardiac pacing. A transcutaneous pacing device can be used under emergent circumstances, and a temporary transvenous system can be used for longer-duration therapy (Table 5-9). A temporary transvenous pacing system should be placed in patients with acute MI if they require transcutaneous pacing or have (1) asystole, (2) symptomatic bradycardia or Mobitz type I second-degree heart block that is unresponsive to atropine, (3) Mobitz type II second-degree heart block, (4) recurrent sinus pauses, (5) incessant VT, or (6) new or age-indeterminate trifascicular block. Patients who are dependent on the atrial contribution to ventricular filling may benefit from atrial or AV sequential pacing. If the rhythm abnormality presents or persists late in the post-MI course, the patient should be evaluated for permanent pacemaker implantation (see Chap. 7, Arrhythmias). Temporary pacing can be considered in patients with a left bundle branch block if placement of a pulmonary

**Table 5-9.** Indications for pacing in acute myocardial infarction

| |
|---|
| **Temporary transcutaneous pacing** |
| Sinus bradycardia with hypotension unresponsive to drug therapy |
| Mobitz II heart block |
| Third-degree heart block |
| New bilateral bundle branch block |
| Newly acquired bundle branch or fascicular block |
| Left or right bundle branch block with first-degree atrioventricular (AV) block |
| **Temporary transvenous pacing** |
| Asystole |
| Symptomatic bradycardia and type 1 second-degree AV block |
| New bilateral bundle branch block |
| New bifascicular bundle branch block with first-degree AV block |
| Mobitz II second-degree AV block |
| **Permanent pacing** |
| Persistent second-degree AV block in the His-Purkinje system with bilateral bundle branch block or complete heart block |
| Transient second- or third-degree AV block associated with bundle branch block |
| Symptomatic AV block at any level |
| Persistent advanced (second or third degree) block at the AV node level |

arterial catheter is indicated, due to the risk of progression to complete heart block with catheter placement. Temporary AV sequential pacing may be helpful in patients with an inferior MI complicated by right ventricular infarction and complete heart block.

7. **Supraventricular tachycardias** (see Chap. 7, Arrhythmias)
   a. **Sinus tachycardia.** This arrhythmia is common in patients with acute MI and is often due to enhanced sympathetic activity resulting from pain, anxiety, hypovolemia, anxiety, heart failure, or fever. Treatment of the underlying contributing factors is indicated. Persistent sinus tachycardia suggests poor underlying ventricular function and is associated with excess mortality. Invasive monitoring of these patients may facilitate choices in volume management and pharmacologic therapy in these individuals.
   b. **Paroxysmal supraventricular tachycardias.** Paroxysmal SVT occurs infrequently in the setting of acute MI. Rate control and rhythm management with beta-blocker or calcium antagonist agents are effective at limiting myocardial oxygen demand in the postinfarction period.
   c. **Atrial fibrillation and flutter.** These arrhythmias are observed in up to 20% of patients with acute MI, with atrial fibrillation occurring more commonly than flutter. Adverse consequences of these rhythms include the loss of AV synchrony and the potential for a rapid ventricular response. Treatment with beta-blockers or calcium antagonists is effective at rate and rhythm control. Because atrial fibrillation and atrial flutter are usually transient in the acute MI period, long-term anticoagulation is often not necessary after documentation of stable sinus rhythm.
   d. **Accelerated junctional rhythm.** Junctional rhythms most commonly occur in conjunction with inferior MI. The rhythm is usually benign

and warrants treatment only if hypotension is present. Digitalis intoxication should be considered in patients with accelerated junctional rhythm.

8. **Ventricular arrhythmias** (see Chap. 7, Arrhythmias)
   a. **Ventricular premature depolarizations (VPDs).** VPDs are common in the course of an acute MI. Beta-blocker therapy used for secondary prevention beginning in the early time period after presentation may reduce the frequency of VPDs and provide symptomatic relief for patients who are aware of the ectopic beats. Prophylactic treatment with lidocaine or other antiarrhythmics has been associated with increased overall mortality and is not recommended.
   b. **Accelerated idioventricular rhythm.** Accelerated idioventricular rhythm, a ventricular rhythm at a rate between 60 and 125 beats/minute, may be seen in up to 20% of patients, often within the first 2 days of the acute MI. It is commonly seen after successful reperfusion with thrombolytic therapy. This rhythm is not associated with an increased incidence of adverse outcomes. Specific treatment is not warranted unless the loss of AV synchrony results in hemodynamic compromise. If needed, sinus activity may be restored with atropine or temporary atrial pacing.
   c. **Nonsustained ventricular tachycardia** (NSVT), defined as three or more consecutive beats greater than 100 beats/minute that last for less than 30 seconds, occur in the majority of patients in the first 24 hours after acute MI. The dysrhythmia may be associated with hemodynamic compromise. The early appearance of this rhythm is not associated with an increase in mortality. Hypokalemia may increase the risk of NSVT. Serum potassium and magnesium should be corrected, as necessary, to values greater than 4.5 mEq/L and 2.0 mEq/L, respectively. NSVT later in the post-MI course should prompt consideration for defibrillator placement in patients with documented ventricular dysfunction.
   d. **VT.** Episodes of sustained VT during the first 48 hours after acute MI are associated with increased in-hospital mortality. Synchronized cardioversion with 200 joules should be used for monomorphic VT, and unsynchronized cardioversion should be used for polymorphic VT. The addition of prophylactic drug therapy is warranted for 24–48 hours (see Chap. 7, Arrhythmias). If VT occurs after appropriate coronary revascularization or later in the post-MI course, long-term antiarrhythmic therapy or defibrillator placement should be considered.
   e. **Ventricular fibrillation.** Primary VF occurs in up to 5% of patients in the early post-MI period. Treatment with immediate unsynchronized cardioversion is appropriate.
9. **Hypertension.** Increased afterload results in elevated myocardial oxygen demand. Patients with hypertension in the setting of an acute MI should be treated initially with short-acting IV agents. Bed rest, pain control, and sedation may facilitate hypertension management.
   a. **β-Adrenergic antagonists.** Beta-blocker therapy is an effective antihypertensive agent that also decreases myocardial oxygen demand by reducing heart rate and contractility. Unless contraindications of hypotension or severe bradycardia exist, beta-blocker therapy should be initiated early in the post-MI course.
   b. **ACE inhibitors.** As with beta-blocker therapy, ACE inhibitors can be used for hypertension management and for secondary prevention after MI. Therapy should be initiated within the first 3 days after MI unless prohibited by contraindications of hypotension or renal dysfunction.
   c. **Calcium channel blockers.** If beta-blocker or ACE inhibitor therapy is contraindicated or not sufficient to manage hypertension, calcium

channel blockers can be used for antihypertensive and for antianginal effects. Short-acting dihydropyridines (nifedipine) are associated with increased in-hospital mortality after acute MI and should be avoided. Although diltiazem and verapamil have not been demonstrated to benefit infarct size or mortality after MI, these agents can be used for BP control and management of supraventricular arrhythmias.

d. **Nitroprusside.** Moderate to severe hypertension can be treated with intravenous nitroprusside (see Chap. 4, Hypertension).

e. **Nitroglycerin.** Predominately a venodilating agent, intravenous nitroglycerin may effectively decrease BP at high doses or in patients with elevated LV filling pressures. Nitroglycerin may also attenuate hypertension through its anti-ischemic effects.

10. **LV failure.** Acute MI may be associated with systolic or diastolic dysfunction, or both. The degree of dysfunction is usually in proportion to the severity of the infarction. The approach to therapy must be individualized to the patient according to etiology, acuity, and extent of the compromise in function. Normotensive patients with pulmonary congestion or a summation gallop on clinical examination can be treated empirically. Cardiac function (ventricular and valvular) can be assessed by echocardiography or at the time of cardiac catheterization, if performed.

a. **Diuretics.** A patient's volume can be controlled, as necessary, with diuretic therapy. Care should be given to avoid intravascular volume depletion.

b. **ACE inhibitors.** Morbidity and mortality after acute MI are clearly favorably affected in patients with documented ventricular dysfunction. This class of medication may also be beneficial in the absence of ventricular dysfunction. If the patient is unable to take an ACE inhibitor, an angiotensin-receptor blocking agent can be substituted; however, the efficacy is less well established.

c. **β-adrenergic antagonists.** Patients should receive beta-blocker therapy after acute MI. In addition to benefits with respect to ischemia and sudden death, this class of medication can be used in the treatment of compensated heart failure.

d. **Digitalis.** Mortality has not been clearly demonstrated to be reduced with digoxin therapy. Improved contractility may be achieved when it is used in patients with severe dysfunction. Digoxin can also be used for rate control in patients with atrial fibrillation in the setting of acute MI. Digitalis, especially in the setting of hypokalemia, may provoke arrhythmias within the first few hours after acute MI.

e. **Nitrates.** Pulmonary congestion may be reduced with nitrate therapy. Intravenous nitroglycerin should be titrated to reduce BP by approximately 10%, but not below 90 mm Hg. Care should be given to avoid a reflex tachycardia. After stabilization, the patient can be converted to an oral preparation.

H. **Hemodynamic monitoring.** Use of a pulmonary artery catheter should be considered in patients with acute MI if their course is complicated by (1) hypotension not corrected by fluid administration; (2) hypotension in the presence of congestive heart failure; (3) cardiogenic shock; (4) potential or confirmed mechanical complications, including VSD, severe mitral regurgitation, and tamponade; (5) unexplained cyanosis or hypoxia; or (6) right ventricular MI. Caution should be used placing a pulmonary artery catheter in patients with a left bundle branch block on ECG because of the risk of inducing complete heart block with the procedure. A temporary pacemaker can be placed prophylactically to obviate this risk.

Patients with MI requiring hemodynamic monitoring can be categorized into one of several groups that are useful for defining treatment strategies. Establishing trends is more important than single absolute values, and therapy must be based on individual responses to initial therapy. All hemodynamic data should be evaluated in terms of the clinical response and viewed critically if they fail to correlate with other physiologic parameters such as urine output. The duration of catheter use should be kept to a minimum.

1. **Hypovolemic hypotension** is characterized by decreased LV filling pressures and systemic hypotension. When accompanied by decreased cardiac index ($<2.5$ L/minute/m$^2$), oliguria, or persistent sinus tachycardia, volume resuscitation with normal saline to a pulmonary arterial wedge pressure of 15–20 mm Hg should be attempted.
2. **Pulmonary congestion** is evident when the pulmonary arterial wedge pressure is elevated ($>20$ mm Hg) in the setting of a normal cardiac index. The condition may be due to volume overload or decreased cardiac compliance. Treatment should consist of intravenous nitroglycerin to reduce preload and diuresis to accomplish more normal cardiac filling pressures.
3. **Peripheral hypoperfusion** is apparent when the BP is maintained but the LV filling pressure is elevated (wedge pressure $>20$ mm Hg) and the cardiac index is depressed ($<2.5$ L/kg/minute). With sufficient BP, the treatment of choice is afterload reduction, initially with intravenous nitroglycerin or nitroprusside. **Nitroglycerin** is preferred early after the onset of MI because it may also induce coronary vasodilation and increase myocardial blood flow to ischemic regions. **Nitroprusside** has less favorable effects than nitroglycerin in terms of coronary blood flow, and its use should be reserved for patients with marked hypertension that is unresponsive to nitroglycerin. The hemodynamic goal should be to reduce the systemic vascular resistance below 1000 dynes/second/cm$^{-5}$. Patients who respond to intravenous therapy can be converted to an oral ACE inhibitor and weaned off the nitroglycerin or nitroprusside. If the BP falls or the cardiac index does not improve with vasodilator therapy, an inotropic agent such as dobutamine should be added.
4. **Cardiogenic shock** is defined as hypotension and cardiac function that are inadequate to meet the metabolic needs of the peripheral tissue. Organ hypoperfusion may be manifest as progressive renal failure or mental status changes. Hemodynamic monitoring reveals elevated filling pressures (wedge pressure $>20$ mm Hg) and a depressed cardiac index ($<2.5$ L/kg/minute) in the setting of a systemic BP of less than 90 mm Hg. Patients with cardiogenic shock in the setting of an MI have a mortality well in excess of 50%. All patients should receive inotropic support. For patients younger than 75 years, an early revascularization strategy decreases 6-month mortality; however, patients older than 75 years benefit from initial medical stabilization (SHOCK Trial, *N Engl J Med* 341:625, 1999). **Dopamine** is the preferred therapeutic agent in patients with a BP of 70–90 mm Hg, but norepinephrine may be required in markedly hypotensive patients (systolic BP $<70$ mm Hg). In patients with a systolic BP near 90 mm Hg, inotropic support with dobutamine is often sufficient and does not adversely affect ventricular afterload. **Milrinone** should be added in patients who are either not responding to or are developing excessive tachycardia in response to dobutamine. These phosphodiesterase inhibitors reduce preload in patients with persistently high filling pressures. Because all inotropes and vasopressors increase myocardial oxygen demand, patients in whom contraindications do not exist should be considered for insertion for an intra-aortic balloon pump. All patients should be evaluated for surgically treatable mechanical complications of MI, such as VSD or severe mitral regurgitation.

5. **Right ventricular MI** is seen in approximately 50% of patients with an acute inferior MI. Roughly half of these patients have hemodynamic compromise as a result of the right ventricular involvement. The LV filling pressures are normal or decreased, the right atrial pressures are elevated (>10 mm Hg), and the cardiac index is depressed. In some patients, elevated right atrial pressures may not be evident until IV fluids are administered. Clinical signs may include hypotension (possibly to the extent of cardiogenic shock), elevated jugular venous pulsation, a Kussmaul's sign (an increase in jugular venous pressures with inspiration), and right-sided third or fourth heart sounds with clear lung fields. Right precordial ECG leads should be obtained and analyzed for ST elevation ($V_4R$ is the most sensitive and specific lead). Initial therapy is intravenous fluids. If hypotension is excessive, inotropic support with dobutamine or an intra-aortic balloon pump may be necessary. In patients with heart block resulting in AV dyssynchrony, sequential AV pacing may have a marked beneficial effect.

I. **Mechanical complications**

1. **Infarct expansion.** Thinning and expansion of the infarct area progress gradually after the acute event. Treatment with ACE inhibitors may limit infarct expansion and prevent remodeling and adverse effects on ventricular geometry. NSAIDs and glucocorticoids should be avoided in patients with acute MI because they promote myocardial thinning.
2. **Aneurysm.** After an MI, the affected area of the myocardium may undergo infarct expansion and thinning. The wall motion may become dyskinetic, and the endocardial surface is at risk for mural thrombus formation. Aneurysm formation is suggested by persistent ST elevation on the ECG and may be diagnosed by imaging studies, including ventriculography or echocardiography. Empiric anticoagulation (warfarin target INR, 2.0–3.0) is warranted to lower the risk of systemic embolization, especially if a mural thrombus is present. Surgical intervention may be appropriate if the aneurysm results in heart failure or ventricular arrhythmias that are not satisfactorily managed with medical therapy.
3. **Pseudoaneurysm.** Incomplete rupture of the myocardial free wall can result in formation of a ventricular pseudoaneurysm in which complete extravasation of blood is prevented by the visceral pericardium. Echocardiography is the preferred diagnostic test to assess for a pseudoaneurysm, often allowing differentiation from a true aneurysm. Prompt surgical intervention for pseudoaneurysms is advised because of the high incidence or myocardial rupture.
4. **Myocardial rupture.** Rupture occurs in an estimated 1–3% of patients with acute MI, most often within the first week after the infarction. The diagnosis is often suggested by a sudden or rapidly progressive hemodynamic decompensation. Rapid evaluation and referral for surgical intervention are necessary because of the high mortality with medical therapy alone.
   a. **Papillary muscle rupture.** Partial or total rupture of the papillary muscle is a rare complication after MI. The posterior medial papillary muscle is most commonly affected due to its isolated vascular supply, but anterolateral and right ventricular papillary rupture has been reported. Acute valvular regurgitation is associated with abrupt clinical deterioration. Papillary muscle rupture may be seen in the setting of a relatively small MI. The diagnostic test of choice is echocardiography with Doppler imaging. The patient can be stabilized with afterload reduction using nitroprusside or nitroglycerin. Inotropic support with dobutamine and intra-aortic balloon pump may also be necessary for hemodynamically unstable patients until definitive therapy with surgical repair can be performed.

**b. VSD.** VSD formation is more commonly associated with anterior MI. The perforation may follow a direct course between the ventricles or a serpiginous route through the septal wall. A new holosystolic murmur often develops. Diagnosis of a VSD can be made by echocardiography with Doppler imaging. In addition, a step-up in hemoglobin oxygen saturation greater than 5% between the right atrium and right ventricle suggests a clinically significant shunt. If a VSD is left untreated, mortality approaches 90%. Initial treatment with nitroprusside or nitroglycerin can be attempted to reduce afterload and decrease the left-to-right shunt. Intra-aortic balloon pump and inotropic support may also be needed to stabilize the patient before definitive surgical repair. In hemodynamically stable patients, surgery is best deferred at least a week to improve patient outcome.

**c. Free wall rupture.** Free wall rupture represents a catastrophic complication of acute MI accounting for 10% of early deaths. This complication can occur after anterior or inferior MI but is more commonly seen in women with a first large transmural MI, with hypertension, treated late with fibrinolytic therapy, and given NSAIDs or glucocorticoids. Rupture typically occurs within the first week after MI. The diagnosis should be suspected in patients who have experienced sudden hemodynamic collapse. Echocardiography may identify patients with particularly thinned ventricular walls at risk for rupture. Pericardiocentesis and intra-aortic balloon pump support may be necessary awaiting emergent surgical correction. Despite optimal intervention, mortality of free wall rupture remains greater than 90%.

**IX. Secondary prevention.** The goal of secondary prevention is to produce a favorable impact on the morbidity and mortality associated with CAD. The strategies outlined for primary prevention and the management of stable angina have also been shown to decrease the rates of repeat infarction, the progression to congestive heart failure, and the incidence of cardiovascular deaths in patients with known CAD who have sustained an MI. The same ABCDE mnemonic can be used as a guide for the approach to therapy.

**A.** Antiplatelet/anticoagulant agents and ACE inhibitors. **Aspirin** is the preferred antiplatelet agent after MI and should be used indefinitely. Doses of 75–325 mg/day have been shown to reduce the chances of recurrent MI, stroke, and cardiac death. **Clopidogrel** (75 mg/day) or **warfarin** (target INR, 2.0–3.0) can be used in patients with contraindications to aspirin therapy, including hypersensitivity reactions or significant gastrointestinal bleeding risk. Clopidogrel is also recommended for a minimum of 4 weeks (in addition to aspirin) after coronary stent placement to reduce the risk of in-stent restenosis. The combination of aspirin and low-dose warfarin is not superior to aspirin alone in reducing cardiac events. Warfarin should be used, however, in patients with atrial fibrillation or a large anterior MI and may be of benefit in patients with severe LV dysfunction. Patients with atrial fibrillation should be treated until at least 3–4 weeks after maintenance of sinus rhythm is ensured. Those with a large anterior MI, LV aneurysm, or documented mural thrombus should receive warfarin for 3–6 months.

**ACE inhibitors** reduce mortality and the incidence of congestive heart failure and recurrent MI. Benefit is seen in asymptomatic patients with LV dysfunction (ejection fraction <40%) and all patients after MI. It is appropriate to titrate therapy to the maximally tolerated dose and to continue treatment indefinitely. Although fewer data are available to demonstrate clear benefit, angiotensin-receptor blockers can be used in patients who are intolerant of ACE inhibitors.

**B. Beta-blockers** and BP control. β-Adrenergic antagonists reduce cardiac events after MI. Treatment with $\beta_1$-selective or nonselective agents is effective (e.g., metoprolol, 100 mg bid; atenolol, 100 mg qd; timolol, 10 mg bid;

propranolol, 80 mg tid). Dosing should be adjusted as necessary if issues of hypotension, bradycardia, or bronchospasm arise. Additional care should be given when using these agents in symptomatic heart failure. Current guidelines favor indefinite treatment after MI. In addition to their role in secondary prevention, beta-blocker agents may also be effective in the treatment of hypertension, angina, and rhythm abnormalities.

C. **Cigarettes** and **cholesterol.** Continued smoking after MI significantly increases the incidence of recurrent ischemic events. Patients should be clearly instructed to quit smoking and attempt to avoid second-hand smoke. Counseling and support group interventions should be used, in addition to pharmacologic therapy. Bupropion (150 mg bid) treatment is needed for a minimum of 7 weeks to be effective, although some patients require up to a year of therapy. After treatment, patients should be slowly tapered off bupropion to reduce the chance of relapse and the risk of seizures. Bupropion is contraindicated in patients with a known seizure disorder or in those taking monoamine oxidase inhibitors. Nicotine patches and gums can be used in conjunction with a supervised smoking cessation program but should be avoided until after the acute hospitalization. Cholesterol-lowering agents should be used to lower cardiovascular event rates after MI (discussed in detail in Hyperlipidemia in Patients with Ischemic Heart Disease, sec. **IV**).

D. **Diet** and **diabetes.** Patients should be counseled about the NCEP-TLC Diet for reducing cholesterol and achieving optimal body weight. A body mass index of less than 25 kg/m$^2$ is desirable. When body mass index is greater than 25 kg/m$^2$, a goal for waist circumference less than 40 inches in men and less than 35 in. in women should be pursued. Although no clear data currently link tight glycemic control with reduced progression of atherosclerotic disease or cardiac events, current recommendations favor appropriate hypoglycemic therapy to achieve near-normal fasting plasma glucose levels and a target hemoglobin $A1_c$ of less than 7%.

E. **Exercise** and **education.** In patients who are physically capable, an exercise stress test can be used for prognostic assessment and to determine functional capacity. A submaximal study can be performed 4–6 days after MI, or symptom-limited study can be performed at 10–14 days. Alternatively, a maximal stress can be administered 3–6 weeks after MI. With an appreciation of the patient's functional exercise capacity, a program of activity can be formulated. The goal is a minimum of 3–4 days per week of 30–60 minutes of activity. Recent studies indicate that a coordinated approach of patient education improves patient compliance with guidelines for post-MI care.

Data on HRT and antioxidant therapy have not clearly demonstrated a benefit in secondary prevention after MI. Current recommendations allow for continued HRT in women who are already taking the medication at the time of MI, but HRT should not be given de novo to postmenopausal women after a cardiac event. Calcium channel blockers and nitrates can be used for anginal relief after MI but do not have a proven mortality benefit in this patient population.

X. **Follow-up care.** Routine office visits every 4–12 months are suggested for the first year after presentation, with an index ischemic event and annual visits thereafter. Five specific questions should be answered during the visits:

1. Has the patient decreased his/her level of physical activity since the last visit?
2. Has the patient's pattern of angina (frequency, severity, or level of activity to provoke) changed since the last visit?
3. How is the patient tolerating therapy?
4. Has the patient attempted to address risk factor modification?
5. What is the status of known or new comorbid illnesses that may affect the patient's ischemic heart disease?

Patients should be instructed to seek more frequent or urgent follow-up evaluation if they experience any noticeable change in their clinical status. Specific plans for a patient's long-term follow-up should be individualized and are affected by their clinical status, anatomy, prior interventions, and any changes in symptoms. Routine testing is not warranted in patients with no change in clinical status or in those with an estimated annual mortality (by prior risk assessment) of less than 1%.

Patients with evidence of new congestive heart failure should be evaluated with a chest x-ray and echocardiogram to assess for changes in ventricular function, for new wall motion abnormalities, and for new or worsening valvular disease. A stress imaging study is appropriate for patients who have a significant change in clinical status (either heart failure or angina). Coronary angiography should be considered for patients with significant ischemic burden on stress testing that is potentially amenable to revascularization or those with marked limitations of ordinary activity despite maximal medical therapy. If new or recurrent coronary disease is identified, options of (repeat) revascularization or other treatments (e.g., transmyocardial laser revascularization or cardiac transplantation) should be considered.

## Hyperlipidemia in Patients with Ischemic Heart Disease

**I. Rationale for therapy.** Lowering cholesterol levels has been shown to decrease the risk of recurrent coronary events and procedures in patients with CAD as well as reduce the risk of developing CAD in people with hypercholesterolemia. Several randomized, placebo-controlled trials have shown decreased mortality and cardiovascular event rates in patients with CAD and a broad range of LDL-cholesterol levels at the time of entry into the studies (*Lancet* 344:1383, 1994; *N Engl J Med* 335:1001, 1996). Data from the Veterans Administration HDL Intervention Trial (*N Engl J Med* 341:410, 1999) suggest that lowering triglycerides and raising HDL may be beneficial in patients with CAD and low HDL-cholesterol levels.

**II. Screening and diagnosis. All patients with evidence of coronary disease** should have lipid profiles performed. For primary prevention of cardiovascular disease, all adults over 20 should have a fasting lipoprotein profile and evaluation of cardiovascular risk factors every 5 years (Table 5-10). The National Cholesterol Education Program has published guidelines for the diagnosis,

**Table 5-10.** National Cholesterol Treatment Program Adult Treatment Panel III guidelines: major risk factors (exclusive of low-density lipoprotein cholesterol) that modify low-density lipoprotein goals

| |
|---|
| Cigarette smoking |
| Hypertension (BP ≥ 140/90 mm Hg or on antihypertensive medication) |
| Family history of premature CHD (CHD in male first-degree relative <55 yr; CHD in female first-degree relative <65 yr) |
| Low HDL cholesterol [<40 mg/dl (1.03 mmol/L)][a] |
| Age: men ≥ 45 yr, women ≥ 55 yr |

CHD, coronary heart disease; HDL, high-density lipoprotein.
[a]HDL-cholesterol level ≥ 60 mg/dl (1.55 mmol/L) counts as a "negative" risk factor; its presence removes one risk factor from the total count.

evaluation, and treatment of high blood cholesterol levels in adults (*JAMA* 285:2486, 2001).

**Lipoprotein analysis** should be performed on serum obtained after a **12-hour fast.** Total cholesterol, triglycerides, and HDL-C are measured, and LDL-C is calculated using the following formula:

$$\text{LDL-C} = \text{total cholesterol} - \text{HDL-C} - (\text{triglyceride}/5)$$

where triglyceride/5 represents the cholesterol contained in very-low-density lipoprotein (VLDL). This formula is not valid when triglyceride levels are greater than 400 mg/dl. In such patients, the most reliable way to ascertain LDL-C is to measure it directly using ultracentrifugation. In patients who have had an acute MI, lipoprotein levels measured within the first 24 hours provide an approximation of their usual levels; otherwise, levels may not be stable for up to 6 weeks.

**Risk assessment** is the first step in the evaluation of patients. Risk is determined based on the lipoprotein profile, the presence or absence of CHD, and other major risk factors (Table 5-10).

A. **Initial classification is based on LDL cholesterol level,** which is the primary target of therapy.
   1. **Optimal LDL-C** is less than 100 mg/dl.
   2. **Near or above optimal LDL-C** is 100–129 mg/dl.
   3. **Borderline-high LDL-C** is 130–159 mg/dl.
   4. **High LDL cholesterol** is 160–189 mg/dl.
   5. **Very-high LDL-C** is greater than or equal to 190 mg/dl.

B. **Total cholesterol and HDL cholesterol classification.**
   1. **Desirable total cholesterol** is less than 200 mg/dl.
   2. **Borderline-high blood cholesterol** is from 200 to 239 mg/dl.
   3. **High blood cholesterol** is greater than or equal to 240 mg/dl.
   4. **Low HDL cholesterol** is less than 40 mg/dl and is counted as a risk factor.
   5. **High HDL-C** is greater than or equal to 60 mg/dl and is a negative risk factor; its presence removes one risk factor from the total count.

C. **Risk categories modify LDL cholesterol goals.**
   1. **Patients in the category of highest risk are those with coronary heart disease (CHD) and CHD risk equivalents.** CHD risk equivalents include clinical CHD, symptomatic carotid artery disease, peripheral vascular disease, and abdominal aortic aneurysm. Other CHD risk equivalents include diabetes mellitus and the presence of multiple risk factors that confer a 10-year risk for CHD greater than 20% (Table 5-11). Patients in this category have an LDL goal of less than 100 mg/dl.
   2. **The next category consists of patients with multiple (2+) risk factors** (Table 5-10). Goal LDL for these patients is less than 130 mg/dl.
   3. **The third category consists of people with 0–1 risk factor.** The goal LDL for this group is less than 160 mg/dl.

D. **The estimation of 10-year risk of CHD** is performed in patients with two or more risk factors using Framingham scoring (*JAMA* 285:2486, 2001).
   1. **A 10-year risk of greater than 20%** is considered a CHD risk equivalent, and the goal LDL is less than 100 mg/dl.
   2. **A 10-year risk of 10–20%** qualifies the patient for a more aggressive approach than a 10-year risk of less than 10% even though the goal LDL is less than 130 mg/dl for both groups.
   3. **A 10-year risk of less than 10%** usually corresponds to fewer than two risk factors.

E. **Classification of patients with CHD.** Patients with CHD or CHD equivalents need aggressive therapy to lower LDL-C.
   1. **Optimal LDL-C** is less than or equal to 100 mg/dl. These patients should have instruction on diet and physical activity. Other lipid and nonlipid risk factors should be treated.

**Table 5-11.** National Cholesterol Education Program Adult Treatment Panel III guidelines: treatment decisions based on low-density lipoprotein (LDL) cholesterol

| Risk category | LDL goal | LDL level at which to initiate TLC | LDL level at which to consider drug therapy |
|---|---|---|---|
| CHD or CHD risk equivalents (10-yr risk >0%) | <100 mg/dl (2.58 mmol/L) | ≥100 mg/dl (2.58 mmol/L) | ≥130 mg/dl (3.36 mmol/L) [100–129 mg/dl (2.58–3.33 mmol/L): drug optional] |
| 2+ Risk factors (10-yr risk ≥20%) | <130 mg/dl (3.36 mmol/L) | ≥130 mg/dl (3.36 mmol/L) | 10-yr risk 10–20%: ≥130 mg/dl (3.36 mmol/L); 10-yr risk <10%: ≥160 mg/dl (4.13 mmol/L) |
| 0–1 Risk factor | <160 mg/dl (4.13 mmol/L) | ≥160 mg/dl (4.13 mmol/L) | ≥190 mg/dl (4.91 mmol/L) [160–189 mg/dl (4.13–4.88 mmol/L): LDL-lowering drug optional] |

CHD, coronary heart disease; TLC, therapeutic lifestyle changes.

2. **Higher than optimal LDL-C** is above 100 mg/dl. Patients with baseline LDL above 130 mg/dl require intensive lifestyle therapy and maximal control of other risk factors. Drug therapy can be started simultaneously with lifestyle therapy. The goal of therapy is less than 100 mg/dl. Patients with LDL-C levels between 100 and 129 mg/dl should have lifestyle therapy started or intensified and should also be considered for initial or intensified drug therapy. The Heart Protection Study included patients with vascular disease and low LDL levels, with benefits from drug therapy shown even in patients whose baseline LDL cholesterol levels were below 115 mg/dl (*Lancet* 360:7, 2002).

F. **Elevated serum triglyceride levels** are an independent risk factor for atherosclerotic disease. They may be associated with increased concentrations of atherogenic particles such as chylomicron remnants, VLDL remnants, and small, dense LDL particles. Patients with hypertriglyceridemia frequently have low levels of HDL-C.
   1. **Normal triglycerides** are less than 150 mg/dl.
   2. **Borderline-high hypertriglyceridemia** levels are between 150 and 199 mg/dl. Nonpharmacologic therapy, including diet, exercise, and weight loss, is the initial form of treatment in these patients. Drug therapy is considered for those who are not at goal level of LDL, which is the first target of therapy in this group of patients.
   3. **High triglycerides** are defined as triglyceride levels between 200 and 499 mg/dl. Nonpharmacologic treatment with diet, exercise, and weight loss is initial therapy. LDL cholesterol remains the primary target of therapy, but non–HDL cholesterol is a secondary target. Non–HDL cholesterol is equal to total cholesterol–HDL. Table 5-12 shows non–HDL cholesterol goals.
   4. **Very-high triglycerides** are greater than 500 mg/dl. These patients are at increased risk for pancreatitis. Nonpharmacologic measures and a search for secondary causes are needed. These patients must be treated aggressively and often require drug therapy. Once triglyceride levels are lowered to less than 500 mg/dl, LDL is again the primary target of therapy.

**Table 5-12.** National Cholesterol Treatment Program Adult Treatment Panel III guidelines: comparison of low-density lipoprotein (LDL) cholesterol and non–high-density lipoprotein (HDL) cholesterol goals for three risk categories

| Risk category | LDL goal (mg/dl) [mmol/L] | Non-HDL goal (mg/dl) [mmol/L] |
|---|---|---|
| CHD and CHD risk equivalent | <100 [2.58] | <130 [3.36] |
| Multiple (2+ risk factors) | <130 [3.36] | <160 [4.13] |
| 0–1 Risk factor | <160 [4.13] | <190 [4.9] |

CHD, coronary heart disease.

## III. Specific disorders

**A. Familial hypercholesterolemia (FH)** is an autosomal-dominant disorder involving the LDL receptor.

1. **Heterozygotes** for FH have 50% of the normal number of LDL receptors, elevated LDL-C levels, and cholesterol levels of 250–500 mg/dl. The incidence is approximately 1 in 500 persons. Affected patients often have premature vascular disease and may have tendon xanthomas. Treatment usually requires drug as well as diet therapy. More severe cases may require the combination of two or more medications, typically a hydroxymethylglutaryl–coenzyme A (HMG-CoA) reductase inhibitor and a bile acid sequestrant resin (see sec. **IV**). Patients with insufficient response to tolerated doses of lipid-lowering medications may be candidates for LDL-apheresis.
2. **Homozygotes** for FH have few or no LDL receptors and thus have markedly elevated LDL-C levels and blood cholesterol levels of 600–1000 mg/dl. The incidence is 1 in 1 million. Heart disease often begins in early childhood, and many patients die of heart disease in their twenties and thirties. Affected children may have plantar and tuberous as well as tendon xanthomas. They respond poorly to diet and drug therapy, although they may have some response to higher doses of potent statins. LDL-apheresis is the preferred therapy. Liver transplantation has been performed in a few patients.

**B. Familial defective apolipoprotein B-100** is an autosomal-dominant disorder caused by an abnormality in the region of the LDL receptor–binding region of apoprotein B-100, the major protein on the surface of LDL particles. It appears to have frequency, clinical features, and lipoprotein levels similar to those of heterozygous FH.

**C. Familial combined hyperlipidemia (FCHL)** is associated with an increased risk of vascular disease. Patients may have elevated cholesterol, triglycerides, or both. The molecular basis of this disorder is unknown; many patients overproduce VLDL. FCHL appears to be an autosomal-dominant disorder and occurs in 1–2% of the population. The diagnosis is made by the presence of multiple lipoprotein abnormalities within one family. Family members may have elevated VLDL, elevated LDL-C, or increased levels of both VLDL and LDL-C. Diet therapy, weight loss, and exercise are useful initial therapies, but many patients require drug therapy aimed at correcting specific lipoprotein abnormalities.

**D. Severe polygenic hypercholesterolemia** is found in adults whose LDL-C is above 220 mg/dl and who do not clearly demonstrate a monogenic inheritance of hypercholesterolemia. These patients are usually at increased risk for premature CHD. Many require medication to achieve LDL-cholesterol goals.

**E. Hypertriglyceridemia** may be secondary to diet, obesity, excess alcohol intake, diabetes mellitus, hypothyroidism, uremia, dysproteinemias, β-adrenergic antagonists, estrogen, oral contraceptive drugs, and retinoids. Triglyceride levels greater than 400 mg/dl are often associated with an underlying genetic disorder. Primary hypertriglyceridemia can be due to FCHL or familial hypertriglyceridemia. Families with familial hypertriglyceridemia have multiple members with elevated triglyceride levels due to increased VLDL levels. Familial hypertriglyceridemia appears to be an autosomal-dominant disorder without a clearly defined molecular basis. Families may show less pronounced risk of CHD than those with FCHL.

F. **Dysbetalipoproteinemia** (type III hyperlipoproteinemia) is a rare (approximately 1 in 5000) disorder caused by an abnormality of apoprotein E, a protein on the surface of VLDL and other lipoproteins, which is important in the uptake of remnant particles by cell surface receptors. Cholesterol-enriched VLDL (beta-VLDL), an atherogenic particle, accumulates in the serum. Cholesterol and triglycerides are both elevated. Isoelectric focusing of plasma proteins shows an abnormal apoprotein E pattern that can be confirmed by specific genotyping. Patients may have palmar or tuberoeruptive xanthomas, and they have an increased risk of vascular disease. Patients with this disorder may respond well to diet and weight loss.

G. **Hyperchylomicronemia** is diagnosed by the presence of a chylomicron layer when plasma is centrifuged or when chylomicrons float to the top of plasma that has been refrigerated overnight. This can be seen when triglyceride levels are in excess of 1000 mg/dl. The patient may have rare syndromes involving absence of lipoprotein lipase activity or absent apoprotein C-II (a cofactor of lipoprotein lipase). Chylomicrons alone may be increased, as in lipoprotein lipase deficiency, or VLDL and chylomicrons may both be elevated. Total cholesterol levels are often markedly elevated because of the presence of large numbers of VLDL particles that contain cholesterol as well as triglycerides. Hyperchylomicronemia may develop in patients with primary hypertriglyceridemia, FCHL, or dysbetalipoproteinemia in the presence of excessive dietary fat intake, uncontrolled diabetes, alcohol excess, obesity, or other secondary causes of hyperlipidemia. The chylomicronemia syndrome may include abdominal pain, hepatomegaly, splenomegaly, eruptive xanthomas, lipemia retinalis, and pancreatitis. Memory loss, paresthesias, and peripheral neuropathy can also occur.

H. **Family members** of patients with hyperlipidemia should be screened to facilitate diagnosis of primary hyperlipidemias as well as to identify other patients in need of treatment.

I. **Secondary causes of hyperlipidemia** include diet, hypothyroidism, diabetes mellitus, nephrotic syndrome, chronic renal failure, and dysproteinemia. Certain **drugs** can have effects on lipids. Thiazide diuretics, β-adrenergic antagonists (particularly less selective ones), glucocorticoids, estrogens, progestins, retinoids, anabolic steroids, protease inhibitors, and alcohol have variable effects on cholesterol, triglycerides, and HDL cholesterol. Treatment of diabetes mellitus with good control of blood sugars is particularly important if reasonable control of hypertriglyceridemia is to be achieved.

J. **Low HDL-C levels (<40 mg/dl)** may be due to a genetic disorder or to secondary causes.
   1. **Primary disorders** include familial hypoalphalipoproteinemia, primary hypertriglyceridemias, and rare disorders such as fish-eye disease, Tangier disease, and lecithin–cholesterol–acyl transferase deficiency.
   2. **Secondary causes** of low HDL-C levels include cigarette smoking, obesity, lack of exercise, androgens, some progestational agents, anabolic steroids, β-adrenergic antagonists, and hypertriglyceridemia.

K. **The metabolic syndrome** is defined by the presence of three of the following:
   - **Abdominal obesity:** waist circumference greater than 102 cm in men and 88 cm in women
   - **Triglycerides** greater than or equal to 150 mg/dl
   - **HDL cholesterol** less than 40 mg/dl in men and 50 mg/dl in women

- **BP** greater than or equal to 130 over greater than or equal to 85 mm Hg
- **Fasting glucose** greater than or equal to 110 mg/dl

**IV. Treatment. Patients who already have coronary disease should have LDL-cholesterol levels reduced to 100 mg/dl or less.** Therapy should begin during hospitalization for an acute coronary event if patients are not already being treated. Patients with coronary disease should be treated with the National Cholesterol Education Program Therapeutic Lifestyle Changes (NCEP-TLC) diet, which restricts saturated fat to 7% of total calories and daily cholesterol intake to less than 200 mg. Patients should see a dietitian for assistance in making diet changes. Patients with elevated triglycerides need to restrict simple sugars and alcohol as well. (**For treatment goals, see** Table 5-11.)

**A. LDL cholesterol** can be lowered with the HMG-CoA reductase inhibitors (statins): lovastatin, pravastatin, simvastatin, fluvastatin, atorvastatin, and rosuvastatin; the bile acid sequestrant drugs cholestyramine, colestipol, and colesevelam; the cholesterol absorption inhibitor, ezetimibe; and nicotinic acid (also called niacin).

1. **The HMG-CoA reductase inhibitors** lower LDL cholesterol well in most patients. These are the drugs of choice for lowering LDL for secondary prevention. LDL cholesterol can drop by 20–60%, depending on the drug and dosage. All the statins are similar in mechanism of actions and side effects. Atorvastatin and rosuvastatin have half-lives of approximately 13 hours and 13–20 hours, respectively. The other reductase inhibitors have half-lives of approximately 2–3 hours. Lovastatin is best given with food, usually with the evening meal; pravastatin, simvastatin, and fluvastatin can be administered without food, preferably in the evening. **Side effects** occur infrequently (approximately 5% of patients) and most commonly include mild gastrointestinal discomfort and myalgias.
   a. **Liver function tests** should be monitored every 6 weeks for the first 3 months, then every 6 months. Approximately 1% of patients have transaminase elevations to greater than three times the upper limit of normal, and the medication should be discontinued. It may be possible to change to a different reductase inhibitor without having a rise in transaminases. Restriction of alcohol intake, if patients are consuming more than two servings a day, may decrease the possibility of transaminase elevation.
   b. **Myopathy** is an infrequent side effect but has been reported more often when the reductase inhibitors are combined with cyclosporine, gemfibrozil, niacin, or erythromycin. Patients with myalgias due to statins may have normal or elevated CK levels. Symptoms usually improve within a few days after the drug is discontinued. Some patients who have myalgias with one statin may be able to tolerate another statin.
   c. **Rhabdomyolysis** is a rare complication of statin use. It is more likely to occur in elderly or debilitated patients, individuals with renal or congestive heart failure, or patients on medications that affect the metabolism of the statins, including fibric acid derivatives (especially gemfibrozil), cyclosporine, macrolide antibiotics, or drugs with significant cytochrome P-450 metabolism such as itraconazole.
2. **Bile acid sequestrant resins** lower LDL by 15–30%. Because the resins can raise triglycerides, they should not be used as monotherapy in patients with triglycerides above 250 mg/dl. Usual dosages are 4–20 g/day cholestyramine or colestipol. Up to 24 g cholestyramine or 30 g colestipol can be used.
   a. **Cholestyramine** and **colestipol** are available in powder form, in bulk, or in single-dose packets. Colestipol is also available in 1-g tablets. Once- or twice-daily dosing close to meals is desirable. A single daily dose of up to 8–12 g may be useful to fit the resin into a medication schedule. Resins can be combined with nicotinic acid or reduc-

tase inhibitors in patients with severe elevations of LDL cholesterol when greater reductions of LDL are required.

b. **Colesevelam** is another bile acid–binding drug. It is available in 625-mg tablets with a recommended dose of six tablets per day and a maximum dose of seven tablets per day. LDL-cholesterol reduction is 15–18%. Interactions with other drugs and gastrointestinal side effects may be less frequent than with the older resins. The addition of bile acid–binding drugs to statins can produce additional reduction of LDL levels that are needed to get to goal in some patients.

c. The most common **side effects** of the resins are bloating, hard stools, and constipation. Initiation of therapy with low doses, patient education, and use of stool softeners or psyllium can increase compliance. Patients with severe constipation and very complicated drug regimens are usually not good candidates for resin therapy. **Other medications must be taken 1 hour before or 4 hours after cholestyramine and colestipol.**

3. **Ezetimibe** is a cholesterol absorption inhibitor. It blocks the absorption of cholesterol at the level of the enterocyte. LDL-cholesterol levels can decrease by approximately 20%. The dose is 10 mg daily, and it is not affected by food. Ezetimibe can be used alone or in combination with statins. The addition of ezetimibe to a given dose of a statin may produce additional lowering of LDL by 20% or more. **Side effects** include diarrhea. Liver enzyme elevations can occur with the combination of ezetimibe and statins, and transaminases should be monitored with the combination as they would be with the statins.

4. **Nicotinic acid** can lower triglycerides, raise HDL, and lower LDL in higher doses. It is particularly useful in combined hyperlipidemia and in patients with low levels of HDL. Niacin requires extensive patient education because of the flushing and other side effects that can occur.

a. **To initiate therapy with nicotinic acid,** patients should begin taking 100 mg/day for 1 day, then increase to 100 mg tid for 1 week, then 200 mg tid the second week, and 300 mg tid the third week, and repeat lipids; serum chemistries should be obtained after another 3 weeks while patients remain on 300 mg tid. The dose can be gradually increased to the highest dose the patient can tolerate that produces desired results, up to 3000 mg/day. Patients should report any nausea or increased fatigue, as these may be signs of toxicity; liver function tests should be measured and the dose decreased if these are elevated. A prescription-only, extended-release formulation can be given once a day at bedtime; significant liver toxicity was not reported at doses up to 2000 mg/day in clinical trials. Thus, the maximum recommended dose is 2000 mg/day. The initial dose is 500 mg at bedtime. The dose can be increased by 500 mg at 4-week intervals up to the maximum dose. The entire dose should be taken at bedtime, and this preparation should not be combined with any other niacin preparations.

b. **Adverse effects. Some over-the-counter sustained-release preparations have been associated with severe liver toxicity;** crystalline or non–time-release preparations should be used. Flushing can be decreased by starting with low doses, use of aspirin before the first few doses, and having the patient take nicotinic acid with meals. Uric acid, blood glucose, and serum transaminases should be monitored every 6–8 weeks during a titration phase. Nicotinic acid should be avoided in patients with a history of gout, active peptic ulcer disease, and liver disease. Diabetic patients should only use niacin if they have hemoglobin $A1_c$ levels of approximately 7% and should monitor blood sugars closely.

B. **Hypertriglyceridemia** usually responds to a combined approach using nonpharmacologic and drug therapy.

1. **Nonpharmacologic therapy.** Patients should be instructed to decrease their intake of alcohol and simple sugars and to exercise regularly. Some patients who markedly increase their carbohydrate intake have increases in triglyceride levels. Hypertriglyceridemic patients should generally not be on diets with fat content less than 25% of calories, except for patients with the chylomicronemia syndrome. The response to very-low-fat diets (i.e., 10% of calories from fat) may be disappointing in patients with impaired glucose tolerance unless the diet is sufficiently hypocaloric. Very-high-carbohydrate diets that are isocaloric may lead to poor glycemic control and increased triglyceride levels. A particular problem is a high intake of nonfat desserts leading to increased calories in an otherwise low-fat diet. Modest amounts of weight loss can be extremely helpful. In addition, patients with diabetes, especially those with very high triglyceride levels, should have good glycemic control. Drugs such as estrogen, retinoids, and thiazides may contribute to hypertriglyceridemia. The use of transdermal estrogen instead of oral estrogen preparations can lead to significant decreases in triglyceride levels in women who are receiving postmenopausal HRT. **Oral estrogen preparations should be avoided in women with triglyceride levels above 500 mg/dl.**
2. **Omega-3 fatty acids,** found in fish oils, can reduce triglyceride levels. Fish oil capsules containing the long-chain fatty acids, **eicosapentaenoic acid and docosahexaenoic acid,** can be used as an adjunct to other therapies in patients with hypertriglyceridemia. At doses of 3–6 g/day of eicosapentaenoic acid plus docosahexaenoic acid, triglycerides may decrease by up to 30%. The major drawbacks to high doses of these fatty acids are the large number of pills to be taken, eructation, and occasional diarrhea. They have a mild antiplatelet effect, which may be of concern in patients who are receiving warfarin or antiplatelet drugs.
3. **Drug therapy. Patients with triglycerides of 400 mg/dl or less** and elevated LDL-cholesterol levels may respond adequately to a statin added to nonpharmacologic measures. **If the triglycerides are above 400 mg/dl** despite adequate dietary modifications and exercise, the choice of medication could include a statin at higher doses, gemfibrozil, fenofibrate, or niacin. For patients with **triglycerides over 1000 mg/dl,** fibrates and niacin are the drugs of choice. If LDL-cholesterol levels remain high after the triglycerides are lowered, combination therapy should be considered. **Gemfibrozil and fenofibrate** are the fibric acid derivatives that are available in the United States.
   a. The usual dose of **gemfibrozil** is 600 mg bid before meals. Triglyceride levels are reduced by 30–50%. The drug should not be used in patients with very low creatinine clearances. Abdominal pain and nausea are the most common side effects. The incidence of gallstones is increased in patients who are receiving the fibric acid derivatives due to the increased cholesterol content of bile. Patients on warfarin need to have their prothrombin time monitored closely after they start taking gemfibrozil.
   b. **The use of fenofibrate** is similar to that of gemfibrozil. Fenofibrate is available in 67-, 134-, and 200-mg capsules and 54- and 160-mg tablets with a usual starting dose of 67 or 54 mg/day. Many patients require the full dose of 160 or 200 mg/day; however, a lower dose should be used in patients with renal insufficiency. It can be given once a day with a meal. Side effects, which occur in 5–10% of patients, are primarily mild GI discomfort and, less frequently, rash and pruritus. Increased transaminases occur in approximately 5% of patients and return to normal when the drug is discontinued. Infrequently, myalgias and increased CK have been reported. In addition

to its use for lowering triglycerides, fenofibrate may be helpful in some patients with combined hyperlipidemia who have moderately elevated LDL-cholesterol levels and high triglycerides.

**C. The chylomicronemia syndrome** requires a diet that is very low in total fat. Patients with triglycerides above 2000 mg/dl should initiate a diet with less than 10% of total calories as fat. It may be possible to increase the fat content gradually as the triglyceride level falls to less than 500 mg/dl. Primary lipoprotein lipase deficiency is treated with fat restriction and does not respond to drug therapy.

**D. The metabolic syndrome is a secondary target of risk-reduction therapy.** It is a constellation of factors, including abdominal obesity, insulin resistance or diabetes, hypertension, and atherogenic lipid profile (elevated triglyceride levels; small, dense LDL; low HDL). **Weight control and increased physical activity** are important in the treatment of the metabolic syndrome. Other risk factors such as hypertension should also be treated. **Elevated triglycerides** or low HDL, or both, should be treated once the LDL goal has been reached.

**E. Low HDL-cholesterol levels** are associated with an increased risk of cardiovascular disease. Attention should be given to factors that lower HDL, such as cigarette smoking and certain medications, including β-adrenergic antagonists, androgenic compounds, and progestins. Nonpharmacologic therapy, such as exercise, weight loss, and smoking cessation, should be stressed. Niacin is the most effective agent for increasing HDL. Some increase (approximately 10–20%) can occur with fibrates.

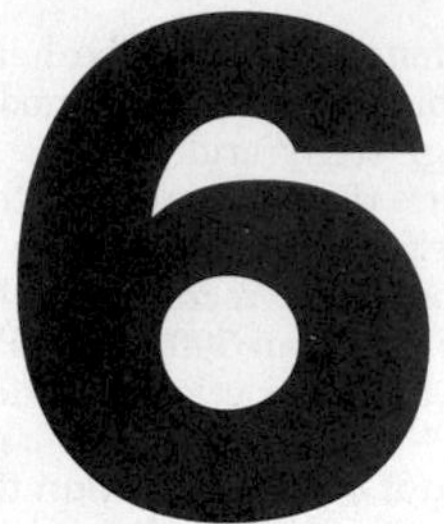

# Heart Failure, Cardiomyopathy, and Valvular Heart Disease

Ioana Dumitru,
Joseph G. Rogers, and
Gregory A. Ewald

## Heart Failure

**I. Clinical diagnosis**

**A. Definition. Heart failure (HF)** is the inability of the heart to maintain an output adequate to meet the metabolic demands of the body. It is an increasingly common condition that affects approximately 5 million Americans and is associated with extremely high morbidity and mortality. It is a syndrome and not a disease.

**B. Etiology.** HF may be secondary to abnormalities in myocardial contraction (systolic dysfunction), ventricular relaxation and filling with normal contractile function (diastolic dysfunction), or both. Hypertension (HTN) and coronary artery disease are the most frequent causes of HF in the United States. Other causes include valvular heart disease, toxic or metabolic disease, infiltrative disease, infections, and drugs, among others.

**C. Pathophysiology.** HF is manifested as organ hypoperfusion and inadequate tissue oxygen delivery due to a low cardiac output and decreased cardiac reserve, as well as pulmonary and systemic venous congestion. A variety of "compensatory adaptations" occur, including (1) increased left ventricular (LV) volume (dilatation) and mass (hypertrophy), (2) increased systemic vascular resistance (SVR) secondary to enhanced activity of the sympathetic nervous system and elevated levels of circulating catecholamines, and (3) activation of the renin-angiotensin-aldosterone and vasopressin (antidiuretic hormone) systems. These secondary mechanisms, in conjunction with pump failure, play an important role in the pathophysiology of HF.

**D. Clinical manifestations** of HF vary depending on the rapidity of cardiac decompensation, underlying etiology, age, and comorbidities of the patient. **Signs and symptoms** of low cardiac output include fatigue, exercise intolerance, and decreased peripheral perfusion. Extreme deterioration in cardiac output and elevated SVR result in hypoperfusion of vital organs such as the kidney (decreased urine output) and brain (confusion and lethargy) and, ultimately, in cardiogenic shock. Elevations in LV diastolic pressure and pulmonary venous pressure result in pulmonary edema. Chronic pulmonary and systemic venous congestion results in orthopnea, dyspnea on exertion, paroxysmal nocturnal dyspnea, peripheral edema, elevated jugular venous pressure, pleural and pericardial effusions, hepatic congestion, and ascites. Associated laboratory abnormalities include elevated levels of BUN and creatinine, hyponatremia, and elevated serum levels of hepatic enzymes.

**E. The diagnosis of HF** should be suspected on the basis of clinical presentation. Radiographic evidence of cardiomegaly and pulmonary vascular redistribution is common. Depressed ventricular function should be confirmed by echocardiography, radionuclide ventriculography, or cardiac catheterization with left ventriculography. Abnormalities in the ECG are common and include supraventricular and ventricular arrhythmias, conduction delays, and nonspecific ST-T changes. **B-type natriuretic peptide** (BNP) is synthe-

**Table 6-1.** American College of Cardiology/American Heart Association guidelines of evaluation and management of chronic heart failure in adults

| Stage | Description | Treatment |
|---|---|---|
| A | No structural heart disease and no symptoms but risk factors: CAD, HTN, DM, cardiotoxins, familial cardiomyopathy | Lifestyle modification—diet, exercise, smoking cessation; treat hyperlipidemia and use ACEI for HTN |
| B | Abnormal LV systolic function, MI, valvular heart disease but no HF symptoms | Lifestyle modifications, ACEI, β-adrenergic blockers |
| C | Structural heart disease and HF symptoms | Lifestyle modifications, ACEI, β-adrenergic blockers, diuretics, digoxin |
| D | Refractory HF symptoms to maximal medical management | Therapy listed under A, B, C and mechanical assist device, heart transplantation, continuous IV inotropic infusion, hospice care in selected patients |

ACEI, angiotensin-converting enzyme inhibitor; CAD, coronary artery disease; DM, diabetes mellitus; HF, heart failure; HTN, hypertension; LV, left ventricular; MI, myocardial infarction.
*Source:* Adapted from SA Hunt, DW Baker, MH Chin, et al. ACC/AHA guidelines for the evaluation and management of chronic heart failure in the adult: executive summary. *J Am Coll Cardiol* 38(7):2102, 2001.

sized by the right and left ventricular myocytes and released in response to stretch, volume overload, and elevated filling pressures. Serum levels of BNP are elevated in patients with asymptomatic LV dysfunction as well as symptomatic HF. A serum BNP of less than 100 pg/ml has a good negative predictive value and typically excludes HF as primary diagnosis in dyspneic patients. BNP levels correlate with the severity of HF and predict survival (*N Engl J Med* 347:161, 2002).

F. **Precipitants** of HF include myocardial ischemia, HTN, arrhythmias, infection, thyroid disease, volume overload, toxins (alcohol, doxorubicin), drugs [nonsteroidal anti-inflammatory drugs (NSAIDs), calcium channel antagonists], pulmonary embolism, and dietary or medical noncompliance.

II. **General principles in the management of HF** (Table 6-1)

A. **Nonpharmacologic therapeutic measures** are used in conjunction with specific pharmacologic treatment.

1. **Exercise training** is recommended in stable HF patients. Ideally, it should be started slowly in a monitored outpatient setting and reach a target of 20–45 minutes a day for 3–5 days a week for a total of 8–12 weeks. Short-term effects of exercise training in chronic stable HF patients are additive to pharmacologic treatment and are associated with a decrease in neurohormonal activation. Patients enrolled in exercise training programs notice increased exercise capacity, decreased symptoms, increased quality of life, and decreased hospitalization rate. However, the effects of long-term exercise training on survival are not defined [*J Am Coll Cardiol* 38(7):2102, 2001]. Restriction of physical activity may be required in acute HF exacerbations to reduce myocardial workload and oxygen consumption.
2. **Weight loss** in obese patients reduces SVR as well as myocardial oxygen demand. However, maintenance of adequate caloric intake in patients with severe HF is necessary to prevent or correct cardiac cachexia.
3. **Dietary sodium restriction** ($Na^+$, ≤ 2 g/day) facilitates control of signs and symptoms of HF and minimizes diuretic requirements.

4. **Fluid and free water restriction** (≤ 1.5 L/day) is especially important in the setting of hyponatremia (serum sodium ≤ 130 mEq/L) and volume overload (see Chap. 3, Fluid and Electrolyte Management).
5. **Minimization of medications with deleterious effects in HF should be attempted. Negative inotropes** (e.g., verapamil, diltiazem) should be avoided in patients with impaired ventricular contractility, as should **over-the-counter beta stimulants** [e.g., compounds containing ephedra, pseudoephedrine hydrochloride (Sudafed)]. **NSAIDs,** which antagonize the effect of angiotensin-converting enzyme (ACE) inhibitors and diuretic therapy, should be avoided if possible.
6. **Administration of oxygen** may relieve dyspnea, improve oxygen delivery, reduce the work of breathing, and limit pulmonary vasoconstriction in patients with hypoxemia. **Sleep apnea** has a prevalence as high as 37% in the HF population. Treatment with nocturnal continuous positive airway pressure improves symptoms and LV ejection fraction (EF) (*Am J Respir Crit Care Med* 160:2147, 1999; *N Engl J Med* 348:1233, 2003).
7. **Dialysis or ultrafiltration** may be necessary in patients with severe HF and renal dysfunction who cannot respond adequately to fluid and sodium restriction and diuretics. Other mechanical methods of fluid removal such as therapeutic thoracentesis and paracentesis may provide temporary symptomatic relief of dyspnea. Care must be taken to avoid rapid fluid removal and hypotension.

B. **Pharmacologic therapy of HF. The general principle** of pharmacologic therapy involves the antagonism of neurohormones that are increased in patients with HF and have deleterious effects on the myocardium and the peripheral vasculature. Vasodilator therapy and β-adrenergic blockade are the cornerstone of therapy for patients with HF. Diuretics are reserved to relieve volume overload. Most patients require a multidrug regimen to control symptoms and prolong survival.

1. **Vasodilator therapy** is the mainstay of treatment in patients with HF. Arterial vasoconstriction (afterload) and venous vasoconstriction (preload) occur in patients with HF as a result of activation of the renin-angiotensin-aldosterone system and adrenergic nervous system, as well as increased secretion of arginine vasopressin. Agents with predominantly venodilatory properties decrease preload and ventricular filling pressures. In the absence of LV outflow tract obstruction, arterial vasodilators reduce afterload by decreasing SVR, resulting in increased cardiac output, decreased ventricular filling pressure, and decreased myocardial wall stress. The efficacy and toxicity of vasodilator therapy depend on intravascular volume status and preload. Vasodilators should be used with caution in patients with a fixed cardiac output [e.g., aortic stenosis (AS) or hypertrophic cardiomyopathy (HCM)] or with predominantly diastolic dysfunction.

   a. **Oral vasodilators** should be the initial therapy in patients with symptomatic chronic HF and in patients in whom parenteral vasodilators are being discontinued. When treatment with oral vasodilators is being initiated in hypotensive patients, it is prudent to use agents with a short half-life.

      (1) **ACE inhibitors** (Table 6-2) attenuate vasoconstriction, vital organ hypoperfusion, hyponatremia, hypokalemia, and fluid retention attributable to compensatory activation of the renin-angiotensin system. Treatment with ACE inhibitors decreases afterload while increasing cardiac output. Large clinical trials have clearly demonstrated that ACE inhibitors improve symptoms and survival in patients with LV systolic dysfunction. ACE inhibitors may also prevent the development of HF in patients with asymptomatic LV dysfunction and in those at high risk of developing structural heart disease or HF symptoms (coronary artery disease, diabetes mellitus,

**Table 6-2.** Drugs commonly used for treatment of heart failure

| Drug | Initial dose | Target |
|---|---|---|
| **Angiotensin-converting enzyme inhibitors** | | |
| Captopril | 6.25–12.5 mg q6–8h | 50 mg tid |
| Enalapril | 2.5 mg bid | 10 mg bid |
| Fosinopril | 5–10 mg qd; can use bid | 20 mg qd |
| Lisinopril | 2.5–5.0 mg qd; can use bid | 10–20 mg bid |
| Quinapril | 2.5–5.0 mg bid | 10 mg bid |
| Ramipril | 1.25–2.5 mg bid | 5 mg bid |
| Trandolapril | 0.5–1.0 mg qd | 4 mg qd |
| **Angiotensin receptor blockers** | | |
| Valsartan[a] | 40 mg bid | 160 mg bid |
| Losartan | 25 mg qd; can use bid | 25–100 mg qd |
| Irbesartan | 75–150 mg qd | 75–300 mg qd |
| Candesartan | 2–16 mg qd | 2–32 mg qd |
| Olmesartan | 20 mg qd | 20–40 mg qd |
| **Thiazide diuretics** | | |
| HCTZ | 25–50 mg qd | 25–50 mg qd |
| Metolazone | 2.5–5.0 mg qd or bid | 10–20 total mg qd |
| **Loop diuretics** | | |
| Bumetanide | 0.5–1.0 mg qd or bid | 10 mg total qd (maximum) |
| Furosemide | 20–40 mg qd or bid | 400 total mg qd (maximum) |
| Torsemide | 10–20 mg qd or bid | 200 total mg qd (maximum) |
| **Aldosterone antagonists** | | |
| Eplerenone | 25 mg qd | 50 mg qd |
| Spironolactone | 12.5–25.0 mg qd | 25 mg qd |
| **Beta-blockers** | | |
| Bisoprolol | 1.25 mg qd | 10 mg qd |
| Carvedilol | 3.125 mg q12h | 25–50 mg q12h |
| Metoprolol succinate | 12.5–25.0 mg qd | 200 mg qd |
| **Digoxin** | 0.125–0.25 mg qd | 0.125–0.25 mg qd |

HCTZ, hydrochlorothiazide.
[a]Valsartan is the only U.S. Food and Drug Administration–approved angiotensin II–receptor blocker in the treatment of heart failure.

HTN). Currently, no consensus has been reached regarding the optimal dosing of ACE inhibitors in HF, although one study suggested that higher doses decrease morbidity without improving overall survival (*Circulation* 100:2312, 1999). Absence of an initial beneficial response to treatment with an ACE inhibitor does not preclude long-term benefit. Most ACE inhibitors are excreted by the kidneys, necessitating careful dose titration in patients with renal insufficiency. Acute renal insufficiency may occur in patients with bilateral renal artery stenosis. Additional adverse effects include rash, angioedema, dysgeusia, increases in serum creatinine, proteinuria, hyperkalemia, leukopenia, and cough. **ACE inhibitors are contraindicated in pregnancy.** Oral potassium supplements, potassium salt substitutes, and potassium-sparing diuretics should be used with caution during treatment with an ACE inhibitor. Agranulocytosis and angioedema are more common with captopril than with other ACE inhibitors, particularly in patients with associated collagen vascular disease or serum creatinine greater than 1.5 mg/dl.

**(2) Angiotensin II–receptor blockers (ARBs)** (Table 6-2) inhibit the renin-angiotensin system via specific blockade of the angiotensin II receptor. In contrast to ACE inhibitors, they do not increase bradykinin levels, which may be responsible for adverse effects such as cough. ARBs reduce mortality and morbidity associated with HF in patients who are not receiving an ACE inhibitor (*Lancet* 355:1582, 2000; *N Engl J Med* 345:1667, 2001; *Lancet* 362:772, 2003). ARBs should be considered in patients who are intolerant to ACE inhibitors due to cough or angioedema. Caution should be exercised when ARBS are used in patients with renal insufficiency and bilateral renal artery stenosis because hyperkalemia and acute renal failure can develop. Renal function and potassium levels should be periodically monitored. ARBs are contraindicated in pregnancy.

**(3) Nitrates** are predominantly venodilators and help relieve symptoms of venous and pulmonary congestion. They reduce myocardial ischemia by decreasing ventricular filling pressures and by directly dilating coronary arteries. Nitrate therapy may precipitate hypotension in patients with reduced preload.

**(4) Hydralazine** acts directly on arterial smooth muscle to produce vasodilation and to reduce afterload. In combination with nitrates, hydralazine improves survival in patients with HF (*N Engl J Med* 314:1547, 1986). Dosage requirements vary widely, but most patients benefit from 25–100 mg PO three or four times a day. Hemodynamic tolerance has been reported and may be reduced by concomitant diuretic use. Reflex tachycardia and increased myocardial oxygen consumption may occur, requiring cautious use in patients with ischemic heart disease. Other adverse effects are described in Chap. 4, Hypertension.

**(5) α-Adrenergic receptor antagonists** such as prazosin and doxazosin have vasodilatory properties and are effective antihypertensive medications (see Chap. 4, Hypertension). α-Adrenergic blockade reduces afterload by antagonizing the effects of norepinephrine. These agents have not been shown to improve survival in HF, and hypertensive patients treated with doxazosin as first-line therapy had an increased risk of developing HF (*JAMA* 283:1967, 2000).

**b. Parenteral vasodilators should be reserved for patients with severe HF** or those who are unable to take oral medications. IV vasodilator therapy may be guided by central hemodynamic monitoring (pulmonary artery catheterization) to assess efficacy and avoid hemodynamic instability. Parenteral agents should be started at low doses, titrated to the desired hemodynamic effect, and discontinued slowly to avoid rebound vasoconstriction.

**(1) Nitroglycerin** is a potent vasodilator, with effects on venous and, to a lesser extent, arterial vascular beds. It relieves pulmonary and systemic venous congestion and is an effective coronary vasodilator. Nitroglycerin is the preferred vasodilator for treatment of HF in the setting of acute myocardial infarction (MI) or unstable angina. (For dosing, see Chap. 5, Ischemic Heart Disease.)

**(2) Sodium nitroprusside** is a direct arterial vasodilator with less potent venodilatory properties. Its predominant effect is to reduce afterload, and it is particularly effective in patients with HF who are hypertensive or who have severe aortic or mitral valvular regurgitation. Nitroprusside should be used cautiously in patients with myocardial ischemia because of a potential reduction in regional myocardial blood flow (coronary steal). The initial dose of 10 μg/minute can be titrated (maximum dose of 300–400 μg/minute) to the desired hemodynamic effect or until hypotension develops. The half-life of nitroprusside is 1–3 minutes, and its metabolism results in the release of cyanide, which is metabolized hepatically to thiocyanate and then is excreted renally. Toxic levels of thiocyanate (>10 mg/dl) may develop in patients with renal insufficiency. Thiocyanate toxicity is manifested as nausea, paresthesias, mental status changes, abdominal pain, and seizures (see Chap. 4, Hypertension). Methemoglobinemia is a rare complication of treatment with nitroprusside.

(3) **Recombinant BNP (nesiritide)** is an arterial and venous vasodilator. Intravenous infusion of nesiritide reduces right atrial and left ventricular end-diastolic pressures (LVEDP) and SVR and results in an increase in cardiac output. It also increases sodium delivery to the distal tubules, which results in diuresis when used in conjunction with a loop diuretic. It is administered as a 2-μg/kg IV bolus followed by a continuous IV infusion of 0.01–0.03 μg/kg/minute. Nesiritide is approved for use in acute HF exacerbations and relieves HF symptoms early after its administration (*JAMA* 287:1531, 2002). Hypotension is the most common side effect of nesiritide, and it should be avoided in patients with systemic hypotension (systolic BP <90 mm Hg) or evidence of cardiogenic shock. Episodes of hypotension should be managed with discontinuation of nesiritide and cautious volume expansion or pressor support if necessary.

(4) **Enalaprilat** is an active metabolite of enalapril that is available for IV administration. Its onset of action is more rapid and its pharmacologic half-life shorter than that of enalapril. The initial dosage is 1.25 mg IV q6h, which can be titrated to a maximum dosage of 5 mg IV q6h. Patients who take diuretics or those with impaired renal function (serum creatinine >3 mg/dl, creatinine clearance <30 ml/minute) initially should receive 0.625 mg IV q6h. When dosing is being converted from IV to PO administration, enalaprilat, 0.625 mg IV q6h, is approximately equivalent to enalapril, 2.5 mg PO daily.

2. **β-Adrenergic receptor antagonists** (see Chap. 4, Hypertension, and Table 6-2) are critical components of HF pharmacotherapy that block the cardiac effects of chronic adrenergic stimulation, including myocyte toxicity. Large randomized trials have documented the beneficial effects of β-adrenergic antagonists on functional status and survival in patients with New York Heart Association (NYHA) class II–IV symptoms. β-Adrenergic antagonists should be added to vasodilator and diuretic therapy for HF patients with stable HF symptoms. Improvement in EF, exercise tolerance, and functional class are common after the institution of a β-adrenergic antagonist. Typically, 2–3 months of therapy is required to observe significant effects on LV function, but reduction of cardiac arrhythmia and incidence of sudden cardiac death may occur much earlier [*JAMA* 289(6):712, 2003]. β-Adrenergic antagonists should be instituted at a low dose and titrated with careful attention to BP and heart rate. Some patients experience volume retention and worsening HF symptoms that typically respond to transient increases in diuretic therapy. Individual β-adrenergic antagonists have unique properties (see Chap. 4, Hypertension), and the beneficial effect of β-adrenergic antagonists in HF may not be a class effect (*Lancet* 362:7, 2003). Therefore, β-adrenergic antagonists

with proven effects on patient survival in large clinical trials (bisoprolol, metoprolol succinate, and carvedilol) should be used.

a. **Bisoprolol** (Table 6-2) (*Lancet* 353:9, 1999)
b. **Carvedilol** (Table 6-2) (*Circulation* 94:2793, 1996; *Circulation* 94:2817, 1996; *N Engl J Med* 344:1651, 2001)
c. **Metoprolol succinate** (Table 6-2) (*JAMA* 283:1295, 2000)

3. **Digitalis glycosides** increase myocardial contractility and may attenuate the neurohormonal activation associated with HF. Digoxin decreases the number of HF hospitalizations without altering overall mortality (*N Engl J Med* 336:525, 1997). Discontinuation of digoxin in patients who are stable on a regimen of digoxin, diuretics, and an ACE inhibitor may result in clinical deterioration (*N Engl J Med* 329:1, 1993). **The toxic-therapeutic ratio is narrow,** and serum levels should be followed closely, particularly in patients with unstable renal function.
   a. **The usual daily dose** is 0.125–0.25 mg and should be decreased in patients with renal insufficiency. Clinical benefits may not be related to the serum levels, and, although serum digoxin levels of 0.8–2.0 ng/ml are considered "therapeutic," toxicity can occur in this range. Observations suggest that women and patients with higher serum digoxin levels (1.2–2.0 ng/ml) have an increased mortality risk [*N Engl J Med* 347:1403, 2002; *JAMA* 289(7):871, 2003].
   b. **Drug interactions with digoxin** are common. Oral antibiotics such as erythromycin and tetracycline may increase digoxin levels by 10–40%. Quinidine, verapamil, flecainide, and amiodarone also increase digoxin levels significantly.
   c. **Digoxin toxicity** may be caused or exacerbated by drug interactions, electrolyte abnormalities (particularly hypokalemia), hypoxemia, hypothyroidism, renal insufficiency, and volume depletion.
      (1) **Clinical manifestations of digoxin toxicity** include all forms of cardiac arrhythmias. Bidirectional ventricular tachycardia (VT), paroxysmal atrial tachycardia with atrioventricular block, and a regular accelerated junctional rhythm in the presence of atrial fibrillation are almost exclusively the result of digoxin toxicity. Noncardiac manifestations of toxicity include GI (anorexia, nausea, vomiting, and diarrhea) and neuropsychiatric symptoms [altered mental status, agitation, lethargy, and visual disturbances (scotomas and color perception changes)].
      (2) **Management of digoxin toxicity** includes discontinuation of the drug, correction of precipitating factors, and continuous ECG monitoring. The serum potassium level should be maintained in the high-normal range but should be replenished cautiously because rapid increases can precipitate complete heart block. Symptomatic bradycardia can be controlled with atropine or temporary pacing; sympathomimetics should be avoided, as they may precipitate or worsen ventricular arrhythmias. Lidocaine or phenytoin should be used to control ventricular and atrial arrhythmias; quinidine should not be used, because it may elevate serum levels further (see Chap. 7, Cardiac Arrhythmias). Cardioversion is contraindicated unless all other measures of controlling hemodynamically significant arrhythmias have been exhausted. **Digoxin-specific Fab antibody fragments** are effective in rapidly reversing life-threatening digoxin intoxication and should be considered when other modes of therapy are inadequate. Digoxin-specific Fab fragment complexes are cleared from the circulation via renal excretion. **Total serum digoxin levels are no longer meaningful after administration of Fab fragments.** Each 40-mg vial of Fab fragments neutralizes approximately 0.6 mg digoxin. Dosage is based on the steady-state serum level (see Table 25-2).

4. The use of **diuretics** (Table 6-2), in conjunction with restriction of dietary sodium and fluids, often leads to clinical improvement in patients with symptomatic HF. Frequent assessment of the patient's weight along with careful observation of fluid intake and output is essential during initiation and maintenance of therapy. Frequent complications of therapy include hypokalemia, hyponatremia, hypomagnesemia, volume contraction alkalosis, intravascular volume depletion, and hypotension. Serum electrolytes, BUN, and creatinine levels should be followed after institution of diuretic therapy. Hypokalemia may be life-threatening in patients who are receiving digoxin or in those who have severe LV dysfunction that predisposes them to ventricular arrhythmias. Potassium supplementation or a potassium-sparing diuretic should be considered in addition to careful monitoring of serum potassium levels.
   a. **Thiazide diuretics** (hydrochlorothiazide, chlorthalidone) can be used as initial agents in patients with normal renal function in whom only a mild diuresis is desired. Metolazone, unlike other thiazides, exerts its action at the proximal as well as the distal tubule and may be useful in combination with a loop diuretic in patients with a low glomerular filtration rate.
   b. **Loop diuretics** should be used in patients who require significant diuresis and in those with markedly decreased renal function. Furosemide reduces preload acutely by causing direct venodilation when administered IV, making it useful for managing severe HF or acute pulmonary edema. Use of loop diuretics may be complicated by hyperuricemia, hypocalcemia, ototoxicity, rash, and vasculitis. Furosemide and bumetanide are sulfa derivatives and may cause drug reactions in sulfa-sensitive patients. Ethacrynic acid can generally be used safely in such patients.
   c. **Potassium-sparing diuretics** do not exert a potent diuretic effect when used alone. Spironolactone (25 mg daily) is an aldosterone receptor antagonist that has been shown to improve survival and decrease hospitalizations in NYHA class III–IV patients (*N Engl J Med* 341:753, 1999). The potential for development of life-threatening hyperkalemia exists with the use of these agents. Gynecomastia may develop in 10–20% of men treated with spironolactone. **Serum potassium** must be monitored closely after initiation; concomitant use of ACE inhibitors and NSAIDs, and the presence of renal insufficiency (creatinine >2.5 mg/dl), increase the risk of hyperkalemia. Eplerenone, a selective aldosterone receptor antagonist without the hormonal side effects of spironolactone, is U.S. Food and Drug Administration approved for treatment of HTN and HF and reduces mortality in patients with HF associated with acute MI (*N Engl J Med* 348:1309, 2003).
5. **Inotropic agents**
   a. **Sympathomimetic agents** (see Appendix D, Intravenous Admixture Preparation and Administration Guide, and Table 6-3) are potent drugs that are primarily used to treat severe HF. Beneficial and adverse effects are mediated by stimulation of myocardial β-adrenergic receptors. The most important adverse effects are related to the arrhythmogenic nature of these agents and the potential for exacerbation of myocardial ischemia. Treatment should be guided by careful hemodynamic and ECG monitoring. Patients with refractory chronic HF may benefit symptomatically from continuous ambulatory administration of IV inotropes as palliative therapy or as a bridge to mechanical ventricular support or cardiac transplantation [*J Am Coll Cardiol* 38(7):2102, 2001]. However, this strategy may increase the risk of life-threatening arrhythmias or indwelling catheter-related infections.
      (1) **Dopamine** (Table 6-3) should be used primarily for stabilization of the hypotensive patient.

**Table 6-3.** Inotropic agents

| Drug | Dose | Mechanism | Effects/side effects |
|---|---|---|---|
| Dopamine | 1–3 μg/kg/min | Dopaminergic receptors | Splanchnic vasodilation |
| | 2–8 μg/kg/min | $\beta_1$-Receptor agonist | +Inotropic |
| | 7–10 μg/kg/min | α-Receptor agonist | ↑ SVR |
| Dobutamine | 2.5–15.0 μg/kg/min | $\beta_1$->$\beta_2$->α-receptor agonist | +Inotropic, ↓ SVR, tachycardia |
| Amrinone[a] | 750-μg/kg bolus IV over 2–3 min, 2.5–10.0 μg/kg/min | ↑ cAMP | ↓ SVR, +inotropic; ↓ platelets; atrial and ventricular tachyarrhythmias |
| Milrinone[a] | 50-μg/kg bolus IV over 10 min, 0.375–0.75 μg/kg/min | ↑ cAMP | ↓ SVR, +inotropic; atrial and ventricular tachyarrhythmias |

cAMP, cyclic adenosine monophosphate; SVR, systemic vascular resistance; ↑, increased; ↓, decreased.
[a]Needs dose adjustment for creatinine clearance.

(2) **Dobutamine** (Table 6-3) is a synthetic analog of dopamine. Dobutamine tolerance has been described, and several studies have demonstrated increased mortality in patients treated with continuous dobutamine. Dobutamine has no significant role in the treatment of HF resulting from diastolic dysfunction or a high-output state.

b. **Phosphodiesterase inhibitors** (see Appendix D, Intravenous Admixture Preparation and Administration Guide, and Table 6-3) increase myocardial contractility and produce vasodilation by increasing intracellular cyclic adenosine monophosphate. Amrinone and milrinone are currently available for clinical use and are indicated for treatment of refractory HF. Hypotension may develop in patients who receive vasodilator therapy or have intravascular volume contraction, or both. Amrinone and milrinone may improve hemodynamics in patients who are treated concurrently with dobutamine or dopamine. Data suggest that in-hospital short-term milrinone administration in addition to standard medical therapy does not reduce the length of hospitalization or the 60-day death or rehospitalization rate when compared with placebo (*JAMA* 287:1541, 2002).

C. **Cardiac resynchronization therapy or biventricular pacing** (see Chap. 7, Cardiac Arrhythmias) appears to be beneficial in patients with NYHA class III–IV HF and conduction abnormalities (left bundle branch block, atrioventricular delay).

D. **Mechanical circulatory support** can be considered for patients in whom other therapeutic modalities have failed, who have transient myocardial dysfunction, or in whom a more definitive procedure, such as transplantation, is planned.

1. **Enhanced external counterpulsation**, initially approved for chronic angina refractory to medical and revascularization therapy, is a pneumatic leg wrap with sequential inflation/deflation that is timed complementary to the cardiac cycle. The treatment consists of 35 1-hour sessions. Studies in patients with stable angina documented a decrease in afterload and LV filling pressures, an increase in coronary perfusion, and improved quality of life. Enhanced external counterpulsation in patients

with stable HF (NYHA II–III, EF <35%) is safe, improves exercise capacity, decreases angina, and improves quality of life at 6 months [*J Am Coll Cardiol* 33(7):1833, 1999; *Congest Heart Fail* 8(4):204, 2002].

2. **The intra-aortic balloon pump** is positioned in the aorta with its tip distal to the left subclavian artery. Balloon inflation is synchronous with the cardiac cycle and results in significant preload and afterload reduction, with decreased myocardial oxygen demand and improved coronary blood flow, resulting in improved cardiac output. Severe aortoiliac atherosclerosis and aortic valve insufficiency are contraindications to intra-aortic balloon pump placement.
3. **Ventricular assist devices** require surgical implantation and are indicated for patients with severe HF after cardiac surgery, for individuals who have intractable cardiogenic shock after acute MI, and for patients whose conditions deteriorate while they await cardiac transplantation. Currently available devices vary with regard to degree of mechanical hemolysis, intensity of anticoagulation required, and difficulty of implantation. Therefore, the decision to institute ventricular assist device circulatory support must be made in consultation with a cardiac surgeon who has experience with this procedure. Ventricular assist devices improve survival in patients with refractory HF who are not candidates for cardiac transplantation ("destination therapy") (*N Engl J Med* 345:1435, 2001).

E. **Cardiac transplantation** is an option for selected patients with severe end-stage HF that has become refractory to aggressive medical therapy and for whom no other conventional treatment options are available.

1. **Candidates considered for transplantation** should be younger than 65 years (although selected older patients may also benefit), have advanced HF (NYHA class III–IV), have a strong psychological support system, have exhausted all other therapeutic options, and be free of irreversible extracardiac organ dysfunction that would limit functional recovery or predispose them to posttransplantation complications (*J Am Coll Cardiol* 22:1, 1993).
2. **Survival rates** of 90% at 1 year and 70% at 5 years have been reported since the introduction of cyclosporine-based immunosuppression. In general, functional capacity and quality of life improve significantly after transplantation.
3. **Immunosuppressive therapy** typically includes cyclosporine or tacrolimus-based regimens in combination with azathioprine, mycophenolate mofetil, sirolimus, and/or glucocorticoids (see Chap. 15, Solid Organ Transplant Medicine).
4. **Posttransplant complications** include acute and chronic rejection, typical and atypical infections, and adverse effects of immunosuppressive agents (see Chap. 15, Solid Organ Transplant Medicine). Cardiac allograft vasculopathy (coronary artery disease/chronic rejection) and malignancy are the leading causes of death after the first posttransplant year.

F. **End-of-life considerations** may be necessary in the patient with advanced HF that is refractory to therapy. Discussions regarding the disease course, treatment options, survival, functional status, and advance directives should be addressed early in the treatment of the patient with HF. For those with end-stage disease (stage D, NYHA class IV) with multiple hospitalizations and severe decline in their functional status and quality of life, hospice and palliative care should be considered.

**III. Acute HF and cardiogenic pulmonary edema (CPE)**

A. **Pathophysiology.** CPE occurs when the pulmonary capillary pressure exceeds the forces (serum oncotic pressure and interstitial hydrostatic pressure) that maintain fluid within the vascular space. Accumulation of fluid in the pulmonary interstitium is followed by alveolar flooding and disturbance of gas exchange. Increased pulmonary capillary pressure may be caused by LV failure of any cause, obstruction to transmitral flow [e.g., mitral stenosis (MS), atrial myxoma], or, rarely, pulmonary veno-occlusive disease.

**B. Diagnosis**

1. **Clinical manifestations** of CPE may occur rapidly and include dyspnea, anxiety, and restlessness. Physical signs of decreased peripheral perfusion, pulmonary congestion, use of accessory respiratory muscles, and wheezing often are present. The patient may expectorate pink frothy fluid.
2. **Radiographic abnormalities** include cardiomegaly, interstitial and perihilar vascular engorgement, Kerley B lines, and pleural effusions. The radiographic abnormalities may follow the development of symptoms by several hours, and their resolution may be out of phase with clinical improvement.

**C. Management**

1. **Initial supportive treatment** of CPE includes administration of oxygen to raise the arterial oxygen tension to greater than 60 mm Hg. Mechanical ventilation is indicated if hypercapnia coexists or if oxygenation is inadequate by other means. A sitting position improves pulmonary function. Placing the patient on strict bed rest and reducing pain and anxiety decrease cardiac workload.
2. **Pharmacologic treatment**
   a. **Morphine sulfate** reduces anxiety and dilates pulmonary and systemic veins. Morphine, 2–5 mg IV, can be given over several minutes and can be repeated every 10–25 minutes until an effect is seen.
   b. **Furosemide** is a venodilator that decreases pulmonary congestion within minutes of IV administration, well before its diuretic action begins. An initial dose of 20–80 mg IV should be given over several minutes and can be increased based on response, to a maximum of 200 mg in subsequent doses.
   c. **Nitroglycerin** is a venodilator that can potentiate the effect of furosemide. IV administration is preferable to oral and transdermal forms because it can be rapidly titrated.
   d. **Nitroprusside** [see sec. **II.B.1.b.(2)**] is an effective adjunct in the treatment of acute CPE. It is useful in CPE that results from acute valvular regurgitation or HTN (see Valvular Heart Disease, sec. **III.B.2.a**). Pulmonary and systemic arterial catheterization should be considered to guide titration of nitroprusside therapy.
   e. **Inotropic agents,** such as dobutamine or phosphodiesterase inhibitors, may be helpful after initial treatment of CPE in patients with concomitant hypotension or shock (see sec. **II.B.5**).
   f. **Recombinant BNP (nesiritide)** is administered as an IV bolus followed by an IV infusion. It reduces intracardiac filling pressures by producing vasodilation and indirectly increases the cardiac output. In conjunction with furosemide (Lasix), nesiritide produces natriuresis and diuresis [see sec. **II.B.1.b.(3)**].
3. **Acute hemodialysis and ultrafiltration** may be effective, especially in the patient with significant renal dysfunction and diuretic resistance.
4. **Right heart catheterization** (e.g., Swan-Ganz catheter) may be helpful in cases in which a prompt response to therapy does not occur. The pulmonary artery catheter allows differentiation between cardiogenic and noncardiogenic causes of pulmonary edema via measurement of central hemodynamics and cardiac output and helps to guide subsequent therapy (see Chap. 9, Pulmonary Disease).
5. **Precipitating factors should be corrected.** Common precipitants of pulmonary edema include severe HTN, MI, or myocardial ischemia (particularly if associated with MR); acute valvular regurgitation; new-onset tachyarrhythmias or bradyarrhythmias; and volume overload in the setting of severe LV dysfunction. Successful resolution of pulmonary edema can often be accomplished only by correction of the underlying process.

# Cardiomyopathy

I. **Dilated cardiomyopathy** is a disease of heart muscle characterized by dilatation of the cardiac chambers and reduction in ventricular contractile function. Dilatation may be secondary to progression of any process that affects the myocardium and is directly related to neurohormonal activation. The majority of cases are idiopathic.

A. **Pathophysiology and clinical features.** Dilatation of the cardiac chambers and varying degrees of hypertrophy are anatomic hallmarks. Symptomatic HF often is present. Tricuspid and mitral regurgitation (MR) are common due to the effect of chamber dilatation on the valvular apparatus. Atrial and ventricular arrhythmias are present in as many as one-half of these patients and probably are responsible for the high incidence of sudden death in this population.

B. **Diagnosis.** The diagnosis can be confirmed with echocardiography or radionuclide ventriculography. Two-dimensional and Doppler echocardiography is helpful in differentiating this condition from hypertrophic or restrictive cardiomyopathy, pericardial disease, and valvular disorders. The ECG is usually abnormal, but changes are typically nonspecific. Endomyocardial biopsy provides little information that affects treatment of patients with dilated cardiomyopathies and is not routinely recommended.

C. **The medical management** of symptomatic patients is identical to that for HF from any cause. The therapeutic strategies include control of total body sodium and volume as well as appropriate preload and afterload reduction using vasodilator therapy. β-Adrenergic antagonists should be used unless contraindicated. Immunizations against influenza and pneumococcal pneumonia are recommended.

1. **Ventricular arrhythmia** (see Chap. 7, Cardiac Arrhythmias) occurs with increased frequency in patients with dilated cardiomyopathy. Sudden cardiac death is relatively more common in patients with mild to moderate symptoms when compared to NYHA class IV HF patients, who are more likely to die of progressive pump failure. Suppression of asymptomatic ventricular premature beats or nonsustained ventricular tachycardia (NSVT) using antiarrhythmic drugs in patients with HF does not improve survival and may increase mortality as a result of the proarrhythmic effects of the drugs (*N Engl J Med* 321:406, 1989; *N Engl J Med* 333:77, 1995).

   Dilated cardiomyopathy (of nonischemic origin) is associated with an increased incidence of sudden cardiac death (SCD). However, there is no benefit from primary prevention of SCD using amiodarone (*N Engl J Med* 333:77,1995), and limited data are available using implantable cardioverter-defibrillator (ICD) implantation as primary prevention. Electrophysiology testing in the absence of sustained VT has limited prognostic value [*J Am Coll Cardiol* 40(9):2155, 2002]. Aggressive HF medical treatment, including β-adrenergic blockade, correction of electrolyte imbalances, and discontinuation of proarrhythmic drugs, is recommended.

2. **Cardiac resynchronization therapy** may be beneficial in selected patients with symptomatic HF (see Chap. 7, Cardiac Arrhythmias).

3. **Chronic oral anticoagulation** has not been shown to decrease the risk of thromboembolism in patients with LV dysfunction. Anticoagulation should be strongly considered in individuals with a history of thromboembolic events, atrial fibrillation, or evidence of an LV thrombus. The level of anticoagulation recommended varies but is generally an international normalized ratio of 2.0–3.0 (see Chap. 18, Disorders of Hemostasis).

4. **Immunosuppressive therapy** with agents such as prednisone, azathioprine, and cyclosporine for biopsy-proven myocarditis has been advocated by some, but efficacy has not been established (*N Engl J Med* 333:269, 1995).

D. **Surgical management.** Primary valvular disease and coronary disease should be evaluated and corrected as indicated (see Valvular Heart Disease and Chap. 5, Ischemic Heart Disease). Coronary revascularization reduces ischemia and may improve systolic function in some patients with coronary artery disease. Intra-aortic balloon counterpulsation or placement of a ventricular assist device may be necessary for stabilization of patients in whom cardiac transplantation is an option or before other definitive surgical therapies. Mitral valve annuloplasty or replacement can be used for symptomatic relief in patients with severe MR. Cardiac transplantation should be considered for selected patients with HF that is refractory to medical therapy (see Heart Failure, sec. **II.E**).

II. **Diastolic dysfunction** accounts for 20–40% of the HF cases. Causes include HTN, ischemia, hypertrophic cardiomyopathy (HCM), restrictive cardiomyopathies, infiltrative disease (amyloidosis, sarcoidosis), and constrictive pericarditis. Diagnosis is often based on two-dimensional echocardiography with Doppler that shows normal LV systolic function with impaired diastolic relaxation. Treatment is directed toward improving the symptoms with diuretic therapy and correcting the precipitating factors (e.g., HTN, coronary artery disease, tachycardia).

III. **HCM** is a myocardial disorder characterized by ventricular hypertrophy, diminished LV cavity dimensions, normal or enhanced contractile function, and impaired ventricular relaxation. The idiopathic form of HCM has an early onset (as early as the first decade of life) without associated HTN. Many cases have a genetic component, with mutations in the myosin heavy-chain gene that follow an autosomal-dominant transmission with variable phenotypic expression and penetrance. An acquired form also occurs in elderly patients with chronic HTN.

A. **The pathophysiologic change** in HCM is myocardial hypertrophy that is typically predominant in the ventricular septum (asymmetric hypertrophy) but may involve all ventricular segments equally. The disease can be classified according to the presence or absence of LV outflow tract obstruction. LV outflow obstruction may occur at rest but is enhanced by factors that increase LV contractility or decrease ventricular volume. Delayed ventricular diastolic relaxation and decreased compliance are common and may lead to pulmonary congestion. Myocardial ischemia is frequently secondary to a myocardial oxygen supply-demand mismatch. **Systolic anterior motion** of the anterior leaflet of the mitral valve often is associated with MR and may contribute to LV outflow tract obstruction.

B. **The clinical presentation** varies but may include dyspnea, angina, arrhythmias, syncope, cardiac failure, or sudden death. Sudden death is most common in children and young adults between the ages of 10 and 35 years and often occurs during periods of strenuous exertion. Physical findings include a bisferious carotid pulse (in the presence of obstruction), a forceful double or triple apical impulse, and a coarse systolic outflow murmur localized along the left sternal border that is accentuated by maneuvers that decrease preload (e.g., standing, Valsalva maneuver).

C. **The diagnosis** is suspected on the basis of clinical presentation or a family history suggestive of familial HCM and is confirmed by two-dimensional echocardiography. Doppler flow studies may be useful in establishing the presence of a significant LV outflow gradient at rest or with provocation. Patients should undergo **risk stratification,** which includes history and physical examination, transthoracic echocardiogram, 24- to 48-hour Holter monitoring, and exercise testing.

D. **Management** is directed toward relief of symptoms and prevention of endocarditis, arrhythmias, and sudden death. Treatment in asymptomatic individuals is controversial, and no conclusive evidence has been found that medical therapy is beneficial. **All individuals with HCM should avoid strenuous physical activity,** including most competitive sports.

1. **Medical therapy**

a. **β-Adrenergic antagonists** may reduce symptoms of HCM by reducing myocardial contractility and heart rate. However, symptoms may recur during long-term therapy.

b. **Calcium channel antagonists,** particularly **verapamil** and **diltiazem,** may improve the symptoms of HCM, primarily by augmentation of diastolic ventricular filling. Dihydropyridines should be avoided in patients with LV outflow tract obstruction as a result of their vasodilatory properties. Therapy should be initiated at low doses, with careful titration in patients with outflow obstruction. The dose should be increased gradually over several days to weeks if symptoms persist.

c. **Diuretics** may improve pulmonary congestive symptoms in patients with elevated pulmonary venous pressures. These agents should be used cautiously in patients with severe LV outflow obstruction because excessive preload reduction worsens the obstruction.

d. **Nitrates and vasodilators should be avoided** because of the risk of increasing the LV outflow gradient.

2. **Atrial and ventricular arrhythmias occur commonly** in patients with HCM. Supraventricular tachyarrhythmias are tolerated poorly and should be treated aggressively; cardioversion is indicated if hemodynamic compromise develops. **Digoxin is relatively contraindicated** because of its positive inotropic properties and potential for exacerbating ventricular outflow obstruction. Atrial fibrillation should be converted to sinus rhythm when possible. Diltiazem, verapamil, or β-adrenergic antagonists can be used to control the ventricular response before cardioversion. Procainamide, disopyramide, or amiodarone (see Chap. 7, Cardiac Arrhythmias) may be effective in the chronic suppression of atrial fibrillation. Patients with NSVT detected on ambulatory monitoring are at increased risk for sudden death. However, the benefit of suppressing these arrhythmias with medical therapy has not been established, and the risk of a proarrhythmic effect of antiarrhythmic drugs exists. The benefit of invasive electrophysiologic testing in predicting patients with HCM who are at high risk for SCD is controversial. ICD placement should be considered in high-risk patients: those with genetic mutations associated with SCD; prior SCD or sustained VT; a history of syncope or near-syncope, recurrent or exertional, in young patients; multiple nonsustained episodes of VT on Holter recordings; hypotensive response to exercise; LV hypertrophy with a wall thickness greater than 30 mm in young patients; and a history of sudden, premature death in close relatives (*N Engl J Med* 342:365, 2000). Symptomatic ventricular arrhythmias should be treated as outlined in Chap. 7, Cardiac Arrhythmias.

3. **Dual-chamber pacing** (see Chap. 7, Cardiac Arrhythmias) improves symptoms in HCM (*Circulation* 85:2149, 1992). Alteration of the ventricular activation sequence via right ventricular (RV) pacing may minimize LV outflow tract obstruction secondary to asymmetric septal hypertrophy. However, only 10% of the patients with HCM meet the criteria for pacemaker implantation, and the effect on decreasing the left ventricular outflow tract (LVOT) gradient is only 25%. The effect of dual-chamber pacing on patient morbidity and mortality is not known.

4. **Prophylaxis for endocarditis** is indicated (see Chap. 13, Treatment of Infectious Diseases).

5. **Anticoagulation** is recommended if paroxysmal or chronic atrial fibrillation develops (see Chap. 18, Disorders of Hemostasis).

6. **Surgical therapy** is useful in the treatment of symptoms but has not been shown to alter the natural history of HCM. The most frequently used operative procedure involves septal myotomy-myectomy with or without mitral valve replacement (MVR). Alcohol septal ablation, a catheter-based alternative to surgical myotomy-myectomy, seems to be equally effective at reducing obstruction and providing symptomatic relief when compared to the gold standard surgical procedure (*Eur Heart J* 23:1617, 2002).

7. **Genetic counseling and family screening** are recommended for first-degree relatives of patients at high risk for SCD, because the disease is transmitted as an autosomal-dominant trait. Screening should include

a careful physical examination and two-dimensional echocardiography with Doppler.

8. **Cardiac transplantation** should be reserved for patients with end-stage HCM with symptomatic HF.

IV. **Restrictive cardiomyopathy** results from pathologic infiltration of the myocardium by amyloidosis or sarcoidosis. Less common causes include glycogen storage diseases, hemochromatosis, endomyocardial fibrosis, and hypereosinophilic syndromes.

A. **Pathophysiology and diagnosis.** Myocardial infiltration results in abnormal diastolic ventricular filling and varying degrees of systolic dysfunction. Echocardiography with Doppler analysis may demonstrate thickened myocardium with normal or abnormal systolic function, abnormal diastolic filling patterns, and elevated intracardiac pressure. The ECG may show conduction system disease or low voltage, in contrast to the increased voltage seen with ventricular hypertrophy. Cardiac catheterization reveals elevated RV and LV filling pressures and a classic dip-and-plateau pattern in the RV and LV pressure tracing. RV endomyocardial biopsy may be diagnostic and should be considered in patients in whom a diagnosis is not established. **It is often difficult to differentiate between restrictive cardiomyopathy and constrictive pericarditis** because of similar clinical presentations and hemodynamics, but this distinction is critical, as surgical therapy may be effective for constrictive pericarditis.

B. **Management**

1. **General measures** include use of diuretics for pulmonary and systemic congestion and digoxin if LV systolic dysfunction is present. **Digoxin should be avoided in patients with cardiac amyloidosis** because of enhanced susceptibility to digoxin toxicity.
2. **Specific therapy aimed at amelioration of the underlying cause should be instituted.** Cardiac hemochromatosis may respond to reduction of total body iron stores via phlebotomy or chelation therapy with deferoxamine. Cardiac sarcoidosis may respond to glucocorticoid therapy, but prolongation of survival with this approach has not been established. No therapy is known to be effective in reversing the progression of cardiac amyloidosis.

## Pericardial Disease

I. **Constrictive pericarditis** may develop as a late complication of pericardial inflammation. Most cases are idiopathic, but pericarditis after cardiac surgery and mediastinal irradiation are important identifiable causes. Tuberculous pericarditis is a leading cause of constrictive pericarditis in some underdeveloped countries.

A. **Pathophysiology and diagnosis.** The noncompliant pericardium causes impairment of ventricular filling and progressive elevation of venous pressure. In contrast to cardiac tamponade, the clinical presentation is characteristically insidious, with gradual development of fatigue, exercise intolerance, and venous congestion. Physical findings include jugular venous distention with prominent X and Y descents, inspiratory elevation of the jugular venous pressure (Kussmaul's sign), peripheral edema, ascites, and a pericardial knock during diastole. Echocardiography may reveal pericardial thickening and diminished diastolic filling. In addition, a chest CT scan or MRI demonstrates pericardial thickening. Cardiac catheterization is usually necessary to demonstrate elevated and equalized diastolic pressures in all four cardiac chambers. Constrictive pericarditis often is difficult to distinguish from restrictive cardiomyopathy (see Cardiomyopathy, sec. **III.A**).

**B. Definitive treatment requires complete pericardiectomy**, which is accompanied by significant perioperative mortality (5–10%) but results in clinical improvement in 90% of patients. Patients who are minimally symptomatic can be managed with judicious sodium and fluid restriction and diuretic therapy but must be followed closely to detect hemodynamic deterioration.

**II. Cardiac tamponade** results from increased intrapericardial pressure secondary to fluid accumulation within the pericardial space. Pericarditis of any cause may lead to cardiac tamponade. Idiopathic (or viral) and neoplastic forms are the most frequent causes.

**A. The diagnosis** should be suspected in patients with elevated jugular venous pressure, hypotension, pulsus paradoxus, tachycardia, evidence of poor peripheral perfusion, and distant heart sounds. The ECG often reveals a tachycardia with low voltage and electrical alternans. Echocardiography can confirm the diagnosis of pericardial effusion and demonstrate hemodynamic significance by right atrial and RV diastolic collapse, increased right-sided flows during inspiration, and respiratory variation of the transmitral flow. Right heart catheterization also is helpful in determining the hemodynamic significance of a pericardial effusion, especially in patients with a subacute or chronic presentation. Hemodynamic findings of elevated, equalized diastolic pressures are present in the patient with cardiac tamponade.

**B. Treatment consists of drainage of the pericardial space** via pericardiocentesis or surgical pericardiotomy. Urgent pericardiocentesis should be performed with echocardiographic guidance, if possible. If pericardial drainage cannot be performed, stabilization with parenteral inotropic support and aggressive administration of IV saline to maintain adequate ventricular filling are indicated. **Diuretics, nitrates, or any other preload-reducing agents are absolutely contraindicated.**

## Valvular Heart Disease

**I. Mitral stenosis (MS)** impedes blood flow from the lungs and left atrium into the left ventricle. Rheumatic heart disease is the most common etiology. MS may result from calcium deposition in the mitral annulus and leaflets, from a congenital valvular malformation, or in association with connective tissue disorders. Left atrial myxoma and cor triatriatum may mimic MS clinically. Prosthetic mitral valves (particularly bioprosthetic valves) may become stenotic late after implantation.

**A. Pathophysiology.** Significant MS results in elevation of left atrial, pulmonary venous, and pulmonary capillary pressures, with consequent pulmonary congestion. The degree of pressure elevation depends on the severity of obstruction, flow across the valve, diastolic filling time, and presence of effective atrial contraction. Therefore, factors that normally augment flow across the mitral valve, such as tachycardia, exercise, fever, and pregnancy, result in a marked increase in left atrial pressure and may exacerbate HF symptoms. Left atrial enlargement and fibrillation may result in atrial thrombus formation, which is primarily responsible for the high incidence (20%) of systemic embolization in patients with MS who are not anticoagulated.

**B. Diagnosis.** Symptoms of pulmonary congestion, such as dyspnea, cough, and, occasionally, hemoptysis are prominent. Physical signs of pulmonary venous congestion and right heart volume and pressure overload often are present. A loud $S_1$, early diastolic opening snap, and rumbling diastolic murmur are present on auscultation. The diagnosis and severity of MS can be confirmed by two-dimensional and Doppler echocardiography. Transesophageal echocardiography (TEE) can also be used to confirm the diagnosis, define the anatomy more fully, and provide diagnostic information in patients in whom transthoracic echocardiography is suboptimal. Cardiac catheterization is indicated in patients in whom there is a likelihood of concomitant coronary artery disease and in whom echocardiographic studies are either technically suboptimal or nondiagnostic.

**C. Medical management**

1. **Factors that increase left atrial pressure,** including tachycardia and fever, should be identified and alleviated. Vigorous physical activity should be avoided in patients with moderate to severe MS.
2. **Diuretics** (see Heart Failure, sec. **II.B.4,** and Table 6-2) are the mainstay of therapy for pulmonary congestion and edema.
3. **Anticoagulant therapy** is indicated for patients with MS and atrial fibrillation (because of the high thromboembolism risk), prior embolic event, or known atrial thrombi. Heparin therapy should be instituted at the onset of atrial fibrillation, followed by long-term warfarin therapy (see Chap. 17, Liver Diseases).
4. **Atrial fibrillation may not be well tolerated.** When the patient is hemodynamically stable, the ventricular response rate to atrial fibrillation can be controlled using digoxin, calcium channel antagonist, or β-adrenergic antagonist (see Chap. 7, Cardiac Arrhythmias). However, synchronized direct current cardioversion should be performed if hemodynamic compromise (hypotension, pulmonary edema, and angina) occurs. An attempt to restore and maintain sinus rhythm may be beneficial. It should be preceded by anticoagulation therapy for at least 3 weeks to minimize the risk of systemic embolization on resumption of normal sinus rhythm. A transesophageal echocardiogram should be performed to evaluate the left atrium for thrombi in patients who require cardioversion before a course of therapeutic anticoagulation. After conversion to sinus rhythm has been accomplished, antiarrhythmics may be beneficial to maintain sinus rhythm.
5. **Infective endocarditis prophylaxis is indicated** (see Chap. 13, Treatment of Infectious Diseases).
6. **Continuous prophylaxis against recurrent rheumatic fever** is indicated in young patients, patients at high risk for streptococcal infection (parents of young children, schoolteachers, medical and military personnel, and those in crowded living conditions), and those who have had acute rheumatic fever within the previous 10 years (see Chap. 13, Treatment of Infectious Diseases).

**D. Surgical considerations**

1. **Patients with severe symptoms** or pulmonary HTN and significant MS (mitral valve area $<1$ cm$^2$/m$^2$) should undergo commissurotomy or MVR.
2. **Patients with mild to moderate symptoms** generally show improvement with diuretic therapy and can be followed with serial echocardiography and clinical evaluation.
3. **A single systemic thromboembolic event** does not necessarily mandate MVR. However, the recurrence rate of systemic thromboembolism in patients with MS is high, even with systemic anticoagulation, and MVR should be strongly considered.
4. **Percutaneous balloon mitral valvuloplasty** can reduce the mitral valve pressure gradient and improve cardiac output in patients with MS. This procedure is an alternative to surgery and carries acceptable morbidity and mortality in select patients without significant MR or severe valvular calcification.

**II. AS** in the adult population may result from (1) calcification and degeneration of a normal valve, (2) calcification and fibrosis of a congenitally bicuspid aortic valve, or (3) rheumatic valvular disease.

**A. Pathophysiology.** AS produces a pressure gradient between the left ventricle and the aorta, causing pressure overload of the left ventricle that leads to concentric hypertrophy. As a result, LV compliance is reduced, LVEDP rises, and myocardial oxygen demand is increased. Elevated LVEDP decreases the perfusion pressure across the myocardium, leading to subendocardial ischemia.

**B. Diagnosis.** The diagnosis of significant AS may be difficult, as the condition may be asymptomatic for a number of years. Clinical suspicion often is raised by the presence of one or more of the classic symptoms in the triad of angina, syncope, and HF. Physical findings include a slowly rising carotid pulse that is sustained (pulsus parvus et tardus) and a mid- to late-peaking systolic murmur that is typically harsh in quality. The pressure gradient across the stenotic aortic valve is directly related to the severity of obstruction and cardiac output. Therefore, the intensity of the systolic murmur may diminish as the cardiac output decreases with increasingly severe AS. In general, murmurs of long duration that peak late in systole indicate severe AS. Doppler echocardiography provides a noninvasive estimation of the aortic valve gradient and aortic valve area, which correlates well with the findings at cardiac catheterization. Most adult patients being considered for aortic valve replacement (AVR) require preoperative cardiac catheterization to determine the extent of concomitant coronary artery disease.

**C. Medical management**

1. **Infective endocarditis** prophylaxis is indicated (see Chap. 13, Treatment of Infectious Diseases).
2. **Vigorous exercise and physical activity** should be avoided in patients with moderate to severe AS.
3. **Atrial (and ventricular) arrhythmias are poorly tolerated** and should be treated (see Chap. 7, Cardiac Arrhythmias).
4. **Digoxin may be useful** in patients with HF in the presence of LV dilatation and impaired systolic function. In severe AS caused by the fixed obstruction of LV outflow, however, inotropic therapy is of little benefit.
5. **Diuretics may be useful** in treating congestive symptoms but must be used with extreme caution. Reduction of LV filling pressure in patients with AS may decrease cardiac output and systemic BP.
6. **Nitrates and other vasodilators should be used with caution** in patients with severe AS, as they may produce severe hypotension and hemodynamic collapse. In patients with severe AS and new-onset angina, nitroglycerin should be initiated cautiously. If nitroglycerin results in hypotension that does not respond to aggressive volume expansion, parenteral inotropic agents (e.g., dobutamine) or vasopressors, or both, should be given.
7. **Asymptomatic patients with mild to moderate AS** can be followed closely with clinical assessment and Doppler echocardiography performed at 6- to 12-month intervals.

**D. Surgical considerations**

1. **Symptomatic patients** should be evaluated for **AVR.** A TEE may be required in patients with suboptimal transthoracic echocardiograms. Coronary arteriography should be performed in men older than 40 years and women older than 50 years, as well as in all patients with anginal symptoms; left ventriculography is indicated in patients with coexistent MR (although a high-quality transthoracic echocardiogram or a TEE may suffice). Symptomatic patients with severe AS (aortic valve area $<1.0$ cm$^2$) and patients with severe AS who are undergoing cardiac or aortic surgery should undergo concomitant AVR. Asymptomatic patients with severe AS should be considered for AVR if LV dilatation or decreased systolic function is present or if they have a hypotensive response to exercise [*J Am Coll Cardiol* 32(5):1486, 1998].
2. **Intra-aortic balloon counterpulsation** may stabilize patients with critical AS and hemodynamic decompensation until AVR can be accomplished. It should not be used when significant aortic insufficiency (AI) coexists with AS.
3. **Percutaneous balloon aortic valvuloplasty** can reduce the aortic valve gradient and improve symptoms and LV function with relatively low morbidity and mortality in selected patients. However, restenosis occurs

in approximately 50% of patients within 6 months. At present, this therapeutic modality is used primarily in patients who require noncardiac surgery before definitive AVR.

**III. MR**

**A. Chronic MR**, as an isolated lesion, is caused most commonly by myxomatous degeneration of the mitral valve. Other etiologies include rheumatic heart disease, calcification of the mitral valve annulus, coronary artery disease with associated papillary muscle dysfunction, infective endocarditis, and connective tissue diseases (e.g., Marfan syndrome, Ehlers-Danlos syndrome). MR may occur as a secondary phenomenon in patients with cardiomyopathy and LV dilatation.

1. **Pathophysiology.** Chronic MR imposes volume overload on the left ventricle as a result of regurgitation of a fraction of the LV blood flow into the left atrium. Normal forward cardiac output is maintained early in the course of the disease, but, with progressive MR, compensatory mechanisms no longer accommodate increasing LV end-diastolic volume. Accordingly, EF falls, and symptoms of right and left HF develop.
2. **Diagnosis.** The diagnosis is suggested by characteristic physical findings of well-preserved carotid pulsations, an enlarged point of maximal impulse, and an apical holosystolic murmur. Doppler and two-dimensional echocardiography confirm the diagnosis, estimate the severity of MR, and provide clues to its etiology. TEE is particularly useful for the evaluation of the mitral valve and is commonly used to evaluate the patient with MR.
3. **Medical management**
   a. **Infective endocarditis prophylaxis** should be given (see Chap. 13, Treatment of Infectious Diseases).
   b. **Anticoagulant therapy** should be considered, particularly in the presence of atrial fibrillation, an enlarged left atrium, or a previous embolic event.
   c. **Vasodilators provide hemodynamic improvement** in MR by reducing SVR, thus decreasing the mitral regurgitant fraction and augmenting forward cardiac output. Beneficial effects have been demonstrated with nitroprusside, captopril, enalapril, and hydralazine.
   d. **Digoxin may be useful** in the presence of impaired LV systolic function.
   e. **Diuretics** are useful for treating congestive symptoms.
   f. **Nitrates** can also be used to reduce preload and ventricular size, which may decrease the severity of MR.
4. **Surgical considerations**
   a. **Patients with moderate to severe symptoms** despite medical therapy should be considered for mitral valve repair or replacement if the LVEF is greater than 40%.
   b. **Patients with severe MR** secondary to LV dilatation associated with depressed LV systolic function (EF <25%) may experience decreased symptoms and demonstrate improved cardiac output after mitral valve repair (*Am Heart J* 129:1165, 1995).
   c. **Patients with minimal or no symptoms** should be followed closely with assessment of LV size and systolic function (by echocardiography or radionuclide ventriculography) every 6–12 months. Patients should be considered for mitral valve repair (or replacement) when the echocardiogram demonstrates an LV end-systolic dimension of less than 45 mm or an LVEF of less than 60%, or both (*J Am Coll Cardiol* 32:1486,1998). Generally, a decreased EF signifies that marked LV dysfunction has occurred and MVR with its attendant increase in LV afterload may be poorly tolerated or may fail to improve the patient's symptoms.

**B. Acute MR** can result from papillary muscle dysfunction or rupture caused by myocardial ischemia or infarction, infective endocarditis with flail or perforated leaflets, severe myxomatous disease with rupture of a chorda that results in a flail leaflet, or trauma.

1. **Pathophysiology.** The pathophysiologic features of acute MR differ from those of chronic MR in that compensatory increases in left atrial and LV compliance do not occur. The result is a sudden increase in pulmonary venous pressure that leads to acute pulmonary edema. Acute MR frequently results in cardiogenic shock.
2. **Medical management**
   a. **Afterload reduction** should be initiated urgently with sodium nitroprusside [see Heart Failure, sec. **II.B.1.b.(2)**] and should be guided by systemic BP and central hemodynamic monitoring. Approximately 50% of patients with acute MR can be stabilized in this manner, allowing MVR to proceed under more controlled conditions.
   b. **Diuretics** (see Heart Failure, sec. **II.B.4**), with or without nitrates, can be used (as the systemic BP tolerates) to relieve pulmonary congestion. However, the direct venodilatory effect of nitroprusside may render other preload-reducing maneuvers unnecessary.
   c. **Intra-aortic balloon counterpulsation** is indicated in cases of severe hemodynamic instability to reduce SVR and improve forward cardiac output.
3. **Surgical therapy.** Surgery is indicated urgently in patients with acute MR and hemodynamic compromise whose condition cannot be stabilized medically. In those with infective endocarditis who are hemodynamically stable, MVR should be delayed for several days while antibiotic therapy is initiated. If refractory hemodynamic deterioration develops, surgery should not be delayed.

**IV. Mitral valve prolapse (MVP)** is characterized by prolapse of one or both MV leaflets into the left atrium more than 2 mm in midsystole. It can be inherited as an autosomal-dominant trait with variable penetrance or may be associated with connective tissue diseases, congenital heart disease, musculoskeletal deformities, MV surgery, or ischemia. MVP may be associated with supraventricular and ventricular tachyarrhythmias such as Wolff-Parkinson-White and long QT syndrome.

**A. Symptoms** are nonspecific, varying from fatigue, anxiety, palpitations, lightheadedness, and chest pain to presyncopal and syncopal episodes. However, most patients are asymptomatic. **Physical examination** reveals a midsystolic click, typically followed by an MR murmur. The early or late occurrence of the click in systole and the duration of the MR murmur are dependent on the LV loading conditions (high LV volume, LV pressures–late midsystolic click).

**B. SBE prophylaxis is indicated** if MR is present or the MV leaflets are thickened, or both (see Chap. 13, Treatment of Infectious Diseases).

**C. If palpitations, near-syncope, or syncope** are of concern, evaluation with Holter monitor and echocardiography is recommended. If there is evidence of NSVT or sustained VT on Holter monitoring, electrophysiologic evaluation is warranted, with possible implantation of a defibrillator if the patient has inducible sustained VT. Symptomatic isolated atrial premature complexes or ventricular premature complexes may respond to treatment with β-adrenergic blockers.

**D. Management of the MR associated with MVP** may require treatment with afterload-reducing agents and possible surgical correction (see sec. **III.A**).

**E. Anticoagulation therapy** is recommended in the presence of atrial fibrillation or previous embolic event (see Chap. 18, Disorders of Hemostasis).

**V. AI** may result from an abnormality of the aortic valve itself, dilatation and distortion of the aortic root, or both. Causes of valvular AI include rheumatic fever, endocarditis, trauma, connective tissue diseases, and congenital bicuspid aortic valve. Dilatation or distortion of the aortic root may be due to systemic HTN, ascending aortic dissection, syphilis, cystic medial necrosis, Marfan syndrome, or ankylosing spondylitis. Chronic AI typically presents insidiously, whereas acute AI usually manifests as severe HF and impending cardiogenic shock.

**A. Pathophysiology.** The diastolic regurgitant flow from the aorta into the left ventricle causes increased LV end-diastolic volume and pressure. In turn, the LV becomes dilated and hypertrophied, which maintains stroke volume and prevents further increase in LVEDP. In acute AI, the chronic compensatory mechanisms are not active, and therefore, the increase in LVEDP is marked. In chronic AI, increases in peripheral resistance (e.g., HTN) lead to increased regurgitant flow and raise diastolic filling pressure and volume.

**B. Diagnosis.** AI may be suspected on the basis of clinical findings, including a wide pulse pressure, bounding pulses, and an aortic diastolic murmur. The presence of AI can be confirmed by two-dimensional and Doppler echocardiography or cardiac catheterization with ascending aortography.

**C. Medical management.** Medical therapy is reserved for patients with chronic stable AI or for stabilization of patients with severe or acute AI before definitive surgical treatment.

1. **Treatment of underlying or precipitating causes**, such as endocarditis, syphilis, and connective tissue diseases, should occur concomitantly with treatment of symptoms.
2. **Patients should receive prophylaxis for endocarditis** (see Chap. 13, Treatment of Infectious Diseases).
3. **Strenuous physical activity should be restricted** in patients with AI and associated LV dysfunction. Activities that involve increases in isometric work (lifting heavy objects) are more detrimental than are activities such as walking or swimming.
4. **Fluid and salt restriction, diuretics, digoxin, and vasodilators** are the cornerstones of therapy for patients with chronic AI who have evidence of LV dysfunction. Nifedipine may reduce the need for AVR in patients with symptomatic AI and normal LV function (*N Engl J Med* 331:689, 1994).
5. **Sodium nitroprusside or positive inotropes** (see Heart Failure, sec. **II.B**) should be used in a patient with acute AI to stabilize his or her condition before AVR.

**D. Surgical treatment**

1. **AVR and repair of associated aortic root abnormalities** should be performed urgently in individuals with acute AI or hemodynamic compromise, or both. In patients with infective endocarditis who are hemodynamically stable with medical therapy, AVR can be deferred for several days while treatment with antibiotics is initiated.
2. **AVR should be recommended in patients with severe chronic AI** in whom signs or symptoms of HF (NYHA class II–III) or LV dysfunction develop. Echocardiography should be performed every 6–12 months and AVR considered when LV dilatation (end-systolic dimension >55 mm or end-diastolic dimension >75 mm) or LV systolic dysfunction develops. The clinical outcome and extent of reversibility of LV dysfunction after AVR depend on the duration of dysfunction, dilatation of the left ventricle (end-systolic diameter and volume), and degree of systolic dysfunction.

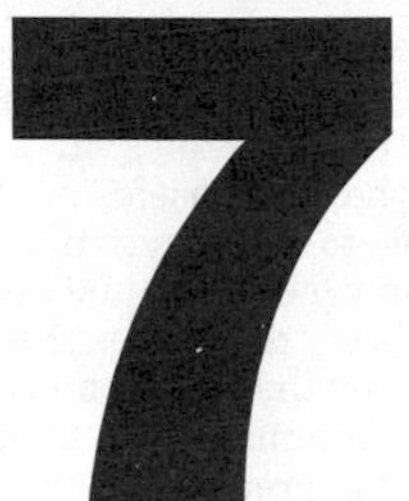

# Cardiac Arrhythmias

Jane Chen

## Recognition and Diagnosis

**I. Clinical history and physical examination.** The treatment of cardiac arrhythmias begins with a thorough understanding of the range of symptoms that can be attributed to an arrhythmia and the manifestations of arrhythmias on physical examination (*N Engl J Med* 338:1369, 1998). Important historical points to elicit include symptoms of palpitations, lightheadedness, dyspnea, angina, or syncope. It is useful to have patients demonstrate their symptoms of palpitations by "tapping out" their arrhythmias. A sudden onset and termination of the palpitations are highly suggestive of a tachyarrhythmia. Many forms of supraventricular tachycardia can be terminated by Valsalva or breath-holding. Patients with a significant bradyarrhythmia may report exercise intolerance, fatigue, lightheadedness, or syncope. A history of familial or congenital causes of arrhythmias [e.g., hypertrophic cardiomyopathy, Wolff-Parkinson-White syndrome (WPW), congenital long QT syndrome, congenital structural heart disease, or maternal systemic lupus erythematosus], organic heart disease (e.g., ischemic, cardiomyopathic, valvular, etc.), or endocrinopathies (e.g., thyroid disease, pheochromocytoma, etc.) should be sought. A thorough history of medications taken, either prescribed, over-the-counter, or herbal, should be investigated. Physical examination should emphasize pulse rate and regularity, as well as evidence of decreased cardiac function, which would raise the suspicion for malignant arrhythmias. BP should be measured supine and standing, with orthostatic changes recorded. A thorough cardiovascular examination should be performed as well as a search for signs of systemic disease. Serum electrolytes, CBC, and a toxicology screen should be considered for all patients under evaluation for a suspected arrhythmia.

**II. Diagnostic tools.** Many diagnostic tools are available to assist in the diagnosis of arrhythmias. Which tool to use should be individualized for each patient, based on the frequency and severity of their symptoms.

**A. A 12-lead ECG** at baseline is critical for the initial evaluation of any patient with a possible cardiac arrhythmia. The tracing should be examined for any evidence of electrical abnormalities, such as preexcitation, or any structural abnormalities, such as prior myocardial infarctions (MIs). If a patient presents with an arrhythmia and is hemodynamically stable, initial data should consist of a standard 12-lead ECG and a continuous rhythm strip with leads that best demonstrate atrial activation (e.g., $V_1$, II, III, aVF). Comparison of a 12-lead ECG at baseline with that obtained during an arrhythmia can highlight subtle features of the QRS deflection that indicate the superposition of atrial and ventricular depolarization. A continuous rhythm strip is very useful to document the response to interventions (e.g., vagal maneuvers, antiarrhythmic drug therapy, electrical cardioversion).

**B. Continuous ambulatory ECG monitoring** for 24–72 hours may be useful for documentation of symptomatic transient arrhythmias that occur with sufficient frequency, such as sinus node dysfunction, or symptomatic ectopic beats. This recording mode is also useful for assessment of a patient's heart rate response to daily activities or response to an antiarrhythmic drug treatment. The correlation between patient-reported symptoms in a time-marked diary and heart rhythm recordings is the most useful method to determine whether the symptoms are attributable to an arrhythmia.

C. **Event recorders** can be kept by patients for a month or more and are more useful than 24- to 72-hour monitors for diagnosis of transient arrhythmias that occur infrequently. A "loop" recorder is worn by the patient and continuously records the ECG. When the patient is symptomatic, the monitor is triggered and the ECG recording is saved with the preceding time period. An "event monitor" is connected only when the patient experiences symptoms. The **implantable loop recorder** is placed surgically, to provide automated or patient-activated recording of significant arrhythmic events that occur infrequently over several months. These recorders are implanted subcutaneously for up to 1–2 years and are useful for patients with very infrequent symptoms or those who are unable to activate external recorders.

D. **Exercise ECG** is useful for studying exercise-induced arrhythmias or to assess the sinus node response to exercise.

E. **Electrophysiology study (EPS)** is an invasive procedure that is used to induce arrhythmias to study their origin. EPS is most useful to induce supraventricular arrhythmias in patients with documented arrhythmia on event recorders or to induce ventricular arrhythmias in patients with prior MIs. The yield of EPS in inducing arrhythmias in patients with normal hearts without a history of palpitations is low. EPS can also be used to assess sinus node function and atrioventricular (AV) conduction; however, the sensitivity and specificity of these data to determine a cause of syncope are low.

## Mechanisms of Arrhythmia

I. **Premature complexes** represent the most common interruption of normal sinus rhythm. **Premature atrial complexes, premature junctional complexes, and premature ventricular complexes (PVCs)** often occur in the absence of structural heart disease and are commonly seen in the clinical settings of infection, inflammation, myocardial ischemia, drug toxicity, catecholamine excess, electrolyte imbalance, or excessive use of tobacco, alcohol, or caffeine. Symptoms range from none to the sensation of "skipped" beats. Premature atrial complexes, premature junctional complexes, and PVCs typically require no therapy. If they are symptomatic, therapy should be directed toward correction or removal of provocative stimuli. β-Adrenergic antagonists or calcium channel antagonists may be useful. **Nonsustained ventricular tachycardia (NSVT)** is defined as three or more consecutive PVCs at a rate of greater than 100 beats/minute that lasts less than 30 seconds (or <30 beats according to some investigators). NSVT in the setting of structurally normal hearts is benign and does not require treatment, unless the patient is very symptomatic. Therapy is the same as for symptomatic PVCs. NSVT in the setting of structurally abnormal hearts is associated with increased mortality (see Treatment, sec. **II.D**).

II. **Bradyarrhythmia** is any rhythm that results in a ventricular rate of less than 60 beats/minute. Mechanisms of bradyarrhythmias include the following.

A. **Sinus bradycardia** is defined as a sinus rate of less than 60 beats/minute with a normal P-wave configuration consistent with an origin in the sinus node area. Increased vagal tone, hypothyroidism, hypothermia, ischemia, and primary sinus node disease are typical causes. Use of drugs that produce sinus node dysfunction, such as digoxin, antiarrhythmic agents (particularly amiodarone), beta-blockers, diltiazem, verapamil, or clonidine, must be sought. Affected patients may be asymptomatic or may complain of fatigue, exercise intolerance, dyspnea or angina with exertion, or confusion in elderly patients. Asymptomatic patients require no therapy. In symptomatic patients, therapy is directed toward the underlying etiology. Acute treatment of very symptomatic patients includes atropine, 0.5–1.0 mg IV every 3–5 minutes to a maximum of 0.04 mg/kg, or cardiac pacing (transcutaneous or transvenous). When no reversible causes are found, permanent pacemakers are indicated (see Treatment, sec. **I.B**).

**B. Sick sinus syndrome (SSS)** is usually a disorder of the elderly and is presumed to arise from intrinsic disease of the sinoatrial node caused by aging, or in association with structural heart disease. The manifestations of SSS are often nonspecific and include palpitations, fatigue, confusion, and syncope. **Chronotropic incompetence** is the inability to increase the heart rate appropriately in response to metabolic need. Typical symptoms are shortness of breath or fatigue with exertion. Exercise testing may be helpful to assess the patient's heart rate and symptoms during activity. Treatment is with a permanent pacemaker with rate response features. **Sinus pause or sinus arrest** occurs when the sinus node intermittently fails to produce an impulse or when sinus node inactivity is prolonged, respectively. Sinus pauses that result in ventricular asystole of greater than 3 seconds in the awake patient are an indication for permanent pacemaker therapy in the absence of reversible causes. **Tachy-brady syndrome** occurs when bradyarrhythmias alternate with tachyarrhythmias, especially atrial fibrillation (AF). Sinus pauses occur after termination of AF as a result of suppression of sinus node function by the rapid atrial rate. Drugs used to treat the tachycardia frequently exacerbate underlying sinus node disease. Treatment frequently requires the concomitant use of drugs to treat the tachycardia and a permanent pacemaker to treat the bradycardia.

**C. AV block** occurs when an atrial impulse is conducted with delay or fails to conduct to the ventricle at a time when the AV node should not be refractory.

1. **First-degree AV block** describes a conduction delay, not actual block, usually within the AV node, that results in a prolonged PR interval on the surface ECG of greater than 200 msec. **Causes** of first-degree AV block include increased vagal tone, drug effect, electrolyte abnormalities, ischemia, and conduction system disease. First-degree block is usually asymptomatic and requires no therapy. However, an excessively prolonged PR interval may cause symptoms from loss of AV synchrony, particularly in patients with cardiomyopathy, who may experience CHF exacerbations. In symptomatic patients, dual-chamber pacemaker therapy can be considered in the absence of treatable causes.
2. **Second-degree AV block** is present when some atrial impulses are not conducted to the ventricle. Distinctions between type I and type II second-degree AV block are important, as they carry different prognostic implications.
   a. **Mobitz type I block (Wenckebach)** is a progressive delay in AV conduction with successive atrial impulses, as evidenced by **progressive PR interval prolongation,** before the block of an atrial impulse. The characteristic ECG pattern is of QRS complexes occurring in regular groupings (grouped beating) separated by the blocked beat. The RR interval progressively shortens before a blocked P wave, and the PR interval just after the block is shorter than the PR interval just before the block. The site of conduction block almost always is within the AV node. **Causes** include increased vagal tone, drug effects, electrolyte abnormalities, myocardial ischemia (typically in an inferior or posterior distribution), and conduction system disease. Mobitz type I block is benign and usually does not portend development of complete heart block. Symptomatic type I AV block is managed initially with atropine, 0.5 mg IV every 2 minutes to a

maximum of 0.04 mg/kg. For persistent symptoms without treatable causes, permanent pacemaker therapy is indicated.

b. **Mobitz type II block** is characterized by abrupt AV conduction block without evidence of progressive conduction delay. The ECG demonstrates no change in PR intervals preceding a nonconducted P wave. The site of block is localized most often to the His-Purkinje system. **Etiologies** include conduction system disease and myocardial ischemia (typically in an anterior distribution). Type II block, especially in the setting of a bundle branch block, often antedates the development of complete heart block, and permanent pacemakers are indicated in symptomatic and in asymptomatic patients. Hemodynamically unstable patients should be treated initially with temporary transvenous pacemakers. **Atropine** is usually not effective in the treatment of Mobitz type II block and may worsen the condition by accelerating the sinus rate, resulting in higher degrees of block.

c. **AV 2:1 block** may be caused by either Mobitz type I or type II mechanisms, and differentiating between the two may be difficult. Mobitz type I 2:1 block often occurs concomitantly with first-degree AV block or AV Wenckebach with grouped beating, or both. An increase in the sinus rate from increased sympathetic input often results in resumption of 1:1 conduction if the mechanism is Mobitz type I. The concomitant presence of bundle branch block or fascicular block suggests the presence of type II second-degree AV block. An increase in the sinus rate frequently worsens the block if Mobitz type II block is present (i.e., 2:1 block may progress to 3:1 or 4:1 block).

3. **Third-degree (complete) AV block** is present when all atrial impulses fail to conduct to the ventricle and the prevailing **ventricular escape rhythm is slower than the atrial rate.** This pattern is distinct from **AV dissociation,** which is present when the ventricular rate exceeds the atrial rate. The ventricular escape rate should be regular in complete heart block. The site of block may be the AV node (as occurs in congenital heart block) or within the His-Purkinje system (typical for acquired heart block). **Etiologies** of acquired complete AV block include ischemia or infarction, drug toxicity, idiopathic degeneration of the conduction system, infiltrative diseases (amyloidosis, sarcoidosis, metastatic disease), rheumatologic disorders (polymyositis, scleroderma, rheumatoid nodules), infectious diseases (Chagas' disease, Lyme disease), calcific aortic stenosis, or endocarditis. Symptoms depend on the degree of bradycardia of the underlying escape rhythm and include lightheadedness, dyspnea, CHF, angina, and syncope. In the absence of reversible causes of complete heart block, permanent pacemaker therapy is indicated for acquired complete heart block. Congenital complete heart block with significant bradycardia (<45 beats/minute) can be treated with permanent pacemaker implantation to prevent a malignant ventricular arrhythmia. **Isorhythmic AV dissociation** describes a condition in which a junctional rhythm is competing with underlying sinus bradycardia. This is a benign condition and is seen typically in young athletes with high vagal tone or in patients who are receiving medications that slow the sinus rate. Treatment is discontinuation of the culprit drugs. In highly trained athletes, a period of "deconditioning" may be needed to increase the sinus rate.

III. **Tachyarrhythmias** are defined as heart rhythms with a rate in excess of 100 beats/minute. These arrhythmias can be further distinguished between supraventricular tachycardia (SVT) or ventricular tachycardia (VT). Initial investigation may allow only for characterization of the tachycardia as either narrow complex (QRS duration <120 msec) or wide complex (QRS duration >120 msec).

A. **SVTs** can be narrow or wide. Wide-complex SVT arises when ventricular activation occurs with bundle branch block aberrancy or in the presence of preexcitation (*N Engl J Med* 332:162, 1995). P waves on a 12-lead ECG should be carefully sought, and their relationship to QRS complexes should be analyzed. A differential diagnosis of tachycardia mechanisms can be generated on the basis of the **R-P interval,** the time interval between the peak of an R wave and the **subsequent** P wave, during the tachycardia.

1. **Short R-P tachycardias** have an R-P interval that is less than 50% of the R-R interval. These include
   a. **"Typical" AV nodal re-entrant tachycardia (AVNRT).** This re-entrant rhythm occurs in patients who have functional dissociation of their AV node into "slow" and "fast" pathways. In typical AVNRT, conduction proceeds antegradely down the slow pathway, with retrograde conduction up the fast pathway. Atrial and ventricular excitation occur concurrently with every tachycardia circuit. On a 12-lead ECG, P waves are often hidden within the QRS complexes and are not visible, or they are buried at the end of the QRS complexes and may be distinguished only by a comparison of the QRS morphologies in tachycardia and in sinus rhythm.
   b. **Orthodromic AV re-entrant tachycardia (O-AVRT)** is an accessory pathway–mediated re-entrant rhythm that occurs when anterograde conduction to the ventricle takes place through the AV node and retrograde conduction to the atrium occurs through an accessory pathway. P waves on a 12-lead ECG are seen shortly after each QRS complex.
   c. **Sinus tachycardia or ectopic atrial tachycardia** associated with first-degree AV block. The two rhythms differ with respect to the P-wave axis and morphology. In these situations, the P wave after each QRS is actually conducting to the subsequent QRS complex with a prolonged PR interval.
   d. **Junctional tachycardia** arises from the AV junction and therefore is usually a narrow-complex tachycardia. The electrical impulses conduct to the ventricle and atrium simultaneously, and therefore, as in typical AVNRT, P waves may not be easily discernible. Junctional tachycardia is commonly seen in children after surgical correction of congenital heart defects. In adults, it is most often seen after mitral or aortic valve surgery, with acute MIs, or in digitalis toxicity.
2. **Long R-P tachycardias** have an R-P interval that is greater than 50% of the RR interval.
   a. **Sinus tachycardia or ectopic atrial tachycardia** (see sec. **III.A.1.c**). The P waves conduct to the subsequent QRS complexes with normal PR intervals.
   b. **"Atypical" AVNRT.** Less common than "typical" AVNRT, this arrhythmia mechanism occurs when anterograde conduction proceeds over the fast AV nodal pathway with retrograde conduction over the slow AV nodal pathway in patients with dual AV nodal physiology (see sec. **III.A.1.a**). Because retrograde conduction to the atrium is slow, the P wave is inscribed well after the QRS complex.
   c. **O-AVRT mediated by an accessory bypass tract with slow or decremental conduction properties.** In this less common form of O-AVRT, retrograde conduction over the accessory pathway to the atrium proceeds slowly enough for atrial activation to occur in the second half of the RR interval. Because the associated tachycardia is often incessant, this arrhythmia may cause a tachycardia-mediated cardiomyopathy.
3. **WPW syndrome** is defined as the presence of preexcitation on 12-lead ECG with symptoms or documentation of SVT. Preexcitation results from anterograde activation of the ventricle via an accessory pathway as well as the AV node, resulting in a short PR interval together with a delta wave slurring the upstroke of the QRS complex. **The most common form of**

**SVT in patients with an accessory pathway, whether or not preexcitation is seen on the baseline 12-lead ECG, is a narrow-complex orthodromic AVRT** (see sec. **III.A.1.b**). Because anterograde conduction during O-AVRT is via the AV node, no preexcitation is seen during SVT.

a. **Antidromic AVRT** occurs when conduction to the ventricle is down the accessory pathway, and the retrograde limb is usually through the His-Purkinje system and the AV node to the atria. The resulting QRS is maximally preexcitated. Antidromic AVRT is seen in fewer than 5% of patients with WPW.

b. **Atrial fibrillation (AF)** in patients with preexcitation is of special concern, as the accessory pathway, which has no decremental properties, may facilitate a very rapid ventricular response to AF that can initiate ventricular fibrillation (VF). The ECG is characterized by an irregular undulating baseline without recognizable P waves, an irregular and typically rapid ventricular rate (180–300 beats/minute), and QRS complexes that demonstrate variable fusion between normal complexes and fully preexcited (wide, bizarre) complexes. The most common cause of AF in patients with WPW is degeneration from orthodromic AVRT.

4. **Multifocal atrial tachycardia** is an irregular SVT that is distinguished by at least three distinct P-wave morphologies apparent on a 12-lead ECG. It often is associated with chronic obstructive pulmonary disease and heart failure and may be potentiated by concomitant therapy with theophylline. Therapy is targeted at treatment of the underlying pathophysiologic process.

5. **Atrial tachycardia with complete heart block** is often a manifestation of digoxin toxicity and should be considered as such until proven otherwise.

B. **AF** is the most common sustained tachyarrhythmia for which patients seek treatment. It is typically a disease of the elderly, affecting more than 10% of those older than 75 years. AF that occurs in patients under 65 years of age, without structural heart disease or hypertension, is termed *lone* AF and is associated with a low risk of stroke (*Chest* 119:194S, 2001). Disease processes that are often associated with AF include valvular, hypertensive, and ischemic heart disease; cardiac surgery; hypertension; acute alcohol ingestion; theophylline or other stimulant toxicity; endocrinopathies (hypothyroidism, hyperthyroidism, pheochromocytoma); pericarditis; and MI. An irregularly fluctuating baseline on the 12-lead ECG with an irregular and frequently rapid ventricular response (>100 beats/minute) is typical of AF. Regularization and slowing of the ventricular rate may be seen in patients with complete heart block, either from conduction disease or from digoxin toxicity. Symptoms of AF may be severe, including acute pulmonary edema, palpitations, angina, and syncope; nonspecific, such as fatigue; or none at all. Most often, symptoms are due to rapid ventricular rates rather than due to the arrhythmia. However, loss of atrial function may cause severe symptoms in some patients, particularly those with significant ventricular dysfunction. Prolonged episodes of rapid ventricular rates may cause a tachycardia-mediated cardiomyopathy. The approach to patients with AF should be focused on relief of symptoms, control of ventricular rates, and prevention of thromboembolic events (see Treatment, sec. **II.B**).

C. **Atrial flutter (AFL)** results from a single re-entrant circuit around functional or structural conduction barriers within the atria. Disease processes associated with AFL are similar to those seen with AF. Prior cardiac surgery that involved an atriotomy incision may promote AFL by providing a nonconductive scar around which re-entry can occur. In typical AFL, flutter waves are negative in the inferior leads (II, III, aVF) of a 12-lead ECG and positive in lead $V_1$, and appear "sawtooth"-like in pattern. Atrial rates in AFL are usually 300 beats/minute, and 2:1 conduction to the ventricle is common. AFL and AF frequently occur in the same patient. In patients with

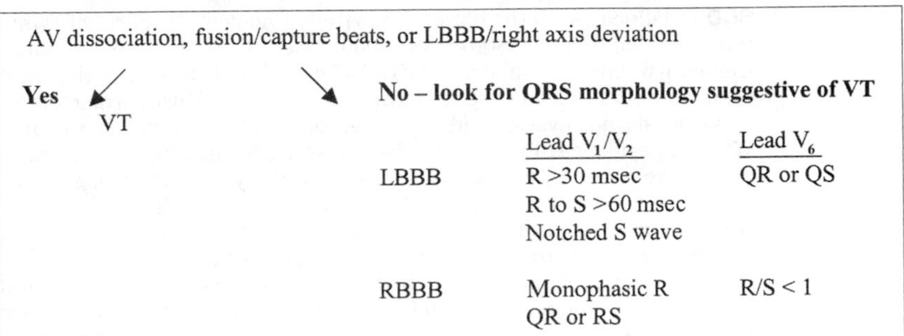


**Fig. 7-1.** Differentiating supraventricular tachycardia from ventricular tachycardia (VT). AV, atrioventricular; LBBB, left bundle branch block; RBBB, right bundle branch block.

pure AFL, stroke risks appear to be higher than previously thought, with an incidence of approximately 5% over a 2.8-year follow-up (*Am J Cardiol* 82:580, 1998). Therefore, recommendations for anticoagulation are the same for patients with AF or flutter (see Treatment, sec. **II.C**).

**D. Ventricular arrhythmias** are the major cause of sudden cardiac death (SCD). **Sustained monomorphic VT** is defined as tachycardia composed of ventricular complexes that last longer than 30 seconds (or 30 beats by some definitions), at a rate of 100–250 beats/minute, with only one QRS morphology throughout the arrhythmia. **Polymorphic VT** is characterized by an ever-changing QRS morphology and is frequently due to ischemia. Torsade de pointes (TdP) is a polymorphic VT that is preceded by a prolonged QT interval in sinus rhythm. **VF** is associated with disorganized mechanical contraction, hemodynamic collapse, and sudden death. The ECG reveals irregular and rapid oscillations (250–400 beats/minute) of highly variable amplitude without uniquely identifiable QRS complexes or T waves.

1. **Differentiation of SVT with aberrancy from VT** on the basis of analysis of the surface ECG is critical in determining appropriate acute and chronic therapy. Acutely, IV adenosine and calcium channel blockers are the mainstay of SVT therapy, but they are contraindicated in VT. Chronically, many SVTs are amenable to radiofrequency ablation, whereas most VTs are malignant and require antiarrhythmic agents or implantable defibrillators, or both. Features that are diagnostic of VT are AV dissociation, capture or fusion beats, and an LBBB morphology with right axis deviation. In the absence of these features, characteristic QRS morphologies that are suggestive of VT must be sought, as shown in Fig. 7-1 (*Circulation* 83:1649, 1991).
2. **Benign VT** is a form of VT that is usually seen in the absence of structural heart disease. The most commonly encountered types are right ventricular outflow tract VT and idiopathic left ventricular (LV) VT. Right ventricular outflow tract VTs occur more frequently in women than in men, are often exercise induced, have an LBBB morphology with an inferior axis, and are responsive to beta-blockers, lidocaine, and adenosine. Idiopathic LV VTs have a right bundle branch block morphology with a superior axis and are frequently responsive to verapamil. Because these patients have structurally normal hearts, they usually tolerate the arrhythmia well, with common symptoms of lightheadedness and palpitations and, rarely, syncope. Both these forms of VTs are benign and are not associated with SCD, and therefore, implantable defibrillators are not indicated. They are focal in origin and are very amenable to treatment with radiofrequency ablation.

3. **SCD** is defined as death that occurs within 1 hour of the onset of symptoms. In the United States, 350,000 cases of SCD occur annually. Among patients with aborted SCD, ischemic heart disease is the most common associated cardiac structural abnormality. Most cardiac arrest survivors do not evolve evidence of an acute MI; however, more than 75% have evidence of previous infarcts. Nonischemic cardiomyopathies; infiltrative diseases; infectious diseases (viral myocarditis, Chagas' disease, Lyme disease); congenital myocardial defects, such as hypertrophic cardiomyopathy or arrhythmogenic right ventricular dysplasia; inflammatory diseases that affect the myocardium (systemic lupus erythematosus, rheumatoid arthritis); surgical repairs for congenital heart disease; and primary and metastatic malignancies that involve the heart also may provide the substrate for ventricular arrhythmias. An underlying pathophysiologic cause should always be corrected, if possible (e.g., aortic valve replacement in critical aortic stenosis, revascularization of critical multivessel coronary artery disease).
4. **Primary electrical disorders. Congenital long QT syndrome** is characterized by considerable genetic and phenotypic heterogeneity. Patients typically have prolonged QT intervals on a baseline 12-lead ECG and recurrent syncope or resuscitated SCD from TdP or VF. Beta-blocker therapy or unilateral sympathectomy has been shown retrospectively to decrease the mortality in patients with congenital long QT syndrome. However, they are now mainly used in conjunction with ICDs in symptomatic patients. Asymptomatic patients are considered to be at high risk for SCD if they have a family history of SCD. Factors that have been associated with the **acquired long QT syndrome** include electrolyte abnormalities (hypokalemia, hypomagnesemia, and, rarely, hypocalcemia), drugs, cardiac disease (ischemia or myocarditis), bradycardia, CNS disease (intracranial trauma, subarachnoid hemorrhage, or cerebrovascular accident), and toxic exposures (organophosphate poisoning, cesium). The **Brugada syndrome** is an inherited disease characterized by typical ECG findings of ST-segment elevation in leads $V_1$–$V_3$ and incomplete right bundle branch block and is associated with an increased risk of SCD from VF. Patients may have SCD or syncope or be asymptomatic. Recurrence rates for patients with resuscitated SCD is high, and an implantable cardioverter-defibrillator (ICD) should be considered. The role of EPS for risk stratification of SCD in asymptomatic patients with ECGs that are consistent with Brugada syndrome is controversial.

**IV. Syncope,** defined as the transient loss of consciousness and postural tone, is common in the general population. Of an unselected population, 40% report at least one lifetime syncopal event. Syncope accounts for approximately 6% of all hospital admissions. Because a syncopal event may herald an otherwise unsuspected, potentially lethal cardiac condition, a careful evaluation of the patient with syncope is warranted. The etiologies of syncope are myriad and can be divided into primary cardiac and noncardiac mechanisms. **Primary cardiac syncope** is caused either by mechanical obstruction of cardiac output (e.g., hypertrophic cardiomyopathy, valvular stenosis, aortic dissection, myxomas, pulmonary embolism) or by brady- or tachyarrhythmias. Most cases of syncope have unknown causes (36.6%). Cardiac causes of syncope account for approximately 9.5% of all identified causes of syncope and are associated with increased mortality. **Neurocardiogenic syncope** is the most commonly diagnosed cause of syncope (21%), particularly in those without underlying heart disease or other comorbidities, and is associated with a benign prognosis. The two components of neurocardiogenic syncope are cardioinhibitory, where significant bradycardia or asystole is the main cause of syncope, or vasodepression, where the main culprit is vasodilation. Most patients have a combination of the two components. Specific stimuli may evoke a neurocardiogenic mechanism, leading to a situational syncope (e.g., micturition, defecation, coughing, swallowing). Other **noncardiac causes of syncope** include orthostatic hypotension, toxic or metabolic influences (e.g., drug toxicities, hypoglycemia, hypoxia, etc.), neurologic etiologies (e.g., seizures or cerebrovascular events), and psychiatric etiologies (e.g., conversion disorders and anxiety disorders) (*N Engl J Med* 347:878, 2002).

**A. History and physical examination.** The clinical history and physical examination have the highest utility for identification of a potential mechanism of a syncopal event. Special attention should be focused on the events or symptoms that precede and follow the syncopal event, the time course of loss and resumption of consciousness (abrupt vs. gradual), and any description of vital signs before, during, and after the event. A characteristic prodrome of nausea, diaphoresis, or flushing preceding loss of consciousness suggests neurocardiogenic syncope, as does the identification of a particular emotional or situational trigger or a postsyncopal sensation of fatigue that lasts for many minutes to hours. Alternatively, an unusual sensory prodrome, incontinence, or a decreased level of consciousness that gradually clears suggests a seizure as a likely diagnosis. With transient ventricular arrhythmias, an abrupt loss of consciousness may occur, with a rapid recovery. A clear history of palpitations preceding syncope is seldom elicited. Physical examination should include assessment of orthostatic vital signs and careful neurologic, pulmonary, and cardiovascular assessment. Bedside manipulations may be useful, including Valsalva maneuvers and squatting, with attention to cardiac auscultatory findings to detect valvular and subvalvular lesions. Carotid sinus massage is contraindicated in patients with a carotid bruit.

**B. Diagnostic testing.** An initial 12-lead ECG and ECG monitoring (24- to 72-hour Holter recordings, patient-activated event recorders, implantable loop recorders) may lead to a diagnosis in only about 10% of cases. Routine laboratory tests are typically unhelpful; however, for patients with comorbid conditions or those who take electrophysiologically active drugs, such screening should be performed. Toxicology screening should be done for suspected illicit drug use or inadvertent drug exposure. Two-dimensional echocardiography with Doppler flow studies should be performed in patients whose history or physical examination suggests the presence of structural heart disease. In the presence of a structurally normal heart, malignant ventricular arrhythmias are an uncommon cause of syncope. Invasive EPS is most useful in patients with syncope and structural heart disease or a documented tachyarrhythmia. Head-up tilt-table testing suffers from a low predictive value in unselected populations but may be useful to distinguish between cardioinhibitory and vasodepressor types of syncope. Neurologic or psychiatric testing is reserved for those with a suggestive clinical history. Routine CT scans, EEGs, or both, in unselected patients with syncope are not supported by available data.

**C. Treatment** of specific arrhythmic causes of syncope is discussed in Treatment, sec. **IV.**

## Treatment

**I. Bradyarrhythmias.** Identification of reversible causes of symptomatic bradycardia should be undertaken immediately after diagnosis. Symptomatic sinus bradycardia, first-degree AV block, or Mobitz I second-degree AV block may respond acutely to atropine treatment, 0.5–2.0 mg IV. For irreversible causes of symptomatic bradycardia, pacemaker therapy should be considered.

**A. Temporary pacemakers.** Temporary pacing is best achieved by insertion of a temporary transvenous pacemaker, although placement of an external

**Table 7-1.** Class I indications for permanent pacemakers

| |
|---|
| Symptomatic sinus bradycardia or atrioventricular (AV) block |
| Sinus bradycardia as a result of necessary drug therapy |
| Symptomatic chronotropic incompetence |
| Advanced AV block with: |
| Asystole ≥ 3 sec in the awake patient |
| Escape rate <40 beats/min |
| Catheter ablation of AV node |
| Neuromuscular disease |
| Postoperative AV block that is not expected to recover |
| Intermittent complete heart block |
| Intermittent type II second-degree block |
| Alternating bundle branch block |
| Recurrent syncope with carotid sinus massage causing asystole ≥ 3 sec |

transthoracic unit can be used. Temporary pacing is indicated for symptomatic second- or third-degree heart block caused by transient drug intoxication or electrolyte imbalance and complete heart block or Mobitz II second-degree AV block in the setting of an acute MI. Sinus bradycardia, AF with a slow ventricular response, or Mobitz I second-degree AV block should be treated with temporary pacemakers only if symptoms or hemodynamic instability is present.

**B. Permanent pacemaker implantation.** Contemporary pacemakers can maintain AV synchrony and adapt the rate of pacing to mimic the normal physiologic heart rate response to exertion. Before a pacemaker is implanted, the patient must be free of any active infections, and anticoagulation issues must be carefully considered. Hematomas over the pacemaker pocket are most often seen in patients who are receiving IV heparin or subcutaneous enoxaparin sodium (Lovenox) and may require surgical evacuation in severe cases.

1. **Indications for permanent pacemakers** are discussed fully in joint recommendations from the American Heart Association, the American College of Cardiology, and the North American Society for Pacing and Electrophysiology (*Circulation* 106:2145, 2002). Class I indications are conditions in which permanent pacing is considered to be acceptable and necessary for adequate treatment and are listed in Table 7-1.
2. **Pacing modalities.** A four-letter alphabetic code is used to identify pacing modalities. The first initial defines the chamber that is paced (**V**entricle, **A**trium, **D**ual chamber, **O** if neither), the second identifies the chamber that is sensed (**V**entricle, **A**trium, **D**ual chamber, **O** for neither), the third indicates the response to a sensed event (**I**nhibited, **T**riggered, **D**ual function, **O** for no response), and the fourth, when present, denotes **R**ate response mode. The VVI and DDD modes are used most commonly. VVI units pace and sense in the ventricle; a sensed (native QRS) event inhibits the ventricular stimulus. DDD units pace and sense in both chambers. Events sensed in the atrium inhibit the atrial stimulus and trigger a ventricular response after an appointed interval (AV delay), whereas ventricle-sensed events inhibit ventricular stimulus. Lower rate limit is the intrinsic heart rate below which the pacemaker begins to pace. Upper rate limit is the maximum heart rate that the pacemaker paces. In patients with atrial arrhythmias (most commonly

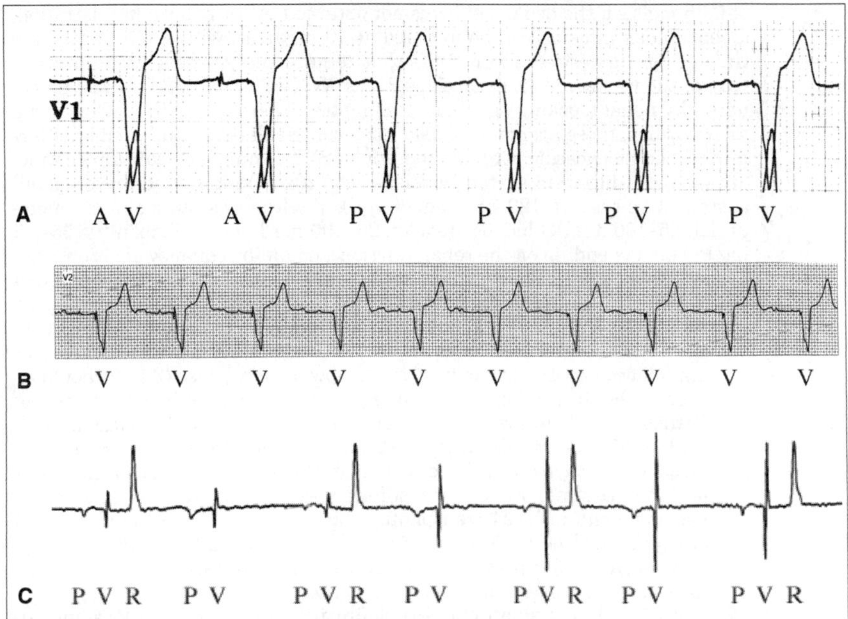


**Fig. 7-2. A:** Normal dual-chamber (DDD) pacing. First two complexes are atrioventricular (AV) sequential pacing, followed by sinus with atrial sensing and ventricular pacing. **B:** Normal single-chamber (VVI) pacing. Underlying rhythm is atrial fibrillation (no distinct P waves), with ventricular pacing at 60 beats/minute. **C:** Pacemaker malfunction. The underlying rhythm is sinus (P) at 80 beats/minute with 2:1 heart block and first-degree AV block (long PR). Ventricular pacing spikes are seen (V) after each P wave, demonstrating appropriate sensing and tracking of the P waves; however, there is failure to capture. A, paced atrial events; V, paced ventricular events; P, sensed atrial events; R, sensed ventricular events.

AF) and AV block, a DDD pacemaker may allow for tracking of AF, resulting in ventricular pacing at the upper rate limit. Pacemakers today have detection protocols that allow automatic switching of pacing modes to prevent rapid ventricular pacing in response to rapid atrial rates ("mode switch"). Application of a magnet to a pacemaker turns off the sensing modality, thereby making a pacemaker asynchronous. For example, VVI mode becomes VOO (ventricular asynchronous pacing), and DDD mode becomes DOO (asynchronous AV pacing). Some examples of normal and abnormal pacing functions are shown in Fig. 7-2.

**II. Tachyarrhythmias.** The acute treatment of symptomatic tachyarrhythmias should follow the protocols of advanced cardiac life support outlined in Chap. 8, Critical Care. Chronic treatment for tachyarrhythmias is aimed at either prevention of recurrence or prevention of the complications associated with the specific tachyarrhythmia.

**A. SVT.** Initial therapy of acute episodes of regular, narrow-complex tachycardias includes vagal maneuvers (e.g., carotid massage, Valsalva maneuver) and, if unsuccessful, bolus administration of short-acting agents that slow or block AV nodal conduction. IV adenosine or metoprolol (5 mg IV q5min) are often the initial agents used. Verapamil is dosed at IV boluses of 5–10 mg over 2–3 minutes and can be repeated after 15–30 minutes, if necessary. Diltiazem can be given as an IV bolus of 0.25 mg/kg over 2 minutes, with a repeat bolus of 0.35 mg/kg if the desired effect is not obtained. After bolus administration, a continuous infusion can be initiated at 10 mg/hour, with the infusion rate titrated to the desired effect. SVTs that require the AV node as an integral part of the re-entrant tachycardia, such as AVNRT or O-AVRT, can be terminated by nodal blocking agents or techniques, whereas in AFL, AF, or atrial tachycardias, these agents would slow the ventricular rate but would not terminate the tachycardia. Chronic therapy of SVT can include calcium channel antagonists (diltiazem sustained release at 120–360 mg PO qd or verapamil sustained release at 120–480 mg PO qd), β-adrenergic antagonists (metoprolol, 25–100 mg PO bid, or atenolol, 25–100 mg PO qd), digoxin (0.125–0.5 mg PO qd, depending on the renal function), or radiofrequency ablation.

1. **Adenosine** is a short-acting agent with a serum half-life of approximately 4–8 seconds. The recommended initial dose is 6 mg given IV as a rapid bolus via an antecubital vein, followed by a 10- to 30-ml saline flush. If within 1–2 minutes SVT is not terminated and AV block is not seen, 12 mg followed by 18 mg can be given. A lower initial dose (3 mg) should be used if the drug is injected through a central venous line. Toxicities of adenosine include precipitation of prolonged asystole in patients with SSS or second- or third-degree AV block. Adenosine effects are antagonized by methylxanthines (caffeine or theophylline), and larger doses may be required. Effects are potentiated by dipyridamole and carbamazepine and in heart transplant recipients, such that a smaller initial dosage should be used. Common side effects, including facial flushing, dyspnea, and chest pressure, usually are of brief duration. Adenosine also rarely may exacerbate bronchoconstriction.
2. **Radiofrequency ablation** offers definitive cure for many SVTs, including AVNRT, accessory pathway–mediated tachycardias, focal atrial tachycardia, and AFL. Complication rates are usually less than 1% and include bleeding, groin hematomas, cardiac perforation or tamponade, strokes, and complete heart block requiring permanent pacemakers. Given the high success rate of ablation procedures, antiarrhythmic drugs are now rarely indicated for the treatments of SVT (*N Engl J Med* 340:534, 1999).
3. **WPW and AF.** For hemodynamically stable preexcited AF, IV procainamide or amiodarone can be used to slow conduction over the accessory pathway, but **AV nodal blocking agents (adenosine, calcium channel antagonists, beta-blockers, or digoxin) must be avoided,** as they may facilitate conduction over the accessory pathway and increase the ventricular rate paradoxically, initiating VF. Hemodynamic compromise or clinical instability should be treated with prompt direct current (DC) cardioversion. Because AF in these patients most commonly results from AVRT, the therapy of choice is ablation of the accessory pathway. Pharmacologic therapy for WPW patients is targeted at slowing conduction and prolonging refractoriness of the accessory bypass tract with an antiarrhythmic agent (class Ia, Ic, and III agents) and is reserved for those who are unable to undergo or who refuse an ablation procedure.

**B. AF.** The management of patients with AF requires careful consideration of three issues: rate control, rhythm control, and anticoagulation (*N Engl J Med* 344:1067, 2001). The Atrial Fibrillation Followup Investigation of Rhythm Management (AFFIRM) trial (*N Engl J Med* 347:1825, 2002) showed no mortality differences between rate and rhythm control groups in asymptomatic patients in AF. Therefore, rhythm control should be reserved for individuals who are symptomatic.

1. **Rate control** of the ventricular response to AF can be achieved with agents that prolong conduction through the AV node. These include diltiazem, verapamil, β-adrenergic blockers, and digoxin (see sec. **II.A**). **Digoxin** is useful in controlling the resting ventricular rate in AF or AFL in the setting of LV dysfunction and CHF, and may be useful as

adjunctive therapy in combination with calcium channel antagonists or β-adrenergic antagonists for optimum rate control of chronic AF (*Am J Cardiol* 69:78G, 1992). Loading regimens for digoxin vary widely, usually 0.25–0.50 mg IV in repeated doses up to 1.0–1.5 mg over 8–24 hours. Usual maintenance doses range between 0.125 and 0.5 mg PO qd, with decreased doses in patients who have renal dysfunction or are receiving other agents that may increase digoxin level, such as amiodarone. **Digitalis toxicity** is usually diagnosed clinically. Paroxysmal atrial tachycardia with varying degrees of AV block and bidirectional VT are the most commonly seen arrhythmias in association with digitalis toxicity. Treatment is supportive, by withholding the drug, insertion of temporary pacemakers for AV block, and IV phenytoin for bidirectional VT (see sec. **II.D.1.a**).

**2. Rhythm control** includes the restoration and the maintenance of sinus rhythm.

**a. Restoration of sinus rhythm** can be achieved with electrical DC cardioversion or with antiarrhythmic agents (chemical cardioversion). With either method, one must consider the potential for a thromboembolic event. AF with a rapid ventricular response in the setting of ongoing myocardial ischemia, MI, hypotension, or marked CHF should receive prompt cardioversion regardless of the anticoagulation status. If the duration of AF is documented to be less than 48 hours, cardioversion may proceed without anticoagulation. If AF has persisted for longer than 48 hours (or for an unknown duration), patients should be anticoagulated with warfarin, with an international normalized ratio of 2.0–3.0, for at least 3 weeks before cardioversion, and anticoagulation should be continued in the same therapeutic range following successful cardioversion (*Circulation* 89:1469, 1994). An alternative to anticoagulation for 3 weeks before cardioversion is to perform a transesophageal echocardiogram to rule out left atrial appendage thrombus before cardioversion (*N Engl J Med* 344:1411, 2001). This method is safe and has the advantage of shorter time to cardioversion than warfarin and therefore is indicated in patients who are not able to wait weeks before cardioversion. Therapeutic anticoagulation with warfarin is indicated after the cardioversion for a minimum of 4 weeks, although the AFFIRM trial suggests that in patients with high risk factors for strokes, warfarin should be continued indefinitely (see sec. **II.B.3**).

**(1) DC cardioversion.** Electrical cardioversion is the safest and most effective method of acutely restoring sinus rhythm. For cardioversion of atrial arrhythmias, the anterior electrode should be positioned just right of the sternum at the level of the third or fourth intercostal space, with the second electrode positioned just below the left scapula. Care should be taken to position electrodes at least 6 cm from permanent pacemaker or defibrillator generators. When practical, sedation should be accomplished with midazolam (1–2 mg IV q2min to a maximum of 5 mg), methohexital (25–75 mg IV), etomidate (0.2–0.6 mg/kg IV), or propofol (initial dose, 5 mg/kg/hour IV). Proper synchronization by the cardioverter-defibrillator should be confirmed by noting the presence of a synchronization marker superimposed on the QRS complex. If electrode paddles are being used, firm pressure should be applied to minimize contact impedance. Direct contact with the patient or the bed should be avoided. Atropine (1 mg IV) should be readily available to treat prolonged pauses. Reports of serious arrhythmias, such as VT, VF, or asystole, are rare and are more likely in the setting of improperly synchronized cardioversion, digitalis toxicity, or concomitant antiarrhythmic drug therapy.

Cardioversion is generally ineffective in multifocal atrial tachycardia unless the underlying cardiopulmonary causes are adequately treated.

**(2) Pharmacologic cardioversion** of AF to sinus rhythm requires similar considerations regarding anticoagulation as for electrical cardioversion. Although oral antiarrhythmics have low rates of conversion, conversions are possible, and patients should be adequately anticoagulated before oral agents are started. **Ibutilide** is the only drug that is U.S. Food and Drug Administration approved for pharmacologic cardioversion. Clinical trials have shown a 45% conversion rate for AF and a 60% conversion rate for AFL. It is a class III agent and is associated with a 4–8% risk for TdP, especially in the first 2–4 hours after administration of the drug. The risk for TdP is higher in patients with cardiomyopathy and congestive heart failure. Ibutilide is given in IV bolus form, at a dosage of 0.01 mg/kg (maximum 1 mg) over 10 minutes, and should be given only under a carefully monitored setting, with an external defibrillator ready in case of TdP. Patients must be monitored on telemetry for at least 4 hours after being given the drug. Intravenous **amiodarone** has a relatively low efficacy for acute conversion of AF and may be associated with hypotension.

**b. Maintenance of normal sinus rhythm** generally requires an antiarrhythmic agent. Maintenance of sinus rhythm has not been shown to reduce mortality or stroke risks, and antiarrhythmic agents are associated with a small risk for life-threatening proarrhythmia (*Circulation* 82:1106, 1990). As a result, antiarrhythmic therapy should be reserved for patients who have highly symptomatic AF. Antiarrhythmic agents are classified according to the Vaughan-Williams classification (*J Clin Pharmacol* 24:129, 1984). Class I agents inhibit the fast sodium channel, class II agents are β-adrenergic antagonists, class III agents primarily block potassium channels, and class IV agents are calcium channel antagonists. Commonly used antiarrhythmic agents, their major route of elimination, and dosing regimen are listed in Table 7-2.

**(1) Class I** antiarrhythmic drugs are subdivided into class Ia, Ib, and Ic. **Class Ia** agents include quinidine, procainamide, and disopyramide, and may cause TdP as a result of QT prolongation. Quinidine and procainamide are rarely used nowadays for the treatment of AF because of their numerous side effects and inconvenient dosing regimen. **Quinidine** is commonly associated with gastrointestinal side effects, including nausea, vomiting, diarrhea, abdominal pain, and anorexia. Long-term use of **procainamide** may be associated with lupus-like reactions (fever, pleuropericarditis, hepatomegaly, arthralgias). In addition, procainamide has an active metabolite, *N*-acetylprocainamide, which exerts an action that is typical of class III agents and can prolong the QT interval. Combined procainamide and *N*-acetylprocainamide levels greater than 30 mg/L are associated with increased toxicity. **Disopyramide** is an effective agent for the treatment of vagally mediated AF. Side effects include urinary retention, dry mouth, and exacerbation of glaucoma and are due to its potent anticholinergic properties. In addition, its negative inotropic effects may worsen congestive heart failure for patients with LV dysfunction. **Class Ib** agents, including lidocaine, mexiletine, tocainide, and phenytoin, have very little effect on atrial tissues and are not used for AF. **Class Ic** agents include flecainide and propafenone and are generally more effective than other class Ia agents in the management of AF. They may cause QRS widening,

**Table 7-2.** Commonly used antiarrhythmic drugs

| Class | Drug | Major route of elimination: renal or hepatic | Oral dosage | IV dosage |
|---|---|---|---|---|
| Ia | Procainamide | R | 1–6 g/d in divided doses | Load: 17 mg/kg up to 50 mg/min; maintenance: 2–5 mg/min |
| | Quinidine | H | Sulfate, 200–400 mg q6h; gluconate, 324–648 mg q8–12h | N/A |
| | Disopyramide | H | 100–300 mg q8h | N/A |
| Ib | Lidocaine | H | N/A | Load: 1 mg/kg, repeat 0.5 mg/kg q8–10min up to 3 mg/kg total; maintenance: 1–4 mg/min |
| | Mexiletine | H | 100–200 mg PO q8–12h | N/A |
| Ic | Flecainide | H (65%); R (35%) | 50–200 mg q12h | N/A |
| | Propafenone | H | 150–300 mg q8h | N/A |
| III | Sotalol | R | 80–320 mg q12h | N/A |
| | Dofetilide | R (70%); H (30%) | 125–500 μg q12h | N/A |
| | Ibutilide | H | N/A | 1 mg (0.01 mg/kg if weight <60 kg) over 10 min; can repeat once after 10 min |
| | Amiodarone | H | Load: 600–1600 mg/d in divided doses | Load: 150-mg bolus, then 1 mg/min for 6 hr, then 0.5 mg/min |

H, hepatic; N/A, not applicable; R, renal.

and the effects are more apparent at higher heart rates (use dependence). Therefore, monitoring for toxicity usually involves an exercise stress test, after a stable dose has been reached, to look for QRS widening at high heart rates. The dose should be reduced or the drug should be discontinued if the QRS duration exceeds 0.2 seconds. Flecainide and propafenone may also cause sinus node depression and AV conduction abnormalities. Both drugs may cause conversion of AF to AFL. The slowing of atrial rate from AF to AFL may result in 1:1 conduction to the ventricle. Therefore, nodal blocking agents, such as beta-blockers or calcium channel blockers, should always be used in conjunction with class Ic agents. Flecainide and propafenone should never be used in post-MI patients, as they are associated with increased mortality in this particular group (*N Engl J Med* 321:406, 1989).

(2) **Class III** agents prolong action potential duration and cause an increase in the QT interval. Ibutilide is a class III agent that is only available in IV form for the acute conversion of AF (see sec. **II.B.2.a**). Oral class III agents that are commonly used for treatment of AF are sotalol and dofetilide. **Sotalol** contains β-antagonistic actions and may result in sinus bradycardia or AV conduction abnormalities. It is generally safe to use in patients with LV dysfunction but should be avoided in individuals who are in active CHF. **Dofetilide** blocks the rapid component of the delayed rectifier potassium current, $I_{Kr}$. As a result of this effect, at clinically effective doses, the QT interval on the 12-lead ECG is usually prolonged, and the main risk of dofetilide is TdP. Dofetilide is contraindicated in patients with a baseline corrected QT ($QT_c$) greater than 440 msec, or 500 msec in patients with bundle branch block. Initial dosing of dofetilide is based on the creatinine clearance. A dose of 500 μg bid is recommended for patients with normal creatinine clearance, 250 μg bid for patients with a creatinine clearance of 40–60 ml/minute, and 125 μg bid for patients with a creatinine clearance of 20–40 ml/minute. It is contraindicated for patients with a creatinine clearance of less than 20 ml/minute. A 12-lead ECG should be obtained before the first dose of dofetilide and 1–2 hours after each dose. If the $QT_c$ interval after the first dose prolongs by 15% of the baseline or exceeds 500 msec, a 50% dosage reduction is indicated. If the $QT_c$ exceeds 500 msec after the second dose, dofetilide must be discontinued. Several medications block the renal secretion of dofetilide (verapamil, cimetidine, prochlorperazine, trimethoprim, megestrol, ketoconazole) and are contraindicated with dofetilide. In patients who previously received amiodarone, dofetilide can be started only after amiodarone has been discontinued for 3 months. The main advantage of dofetilide is that it is not associated with increased CHF or mortality in patients with LV dysfunction (*N Engl J Med* 341:857, 1999).

(3) **Class II and IV** are β antagonists and calcium channel antagonists, respectively. Their use in the treatment of AF is mainly for rate control. These agents are not effective in the conversion or maintenance of sinus rhythm. Commonly used class II agents are metoprolol (25–100 mg PO bid; a sustained-release preparation can be given qd) and atenolol (25–100 mg PO qd). Commonly used class IV agents are diltiazem (30–90 mg PO qid, or 120–360 mg PO qd of the sustained-release form) or verapamil (80–120 mg tid, or 180–480 mg PO qd of the sustained-release form).

(4) **Amiodarone** has the properties of class I, II, III, and IV drugs, and is arguably the most effective antiarrhythmic agent for maintenance of sinus rhythm. Intravenous amiodarone has low efficacy for acute conversion of AF, although conversion after several days of IV amiodarone has been observed. Adverse effects of oral amiodarone are partially dose dependent and may occur in up to 75% of patients treated at high doses for 5 years. At lower dosages (200–300 mg/day), adverse effects that require discontinuation occur in approximately 5–10% of patients per year. Specific toxicity syndromes include the following: (1) **Pulmonary toxicity** occurs in 1–15% of treated patients but appears less likely in those who receive less than 300 mg/day (*Circulation* 82:51, 1990). Patients characteristically have a dry cough and dyspnea associated with pulmonary infiltrates and rales. The

process appears to be reversible if detected early, but undetected cases may result in a mortality of up to 10% of those affected. A chest radiograph and pulmonary function tests should be obtained at baseline and every 12 months or when patients complain of shortness of breath. The presence of interstitial infiltrates on the chest radiograph and decreased diffusing capacity raise concern of amiodarone pulmonary toxicity. (2) **Photosensitivity** is a common adverse reaction, and, in some patients, a violaceous skin discoloration develops in sun-exposed areas. The blue-gray discoloration may not resolve completely with discontinuation of therapy. (3) **Thyroid dysfunction** is a common adverse effect. Hypothyroidism and hyperthyroidism have been reported, with an incidence of 2–5% per year. Thyroid-stimulating hormone should be obtained at baseline and monitored every 6 months. If hypothyroidism develops, concurrent treatment with levothyroxine may allow continued amiodarone use. (4) **Corneal microdeposits,** detectable on slit-lamp examination, develop in virtually all patients. These deposits rarely interfere with vision and are not an indication for discontinuation of the drug. Optic neuritis, leading to blindness, is rare but has been reported in association with amiodarone. (5) The most common **ECG changes** are lengthened PR intervals and bradycardia; however, high-grade AV block may occur in patients who have preexisting conduction abnormalities. Amiodarone may prolong QT intervals, although usually not extensively, and TdP is rare. Other agents that prolong the QT interval, however, should be avoided in patients who are taking amiodarone. (6) **Liver dysfunction** usually manifests in an asymptomatic and transient rise in hepatic transaminases. If the increase exceeds three times normal or doubles in a patient with an elevated baseline level, amiodarone should be discontinued or the dose should be reduced. AST and ALT should be monitored every 6 months in patients who are receiving amiodarone. (7) **Drug interactions:** Amiodarone may raise the blood levels of warfarin and digoxin; therefore, these drugs should be reduced routinely by one-half when amiodarone is started, and levels should be followed closely.

**(5) Choosing and monitoring antiarrhythmic agents.** A reasonable outline for the management of AF and the choice of commonly used antiarrhythmic agents is shown in Fig. 7-3. In general, loading of antiarrhythmic drugs should be performed in an inpatient setting for four to five doses, with daily ECGs performed to check QT and QRS intervals, and continuous telemetry to monitor for the development of bradycardia and TdP. Renal function must be carefully assessed and followed for patients who are receiving renally cleared drugs. The loading of dofetilide requires a mandatory 3-day hospitalization for monitoring. Outpatient loading of antiarrhythmic drugs is acceptable in limited circumstances, generally for patients without any structural cardiac diseases or conduction abnormalities. Event monitors are recommended in these cases, as recordings can be sent by patients daily to monitor for bradyarrhythmias and QT/QRS intervals.

**3. Indications for anticoagulation.** Chronic warfarin anticoagulation is the most effective therapy for attenuating the risk of stroke associated with AF. The decision to anticoagulate a patient and which anticoagulants to use should be based on the patient's risk factors for thromboembolic events, balanced by the risk for significant hemorrhagic events. Patients with paroxysmal AF have the same risk for stroke as those with persistent AF (*J Am Coll Cardiol* 35:183, 2000). **High risk**

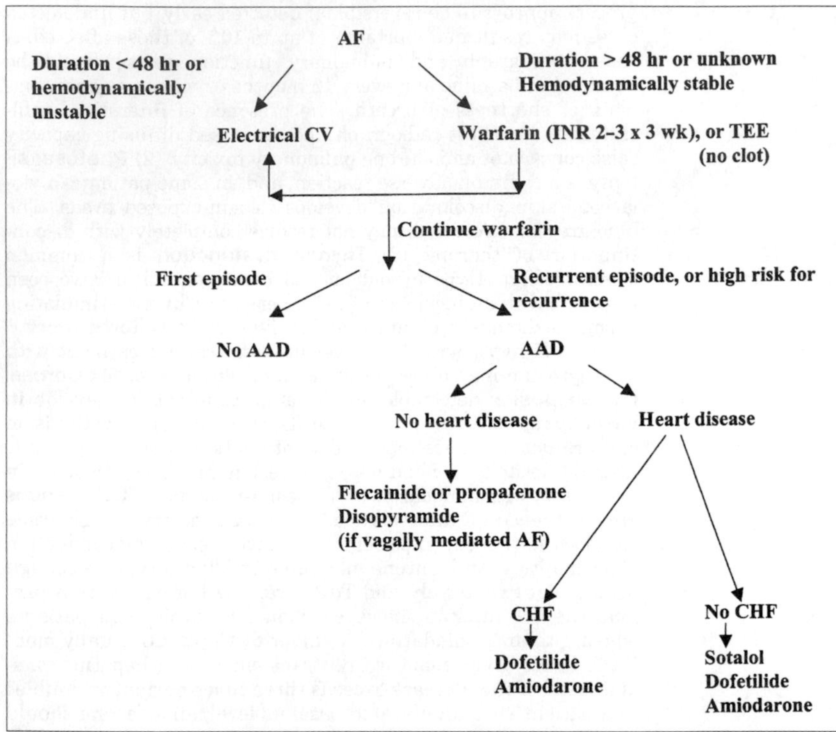


**Fig. 7-3.** Recommendations for the management of atrial fibrillation (AF). AAD, antiarrhythmic drug; CV, cardioversion; INR, international normalized ratio; TEE, transesophageal ECG.

**factors for thromboembolic events** include age greater than 75 years, previous stroke/transient ischemic attack or systemic embolus, valvular heart disease, and poor LV systolic function. Patients with high risk factors face a greater than 7% per year risk of stroke. Moderate risk factors include age between 65 and 75 years old, hypertension, diabetes, and coronary artery disease with normal LV function. Moderate-risk patients have a 2.5% per year risk of stroke. Patients with neither high nor moderate risks are defined as having "lone" AF, and their risk of stroke is on the order of 1% per year (*Chest* 119:194S, 2001). Left atrial spontaneous echo contrast also appears to identify those at increased risk, although large clinical studies are lacking (*J Am Coll Cardiol* 24:755, 1994). Aspirin at 325 mg/day reduces the risk of stroke in high-risk patients from 6.3% per year to 3.6% per year, but warfarin with international normalized ratio 2.0–4.5 reduces stroke risk even more, to 2.3% per year (*Circulation* 84:527, 1991). **Current recommendations for anticoagulation** are to use warfarin, international normalized ratio 2.0–3.0, in patients with any one high risk factor or two or more moderate risk factors. Anticoagulation with aspirin alone at 325 mg is adequate for patients without any risk factors and who are less than 65 years old, or who have absolute contraindications to warfarin therapy (*Circulation* 104:2118, 2001). It is important to continue warfarin therapy even after rhythm control has been achieved, because patients often have asymptomatic episodes of AF, and achievement of sinus rhythm has not been proven to be associated with a reduction in strokes. No trials are available on the efficacy of other anticoagulants, such as low-molecular-weight heparin or clopidogrel, on decreasing the risk of strokes.

4. **Postoperative AF** occurs in 11–40% of patients after coronary artery bypass surgery and in more than 50% after valvular surgery (*N Engl J Med* 336:1429, 1997). It is often transient; however, patients with a history of AF or valvular heart disease are at high risk for recurrence. **Beta-blockers** have been shown to be effective in preventing postoperative AF and should be started preoperatively, if possible. Preoperative administration of oral amiodarone has also been shown to reduce the incidence of postoperative AF (*N Engl J Med* 337:1785, 1997). Patients in whom AF develops after heart surgery should be treated with rate control, and prompt cardioversion within 48 hours after onset of AF is recommended. If AF recurs, or if cardioversion is not performed within 48 hours after onset, treatment is the same as that outlined for AF in Fig. 7-3. For postoperative AF in patients without significant risk factors for recurrence, antiarrhythmic therapy and warfarin can be discontinued in 1–3 months if no recurrence is noted.
5. **Nonpharmacologic therapies. Catheter ablation of the AV node with pacemaker implantation** can be performed for ventricular rate control when drug therapy is ineffective or if high doses of nodal blocking drugs cause hypotension or congestive heart failure. It is a method of rate control, not rhythm control, and patients continue to require anticoagulation for stroke prevention. This method has no effect on long-term survival but is associated with an improved sense of well-being (*N Engl J Med* 344:1043, 2001). A small subset of AF has been shown to initiate from focal sites within the pulmonary veins (*N Engl J Med* 339:659, 1998). **Ablation of these trigger foci, or circumferential ablation and isolation of pulmonary veins** from the left atrium, are now performed in multiple centers. This procedure is associated with complications of stroke, pulmonary hemorrhage, and pulmonary vein stenoses, and long-term efficacy remains unclear. It should be reserved for extremely symptomatic patients in whom no other therapeutic options are available. The **Maze procedure** involves multiple incisions in the right and left atrium, creating "dead-end" corridors so that atrial fibrillatory waves can be extinguished. It requires cardiopulmonary bypass and has been used successfully in conjunction with other heart operations, in particular mitral valve surgery. Atrial defibrillators are devices that use low energy to cardiovert AF. They are most useful in patients with infrequent episodes of persistent AF. Their main limitation is that the shocks are painful to patients, and they currently have a limited role as a sole method of therapy for patients with AF (*N Engl J Med* 346:2062, 2002). Hybrid therapy is a combination of pharmacologic and nonpharmacologic therapy. Some antiarrhythmic agents, specifically amiodarone, flecainide, and propafenone, have been known to convert AF to AFL. The AFL can then be ablated. Antiarrhythmic drugs must be continued after ablation of AFL to prevent the recurrence of AF.

C. **AFL** is treated similarly to AF. Although data for thromboembolic risks in patients with AFL are not as extensive as those for AF, several reports have shown embolizations in patients with pure AFL (*Am J Cardiol* 82:580, 1998). Often, patients with AFL also have undiagnosed AF, which may contribute to the risks of embolization. Therefore, the general consensus is that **patients with AFL should be anticoagulated in the same manner as patients with AF.** The main difference in the pathophysiology of AFL compared to AF is that AFL results from an organized macro–re-entrant circuit and therefore is usually amenable to overdrive atrial pacing and to catheter ablation. Overdrive atrial pace-termination of AFL is most often performed in patients with permanent pacemakers that allow temporary programming of high atrial rates or in post–heart surgery patients with atrial epicardial wires. Catheter ablation of typical AFL can replace antiarrhythmic drug therapy as a means to restore and maintain sinus rhythm (*Circulation* 86:1233, 1992). It is associated with potential complications of complete heart block and, rarely, injury to the right coronary artery with inferior MI. Ablation of AFL involving prior cardiotomy scars is associated with a lower rate of success. Similar considerations regarding anticoagulation for electrical or pharmacologic cardioversion should be observed before an attempt is made at overdrive pace-termination or catheter ablation of AFL.

**D. VT and VF.** Immediate unsynchronized DC cardioversion is the primary therapy for pulseless VT and VF (see Chap. 8, Critical Care). VF that is resistant to external defibrillation requires the addition of IV antiarrhythmic agents. Intravenous lidocaine is frequently used; however, IV amiodarone appears to be more effective in increasing survival of VF when used in conjunction with defibrillation (*N Engl J Med* 346:884, 2002). After successful cardioversion, continuous IV infusion of effective antiarrhythmic therapy should be maintained until any reversible causes have been corrected. In the case of **TdP associated with long QT syndrome,** acute therapy is immediate DC cardioversion. Bolus administration of magnesium sulfate in 1- to 2-g increments up to 4–6 g IV is highly effective. In cases of acquired long QT syndrome, identification and treatment of the underlying condition should be undertaken, if possible. Elimination of long-short triggering sequences and shortening of the QT interval can be achieved by increasing the heart rate to the range of 90–120 beats/minute by either IV isoproterenol infusion (initial rate at 1–2 μg/minute) or temporary transvenous pacing. **Primary VF that occurs within the first 72 hours of an acute MI** is not associated with an elevated risk of recurrence and does not require chronic antiarrhythmic therapy. In patients with resuscitated VF arrests without an identifiable and reversible cause, ICD implantation has been demonstrated to provide a survival benefit when compared to antiarrhythmic drug therapy (*N Engl J Med* 337:1576, 1997).

1. **Antiarrhythmic drug therapy.** Chronic antiarrhythmic drug therapy is indicated for the treatment of recurrent symptomatic ventricular arrhythmias. In the setting of hemodynamically unstable ventricular arrhythmias treated with an ICD, antiarrhythmic drug therapy is often necessary to suppress frequent device discharges.

   a. **Class I** agents in general have not been shown to reduce mortality in patients with VT/VF. Class Ic agents, such as **flecainide and encainide** (now off the market), are associated with increased mortality when used prophylactically for ventricular ectopy suppression in the post-MI patient, as demonstrated in the Cardiac Arrhythmia Suppression Trial (CAST) (*N Engl J Med* 324:781, 1991). **Lidocaine** is a class Ib agent that is available only in IV form and is very effective in the management of sustained and recurrent VT/VF, particularly in the setting of an acute MI. The prophylactic use of lidocaine for suppression of PVCs and NSVT in the otherwise uncomplicated post-MI setting is **not** indicated and may lead to an increase in mortality from bradyarrhythmias (*Arch Intern Med* 149:2694, 1989). Toxicities of lidocaine include CNS effects (convulsions, confusion, stupor, and, rarely, respiratory arrest), all of which resolve with discontinuation of therapy. Negative inotropic effects are seen only at high drug levels. **Mexiletine** is similar to lidocaine but is available in oral form. Mexiletine is most often used in combination with either amiodarone or sotalol for treatment of refractory ventricular arrhythmias. It may have a limited role in the treatment of some patients with congenital long QT syndromes. CNS toxicity includes tremor, dizziness, and blurred vision. Higher levels may result in dysarthria, diplopia, nystagmus, and an impaired level of consciousness. Nausea and vomiting are common. **Tocainide** has not been shown to be effective in preventing recurrences of sustained life-threatening ventricular arrhythmias and is rarely used. **Phenytoin** is used primarily in the treatment of digitalis-induced ventricular arrhythmias. It may have a limited role in the treatment of ventricular arrhythmias associated with congenital long QT syndromes. The IV loading dose is 250 mg given over 10 minutes (maximum rate of 50 mg/minute). Subsequent doses of 100 mg can be given q5min as necessary and as BP tolerates, to a total of 1000 mg. Frequent monitoring of the ECG, BP, and neurologic status is required. Continuous infusion is not recommended (see Chap. 24, Neurologic Disorders).

b. **Class II** agents, the β-adrenergic antagonists, are the only class of antiarrhythmic agent to have consistently shown improved survival in post-MI patients. Beta-blockers reduce postinfarction total mortality by 25–40% and SCD by 32–50% (*Lancet* 2:823, 1981).

c. **Class III** agents used for VT/VF include bretylium and sotalol. **Bretylium** is available in IV form and is used for the treatment of VF and hemodynamically unstable VF. The initial dose is 5 mg/kg, with repeat boluses as needed to a maximum of 35 mg/kg total. Rapid infusion is associated with hypotension. With the availability and efficacy of IV amiodarone, bretylium is no longer a first-line agent used in the acute treatment of VT/VF (see Appendix H, Advanced Cardiac Life Support Algorithms). **Sotalol** prevents the recurrence of sustained VT and VF in 70% of patients (*N Engl J Med* 329:452, 1993) but must be used with caution in individuals with congestive heart failure. Sotalol is available today as d,l-sotalol, a racemic mixture that contains β-antagonist properties. The pure form of sotalol, d-sotalol, which has no beta-blocking activities, was shown to have increased mortality compared to placebo and thus is not clinically available (*Lancet* 348:7, 1996). Dofetilide has not been shown to have efficacy in the treatment of ventricular arrhythmias.

d. **Class IV agents** have no role in the chronic management of VT. Intravenous calcium channel blockers should never be used in the acute management of VT, as they may cause hemodynamic collapse (see Chap. 8, Critical Care). Oral calcium channel blockers are not effective in the management of VT. Short-acting nifedipine is associated with a trend toward increasing mortality when used in the post-MI patient (*Arch Intern Med* 153:345, 1993).

e. **Amiodarone** is safe and well tolerated, and has a hemodynamic profile that is suitable for patients with low ejection fractions (EF). It has complex pharmacokinetics and is associated with significant toxicities (*Am Heart J* 125:109, 1993). After oral loading, amiodarone prevents the recurrence of sustained VT or VF in up to 60% of patients. A therapeutic latency of more than 5 days exists before beneficial antiarrhythmic effects are observed with oral dosing, and full suppression of arrhythmias may not occur for 4–6 weeks after therapy is initiated. Amiodarone has become the most well-studied antiarrhythmic agent in the treatment of SCD and the main drug against which ICDs are compared, in secondary and in primary prevention trials (see sec. **II.D.2**). Amiodarone, when used prophylactically in post-MI patients, is associated with a reduction in ventricular ectopy and arrhythmic deaths but is not associated with a reduction in total mortality (*Lancet* 349:667, 1997; *Lancet* 349:675, 1997). In patients with nonischemic cardiomyopathy, amiodarone appears to have some benefit in the reduction of total mortality (*Lancet* 344:493, 1994).

**Table 7-3.** Class I indications for implantable cardioverter-defibrillator therapy

| |
|---|
| Resuscitated ventricular fibrillation/ventricular tachycardia (VF/VT) arrest not due to reversible cause |
| Spontaneous VT with structural heart disease |
| Syncope of unknown etiology with relevant VT/VF induced at electrophysiologic study |
| Inducible VT in asymptomatic patients with nonsustained ventricular tachycardia, coronary artery disease, and left ventricular dysfunction that is not suppressible by class I antiarrhythmic drugs |
| Spontaneous VT in patients without structural heart disease that is not amenable to other treatments |

2. **ICDs** provide automatic recognition and treatment of ventricular arrhythmias. ICD implantation improves survival in patients resuscitated from ventricular arrhythmias (secondary prevention of SCD) and in individuals without prior symptoms who are at high risk for SCD (primary prevention of SCD). Techniques for implantation of transvenous ICDs are the same as for pacemaker implantation, with the exception of the need for defibrillation threshold testing. Defibrillation threshold testing is performed by induction of VF after implantation of the ICD, before closure of the pocket. The energy required to defibrillate VF successfully is then determined to ensure an adequate safety margin. VT and VF zones can be programmed independently, and therapies are programmed independently in each zone. The therapies available include (1) high-energy defibrillation for VF or rapid VT, (2) low-energy cardioversion for stable VT, (3) antitachycardia pacing algorithms to terminate VT, and (4) ventricular or dual-chamber bradycardia pacing. ICD detects an arrhythmia based mainly on the ventricular rate. Inappropriate therapy for SVT, most often AF with rapid ventricular rate, is therefore not uncommon. A magnet applied over the ICD turns off detection, and therefore, without detection of arrhythmias, no therapies can be delivered. A magnet over the ICD does **not** turn the pacemaker function of the ICD into asynchronous pacing mode, unlike the effect of a magnet over a pacemaker. Class I indications for ICD implantation are listed in Table 7-3.
   a. **Secondary prevention of SCD** attempts to prevent recurrent SCD in patients who have already survived an episode of SCD. Multiple studies have shown the superiority of ICDs compared to antiarrhythmic agents, in particular sotalol and amiodarone, in the secondary prevention of SCD (AVID trial, *N Engl J Med* 337:1576, 1997). ICD is thus indicated for patients who have survived a cardiac arrest due to VF/VT that is not due to a reversible cause, or in patients in whom spontaneous VT develops in the setting of structural heart disease.
   b. **Primary prevention of SCD** is aimed at patients who are at high risk of SCD, to prevent an initial episode of SCD. In patients with a history of coronary artery disease, those with depressed LV function with an EF of less than 35%, and patients with asymptomatic nonsustained VT who had inducible VT during an EPS that was not suppressed with IV procainamide, ICD decreased mortality to 16% compared with 39% in the group treated with antiarrhythmic drugs over a 5-year follow-up period [Multicenter Automatic Defibrillator Implantation Trial (MADIT), *N Engl J Med* 335:1933, 1996]. The results were corroborated by the data from the Multicenter UnSustained Tachycardia Trial (MUSTT) (*N Engl J Med* 341:1882, 1999).

The MADIT II data (*N Engl J Med* 346:877, 2002) showed that in patients with coronary artery disease and EF of 30% or less (no NSVT or EP study was required in this study), prophylactic implantation of an ICD was associated with a mortality of 14.2% compared to 19.8% in the conventionally treated group over an average follow-up of 20 months. In all of these studies, patients with severe heart failure or those who had recent MIs, coronary artery bypass grafting, or percutaneous angioplasties were excluded.

c. **Other indications for ICD.** For patients with hypertrophic cardiomyopathy, arrhythmogenic right ventricular dysplasia, congenital long QT syndrome, or Brugada syndrome, ICDs are indicated if they have had a resuscitated cardiac arrest or documented ventricular arrhythmias. Prophylactic implantation for patients with these cardiac abnormalities but no symptoms is controversial, and the consensus is to implant ICDs in patients who are at high risk for SCD. In general, the risk factors are a family history of SCD or a personal history of syncope suspicious for ventricular arrhythmias. Patients who are awaiting cardiac transplantation are at high risk for SCD, especially if they are receiving inotropic agents. ICD is indicated if they have ventricular arrhythmias. However, there are currently no data supporting the prophylactic implantation of ICD in patients without known ventricular arrhythmias. ICDs are contraindicated in patients who have incessant VT, significant psychiatric illnesses, or life expectancy of less than 6 months (*Circulation* 106:2145, 2002).

3. **Radiofrequency catheter ablation of VT** is most successfully performed in patients with hemodynamically stable forms of VT without structural heart disease, such as right ventricular outflow tract and idiopathic LV VT. Long-term cure rates are similar to those achieved for catheter ablation of SVT. Bundle branch re-entry VT is a form of VT that involves the His-Purkinje system in its re-entrant circuit. It can be treated successfully by catheter ablation of the right bundle branch. Because it usually occurs in patients with cardiomyopathy and an abnormal conduction system, an ICD is generally implanted in conjunction with ablation. VT associated with ischemic heart disease can also be treated by catheter ablation; however, success rates are significantly lower. The reasons for the lower success rate include the hemodynamic instability of VT and the multiple different VT circuits (due to multiple areas of scars from prior MIs) that are often present. Catheter ablation of ischemic VT in patients with antiarrhythmic drug-refractory VT and an implanted ICD has been successful in reducing frequent ICD shocks (*Circulation* 96:1525, 1997). Ablation of VT in nonischemic cardiomyopathy is more difficult and is associated with an even lower success rate, because these VTs are not caused by scar tissues, thus making target sites for ablation difficult to locate.

III. **Device therapy for heart failure.** Patients with severe heart failure [New York Heart Association (NYHA) class III or IV] are at significant risk of SCD. These patients were excluded from all primary prevention studies on SCD, although many multicenter trials are now under way. Contractile dyssynchrony, such as is seen in patients with bundle branch block or those in whom right ventricular pacing results in effective LBBB, is thought to be associated with increased mortality and morbidity in patients with heart failure. **Cardiac resynchronization therapy** describes pacing from the right and the left ventricle, in an attempt to restore biventricular synchrony. The left ventricle is paced via a lead placed in a branch of the coronary sinus. Cardiac resynchronization therapy has been shown to be associated with an improvement in the 6-minute walk test, quality-of-life score, and NYHA functional class (*N Engl J Med* 346:884, 2002), although no mortality benefit has been shown. The target patients generally had NYHA class III or IV, EF less than 20%, and bundle branch block (mostly left) with QRS durations of 150 msec or greater. Combining biventricular pacing with ICD may decrease firing from the ICD (*J Am Coll Cardiol* 36:824, 2000). Larger trials addressing whether this translates to an improvement in mortality are under way.

**IV. Syncope.** Appropriate therapy for patients with syncope is determined by the underlying etiology. Syncope in the setting of ischemic or nonischemic cardiomyopathy carries a poor prognosis, and the implantation of ICDs is appropriate when no reversible causes are found. Syncope due to reversible causes, whether cardiac, neurologic, or medication related, should be appropriately treated. When the clinical history or diagnostic testing is suggestive of a **neurocardiogenic mechanism,** initial treatment is targeted at counseling patients to take precautionary steps to avoid injury. Patients should be aware of their prodromal symptoms and maintain horizontal positions at those times, increase fluid uptake, keep their feet elevated, and use support stockings to minimize the impact of peripheral vasodilatation. Medical therapy begins with **β-adrenergic antagonists,** which block peripheral adrenergic-mediated vasodilatation and decrease cardiac inotropy, or volume expansion with salt tablets or fludrocortisone, or both. Metoprolol and atenolol are commonly used beta-blockers. In patients with baseline sinus bradycardia, the use of beta-blockers with intrinsic sympathomimetic activities (pindolol, 5–10 mg bid, or acebutolol, 200–400 mg bid) may prevent worsening bradycardia. **Midodrine,** an $\alpha_1$-adrenergic agonist that induces venous and arterial vasoconstriction, appears to be effective in patients with vasodepressor syncope (*Am J Cardiol* 88:80, 2001). Midodrine is given 5 mg PO tid and can be increased as needed to 15 mg tid. As with salt tablets and fludrocortisone, midodrine may cause hypertension. **Disopyramide** may have utility to prevent neurocardiogenic syncope, probably through its strong negative inotropic action in reducing stimulation of ventricular mechanoreceptors. However, given its antiarrhythmic properties and potential for causing malignant arrhythmias, it is rarely used to treat benign vasovagal syncope. Centrally acting agents such as selective serotonin-reuptake inhibitors or yohimbine may be useful to attenuate central reflex centers involved in neurocardiogenic mechanisms. **Permanent dual-chamber pacemakers** with a hysteresis function (high-rate pacing in response to a detected sudden drop in heart rate) have been shown to be useful in highly selected patients with recurrent neurocardiogenic syncope with a prominent cardioinhibitory component (*J Am Coll Cardiol* 33:16, 1999).

# 8 Critical Care

Marin H. Kollef

The goals of critical care medicine are to save the lives of patients with life-threatening but reversible medical or surgical conditions and to offer the dying a peaceful and dignified death. Open discussions between physicians and patients and their family members ensure that critical care is provided in a manner that is most consistent with the patient's wishes.

## Respiratory Failure

**I. General considerations.** Hypercapnic respiratory failure occurs with acute carbon dioxide retention [arterial carbon dioxide tension ($PaCO_2$) >45–55 mm Hg], producing a respiratory acidosis (pH <7.35). Hypoxic respiratory failure occurs when normal gas exchange is seriously impaired, resulting in hypoxemia [arterial oxygen tension ($PaO_2$) <60 mm Hg or arterial oxygen saturation ($SaO_2$) <90%]. Usually, this type of respiratory failure is associated with tachypnea and hypocapnia; however, its progression can lead to hypercapnia as well. Hypoxic respiratory failure can result from a variety of insults, as shown in Table 8-1. The acute respiratory distress syndrome (ARDS) is a form of hypoxic respiratory failure caused by acute lung injury. The common end result is disruption of the alveolar capillary membrane, leading to increased vascular permeability and accumulation of inflammatory cells and protein-rich edema fluid within the alveolar space. The American-European Consensus Conference has defined ARDS as follows: (1) acute bilateral pulmonary infiltrates, (2) ratio of $PaO_2$ to inspired oxygen concentration ($FIO_2$) less than 200, and (3) no evidence for heart failure or volume overload as the principal cause of the pulmonary infiltrates (*Am J Respir Crit Care Med* 149:818, 1994).

**II. Pathophysiology**

**A. Hypoxic respiratory failure** usually is the result of the lung's reduced ability to deliver oxygen into the bloodstream, owing to one of the following six processes.

**1. Shunt.** This term refers to the fraction of mixed venous blood that passes into the systemic arterial circulation after bypassing functioning lung units. Congenital shunts are due to developmental anomalies of the heart and great vessels. Acquired shunts usually result from diseases that affect lung units, although acquired cardiac and peripheral vascular shunts also can occur. Table 8-1 lists some of the more common disease processes that produce clinically significant pulmonary shunts. Shunts are associated with a widened alveolar-arterial oxygen tension [$P(A\text{-}a)O_2$] gradient, and the resultant hypoxemia is resistant to correction with supplemental oxygen alone when the shunt fraction of the cardiac output (CO) is greater than 30%.

**2. Ventilation-perfusion mismatch.** Diseases associated with airflow obstruction [e.g., chronic obstructive pulmonary disease (COPD),

**Table 8-1.** Causes of shunts and hypoxic respiratory failure

| Clinical presentation | Causes |
|---|---|
| Cardiogenic pulmonary edema (low permeability, high hydrostatic pressure) | Acute myocardial infarction<br>Left ventricular failure<br>Mitral regurgitation<br>Mitral stenosis<br>Diastolic dysfunction |
| Noncardiogenic pulmonary edema/ ARDS (high permeability, low hydrostatic pressure) | Aspiration<br>Sepsis<br>Multiple trauma<br>Pancreatitis<br>Near-drowning<br>Pneumonia<br>Reperfusion injury<br>Inhalational injury<br>Drug reaction (aspirin, narcotics, interleukin-2) |
| Mixed pulmonary edema (high permeability, high hydrostatic pressure) | Myocardial ischemia or volume overload associated with sepsis, aspiration, etc.<br>High-altitude exposure |
| Pulmonary edema of unclear etiology | Upper airway obstruction<br>Neurogenic cause<br>Lung re-expansion |

ARDS, acute respiratory distress syndrome.

asthma], interstitial inflammation (e.g., pneumonia, sarcoidosis), or vascular obstruction (e.g., pulmonary embolism) often produce lung regions with abnormal ventilation-to-perfusion relationships. In ventilation-perfusion mismatch, unlike shunt physiology, increases in $FIO_2$ result in increases in $PaO_2$.

3. **Low inspired oxygen.** Usually, $FIO_2$ is reduced at high altitudes or when toxic gases are inhaled. In patients with other cardiopulmonary disease processes, an inappropriately low $FIO_2$ can contribute to hypoxic respiratory failure.
4. **Hypoventilation.** This condition is associated with elevated $PaCO_2$ values, and the resultant hypoxemia is due to increased alveolar carbon dioxide, which displaces oxygen. Usually, oxygen therapy improves hypoxemia as a result of hypoventilation but may worsen the overall degree of hypoventilation, especially in patients with chronic airflow obstruction. Primary treatment is directed at correcting the cause of the hypoventilation.
5. **Diffusion impairment.** Hypoxemia due to diffusion impairments usually responds to supplemental oxygen therapy, as is seen in patients with interstitial lung diseases.
6. **Low mixed venous oxygenation.** Normally, the lungs fully oxygenate pulmonary arterial blood, and mixed venous oxygen tension ($P\bar{v}O_2$) does not affect $PaO_2$ significantly. However, a decreased $P\bar{v}O_2$ can lower the $PaO_2$ significantly when either intrapulmonary shunting or ventilation-perfusion mismatch is present. Factors that can contribute to low mixed venous oxygenation include anemia, hypoxemia, inadequate CO,

and increased oxygen consumption. Improving oxygen delivery to tissues by increasing hemoglobin or CO usually decreases oxygen extraction and improves mixed venous oxygen saturation ($SvO_2$).

B. **Hypercapnic respiratory failure** usually involves some combination of the following three processes.

   1. **Increased carbon dioxide production** (i.e., respiratory acidosis) can be precipitated by fever, sepsis, seizures, and excessive carbohydrate loads in patients with underlying lung disease. The oxidation of carbohydrate fuels is associated with more carbon dioxide production per molecule of oxygen consumed as compared to the oxidation of fat fuels.
   2. **Increased dead space** occurs when areas of the lung are ventilated but not perfused or when decreases in regional perfusion exceed decreases in ventilation. Examples include intrinsic lung diseases (e.g., COPD, asthma, cystic fibrosis, pulmonary fibrosis) and chest wall disorders associated with parenchymal abnormalities (e.g., scoliosis). Usually, these disorders are associated with widened $P(A\text{-}a)O_2$ gradients.
   3. **Decreased minute ventilation** can result from CNS disorders (e.g., spinal cord lesions), peripheral nerve diseases (e.g., Guillain-Barré syndrome, botulism, myasthenia gravis, amyotrophic lateral sclerosis), muscle disorders (e.g., polymyositis, muscular dystrophy), chest wall abnormalities (e.g., thoracoplasty, scoliosis), drug overdoses, metabolic abnormalities (e.g., myxedema, hypokalemia), and upper airway obstruction. These disorders usually are associated with a normal $P(A\text{-}a)O_2$ gradient unless accompanying lung disease is also present.

C. **Mixed respiratory failure** is seen most commonly after surgery, particularly in patients with underlying lung disease who are undergoing upper abdominal procedures. Abnormalities in oxygenation usually occur on the basis of atelectasis, which often is multifactorial in origin (decreased lung volumes and cough due to the effects of anesthesia, abnormal diaphragmatic function resulting from the surgery or associated pain, and interstitial edema causing small airways to close). Hypoventilation can also result from abnormal diaphragmatic function, particularly when complete paralysis occurs, as with phrenic nerve injury.

III. **Blood gas analysis** (see Acid-Base Disturbances in Chap. 3, Fluid and Electrolyte Management)

## Oxygen Therapy

The goal of oxygen administration is to facilitate adequate uptake of oxygen into the blood to meet the needs of peripheral tissues. When this goal cannot be accomplished with the methods outlined in secs. **I–V,** endotracheal intubation may be necessary.

I. **Nasal prongs** allow patients to eat, drink, and speak during oxygen administration. Their disadvantage is that the exact $FIO_2$ delivered is not known, as it is influenced by the patient's peak inspiratory flow demand. As an approximation, the following guide can be used: 1 L/minute of nasal prong oxygen flow is approximately equivalent to an $FIO_2$ of 24%, with each additional liter of flow increasing the $FIO_2$ by approximately 4%. Flow rates should be limited to less than 5 L/minute.

II. **Venturi masks** allow the precise administration of oxygen. Usual $FIO_2$ values delivered with these masks are 24%, 28%, 31%, 35%, 40%, and 50%. Often, Venturi masks are useful in patients with COPD and hypercapnia because one can titrate the $PaO_2$ to minimize carbon dioxide retention.

III. **Nonrebreathing masks** achieve higher oxygen concentrations (approximately 80–90%) than do partial rebreathing systems. A one-way valve prevents exhaled gases from entering the reservoir bag in a nonrebreathing system, thereby maximizing the $FIO_2$.

IV. **A continuous positive airway pressure (CPAP) mask** can be used if the $PaO_2$ is less than 60–65 mm Hg during use of a nonrebreathing mask and the patient is conscious and cooperative, able to protect the lower airway, and hemodynamically stable (*N Engl J Med* 339:429, 1998). CPAP is delivered by a tight-fitting mask equipped with pressure-limiting valves. Many patients cannot tolerate a CPAP mask because of persistent hypoxemia, hemodynamic instability, or feelings of claustrophobia or aerophagia. In these patients, endotracheal intubation should be performed. Initially, 3–5 cm $H_2O$ of CPAP should be applied while the $PaO_2$ or $SaO_2$ is monitored. If the $PaO_2$ is still less than 60 mm Hg ($SaO_2$ <90%), the level of CPAP should be increased in steps of 3–5 cm $H_2O$ up to a level of 10–15 cm $H_2O$.

V. **Bilevel positive airway pressure (BiPAP)** is a method of noninvasive ventilation whereby inspiratory and expiratory pressure can be applied by a mask during the patient's respiratory cycle. The inspiratory support decreases the patient's work of breathing. The expiratory support (CPAP) improves gas exchange by preventing alveolar collapse. Noninvasive ventilation using face or nasal masks has been successfully performed in patients with neuromuscular disease, COPD, and postoperative respiratory insufficiency as a means of decreasing the need for endotracheal intubation and mechanical ventilation (*Ann Intern Med* 128:721, 1998). In using BiPAP, a pressure-support ventilation (PSV) level of 5–10 cm $H_2O$ and a CPAP level of 3–5 cm $H_2O$ are reasonable starting points. The PSV level can be increased in increments of 3–5 cm $H_2O$, using the patient's respiratory rate as a guide of effectiveness.

## Airway Management and Tracheal Intubation

Establishment of a patent airway and ventilatory support are required by many ICU patients. Specific indications for airway support in the form of endotracheal intubation include (1) initiation of mechanical ventilation, (2) airway protection, (3) inadequate oxygenation using less invasive methods, (4) prevention of aspiration and allowing for the suctioning of pulmonary secretions, and (5) hyperventilation for the treatment of increased intracranial pressure. In an emergency situation, such simple maneuvers as a jaw thrust with mask-to-face ventilation may assist the patient in clearing an obstructed airway and in maintaining adequate ventilation until endotracheal intubation can be performed.

I. **Airway management**

A. **Head and jaw positioning.** The oropharynx should be inspected, and all foreign bodies should be removed. For patients with inadequate respirations, the jaw thrust or head tilt–chin lift maneuvers should be performed (see Acute Upper Airway Obstruction in Chap. 25, Medical Emergencies).

B. **Oral and nasopharyngeal airways.** When head and jaw positioning fail to establish a patent airway or when more permanent airway maintenance is desired, an oral or nasopharyngeal airway can be used. Initially, oral airways are positioned with the concave curve of the airway facing up into the roof of the mouth. The oral airway then is turned 180 degrees so that the concave curve of the airway follows the natural curve of the tongue. A tongue depressor can also be used to displace the tongue inferiorly and laterally to allow direct positioning of the oral airway. Careful monitoring of airway patency is required, as malpositioning of oral airways can push the tongue posteriorly and can result in obstruction of the oropharynx. Nasopharyngeal airways are made of soft plastic. These airways are passed easily down one of the nasal passages to the posterior pharynx after topical nasal lubrication and anesthesia with viscous lidocaine jelly.

**C. Laryngeal mask airway (LMA).** The LMA is an endotracheal tube with a small mask on one end that can be passed orally over the larynx to provide ventilatory assistance and prevent aspiration. Placement of the LMA is more easily performed than endotracheal intubation. However, it should be considered a temporary airway for patients who require prolonged ventilatory support.

**D. Mask-to-face ventilation.** After an airway is established, respiratory efforts should be evaluated and monitored closely. Ineffective respiratory efforts can be augmented with simple mask-to-face ventilation. Proper fitting and positioning of the mask ensure a tight seal around the mouth and nose, optimizing ventilation. Additionally, proper head positioning (see sec. **II.A**) and the use of airway adjuncts (e.g., oral or nasopharyngeal airways) optimize ventilation with a mask-to-face system.

## II. Endotracheal intubation (*Respir Care* 44:615, 1999)

**A. Technique.** Depending on the skill of the operator and the urgency of the situation, one of several techniques can be selected for intubation of the trachea. Such techniques include (1) direct laryngoscopic orotracheal intubation, (2) blind nasotracheal intubation, and (3) flexible fiberoptically guided orotracheal or nasotracheal intubation. In emergency situations, the direct laryngoscopic technique allows for the most rapid intubation of the trachea with the largest endotracheal tube. Nasotracheal intubation often requires smaller endotracheal tubes that are more susceptible to kinking and obstruction and is associated with a higher incidence of otitis media and sinusitis. Before endotracheal intubation is attempted, a systematic evaluation of the patient's head and neck positioning must be performed. The oral, pharyngeal, and tracheal axes should be aligned before any intubation attempts. This "sniffing" position is achieved by flexing the patient's neck and extending the head. A small pillow or several towels placed under the occiput can assist in maintaining this position. Table 8-2 offers a step-by-step approach to performing successful orotracheal intubation. After successful intubation of the trachea, the tracheal tube cuff pressures should be monitored at regular intervals and should be maintained below capillary filling pressure (i.e., <25 mm Hg) to prevent ischemic mucosal injury.

**B. Verification of correct endotracheal tube positioning.** Proper tube positioning must be ensured by (1) direct view of the endotracheal tube entering the trachea through the vocal cords, (2) fiberoptic inspection of the airways through the endotracheal tube, or (3) use of an end-tidal carbon dioxide monitor. Clinical evaluation of the patient (i.e., listening for bilateral breath sounds over the chest and the absence of ventilation over the stomach) and radiographic evaluation (e.g., standard portable chest radiograph) can be unreliable for establishing correct endotracheal tube positioning. If uncertainty exists regarding the positioning of the endotracheal tube, it should be withdrawn and the patient reintubated.

**C. Complications.** Improper endotracheal tube positioning is the most important immediate complication to be recognized and corrected. Ideally, the tip of the endotracheal tube should be 3–5 cm above the carina, depending on head and neck positioning. Esophageal or right main-stem intubation should be suspected if hypoxemia, hypoventilation, barotrauma, or cardiac decompensation occurs. Abdominal distention, lack of breath sounds over the thorax, and regurgitation of stomach contents through the endotracheal tube indicate an esophageal intubation. Any uncertainty regarding the possibility of an esophageal intubation calls for immediate verification of tube positioning or reintubation of the patient, with direct confirmation of endotracheal tube positioning. Other complications associated with endotracheal intubation include dislodgment of teeth, trauma to the upper airway, and increased intracranial pressure.

**Table 8-2.** Procedure for direct orotracheal intubation

Administer oxygen by face mask.

Ensure that basic equipment is present and easily accessible [oxygen source, bag-valve device, suctioning device, endotracheal (ET) tube, blunt stylet, laryngoscope, 20-ml syringe].

Place patient on nonmobile rigid surface.

If patient is in hospital bed, remove backboard and adjust bed height.

Depress patient's tongue with tongue depressor and administer topical anesthesia to patient's pharynx.

Position patient's head in sniffing position (see Airway Management and Tracheal Intubation, sec. **II.A**).

Administer IV sedation and neuromuscular blocker if necessary.[a]

Have assistant apply Sellick maneuver (compressing cricothyroid cartilage posteriorly against vertebral bodies) to prevent regurgitation and aspiration of stomach contents from esophagus.

Grasp laryngoscope handle in left hand while opening patient's mouth with gloved right hand.

Insert laryngoscope blade on right side of patient's mouth and advance to base of tongue, displacing tongue to the left.

Lift laryngoscope away from patient at a 45-degree angle using arm and shoulder strength. Do not use patient's teeth as a fulcrum.

Suction oropharynx and hypopharynx if necessary.

Grasp ET tube with inserted stylet in right hand and insert it into right corner of patient's mouth, avoiding obscuration of epiglottis and vocal cords.

Advance ET tube through vocal cords until cuff is no longer visible and remove stylet.

Inflate cuff with enough air to prevent significant air leakage.

Verify correct ET tube positioning by auscultation of both lungs and the abdomen.

Obtain a chest radiograph or use end-tidal $CO_2$ monitor to verify correct position of the ET tube.

[a]Neuromuscular blockade can result in complete airway collapse and airway obstruction. Personnel who are skillful in establishment of an emergency surgical airway should be available if paralysis is used.

## III. Surgical airways

**A. Tracheostomy.** The main indications for surgical tracheostomy are (1) the need for prolonged respiratory support, (2) potentially life-threatening upper airway obstruction (due to epiglottitis, facial burns, or worsening laryngeal edema), (3) obstructive sleep apnea that is unresponsive to less invasive therapies, and (4) congenital abnormalities (e.g., Pierre-Robin syndrome). Tracheostomy sites usually require at least 72 hours to mature. Tube dislodgment before site maturation, followed by blind attempts at tube reinsertion, can lead to tube malpositioning within a false channel in the pretracheal space; this misplacement can result in complete loss of the airway followed by progressive hypoxemia and hypotension. If a tracheostomy tube cannot be reinserted easily, standard direct orotracheal intubation should be performed (Table 8-2). Optimal timing of surgical tracheostomy is controversial but should be considered after 10–14 days of mechanical ventilation if prolonged ventilation is anticipated (*Chest* 114:605, 1998).

1. **Cricothyrotomy.** This procedure is indicated for the establishment of an emergency airway when direct tracheal intubation cannot be performed owing to upper airway obstruction. A pillow or towel roll should be placed under the patient's shoulders to extend the neck. The thyroid cartilage superiorly and the cricoid cartilage inferiorly should be located where they border the cricothyroid membrane. The thumb and second finger of the surgeon's nondominant hand should grasp and stabilize the lateral aspects of the cricothyroid membrane. With a scalpel, a transverse skin incision is made over the entire distance of the membrane. The incision then is deepened to the cricothyroid membrane, avoiding injury to surrounding structures. Standard tracheostomy tubes or endotracheal tubes can be inserted into the stoma to ventilate the patient. Alternatively, prepackaged kits using the Seldinger technique with progressive dilatation of the stoma can be used.
2. **Cricothyroid needle cannulation.** In emergency settings when standard endotracheal intubation cannot be performed and placement of a surgical airway is not immediately possible, needle cannulation of the cricothyroid membrane can be performed as an intermediate procedure until a more definitive airway can be established. The ends of the cricothyroid membrane are grasped with the nondominant hand and a 22-gauge needle is inserted into the airway, aspirating air to confirm positioning. Lidocaine then is injected into the trachea to blunt the patient's cough reflex before the needle is withdrawn. By the same technique, a 14-gauge (or larger) needle-through-cannula device can be passed through the cricothyroid membrane at a 45-degree angle to the skin. When air is aspirated freely, the outer cannula is passed into the airway caudally, and the needle is removed. A 3-ml syringe barrel then can be attached to the catheter and a 7-mm inner-diameter endotracheal tube adapter attached to the syringe to allow bag-valve ventilation. Alternatively, the cannula can be attached directly to high-flow oxygen (i.e., 10–15 L/minute).

## Mechanical Ventilation

I. **Indications.** The decision to begin mechanical ventilation is a clinical judgment that should take into account the reversibility of the underlying disease process as well as the patient's overall medical condition. Usual indications include severely impaired gas exchange, rapid onset of respiratory failure, an inadequate response to less invasive medical treatments, and increased work of breathing with evidence of respiratory muscle fatigue. Parameters that can help to guide the decision as to whether mechanical ventilation is needed include respiratory rate (>35), inspiratory force ($\leq$ 25 cm $H_2O$), vital capacity (<10–15 ml/kg), $PaO_2$ (<60 mm Hg with $FIO_2$ >60%), $PaCO_2$ (>50 mm Hg with pH <7.35), and an absent gag or cough reflex.

II. **Initiation of mechanical ventilation.** Certain variables should be considered when initiating mechanical ventilation.

A. **Ventilator type.** Often, ventilator selection is dictated by what is available at a particular hospital. A volume-cycled ventilator is used in most clinical circumstances.

B. **Mode of ventilation.** Several modes of mechanical ventilation are available. General guidelines for the use of the more commonly administered or referred to modes are provided.

1. **Assist-control ventilation (ACV)** should be the initial mode of ventilation used in most patients with respiratory failure. It produces a ventilator-delivered breath for every patient-initiated inspiratory effort.

Controlled ventilator-initiated breaths are delivered automatically when the patient's spontaneous rate falls below the selected backup rate. Respiratory alkalosis is a potential concern when using ACV for patients with tachypnea.

2. **Intermittent mandatory ventilation (IMV)** allows patients to breathe at a spontaneous rate and tidal volume without triggering the ventilator, while the ventilator adds additional mechanical breaths at a preset rate and tidal volume. **Synchronized intermittent mandatory ventilation (SIMV)** allows the ventilator to become sensitized to the patient's respiratory efforts at intervals determined by the frequency setting. This capability allows coordination of the delivery of the ventilator-driven breath with the respiratory cycle of the patient to prevent inadvertent stacking of a mechanical breath on top of a spontaneous inspiration. Potential advantages of SIMV include less respiratory alkalosis, fewer adverse cardiovascular effects due to lower intrathoracic pressures, less requirement for sedation and paralysis, maintenance of respiratory muscle function, and facilitation of long-term weaning. However, considerable patient-initiated respiratory muscle work may contribute to respiratory muscle fatigue and failure to wean from mechanical ventilation in some patients. This nonphysiologic work of spontaneous breathing can be alleviated by the addition of low levels of PSV (4–8 cm $H_2O$) or the addition of flow-by, or both (see sec. **II.C.6**).
3. **PSV** augments each patient-triggered respiratory effort by an operator-specified amount of pressure that is usually between 5 and 50 cm $H_2O$. PSV is used primarily to augment spontaneous respiratory efforts during IMV modes of ventilation or during weaning trials (see sec. **IV**). PSV can also be used as a primary form of ventilation in patients who can trigger the ventilator spontaneously. Increased airway resistance, decreased lung compliance, and decreased patient effort result in diminished tidal volumes and, frequently, in decreased minute ventilation. PSV is not recommended as a primary ventilatory mode in patients in whom any of the aforementioned parameters are expected to fluctuate widely.
4. **Inverse ratio ventilation (IRV)** uses an inspiratory-to-expiratory ratio that is greater than the standard 1:2–1:3 ratio (i.e., $\geq$ 1:1) to stabilize terminal respiratory units (i.e., alveolar recruitment) and to improve gas exchange primarily for patients with ARDS (*Crit Care Clin* 14:707, 1998). The goals of IRV are to decrease peak airway pressures, to maintain adequate alveolar ventilation, and to improve oxygenation. The use of IRV can be considered in patients with a $PaO_2$ of less than 60 mm Hg despite an $FIO_2$ of greater than 60%, peak airway pressures greater than 40–45 cm $H_2O$, or the need for positive end-expiratory pressure (PEEP) of greater than 15 cm $H_2O$. Most patients need heavy sedation and often muscle paralysis during the implementation of IRV.
5. **Lung-protective, pressure-targeted ventilation** (i.e., permissive hypercapnia) is a method whereby controlled hypoventilation is allowed to occur with elevation of the $PaCO_2$ to minimize the detrimental effects of excessive airway pressures. This form of ventilation has been used in patients with respiratory failure due to asthma and ARDS. In patients with ARDS the application of tidal volumes less than or equal to 6 ml/kg has been used as a lung-protective strategy and has been associated with improved outcomes (*N Engl J Med* 342:1301, 2000). The use of smaller tidal volumes is thought to prevent ventilator-induced lung injury. Additional methods for improving oxygenation while minimizing lung injury during mechanical ventilation in ARDS include prone positioning (*N Engl J Med* 345:568, 2001) and the administration of nitric oxide (NO) (see sec. **II.B.9**), although these interventions have not been associated with a survival advantage. The administration of corticoster-

oids for established ARDS has been associated with improved survival in one small randomized controlled trial of ARDS (*JAMA* 280:159, 1998). For patients with asthma, the use of a helium-oxygen mixture may result in improved lung mechanics compared to the use of oxygen alone (*Am J Respir Crit Care Med* 165:1317, 2002).

6. **Independent lung ventilation** uses two independent ventilators and a double-lumen endotracheal tube. Usually, this modality is reserved for severe unilateral lung disease, such as unilateral pneumonia, respiratory failure associated with hemoptysis, or a bronchopleural fistula.
7. **High-frequency ventilation** uses rates that are substantially faster (60–300 breaths/minute) than conventional ventilation with small tidal volumes (2–4 ml/kg). The use of high-frequency ventilation is controversial except during upper airway surgery.
8. **Partial liquid ventilation** involves the partial filling of the lung with a perfluorocarbon solution. This type of ventilation has been demonstrated to improve pulmonary mechanics, oxygenation, and ventilation and perfusion matching in patients with ARDS. Partial liquid ventilation appears to improve gas exchange by recruiting previously atelectatic lung regions and by facilitating the transport of oxygen to all lung regions.
9. **Mechanical ventilation with inhaled NO** has been demonstrated to improve gas exchange in adults and children with respiratory failure, including patients with ARDS, primary pulmonary hypertension, or cor pulmonale secondary to congenital heart disease, and after cardiac surgery or heart or lung transplantation. Inhaled NO acts as a selective pulmonary artery (PA) vasodilator, decreasing PA pressures (without decreasing systemic BP or CO) and improving oxygenation by reducing intrapulmonary shunt (*Crit Care Med* 26:15, 1998). Generally, 5–20 ppm NO is administered, and the level of methemoglobin is monitored periodically.

**C. Ventilator management**

1. **$FIO_2$.** Hypoxemia is more dangerous than is brief exposure to high inspired levels of oxygen. The initial $FIO_2$ should be 100%. Adjustments in the $FIO_2$ can be made to achieve a $PaO_2$ of greater than 60 mm Hg or an $SaO_2$ of greater than 90%.
2. **Minute ventilation.** Minute ventilation is determined by the respiratory rate and the tidal volume. In general, a respiratory rate of 10–15 breaths/minute is an appropriate rate with which to begin. Close monitoring of minute ventilation is especially important in ventilating patients with COPD and carbon dioxide retention. In these individuals, the minute ventilation should be adjusted to achieve the patient's baseline $PaCO_2$ and not necessarily a normal $PaCO_2$. Inadvertent hyperventilation with resultant metabolic alkalosis in these patients may be associated with serious serum electrolyte shifts and arrhythmias. Initial tidal volumes usually can be set at 10–12 ml/kg. Patients with decreased lung compliance (e.g., ARDS) often need smaller lung volumes (6–8 ml/kg) to minimize peak airway pressures and iatrogenic morbidity.
3. **PEEP** is defined as the maintenance of positive airway pressure at the end of expiration. It can be applied to the spontaneously breathing patient in the form of CPAP or to the patient who is receiving mechanical ventilation. The appropriate application of PEEP usually increases lung compliance and oxygenation while decreasing the shunt fraction and the work of breathing. PEEP increases peak and mean airway pressures, which can increase the likelihood of barotrauma and cardiovascular compromise. PEEP is used primarily in patients with hypoxic respiratory failure (e.g., ARDS, cardiogenic pulmonary edema). Low levels of PEEP (3–5 cm $H_2O$) may also be useful in patients with COPD, to prevent dynamic airway collapse from occurring during expiration.

The main goal of PEEP is to achieve a $PaO_2$ of greater than 55–60 mm Hg with an $FIO_2$ of less than or equal to 60% while avoiding significant cardiovascular sequelae. Usually, PEEP is applied in 3- to 5-cm $H_2O$ increments during monitoring of oxygenation, organ perfusion, and hemodynamic parameters. Patients who receive significant levels of PEEP (i.e., >10 cm $H_2O$) should not have their PEEP removed abruptly, because removal can result in collapse of distal lung units, the worsening of shunt, and potentially life-threatening hypoxemia. PEEP should be weaned in 3- to 5-cm $H_2O$ increments while oxygenation is monitored closely.

4. **Inspiratory flow rate.** Flow rates set inappropriately low can be associated with prolonged inspiratory times that can lead to the development of auto-PEEP (see sec. **III.G**). The resultant lung hyperinflation can affect patient hemodynamics adversely by impairing venous return to the heart. Patients with severe airflow obstruction are at the greatest risk for development of lung hyperinflation when improper flow rates are used. Increasing the inspiratory flow rate usually allows for longer expiratory times that help to reverse this process.
5. **Trigger sensitivity.** Most mechanical ventilators use pressure triggering either to initiate a machine-assisted breath or to permit spontaneous breathing between IMV breaths, or during trials of CPAP. The patient must generate a decrease in the airway circuit pressure equal to the selected pressure sensitivity. Most patients do not tolerate a trigger sensitivity of less than –1 or –2 cm $H_2O$ because of autocycling of the ventilator. Alternatively, excessive trigger sensitivity can increase the patient's work of breathing, contributing to failure to wean from mechanical ventilation. In general, the smallest trigger sensitivity should be selected, allowing the patient to initiate mechanical or spontaneous breaths without causing the ventilator to autocycle.
6. **Flow-by.** To decrease the patient work of breathing, flow-by can be used as an adjunct to conventional modes of mechanical ventilation. Flow-by refers to triggering of the ventilator by changes in airflow as opposed to changes in airway pressures. A continuous base flow of gas is provided through the ventilator circuit at a preselected flow rate (5–20 L/minute). A flow sensitivity (i.e., patient rate of inhaled flow that triggers the ventilator to switch from base flow to either a machine-delivered or a spontaneous breath) is selected (usually 2 L/minute). Flow-triggered systems are more responsive than are pressure-triggered systems and result in a decreased work of breathing.

**III. Management of problems and complications**

**A. Airway malpositioning and occlusion** (see Airway Management and Tracheal Intubation, sec. **II.C**).

**B. Worsening respiratory distress or arterial oxygen desaturation** may develop suddenly as a result of changes in the patient's cardiopulmonary status or secondary to a mechanical malfunction. The first priority is to ensure patency and correct positioning of the patient's airway so that adequate oxygenation and ventilation can be administered during the ensuing evaluation.

1. **Briefly note ventilator alarms, airway pressures, and tidal volume.** Low-pressure alarms with decreased exhaled tidal volumes may suggest a leak in the ventilator circuit.
2. **Disconnect the patient from the ventilator and manually ventilate with an anesthesia bag using 100% oxygen.** For patients receiving PEEP, manual ventilation with a PEEP valve should be used to prevent atelectasis and hypoxemia.
3. **If manual ventilation is difficult, check airway patency by passing a suction catheter through the endotracheal tube or tracheostomy.** Additionally, listen for prolonged expiration continuing up to the point

of the next manual breath. This suggests the presence of gas trapping and auto-PEEP.

4. **Check vital signs and perform a rapid physical examination with attention to the patient's cardiopulmonary status.** Be attentive to asymmetry in breath sounds or tracheal deviation suggesting tension pneumothorax. Note other parameters, including cardiac rhythm and hemodynamics.
5. **Treat appropriately on the basis of the foregoing evaluation.** Treatment should be specific to the identified problems. If the presence of gas trapping and auto-PEEP is suspected, a reduction in the minute ventilation is appropriate. In some circumstances, periods of hypoventilation (4–6 breaths/minute) or even apnea for 30–60 seconds may be necessary to reverse the hemodynamic sequelae of auto-PEEP (e.g., shock, electromechanical dissociation).
6. **Return the patient to the ventilator only after checking its function.** Increase the level of support provided by the ventilator to the patient after an episode of respiratory distress or arterial oxygen desaturation. Usually, this adjustment means increasing the $FIO_2$ and the delivered minute ventilation unless significant auto-PEEP is present.

C. An **acute increase** in the **peak airway pressure** usually implies either a decrease in lung compliance or an increase in airway resistance. At a minimum, considerations that should be entertained as causes of increased airway pressure include (1) pneumothorax, hemothorax, or hydropneumothorax; (2) occlusion of the patient's airway; (3) bronchospasm; (4) increased accumulation of condensate in the ventilator circuit tubing; (5) main-stem intubation; (6) worsening pulmonary edema; or (7) the development of gas trapping with auto-PEEP.

D. **Loss of tidal volume,** as evidenced by a difference between the tidal volume setting and the delivered tidal volume, implies a leak in either the ventilator or the inspiratory limb of the circuit tubing. A difference between the delivered tidal volume and the expired tidal volume implies the presence of a leak at the patient's airway due either to cuff malfunction or to malpositioning of the airway (e.g., positioning of the cuff at or above the level of the glottis) or a leak within the patient (e.g., presence of a bronchopleural fistula in a patient with a chest tube).

E. **Asynchronous breathing ("fighting" or "bucking" the ventilator)** occurs when a patient's breathing coordinates poorly with the ventilator. This difficulty may indicate unmet respiratory demands. A careful evaluation is mandated, with attention focused at the identification of leaks in the ventilator system or airway, inadequate $FIO_2$, or inadequate ventilatory support. The problem can be alleviated by adjustments in the mode of mechanical ventilation, rate, tidal volume, inspiratory flow rate, and level of PEEP. The identification of gas trapping with auto-PEEP may require changing multiple settings to allow adequate time for exhalation (e.g., decreasing rate and tidal volume, increasing inspiratory flow rate, switching from assist-control to SIMV in selected cases). Additionally, measures aimed at reducing the work of breathing with mechanical ventilation also may resolve the problem (addition of flow-by triggering or low levels of PSV to patients taking spontaneous breaths). If these adjustments are unsuccessful, sedation should be attempted. Muscle paralysis should be reserved for patients in whom effective gas exchange and ventilation cannot be achieved with other measures.

F. **Organ hypoperfusion or hypotension** can occur. Positive-pressure ventilation can result in decreased CO and BP by decreasing venous return to the right ventricle, increasing pulmonary vascular resistance, and impairing diastolic filling of the left ventricle because of increased right-sided heart pressures. Increasing the preload to the left ventricle with fluid administration should increase stroke volume and CO in most cases. Occasionally, the administration of dobutamine (after appropriate preload replacement) or vasopressors becomes necessary. Under these circumstances, consideration should be given to reducing airway pressures (peak airway pressures <40 cm $H_2O$) at the expense of relative hypoventilation (i.e., pressure-targeted ventilation).

G. **Auto-PEEP** is the development of end-expiratory pressure caused by airflow limitation in patients with airway disease (emphysema, asthma), excessive minute ventilation, or an inadequate expiratory time. Graphic tracings on modern ventilators can suggest the presence of gas trapping by demonstrating persistent airflow at end expiration. The level of auto-PEEP can be estimated in the spontaneously breathing patient by occluding the expiratory port of the ventilator briefly just before inspiration and measuring the end-expiratory pressure reading on the ventilator's manometer. The presence of auto-PEEP can increase the work of breathing, contribute to barotrauma, and result in organ hypoperfusion by impairing CO. Appropriate adjustments to the ventilator can reduce or eliminate the presence of auto-PEEP (see sec. **II.C**).

H. **Barotrauma or volutrauma** in the form of subcutaneous emphysema, pneumoperitoneum, pneumomediastinum, pneumopericardium, air embolism, and pneumothorax is associated with high peak airway pressures, PEEP, and auto-PEEP. Subcutaneous emphysema, pneumomediastinum, and pneumoperitoneum seldom threaten the patient's well-being. However, the occurrence of these disorders usually indicates a need to reduce peak airway pressures and the total level of PEEP. The occurrence of a pneumothorax is a potentially life-threatening complication and should be considered whenever airway pressure rises acutely, breath sounds are diminished unilaterally, or BP falls abruptly (see Pneumothorax in Chap. 25, Medical Emergencies). In most cases, acute tension pneumothorax should be treated as an emergency by inserting a 14-gauge catheter-over-needle device into the pleural space at the xiphoid level in the midaxillary line or anteriorly into the second or third intercostal space in the midclavicular line. Chest tube insertion should follow.

I. **Positive fluid balance and hyponatremia** in mechanically ventilated patients often develop from several factors, including applied PEEP, humidification of inspired gases, administration of hypotonic fluids and diuretics, and increased levels of circulating antidiuretic hormone.

J. **Cardiac arrhythmias,** particularly multifocal atrial tachycardia and atrial fibrillation, are common in respiratory failure and should be treated as outlined in Chap. 7, Cardiac Arrhythmias.

K. **Aspiration** commonly occurs despite the use of a cuffed endotracheal tube, especially in patients who are receiving enteral nutrition. Elevating the head of the bed and avoiding excessive gastric distention help to minimize the occurrence of aspiration. Additionally, pooling of secretions around the cuff of the endotracheal tube requires suctioning of these secretions before deflation or manipulation of the cuff.

L. **Ventilator-associated pneumonia** is a frequent complication connected with increased patient morbidity and mortality. Prevention of ventilator-associated pneumonia is aimed at avoiding colonization in the patient of pathogenic bacteria and their subsequent aspiration into the lower airway (*N Engl J Med* 340:627, 1999).

M. **Upper GI hemorrhage** may develop secondary to gastritis or ulceration. The prevention of stress bleeding requires ensuring hemodynamic stability and, in high-risk patients [e.g., those receiving prolonged mechanical ventilation (>48–72 hours) or with a coagulopathy], the administration of $H_2$-receptor antagonists, antacids, or sucralfate.

N. **Thromboembolism** (deep venous thrombosis and pulmonary embolism) may complicate the clinical course of patients who require mechanical ventilation. This disorder can be prevented in most patients by the prophylactic administration of SC heparin, 5000 U q8–12h, or the use of intermittent pneumatic compression devices (see Chap. 1, Patient Care in Internal Medicine).

O. **Acid-base complications** are common in the critically ill patient (see also Chap. 3, Fluid and Electrolyte Management).

1. **Nonanion gap metabolic acidosis** may render weaning difficult, as minute ventilation must increase to normalize pH.
2. **Metabolic alkalosis** may compromise weaning by blunting ventilatory drive to maintain a normal pH. In patients with chronic ventilatory insufficiency (e.g., emphysema, cystic fibrosis), correction of metabolic alkalosis usually is inappropriate and can cause an unsustainable minute ventilation requirement. Under these circumstances, a patient should be allowed to slow minute ventilation gradually to a more appropriate level. This change may be facilitated by switching from ACV to SIMV or PSV.
3. **Respiratory alkalosis** may develop rapidly during mechanical ventilation. When severe, it can lead to arrhythmias, CNS disturbances (including seizures), and a decrease in CO. Changing the ventilator settings to reduce the minute ventilation or changing the mode of ventilation (ACV to SIMV) usually corrects the alkalosis. However, some patients (such as those with ARDS, interstitial lung disease, pulmonary embolism, asthma) are driven to high respiratory rates by local pulmonary stimuli. In such patients, sedation with or without paralysis may be indicated briefly during the acute phase of the respiratory compromise.

P. **Oxygen toxicity** commonly is accepted to occur when an $FIO_2$ of greater than 0.6 is administered, particularly for more than 48 hours. However, the highest $FIO_2$ necessary should be used initially to maintain the $SaO_2$ at more than 0.9. The application of PEEP or other maneuvers that increase mean airway pressure (e.g., IRV) can be used to reduce $FIO_2$ requirements. However, an $FIO_2$ of 0.6–0.8 should be accepted before a plateau pressure above 30 cm $H_2O$ is accepted. This cautionary note is due to the greater risk of morbidity associated with plateau pressures above this level (*N Engl J Med* 338:347, 1998).

IV. **Weaning from mechanical ventilation.** Weaning is the gradual withdrawal of mechanical ventilatory support (*Chest* 114:886, 1998). Successful weaning depends on the condition of the patient and on the status of the cardiovascular and respiratory systems. In patients who have had brief periods of mechanical ventilation, the manner in which ventilatory support is discontinued often is not crucial. In patients with marginal respiratory function, chronic underlying lung disease, or incompletely resolved respiratory impairment, the approach to weaning may be critical to obtaining a favorable outcome.

A. **Weaning strategies.** In general, the level of supported ventilation (minute ventilation) is decreased gradually, and the patient assumes more of the work of ventilation with each of the techniques described. However, it is important during the weaning process not to fatigue the patient excessively, which can prolong the duration of mechanical ventilation.

1. **IMV** allows a progressive change from mechanical ventilation to spontaneous breathing by decreasing the ventilator rate gradually. However, the weaning process may be prolonged if ventilator changes are not made often enough. Prolonged periods at low rates (<6 breaths/minute) may promote a state of respiratory muscle fatigue because of the imposed work of breathing through a high-resistance ventilator circuit. The addition of PSV (see sec. **II.B.3**) may alleviate this fatigue but can prolong the weaning process if not titrated appropriately. Very often, tachypnea that occurs during weaning of the IMV rate represents a problem related to the imposed work from the ventilator circuit and the endotracheal tube rather than a diagnosis of persistent respiratory failure. In circumstances in which this problem is suspected, a trial of extubation may be appropriate.
2. **T-tube technique** intersperses periods of unassisted spontaneous breathing through a T tube (or other continuous-flow circuit) with periods of ventilator support (*N Engl J Med* 332:345, 1995). Short daytime periods (5–15 minutes two to four times/day) are used initially and then are increased progressively in duration. Small amounts of CPAP (3–5 cm

**Table 8-3.** Factors to be considered in the weaning process

| |
|---|
| **W**eaning parameters |
| See Table 8-4 |
| **E**ndotracheal tube |
| Use largest tube possible |
| Consider use of supplemental pressure-support ventilation |
| Suction secretions |
| **A**rterial blood gases |
| Avoid or treat metabolic alkalosis |
| Maintain $PaO_2$ at 60–65 mm Hg to avoid blunting of respiratory drive |
| For patients with carbon dioxide retention, keep $PaCO_2$ at or above the baseline level |
| **N**utrition |
| Ensure adequate nutritional support |
| Avoid electrolyte deficiencies |
| Avoid excessive calories |
| **S**ecretions |
| Clear regularly |
| Avoid excessive dehydration |
| **N**euromuscular factors |
| Avoid neuromuscular-depressing drugs |
| Avoid unnecessary corticosteroids |
| **O**bstruction of airways |
| Use bronchodilators when appropriate |
| Exclude foreign bodies within the airway |
| **W**akefulness |
| Avoid oversedation |
| Wean in morning or when patient is most awake |

$H_2O$) during these periods may prevent distal airway closure and atelectasis, although the effects on weaning success appear to be negligible (*Chest* 100:1655, 1991). Similar to IMV weaning, small amounts of pressure support (4–8 cm $H_2O$) can be used to decrease inspiratory resistance imposed by the ventilator circuit and the endotracheal tube. Extubation may be appropriate when the patient can comfortably tolerate more than 30–90 minutes of T-tube ventilation. More prolonged periods of T-tube breathing may produce fatigue, especially when small endotracheal tubes (i.e., <8 mm internal diameter) are used.

3. **PSV** is preferred by some practitioners when respiratory muscle weakness appears to be compromising weaning success (*Am J Respir Crit Care Med* 150:896, 1994). PSV can reduce the patient's work of breathing through the endotracheal tube and the ventilator circuit. The optimal level of PSV is selected by increasing the PSV level from a baseline of 15–20 cm $H_2O$ in increments of 3–5 cm $H_2O$. A decrease in respiratory rate with achieved tidal volumes of 10–12 ml/kg signals that the optimal PSV level has been reached. When the patient is ready to begin weaning, the level of PSV is reduced gradually by 3- to 5-cm $H_2O$ incre-

**Table 8-4.** Guidelines for assessing withdrawal of mechanical ventilation

| |
|---|
| Patient's mental status: awake, alert, cooperative |
| $PaO_2$ >60 mm Hg with an $FIO_2$ <50% |
| PEEP ≤ 5 cm $H_2O$ |
| $PaCO_2$ and pH acceptable |
| Spontaneous tidal volume >5 ml/kg |
| Vital capacity >10 ml/kg |
| MV <10 L/min |
| Maximum voluntary ventilation double of MV |
| Maximum negative inspiratory pressure ≥ 25 cm $H_2O$ |
| Respiratory rate <30 breaths/min |
| Static compliance >30 ml/cm $H_2O$ |
| Rapid shallow breathing index (ratio of respiratory rate to tidal volume) <100 breaths/min/L |
| Stable vital signs after a 1- to 2-hr spontaneous breathing trial |

$FIO_2$, inspired oxygen concentration; MV, minute ventilation; $PaCO_2$, arterial carbon dioxide tension; $PaO_2$, arterial oxygen tension; PEEP, positive end-expiratory pressure.
*Source:* From KL Yang, MJ Tobin. A prospective study of indexes predicting the outcome of trials of weaning from mechanical ventilation. *N Engl J Med* 324:1445, 1991; and EW Ely, AM Baker, DP Dunagan, et al. Effect on the duration of mechanical ventilation of identifying patients capable of breathing spontaneously. *N Engl J Med* 335:1864, 1996, with permission.

ments. Once a PSV level of 5–8 cm $H_2O$ is reached, the patient can be extubated without further decreases in PSV.

4. **Protocol-guided weaning of mechanical ventilation** has been safely and successfully used by nonphysicians (*Crit Care Med* 25:567, 1997). The use of protocols or guidelines can reduce the duration of mechanical ventilation by expediting the weaning process.

B. **Failure to wean.** Patients who do not wean from mechanical ventilation after 48–72 hours of the resolution of their underlying disease process need further investigation. Table 8-3 lists the factors that should be considered when weaning failure occurs. The acronym "WEANS NOW" has been developed to aid in addressing each of these factors (*J Respir Dis* 6:80, 1985). Commonly used parameters that can be assessed in predicting weaning success are listed in Table 8-4.

C. **Extubation.** Usually, extubation should be performed early in the day, when full ancillary staff are available. The patient should be clearly educated about the procedure, the need to cough, and the possible need for reintubation. Elevation of the head and trunk to more than 30–45 degrees improves diaphragmatic function. Equipment for reintubation should be available, and a high-humidity, oxygen-enriched gas source with a higher-than-current $FIO_2$ setting should be available at the bedside. The patient's airway and the oropharynx above the cuff should be suctioned. The cuff of the endotracheal tube should be deflated partially, and airflow around the outside of the tube—indicating the absence of airway obstruction—should be detected. After the cuff is deflated completely, the patient should be extubated, and high-humidity oxygen should be administered by a face mask. Coughing and deep breathing should be encouraged while the examiner monitors the patient's vital signs and upper airway for stridor. Inspiratory stridor may result from glottic and subglottic edema. If clinical status permits, treatment with nebulized 2.5% racemic epinephrine (0.5 ml in 3 ml normal saline) should be administered. If upper airway obstruction persists

**Table 8-5.** ICU drugs to facilitate endotracheal intubation and mechanical ventilation

| Drug | Bolus dosages (IV) | Continuous-infusion dosages[a] | Onset | Duration after single dose |
|---|---|---|---|---|
| Succinylcholine | 0.3–1 mg/kg | — | 45–60 sec | 2–10 min |
| Pancuronium | 0.05–0.08 mg/kg | 0.2–0.6 μg/kg/min | 2–4 min | 40–60 min |
| Vecuronium | 0.08–0.10 mg/kg | 0.3–1.0 μg/kg/min | 2–4 min | 30–45 min |
| Atracurium | 0.4–0.5 mg/kg | 5–10 μg/kg/min | 2–4 min | 20–45 min |
| Diazepam | 2.5–5.0 mg up to 20–30 mg | 1–10 mg/hr or titrate to effect | 1–5 min | 30–90 min[b] |
| Midazolam | 1–4 mg | 1–10 mg/hr or titrate to effect | 1–5 min | 30–60 min[b] |
| Morphine | 2–5 mg | 1–10 mg/hr or titrate to effect | 2–10 min | 2–4 hr[b] |
| Fentanyl | 0.5–1.0 μg/kg | 1–2 μg/kg/hr or titrate to effect | 30–60 sec | 30–60 min[b] |
| Thiopental | 50–100 mg; repeat up to 20 mg/kg | — | 20 sec | 10–20 min[b] |
| Methohexital | 1–1.5 mg/kg | — | 15–45 sec | 5–20 min[b] |
| Etomidate | 0.3–0.4 mg/kg | — | 10–20 sec | 4–10 min |
| Propofol | 0.25–1.00 mg/kg | 50–100 μg/kg/min | 15–60 sec | 3–10 min[b] |

[a]A continuous infusion should be started or titrated upward only after the desired level of sedation is achieved with bolus administration.
[b]Duration is prolonged with continued use either as repeated boluses or continuous IV administration. Frequent titration to the minimum effective dose is required to prevent accumulation of drug.

or worsens, reintubation should be performed. Extubation should not be reattempted for 24–72 hours after reintubation for upper airway obstruction. Otolaryngology consultation may be beneficial to exclude other causes of upper airway obstruction and to perform tracheostomy if upper airway obstruction persists.

V. **Drugs** are commonly used in the ICU to facilitate tracheal intubation and mechanical ventilation (Table 8-5). Nondepolarizing muscle relaxants have been implicated in muscle dysfunction and prolonged weakness after their use in ICU patients (*Am Rev Respir Dis* 147:234, 1993). Some reports suggest a drug interaction between muscle relaxants and glucocorticoids, potentiating this effect. To minimize the chances of this complication, the continuous use of muscle relaxants should be limited to as brief a period as possible. Peripheral nerve stimulators should be used to titrate the dose of the muscle relaxant to the lowest effective dose. Finally, glucocorticoids should be avoided in patients who are receiving muscle relaxants unless their use is clearly indicated (e.g., for status asthmaticus, anaphylactic shock).

## Shock

Circulatory shock is a process in which blood flow and oxygen delivery to tissues are disturbed; this event leads to tissue hypoxia, with resultant compromise of cellular metabolic activity and organ function. Oliguria, decreased mental status, decreased peripheral pulses, and diaphoresis represent the major clinical manifestations of circulatory shock. Survival from shock is related to the adequacy of the initial resuscitation and the degree of subsequent organ system dysfunction. The main goal of therapy is rapid cardiovascular resuscitation with the re-establishment of tissue perfusion using fluid therapy and vasoactive drugs. The definitive treatment of shock requires reversal of the underlying etiologic process.

**I. Resuscitative principles**

**A. Fluid resuscitation** is usually the first treatment used. All patients in shock should receive an initial IV fluid challenge. The amount of fluid necessary is unpredictable but should be based on changes in clinical parameters, including arterial BP, urine output, cardiac filling pressures, and CO. Crystalloid fluid solutions (0.9% sodium chloride or Ringer's lactate) usually are administered, owing to their lower cost and comparable efficacy compared to colloid solutions (5% and 25% albumin, 6% hetastarch, dextran 40, and dextran 70). Blood products should be administered to patients with significant anemia or active hemorrhage. Young, adequately resuscitated patients usually tolerate hematocrits of 20–25%. In older patients, individuals with atherosclerosis, and patients who exhibit ongoing anaerobic metabolism, hematocrits of 30% or greater may be required to optimize oxygen transport to tissues.

**B. Vasopressors and inotropes** play a crucial role in the management of shock states. Their use usually requires monitoring with intra-arterial and PA catheters. **Dopamine** is capable of stimulating cardiac $\beta_1$-receptors, peripheral α-receptors, and dopaminergic receptors in renal, splanchnic, and other vascular beds. The effects of dopamine are dose dependent. At dosages of 2–3 μg/kg/minute, dopamine primarily acts as a vasodilator, increasing renal and splanchnic blood flow. At dosages of 4–8 μg/kg/minute, dopamine increases cardiac contractility and CO via the activation of cardiac $\beta_1$-receptors. At higher dosages (>10 μg/kg/minute), dopamine increases BP by activation of peripheral α-receptors. **Dobutamine** is an inotropic agent that activates the $\alpha_1$-, $\beta_1$-, and $\beta_2$-receptors. It exerts powerful inotropic effects, reduces afterload by indirect (reflex) peripheral vasodilation, and is a relatively weak chronotropic agent, accounting for its favorable hemodynamic response (increased stroke volume with modest increases in heart rate unless used in high dose or in the setting of hypovolemia). **Epinephrine** has α- and β-adrenergic activity. It is the agent of choice for anaphylactic shock. Like dopamine, its relative effects are dose dependent. **Norepinephrine** also has α- and β-adrenergic activity but primarily is a potent vasoconstricting agent. **Vasopressin** is a vasoconstrictor mediated by three different G-peptide receptors called $V_{1a}$, $V_{1b}$, and $V_2$ (*Am J Med Sci* 324:146, 2002). The usual dose of vasopressin for hypotension is 0.04 U/minute. **Amrinone and milrinone** are noncatecholamine inhibitors of phosphodiesterase III that act as inotropes and as direct peripheral vasodilators to increase CO.

**II. Individual shock states** usually can be classified into four broad categories. These categories include hypovolemic shock (e.g., hemorrhage, dehydration), cardiogenic shock (e.g., acute myocardial infarction, cardiac tamponade), obstructive shock (e.g., acute pulmonary embolism), and distributive shock (septic shock and anaphylactic shock). Table 8-6 gives the main hemodynamic patterns seen with each of these shock states.

**A. Hypovolemic shock** results from a decrease in effective intravascular volume that decreases venous return to the right ventricle. Significant hypovolemic shock (i.e., >40% loss of intravascular volume) that lasts for more than several hours is often associated with a fatal outcome despite resuscitative efforts. Therapy of hypovolemic shock usually is aimed at re-establishing the adequacy of the intravascular volume. At the same time, ongoing sources of

**Table 8-6.** Hemodynamic patterns associated with specific shock states

| Type of shock | CI | SVR | PVR | $SvO_2$ | RAP | RVP | PAP | PAOP |
|---|---|---|---|---|---|---|---|---|
| Cardiogenic (e.g., MI, cardiac tamponade[a]) | ↓ | ↑ | N | ↓ | ↑ | ↑ | ↑ | ↑ |
| Hypovolemic (e.g., hemorrhage) | ↓ | ↑ | N | ↓ | ↓ | ↓ | ↓ | ↓ |
| Distributive (e.g., septic) | — | ↓ | N | N–↑ | N–↓ | N–↓ | N–↓ | N–↓ |
| Obstructive (e.g., massive pulmonary embolism) | ↓ | ↑–N | ↓ | ↑ | ↑ | ↑ | ↑ | N–↓ |

CI, cardiac index; MI, myocardial infarction; N, normal; PAOP, pulmonary artery occlusion pressure; PAP, pulmonary artery pressure; PVR, pulmonary vascular resistance; RAP, right atrial pressure; RVP, right ventricular pressure; $SvO_2$, mixed venous oxygen saturation; SVR, systemic vascular resistance; ↑, increased; ↓, decreased.
[a]Equalization of RAP, PAOP, diastolic PAP, and diastolic RVP establishes a diagnosis of cardiac tamponade.

volume loss, such as a bleeding vessel, may require surgical intervention. Crystalloid solutions are used initially for the resuscitation of patients in hypovolemic shock. Fluid resuscitation must be prompt and should be given through large-bore catheters placed in large peripheral veins. **Rapid infusers or pumps** are available to increase the rate of fluid resuscitation. In the absence of overt signs of CHF, the patient should receive a 500- to 1000-ml initial bolus of normal saline or Ringer's lactate, with further infusions adjusted to achieve adequate BP and tissue perfusion. When shock is due to hemorrhage, packed RBCs should be given as soon as feasible. When hemorrhage is massive, type-specific unmatched blood can be given safely. Rarely, type O-negative blood is needed.

**B. Cardiogenic shock** is seen most commonly after acute myocardial infarction (see Chap. 5, Ischemic Heart Disease) and usually is the result of pump failure. Other causes of cardiogenic shock include septal wall rupture, acute mitral regurgitation, myocarditis, dilated cardiomyopathy, arrhythmias, pericardial tamponade, and right ventricular failure due to pulmonary embolism. Cardiogenic shock secondary to acute myocardial infarction usually is associated with hypotension (mean arterial BP <60 mm Hg), decreased cardiac index (<2.0 L/minute/$m^2$), elevated intracardiac pressures [pulmonary artery occlusive pressure (PAOP) >18 mm Hg], increased peripheral vascular resistance, and organ hypoperfusion (e.g., decreased urine output, altered mentation) (Table 8-6).

1. Certain **general measures** should be undertaken. A $PaO_2$ of greater than 60 mm Hg should be achieved, and the hematocrit should be maintained at equal to or greater than 30%. Endotracheal intubation and mechanical ventilation should be considered to reduce the work of breathing (and therefore oxygen requirements) and to increase juxtacardiac pressures ($P_{JC}$), which may improve cardiac function. Noninvasive mechanical ventilation with BiPAP can be used to accomplish similar end points in patients who are able to sustain spontaneous breathing. Careful attention to fluid management is necessary to ensure that an adequate preload is present to optimize ventricular function (especially in the presence of right ventricular infarction) and to avoid excessive volume administration with resultant pulmonary edema.
2. **Pharmacologic treatment** usually involves two classes of drugs: inotropes and vasopressors. Vasodilators generally are not used in patients

with cardiogenic shock due to severe hypotension. The use of vasodilators can be considered after the patient's hemodynamics have stabilized as a means of improving left ventricular function. **Dopamine** usually is administered first in patients with cardiogenic shock because it has inotropic and vasopressor properties. Typically, the dose is titrated to maintain a mean arterial BP of 60 mm Hg or greater. Subsequent guidance using a PA catheter helps to define what further measures are required, including inotropic support (dobutamine, amrinone), afterload reduction (nitroprusside), and changes in intravascular volume (fluid administration vs. diuresis).

3. **Mechanical circulatory assist devices** are required in patients who do not respond to medical therapy or who have specific conditions identified as the cause of shock (e.g., acute mitral valve insufficiency, ventricular septal defect). Intra-aortic balloon counterpulsation (see Chap. 5, Ischemic Heart Disease) usually is performed with the device inserted percutaneously. The balloon filling is controlled electronically so that it is synchronized with the patient's ECG. The balloon inflates during diastole and deflates during systole, thus reducing afterload and improving CO. Additionally, coronary artery blood flow is improved during diastolic inflation. Intra-aortic balloon pumps should be considered only as an interim step to more definitive therapy.
4. **Definitive treatment** must be considered for any patient with cardiogenic shock. This treatment can take the form of relatively noninvasive procedures (e.g., angioplasty) or more invasive surgical procedures (e.g., coronary artery bypass surgery, valve replacement, heart transplantation).

C. **Obstructive shock** usually is caused by massive pulmonary embolism. Occasionally, air embolism, amniotic fluid embolism, or tumor embolism also may cause obstructive shock. When shock complicates pulmonary embolism, therapy is directed toward preserving peripheral organ perfusion and removing the vascular obstruction. Fluid administration and the use of vasoconstrictors (e.g., norepinephrine, dopamine) may preserve BP while more definitive measures, such as thrombolytic therapy (e.g., streptokinase, alteplase, reteplase) or surgical embolectomy, are considered.

D. **Distributive shock** occurs primarily as septic shock or anaphylactic shock. These two forms are associated with significant decreases in vascular tone.

1. **Septic shock** is caused by the systemic release of mediators that usually are triggered by circulating bacteria or their products, although the systemic inflammatory response syndrome can be seen without evidence of infection (e.g., pancreatitis, crush injuries, and certain drug ingestions such as salicylates) (*N Engl J Med* 344:759, 2001). Septic shock is characterized primarily by hypotension due to decreased vascular tone. CO also is increased, owing to increased heart rate and end-diastolic volumes despite overall myocardial depression. The main goals of treatment of septic shock include initial fluid resuscitation, adequate treatment of the underlying infection, and interruption of the mediator-associated systemic inflammatory response. **Initial resuscitation** includes appropriate large-volume fluid administration to compensate for the decrease in vascular tone and dilated ventricular capacity. PA catheter–directed therapy may be important in such patients to determine the adequacy of preload and the need for inotropic or vasoconstrictor agents. A new therapy for septic shock has been developed. **Drotrecogin alfa** (activated), or **recombinant human activated protein C,** has antithrombotic, anti-inflammatory, and profibrinolytic properties. It has been shown to reduce mortality significantly in patients with severe sepsis (*N Engl J Med* 344:699, 2001). The usual dosage of drotrecogin alfa is an infusion of 24 μg/kg body weight/hour. The main contraindication to its use is an increased risk of hemorrhage (e.g., recent invasive procedure, severe thrombocytopenia). Septic shock can also be associ-

ated with relative adrenal insufficiency. Among patients with septic shock who were classified as nonresponders to a corticotropin test (i.e., an increase in the serum cortisol level of ≤ 9 μg/dl), a 7-day course of hydrocortisone (50 mg q6h IV) and fludrocortisone (50-μg tablet once a day) was associated with a significant 28-day survival advantage (*JAMA* 288:862, 2002).

2. **Anaphylactic shock** is discussed further in the section Anaphylaxis in Chap. 10, Allergy and Immunology.

## Hemodynamic Monitoring and Pulmonary Artery Catheterization

I. **Indications.** A PA catheter can be placed to differentiate between cardiogenic and noncardiogenic forms of pulmonary edema, to identify the etiology of shock (Table 8-6), for the evaluation of acute renal failure or unexplained acidosis, for the evaluation of cardiac disorders, or to monitor high-risk surgical patients in the perioperative setting. The PA catheter allows measurement of intravascular and intracardiac pressures, CO, and $P\bar{v}O_2$ and $SvO_2$.

II. **Obtaining a PAOP "wedge pressure" tracing.** The PA catheter is advanced through a central vein after the distal balloon is inflated. Bedside waveform analysis is used to determine successful passage of the catheter through the right atrium, right ventricle, and PA into a PAOP position. Fluoroscopy should be used when difficulty is encountered in positioning the PA catheter. If, at any time after passage into the PA, the tracing is found to move off the scale of the graph, overwedging of the catheter has occurred. An overwedged catheter should be withdrawn immediately 2–3 cm after balloon deflation, and catheter positioning should then be rechecked with reinflation of the balloon. Overwedging of a PA catheter increases the likelihood of serious complications (e.g., PA rupture).

III. **Acceptance of PAOP readings.** Respiratory variation on the waveform, atrial pressure characteristics (including *a* and *v* waves), mean value of the PAOP tracing obtained at end expiration at less than the mean value of the PA pressure measurement, and the aspiration of highly oxygenated blood with the catheter in the PAOP position all indicate an accurate reading.

IV. **Transmural pressure.** When PEEP is present (applied or auto-PEEP), the positive intra-alveolar pressure at end expiration is transmitted through the lung to the pleural space. In these circumstances, the measured PAOP reflects the sum of the hydrostatic pressure within the vessel and the $P_{JC}$. When significant levels of total PEEP are present (>10 cm $H_2O$), it is more appropriate to use the transmural pressure as a measure of left ventricular filling (transmural pressure = PAOP – $P_{JC}$). For patients with normal lung compliance, one-half of the total PEEP can be used as an estimate of $P_{JC}$. When lung compliance is depressed significantly (e.g., in ARDS), one-third of the total PEEP can be used as an estimate for $P_{JC}$.

V. **CO.** PA catheters are equipped with a thermistor to measure CO. At least two measurements that differ by less than 10–15% should be obtained. Injections should be synchronized with the respiratory cycle to minimize variability between results. Often, thermodilution measurements of CO are inaccurate at an extremely low CO (e.g., <1.5 L/minute) or an extremely high CO (e.g., >7.0 L/minute), in the presence of significant valvular disease (e.g., severe tricuspid insufficiency), and when large intracardiac shunts are present. Calculation of the CO using the Fick formula may be more accurate in these circumstances.

**VI. Interpretation of hemodynamic readings.** PAOP can be used as an index of left ventricular filling (preload) and as an index of the patient's propensity for development of pulmonary edema.

**A. Optimizing cardiac function.** Improving cardiac function by optimizing preload is more efficient in terms of myocardial oxygen consumption than similar improvements in cardiac function by use of inotropes when preload is inadequate. As a general rule, preload should be optimized before inotropic agents (which can increase myocardial oxygen consumption) or vasodilators (which can cause hypotension when preload is inadequate) are used. Fluid boluses should be administered in patients who are suspected of having inadequate cardiac filling pressures (i.e., inadequate preload) and should be followed by repeat measurements of PAOP, CO, heart rate, and stroke volume. In low CO states, if the PAOP increases by less than 5 mm Hg without significant changes in heart rate, CO, and stroke volume, additional fluid boluses may have to be given. An increase in the PAOP by more than 5 mm Hg usually signals that adequate ventricular filling is being achieved. Once the patient's preload has been optimized, cardiac performance can be reassessed and, if necessary, further therapy with inotropes (e.g., dobutamine, amrinone) or with vasodilators (e.g., nitroprusside, hydralazine, angiotensin-converting enzyme inhibitors) can be initiated to achieve further improvements in cardiac performance and tissue perfusion.

**B. Reducing unnecessary lung water.** PAOP is a reflection of the lung's tendency to develop pulmonary edema. Decreased left ventricular compliance results in a "critical pressure" being reached sooner for similar volume changes as compared to a normally compliant left ventricle. This difference is due to the increased stiffness of the noncompliant ventricle that causes higher pressures to be achieved for similar changes in volume. To optimize cardiac performance and to minimize the tendency for pulmonary edema formation, PAOP should be kept at the lowest point at which cardiac performance is acceptable.

**C. Differentiating hydrostatic from nonhydrostatic pulmonary edema.** The management of pulmonary edema depends in large part on whether the excessive accumulation of lung water is due to increased hydrostatic pressures (e.g., left ventricular failure, mitral stenosis, acute volume overload), increased permeability of the alveolocapillary barrier (e.g., ARDS due to sepsis, aspiration, or trauma), or a combination of these factors. Clinical and radiographic criteria alone often are insufficient to determine the underlying mechanisms of pulmonary edema. Therefore, less than optimal management of the patient's underlying disease process may occur. In general, a PAOP of less than 18 mm Hg suggests that the primary mechanism of pulmonary edema is nonhydrostatic. Values above 18 mm Hg support a hydrostatic cause for the increased lung water.

**D. Adequacy of organ perfusion.** Oxygen delivery to tissues depends on (1) an intact respiratory system to provide oxygen for hemoglobin saturation, (2) the concentration of hemoglobin, (3) CO, (4) tissue microcirculation, and (5) the unloading of oxygen from hemoglobin for diffusion into the tissue beds. Oxygen delivery can be measured as the product of CO and arterial oxygen content ($CaO_2$). $CaO_2$ is the sum of hemoglobin-bound and dissolved oxygen. Inadequate organ perfusion generally is associated with elevated blood lactate levels and decreased $SvO_2$ (usually $<0.6$). Factors that contribute to a low $SvO_2$ include anemia, hypoxemia, inadequate CO, and increased oxygen consumption. Factors that may elevate measured $SvO_2$ despite tissue hypoxia include peripheral arteriovenous shunting, the blood flow maldistribution of sepsis or cirrhosis, and cellular poisoning, such as that associated with cyanide toxicity. In general, optimization of gas exchange and CO along with an adequate hemoglobin (usually $\geq$ 10 g/dl) results in improved oxygen delivery to tissues.

# 9 Pulmonary Disease

Roger D. Yusen

## Pulmonary Hypertension

**I. Pulmonary hypertension (PH)** is defined as sustained elevation of the mean pulmonary artery pressure (>25 mm Hg at rest or 30 mm Hg during exertion) or of the systolic pulmonary artery pressure (>40 mm Hg). Cardiac disease, respiratory disease and hypoxemia, venous thromboembolic disease, and pulmonary vascular disease cause PH. **Pulmonary venous hypertension** is defined by the presence of a pulmonary capillary wedge pressure of greater than 15 mm Hg. This increased intravascular pressure distal to the pulmonary arterioles, either in the pulmonary veins or in the left heart (i.e., left ventricular dysfunction), may lead to **pulmonary arterial hypertension (PAH).** The World Symposium on Primary Pulmonary Hypertension 1998 (World Health Organization 1999, http://www.who.int/ncd/cvd/pph.html) suggested classifying PH based on its clinical features (Table 9-1).

PAH represents a heterogeneous group of disorders. **Primary PH (PPH)** is an uncommon disease of unclear etiology, and 10% of patients with PPH may have familial disease. Risk factors or possible triggers for the development of PPH have been identified, such as use of diet pills, including fenfluramine and dexfenfluramine. The cause of death in patients with PPH is usually right heart failure. The median survival in the United States registry was 2.8 years (*Ann Intern Med* 107:216–223, 1987) before the institution of currently available therapies.

**II.** The **diagnosis** of PH is usually based on **symptoms** of dyspnea (especially on exertion), fatigue, palpitations, presyncope, syncope, chest pain, hemoptysis, and cough. **Signs** of PH include a right ventricular heave, a widened splitting of the $S_2$, a prominent $P_2$, a right ventricular $S_4$, and a tricuspid regurgitation murmur. When **right heart failure** develops, elevated jugular venous pressure, a right ventricular $S_3$, a pulsatile liver, pedal edema, and sometimes ascites occur.

Raynaud's phenomenon is associated with PPH, but it is also associated with scleroderma and other collagen vascular diseases. Clubbing is not associated with PPH. Telangiectasias and sclerodactyly suggest the presence of other underlying illnesses, such as scleroderma (see Chap. 23, Arthritis and Rheumatologic Diseases). **A modified New York Heart Association (NYHA) classification** is often used to define the clinical severity of PH based on functional limitations (Table 9-2).

**III. Diagnostic testing** should be undertaken once signs and symptoms suggestive of PH develop. However, acute illnesses with reversible PH (pneumonia, pulmonary edema, etc.) should be treated and resolved before one embarks on an exhaustive evaluation for chronic etiologies.

**A.** A **transthoracic echocardiogram** is the preferred test for the initial evaluation of suspected PH because noninvasive Doppler techniques estimate the pulmonary artery systolic pressure. The absence of tricuspid regurgitation precludes estimation of the pulmonary artery systolic pressure but does not

**Table 9-1.** Diagnostic classification of pulmonary hypertension

- Pulmonary arterial hypertension
  - Primary pulmonary hypertension
    - Sporadic
    - Familial
  - Related to:
    - Collagen vascular disease
    - Congenital systemic-to-pulmonary shunts
    - Portal hypertension
    - HIV infection
    - Drugs/toxins
      - Anorexigens
      - Other
    - Persistent pulmonary hypertension of the newborn
    - Other
- Pulmonary venous hypertension
  - Left-sided atrial or ventricular heart disease
  - Left-sided valvular heart disease
  - Extrinsic compression of central pulmonary veins
    - Fibrosing mediastinitis
    - Adenopathy/tumors
  - Pulmonary veno-occlusive disease
  - Other
- Pulmonary hypertension associated with disorders of the respiratory system and/or hypoxemia
  - Chronic obstructive pulmonary disease
  - Interstitial lung disease
  - Sleep-disordered breathing
  - Alveolar hypoventilation disorders
  - Chronic exposure to high altitude
  - Neonatal lung disease
  - Alveolar-capillary dysplasia
  - Other
- Pulmonary hypertension due to chronic thrombotic and/or embolic disease
  - Thromboembolic obstruction of proximal arteries
  - Obstruction of distal pulmonary arteries
    - Pulmonary embolism (thrombus, tumor, ova and/or parasites, foreign material)
    - In situ thrombosis
    - Sickle cell disease
- Pulmonary hypertension due to disorders that directly affect the pulmonary vasculature
  - Inflammatory
    - Schistosomiasis
    - Sarcoidosis
    - Other
  - Pulmonary capillary hemangiomatosis

*Source:* World Health Organization, 1999.

**Table 9-2.** Functional assessment

| | |
|---|---|
| Class I | No limitation of physical activity. Ordinary physical activity does not cause undue dyspnea or fatigue, chest pain, or near syncope. |
| Class II | Slight limitation of physical activity. Comfortable at rest. Ordinary physical activity causes undue dyspnea or fatigue, chest pain, or near syncope. |
| Class III | Marked limitation of physical activity. Comfortable at rest. Less than ordinary activity causes undue dyspnea or fatigue, chest pain, or near syncope. |
| Class IV | Unable to carry out any physical activity without symptoms. Dyspnea and/or fatigue may be present at rest. Discomfort is increased by any physical activity. Signs of right heart failure are present. |

*Source:* Modified after the New York Heart Association Functional Classification; World Health Organization, 1999.

assure normal pulmonary artery pressures. Signs of elevated right ventricular pressure (e.g., dilated or hypokinetic right ventricle, paradoxical septal motion, or a "D"-shaped right ventricle) may indirectly suggest the presence of PH. Transthoracic echocardiography usually demonstrates the presence of left ventricular dysfunction or valvular heart disease in patients with pulmonary venous hypertension secondary to cardiac disease, a common cause of PH. Patients with PAH should undergo an evaluation for the presence of a **right-to-left shunt** (i.e., patent foramen ovale, atrial septal defect, etc.) with an echocardiogram bubble or contrast study (or a radionuclide lung perfusion scan that looks for abnormal accumulation of tracer in the brain or kidneys).

Once PH is diagnosed, patients should undergo a thorough evaluation for causes. The type of PH (Table 9-1) assists in directing the evaluation described below.

**B. Chest radiography** often shows enlarged pulmonary arteries, decreased vascular markings in the periphery, and right ventricular enlargement, and may suggest secondary causes of PH [e.g., interstitial lung disease (ILD), chronic obstructive pulmonary disease (COPD), etc.].

**C. Pulmonary function testing** often shows a mild-moderate reduction in the diffusing capacity for carbon monoxide (DLCO), although a normal value does not exclude the presence of PH. A decreased DLCO is often the sole pulmonary function testing abnormality of patients with PPH. Additional abnormalities of airflow and lung volumes may suggest the presence of secondary causes of PH.

**D. Arterial blood gas (ABG) measurement** may show hypoxemia and oxyhemoglobin desaturation with exertion. A normal arterial oxygen tension ($PaO_2$) does not exclude the presence of PH. Hypercapnia is an important clue for a hypoventilation syndrome.

**E. Six-minute walk test.** In addition to demonstrating oxyhemoglobin desaturation with exertion, the distance achieved may be lower than expected. The distance covered during the 6-minute walk assists in quantifying functional limitations within the modified NYHA classification (Table 9-2) (*Am J Respir Crit Care Med* 161:487, 2000).

**F. Electrocardiography** may demonstrate signs of right ventricular and right atrial hypertrophy. Other findings suggestive of cardiovascular disease may be present.

**G.** A **cardiopulmonary exercise test should be performed with caution,** and only if necessary. Exercise is usually limited by cardiovascular function, especially if oxyhemoglobin saturation is maintained with oxygen supplementation.

**H. Ventilation-perfusion ($\dot{V}/\dot{Q}$) lung scanning** should be performed to evaluate for the presence of chronic thromboembolic disease (see the section Thromboembolic Disorders in Chap. 18). In the presence of chronic thromboembolic PH, the $\dot{V}/\dot{Q}$ scan is usually interpreted as high probability for pulmonary embolism (PE). Although the perfusion scan is often described as "heterogeneous" in the setting of PH, the presence of any segmental defects should be further explored with pulmonary angiography. The detection of radiolabeled tracer in the brain suggests the presence of a right-to-left shunt, most likely within the heart.

I. **Contrast-enhanced helical chest CT (PE protocol)/high-resolution CT.** In addition to the assessment for thromboembolic disease, the CT can be used to look for signs of secondary causes of PH, such as fibrosing mediastinitis, ILD, and emphysema. CT cannot definitively exclude the presence of any chronic thromboembolic disease, but the absence of thrombotic changes within the larger central vessels decreases the likelihood of surgically accessible chronic thromboembolic disease.

J. **Pulmonary arteriography** is indicated if chronic thromboembolic disease cannot be sufficiently excluded by $\dot{V}/\dot{Q}$ scan or CT scan or if thromboendarterectomy is being considered. Patients with chronic thromboemboli should be referred for a thromboendarterectomy evaluation at an experienced center.

K. **Lung biopsy** is indicated only when a lung disease that requires a tissue diagnosis for confirmation is suspected (e.g., pulmonary vasculitis or veno-occlusive disease).

L. **Radionuclide ventriculography** assesses function of the right and left heart, including ventricular ejection fraction and wall motion.

M. **Sleep study** is indicated in patients with signs or symptoms of sleep apnea (see the section Obstructive Sleep Apnea–Hypopnea Syndrome).

N. **Screening laboratory tests** may detect **underlying** liver disease, collagen vascular disease, and HIV infection, as well as **secondary** polycythemia. Patients should undergo assessment for thyroid disease because of its frequent association with PPH and its propensity to aggravate underlying cardiopulmonary dysfunction (*Chest* 122:1668–1673, 2002). **Other signs of systemic diseases** may include anemia, thrombocytopenia, leukopenia, renal dysfunction, hematuria, and proteinuria.

O. **Right heart catheterization** should be performed to further evaluate echocardiographic findings of PAH or to evaluate patients who have clinical signs of PAH that are not confirmed by echocardiogram. Echocardiographic estimates of pulmonary artery pressures can be significantly lower than those found with right heart catheterization (*Circulation* 95:1479, 1997). If the catheterization does not reveal PAH, pulmonary hemodynamics should be measured during exercise. Right heart catheterization may also help to determine the cause of the PAH (i.e., pulmonary venous hypertension due to left ventricular dysfunction, **left-to-right shunt,** etc.). In addition, right heart catheterization measurements have important prognostic information in the setting of PAH (*Ann Intern Med* 115:343, 1991). Ideally, thermodilution and (measured or estimated) Fick cardiac output should be measured because significant tricuspid insufficiency may lead to underestimation of the cardiac output via the thermodilution technique (see Chap. 8, Critical Care, the section Hemodynamic Monitoring and Pulmonary Artery Catheterization).

P. If PAH is confirmed with right heart catheterization, patients should undergo **vasodilator testing** with short-acting IV adenosine, IV epoprostenol sodium (Flolan), or inhaled nitric oxide (NO). Calcium channel blockers (CCBs) are no longer recommended for determination of vasoreactivity, because they may induce prolonged systemic hypotension, syncope, and cardiovascular collapse. Patients with severe right heart failure (i.e., mean right atrial pressure >15 mm Hg) may be at higher risk for circulatory collapse during vasodilator testing. One definition of vasodilator responsiveness is (1) a reduction in the mean pulmonary artery pressure of at least 10 mm Hg and (2) no change or an increase in the cardiac output (World Symposium on Primary Pulmonary Hypertension, 1998). One study demonstrated that patients with an acute vasodilator response of more than a 20% decrease in mean pulmonary artery pressure and more than a 20% decrease in pulmonary vascular resistance had a favorable response to treatment with PO CCBs (*N Engl J Med* 327:76–81, 1992).

**IV. Therapeutics and management of PH** depend on the underlying cause. For example, PH in patients with COPD and untreated hypoxemia is often due to hypoxic vasoconstriction, and treatment should include oxygen supplementation. PH secondary to left heart failure requires treatment of the left heart failure and its causes. This section focuses on the treatment of PAH, especially PPH.

**A. Pharmacologic treatment**

**1. Vasodilator therapy** has been demonstrated to improve pulmonary hemodynamics, right ventricular function, cardiac output, oxygen delivery, symptoms, functioning, and survival (*N Engl J Med* 327:76, 1992; *N Engl J Med* 334:296, 1996). Individual responses to vasodilators are variable and often difficult to predict. Systemic hypotension is the most common complication of therapy, and other adverse effects include a drop in the $PaO_2$. **During chronic use of vasodilator therapy, abrupt discontinuation can result in rebound PH and death.**

**a. CCBs** vasodilate the pulmonary and systemic vascular smooth muscle. In **vasodilator-responsive patients** (see sec. **III.P**), PO CCBs improve symptoms, exercise tolerance, hemodynamics (decreased pulmonary artery pressure and increased cardiac output), and survival. Because CCBs also possess negative inotropic properties and reflexively increase β-adrenergic tone, these agents should be used cautiously. Only the minority (10–20%) of patients who respond to vasodilator therapy during the acute challenge should receive CCB therapy. Nifedipine is commonly used, and diltiazem may be more appropriate for patients with resting tachycardia. CCB therapy should be titrated according to a protocol (*N Engl J Med* 334:296–301, 1996), typically guided by right heart catheterization. Vasodilator responders are started with low-dose CCB therapy, and doses are cautiously advanced until a significant improvement in hemodynamic parameters is reached, as tolerated by BP. Over time, dosing is regulated based on symptoms, as tolerated by BP. Large doses of CCBs (i.e., nifedipine, 240 mg/day, or diltiazem, 720 mg/day, in divided doses) are well tolerated. Patients without evidence of a hemodynamic response to CCBs during the vasodilator challenge are unlikely to benefit from chronic therapy. In addition, CCBs may cause systemic hypotension, pulmonary edema, right ventricular failure, and death in **nonresponders.** Patients who do not respond to vasodilator therapy during the acute challenge should be considered for continuous IV epoprostenol and other therapies.

**b. Prostaglandins.** Continuous IV **prostacyclin (epoprostenol)** therapy is indicated for patients with PAH. Prostacyclin has been demonstrated in a prospective randomized clinical trial of PPH to improve exercise tolerance, hemodynamics, and survival in patients with a modified NYHA (Table 9-2) functional class III or IV status (*N Engl J Med* 334:296–301, 1996). Similar benefits, excluding an improvement in survival, have also been demonstrated in patients with scleroderma (*Ann Intern Med* 132:425, 2000). Studies have also demonstrated that lack of an acute response to prostacyclin does not preclude a chronic beneficial response. Prostacyclin therapy should be instituted in the hospital, and initial dosing is typically limited by side effects, such as jaw pain, headache, diarrhea, and musculoskeletal pain. The development of tolerance to the effects of IV prostacyclin is common but often responds to dose escalation. However, overmedication with prostacyclin can occur, requiring gradual dose reduction. **Sudden discontinuation of therapy can be dangerous,** and this may be due to accidental kinking or disconnection of the infusion catheter. Catheter-related infections can be problematic as well. The optimal dosing and frequency of dose changes of IV prostacyclin for PPH remain uncertain.

**Analog molecules of prostacyclin** that can be inhaled [e.g., iloprost (*N Engl J Med* 342:1866, 2000)] or taken orally [e.g., beraprost (*Lancet* 349:1365, 1997)] have been studied, but their efficacy remains to be demonstrated in adequately sized, randomized, placebo-controlled trials.

In a 12-week study, **treprostinil sodium** (Remodulin) led to statistically significant but small clinical improvements in dyspnea, exercise capacity, and hemodynamics in patients with primary and secondary PH who were NYHA functional class II–IV (*Am J Respir Crit Care Med* 165:800, 2002). A survival benefit was not demonstrated. Treprostinil was administered subcutaneously via an infusion device, and 85% of patients experienced infusion site pain, leading to discontinuation of treprostinil in 8% of patients.

**c.** A **PO endothelin receptor antagonist,** bosentan (Tracleer), was studied in patients with symptomatic severe PAH who were NYHA functional class III or IV (*N Engl J Med* 346:896, 2002). Patients had PPH or PH due to scleroderma or systemic lupus erythematosus. Bosentan significantly improved exercise capacity and prolonged time to clinical worsening as compared to placebo over a 3-month period, although a survival benefit was not demonstrated. Drug side effects were similar to those of placebo, although liver function abnormalities are common.

**d. Inhaled NO** causes pulmonary vasodilation, but any NO that diffuses into the blood is inactivated by hemoglobin, thereby preventing systemic vasodilation. The role of NO for PPH remains investigational.

**2. Inotropic therapy** may modestly improve right heart function, cardiac output, and symptoms (*Chest* 114:792–797, 1998), but data are lacking in terms of effect on survival.

**3. Anticoagulation** with PO warfarin therapy may improve survival, although a large, definitive, randomized controlled trial has not been performed. Warfarin is dosed (see the section Anticoagulants, sec. **IV** in Chap. 18) with a goal international normalized ratio (INR) of 1.5–2.0, lower than that typically used for treatment of venous thrombosis. Patients with recurrent syncope or hemoptysis may not be good candidates for anticoagulation therapy.

**4. Diuretic therapy** is indicated for the treatment of the consequences of right heart failure, such as peripheral edema and ascites, although overdiuresis can affect the preload dependent right ventricle and lead to decreased cardiac output and systemic hypotension.

**5. Other medications** can be used to treat problems that may lead to increased intrathoracic pressure, decreased cardiac output, and syncope (e.g., stool softeners for constipation or antitussives for chronic cough).

**6. Patients should avoid vasoactive drugs and activities:** nasal decongestants; sedatives that can lower BP; narcotics, nitrates, and other agents that decrease preload and right ventricular filling; barbiturates and other drugs that depress cardiac output; platelet and fresh frozen plasma transfusions because of their volume load and presence of vasoactive compounds; vigorous exercise because of the risk of developing cardiovascular collapse; high altitudes because of the low inspired concentration of oxygen; and cigarette smoking and illicit drug use. Pregnancy should usually be avoided, although the use of estrogen-based contraception is normally not recommended because it may exacerbate the symptoms or increase the risk of thrombosis.

**B.** An **IV filter** put inline in patients with documented right-to-left shunt may prevent air embolism.

C. **Supplemental oxygen therapy** is indicated, based on standard **recommendations** (see the section Chronic Obstructive Pulmonary Disease, sec. **III.B**), to avoid hypoxic vasoconstriction. However, a significant right-to-left shunt may not allow the generation of a normal arterial oxygen saturation ($SaO_2$) despite oxygen supplementation. Rest, exertion, and sleep oxygen assessments should be performed as clinically indicated.

D. **Vaccinations** for influenza and *Streptococcus pneumoniae* may provide benefit (see Appendix F, Immunizations and Post-Exposure Therapies).

E. **Surgical therapy**

1. **Lung transplantation or heart-lung transplantation** is a viable option for patients with PPH or PAH secondary to congenital heart defects when medical therapy has been exhausted. Heart transplantation is usually not necessary in PPH because the right ventricle recovers after isolated lung transplantation. Patients should be referred early for transplantation because of long wait-list times and the fast rate of deterioration of PPH, especially in patients with NYHA functional class III–IV, mean right atrial pressure greater than 15 mm Hg, mean pulmonary artery pressure greater than 55 mm Hg, or a cardiac index of less than 2 L/minute/$m^2$ (*Am J Respir Crit Care Med* 158:335, 1998). A randomized trial of medical versus transplant therapy has not been conducted, but lung transplant is thought to prolong survival in select patients with modified NYHA functional class III–IV status and PPH. The 5-year survival of patients with PPH who are undergoing lung transplantation is less than 50%.
2. **Atrial septostomy** allows decompression of the right heart by creating a hole between the right and left atrium, leading to right-to-left shunting in patients with right heart pressures greater than left. Left ventricular filling and cardiac output subsequently improve. Atrial septostomy is considered a palliative procedure. Indications for atrial septostomy include severe PPH refractory to maximal medical therapy with recurrent syncope or ascites. Atrial septostomy may also serve as a bridge to transplantation in patients whose conditions are deteriorating despite all medical efforts. The procedure-induced shunt produces hypoxemia. Only highly experienced centers should perform this procedure because of its risk of high mortality.

## Pleural Effusion

I. Normally, the pleural space only contains a small amount of fluid that is not radiologically detected. Alteration of hydrostatic and oncotic factors that increase the formation or decrease the absorption of pleural fluid [e.g., increased mean capillary pressure (heart failure) or decreased oncotic pressure (cirrhosis or nephrotic syndrome)] produces **transudative pleural effusions.** Damage or disruption of the normal parietal pleural membranes or vasculature (e.g., tumor involvement of the pleural space, infection, inflammatory conditions, or trauma) leads to increased capillary permeability or decreased lymphatic drainage and **exudative pleural effusions.**

II. **Diagnosis.** The underlying cause of the effusion usually dictates the symptoms, although patients may be asymptomatic. Pleural inflammation, abnormal pulmonary mechanics, and worsened alveolar gas exchange produce **symptoms and signs** of disease. Inflammation of the parietal pleura leads to pain in local (intercostal) involved areas or referred (phrenic) distributions (shoulder). Cough is frequent. Dyspnea may be present and out of proportion to the size of the effusion. Chest examination is notable for dullness to percussion, decreased or absent tactile fremitus, and decreased breath sounds. A shifted trachea or a pleural rub may be present. Other findings in the history and examination, such as classic findings of CHF, cirrhosis, or rheumatoid arthritis, may provide clues to the diagnosis.

**A.** If a pleural effusion is visible on imaging studies, further evaluation is warranted unless the origin is clear (e.g., heart failure) and the patient is responding well to therapy (*Am Rev Respir Dis* 140:257, 1989). **Thoracentesis** can be performed safely, in the absence of disorders of hemostasis, on effusions that extend greater than 10 mm from the inner chest wall on a lateral decubitus film. Loculated effusions can be localized with ultrasonography or CT scan. Proper technique and sonographic guidance minimize the risk of pneumothorax and other complications. The transudate/exudate classification system narrows the **differential diagnosis** for pleural effusion.

**1. Transudative pleural effusions** have low protein and lactate dehydrogenase (LDH) laboratory values. **Exudative pleural effusions** have high protein or LDH values. Specifically, pleural effusions that meet any of **Light's criteria** of (1) a pleural fluid serum **protein** ratio of greater than 0.5, (2) a pleural fluid–serum **LDH** ratio of greater than 0.6, or (3) a pleural fluid LDH of more than two-thirds of the upper limit of normal for serum LDH are exudates, whereas transudative pleural effusions do not meet any of Light's criteria (*Ann Intern Med* 77:507, 1972). In addition to testing pleural fluid for LDH and protein, **other useful tests** of pleural fluid include cell count and differential, amylase, triglycerides, microbiologic stains, cultures, and cytology. Serum LDH, protein, and pH should be measured within hours of the thoracentesis to allow appropriate comparisons.

Most **transudates** are clear, straw-colored, nonviscid, and without odor. The WBC count is usually less than 100/mm$^3$, and the RBC count is generally less than 10,000/mm$^3$. The pleural fluid glucose level is usually similar to the serum level, and the pleural fluid pH is higher than the blood pH. Transudates should lead to further evaluation of the heart, liver, and kidneys, and therapy is directed accordingly.

**2. Exudative pleural effusions** are defined by Light's criteria (see sec. **II.A.1**). If a patient surprisingly has an exudative effusion according to Light's criteria, a serum to pleural fluid albumin gradient should be checked. A gradient of greater than 1.2 g/dl suggests that the pleural fluid is really transudative. Exudates have a broad differential diagnosis. Other test characteristics of the fluid can be diagnostic.

**a. Red-tinged pleural effusions** indicate the presence of blood. In exudative pleural effusions, **serosanguineous** fluid is not extremely helpful in narrowing the diagnosis. If the blood is due to the procedure, the degree of discoloration should clear during the aspiration. **Bloody pleural fluid** usually indicates the presence of malignancy, PE, or trauma. The presence of gross blood should lead to the measurement of a pleural fluid hematocrit. **Hemothorax** is defined as a pleural fluid–blood hematocrit ratio of more than 0.5, and chest tube drainage should be considered.

**b.** For exudative pleural effusions, the **WBC differential** is often not diagnostic, although **neutrophilia** is suggestive of infection. **Eosinophilia** (>10% of total nucleated cell count) is suggestive of air or blood in the pleural space. If air or blood is not present in the pleural space, consideration should be given to fungal and parasitic infection, drug-induced disease, PE, asbestos-related disease, and Churg-Strauss syndrome. If more than 50% of WBC are small **lymphocytes,** malignancy or tuberculosis is likely. The presence of **mesothelial cells** argues against the diagnosis of tuberculosis. Many **plasma cells** suggest the diagnosis of multiple myeloma.

**c.** Exudative effusions with **normal protein but high LDH** are likely to be parapneumonic (see sec. **II.A.3**) or secondary to malignancy. LDH is an indicator of the degree of pleural inflammation.

   **d.** A **glucose** concentration of less than 60 mg/dl is probably due to tuberculosis, malignancy, rheumatoid arthritis, or parapneumonic effusion. For parapneumonic pleural effusions with a glucose of less than 40–60 mg/dl, tube thoracostomy should be considered (Table 9-3).
   **e.** **Pleural fluid with a low pH** usually has a low glucose and a high LDH; otherwise, the low pH may be due to poor sample collection technique. A pH of less than 7.3 is seen with empyema, tuberculosis, malignancy, collagen vascular disease, or esophageal rupture. For parapneumonic pleural effusions with a pH of less than 7.00–7.20, tube thoracostomy should be considered (Table 9-3). Pleural fluid for pH testing should be collected anaerobically in a heparinized syringe and placed on ice.
   **f.** An elevation of **amylase** suggests that the patient has pancreatic disease, malignancy, or esophageal rupture. Malignancy and esophageal rupture have salivary amylase elevations and not pancreatic amylase elevations.
   **g.** **Turbid or milky fluid** should be centrifuged. If the supernatant clears, the cloudiness is likely due to cells and debris. If the supernatant remains turbid, pleural lipids should be measured. Elevation of triglycerides (>110 mg/dl) suggests that a chylothorax is present, usually due to thoracic duct rupture from trauma, surgery, or malignancy (i.e., lymphoma).
   **h.** **Cytology** is positive in approximately 60% of malignant effusions. Priming the fluid collection bag with unfractionated heparin (UFH; e.g., 1000 IU) and submitting a large pleural fluid volume maximize the diagnostic yield for cytologic diagnosis. **Repeat thoracentesis** increases the diagnostic yield. **Closed pleural biopsy** can be performed when the cause of an exudative pleural effusion cannot be determined by thoracentesis. **Thoracoscopy** has largely replaced closed pleural biopsy. For tuberculous effusions, pleural fluid cultures alone are positive in only 20–25% of cases. However, the combination of pleural fluid studies and pleural biopsy (demonstrating granulomas or organisms) is 90% sensitive in establishing tuberculosis as the etiology of the effusion. For malignant effusions, pleural biopsies add a small but significant diagnostic yield to fluid cytology alone.

  **3.** **Parapneumonic effusions** are exudates that develop secondary to pulmonary infections. Patients with pneumonia and a pleural effusion should undergo **rapid diagnostic testing** because an infected pleural space (empyema) needs to be **treated without delay.** Pleural fluid LDH, protein, pH, and Gram stain/culture are used to define complicated parapneumonic effusions and to guide treatment (Table 9-3; Chest 18:1158, 2000).

 **B.** **Other diagnostic procedures** that are useful in establishing the etiology of a pleural effusion when the aforementioned tests are nondiagnostic include biopsy of other abnormal sites (e.g., a mediastinal or lung mass), diagnostic thoracoscopy, and testing for PE (see the section Thromboembolic Disorders in Chap. 18).

**III.** **Treatment.** Most transudates resolve with treatment of the underlying heart, kidney, or liver disease. Occasionally, more aggressive approaches including pleurodesis and shunts are required.

 **A.** **Symptomatic pleural effusions** may require removal of large amounts of pleural fluid. The rapid removal of more than 1 L of pleural fluid may rarely result in re-expansion pulmonary edema, especially if an airway obstruction is present (i.e., endobronchial tumor). When frequent or repeated thoracentesis is required for effusions that reaccumulate, early consideration should be given to tube drainage and pleurodesis.

 **B.** Appropriate management of **parapneumonic effusions and empyema** should be instituted based on the size of the effusions, the gross characteristics of the pleural fluid, the biochemical analysis, and the presence of loculations (Table 9-3; Chest 18:1158, 2000).

**Table 9-3.** Categorizing risk for poor outcome in patients with parapneumonic pleural effusion

| Pleural space anatomy | | Pleural fluid bacteriology | | Pleural fluid chemistry[a] | Category | Risk of poor outcome | Drainage |
|---|---|---|---|---|---|---|---|
| $A_0$ minimal, free-flowing effusion (<10 mm on lateral decubitus)[b] | *And* | $B_x$ culture and Gram stain results unknown | *And* | $C_x$ pH unknown | 1 | Very low | No[c] |
| $A_1$ small to moderate free-flowing effusion (>10 mm and <1/2 hemithorax) | *And* | $B_0$ negative culture and Gram stain[d] | *And* | $C_0$ pH ≥7.20 | 2 | Low | No[e] |
| $A_2$ large, free-flowing effusion (≥1/2 hemithorax),[f] loculated effusion,[g] or effusion with thickened parietal pleura[h] | *Or* | $B_1$-positive culture or Gram stain | *Or* | $C_1$ pH <7.20 | 3 | Moderate | Yes |
| | | $B_2$ pus | | | 4 | High | Yes |

[a]pH is the preferred pleural fluid chemistry test, and pH must be determined using a blood gas analyzer. If a blood gas analyzer is not available, pleural fluid glucose should be used ($P_0$ glucose ≥60 mg/dl; $P_1$ glucose <60 mg/dl). The panel cautions that the clinical utility and decision thresholds for pH and glucose have not been well established.

[b]Clinical experience indicates that effusions of this size do not require thoracentesis for evaluation, but will resolve.

[c]If thoracentesis were performed in a patient with $A_0$ category pleural anatomy and $P_1$ or $B_1$ status found, clinical experience suggests that the $P_1$ or $B_1$ findings might be a false-positive. Repeat thoracentesis should be considered if effusion enlarges and/or clinical condition deteriorates.

[d]Regardless of prior use of antibiotics.

[e]If clinical condition deteriorates, repeat thoracentesis and drainage should be considered.

[f]Larger effusions are more resistant to effective drainage, possibly because of the increased likelihood that large effusions will also be loculated.

[g]Pleural loculations suggest a worse prognosis.

[h]Thickened parietal pleura on contrast-enhanced CT suggests the presence of empyema.

*Source:* From GL Colice, A Curtis, J Deslauriers, et al. Medical and surgical treatment of parapneumonic effusions: an evidence-based guide. *Chest* 118:1158–1171, 2000, with permission.

C. **Malignant pleural effusions** arise from tumor involvement of the pleura or mediastinum. Patients with malignancy are also at increased risk for pleural effusions from postobstructive pneumonia, pulmonary emboli, chylothorax, and drug or radiation reactions. Several therapeutic options exist (*Clin Chest Med* 14:189, 1993).

1. **Observation** without invasive interventions may be appropriate for some patients.
2. **Therapeutic thoracentesis** may improve patient comfort and relieve dyspnea. The subjective response to drainage and the rate of fluid reaccumulation should be monitored. Repeated thoracenteses are reasonable if they achieve symptomatic relief and if fluid reaccumulation is slow.
3. **Chemical pleurodesis** is an effective therapy for recurrent effusions. This treatment is recommended in patients whose symptoms are relieved with initial drainage but who have rapid reaccumulation of fluid. Talc pleurodesis appears to be the most effective and least expensive agent, particularly in malignant pleural effusions with a pH of less than 7.30 (*Chest* 113:1007, 1998). However, talc pleurodesis requires thoracoscopy and general anesthesia. Doxycycline or minocycline can be instilled in the pleural space at the bedside without thoracoscopy or general anesthesia. If the chest tube drainage remains high (>100 ml/day) more than 2 days after the initial pleurodesis, a second dose of the sclerosing agent can be administered. Bleomycin appears to be less effective and more expensive than other drugs. Systemic analgesics and the administration of lidocaine in the sclerosing agent solution help to decrease the appreciable discomfort associated with the procedure (*Ann Intern Med* 120:56, 1994).
4. **Pleurectomy or pleural abrasion** requires thoracic surgery and should be reserved for patients with a good prognosis who have had an ineffective pleurodesis.
5. **Chemotherapy and mediastinal radiotherapy** may control effusions in responsive tumors, such as lymphoma or small-cell bronchogenic carcinoma, although it has poor efficacy in metastatic carcinoma.

## Obstructive Sleep Apnea–Hypopnea Syndrome

I. **Introduction. Obstructive sleep apnea–hypopnea syndrome (OSAHS)** is a disorder of sleep that produces excessive daytime sleepiness (hypersomnolence) (*Sleep* 22:667–689, 1999) and consequences such as motor vehicle accidents (*Sleep* 20:608–613, 1997). Patients with OSAHS have an increased risk of death (*Chest* 97:27, 1990), mainly due to cardiovascular events (*Eur Respir J* 13:179, 1999). Of middle-aged adults, 2–4% have OSAHS (*N Engl J Med* 328:1230, 1993). **Lack of recognition and diagnosis** of OSAHS is a significant problem.

II. **Pathophysiology.** Sleep apnea may be central, obstructive, or a combination of both. In **central** sleep apnea, the absent central drive to breathe results in no respiratory effort and no airflow, despite adequate airway patency. However, most cases of sleep apnea are **obstructive** sleep apnea (**OSA**) and result from decreased or absent respiratory airflow due to narrowing or collapse of the upper airway. OSA with symptoms of excessive daytime sleepiness results in **OSAHS.**

III. **Diagnosis of OSAHS**

A. **Symptoms of OSAHS** (Table 9-4). Habitual loud snoring is the most common symptom of OSAHS, although not all people who snore have this syndrome. Excessive daytime sleepiness (daytime hypersomnolence) is a classic symptom of OSAHS. Patients may describe falling asleep while driving or having difficulty concentrating at work. They may complain also of personality changes, intellectual deterioration, morning headaches, automatic behav-

**Table 9-4.** Symptoms associated with obstructive sleep apnea–hypopnea syndrome

| | |
|---|---|
| Excessive daytime sleepiness | Enuresis |
| Snoring | Awakening unrefreshed |
| Nocturnal arousals | Morning headaches |
| Apneas | Impaired memory and concentration |
| Nocturnal gasping, grunting, and choking | Irritability and depression |
| Nocturia | Impotence |

ior, and loss of libido. Subjective sleepiness can be assessed by a validated scale, such as the **Epworth Sleepiness Scale** (Table 9-5; *Sleep* 14:40, 1991).

**B. Signs.** Disorders commonly associated with OSA include obesity, nasal obstruction, adenoidal or tonsillar hypertrophy, micrognathia, retrognathia, macroglossia, acromegaly, hypothyroidism, vocal cord paralysis, and bulbar involvement from neuromuscular disease (*Otolaryngol Clin North Am* 23:727, 1990). All patients should have a thorough **nose and throat examination** to detect sources of upper airway obstruction that are surgically correctable (e.g., septal deviation, enlarged tonsils, enlarged uvula), especially if continuous positive airway pressure (CPAP; see sec. **V.B.1**) is poorly tolerated. Patients with OSAHS often have associated cardiovascular disease, including systemic hypertension (*N Engl J Med* 342:1378–1384, 2000; *JAMA* 283:1829–1836, 2000) and CHF (*Clin Chest Med* 19:99, 1998). When OSAHS is associated with disorders, such as obesity and chronic lung disease, hypoxemia, hypercapnia, polycythemia, and cor pulmonale may develop (*Mayo Clin Proc* 65:1087, 1990).

**Table 9-5.** Epworth Sleepiness Scale

How likely are you to doze off or fall asleep in the following situations, in contrast to just feeling tired? This refers to your usual way of life in recent times. Even if you have not done some of these things recently, try to work out how they would have affected you. Use the following scale to choose the most appropriate number for each situation:

| | |
|---|---|
| 0 = would never doze | 2 = moderate chance of dozing |
| 1 = slight chance of dozing | 3 = high chance of dozing |

| Situation |
|---|
| Sitting and reading |
| Watching TV |
| Sitting, inactive, in a public place |
| As a passenger in a car for an hour |
| Lying down in the afternoon |
| Sitting and talking to someone |
| Sitting quietly after a lunch without alcohol |
| In a car, while stopped for a few minutes in traffic |

*Note:* The scores for each situation are summed to obtain the Epworth score. An Epworth score greater than 10 suggests that significant daytime sleepiness is present.
*Source:* Adapted from MW Johns. A new method for measuring daytime sleepiness: the Epworth sleepiness scale. *Sleep* 14:541, 1991.

**IV. Testing.** Patients with risk factors and symptoms or sequelae of OSAHS should be referred to a sleep specialist and sleep laboratory for further evaluation. The gold standard for the diagnosis of OSAHS is overnight **polysomnography** (**PSG** or "sleep study") (*Am Rev Respir Dis* 139:559, 1989) with direct observation by a qualified technician. Typical indications for a sleep study include snoring with excessive daytime sleepiness, titration of optimal nasal CPAP therapy, and assessment of objective response to therapeutic interventions. Other indications include unexplained PH, polycythemia, and daytime hypercapnia. Sleep studies are typically performed in the outpatient setting. PSG stages sleep using EEG, electromyography, and electrooculography. PSG assesses respiratory airflow and effort, oxyhemoglobin saturation, heart electrical activity (ECG), and body position.

**A.** The sleep study is analyzed for sleep staging and for the frequency of respiratory events. Events are categorized as

1. **Obstructive.** Airflow is absent or reduced despite continuous respiratory efforts.
2. **Central.** Airflow and respiratory effort are absent.

**B.** The **respiratory disturbance index** or the **apnea-hypopnea index (AHI)** is used to diagnose sleep-disordered breathing and to quantify its severity. **Apnea** is defined as a prolonged complete cessation of airflow. **Hypopnea** is defined as a significant reduction in baseline airflow for at least 10 seconds, associated with an arousal from sleep or a significant reduction in oxyhemoglobin saturation (i.e., $\geq 3\%$). The **AHI** is the sum of apneic and hypopneic episodes per hour of sleep. **OSA** is present when a sleep study shows an AHI of at least five events per hour in a symptomatic patient. Mild OSA has an AHI of 5–15, moderate OSA has an AHI of 16–30, and severe OSA has an AHI of more than 30 (*Sleep* 22:667–668, 1999). The risk of death, hypertension, and poor neuropsychological functioning rises as the AHI increases.

**C.** A single sleep study is usually sufficient to diagnose OSAHS. A second study should be performed for treatment titration (see sec. **V.B.1**). However, if classic symptoms of OSAHS are present and if the diagnosis of severe OSAHS is made early in the first study, a "split-night" study can be performed, whereby the first half is done to make the diagnosis of OSAHS and the second half is used to titrate positive airway pressure and supplemental oxygen treatment.

**V. Therapeutics and management of OSAHS.** The therapeutic approach to OSAHS depends on the severity of the disease, the underlying medical condition, the cardiopulmonary sequelae, and the expected degree of patient compliance. The treatment must be highly individualized, with special attention to correcting potentially reversible exacerbating factors.

**A.** Treatments include **weight reduction** for the obese (*Chest* 92:631–637, 1987), avoidance of alcohol and sedatives, nasal decongestants if needed, oxygen supplementation when needed, and specific therapy for other conditions (e.g., COPD, hypertension, hypothyroidism).

**B. Positive airway pressure**

1. **CPAP** is used to deliver air via a nasal or oral mask. **Nasal continuous positive airway pressure (nCPAP)** is the current **treatment of choice** for most patients with OSAHS. nCPAP pneumatically splints open the upper airway and prevents collapse. The sleep study determines the airway pressure (cm $H_2O$) required to optimize airflow; the nCPAP pressure is gradually increased until obstructive events, snoring, and oxygen desaturations are minimized. Some patients, such as those with COPD, require **supplemental oxygen** to maintain adequate oxygen saturations ($SaO_2 \geq 90\%$).

   CPAP leads to consolidated sleep and decreased daytime hypersomnolence in almost all patients. BP, nocturia, peripheral edema, polycythemia, and PH may improve.

2. **Bilevel positive airway pressure (BiPAP)** can be used to treat patients with OSAHS. BiPAP is more expensive than CPAP and does not improve patient compliance. Patients with intolerance of very high levels of CPAP, a poor response to CPAP, or concomitant alveolar hypoventilation may respond well to noninvasive mechanical ventilation with BiPAP or volume ventilation. **Autotitrating** or "smart" CPAP machines use flow and pressure transducers to sense airflow patterns and then automatically adjust the CPAP, but their effectiveness has not been well studied.
3. **Adverse effects of CPAP or BiPAP.** All noninvasive positive pressure or mechanical ventilation devices may induce dryness of the airway, nasal congestion, rhinorrhea, epistaxis, skin reactions to the mask, nasal bridge abrasions, and aerophagia.
4. **Compliance.** The compliance rate with nasal CPAP is approximately 50%. Compliance can be improved with education, instruction, follow-up, adjustment of the mask for fit and comfort, humidification of the air to decrease dryness, and treatment of nasal or sinus symptoms. Use of a full mask (oronasal) has not improved compliance compared to the use of nasal masks.

C. **Oral appliances** for mild OSAHS, such as the mandibular repositioning device, aim to increase airway size to improve airflow. The devices can be fixed or adjustable, and most require customized fitting. Many devices have not been well studied.

D. **Surgical treatment**

1. For patients with OSAHS, **tracheostomy** has been consistently effective, but it is rarely used since the advent of positive airway pressure therapy. Tracheostomy should be reserved for patients with life-threatening disease (cor pulmonale, arrhythmias, or severe hypoxemia) or significant alveolar hypoventilation that cannot be controlled with other measures.
2. **Uvulopalatopharyngoplasty (UPPP)** is the most common surgical treatment of **mild to moderate OSAHS** in patients who do not respond to medical therapy. UPPP enlarges the airway by removing tissue from the tonsils, tonsillar pillars, uvula, and posterior palate. UPPP may be complicated by change in voice, nasopharyngeal stenosis, foreign body sensation, and velopharyngeal insufficiency with associated nasal regurgitation during swallowing, and CPAP tolerance problems. UPPP's success rate for treatment of OSAHS is only 50%, and improvements related to UPPP may diminish over time. Thus, UPPP is considered a second-line treatment for patients with mild to moderate OSAHS who cannot successfully use CPAP and who have retropalatal obstruction. Other surgical procedures have shown promise and may be best for patients with retroglossal obstruction.

E. **Pharmacologic treatment.** At this time, medications have a minimal role in the treatment of OSAHS, except for nasal saline and decongestants. Patients should be assessed and treated for hypothyroidism. They should **avoid use of alcohol, tobacco, and sedatives.**

## Cystic Fibrosis

I. **Cystic fibrosis (CF)** is the most common lethal genetic disease in whites, with an incidence of 1 in 3200 live births in the United States (*J Pediatr* 132:255, 1998). Although CF is less common in nonwhites, the diagnosis needs to be considered in patients of diverse backgrounds. The diagnosis of CF is typically made during childhood, but 8% of patients are diagnosed during adolescence or adulthood (*J Pediatr* 122:1, 1993). With improved therapy, the median survival has been extended to approximately 33 years (CFF Patient Registry, *2001 Annual data report*). Predictors of increased mortality include age, female gender, low weight, low forced expiratory volume in 1 second ($FEV_1$), pancreatic insufficiency, diabetes mellitus, infections with *Staphylococcus aureus* or *Burkholderia cepacia*, and the number of acute exacerbations (*JAMA* 286:2683, 2001).

II. **Pathophysiology.** CF is an autosomal-recessive disorder caused by mutations of the cystic fibrosis transmembrane conductance regulator (**CFTR**), a gene located on chromosome 7. CFTR normally regulates and participates in the transport of electrolytes across epithelial cell and intracellular membranes (*Science* 245:1073, 1989). The primary pulmonary manifestations of disease are thought to be related to abnormal electrolyte transport in the airway, which results in desiccated airway secretions and impaired mucociliary clearance. Secretions become infected, and a vicious cycle of infection, inflammation, and chronic airways obstruction ensues, resulting in bronchiectasis, chronic infection, and ultimately premature death.

III. The **diagnosis** of CF is based on (1) a compatible clinical and family history and (2) persistently elevated concentrations of sweat chloride, two known disease-causing CF mutations, or nasal transepithelial potential difference measurements that are typical of CF. Atypical patients may lack classic symptoms and signs or have normal sweat tests. Although genotyping may assist in the diagnosis, it alone cannot establish or rule out the diagnosis of CF, and the initial test of choice remains the sweat test.

A. **Clinical manifestations**

1. **Pulmonary symptoms** lead to consideration of the diagnosis of CF in 50% of cases (*J Pediatr* 122:1, 1993). In almost all patients, chronic (sino) pulmonary disease eventually develops, most notable for bronchiectasis and chronic airflow obstruction. Symptoms initially include cough and purulent sputum production. Dyspnea ensues as the disease progresses. Acute pulmonary disease exacerbations may lead to significant deterioration and subsequent hospitalization. Isolation of a mucoid variant of *Pseudomonas aeruginosa* from the respiratory tract occurs frequently. Other pulmonary complications may include allergic bronchopulmonary aspergillosis, hemoptysis, and pneumothorax.
2. **Extrapulmonary manifestations** of CF include pancreatic exocrine insufficiency, which is seen in 90% of patients and leads to fat malabsorption and malnutrition. Pancreatitis occasionally develops. GI complications include distal intestinal obstruction syndrome, volvulus, intussusception, and rectal prolapse. CF also affects the endocrine pancreatic (diabetes mellitus), the hepatobiliary (fatty liver, cirrhosis, portal hypertension, cholelithiasis, and cholecystitis), the genitourinary (male infertility and epididymitis), and the skeletal (retardation of growth, demineralization, and osteoarthropathy) systems. Digital clubbing appears in childhood in virtually all symptomatic patients. Although fertility may be decreased in women with CF secondary to thickened cervical mucus, many women with CF have tolerated pregnancy well (*Thorax* 50:170, 1995).

B. **Differential diagnosis. Primary ciliary dyskinesia** or **immunoglobulin deficiency** may lead to bronchiectasis, sinusitis, and infertility. However, limited GI symptoms and normal sweat electrolytes distinguish these diseases from CF. **Shwachman syndrome,** consisting of pancreatic insufficiency and cyclic neutropenia, may also lead to lung disease, but sweat chloride concentrations are normal and the neutropenia is distinguishing. Men with **Young's syndrome** have bronchiectasis, sinusitis, and azoospermia, but this disorder only has mild respiratory symptoms, lacks GI symptoms, and has normal sweat chloride levels.

C. **Testing**

1. **Skin sweat testing** with a standardized quantitative pilocarpine iontophoresis method remains the gold standard for the diagnosis of CF. **A sweat chloride concentration of greater than 60 mmol/L** is consistent with the diagnosis of CF. However, the diagnosis requires an elevated sweat chloride concentration on two separate occasions in a patient with a typical phenotype or with a history of CF in a sibling. Borderline sweat test results (40–60 mmol/L sweat chloride) or nondiagnostic results in the setting of high clinical suspicion should also lead to repeat sweat testing, nasal potential difference testing, or genetic testing. Abnormal sweat chloride concentrations are rarely detected in non-CF patients (e.g., Addison's disease and untreated hypothyroidism).
2. **Genetic tests** have detected more than 900 putative CF mutations. Patients with CF most commonly have the ΔF508 CFTR mutation. Two recessive genes must be abnormal to cause CF. Commercially available probes identify more than 90% of the abnormal genes in a white Northern European population, although they test for only a minority of the known CF genes.
3. **Other tests** may support the diagnosis of CF. Typically, **chest radiography** eventually shows enlarged lung volumes, with cystic lung disease and bronchiectasis, especially in the upper lobes. **Pulmonary function tests** eventually show expiratory airflow obstruction with increased residual volume and total lung capacity. Impairment of alveolar gas exchange may be present as well, progressing to oxyhemoglobin desaturation with exertion, hypoxemia, and hypercapnia. **Sputum cultures** typically identify *P. aeruginosa* or *S. aureus*, or both, and **sputum sensitivity testing** may direct therapy. **Testing for malabsorption due to pancreatic exocrine insufficiency** is often not formally performed, because clinical evidence [the presence of foul-smelling, bulky, and loose stools; **low fat-soluble vitamin levels (vitamins A, D, and E);** and a **prolonged prothrombin time** (vitamin K–dependent)] and a clear response to pancreatic enzyme treatment are usually considered sufficient for the diagnosis. Tests that identify sinusitis or infertility, especially obstructive azoospermia in men, would also support the diagnosis of CF.

IV. **Therapeutics and management.** CF therapy aims to improve quality of life and functioning, decrease the number of exacerbations and hospitalizations, avoid complications associated with therapy, and decrease mortality. A comprehensive program addressing multiple organ/system derangements, as provided at CF care centers, is recommended. The greatest number of adults with CF have significant lung disease and a large portion of therapy is focused on clearing pulmonary mucus and controlling infection.

A. **Pulmonary disease**

1. **Nonpharmacologic treatment**
   a. **Mucus mobilization** may be accomplished by various airway clearance techniques, including postural drainage with chest percussion and vibration, with or without mechanical devices (flutter valves, high-frequency chest oscillation vests, low- and high-pressure positive expiratory pressure devices, etc.), and breathing and coughing exercises.
   b. **Pulmonary rehabilitation** that includes exercise rehabilitation may improve functioning.
   c. **Oxygen therapy** is indicated based on standard recommendations (see Chronic Obstructive Pulmonary Disease, sec. **III.B**). Rest and exercise oxygen assessments should be performed as clinically indicated.
   d. **Vaccinations.** Yearly influenza vaccination (0.5 ml IM) decreases the incidence of infection and subsequent deterioration (*N Engl J Med* 311:1653, 1984). Pneumovax (0.5 ml IM) may also provide benefit (see App. F, Immunizations and Post-Exposure Therapies).

2. **Pharmacologic treatment**
   a. **Bronchodilators** such as β-adrenergic agonists [albuterol metered-dose inhaler (MDI), 2–4 puffs bid–qid; salmeterol or formoterol, 1 dry powder inhalation bid] or cholinergic blockers (ipratropium bromide MDI, 2–4 puffs bid–qid) are used to treat the reversible components of airflow obstruction and facilitate mucus clearance (see Chronic Obstructive Pulmonary Disease, sec. **II.B**). These agents are contraindicated in the rare patient with associated paradoxical deterioration of airflow after their use.
   b. **Recombinant human deoxyribonuclease (Dnase, dornase alpha, Pulmozyme)** digests extracellular DNA, decreasing the viscoelasticity of the sputum. It improves pulmonary function and decreases the incidence of respiratory tract infections that require parenteral antibiotics (*N Engl J Med* 326:812, 1992; *Am Rev Respir Dis* 148:145, 1993). The recommended dose is 2.5 mg (1 ampule)/day inhaled using a jet nebulizer. Adverse effects may include pharyngitis, laryngitis, rash, chest pain, and conjunctivitis.
   c. **Antibiotics.** *P. aeruginosa* is the most frequent pulmonary pathogen. A combination of an IV semisynthetic penicillin, a third- or fourth-generation cephalosporin, or a quinolone and an aminoglycoside is typically recommended during acute exacerbations. Sputum culture sensitivities should guide therapy. The duration of antibiotic therapy is dictated by the clinical response. At least 10 to 14 days of antibiotics is typically given to treat an exacerbation. Home IV antibiotic therapy is common, but hospitalization may allow better access to comprehensive therapy and diagnostic testing. PO antibiotics are recommended only for mild exacerbations. The use of chronic or intermittent prophylactic antibiotics can be considered, especially in patients with frequent recurrent exacerbations, but antimicrobial resistance may develop. Inhaled aerosolized tobramycin (300 mg nebulized bid, 28 days on alternating with 28 days off, using appropriate nebulizer and compressor) improves pulmonary function, decreases the density of *P. aeruginosa*, and decreases the risk of hospitalization (*N Engl J Med* 340:23, 1999). Voice alteration (13%) and tinnitus (3%) are potential adverse events associated with long-term inhaled tobramycin (*N Engl J Med* 340:23, 1999).
   d. **Laboratory monitoring.** Patients with CF have atypical pharmacokinetics and often require higher drug doses at more frequent intervals. In patients with CF, for example, cefepime is often dosed at 2 g IV q8h and gentamicin or tobramycin is often dosed at 3 mg/kg IV q8h (aiming for peak levels of 9–10 mg/ml and trough levels of <2 mg/ml). Monitoring levels (peaks and troughs) of drugs such as aminoglycosides helps to assure therapeutic levels and decrease the risk of toxicity (see Antibacterial Agents, sec. **V** in Chap. 12). Monitoring of electrolytes is indicated in patients with a history of electrolyte abnormalities or renal insufficiency.
   e. **Glucocorticoids.** The anti-inflammatory effects of short courses of glucocorticoid therapy may be helpful to some patients, but long-term therapy should be avoided to minimize the side effects that include glucose intolerance, osteopenia, and growth retardation.
   f. **Azithromycin.** Recent studies have shown that PO azithromycin mildly improves lung function and reduces days in the hospital for treatment of respiratory exacerbations in patients who are chronically infected with *P. aeruginosa*.
3. **Other treatments**
   a. **Lung transplantation.** The majority of patients with CF die from pulmonary disease. $FEV_1$ is a strong predictor of mortality (*N Engl J Med* 326:1187, 1992), and it is helpful in deciding when to refer patients for lung transplantation. An $FEV_1$ that is less than 30% of

the predicted normal value, marked alveolar gas exchange abnormalities (resting hypoxemia or hypercapnia), evidence of PH, or increased frequency or severity of pulmonary exacerbations should lead to consideration of lung transplantation as a treatment option (*Am J Respir Crit Care Med* 155:789–818, 1997).

b. **Noninvasive ventilation** for chronic respiratory failure due to CF-related bronchiectasis has not been clearly demonstrated to provide a survival benefit, although it may provide symptomatic relief or it can be used as a bridge to transplantation.

c. **Avoidance of irritating inhaled fumes, dusts, or chemicals** is recommended.

**B. Extrapulmonary disease**

1. **Pancreatic enzyme supplementation** should be instituted for pancreatic insufficiency and malabsorption, titrating enzyme dose to achieve one to two semisolid stools per day. Enzymes are taken immediately before meals and snacks. Dosing of pancreatic enzymes should be initiated at 500 U lipase/kg/meal and should not exceed 2500 U lipase/kg/meal. High doses (6000 U lipase/kg/meal) have been associated with chronic intestinal strictures (*N Engl J Med* 336:1283–1289, 1997). **Generic** enzyme substitutes may not provide adequate lipase needed for absorption.
2. **Vitamin supplementation** is recommended, especially the fat-soluble vitamins that are not well absorbed in the setting of pancreatic insufficiency. Vitamins A, D, E, and K can all be taken orally on a regular basis (see Table 2-4 in Chap. 2). Iron-deficiency anemia requires iron supplementation. Osteopenia from chronic steroid use should be treated.
3. **Sinusitis regimens** are used in the typical fashion.
4. **Treatment of pancreatic endocrine dysfunction,** specifically diabetes mellitus, is usually done with **insulin** (see Chap. 21, Diabetes Mellitus and Related Disorders), but typical diabetic dietary restrictions are liberalized (high-calorie diet with unrestricted fat) to encourage appropriate growth and weight maintenance.

## Chronic Obstructive Pulmonary Disease

The hallmark of **COPD** is expiratory airflow obstruction that is not fully reversible. The airflow obstruction is associated with an abnormal inflammatory response, and it usually progresses. Chronic bronchitis and emphysema may produce COPD. **Emphysema** is defined as enlargement of the distal airways with destruction of the acinus, without associated fibrosis. **Chronic bronchitis** is defined clinically as cough, productive of at least 2 tablespoons of sputum (not postnasal drip) on most days of 3 consecutive months in 2 consecutive years, in the absence of other lung diseases, such as bronchiectasis or CF. Although asthma (see Chap. 10, Allergy and Immunology), bronchiolitis, tumors, sarcoidosis, and lung damage from previous infections are associated with expiratory airflow obstruction, they are not classified as COPD.

Most cases of COPD are attributable to cigarette smoking, although COPD does not develop in the majority of smokers. Occupational and environmental dusts and gases are other known risk factors for COPD. Chronic respiratory diseases and allied conditions affect approximately 15 million people and are the fourth leading cause of death in the United States.

**I. Diagnosis and evaluation** (*Am J Respir Crit Care Med* 152:77S, 1995; *Am J Respir Crit Care Med* 163:1256, 2001)

**A. History and physical examination.** Exposure to cigarette smoking should be quantified. **$\alpha_1$-Antitrypsin deficiency** should be considered in a patient with emphysema who has (1) a minimal smoking history, (2) early-onset COPD, (3) a family history of lung disease, or (4) a predominance of lower lobe emphysema. **Symptoms** of dyspnea on exertion that progress over time gradually develop in patients with COPD. Nocturnal symptoms are unusual in COPD, except in patients with comorbidities such as cardiac disease, sleep-disordered breathing, gastroesophageal reflux, or a marked reactive airway component. Weight loss occurs in patients with end-stage emphysema, but other etiologies, such as malignancy, should be sought. Worsened dyspnea, cough, and sputum production often characterize exacerbations of COPD. On **physical examination,** patients with marked COPD show prolonged exhalation, use of accessory muscles of respiration, chest hyperresonance to percussion, enlarged thoracic volume, and decreased breath sounds. Signs of cor pulmonale may be present (see the section Pulmonary Hypertension, sec. **II**). Clubbing is not a feature of COPD, and its presence should prompt an evaluation for etiologies such as lung cancer. More marked abnormalities on physical examination characterize COPD exacerbations. Marked tachypnea, cyanosis, and signs of increased work of breathing, such as paradoxical abdominal motion, may signify the need for assisted ventilation.

**B. Chest radiographs** are not sensitive for the diagnosis of COPD. With increasing disease severity, thoracic hyperinflation with flattening of the diaphragm and hyperlucency with diminished vascular markings develop. Bullae may be visible. Usually, emphysema is most prominent in the upper lung zones. However, in $\alpha_1$-antitrypsin deficiency, emphysema usually shows a basilar predominance. Chest radiographs are valuable during an acute exacerbation to exclude such complications as pneumonia and pneumothorax.

**C. Pulmonary function testing.** Spirometry is the only reliable means for diagnosing COPD, although it has limited utility during an acute illness in a patient already diagnosed with COPD. A diagnosis of COPD requires the presence of expiratory airflow obstruction, defined as a low $FEV_1$/forced vital capacity ratio (<0.7). The $FEV_1$ defines the severity of the expiratory airflow obstruction. Smoking cessation for more than a year leads to an improvement in lung function, and an $FEV_1$ decline equal to that of nonsmokers (*JAMA* 272:1497, 1994). The $FEV_1$ is often used to assess the clinical course and response to therapy, and it is an important predictor of prognosis and mortality in patients with COPD (Table 9-6). When the $FEV_1$ falls to less than 1 L, the 5-year survival is approximately 50%.

Total lung capacity, functional residual capacity, and residual volume increase to supranormal values in patients with COPD, indicating thoracic hyperinflation and air trapping. Emphysema and many other diseases produce a reduction in the diffusing capacity of the lung (DLCO).

**D. ABG** should be obtained in patients with COPD and acute respiratory illness, because measurement of oxyhemoglobin saturation with a pulse oximeter neglects to provide information about alveolar ventilation (arterial carbon dioxide tension, or $Paco_2$). ABGs detect acute and chronic hypercapnia, and the development of acute respiratory acidosis may signal acute respiratory failure and the need for assisted ventilation.

**II. Treatment of acute COPD exacerbations.** A variety of insults may provoke a COPD exacerbation, which consists of some combination of increased dyspnea, sputum purulence, and sputum volume, often associated with wheezing. The most common identifiable causes of acute exacerbations are infections, typically due to viruses (e.g., influenza and adenovirus) or bacteria (e.g., *Haemophilus influenzae*, *S. pneumoniae*, *Moraxella catarrhalis*, and *Mycoplasma pneumoniae*). The differential diagnosis list for the decompensation should include pneumothorax, pneumonia, CHF, volume overload, cardiac ischemia, oversedation, and PE.

**Table 9-6.** GOLD classification of chronic obstructive pulmonary disease by severity

| Stage | Characteristics |
|---|---|
| 0: At risk | Normal spirometry<br>Chronic symptoms (cough, sputum production) |
| I: Mild COPD | $FEV_1/FVC < 70\%$<br>$FEV_1 \geq 80\%$ predicted<br>With or without chronic symptoms (cough, sputum production) |
| II: Moderate COPD | $FEV_1/FVC < 70\%$<br>$30\% \leq FEV_1 < 80\%$ predicted<br>(IIA: $50\% \leq FEV_1 < 80\%$ predicted)<br>(IIB: $30\% \leq FEV_1 < 50\%$ predicted)<br>With or without chronic symptoms (cough, sputum production, dyspnea) |
| III: Severe COPD | $FEV_1/FVC < 70\%$<br>$FEV_1 < 30\%$ predicted, or the presence of respiratory failure,[a] or clinical signs of right heart failure |

COPD, chronic obstructive pulmonary disease; $FEV_1$, forced expiratory volume in 1 second; FVC, forced vital capacity; GOLD, Global Initiative for Chronic Obstructive Lung Disease.
[a]Respiratory failure: $PaO_2$ <8.0 kPa (60 mm Hg) with or without $PaCO_2$ >6.7 kPa (50 mm Hg) while breathing air at sea level.
*Source:* From RA Pauwels, AS Buist, PM Calverley, et al. Global strategy for the diagnosis, management, and prevention of chronic obstructive pulmonary disease. National Heart, Lung, and Blood Institute/World Health Organization Global Initiative for Chronic Obstructive Lung Disease (GOLD) workshop summary. *Am J Respir Crit Care Med* 163:1257, 2001, with permission.

A. **Oxygen** (see sec. **III.B**) should be administered to achieve and maintain a $PaO_2$ of greater than 55–60 mm Hg (≥ 89% oxyhemoglobin saturation). Adequate oxygenation must be maintained, despite the presence of hypercapnia. Increasing requirements of supplemental oxygen suggest that a complicating condition exists (e.g., PE, pneumonia, pneumothorax, or right-to-left shunt).

B. **Inhaled bronchodilators** (Table 9-7)

1. **Short-acting inhaled $\beta_2$-adrenergic agonists** are the first-line therapy for COPD exacerbations. Inhaled $\beta_2$-adrenergic agonists, such as albuterol, have a reduced duration of action in acute exacerbations of COPD, allowing a treatment frequency of q30–60min as tolerated (*Am J Respir Crit Care Med* 152:577, 1995); subsequent treatments can be decreased to 2–4 puffs q4h as the acute exacerbation of COPD starts resolving. Use of an **MDI** with a **spacer device or reservoir** is as effective as delivery of the drug by a **nebulizer** in most patients (*Chest* 98:822, 1987). Patient instruction and supervised administration are essential to ensure effective delivery. Long-acting β agonists, salmeterol and formoterol, are most useful during maintenance therapy. $\beta_2$-Adrenergic agonists may cause tremor, nervousness, tachycardia, and tachyarrhythmias.

2. **Short-acting inhaled anticholinergic agents,** such as ipratropium bromide, have similar efficacy to short-acting $\beta_2$-adrenergic agonists in the treatment of acute exacerbations of COPD. However, anticholinergic agents have less tendency to produce hypoxemia and other side effects of $\beta_2$-adrenergic agents (*Am Rev Respir Dis* 136:1091, 1987).

**Table 9-7.** Inhaled drugs for the treatment of chronic obstructive pulmonary disease

| Generic name | Brand name | Dose |
|---|---|---|
| Sympathomimetic bronchodilators[a] | | |
| Albuterol | | MDI: 90 µg |
| | | Nebulizer: 0.5% solution, 2.5–5.0 mg; (0.5–1.0 ml) diluted in 1.0–2.5 ml of NS |
| | | Rotocaps inhalation powder: 200 µg |
| Metaproterenol | | MDI: 650 µg |
| | | 5% solution, 0.2–0.3 ml diluted in 2–5 ml of NS |
| Terbutaline sulfate | | Nebulizer: 0.01–0.03 mg/kg |
| Pirbuterol acetate | | Autohaler: 200 µg |
| Bitolterol mesylate | | MDI: 370 µg |
| | | Nebulizer: 0.2% solution |
| Isoetharine HCl | | Nebulizer: 1% 0.3–0.5 ml |
| Formoterol fumarate[b] | Foradil | Inhalation powder: 1 cap = 12 µg |
| Salmeterol xinafoate[b] | Serevent | Diskus: 50 µg |
| Combination drugs | | |
| Ipratropium/albuterol | Combivent | MDI: ipratropium, 18 µg/albuterol, 103 µg/puff |
| | DuoNeb | Nebulizer: 0.5 mg ipratropium, 2.5 mg albuterol |
| Salmeterol/fluticasone[b] | Advair | Diskus (inhalation powder): |
| | | Fluticasone, 100 µg/salmeterol, 50 µg/inhalation |
| | | Fluticasone, 250 µg/salmeterol, 50 µg/inhalation |
| | | Fluticasone, 500 µg/salmeterol, 50 µg/inhalation |
| Anticholinergic bronchodilators[a] | | |
| Atropine | Atropine | Nebulizer: 0.025 mg/kg diluted to 3–5 ml with saline |
| Glycopyrrolate | Robinul | Nebulizer: 0.3–2.0 mg; 1.5–10.0 ml |
| Ipratropium bromide | Atrovent | MDI: 18 µg |
| | | Nebulizer: 0.02% solution 2.5 ml |
| Corticosteroid anti-inflammatory drugs[c] | | See Table 10-5 |

MDI, metered-dose inhaler.
[a]Usual dosing qid, although more frequent dosing can be used during acute exacerbations.
[b]Maximum frequency q12h.
[c]Usual dosing bid–qid.

During acute exacerbations, the usual dose of ipratropium, 2 puffs qid, can be increased to 4–6 puffs q4–6h to produce maximal bronchodilation. Ipratropium and glycopyrrolate are available in solution for nebulization. Anticholinergic agents often cause dry mouth and may result in bladder outlet obstruction or an exacerbation of acute angle glaucoma.

3. **Combination agents.** Short-acting β-agonists and anticholinergic agents can be nebulized together or used together in an MDI (Combivent) for synergistic bronchodilation (*Chest* 109:294, 1996). Combination therapy may have other advantages that include a rapid onset of action and a long duration of action and fewer side effects (compared to sole use of large doses of $\beta_2$-adrenergic agonists). The long-acting agent salmeterol combined with fluticasone (Advair) has a role in chronic therapy, but it is not a first-line therapy in acute exacerbations of COPD.

C. **Systemic bronchodilators (methylxanthines),** such as PO theophylline or IV aminophylline, can be tried if the patient's condition does not improve with the repetitive administration of inhaled $\beta_2$-agonist bronchodilators. IV methylxanthines have a higher risk of acute side effects than the oral form. Theophylline and a number of other drugs interact, which may increase or decrease the dosage requirements and the incidence of toxicity (see Appendix C, Drug Interactions). Continued inhalation of tobacco smoke lowers theophylline levels. Sustained-release theophylline is dosed once or twice a day. Levels should be maintained below 20 mg/L (between 6 and 12 mg/L) to avoid toxicity. If symptoms of **toxicity** develop, including anxiety, tremor, nausea, vomiting, tachycardia, and tachyarrhythmias, the drug should be stopped and a level should be measured. Toxic levels may lead to seizures and death.

D. **Glucocorticoids,** such as methylprednisolone, 125 mg IV q6h for 3 days, are indicated for COPD exacerbations that require hospitalization. Improvement in hospital length of stay, lung function, and the incidence of relapse has been demonstrated compared with placebo, although IV high-dose glucocorticoids increase the risk of hyperglycemia (*N Engl J Med* 340:1941, 1999). PO prednisone, 40–60 mg PO qd, usually replaces IV glucocorticoids after a few days, and the therapy should be tapered as tolerated. Patients who use long-term PO steroids or high-dose inhaled steroid therapy might require a longer tapering period. The role of glucocorticoids for acute exacerbations in outpatients with COPD is controversial. However, in patients with moderate to severe COPD, short courses of PO steroids in combination with other medical therapy can improve outcomes of those with COPD exacerbations who are discharged from the emergency department (*N Engl J Med* 348:2618, 2003). Inhaled steroids currently do not have a role in treatment of an acute COPD exacerbation.

E. Controversy surrounds the role of **antimicrobial therapy** for COPD exacerbations. For routine exacerbations of COPD in the absence of pneumonia, current methods do not reliably differentiate exacerbations caused by bacteria versus those produced by other agents. Antibiotic therapy most often benefits patients who have more severe underlying lung disease and those who experience more severe exacerbations (*JAMA* 273:957, 1995). Traditional first-line antibiotic regimens for acute bacterial exacerbations of chronic bronchitis (**ABECB**) consist of a 7- to 10-day course of PO therapy [e.g., trimethoprim/sulfamethoxazole, 160 mg/800 mg (one double-strength tablet) PO bid; amoxicillin, 250 mg PO tid; doxycycline, 100 mg PO bid; or a PO cephalosporin]. For more severe exacerbations, recommended antibiotics include azithromycin (500 mg PO on day 1 and 250 mg PO on days 2–5), clarithromycin (500 mg PO bid or extended-release, 1 g PO qd), amoxicillin/clavulanate (500 mg PO tid or 875 mg PO bid), or newer quinolones with enhanced activity against penicillin-resistant *S. pneumoniae*, such as levofloxacin (500 mg PO qd), gatifloxacin (400 mg PO qd), or moxifloxacin (400 mg PO qd).

F. **Psychoactive drugs,** including benzodiazepines and narcotics, should be used with caution in patients with COPD. Low-dose anxiolytics may reduce anxiety. The anxiolytic buspirone (5–10 mg PO tid) is usually well tolerated; however, it requires several weeks to become effective. Selective serotonin reuptake inhibitors may be a reasonable choice given their low side effect profile. However, caution is advised in patients who are receiving theophylline, as some serotonin reuptake inhibitors prolong its elimination (*Can Med Assoc J* 151:1289, 1994) (see Appendix C, Drug Interactions).

G. **Chest physiotherapy** and mechanical clearance devices may improve clearance of secretions in patients with copious respiratory secretions (>50 ml/day), although they are not routinely recommended during acute COPD exacerbations. Chest percussion or postural drainage may produce or worsen hypoxemia.

H. **Indications for ICU admission** include severe dyspnea, mental status changes, persistent or worsening hypoxemia, hypercapnia, or respiratory acidosis, despite medical therapy.

I. **Mechanical ventilation** should be considered in patients with acute ventilatory failure. **Indications for invasive mechanical ventilation** include severe dyspnea with use of accessory muscles and paradoxical abdominal motion, marked tachypnea, life-threatening hypoxemia, severe acidosis, respiratory arrest, impaired mental status, cardiovascular complications, and other major complicating conditions. **Noninvasive ventilation** with positive pressure delivered via a nasal or face mask is an alternative to intubation in selected patients with acute exacerbation of COPD (*N Engl J Med* 333:817, 1995). **Exclusion criteria for noninvasive positive pressure ventilation** include respiratory arrest, cardiovascular instability, impaired mental status, high aspiration risk, copious secretions, facial/gastroesophageal/craniofacial/nasal pharyngeal disease, and extreme obesity (*Am J Respir Crit Care Med* 151:1799, 1995).

J. **Discharge criteria** for patients with acute exacerbations of COPD include use of inhaled bronchodilators less frequently than every 4 hours, clinical and ABG stability for at least 12–24 hours, and an acceptable ability to eat, sleep, and ambulate.

III. **Long-term management** (*Am J Respir Crit Care Med* 152:77S, 1995; *Am J Respir Crit Care Med* 163:1256, 2001) should aim to relieve symptoms, decrease the frequency and the severity of acute exacerbations, slow the progression of disease, prevent morbidity, and prolong survival. Although an extensive therapeutic armamentarium exists, smoking cessation and the correction of hypoxemia with supplemental oxygen are the only medical therapies that have been shown to improve survival in randomized controlled trials. Long-term management with bronchodilators, steroids, vaccinations, and so forth are not discussed in this chapter.

A. **Strategies to help the patient who is willing to quit smoking** include **asking** about tobacco use, **advising** quitting, **assessing** willingness to quit, **assisting** the patient in quitting, and **arranging** follow-up (*JAMA* 283:3244, 2000). Standard interventions include (1) pharmacotherapy, (2) counseling (on the preventable health risks of smoking, providing advice to stop smoking, and encouraging patients to make further attempts to stop smoking even after previous failures), and (3) providing smoking cessation materials to patients (*JAMA* 275:1270, 1996). Pharmacotherapy doubles the quit rate. Current U.S. Food and Drug Administration–approved medications for smoking cessation include nicotine replacement therapy and bupropion.

1. **Nicotine replacement therapy** is most effective when used in **conjunction with formal smoking cessation programs** or close medical follow-up (*JAMA* 281:72, 1999). Nicotine therapy **side effects** may include headache, insomnia, nightmares, nausea, dizziness, and blurred vision. **Contraindications** to nicotine use include significant vascular disease, pregnancy, breast-feeding, and allergy to the drug. Heavy smokers typically require combination therapy with the long-acting patch and a short-acting nicotine product to decrease cravings and improve efficacy. Nonheavy smokers often do not require nicotine patch therapy during sleep.

a. **Nicotine-containing chewing gum** (2- or 4-mg pieces) One piece is chewed for a few minutes until a tingling sensation arises, and then it is "parked" between the cheek and the gums for 20–30 minutes until the craving returns, repeating the process, as needed, up to 60 mg/day.
b. The **transdermal nicotine patch** regimen usually consists of 6 weeks of a high-dose patch (21 mg/day) followed by 2–4 weeks of an intermediate-dose patch (14 mg/day) and then 2–4 weeks of a low-dose patch (7 mg/day). Redness and pruritus at the patch site might develop.
c. The **nicotine nasal spray** regimen consists of one (0.5-mg) spray to each nostril q1–2h prn, not to exceed 5 doses/hour or 40 doses/day. Side effects may also include sneezing, excess lacrimation, and cough.
d. The **nicotine inhaler** (10 mg/cartridge) is used over 20 minutes, 6–16 cartridges/day for 12 weeks, followed by tapering over 6–12 weeks. Side effects may also include cough and irritation of the mouth.
e. **Nicotine lozenges** (2 mg) are used q1–2h prn, not to exceed 20 lozenges over 24 hours.
f. **Bupropion hydrochloride SR (Zyban)** started 1 week before quitting smoking (150 mg PO qd for 3 days, then 150 mg PO bid for 7–12 weeks) increases the smoking cessation rate when used with a behavior modification program. Bupropion combined with nicotine replacement may improve efficacy (*N Engl J Med* 340:685, 1999). Longer-duration (e.g., 6 months) use of bupropion has been recommended to improve long-term cessation rates.

B. **Oxygen therapy** has been shown to decrease mortality and improve physical and mental function in hypoxemic patients with COPD. After return to baseline from a COPD exacerbation, patients with increased supplemental oxygen requirements should undergo an oxygen reassessment to redefine the appropriate oxygen needs. A **room air resting ABG** is the gold standard test for determining the need for supplemental oxygen. Pulse oximetry may be useful for routine checks after a baseline measured oxyhemoglobin saturation is determined. Oxygen therapy is indicated for any patient with a $Pao_2$ of 55 mm Hg or less or an $Sao_2$ of 88% or less. If a patient has a $Pao_2$ of 56–59 mm Hg or an $Sao_2$ of 89% or less, and evidence of PH, polycythemia (hematocrit >55%), or heart failure, oxygen therapy is indicated. Supplemental oxygen requirements are typically greatest during exertion and least at rest while awake. Patients who require supplemental oxygen during exertion often need it during sleep. Although the exact amount required nocturnally might be measured with pulse oximetry, it is not unreasonable to set the oxygen to be delivered during sleep as 1 L/minute greater than that required during rest when awake. Stable patients receiving long-term oxygen therapy should undergo routine re-evaluation no less than once a year (*Chest* 107:358, 1995). The **oxygen prescription** should state the delivery system required (compressed gas, liquid, or concentrator) and the required oxygen flow rates (L/minute) for rest, sleep, and exercise.

C. **Pulmonary rehabilitation** has been defined by the American Thoracic Society as a multidisciplinary program of care for patients with chronic respiratory impairment that is individually tailored and designed to optimize physical and social performance and autonomy (*Am J Respir Crit Care Med* 159:1666, 1999). Pulmonary rehabilitation improves exercise tolerance and dyspnea, and may improve quality of life and decrease the frequency of exacerbations in patients with COPD. Patients with COPD who should be referred to a comprehensive rehabilitation program include those who (1) have severe dyspnea despite optimal medical management, (2) have reduced exercise tolerance, and (3) experience a restriction in activities.

IV. **Surgery in patients with COPD**

A. Three **surgical treatment options** exist for carefully selected patients with COPD, and referral to experienced centers should be considered in individuals with severe dyspnea. **Lung transplantation** is an alternative for patients with marked expiratory airflow obstruction ($FEV_1$ <25% predicted) and severe limitations in quality of life, especially individuals with hypercapnia, marked hypoxemia, or PH. Lung transplantation is typically not an option for elderly patients or those with significant comorbidities (*Am J Respir Crit Care Med* 158:335, 1998). **Bullectomy** is considered in patients with COPD and dyspnea in whom a bulla or bullae occupy approximately 50% of the hemithorax. **Lung volume reduction surgery** has had excellent results in highly selected patients with severe COPD due to emphysema (*Chest* 123:1026, 2003; *N Engl J Med* 348:2059, 2003). Target areas for surgical resection consist of focal areas of emphysematous lung that are accessible to surgical resection. Poor candidates for lung volume reduction surgery include patients with (1) very low (≤ 20% of the predicted normal value) $FEV_1$ and DLCO, (2) very low $FEV_1$ and homogeneous disease, or (3) non–upper lobe predominant emphysema and high exercise capacity.

B. **Lung resection** for diagnostic or therapeutic indications is relatively common in individuals with COPD. In evaluating patients for lung resection, one should estimate the lung function that will remain after surgery and the likelihood of morbidity, mortality, and respiratory disability. Quantitative lung scan, pulmonary function, blood gas, and exercise testing assist in the evaluation of lung resection candidacy. Decisions must be individualized (*Am J Respir Crit Care Med* 153:1201, 1996), especially because some lung resections might actually lead to improvement in lung function related to a lung volume reduction surgery effect.

C. **Perioperative management of COPD patients undergoing nonpulmonary surgery** is discussed in Chap. 1, Patient Care in Internal Medicine, Perioperative Medicine section, sec. **II**).

## Hemoptysis

**Hemoptysis,** the expectoration of blood, is a nonspecific sign associated with many pulmonary diseases, including infection (e.g., acute bronchitis, lung abscess, tuberculosis, aspergilloma, pneumonia, bronchiectasis), neoplasm, cardiovascular disease (e.g., mitral stenosis, pulmonary embolus, pulmonary vascular malformations), trauma, autoimmune disorders (e.g., Wegener's granulomatosis, Goodpasture's syndrome, systemic lupus erythematosus), and drugs or toxins (e.g., cocaine, anticoagulants, thrombolytic agents, penicillamine, solvents). Often, the specific etiology of hemoptysis is never determined.

I. **Diagnosis**

A. **History and physical examination** should confirm that the source of bleeding is located in the respiratory tract and not in the GI tract or nasopharynx. An attempt should be made to estimate the amount of bleeding. The clinician should assess the patient for symptoms and signs of underlying diseases.

B. **Laboratory studies** include a chest radiograph, tests of hemostasis (INR and partial thromboplastin time), CBC to look for anemia and thrombocytopenia, liver function tests to evaluate for hepatic dysfunction if the platelet count is low or the INR is prolonged, creatinine to evaluate for renal dysfunction, sputum bacterial and mycobacterial (and sometimes fungal) stains and cultures, sputum cytology, urinalysis to evaluate for RBCs or RBC casts that may be associated with Wegener's granulomatosis or Goodpasture's syndrome, and an ABG.

**C. Chest radiography** should be performed to look for the cause of hemoptysis, such as pneumonia or lung cancer. PE evaluation (see Thromboembolic Disorders in Chap. 18) should be performed, if indicated, preferentially using CT scan over $\dot{V}/\dot{Q}$ because alternative etiologies are best detected with CT. Chest CT scan is also indicated if there is concern for underlying parenchymal disease.

**D. Bronchoscopy** is indicated in patients who have hemoptysis and a risk factor for carcinoma, even if the hemoptysis is minor and the radiograph is normal. Risk factors for carcinoma include (1) age greater than 40 years, (2) significant smoking history, (3) hemoptysis of more than 1 week's duration, and (4) unexplained abnormality on chest radiograph. If bleeding is brisk, rigid bronchoscopy may be required. Bronchoalveolar lavage (BAL) fluid should be sent for cytology and culture (e.g., mycobacterial, fungal, bacterial). Alveolar hemorrhage can be detected on BAL, where the returned fluid becomes progressively bloody.

**II. Therapy is tailored to the severity of the episode and to the underlying cause. Massive hemoptysis** is defined as more than 600 ml blood over 48 hours or quantities that are sufficient to impair alveolar gas exchange. The primary immediate goals of therapy are to maintain the airway, optimize oxygenation, stabilize the hemodynamic status, and cease the bleeding. Therapy for minor bleeding or blood-streaked sputum should be directed at the specific etiology.

**A. Supportive care.** Causal laboratory abnormalities should be corrected: fresh frozen plasma for elevated INR or partial thromboplastin time, platelets for thrombocytopenia or platelet dysfunction (due to aspirin or other nonsteroidal anti-inflammatory drugs), and desmopressin acetate in the setting of uremia (see Chap. 18, Disorders of Hemostasis). Bed rest, mild cough suppression, and avoidance of excessive thoracic manipulation (e.g., chest percussion, incentive spirometry) are helpful. Patients should undergo pulse oximetry monitoring and should receive supplemental oxygen for oxyhemoglobin desaturation. Sedatives aid patient cooperation, but excessive sedation may suppress airway protection and mask signs of respiratory decompensation. For massive hemoptysis, while awaiting surgical consultation, clinically stable patients should be positioned with the bleeding side in a dependent position to reduce aspiration of blood into the contralateral lung.

**B. Definitive therapy.** Once stabilization is accomplished, diagnostic and therapeutic interventions should be performed promptly, because recurrent bleeding occurs unpredictably.

1. **Early fiberoptic bronchoscopy,** especially during active bleeding, may localize the specific site and identify the cause of the bleeding. Immediate control of the airway can sometimes be obtained with endobronchial tamponade or unilateral intubation of the nonbleeding lung.
2. **If bleeding continues,** but the site of origin is uncertain, lung isolation or use of a double-lumen tube should be considered, provided that the staff is skilled in this procedure. If the bleeding cannot be localized because the rate of hemorrhage does not allow adequate visualization of the airway, emergency rigid bronchoscopy or arteriography and embolization are indicated.
3. **Urgent surgical intervention** should be considered in operative candidates with unilateral bleeding when embolization is unavailable or unfeasible, when bleeding continues despite embolization, or when bleeding is associated with persistent hemodynamic and respiratory compromise. Contraindications to surgical treatment may include inoperable lung cancer and previous pulmonary function studies precluding pulmonary resection.

## Interstitial Lung Disease

**I. Introduction. ILDs** are a heterogeneous group of disorders, pathologically characterized by infiltration of the alveolar walls by cells, fluid, and connective tissue. The most common **acute** presentations are due to infection and cardiogenic pulmonary edema. This section mainly focuses on subacute and chronic **ILD.** Approximately 30% of patients with chronic ILD have idiopathic pulmonary fibrosis (IPF), a primary lung disease. The **differential diagnosis** of ILD is extensive (Table 9-8).

**II. Pathophysiology.** Inflammation (infectious or not), increased lung water, or infiltrative material causes ILD. The decreased distensibility of the lung produces a restrictive pulmonary function pattern and dyspnea. With long-standing disease, PH may develop late in the course.

**III. Diagnosis.** Clues about the etiology come from assessment of **chronicity** of disease, **underlying systemic disease** or **exposure,** and **immune status.** If the patient is known to be immunosuppressed and acutely ill, urgent evaluation is warranted.

**A.** The **history** should focus on possible reversible causes of lung injury, giving particular attention to **exposure** to infections, dusts, fumes, and drugs with known pulmonary toxicity. Patients with acute and chronic ILD typically present with dyspnea on exertion and cough. Chest pain, wheezing, and hemoptysis are less common. The occupational and family history provide useful information.

**B.** The **physical examination** often demonstrates bibasilar inspiratory crackles. IPF and bronchogenic carcinoma are associated with clubbing of the digits. Signs of PH develop with severe disease. Extrapulmonary findings may assist with the diagnosis. For example, erythema nodosum is highly suggestive of sarcoidosis and telangiectasias are suggestive of scleroderma.

**C.** All stable patients who present with ILD should undergo (1) **pulmonary function testing** (spirometry, lung volumes, and diffusing capacity); (2) a resting ABG; and (3) an exercise assessment of arterial oxygenation. Most patients with ILD have abnormal routine pulmonary function tests, although some are initially normal. As the lungs become stiffer, the vital capacity and total lung capacity decrease, producing a restrictive pulmonary function pattern. The restriction is often accompanied by a decrease in the diffusing capacity for DLCO, a widening of the alveolar-arterial difference for oxygen at rest, and at times a dramatic fall in the $SaO_2$ with exercise. Most patients present with a respiratory alkalosis. Carbon dioxide retention occurs only in very severe and terminal disease. With long-standing or far-advanced disease, distortion of the small airways may produce concomitant airway obstruction.

**D. Laboratory evaluation.** Routine blood testing is **rarely diagnostic,** although certain abnormalities may define the underlying disorder: iron-deficiency anemia due to alveolar hemorrhage, eosinophilia due to eosinophilic pneumonia or drug reaction, thrombocytopenia due to collagen vascular disease, and hypercalcemia due to sarcoid. Rheumatoid factor and antinuclear antigen are present in high titers in rheumatoid arthritis and systemic lupus erythematosus, although they are nonspecifically present in lower titers in other diseases, such as IPF and silicosis. The presence of antineutrophil cytoplasmic antibody provides evidence for Wegener's granulomatosis, necrotizing vasculitis, and pulmonary capillaritis. A positive assay for anti–Jo 1 is helpful in diagnosing polymyositis. Serum precipitating antibody testing may support the presence of extrinsic allergic alveolitis related to farming or pigeon breeding. The angiotensin-converting enzyme level is neither sensitive nor specific for the diagnosis of sarcoidosis.

**Table 9-8.** Classification of interstitial lung disease

| Category | Examples |
|---|---|
| Granulomatous disease | Sarcoidosis |
| | Berylliosis |
| | Hypersensitivity pneumonitis |
| Connective tissue diseases | Scleroderma |
| | Rheumatoid arthritis |
| | Polymyositis-dermatomyositis |
| | Systemic lupus erythematosus |
| | Mixed connective tissue disease |
| | Ankylosing spondylitis |
| | Sjögren's syndrome |
| | Psoriatic arthritis |
| | Behçet's disease |
| | Relapsing polychondritis |
| Iatrogenic | Drug induced |
| | Antibiotics |
| | Nitrofurantoin |
| | Sulfasalazine |
| | Antiarrhythmics |
| | Amiodarone |
| | Chemotherapeutic agents |
| | Bleomycin |
| | Methotrexate |
| | Azathioprine |
| | Illicit |
| | Crack cocaine (inhaled) |
| | Radiation |
| | Bone marrow transplantation |
| | Vitamins |
| | L-tryptophan |
| Familial | Tuberous sclerosis/neurofibromatosis |
| | Idiopathic pulmonary fibrosis |
| | Sarcoidosis |
| Occupational and environmental | Inorganic dusts |
| | Asbestos |
| | Hard metals |
| | Silicates |
| | Talc |

*continued*

**Table 9-8.** Continued

| Category | Examples |
|---|---|
| | Organic dusts (hypersensitivity pneumonitis) |
| | Bird breeder's lung |
| | Farmer's lung |
| | Fumes |
| Idiopathic | Idiopathic pulmonary fibrosis |
| | Autoimmune-associated pulmonary fibrosis (see Connective tissue diseases) |
| | Nonspecific interstitial pneumonitis |
| | Acute interstitial pneumonitis/Hamman-Rich syndrome |
| | Lymphocytic interstitial pneumonia |
| | Respiratory bronchiolitis |
| | Lymphangioleiomyomatosis |
| | Eosinophilic granuloma (EG) |
| | Chronic eosinophilic pneumonia |
| | Eosinophilic pneumonia |
| | Bronchiolitis obliterans and organizing pneumonia |
| | Pulmonary hemorrhage syndromes |
| | Amyloidosis |
| | Alveolar microlithiasis |
| | Metastatic calcification |
| | Acute respiratory distress syndrome |
| | Postinfectious |
| | Pulmonary alveolar proteinosis |
| Neoplasm | Lymphangitic carcinoma |
| | Bronchoalveolar carcinoma |
| | Lymphoma |
| Lung water | Pulmonary edema |
| | Cardiogenic |
| | Noncardiogenic |
| Infectious | Mycobacteriosis |
| | Fungal |
| | *Pneumocystis carinii/jiroveci* |
| | Viral |
| | Parasitic |
| | Bacterial |
| Chemical | Aspiration |
| | Lipoid pneumonia |

E. **Imaging evaluations** with **chest radiograph or CT scan** are usually abnormal, although some patients initially have normal tests. Imaging studies most often provide nonspecific but useful information (Table 9-9). All patients should undergo chest radiography. If infection or pulmonary edema is not likely, further imaging is appropriate. The CT scan, including high-resolution CT (HRCT), although more sensitive than chest radiography, usually does not provide specific diagnostic information that obviates the need for further testing, except in rare situations such as lymphangioleiomyomatosis. Perhaps the strongest reason for obtaining an HRCT is to provide guidance for obtaining tissue from the most active sites of parenchymal disease and to detect associated findings such as mediastinal lymphadenopathy.

F. **Invasive diagnostic studies.** When biologic specimens are needed to make a diagnosis, three types of tests can be considered. The clinician should exclude pulmonary edema as the cause of the ILD before embarking on invasive testing.

1. **BAL** obtains cells and material from the periphery of the airways during bronchoscopy. It is most useful in patients with infections, particularly in those who are immunosuppressed, and in those with alveolar hemorrhage. The role of BAL as a diagnostic tool in other patients with ILD is so limited as to almost never be worthwhile as a sole procedure.
2. **Transbronchial lung biopsy (TBBx)** obtains small pieces of lung tissue close to the bronchiolar areas. It is most useful in diseases that follow

**Table 9-9.** Chest radiograph patterns in diffuse interstitial lung disease

| Category | Example |
|---|---|
| Lower lobe predominance | Idiopathic pulmonary fibrosis |
| | Collagen vascular disease (scleroderma) |
| | Asbestosis |
| | Hypersensitivity pneumonitis |
| Upper lobe predominance | Pneumoconiosis (silicosis) |
| | Ankylosing spondylitis |
| | Eosinophilic granuloma (EG; Langerhan's cell granulomatosis) |
| | Sarcoid |
| Hilar adenopathy | Sarcoid |
| | Hypersensitivity pneumonitis, including some drugs (e.g., methotrexate) |
| Associated pneumothorax | EG |
| | Lymphangioleiomyomatosis (LAM)/tuberous sclerosis |
| Increased lung volumes | EG |
| | LAM |
| | Sarcoidosis |
| Eggshell calcification of lymph nodes | Silicosis |
| | Sarcoidosis |
| | Radiation |

that distribution, especially sarcoid and lymphangitic carcinoma. With the exception of infection, TBBx is much less useful and may be inadequate if a large amount of tissue is needed to make a diagnosis of other types of ILD (*Am J Respir Crit Care Med* 151:909, 1995). The finding of inflammation or fibrosis is considered nondiagnostic.

3. **Surgical lung biopsy (video-assisted thoracoscopic surgery or thoracotomy)** is the procedure of choice to obtain lung tissue that is sufficient for diagnosis. Pathologic classification of ILD aids in assessing prognosis and choosing therapy (*Am J Respir Crit Care Med* 157:1301, 1998). The surgical biopsy should be directed toward the most active sites of inflammation as determined by HRCT and not routinely directed at only end-stage fibrotic areas or the easily accessible right middle lobe or lingula. Patients with rapidly advancing disease, suspicion of vasculitis, marked systemic symptoms, or atypical imaging findings should receive strong consideration for surgical biopsy. The risks of a biopsy may exceed the benefits in patients with advanced age, severe comorbidity, stable or very slowly progressive disease, known collagen vascular disease, and typical imaging and functional abnormalities.

G. **Monitoring.** Serial evaluation of symptoms (e.g., dyspnea), pulmonary function, exercise tolerance, oxygenation, and radiographic changes (including HRCT scan) is used to assess the rate of progression of disease and to facilitate decisions concerning therapy.

## IV. Treatment

A. **General.** Treatment of ILD varies depending on the underlying etiology. Before embarking on a course of treatment, the physician likely needs to exclude the presence of infection and pulmonary edema and then obtain lung fluid and tissue for as accurate a diagnosis as possible. Depending on the etiology, treatment might include antibiotics, immunosuppression, or avoidance of exposures to offending agents. In many cases, particularly those of sarcoid, bronchiolitis obliterans organizing pneumonia, and chronic eosinophilic pneumonia, various regimens of corticosteroids can be used effectively. Treatment of three common ILDs is discussed below.

B. **Sarcoidosis** is a syndrome of unknown etiology, consisting of multiorgan involvement with noncaseating granulomas. Patients typically develop sarcoidosis before the age of 40 years. The lungs and thoracic lymph nodes are involved in more than 90% of patients. Half of the patients present with asymptomatic abnormalities incidentally noted on chest radiographs. The most common pulmonary symptoms include cough, dyspnea, and chest pain. Skin and eyes are each involved in approximately 20% of the cases. Cardiac involvement is clinically evident in only 5% of the patients, most of whom have extensive extracardiac disease. Cardiac disease is frequently unrecognized antemortem and is the most common cause of death attributed to sarcoidosis (*Chest* 103:253, 1993). Sarcoid may involve multiple other organs.

Sarcoid is most often diagnosed by demonstrating characteristic noncaseating granulomas in the affected organs and ruling out other etiologies of granulomatous disease such as infection with fungi or tuberculosis. Although skin and lymph nodes are easily accessible, TBBx is often used to make the diagnosis because of the high frequency of pulmonary involvement.

1. **Staging and prognosis.** Five percent to 10% of patients have a normal chest radiograph (stage 0). Patients with bilateral hilar lymphadenopathy (stage I) usually experience stability or resolution without therapy within a few years of diagnosis. Two-thirds of patients with pulmonary infiltrates and hilar lymphadenopathy (stage II) undergo spontaneous resolution. Therapy for patients with pulmonary infiltrates but no hilar lymphadenopathy (stage III) is controversial, because about half of patients experience improvement without therapy within 2 years. **Asymptomatic patients** without evidence of clinical or radiologic pro-

gression could be followed closely without treatment. Decisions regarding initiation of therapy should be individualized in patients with parenchymal infiltrates and a mild to moderate restrictive defect. Patients with fibrotic lung disease (stage IV) may not benefit from therapy other than lung transplantation.

2. **Treatment. Corticosteroids** are the mainstay of treatment for patients with progressive impairment of pulmonary function, vital organ dysfunction (eye, CNS, heart, kidney), or persistent hypercalcemia.
   a. **Lung involvement.** Although there is still debate as to their long-term effectiveness, corticosteroids may reverse the early changes of pulmonary parenchymal involvement. Corticosteroid therapy is a long-term commitment, as the patient will likely require it for at least 1 year to prevent relapse. The lowest dose that will continue to suppress the patient's symptoms should be maintained, while monitoring for toxicity. The efficacy of other immunosuppressive agents in sarcoid has not been clearly defined, although they may allow treatment with a lower dose of steroids.
   b. **Other organ involvement.** Because untreated uveitis can lead to blindness, all patients with sarcoid should regularly receive a detailed ophthalmologic evaluation. CNS and cardiac involvement respond poorly to therapy. Hypercalcemia due to sarcoid responds well to corticosteroids and avoidance of ultraviolet light exposure.

C. **Idiopathic pulmonary fibrosis** is a relatively uncommon chronic lung disease. Lung inflammation leads to injury and then fibrosis. The classic histologic appearance consists of usual interstitial pneumonitis, although other diseases may show similar biopsy findings. IPF occurs more frequently in men than in women, with onset typically occurring in middle age. IPF has a highly variable but progressive course. Spontaneous remissions do not occur. Patients usually do not significantly improve with therapy, although it may slow the progression of disease. From the time of diagnosis, patients with IPF have a median survival of less than 5 years. Relatively good prognostic factors include young age, female gender, recent onset of symptoms, less severe breathlessness, infiltrates at presentation, predominantly cellular histology (as opposed to fibrosis), and initial responsiveness to glucocorticoids (*Am J Respir Crit Care Med* 149:450, 1994; *Am J Respir Crit Care Med* 161:646, 2000).

Typically, radiologic studies show lower lobe–predominant patchy peripheral and subpleural basal reticular abnormalities, often with traction bronchiectasis and honeycombing. HRCT increases the accuracy of the diagnosis compared to chest radiography. However, a definitive diagnosis relies on obtaining lung tissue. Bronchoscopy with TBBx does not obtain sufficient lung tissue to define the disease process adequately, and a diagnostic surgical biopsy should be considered.

1. **Treatment** options include corticosteroids, immunosuppressive/cytotoxic agents, antifibrotic agents, and lung transplantation. Small studies have suggested that the minority of patients experience modest and limited benefit from medical therapy. Few large clinical trials have been conducted. Given the poor efficacy and the high risk of complications of treatment, the American Thoracic Society (*Am J Respir Crit Care Med* 161:646, 2000) recommends a cautious undertaking of treatment in patients with advanced age, extreme obesity, severe comorbidity (e.g., diabetes mellitus, cardiac disease, osteoporosis), or end-stage honeycomb lung on HRCT examination. For patients who are undergoing therapy, the American Thoracic Society recommends combined therapy with corticosteroids and either azathioprine or cyclophosphamide. Supplemental oxygen (see Chronic Obstructive Pulmonary Disease, sec. **III.B**) requirements should be assessed and treated accordingly. Contraindications and side effects of immunosuppressive agents are discussed in Chap. 23, Arthritis and Rheumatologic Diseases.

a. **Corticosteroids** (prednisone, 0.5–1.0 mg/kg PO qd) should be initiated early in the course of the illness. If an objective response occurs within 3 months, therapy should be continued. The steroid dosage should be gradually decreased to 0.25–0.5 mg/kg PO qd over the next few months. Eventually, prednisone is tapered slowly to the minimal dosage that maintains clinical stability, such as 10–15 mg PO every other day (*J Respir Dis* 14:1244, 1993).

b. **Azathioprine,** 2–3 mg/kg PO qd, not to exceed 150 mg/day, or **cyclophosphamide,** 2 mg/kg (lean body weight) PO qd, not to exceed 150 mg/day, in combination with low-dose glucocorticoids, may result in improvement in some cases that are unresponsive to glucocorticoids alone (*Am Rev Respir Dis* 144:291, 1991; *Chest* 102:1090, 1992). Dosing of either can begin at 25–50 mg/day and increase by 25-mg increments every 1–2 weeks until the maximum dose is reached (as tolerated by WBC and platelet count). *Pneumocystis carinii* pneumonia prophylaxis should be considered.

c. **Other drug therapies,** including colchicine, methotrexate, penicillamine, pirfenidone, interferon-gamma, interferon-beta, and thalidomide, have not clearly demonstrated efficacy. Interferon gamma-1b may improve lung function and oxygenation in patients with IPF who had no response to glucocorticoids alone (*N Engl J Med* 341:1264, 1999). Colchicine (0.6 mg PO qd or bid) might have similar efficacy to corticosteroids with fewer side effects.

2. **Treatment should be continued for at least 6 months.** Studies should be performed to evaluate response (see secs. **III.G** and **IV.C.3**). If the patient's condition is improved or stable, the drugs should be maintained at the same dose, although therapy should be individualized. If the patient's condition worsens, as is frequently the case, the drugs can be tapered and stopped or changed.

3. **Monitoring** of the clinical course with clinical, radiographic, and physiologic parameters may be useful, especially if the patient is being treated. A battery of information should be obtained at baseline and at regular intervals to assess progression or remission.

D. **Radiation pneumonitis** is a subacute inflammatory pneumonitis that occurs in response to radiation exposure to the lung.

1. **Symptoms** include cough, dyspnea, and fever. The incidence, severity, and time of onset of symptoms depend on several factors, the most important of which are the total radiation dose, the fractionation schedule, the volume of lung irradiated, and the concomitant administration of cytotoxic therapy. In general, the onset of symptoms occurs within  weeks after completion of radiotherapy, although disease can develop as late as 6 months after radiation therapy. The classic **radiograph** shows the presence of an infiltrate corresponding to the region of radiation exposure.

2. **Management** includes the exclusion of other causes of pulmonary infiltrates, especially infections, recurrent tumors, and lymphangitic carcinomatosis. Mild symptoms can be managed with cough suppressants, antipyretics, and rest. Moderate to severe symptoms or a deterioration in oxygenation should be treated with glucocorticoids, although only half of patients respond. Prednisone is started at 60–100 mg/day, continued until symptoms and hypoxemia improve (usually 3–5 days), and then tapered to 20–40 mg PO qd. After 4 weeks of treatment, the prednisone dose should be tapered and eventually discontinued.

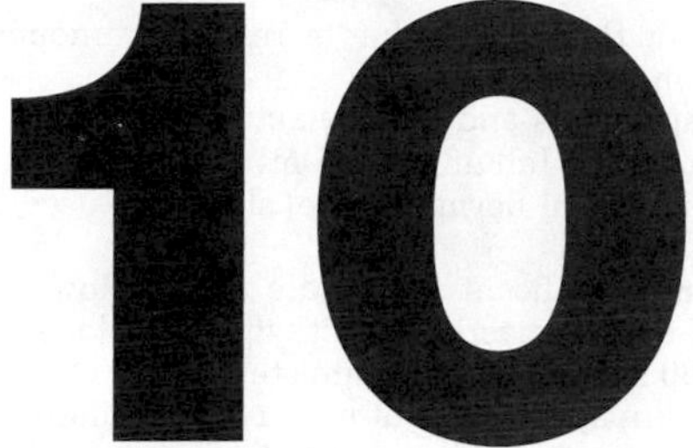

# Allergy and Immunology

Alpa Jani, Adrian Shifren, Mitchell Grayson, and Mario Castro

## Anaphylaxis

Anaphylaxis is an IgE-mediated, rapidly developing, systemic allergic reaction. Anaphylactoid reactions result from the direct release of mast cell mediators.

I. **The clinical manifestations of anaphylaxis and anaphylactoid reactions** are the same. Most serious reactions occur within minutes after exposure to the antigen. However, the reaction may be delayed for hours. Some patients experience a biphasic reaction characterized by a recurrence of symptoms after 4–8 hours. A few patients have a protracted course that requires several hours of continuous treatment.

   A. **Manifestations** include pruritus, urticaria, angioedema, respiratory distress (due to laryngeal edema, laryngospasm, or bronchospasm), hypotension, abdominal cramping, and diarrhea. The most common cause of death is airway obstruction, followed by hypotension. The spectrum of reactions ranges from very severe and life-threatening to mild. However, left untreated, all reactions have the potential to become severe very rapidly. **A previous mild reaction does not predict the severity of future reactions with re-exposure to the offending agent.**

   B. **Immediate treatment of anaphylaxis and anaphylactoid reactions**

      1. **Epinephrine** is the mainstay of therapy and should be administered immediately. A dose of **0.3–0.5 mg (0.3–0.5 ml of a 1:1000 solution) IM or SC** should be administered and repeated at 20-minute intervals if necessary. Patients with major airway compromise or hypotension can be given epinephrine sublingually (0.5 ml of a 1:1000 solution), via a femoral or internal jugular vein (3–5 ml of a 1:10,000 solution) or via an endotracheal tube (3–5 ml of a 1:10,000 solution diluted to 10 ml with normal saline). For protracted anaphylaxis that requires multiple doses of epinephrine, an IV epinephrine drip may be useful. The infusion is titrated to BP (see Appendix D, Intravenous Admixture Preparation and Administration Guide).

      2. **Airway management** should be a priority. Supplemental 100% oxygen therapy should be administered. Endotracheal intubation may be necessary. If laryngeal edema is not rapidly responsive to epinephrine, cricothyroidotomy or tracheotomy may be required.

      3. **Volume expansion** with IV fluids may be necessary. An initial bolus of 500–1000 ml normal saline should be followed by an infusion that is titrated to BP and urine output.

      4. **β-Adrenergic antagonist therapy increases the risk of anaphylactoid reaction and anaphylaxis** and renders the reaction more difficult to treat (*Ann Intern Med* 115:270, 1991). Therefore, glucagon, given as a 1-mg (1 ampule) bolus and followed by a drip of up to 1 mg/hour, can be used to provide inotropic support for patients who are taking β-adrenergic antagonists. **α-Adrenergic or mixed-adrenergic agonist vasopres-**

**sors must be avoided** in this setting due to resultant unopposed α-mediated vasoconstriction.

C. **Additional treatment of anaphylaxis and anaphylactoid reactions**
   1. **Inhaled β-adrenergic agonists** [albuterol, 0.5 ml (2.5 mg), or metaproterenol, 0.3 ml (15 mg) in 2.5 ml normal saline] should be used to treat resistant bronchospasm.
   2. **Glucocorticoids** have no significant immediate effect. However, they may prevent relapse of severe reactions. Methylprednisolone, 125 mg IV, or hydrocortisone, 500 mg IV, can be administered.
   3. **Antihistamines** relieve skin symptoms but have no immediate effect on the reaction. They may shorten the duration of the reaction. The addition of an $H_2$ antagonist may be useful.

II. **Observation** for a minimum of 6 hours is indicated for patients with mild reactions limited to urticaria, angioedema, or mild bronchospasm. Patients with moderate to severe reactions should be admitted to the hospital for close observation of a possible biphasic reaction.

III. **Recurrent anaphylaxis. Prevention of recurrent episodes** requires identification and avoidance of the offending antigen. Medications, *Hymenoptera* stings, and foods are the most common causes of anaphylaxis. Radiocontrast medium is the most common cause of anaphylactoid reactions. An exhaustive diagnostic evaluation is not indicated after a single episode of anaphylaxis if a cause is not suggested by the history. In patients with recurrent episodes and no obvious etiologic finding, other possible diagnoses should be considered. An elevated serum β-tryptase during an episode confirms the diagnosis of anaphylaxis.

A. **Self-administered epinephrine** should be prescribed for all patients with a history of anaphylaxis to a food or *Hymenoptera* sting. The patient should be instructed in its use. Patients with a history of anaphylaxis to *Hymenoptera* also should be referred to an allergist for venom immunotherapy.

B. **Mastocytosis** should be considered in patients with recurrent, unexplained anaphylaxis or flushing. The diagnosis is confirmed by demonstration of persistently elevated levels of mast cell mediators, such as serum α-tryptase, even when the patient is asymptomatic.

## Drug Reactions

Adverse reactions to drugs are a very common problem. Only a subset of reactions are mediated immunologically; other drug reactions may be toxic or idiosyncratic. Many different mechanisms can account for immunologically mediated drug reactions (Table 10-1). These reactions can occur with relatively low doses of the drug, usually on re-exposure after an initial sensitization to the drug.

I. **Beta-lactam sensitivity.** Penicillins and other beta-lactam antibiotics are commonly associated with immunologically mediated drug reactions.

A. **Penicillins** have a high incidence of immunologic reactivity as a result of their chemical structure. The core structure consists of a reactive bicyclic beta-lactam ring that serves as a hapten by covalently binding to tissue carrier proteins. Ninety-five percent of tissue-bound penicillin is haptenated as the benzylpenicilloyl form and is called the **major determinant.** Five percent of tissue-bound penicillin consists of three non–cross-reactive metabolites, termed the **minor determinants.** Immediate allergic reactions are most often related to the major determinant. In addition, some modified penicillins, such as ampicillin, can produce allergic reactions in which the antigenic determinant is the side chain. Skin testing is available if there is a

**Table 10-1.** Immunologically mediated drug reactions

| Type of reaction | Representative examples | Mechanism |
|---|---|---|
| Anaphylactic | Anaphylaxis<br>Urticaria<br>Angioedema | IgE-mediated degranulation of mast cell with resultant mediator release |
| Cytotoxic | Autoimmune hemolytic anemia<br>Interstitial nephritis | IgG or IgM antibodies against cell antigens and complement activation |
| Immune complex | Serum sickness<br>Vasculitis | Immune complex deposition and subsequent complement activation |
| Cell mediated | Contact dermatitis<br>Photosensitivity dermatitis | Activated T cells against cell surface–bound antigens |

question of immediate hypersensitivity to penicillin. In 97% of patients with a negative skin test to penicillin, a significant immediate hypersensitivity reaction to penicillin will not develop. A delayed, non-IgE–mediated reaction (e.g., a morbilliform rash or serum sickness) may still develop in these patients. **No case of penicillin-induced anaphylaxis has been reported in a patient who is skin test negative.** Seventy-five percent of patients who report a history of penicillin sensitivity are negative on skin testing and are not at risk for anaphylaxis. However, 4% of patients with unknown or negative histories of penicillin reactions have positive skin tests and are at risk for having an IgE-mediated event. Skin testing should only be performed by an allergist who has been appropriately trained to perform these tests.

**B. Cephalosporins** share cross reactivity with penicillins because of their related structure. Studies report a fourfold increased risk of hypersensitivity reactions to cephalosporins in penicillin-allergic patients as compared to the general population (8% vs. 2%) (*J Infect Dis* 137:S74–S79, 1978). The degree of cross reactivity is related to the generation of the cephalosporin (first greater than second greater than third generation). Although many of the reactions to second- and third-generation cephalosporins are directed at the side chains, skin testing to penicillin in these patients can be helpful, as most severe anaphylactic reactions are directed at the reactive bicyclic core. Patients with a history of a severe reaction to penicillin should be considered sensitive to cephalosporin unless they are skin test negative. Although patients with a history of a nonanaphylactic reaction to penicillin can often be given a second- or third-generation cephalosporin safely, it is advisable to precede the dose with an oral provocation dose challenge.

**C. Other related antibiotics**

1. **Monobactams. Aztreonam** is the prototypical antibiotic with a monocyclic structure. No significant cross reactivity is found between this group and the beta-lactams.
2. **Carbapenems. Imipenem** is the prototypical member of this antibiotic group. A very high degree of cross reactivity (50%) is found between imipenem determinants and penicillin determinants.
3. **Carbacephems** (e.g., loracarbef) are structurally related to cephalosporins. Few data exist in regard to cross reactivity, but they are assumed to be related antigenically and should be avoided in severely penicillin-sensitive patients.

**II. Anaphylactoid reactions to drugs** mimic anaphylaxis but are not IgE mediated. They are due to the degranulation of mast cells induced directly by the offending drug.

**A. Radiocontrast sensitivity reactions** mimic anaphylaxis but are not IgE mediated. As a result of osmotic shifts, the contrast medium probably causes a direct degranulation of mast cells in susceptible patients. Reactions can occur in 5–10% of patients, with a fatal reaction occurring in 1 in 40,000 procedures. The following **risk factors** have been identified: age greater than 50 years, preexisting cardiovascular or renal disease, a personal history of allergy, and a history of a radiocontrast reaction. No evidence has been found that sensitivity to seafood or iodine predisposes to reactions to radiocontrast media. Although no predictive tests are available, if patients have a history of a reaction, the use of a low-ionic-strength contrast medium and premedication is strongly suggested. The **premedication regimen** includes prednisone (50 mg PO) given 13 hours, 7 hours, and 1 hour before the procedure and diphenhydramine (50 mg PO) given 1 hour before the procedure. An $H_2$ blocker can be given 1 hour before the procedure as well. It is important to remember that premedication is not 100% effective and that appropriate precautions for handling a reaction should be taken.

**B. Red man's syndrome** from vancomycin consists of pruritus and flushing of the neck and face. It can be prevented by slowing the rate of infusion and premedicating with diphenhydramine (50 mg PO) 30 minutes before the infusion.

**C.** Other drugs, including **opiates and fluoroquinolones,** may cause anaphylactoid reactions.

**III. Erythema multiforme, Stevens-Johnson syndrome (SJS), and toxic epidermal necrolysis (TEN)** are all serious drug reactions that primarily involve the skin. Erythema multiforme is characterized most typically by target lesions. SJS and TEN manifest with varying degrees of sloughing of the epidermis and mucous membranes (<10% of total body surface area in SJS, 10–30% in SJS-TEN overlap, and >30% in TEN). Treatment focuses on the discontinuation of suspected drugs and treating any underlying infection. Other therapeutic maneuvers are directed to symptoms and may include hydration to maintain fluid balance, antihistamines to decrease pruritus, analgesics to relieve pain, and wet dressings to débride crusted erosions. Care in a burn unit or ICU may be required. Systemic corticosteroids are often used, but their efficacy is unproven. **Re-administration or future skin testing with the offending drug is absolutely contraindicated.**

**IV. Management of the patient with a history of drug reactions.** Use of the drug in question should always be avoided unless a definite medical indication exists. If use of the drug must be considered, a careful history of the reaction is helpful in defining the potential risk. The date of a reaction is useful given that patients may lose their sensitivity to a drug over time. Timing of symptoms is important; symptoms occurring with the onset of a drug course are more likely to be IgE mediated than are symptoms that develop several days after the completion of a course. On occasion, a history of an unrecognized, inadvertent re-exposure to a drug that had previously caused a reaction may be elicited. If this re-exposure was not associated with any reaction, a lack of true IgE-mediated hypersensitivity or a loss of sensitivity may have developed. Finally, the type of symptoms must be detailed. **Toxic reactions** (e.g., nausea secondary to macrolide antibiotics or codeine) are not immunologic reactions and do not necessarily predict problems with other members in their respective class. However, a history of **a true IgE-mediated reaction (anaphylaxis)** does increase the likelihood of further IgE-mediated reactions. If no alternative drug is available and the patient gives a history of an IgE-mediated reaction, **skin testing** should first be performed. Skin testing is standardized only for penicillin but may be useful for beta-lactam–related antibiotics and cephalosporins. If the patient has a positive skin test to penicillin, desensitization by an allergist should be performed. Results of testing to drugs other than penicillin must be interpreted within the clinical context of the case, and management may include a graded dose challenge under the direction of an allergist. A successful desensitization or graded challenge does not preclude the development of a non-IgE–mediated, delayed reaction (e.g., rash). Furthermore, if a dose of drug is missed following a desensitization procedure, the patient often needs to undergo a repeat desensitization.

V. **Treatment of drug reactions.** Discontinuation of the suspected drug or drugs is the most important initial approach in managing an allergic reaction. If the patient is taking the drug for a life-threatening illness (e.g., meningitis) and the reaction is a mild skin reaction, it may be reasonable to continue the medication and treat the reaction symptomatically. However, if the rash is progressive, the drug must be discontinued to avoid a desquamative process such as SJS.

## Eosinophilia

Peripheral blood **eosinophilia** is defined as an absolute eosinophil count greater than 450/µl. Eosinophils are tissue-dwelling cells, most abundant in mucosal tissues such as the respiratory and GI tracts. Activation of eosinophils leads to the release of stored granular components, which are believed to be responsible for the tissue damage ascribed to these cells.

I. The **etiology** of eosinophilia can be classified by associated clinical context, as shown in Table 10-2. In industrialized nations, peripheral blood eosinophilia is most often due to atopic disease, whereas helminthic infections are the most common cause of eosinophilia in the rest of the world.
   A. **Eosinophilia associated with atopic disease.** Modest peripheral blood levels of eosinophils are often found in patients with allergic rhinitis, asthma, or atopic dermatitis.
   B. **Eosinophilia associated with pulmonary infiltrates.** This classification is inclusive of those diseases with pulmonary infiltrates and lung tissue eosinophilia, with or without blood eosinophilia (eosinophilic pneumonias), and those disorders with pulmonary infiltrates and blood eosinophilia (pulmonary infiltrates with eosinophilia syndromes). The pulmonary infiltrates with eosinophilia syndromes include allergic bronchopulmonary aspergillosis (ABPA), an immunologic reaction to *Aspergillus fumigatus* that causes pulmonary infiltrates, proximal bronchiectasis and asthma and drug-induced pneumonitis (see sec. **I.E.1**). The eosinophilic pneumonias include acute and chronic eosinophilic pneumonia, both idiopathic diseases presenting with fever, cough, and dyspnea; Loeffler's syndrome, the combination of blood eosinophilia and transient pulmonary infiltrates from passage of helminthic larvae, usually *Ascaris lumbricoides*, through the lung; and tropical pulmonary eosinophilia, a hypersensitivity response in the lung to lymphatic filariae.
   C. **Eosinophilia associated with parasitic infection.** Various multicellular parasites, or helminths, can induce eosinophilia, whereas single-celled protozoan parasites, such as *Giardia lamblia*, do not. *Strongyloides stercoralis* infection must be excluded, as this helminth can set up a cycle of autoinfection that leads to chronic infection, with intermittent, sometimes marked, eosinophilia.
   D. **Eosinophilia associated with cutaneous disease.** Atopic dermatitis is classically associated with blood and tissue eosinophilia. Eosinophilic fasciitis is characterized by acute erythema, swelling and induration of the extremities progressing to symmetric induration of the skin, sparing the fingers, feet, and face. Antibiotic therapy failure and recurrent swelling of an extremity without tactile warmth are characteristic of eosinophilic cellulitis. Patients

**Table 10-2.** Causes of eosinophilia

| | |
|---|---|
| Eosinophilia associated with atopic disease | Eosinophilia associated with primary cutaneous disease |
| Allergic rhinitis | Atopic dermatitis |
| Asthma | Eosinophilic fasciitis |
| Atopic dermatitis | Eosinophilic cellulitis |
| Eosinophilia associated with pulmonary infiltrates | Eosinophilic folliculitis |
| Passage of larvae through the lung (Loeffler's syndrome) | Episodic angioedema with anaphylaxis |
| Chronic eosinophilic pneumonia | Eosinophilia associated with multiorgan involvement |
| Acute eosinophilic pneumonia | Drug-induced eosinophilia |
| Tropical pulmonary eosinophilia | Churg-Strauss syndrome |
| Allergic bronchopulmonary aspergillosis | Idiopathic hypereosinophilic syndrome |
| Coccidiomycosis | Eosinophilic leukemia |
| Eosinophilia associated with parasitic infection | Miscellaneous causes |
| Helminths (*Ascaris lumbricoides*, *Strongyloides stercoralis*, hookworm, *Toxocara canis* or *cati*, *Trichinella*) | Eosinophilic gastroenteritis |
| Protozoa (only *Dientamoeba fragilis* and *Isospora belli*) | Interstitial nephritis |
| | HIV infection |
| | Eosinophilia myalgia syndrome |
| | Transplant rejection |
| | Atheroembolic disease |

with HIV are at risk for eosinophilic pustular folliculitis. A rare disease, episodic angioedema with eosinophilia, leads to recurrent attacks of fever, angioedema, and blood eosinophilia without other organ damage.

**E. Eosinophilia associated with multiorgan involvement**

1. **Drug-induced eosinophilia.** Numerous drugs can cause blood eosinophilia or tissue eosinophilia, or both. Drug-induced eosinophilia typically responds to cessation of the culprit medication. Asymptomatic drug-induced eosinophilia does not necessitate cessation of therapy.
2. **Churg-Strauss syndrome** (CSS) is a small-vessel vasculitis that is distinguished from other vasculitides by intravascular and extravascular eosinophilic granuloma formation, tissue and blood eosinophilia, frequent lung involvement with transient infiltrates on chest radiograph, and association with asthma. The onset of asthma and eosinophilia may precede the development of CSS by several years. Other manifestations include sinusitis, mono- or polyneuropathy, and rash. Half of patients have antineutrophil cytoplasmic antibodies directed against myeloperoxidase (p-ANCA). Biopsy of affected tissue reveals a necrotizing vasculitis with extravascular granulomas and tissue eosinophilia. Initial treatment involves high-dose glucocorticoids with the addition of cyclophosphamide, if necessary. Leukotriene modifiers, like all systemic steroid-sparing agents (including inhaled steroids), have been associated with unmasking of CSS due to a decrease in systemic steroid therapy; however, there is no evidence that these drugs cause CSS (*Chest* 117:708, 2000).
3. Idiopathic **hypereosinophilic syndrome** (HES) is a proliferative disorder of eosinophils characterized by specific organ damage due to infiltra-

tion of eosinophils, most notably in the heart. HES occurs predominantly in men between the ages of 20 and 50 years and presents with insidious onset of fatigue, cough, and dyspnea and an associated eosinophil count of greater than 1500/µl. At presentation, patients typically are in the late thrombotic and fibrotic stages of eosinophil-mediated cardiac damage with signs of a restrictive cardiomyopathy, including CHF and mitral regurgitation. An echocardiogram may detect intracardiac thrombi, endomyocardial fibrosis, or thickening of the posterior mitral valve leaflet. Neurologic manifestations range from peripheral neuropathy to stroke or encephalopathy. Bone marrow examination reveals increased eosinophil precursors. Treatment is with prednisone at 1 mg/kg/day; interferon-alpha has been shown to be effective as well (*Br J Haematol* 92:176, 1996).

4. **Acute eosinophilic leukemia** is a very rare myeloproliferative disorder that is distinguished from HES by several factors: an increased number of immature eosinophils in the blood or marrow, or both; greater than 10% blast forms in the marrow; and symptoms and signs that are compatible with an acute leukemia. Treatment is similar to that for other leukemias (see Chap. 20, Medical Management of Malignant Disease).

II. **History and physical examination.** The presence of cough, dyspnea, fever, or any symptoms of cancer should be determined, as should any history of rhinitis, wheezing, or rash. A complete medication list, including over-the-counter supplements, should be recorded, as should a full travel history (focusing on countries where filariasis may be endemic, e.g., southeast Asia, Africa, South America, or the Caribbean). Any contact with pets should be ascertained for possible exposure to *Toxocara*. Physical examination should be guided by the history, with special focus on the skin, upper and lower respiratory tracts, and cardiovascular and neurologic systems.

III. **Diagnosis.** Two approaches are useful for evaluating eosinophilia, either by associated clinical context (Table 10-2) or by degree of eosinophilia (Table 10-3).

A. Mild **eosinophilia associated with symptoms of rhinitis or asthma** is indicative of underlying atopic disease, which can be confirmed by skin testing.

B. **Eosinophilia associated with pulmonary infiltrates** has a wide differential diagnosis. The presence of asthma should lead to consideration of ABPA, CSS, or tropical pulmonary eosinophilia. Specific tests for parasitic infection should also be performed (see sec. **III.C**). Diagnosis at the time of presenta-

**Table 10-3.** Classification of eosinophilia based on the peripheral blood eosinophil count

| | Peripheral blood eosinophil count (cells/µl) | |
|---|---|---|
| 500–2000 | 2000–5000 | >5000 |
| Allergic rhinitis | Intrinsic asthma | Eosinophilia-myalgia syndrome |
| Allergic asthma | ABPA | Idiopathic hypereosinophilic syndrome |
| Food allergy | Helminthiasis | Episodic angioedema with eosinophilia |
| Urticaria | Churg-Strauss syndrome | Leukemia |
| Addison's disease | Drug reactions | |
| PIE syndromes | Vascular neoplasms | |
| Solid neoplasms | Eosinophilic fasciitis | |
| Nasal polyposis | HIV | |

ABPA, allergic bronchopulmonary aspergillosis; PIE, pulmonary infiltrates with eosinophilia.

tion with Loeffler's syndrome can be made by detection of *Ascaris* larvae in respiratory secretions or gastric aspirates (but not stool). **Chest x-ray** findings may also help narrow the differential diagnosis. Peripheral infiltrates with central clearing are indicative of chronic eosinophilic pneumonia. Diffuse infiltrates in an interstitial, alveolar, or mixed pattern may be seen in acute eosinophilic pneumonia as well as drug-induced eosinophilia with pulmonary involvement. Transient infiltrates may be seen in Loeffler's syndrome, CSS, or ABPA. Central bronchiectasis is a major criterion in the diagnosis of ABPA. A diffuse miliary or nodular pattern, consolidation, or cavitation may be found in cases of tropical pulmonary eosinophilia. If no other cause of pulmonary infiltrates has been identified, a **bronchoscopy** may be necessary for analysis of bronchoalveolar lavage fluid and lung tissue. The presence of eosinophils in bronchoalveolar lavage fluid or sputum with eosinophilic infiltration of the parenchyma is most typical of acute or chronic eosinophilic pneumonia.

C. **Eosinophilia associated with parasitic infection. Stool examination** for ova and parasites should be done on three separate occasions. Because only small numbers of helminths may pass in the stool, and because tissue or blood-dwelling helminths are not found in the stool, **serologic tests** for antiparasite antibodies should also be sent. Currently, such tests are available for *Strongyloides*, *Toxocara*, and *Trichinella*.
D. The diagnosis of **eosinophilia associated with cutaneous lesions** is guided by the appearance of the lesions and by results of skin biopsy.
E. **Eosinophilia with multiorgan involvement.** When a drug reaction is suspected, discontinuation of the drug is a diagnostic and a therapeutic maneuver. A history of asthma, significant peripheral blood eosinophilia (>10% of the leukocyte count), and pulmonary infiltrates suggests CSS. In this case, a sinus CT, nerve conduction studies, and testing for p-ANCA may aid in diagnosis. However, the diagnosis of CSS cannot be made without a tissue biopsy showing infiltrating eosinophils and granulomas. When eosinophilia is marked and all other causes have been ruled out, the diagnosis of idiopathic HES should be considered. Diagnosis requires a blood eosinophilia of greater than 1500/µl for more than 6 months with associated organ involvement. No specific test exists to identify these patients, and, in general, this is a diagnosis of exclusion.

## Asthma

Asthma is a disease of the airways characterized by airway inflammation and increased responsiveness (hyperreactivity) to a wide variety of stimuli (triggers). This hyperreactivity leads to obstruction of the airways, the severity of which may be widely variable in the same individual. As a consequence, patients have paroxysms of cough, dyspnea, chest tightness, and wheezing. Asthma is an episodic disease, with acute exacerbations that are interspersed with symptom-free periods. Other conditions may present with wheezing and must be considered, especially in patients who are not responsive to therapy (Table 10-4).

### I. Clinical manifestations and evaluation of asthma

A. **Attacks** are episodes of shortness of breath or wheezing that last minutes to hours. Patients may be completely symptom free between attacks. Typically, attacks are triggered by acute exposure to irritants (e.g., smoke) or allergens.
B. **Exacerbations** occur when airway reactivity is increased and lung function becomes unstable. During an exacerbation, attacks occur more easily and are more severe and persistent. Exacerbations are associated with factors

**Table 10-4.** Conditions that can present as refractory asthma

| | |
|---|---|
| Upper airway obstruction | Sinusitis |
| Tumor | Herpetic tracheobronchitis |
| Epiglottitis | Adverse drug reaction |
| Vocal cord dysfunction | Aspirin |
| Obstructive sleep apnea | β-Adrenergic antagonist |
| Tracheomalacia | Angiotensin-converting enzyme inhibitors |
| Endobronchial lesion | Inhaled pentamidine |
| Foreign body | Allergic bronchopulmonary aspergillosis |
| CHF | Hyperventilation with panic attacks |
| Gastroesophageal reflux | |

that increase airway hyperreactivity, such as viral infections, allergens, and occupational exposures.

C. **Nasal polyps.** Patients with asthma and nasal polyps should avoid aspirin and all nonsteroidal anti-inflammatory drugs (NSAIDs) because of the possibility of a severe systemic reaction.

D. **Pulmonary function tests (PFTs)** are essential to diagnose asthma. In patients with asthma, PFTs demonstrate an obstructive pattern, the hallmark of which is a decrease in expiratory flow rates. A reduction in the forced expiratory volume over 1 second ($FEV_1$) and a proportionally smaller reduction in the forced vital capacity (FVC) occur. This produces a decreased $FEV_1$/FVC ratio (generally <0.75). With mild obstructive disease that involves only the small airways, the $FEV_1$/FVC ratio may be normal, with the only abnormality being a decrease in airflow at midlung volumes (forced expiratory flow 25–75%). The clinical diagnosis of asthma is supported by an obstructive pattern that improves after bronchodilator therapy. Improvement is defined as **an increase in $FEV_1$ of more than 12% and 200 cc** after 2–3 puffs of a short-acting bronchodilator. In patients with chronic, severe asthma, the airflow obstruction may no longer be completely reversible. In these patients, the most effective way to establish the maximal degree of airway reversibility is to repeat PFTs after a course of oral corticosteroids (usually 40 mg/day for 10 days). The lack of demonstrable airway obstruction or reactivity does not rule out a diagnosis of asthma. In cases in which spirometry is normal, the diagnosis can be made by showing heightened airway responsiveness to a methacholine or histamine challenge.

E. **A chest radiograph** should be obtained to eliminate other causes of dyspnea, cough, or wheezing in patients being evaluated for asthma.

## II. Evaluation and treatment of an acute asthma attack

### A. Assessment of severity

1. **History.** Recent emergency room visits and current oral corticosteroid use may indicate an exacerbation that has become refractory to outpatient management. Previous attacks that have required the use of oral corticosteroids, a previous episode of respiratory failure, use of more than two canisters per month of inhaled short-acting bronchodilator, and seizures with asthma attacks have been associated with severe and potentially fatal asthma. Most patients have a progressive worsening of symptoms over a period of days or weeks. A precipitous onset of symptoms should raise the possibility of gastroesophageal reflux or a reaction to acute ingestion of aspirin or an NSAID.
2. **Physical examination.** A rapid assessment should be performed to identify those patients who require immediate intervention. **The presence**

**or intensity of wheezing is an unreliable indicator of the severity of an attack.** A severe attack is suggested by respiratory distress at rest, difficulty in speaking in sentences, diaphoresis, or agitation. A respiratory rate greater than 28 breaths/minute, a pulse greater than 110 beats/minute, or a pulsus paradoxus greater than 25 mm Hg also indicates a severe episode. Patients with depressed mental status require intubation. **Subcutaneous emphysema** should alert the examiner to the presence of a pneumothorax or pneumomediastinum. Impending respiratory muscle fatigue may cause a depressed respiratory effort and paradoxical diaphragmatic movement.

3. **Laboratory evaluation**
   a. **An objective measurement of airflow obstruction** is essential to the evaluation of an asthma attack. The severity of the exacerbation should be classified as **mild-moderate** [peak expiratory flow (PEF) or $FEV_1$ >50% of predicted], **severe** (PEF or $FEV_1$ <50%), or impending or actual respiratory arrest. Hospitalization is recommended if the response to treatment is poor or incomplete. A low threshold for admission is appropriate for patients with recent hospitalization, a failure of aggressive outpatient management (with oral corticosteroids), or a previous life-threatening attack. When spirometry is not available, peak flow rates can be obtained easily with a peak flowmeter. Generally, hospitalization is recommended if the PEF or $FEV_1$ is less than 50% of predicted, arterial carbon dioxide tension ($PaCO_2$) is greater than 42 mm Hg, the symptoms are severe, or the patient is drowsy or confused. The response to initial treatment (60–90 minutes after three treatments with a short-acting bronchodilator) is a better predictor of the need for hospitalization than is the severity of an exacerbation.
   b. **Arterial blood gas measurement** should be considered in patients in severe distress or with an $FEV_1$ of less than 30% of predicted values after initial treatment. An arterial oxygen tension of less than 60 mm Hg is a sign of severe bronchoconstriction or of a complicating condition. Initially, the $PaCO_2$ is low, owing to an increase in respiratory rate. With a prolonged attack, the $PaCO_2$ may rise as a result of severe airway obstruction, increased dead-space ventilation, and respiratory muscle fatigue. **A normal or increased $PaCO_2$ is a sign of impending respiratory failure and necessitates hospitalization.** The patient requires aggressive bronchodilator therapy and should be monitored closely (often in an ICU) to assess the need for mechanical ventilation.
   c. **Chest radiograph** is not routinely required and is performed only if a complicating pulmonary process, such as pneumonia, is suspected.

B. **Therapy**

1. **Supplemental oxygen** should be administered to the patient who is awaiting an assessment of arterial oxygen tension and should be continued to maintain an oxygen saturation of greater than 90% (95% in patients with coexisting cardiac disease or pregnancy).
2. **Bronchodilators** are first-line therapy in an asthma attack. Reversal of airflow obstruction is achieved most effectively by frequent administration of inhaled $\beta_2$-adrenergic agonists.
   a. **Albuterol** is administered either via metered-dose inhaler (MDI) or nebulizer. For a **mild-moderate exacerbation,** initial treatment starts with 6–12 puffs of albuterol via MDI or 2.5 mg via nebulizer and is repeated q20min until improvement is obtained or toxicity is noted. For a **severe exacerbation,** albuterol, 2.5–5.0 mg q20min, and ipratropium bromide 0.5 mg q3–4h, should be administered via nebulizer. Alternatively, albuterol, 10.0–15.0 mg, administered continuously over an hour, may be more effective in severely obstructed

adults. The subsequent dosing schedule is adjusted according to the patient's symptoms and clinical presentation. Often, patients require a $\beta_2$-adrenergic agonist q2–4h during an acute attack. The use of an MDI with a spacer device under supervision of trained personnel is as effective as aerosolized solution by nebulizer. Cooperation may not be possible in the patient with severe airflow obstruction.

b. **Parenteral administration of bronchodilators** is unnecessary if inhaled medications can be administered quickly. In rare settings, aqueous epinephrine (0.3 ml of a 1:1000 solution SC q20min) for up to three doses can be used. If epinephrine is administered, ECG monitoring is necessary.

3. **Systemic corticosteroids** speed the resolution of exacerbations of asthma and should be administered to all patients with a moderate or severe exacerbation.
   a. **Methylprednisolone** is the drug of choice for therapy. IV methylprednisolone, 125 mg, given on initial presentation decreases the rate of return to the emergency room of those patients who are discharged.
   b. **The ideal dose of corticosteroid** needed to speed recovery and limit symptoms is still not well defined. Currently, methylprednisolone, 40–60 mg IV q6h, is recommended. Oral corticosteroid administration may be as effective if given in equivalent doses (prednisone, 60 mg PO q6–8h).
   c. For maximal therapeutic response, **tapering of high-dose corticosteroids** should not take place until objective evidence of clinical improvement is observed (usually 36–48 hours). Initially, patients are given a daily dose of oral prednisone, which is then reduced slowly. Dosing oral steroids twice a day may minimize symptoms. A 7- to 14-day tapering dosage of prednisone usually is successful in combination with an inhaled corticosteroid that has been instituted at the beginning of the tapering schedule. In patients with severe disease or with a history of respiratory failure, a slower reduction in dosage is appropriate.
   d. **Patients discharged from the emergency room should receive oral corticosteroids.** A dose of prednisone, 40 mg/day for 5 days, can be substituted for a tapering schedule in selected patients. Either regimen should be accompanied by the initiation of an inhaled corticosteroid (or an increase in the previous dose of inhaled corticosteroid).
4. **Methylxanthines** are generally not recommended for acute asthma attacks.
5. **Antibiotics** have not been shown to have any benefit when administered routinely for acute asthma exacerbations. They can only be recommended as needed for treatment of comorbid conditions, such as pneumonia or bacterial sinusitis (*NHBLI*, NIH publication 02-5075, July 2002).
6. **Close follow-up** is required for patients discharged from the hospital or emergency room, because increased airway hyperreactivity persists for 4–6 weeks after an asthma exacerbation. A return visit to the physician should be scheduled for 5–7 days after discharge.

**III. Daily asthma management**

**A. The goals of daily management** are to control symptoms while maintaining normal activity and pulmonary function, to prevent exacerbations, and to minimize medication toxicity. Successful management requires patient education, objective measurement of airflow obstruction, and a medication plan for daily use and for exacerbations.

1. **Patient education** should focus on the chronic and inflammatory nature of asthma, with identification of factors that contribute to

increased inflammation. The consequences of ongoing exposure to chronic irritants or allergens and the rationale for therapy should be explained. Patients should be instructed to avoid factors that aggravate their disease, how to manage their daily medications, and how to recognize and deal with acute exacerbations (known as an **asthma action plan**). The use of a *written* daily management plan, as part of the education strategy, is recommended in all patients with persistent asthma.

2. A number of factors **increase airway hyperresponsiveness** and cause an acute and chronic increase in the severity of the disease.
   a. **Allergens,** such as dust mites, cockroaches, and pet dander, cause an increase in airway inflammation and symptoms in allergic patients. Many occupational allergens and irritants cause asthma, even in small doses.
   b. **Viral upper respiratory tract infections and sinusitis** are important causes of asthma exacerbations.
   c. **Gastroesophageal reflux** can cause cough and wheezing in some patients. Some factors, such as tobacco and wood smoke, trigger acute bronchospasm and should be avoided by all patients.
   d. **Cold air and exercise** can increase symptoms. Prophylactic use of cromolyn, nedocromil, or an inhaled $\beta_2$-adrenergic agonist (3 puffs 20 minutes before exposure) can minimize exercise-induced symptoms.
   e. **Aspirin and nonsteroidal anti-inflammatory medications** can cause the sudden onset of severe airway obstruction. Patients with aspirin sensitivity and nasal polyps typically have the onset of asthma in the third or fourth decade of life.
3. **PEF monitoring** provides an objective measurement of airflow obstruction and should be considered in patients with moderate to severe persistent asthma. Ideally, the PEF should be measured in the early morning and again after 12 hours, with additional measurements taken before and 20 minutes after bronchodilator therapy. The personal best PEF (the highest PEF obtained when the disease is under control) is identified, and the PEF is checked when symptoms escalate or in the setting of an asthma trigger. This should be incorporated into an asthma action plan, setting 80–100% of personal best PEF as the "green" zone, 50–80% as the "yellow" zone, and less than 50% as the "red" zone. Patients should learn to anticipate situations that cause increased symptoms. For many individuals, monitoring symptoms instead of PEF is sufficient. In addition, it is useful for patients to monitor their PEF during times in which medications are changed.
4. It is important for patients to recognize **signs of poorly controlled disease.** These signs include an increased or daily need for $\beta_2$-adrenergic agonists, limitation of activity, waking at night because of asthma symptoms, and variability in the PEF. Poorly controlled asthma is characterized by a greater response to bronchodilator therapy (increased difference between PEF before and after bronchodilator) and by an increase in the circadian variation in PEF. Specific instructions about handling these symptoms, including criteria for seeking emergency care, should be provided.

B. **Medical management** involves chronic management and a plan for acute exacerbations. Most often it includes the daily use of an anti-inflammatory, disease-modifying medication **(long-term-control medications)** and as-needed use of a short-acting bronchodilator **(quick-relief medications)**.
   1. The **severity** of asthma varies over time in individual patients. Consequently, medication requirements vary over time. The National Heart, Lung, and Blood Institute consensus report classifies asthma into four

different steps (mild intermittent, mild, moderate, and severe persistent) (*NHBLI*, NIH publication 02-5075, July 2002). The goal of the stepwise approach is to gain control of symptoms as quickly as possible by assigning the patient to the most severe step in which any one feature occurs. Therapy is started at a level higher than the patient's severity to gain control and then decreased in follow-up once control has been achieved. Therapy should be reviewed every 1–6 months to check if stepwise reduction is possible.

a. **Mild intermittent asthma.** This is characterized by mild asthma symptoms two or fewer times a week, nocturnal awakening fewer than two times a month, a PEF of more than 80% of personal best, and an $FEV_1$ of greater than 80% predicted. In this setting, a short-acting $\beta_2$-adrenergic agonist used on an as-needed basis (e.g., albuterol, 2–3 puffs) is appropriate.
b. **Mild persistent asthma.** These patients have asthma symptoms more than two times a week, nocturnal awakening more than two times a month but less than once per week, a PEF greater than 80% of personal best, and an $FEV_1$ greater than 80% predicted. In addition to the short-acting $\beta_2$-adrenergic agonist, a long-term controller medication is required. A **low dose of inhaled corticosteroid** (Table 10-5) is the recommended long-term controller medication for this severity. Alternative therapies, which are less effective, include a leukotriene antagonist, cromolyn, nedocromil, or theophylline.
c. **Moderate persistent asthma.** These patients have asthma symptoms daily, nocturnal awakening more than one time a week, a PEF of less than 60% to less than 80% of personal best, and an $FEV_1$ of greater than 60% to greater than 80% of predicted. The use of a **low-medium dose inhaled corticosteroid together with a long-acting bronchodilator** (salmeterol, 2 puffs bid) is the preferred therapy. Alternatives include increasing to a medium dose of inhaled cortico-

**Table 10-5.** Comparative daily dosages for inhaled corticosteroids

| Drug | Low dose | Medium dose | High dose |
|---|---|---|---|
| Triamcinolone (100 μg/puff) | 4–10 puffs | 10–20 puffs | >20 puffs |
| Beclomethasone dipropionate (42, 84 μg/puff) | 4–12 puffs: 42 μg<br>2–6 puffs: 84 μg | 12–20 puffs: 42 μg<br>6–8 puffs: 84 μg | >20 puffs: 42 μg<br>>10 puffs: 84 μg |
| Budesonide Turbuhaler (DPI: 200 μg/dose) | 1–2 inhalations | 2–3 inhalations | >3 inhalations |
| Flunisolide (250 μg/puff) | 2–4 puffs | 4–8 puffs | >8 puffs |
| Fluticasone (MDI: 44, 110, 220 μg/puff) | 2–6 puffs: 44 μg<br>2 puffs: 110 μg | 2–6 puffs: 110 μg | >6 puffs: 110 μg<br>>3 puffs: 220 μg |
| DPI: 50, 100, 250 μg/dose | 2–6 inhalations: 50 μg | 3–6 inhalations: 100 μg | >6 inhalations: 100 μg<br>>2 inhalations: 250 μg |

DPI, dry powder inhaler; MDI, metered-dose inhaler.

steroid (Table 10-5) or the addition of a leukotriene antagonist or theophylline to low-medium doses of inhaled corticosteroid.

d. **Severe persistent asthma.** These patients have asthma symptoms continuously, frequent nocturnal awakenings, PEF of less than 60% of personal best or $FEV_1$ of less than 60% predicted or are limited in their physical activity. A **high dose of inhaled corticosteroid** (Table 10-5) **and a long-acting bronchodilator** are the recommended therapies. These patients may require long-term oral corticosteroids (started at 2 mg/kg/day, not to exceed 60 mg/day), although repeated attempts should be made to reduce the dose while they are receiving high-dose inhaled corticosteroids. Patients who have severe persistent asthma in whom control is inadequate despite the use of oral or high-dose inhaled corticosteroids typically have chronic limitation of activity and require frequent bronchodilator use. These patients should be referred to an asthma specialist. The goal of therapy is to minimize symptoms and the need for oral corticosteroids.

e. **Nocturnal symptoms.** These symptoms may necessitate the addition at night of either a long-acting inhaled β-adrenergic agonist (e.g., salmeterol, 2 puffs qhs) or sustained-release theophylline. Increased circadian variability in airflow obstruction (nighttime awakening) is a sign of heightened airway hyperreactivity; thus, an increase in the dose of anti-inflammatory medication also should be considered in these patients.

## IV. Medications

A. **Inhaled corticosteroids** are safe and effective for the treatment of chronic asthma (Table 10-5). They should be administered with a spacing device, and patients should be instructed to rinse their mouth with water after each administration to reduce the possibility of oral candidiasis and hoarseness. The dose is increased as necessary according to symptoms and PEF. In patients with frequent $\beta_2$-adrenergic agonist use or other signs of poorly controlled disease, the dose should be increased by 50–100% until symptoms are controlled. If symptoms are severe, accompanied by nighttime awakening, or PEF is less than 65% of predicted values, a short course of oral corticosteroid (40–60 mg/day for 5–7 days) might be necessary to get control of the disease quickly. Attempts should be made to decrease the dose of inhaled corticosteroid by 25% every 2–3 months to the lowest possible dose to maintain control.

1. In patients who require regular use of oral corticosteroid, both **fluticasone,** 8 puffs/day (220 μg/puff), and **budesonide,** 8–16 puffs/day (200 μg/puff), are very effective in reducing symptoms and in minimizing the effects of oral corticosteroid use.
2. **Systemic corticosteroid absorption** can occur in patients who use high doses of inhaled corticosteroids. Consequently, prolonged therapy with high-dose inhaled corticosteroids should be reserved for patients with severe disease or for those who otherwise require oral corticosteroids. Repeated efforts should be made at tapering the dose.

B. **Cromolyn sodium** and **nedocromil sodium** are anti-inflammatory inhaled medications that are alternatives to inhaled corticosteroids in children with mild persistent asthma. The usual dosage is 8–12 puffs/day in three to four divided doses. Maximum improvement may be delayed for 4–6 weeks after initiation of therapy. Little additional benefit accrues from using these medications with an inhaled corticosteroid.

C. **Leukotriene antagonists.** Montelukast (10 mg PO qd) and zafirlukast (20 mg PO bid) are oral leukotriene-receptor antagonists. These agents provide effective control of mild persistent asthma in the majority of patients. However, in comparison with inhaled corticosteroids, they are not as effective in improving asthma outcomes. Leukotriene antagonists should be strongly considered for patients with aspirin-induced asthma or for individuals who cannot master the use of an inhaler.

**D. Methylxanthines.** Theophylline provides mild bronchodilation in asthmatics. Sustained-release theophylline may be useful as adjuvant therapy to an anti-inflammatory agent in persistent asthma, especially for controlling nighttime symptoms. It is essential that serum concentrations of theophylline be monitored on a regular basis, aiming for a level of 5–15 μg/ml, because theophylline has a narrow therapeutic range with significant toxicities. Theophylline has many potential drug interactions, especially with antibiotics (see Appendix C, Drug Interactions).

**E. Long-acting $\beta_2$-adrenergic agonists,** such as salmeterol (2 puffs bid), added to low- or medium-dose inhaled corticosteroids have consistently been shown to improve lung function and symptoms. Limited evidence shows that their addition can also reduce the required dose of inhaled corticosteroids in patients with moderate persistent asthma (*AHRQ*, AHRQ publication 01-E044, September 2001). The benefits of adding long-acting $\beta_2$-adrenergic agonists are more substantial than those achieved by leukotriene antagonists, theophylline, or increased doses of inhaled corticosteroid (*NHBLI*, NIH publication 02-5075, July 2002). Inhaled, short-acting, $\beta_2$-adrenergic agonists should continue to be used on an as-needed basis.

**F. Medications to reduce the need for oral corticosteroids,** such as methotrexate, cyclosporine, or troleandomycin, have been studied and may be useful in some patients. These individuals should be evaluated by an asthma specialist.

## Urticaria and Angioedema

**Urticaria** (hives) are raised, flat-topped, well-demarcated skin lesions with surrounding erythema. Central clearing can cause an annular lesion and is often seen after antihistamine use. An individual lesion usually lasts minutes to hours. **Angioedema** is a deeper lesion causing areas of skin-colored, localized swelling. It can be found anywhere on the body but most often involves the tongue, lips, or eyelids. In 50% of cases, patients have angioedema and urticaria at the same time. When angioedema occurs without urticaria, specific diagnoses must be entertained (see sec. **III**).

**I. Acute urticaria and angioedema**

**A. Acute urticaria (with or without angioedema)** is defined as an episode that lasts for less than 6 weeks. Usually, it is caused by an allergic reaction to a medication or food, but it may be related to underlying infection, recent insect sting, or exposure (contact or inhalation) to an allergen. A hypersensitivity can develop to a food, medication, or self-care product that previously had been used without difficulty.

**B. Treatment**

1. **In the presence of systemic symptoms** that suggest hypotension, laryngeal edema, or bronchospasm, the patient is experiencing anaphylaxis and the reaction should be treated as such with **epinephrine** (0.3–0.5 ml of a 1:1000 solution IM or SC). See the section on Anaphylaxis for additional treatment.
2. The ideal treatment of acute urticaria with or without angioedema is **identification and avoidance of the specific cause.** All potential causes should be eliminated. Most cases resolve within 1 week. In some instances, it is possible to reintroduce an agent cautiously if it is believed not to be the cause. This trial should be done in the presence of a physician, with epinephrine readily available.
   a. **Medications,** especially antibiotics, are common offenders and should be discontinued when possible. Agents such as aspirin, NSAIDs, opiates, and alcohol should be avoided, as they can induce nonspecific mast cell degranulation and exacerbate urticaria caused by other agents.

b. **Foods** that commonly cause a reaction include peanuts, tree nuts, shellfish and fish, milk, eggs, wheat, soy, and fruits. However, any food can cause an allergic reaction and should be avoided if suspected.
c. In hospitalized patients, medications, **IV contrast media,** and **latex** should be considered as possible causes.

3. **Second-generation oral antihistamines** (e.g., cetirizine, fexofenadine, desloratadine, or loratadine) should be administered to patients until the hives have cleared. A first-generation antihistamine such as hydroxyzine can be added as an evening dose to obtain control in refractory cases.
4. **Oral corticosteroids** should be reserved for patients with laryngeal edema or systemic symptoms of anaphylaxis, after treatment with epinephrine. Corticosteroids do not have an immediate effect but may prevent relapse. They may also be helpful for those with severe symptoms that have not responded to antihistamines.
5. If a patient has presented with systemic symptoms, **self-administered epinephrine** should be prescribed for use in the case of accidental exposure to the same trigger in the future.

**II. Chronic urticaria and angioedema**

**A. Chronic urticaria (with or without angioedema)** is defined as episodes that persist for longer than 6 weeks. There are innumerable possible causes of chronic urticaria and angioedema, including medications, autoimmune causes, self-care products, and physical triggers. However, the etiology remains unidentified in more than 80% of cases.

**B. Evaluation of chronic urticaria.** A complete history and physical examination should elicit any identifiable triggers, including physical triggers, such as pressure, cold, or heat. The examiner should check for dermographism, an immediate wheal-and-flare response on stroking the skin. The history should also aim to rule out systemic causes. This includes determining if any individual lesion lasts for greater than 24 hours, in which case the diagnosis of urticarial vasculitis must be investigated by skin biopsy. A laboratory screen for underlying disease may include a CBC, erythrocyte sedimentation rate, urinalysis, and liver function tests to evaluate for systemic etiologies of chronic urticaria: hematologic malignancies, autoimmune phenomena, and occult infections (including hepatitis). Mast cell releasability syndromes such as systemic mastocytosis and cutaneous mastocytosis, including urticaria pigmentosa, should also be considered. If no cause is identified, the patient should be referred to an allergist for evaluation of autoimmune triggers, including the presence of antithyroid antibodies or antibodies against the IgE receptor.

**C. Treatment of chronic urticaria**

1. **Resolution of the underlying disease condition** leads to abatement of the urticarial rash.
2. Careful consideration should be given to the **elimination or substitution of each prescription or over-the-counter medication** or supplement. If a patient reacts to one medication in a class, the reaction likely will be triggered by all medications in that class. Exacerbating agents (aspirin, NSAIDs, opiates, alcohol) should be avoided.
3. **Elimination of all self-care products,** with the exception of those that contain no methylparaben, fragrance, or preservative, is useful when sensitivity to these products is possible.
4. **Antihistamines** for symptom control are the mainstay of treatment. Treatment should be continued for a period of 6 months, then tapered to the amount necessary for symptom control.
   a. **Second-generation antihistamines,** such as cetirizine, fexofenadine, loratadine, and desloratadine, are well tolerated and should be used as first-line agents. Cetirizine may be minimally sedating. Loratadine is available over-the-counter.
   b. **Classic antihistamines,** such as hydroxyzine, 25 mg PO q4–6h or prn, can be added for better control of lesions or for breakthrough lesions. The dose usually is limited by sedation.

c. **Doxepin,** an antidepressant with $H_1$- and $H_2$-blocking effects, is a useful addition and often is less sedating than hydroxyzine.
d. **$H_2$-blocking agents** may be helpful in addition to $H_1$ antihistamines to control breakthrough hives.
e. **Oral corticosteroids** should be reserved for patients in whom adequate control cannot be achieved with a combination of the aforementioned agents. Steroids should be used only for short periods.

III. **Angioedema without urticaria** should lead to consideration of specific entities.

A. Use of **angiotensin-converting enzyme inhibitors** or angiotensin II–receptor blockers can be associated with angioedema at any point in the course of therapy. Substitution with a different class of drug should be made, as both angiotensin-converting enzyme inhibitors and angiotensin II–receptor blockers should be avoided.

B. **Hereditary angioedema (HAE), or C1 esterase inhibitor (C1 INH) deficiency** is inherited in an autosomal-dominant pattern. Patients present with angioedema of any part of the body, but never with urticaria. Angioedema of the intestinal tract may cause episodic abdominal pain. All patients with angioedema without urticaria should be screened with a C4 level, which is reduced during and between attacks of HAE. If the C4 level is reduced, a quantitative and functional C1 INH assay should be performed. A quantitative level is not sufficient, as 15% of patients have normal levels of a dysfunctional C1 INH protein. Treatment of attacks is supportive but may be difficult given the involvement of mediators other than histamine. Prophylactic treatment with anabolic steroids should be directed by an allergist.

C. **Acquired C1 INH deficiency** presents similarly to HAE but is typically associated with an underlying lymphoproliferative disorder or connective tissue disease. These patients have reduced C1q, C1 INH, and C4 levels. Other patients with the acquired form have an autoantibody to C1 INH, with low C4 and C1 INH levels but a normal C1 level.

## Immunodeficiency

Immunodeficiency diseases are characterized by an increased susceptibility to infection. The type of infection and age of onset provide the first clues as to the type of immune defect. The most common disease of immune deficiency is AIDS (see Chap. 14, Human Immunodeficiency Virus Infection and Acquired Immunodeficiency Syndrome). Children and young adults present with abnormalities in T and B cells and are at risk for severe viral and bacterial infections. Adults usually present with defects in humoral immunity and are at increased risk of sinus or pulmonary infection from encapsulated bacteria.

I. **Humoral immunodeficiency**

A. **IgA deficiency** is the most common immune deficiency, with a prevalence of 1 in 500 people. Patients may be asymptomatic or present with recurrent sinus and pulmonary infections. Therapy is directed at early treatment with antibiotics because IgA replacement is not available. In 15% of cases an associated IgG subclass deficiency is present. Absolute IgA-deficient patients are at risk for development of a severe transfusion reaction because of the presence in some individuals of anti-IgA IgE antibodies; therefore, these patients should be transfused with washed RBCs or receive blood products only from IgA-deficient donors.

B. **Common variable immunodeficiency (CVID).** This diagnosis includes a heterogeneous group of disorders in which patients present in the second to fourth decade of life with recurrent sinus and pulmonary infections and are discovered to have low or dysfunctional IgG, IgA, and IgM antibodies. B-cell numbers are usually normal, but there is a decreased ability to produce immunoglobulin after immunization. Some patients may also exhibit T-cell dysfunction and be anergic. Patients may have associated GI disease or autoimmune abnormalities, most commonly autoimmune hemolytic anemia, idiopathic thrombocytopenic purpura, pernicious anemia, and rheumatoid arthritis. The incidence of malignancy, especially lymphoid and GI, is increased. Therapy consists of IV immunoglobulin (IVIG) replacement therapy (see sec. **III**) as well as prompt treatment of infections with antibiotics.

**C. Subclass deficiency.** Deficiencies of each of the IgG subclasses ($IgG_1$, $IgG_2$, $IgG_3$, and $IgG_4$) have been described. These patients present with complaints similar to those of CVID patients. Total IgG levels may be normal. A strong association with IgA deficiency exists (see sec. **I.A**).

**D. Hyper-IgE syndrome** (Job's syndrome) is characterized by recurrent pyogenic infections of the skin and lower respiratory tract. This infection can result in severe abscess and empyema formation. The most common organism is *Staphylococcus aureus*, but other bacteria and fungi have been reported. Patients present with recurrent infections and have an associated pruritic dermatitis, coarse facies, growth retardation, and hyperkeratotic nails. Laboratory data reveal the presence of normal levels of IgG, IgA, and IgM but markedly elevated levels of IgE. A marked increase in tissue and blood eosinophils also may be observed. The pathogenesis of the disorder is unknown, but it appears to be transmitted in an autosomal mode of inheritance with variable penetrance. No specific therapy exists except for early treatment of infection with antibiotics.

**E.** Immunodeficiency may be caused by **hypercatabolism of immunoglobulin proteins.** The majority of immune defects of humoral immunity represent disorders in synthesis. However, there are states associated with infection that represent increased degradation or catabolism of immunoglobulin. Increased utilization of immunoglobulin may be seen in patients with severe underlying infection. Therefore, any formal diagnosis and evaluation of humoral immunodeficiency should be postponed until infections are adequately treated. Protein-losing gastroenteropathy and renal glomerular defects, such as nephrotic syndrome, can result in the loss of large amounts of serum proteins, giving rise to hypogammaglobulinemia in addition to hypoalbuminemia.

**II. Evaluation of suspected immunodeficiency.** Increased frequency of sinopulmonary infections is the most common problem confronted in clinical practice that requires an evaluation for possible humoral immunodeficiency. Workup begins with a CBC with differential, quantitative immunoglobulin levels, complement levels, and an HIV test. If levels of immunoglobulin are normal and other possible precipitating factors such as allergy and anatomic abnormalities are ruled out, further evaluation should be pursued, including an evaluation of B-cell function. B-cell response to immunization with a protein antigen, such as tetanus, and a polysaccharide antigen, such as pneumococcus (using the unconjugated 23-valent vaccine), is tested because of the differences in the way in which proteins and polysaccharides are handled by the immune system. Titers of specific antibody are measured before and 4 weeks after immunization, with a good response being a fourfold increase in antibody titer. Multiple serotypes of pneumococcus should be evaluated. A good response would be expected in greater than three of the serotypes. A patient with normal or low immunoglobulin and a poor response to immunization is classified as having CVID.

**III. Treatment of humoral immunodeficiency.** Specific replacement therapy does not exist for the treatment of IgA deficiency. These patients should be treated promptly at the first sign of infection with an antibiotic that covers *Streptococcus pneumoniae* or *Haemophilus influenzae*. Patients with subclass deficiency or CVID can be treated with IVIG. Numerous preparations of IVIG are available, all of which are treated with viral inactivation steps. Replacement should be initiated with 400 mg/kg and infused slowly according to the manufacturer's suggestions (for most preparations, begin at 30 ml/hour and increase by 30 ml/hour every 15 minutes as tolerated to a maximum rate of 210 ml/hour). Possible side effects include myalgias, vomiting, chills, or lingering headache (due to immune complex–mediated aseptic meningitis). Patients, especially those with no detectable IgA, need to have vital signs monitored q15min initially, as **anaphylaxis from anti-IgA IgE antibodies** can develop in these individuals. In patients with low or absent IgA, it is best to use an IVIG preparation that is documented to contain very little IgA, such as Gammagard. Infusions generally are done at monthly intervals, but it is best to document that adequate IgG levels are maintained between infusions. This is achieved by obtaining a quantitative IgG level just before the next infusion. The dose or the frequency of the IVIG is then altered to reach low normal levels of IgG at the nadir before the next dose.

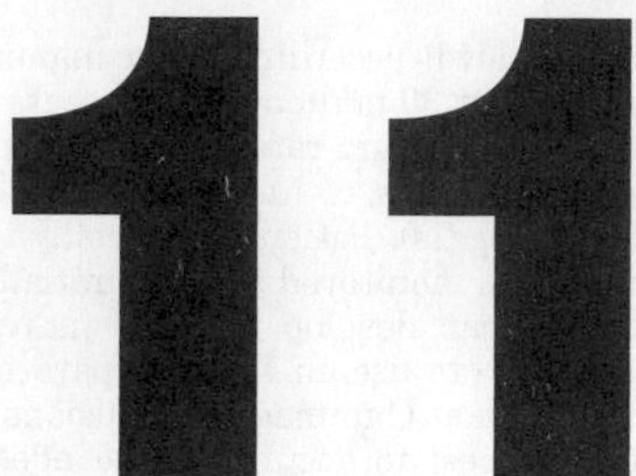

# Renal Diseases

Gopa B. Green and
Daniel W. Coyne

## Evaluation of the Patient with Renal Disease

Chronic kidney disease (CKD) frequently presents as abnormal routine laboratory data, such as an elevated serum creatinine (Cr) level (>1.0 mg/dl in women, or >1.5 mg/dl in men) or an abnormal urinalysis with proteinuria, hematuria, or pyuria. Acute renal failure (ARF) may manifest as abrupt onset of edema, malaise, oliguria, or hematuria, or may be detected as an asymptomatic laboratory finding. Initial evaluation should determine the need for emergent dialysis and then be directed at identifying reversible causes of renal dysfunction.

I. **Initial studies** in the evaluation of patients with suspected renal disease should include the following:

A. **Serum chemistries,** including electrolytes, Cr, BUN, calcium, magnesium, phosphate, uric acid, and albumin. If the serum Cr is stable, the glomerular filtration rate (GFR) can be estimated by using the **Cockcroft-Gault formula for Cr clearance ($Cl_{Cr}$):**

$$Cl_{Cr}(\text{ml/min}) = \frac{[(140 - \text{age}) \times \text{weight (kg)}]}{[72 \times \text{serum Cr (mg/dl)}]} \times 0.85 \text{ (for women)}$$

Weight should reflect ideal body weight.

B. **Urine dipstick** for protein, occult blood, leukocytes, and pH, and microscopic examination of a freshly voided specimen for formed elements, such as crystals, RBCs, WBCs, and casts. Proteinuria (g/1.73 $m^2$ body surface area/day) can be roughly quantitated by a **spot urine protein (mg/dl)-to-Cr (mg/dl) ratio** in a random urine specimen; a ratio of greater than 3:1 suggests nephrotic-range proteinuria. Hematuria may reflect a variety of conditions, including infection or inflammation of the prostate or bladder, malignancy (e.g., bladder or renal cell carcinoma), renal stones (see the section Nephrolithiasis), polycystic kidney disease, trauma with or without the presence of a bleeding diathesis, papillary necrosis, or glomerular disease (see the section Glomerulopathies). Urine sediment with epithelial cells and "muddy brown" granular casts is seen with ischemic damage of the tubules. Pyuria is seen with urinary tract infection or interstitial nephritis. WBC casts may be seen in pyelonephritis and interstitial nephritis, and RBC casts are indicative of glomerulonephritis (GN). The presence of crystals may indicate stone disease or certain alcohol poisonings (see Chap. 25, Medical Emergencies).

II. **Supplementary studies** can be useful to assess renal function further and may aid in identifying specific disorders.

A. **Twenty-four–hour urine studies** include measurement of urine volume, Cr, and protein. The GFR can be estimated by calculation of the $Cl_{Cr}$:

$$Cl_{Cr}(\text{ml/min}) = \frac{[\text{urine Cr (mg/dl)} \times \text{volume (ml)}]}{[\text{serum Cr (mg/dl)} \times \text{time (minutes)}]}$$

This value is useful in adjusting drug dosage in renal insufficiency, in predicting remaining renal function, and in timing the placement of dialysis access. In adults under the age of 50 years, if the 24-hour Cr for women is less than 15–20 mg/kg lean body weight and for men is less than 20–25 mg/kg lean body weight, the collection may be incomplete, leading to an underestimation of the GFR. In severe renal failure, the measured $Cl_{Cr}$ may overestimate the true GFR. In this setting, the mean of the $Cl_{Cr}$ and urea clearance is a more accurate reflection of GFR. Twenty-four–hour protein quantitation is necessary for confirmation of the nephrotic syndrome and is useful for following the response to treatment of certain glomerular diseases. Measurements of 24-hour urinary volume, Cr, sodium, citrate, calcium, phosphate, oxalate, and uric acid are indicated in the evaluation of some patients with nephrolithiasis; this evaluation is best performed in the outpatient setting when the patient is on his or her usual diet.

**B. Other laboratory evaluations.** Blood tests—including the erythrocyte sedimentation rate; antinuclear, anti–glomerular basement membrane (anti-GBM), and antineutrophil cytoplasmic antibodies; complement levels; cryoglobulin studies; hepatitis B and C serologies; and antistreptococcal antibody titers—may be useful in evaluating glomerular disease. Serum and urine protein electrophoresis should be performed in selected patients with proteinuria to exclude multiple myeloma and amyloid disease. Of note, a routine dipstick urinalysis is less sensitive to proteins other than albumin. Urine eosinophils are seen in allergic interstitial nephritis, rapidly progressive glomerulonephritis (RPGN), acute prostatitis, and renal atheroemboli. Urine osmolality may be useful in the evaluation of hyponatremia.

**C. Renal ultrasonography** can assess kidney size, determine the presence of hydronephrosis, and identify renal cysts. Small kidneys (<9 cm) generally reflect chronic renal disease, although kidney size may not be diminished in some common chronic processes, such as diabetes, HIV, amyloidosis, and multiple myeloma. A discrepancy in kidney size of greater than 2 cm may suggest unilateral renal artery stenosis, with atrophy of the kidney on the stenotic side. The presence of hydronephrosis suggests obstructive nephropathy that may be chronic or acute in nature. Multiple bilateral cortical cysts are suggestive of autosomal-dominant polycystic kidney disease.

**D. IV urography** is useful in the evaluation of nonglomerular hematuria, stone disease, and voiding disorders.

**E. Radionuclide scanning** uses technetium isotopes to assess the relative contribution of each kidney to overall renal function and provides important information if unilateral nephrectomy is being considered. Renal scanning is useful when disruption of renal blood flow is suspected; the absence of perfusion to either kidney should prompt further investigation of the renal vasculature. In addition, radionuclide studies can be used to follow renal function, leaks, and rejection in transplanted kidneys.

**F. MRI and magnetic resonance angiography** can be helpful in evaluating renal masses, detecting main renal artery stenosis, and diagnosing renal vein thrombosis. Unlike **standard arteriography,** magnetic resonance angiography does not require the administration of nephrotoxic contrast agents and possesses high sensitivity and specificity for atherosclerotic disease involving the proximal renal arteries.

**G. Renal biopsy** can determine diagnosis, guide therapy, and provide prognostic information in many settings, particularly in the evaluation of the nephrotic syndrome or glomerular hematuria.

1. **Biopsy may be indicated** in adults with glomerular diseases that present with proteinuria greater than 2 g/day, hematuria, or RBC casts. It can be helpful in diseases such as systemic lupus erythematosus (SLE), pulmonary-renal syndromes, and paraproteinemias with renal involvement. Biopsy should also be considered in patients with renal failure and kidneys of normal size when other studies are nondiagnostic.

2. **Preparative measures for biopsy** include ultrasound imaging to establish the presence of two kidneys, urinalysis and culture to exclude urinary tract infection before biopsy, adequate BP control, and correction of coagulation parameters. If renal function is significantly impaired, uremic platelet dysfunction may result in abnormal bleeding time (>10 minutes), which may increase the risk of significant postprocedure hemorrhage. IV desmopressin acetate (ddAVP; 0.3 µg/kg) can be infused over 30 minutes before biopsy to correct an abnormal bleeding time. Packed RBCs should be available for transfusion. The patient should not take medications that interfere with platelet function (e.g., aspirin) before or immediately after the biopsy. Patients on dialysis who require a biopsy should have their dialysis sessions scheduled so as to avoid heparin anticoagulation immediately after the biopsy.

## Acute Renal Failure

ARF presents clinically as a rapidly rising Cr level or a decline in urine output over several hours to days. It is incited by many causes (Table 11-1), but all result in a sudden decline in the ability of the kidney to maintain fluid and electrolyte homeostasis. Renal failure may be oliguric (urine output <500 ml/day) or nonoliguric. **ARF may be classified as prerenal, intrinsic, or postrenal (obstructive).** Table 11-2 includes laboratory tests that are helpful in differentiating oliguric prerenal azotemia from oliguric, intrinsic acute tubular necrosis (ATN). Serum and urine samples should be obtained simultaneously before a fluid challenge or diuretic use is initiated. **Microscopic examination of a fresh urine sample is essential.**

I. **Prerenal azotemia** is the clinical result of renal hypoperfusion due to a decrease in effective arterial blood volume. Decreased effective circulating volume may result from volume depletion, peripheral vasodilation, or low cardiac output.
   A. The prerenal state can be suggested by the presence of orthostasis or other signs of volume depletion on examination, by careful review of the patient's intake and urine output history, or by the presence of heart failure or liver failure, which may compromise effective circulating volume. Volume expansion, BP support, or treatment of heart failure may result in reversal of renal insufficiency.
   B. In prerenal states, the kidney avidly retains sodium, usually resulting in low urine sodium and a **fractional excretion of sodium ($FE_{Na}$)** of less than 1%. Other conditions in which an $FE_{Na}$ of less than 1% may be observed are radiocontrast-induced renal failure, acute GN, liver failure (see Chap. 17, Liver Diseases), pigment-induced nephrotoxicity, early obstructive nephropathy, vasculitis, and normal renal function. $FE_{Na}$ is particularly helpful in oliguric ARF. $FE_{Na}$ is calculated as follows:

$$FE_{Na} = [(U_{Na} \times P_{Cr})/(P_{Na} \times U_{Cr})] \times 100$$

   where U = urine and P = plasma. Because loop diuretics force natriuresis, calculation of the $FE_{Na}$ is misleading in patients who are taking these agents. The fractional excretion of urea ($FE_{urea}$) can be used to confirm the prerenal state in the presence of recent diuretic use, with an $FE_{urea}$ of less than 30% suggestive of prerenal azotemia. $FE_{urea}$ can be calculated as follows:

$$FE_{urea} = \frac{(U_{urea} \times P_{Cr})}{(BUN \times U_{Cr})} \times 100$$

   where $U_{urea}$ = urine urea concentration (mg/dl) and BUN = blood urea nitrogen concentration (mg/dl).

**Table 11-1.** Causes of acute renal failure

**Prerenal failure**

Volume contraction

Hypotension

Heart failure (severe)

Liver failure (see Chap. 17, Liver Diseases)

**Intrinsic renal failure**

Acute tubular necrosis (prolonged ischemia; nephrotoxic agents, such as heavy metals, aminoglycosides, radiographic contrast media)

Arteriolar injury

Accelerated hypertension

Vasculitis

Microangiopathic disorder (thrombotic thrombocytopenic purpura, hemolytic-uremic syndrome)

Glomerulonephritis

Acute interstitial nephritis (drug induced)

Intrarenal deposition or sludging (uric acid, myeloma)

Cholesterol embolization (especially after an arterial procedure)

**Postobstructive failure**

Ureteral obstruction (clot, calculus, tumor, sloughed papillae, external compression)

Bladder outlet obstruction (neurogenic bladder, prostatic hypertrophy, carcinoma, calculus, clot, urethral stricture)

C. **Hemodynamic monitoring** may be of value to assure adequate volume expansion while avoiding overexpansion and to assess and manage poor cardiac function. Invasive monitoring with a central venous pressure or pulmonary artery catheter is indicated if an accurate assessment of intravascular volume cannot be determined by physical examination or an initial volume challenge.

II. **Obstruction** of the upper or lower urinary tract may incite ARF. **Early diagnosis and relief of obstruction** are essential to prevent permanent renal damage.

A. **Lower urinary tract obstruction** is common in older men with enlarged prostates that cause bladder outlet obstruction. It can be assessed (and relieved) by temporary bladder catheterization and measurement of postvoid residual (>300 ml urine remaining in the bladder postvoid is highly suggestive of bladder outlet obstruction).

B. Renal ultrasonography usually identifies hydronephrosis in lower and **upper tract obstruction,** which may result from nephrolithiasis, tumor mass, retroperitoneal fibrosis, or other etiologies. Urine flow often increases

**Table 11-2.** Laboratory examination in oliguric acute renal failure

| Diagnosis | $U/P_{Cr}$ | $U_{Na}$ | $FE_{Na}$ (%) | U osmolality |
|---|---|---|---|---|
| Prerenal azotemia | >40 | <20 | <1 | >500 |
| Oliguric ATN | <20 | >40 | >1 | <350 |

ATN, acute tubular necrosis; $FE_{Na}$, fractional excretion of sodium; P, plasma; U, urine.

dramatically after relief of bilateral obstruction. This postobstructive diuresis frequently is physiologic and reflects excretion of fluid, urea, and sodium accumulated during the period of obstruction. If the postobstructive diuresis appears excessive, fluid and electrolytes can be replaced with 0.45% saline.

C. **Micro-obstructive uropathy** with associated pyuria and eosinophiluria may be caused by **indinavir,** a protease inhibitor used in the treatment of HIV disease. Discontinuation of the drug can restore renal function.

III. **Intrinsic renal failure** results from a variety of injuries to the renal blood vessels, glomeruli, tubules, or interstitium (Table 11-1). These insults may be toxic, immunologic, or idiopathic. They may be iatrogenic or develop as part of a systemic disorder or as a primary renal disease.

A. **Ischemic ATN** may occur with decreased renal perfusion from any cause that results in ischemic damage and sloughing of the renal tubular epithelium. ATN is the most common cause of ARF in hospitalized patients and may frequently present postoperatively, after a hypotensive episode from sepsis or profound volume depletion, or may be induced by medications that cause renal arterial vasoconstriction or direct tubular toxicity.

1. The classic findings in ATN may include evidence of a hypotensive episode, oliguria, rising serum Cr, "muddy brown" coarse granular casts on examination of the urine sediment, and $FE_{Na}$ of greater than 1%, reflecting tubular damage and inability to conserve sodium.
2. **Management of ATN** is supportive, with volume repletion only until the patient is euvolemic, restriction of potassium-containing fluids, and close observation for the need to initiate dialytic support for electrolyte abnormalities, volume overload, acidosis, or uremia.
3. If volume overload becomes evident, a **diuretic challenge** is reasonable, with a combination of loop and thiazide diuretics. Because diuretics must be filtered and secreted to achieve efficacy, a high dose must be administered in the setting of decreased GFR (for furosemide, a rule of thumb is to administer 20 times the serum Cr as an initial dose challenge). If urine output improves after administration of a bolus dose of loop diuretics, fluid management may be easier to achieve with a continuous infusion of loop diuretics (i.e., furosemide at 10–20 mg/hour) or with repeated bolus doses every 6–8 hours to convert the oliguric state to nonoliguric. However, it should be emphasized that this approach likely does not change outcome and may not always be successful in preventing the other complications of ARF, such as hyperkalemia and uremia.
4. In all cases of ATN, **supportive care** should focus on minimizing additional renal insults (avoidance of volume depletion, further hypotension, nonsteroidal anti-inflammatory drugs, radiocontrast, aminoglycosides, and other nephrotoxins) and carefully assessing the need for dialytic intervention if volume overload, acidosis, uremia, or hyperkalemia cannot be managed otherwise.
5. The natural history of most cases of ischemic ATN is eventual recovery of renal function over 1–6 weeks, although the patient may be left with some degree of CKD. However, if a patient has become dialysis dependent for longer than 6 weeks, prognosis for renal recovery is usually poor.

B. **Radiocontrast nephropathy** occurs with increased frequency in patients with preexisting renal insufficiency (Cr >2.5 mg/dl), particularly in the setting of diabetes mellitus. Volume depletion, multiple myeloma, heart failure, and age greater than 65 years may also be risk factors. The ARF of contrast nephropathy tends to be oliguric, and the serum Cr peaks in the first 72 hours after contrast exposure. Patients often recover renal function over 7–14 days. To reduce the incidence of ARF, patients at risk should be hydrated with 75–150 ml/hour of 0.45% saline beginning 12–24 hours before the contrast study and ending 12 hours after the study. Furosemide should be reserved for patients in whom volume overload develops during hydration.

Acetylcysteine (600 mg PO bid; 4 doses total, starting 1 day before the procedure) may reduce the incidence and severity of contrast nephropathy (*N Engl J Med* 343:180, 2000).

C. **Aminoglycoside nephrotoxicity** may cause ARF that is often nonoliguric and results from direct toxicity to the proximal tubules. Predisposing factors include prolonged exposure (usually >5 days) to these drugs, advanced age, volume depletion, liver disease, and preexisting renal disease. The risk of aminoglycoside nephrotoxicity appears to be lower when the extended-interval dosing method is used (see Chap. 12, Antimicrobials), although this method should be avoided in patients with preexisting renal insufficiency.

D. **Pigment-induced renal injury** occurs during hemolysis or rhabdomyolysis. In **rhabdomyolysis,** aggressive IV fluid administration should be initiated to replace the fluid that is lost into necrotic muscle and to establish high urine flow. If sufficient urine flow can be established, alkalinization of the urine (urine pH >6.5) by IV infusion of 2–3 ampules of $NaHCO_3$ in 1 L 5% dextrose in water increases the solubility of heme pigments and may hasten recovery.

E. **Acute uric acid nephropathy (tumor lysis syndrome)** may occur from cell lysis, with consequent hyperuricemia during cytotoxic therapy for hematologic malignancies. Uric acid production can be decreased by administration of allopurinol, 600 mg PO, before cytotoxic therapy, followed by 100–300 mg/day. The dosage should be adjusted for renal function (see Appendix E, Dosage Adjustment of Drugs in Renal Failure). Forced alkaline diuresis to maintain a urine pH of 6.5–7.0 also helps to prevent uric acid precipitation; this can be accomplished with acetazolamide, 250 mg PO qid, or with IV infusion of 2–3 ampules of $NaHCO_3$ in 1 L 5% dextrose in water. If tumor lysis results in hyperphosphatemia, urine alkalinization greater than pH 7.0 increases the risk of calcium phosphate precipitation and thus should be avoided.

F. **Acute interstitial nephritis** secondary to drugs may present with the classic signs of fever, rash, and renal dysfunction. When present, eosinophilia and eosinophiluria suggest the diagnosis. A high index of suspicion for interstitial nephritis must be maintained in patients who are taking drugs such as penicillins, sulfonamides, quinolones, and nonsteroidal anti-inflammatory drugs. In most cases, renal insufficiency resolves with discontinuation of the offending agent. A 1-week course of prednisone, 60 mg PO qd, may hasten recovery. Streptococcal infections, leptospirosis, viral infections, and sarcoidosis have also been implicated as causes of interstitial nephritis.

G. **Hemolytic-uremic syndrome/thrombotic thrombocytopenic purpura** may be induced by bacterial toxins, medications such as mitomycin-C, cyclosporine, tacrolimus (see Chap. 15, Solid Organ Transplant Medicine), OKT3, or radiation therapy, or may be associated with pregnancy or certain malignancies of the GI tract. Diagnosis and therapy are discussed in Chap. 18, Disorders of Hemostasis.

H. **Bone marrow transplant (BMT)–associated nephropathy** refers to renal failure that develops at least 3 months after autologous or allogeneic BMT. **Acute BMT nephropathy** presents with marked hypertension, peripheral edema, microangiopathic hemolytic anemia, thrombocytopenia, and elevated lactic acid dehydrogenase. Renal function typically declines rapidly and is often associated with severe proteinuria. **Chronic BMT nephropathy** is characterized by less severe manifestations of the acute form, with initial steady reduction in renal function within the first 12–24 months followed by stabilization. Radiation is frequently implicated in the pathogenesis of the disease. Treatment is generally supportive and includes good BP control.

I. **Cholesterol emboli** are seen in patients with diffuse atherosclerotic disease who undergo aortic or other large arterial manipulation or who are receiving warfarin or thrombolytic therapy. Physical findings may include retinal arteriolar plaques, lower extremity livedo reticularis, or necrotic areas of the distal digits. Laboratory findings that may aid in the diagnosis include eosinophilia, eosinophiluria, and hypocomplementemia. Renal cholesterol embolization frequently progresses to CKD and possible end-stage renal disease (ESRD). No specific therapy is available; anticoagulation can worsen embolic disease.

**J. Acute GN** can result in ARF. **RPGN** presents with an acute deterioration in renal function, nephrotic or non-nephrotic proteinuria, and an active urinary sediment with hematuria and RBC casts (nephritic syndrome). Oliguria may be present. Many patients with idiopathic RPGN note a preceding viral-like illness. RPGN can be further characterized by the presence of immune complex deposition [e.g., SLE, poststreptococcal GN, IgA nephropathy, endocarditis], the paucity of immune complex deposition (e.g., Wegener's granulomatosis, microscopic polyangiitis, Churg-Strauss syndrome, idiopathic), or the presence of anti-GBM disease (see the section Glomerulopathies). Pathology is notable for crescent formation in more than 50% of glomeruli on renal biopsy. As many as 75% of patients with idiopathic RPGN may respond to high-dose, pulse glucocorticoid therapy—methylprednisolone, 7–15 mg/kg/day in divided doses for 3 days, followed by prednisone, 1 mg/kg/day for 1 month, gradually tapered over the next 6–12 months. In patients with extrarenal disease that is suggestive of vasculitis or a renal biopsy that demonstrates necrotizing GN, the addition of cyclophosphamide, 2 mg/kg/day PO, may be beneficial.

**IV. Management of ARF** requires repeated assessment of clinical and laboratory data and appropriate interventions to maintain fluid and electrolyte homeostasis.

**A. Conservative medical management** of ARF requires complete fluid intake and output records, daily weights, and frequent (at least 3 times/week) measurements of serum electrolytes, BUN, Cr, calcium, and phosphate. Intravascular volume should be clinically assessed at least daily.

**B. Fluid management** is essential to avoid volume depletion, which may contribute to ARF by decreasing renal perfusion. When clinical assessment is unclear, invasive hemodynamic monitoring may be required. Once any volume deficit has been corrected, fluid and sodium balance must be carefully regulated to avoid volume overload. Fluid replacement (usually 0.45% saline if IV) should be equal to insensible losses (approximately 500 ml/day in afebrile patients) plus urinary and other drainage losses. Increased urine output and diuretic responsiveness in nonoliguric ARF allow more liberal administration of fluids (and nutrients). Because patients with nonoliguric ARF may lose significant amounts of fluid and electrolytes in the urine, careful attention to volume status and serum electrolyte levels is necessary to avoid electrolyte and water depletion. Hyponatremia in patients with ARF usually is secondary to volume expansion with hypotonic fluid, whereas hypernatremia is caused most often by overly aggressive diuresis in combination with inadequate intake of free water. **Fluid challenge** may be appropriate in oliguric patients who are not volume overloaded. The quantity of fluid to be given must be determined on an individual basis, but typically 500–1000 ml normal saline is infused over 30–60 minutes. Frequent cardiopulmonary examination is necessary. Diuretic challenge may be appropriate if volume overload occurs in the setting of intrinsic renal failure (see sec. **III.A.3**). **Dopamine** (<3 μg/kg/minute, a dosage that preferentially dilates the renal vasculature) occasionally initiates natriuresis and diuresis. However, clear evidence for a renal protective effect of dopamine is lacking and hence it is not routinely recommended in ARF (*Kidney Int* 50:4, 1996).

**C. Dietary modification. Total enteral caloric intake** should be 35–50 kcal/kg/day to avoid catabolism. Patients who are highly catabolic (e.g., postsurgical and burn patients) or malnourished require higher protein intake and should be considered for early institution of dialysis (see sec. **IV.K**). **Salt intake** should be restricted to 2–4 g/day to facilitate volume management. **Potassium intake** should be restricted to 40 mEq/day, and **phosphorus intake** should be restricted to 800 mg/day. Ingestion of magnesium-containing compounds should be avoided.

D. **Hyperkalemia** is common and, if mild (<6 mEq/L), can be treated with dietary restriction (see sec. **IV.C**) and potassium-binding resins (e.g., sodium polystyrene sulfonate). Marked hyperkalemia or hyperkalemia accompanied by ECG abnormalities requires immediate medical therapy (e.g., calcium gluconate, insulin, glucose, and bicarbonate; see Chap. 3, Fluid and Electrolyte Management). **Hyperkalemia that is refractory to medical therapy is an indication for urgent dialysis.**

E. **Phosphorus and calcium levels** are frequently abnormal in renal failure due to reduced renal excretion and excess release of cellular phosphate, despite dietary restriction. Serum calcium often is low but rarely requires specific treatment. The calcium-phosphate product should be kept at less than 60 to avoid metastatic calcification (see the section Chronic Kidney Disease for therapy).

F. **Metabolic acidosis** that is mild (serum bicarbonate level ≥ 16 mEq/L) does not require therapy. More marked acidosis should be corrected with sodium bicarbonate, 650–1300 mg PO tid. Severe uncompensated acidosis (serum pH <7.2) requires prompt medical therapy with parenteral sodium bicarbonate (see Chap. 3, Fluid and Electrolyte Management) and a search for the underlying etiology. Sodium bicarbonate therapy should be used with care, as it may exacerbate volume overload and cause tetany by decreasing the ionized calcium concentration. **Acidosis that is unresponsive to medical therapy is an indication for dialysis** (see sec. **IV.K**).

G. **Hypotension** should be promptly evaluated and corrected with volume expansion or vasopressors, depending on the patient's intravascular volume status. **Hypertension** should be managed aggressively. Volume overload frequently contributes to hypertension. Antihypertensive medications that do not decrease renal blood flow (e.g., clonidine, prazosin, or calcium channel antagonists) are preferred. Hypertensive crisis can be managed with IV labetalol or IV sodium nitroprusside, with monitoring of thiocyanate levels in patients with renal insufficiency (see Chap. 4, Hypertension). **Fenoldopam** (starting dose of 0.1 μg/kg/minute with dose titration at 15-minute intervals), a peripheral dopamine-1–receptor agonist, maintains or increases renal perfusion while it lowers BP and may be particularly beneficial in patients with renal insufficiency who present in hypertensive crisis.

H. **Drug dosages** of agents excreted by the kidney must be adjusted for the level of renal function (see Appendix E, Dosage Adjustments of Drugs in Renal Failure).

I. **Anemia** is common in ARF and usually is caused by decreased RBC production and increased blood loss. GI bleeding is common in ARF, probably due to uremic platelet dysfunction and GI mucosal changes. Major bleeding sources should be excluded. ddAVP, 0.3 μg/kg IV over 30 minutes may correct abnormal bleeding times. Transfusion is appropriate for patients with active bleeding or symptoms referable to anemia (see Chap. 19, Anemia and Transfusion Therapy). Erythropoietin is expensive and not effective as short-term therapy for anemia; data are lacking to support its use in ARF.

J. **Infection** is the most common cause of death in patients with ARF. Antimicrobial therapy is dictated by the infectious process, and potentially nephrotoxic agents should not be withheld if their use is otherwise indicated. Most antimicrobial dosages need to be adjusted for the degree of renal failure (see Appendix E, Dosage Adjustments of Drugs in Renal Failure).

K. **Indications for dialysis.** All patients with ARF should be evaluated daily to assess the need for dialysis. Technical aspects of dialysis are considered under the section Renal Replacement Therapies.

   1. **Severe hyperkalemia, acidosis, or volume overload refractory to conservative therapy** mandates the initiation of dialysis.
   2. **Additional indications** for initiation of dialysis include uremic pericarditis, encephalopathy, neuropathy, and nutritional requirements (e.g., hyper-

alimentation) that may precipitate volume overload or uremia, and certain alcohol and drug intoxications (see Chap. 25, Medical Emergencies).

3. **Uremic signs and symptoms** become prominent as BUN rises. Neurologic manifestations, such as lethargy, seizures, myoclonus, asterixis, and peripheral polyneuropathies, may develop with uremia and are an indication for dialysis. **Uremic pericarditis** often manifests only as a pericardial friction rub and should be treated with intensive dialysis; heparin use during dialysis should be minimized in these patients. If pericarditis fails to resolve with dialysis, or if signs of pericardial tamponade develop, pericardial drainage is indicated.

**V. Management of the recovery phase of ARF** usually requires careful monitoring of serum electrolytes, volume status, and urinary fluid and electrolyte losses. As with obstructive nephropathy, a diuretic phase may occur during recovery. Management is similar to that for postobstructive diuresis (see sec. **II**). Renal function may continue to improve over weeks to months.

## Glomerulopathies

### I. General considerations

**A. Glomerular disease** may be primary or secondary to a systemic process and may present with isolated hematuria or proteinuria, nephritic syndrome, or nephrotic syndrome. The **nephritic syndrome** is characterized by hematuria, RBC casts, proteinuria, hypertension, edema, and deteriorating renal function. The **nephrotic syndrome** is characterized by proteinuria (>3.5 g/day), hypoalbuminemia, hyperlipidemia, and edema. These syndromes may appear as a manifestation of primary glomerular disease or may be associated with systemic diseases, such as diabetes mellitus, amyloidosis, multiple myeloma, SLE, or other disorders. Renal biopsy often provides useful diagnostic, therapeutic, and prognostic information.

**B. General principles in the treatment of glomerular disease**

1. **Edema and volume overload** can usually be managed with diuretics, as appropriate, and dietary sodium restriction.
2. **Aggressive treatment of hypertension** with a goal BP of less than 125/75 in most cases has been associated with decreased proteinuria and slower progression of disease.
3. **Management of proteinuria** with angiotensin-converting enzyme (ACE) inhibitors or angiotensin-receptor blockers (ARBs) to reduce intraglomerular pressure is beneficial in proteinuric renal diseases. Use caution with these agents in patients with accelerating renal failure or a tendency toward hyperkalemia. Serum chemistries, including potassium and Cr, should be monitored within 1–2 weeks of initiation of therapy.
4. **Treatment of hyperlipidemia,** usually with HMG-CoA (hydroxymethylglutaryl–coenzyme A) reductase inhibitors (statins) to normalize serum cholesterol, may reduce cardiovascular risk.
5. **Dietary modifications** include modest dietary protein restriction (controversial) and dietary salt restriction.

**C. Disease-specific therapy** is most often guided by results of renal biopsy and supplemental laboratory evaluation but frequently involves corticosteroid-based therapy for primarily nephrotic disorders and cytotoxic agents plus corticosteroids for primarily proliferative or nephritic disorders. The use of such agents should be considered only in consultation with a nephrologist or other experienced physician. Initial dosages of cytotoxic drugs are suggested but may require adjustment to keep the WBC count above 3000–3500 cells/μl. WBC counts should initially be checked at least weekly during the administration of cytotoxic agents.

## II. Primary glomerulopathies

**A. Minimal-change disease (MCD)** presents with nephrotic syndrome. Certain neoplastic disorders, such as Hodgkin's disease and non-Hodgkin's lymphoma, have been associated with the development of MCD and should be considered in the appropriate setting. Progression to CKD is rare.

1. The **pathologic diagnosis** is made by normal light microscopy, negative immunofluorescence, and foot process fusion on electron microscopy.
2. **Therapy.** Approximately 80% of adults with MCD respond to prednisone, 1 mg/kg/day PO, with a decrease in proteinuria to less than 3 g/day or a remission of the nephrotic syndrome. In patients who respond, steroids should be tapered over 3 months and then discontinued. Failure to respond may reflect an error in diagnosis; MCD is most commonly confused with early focal segmental glomerulosclerosis. Urinary protein excretion should be carefully monitored during steroid taper. If relapse is documented, reinstitution of prednisone often is effective. Treatment with cytotoxic agents may be indicated in patients who are deemed steroid dependent, steroid resistant, or frequent relapsers. Cyclophosphamide, 2 mg/kg/day PO for 8 weeks; chlorambucil, 0.2 mg/kg/day PO for 8–12 weeks; or cyclosporine, 5 mg/kg/day PO for 6–12 months, are typical regimens (*Kidney Int* S70:1, 1999).

**B. Focal segmental glomerulosclerosis** is an idiopathic glomerular disorder that is usually characterized by hypertension, hematuria, renal insufficiency, and nephrotic syndrome. The disease frequently progresses to CKD and ESRD within 5–10 years of diagnosis.

1. **Pathology** reveals focal and segmental sclerosis of glomeruli.
2. **Therapy** has generally not proved to be effective in the treatment of this disorder, but a trial of prednisone, 60 mg PO qd for at least 2–3 months, may be appropriate in an effort to reduce proteinuria and slow progression to ESRD. Some authors recommend a combination of glucocorticoids and agents such as cyclosporine, 5 mg/kg/day PO, or cyclophosphamide, 2 mg/kg/day PO, to induce remission (*Kidney Int* S70:26, 1999).

**C. Membranous nephropathy** usually presents with the nephrotic syndrome, although some patients have isolated proteinuria. Membranous nephropathy may be a primary renal disease or associated with a systemic disease (e.g., malignancy, SLE, or infections such as hepatitis B, syphilis, hepatitis C, or schistosomiasis) or drug ingestions (e.g., penicillamine, gold). The GFR generally is normal or near normal, and the urinary sediment often is unremarkable. Approximately one-third of patients with membranous nephropathy progress to ESRD; the remainder enter remission or have stable or very slowly declining renal function. Because of the generally good outcome, treatment usually is reserved for patients with poor prognostic factors (age >50, male gender, hypertension, reduced GFR, proteinuria >10 g/day, or marked interstitial fibrosis on renal biopsy).

1. **Pathologic examination** demonstrates thickening of the GBM and subepithelial deposits of IgG and C3 on electron microscopy.
2. **Treatment** options include high-dose alternate-day glucocorticoids in conjunction with a cytotoxic agent (e.g., chlorambucil, 0.2 mg/kg/day, or cyclophosphamide, 1.5–2.5 mg/kg/day) for 6–12 months and, in nonresponders, cyclosporine, 3.5 mg/kg/day for 12 months.

**D. IgA nephropathy** is most often an idiopathic disorder that is characterized by asymptomatic microscopic hematuria with mild proteinuria or recurrent episodes of gross hematuria that may be concomitant with an upper respiratory infection. Renal biopsy may be indicated if evidence of renal insufficiency or proteinuria greater than 1 g/day is found. IgA nephropathy may be associated with hepatic cirrhosis, gluten enteropathy, or dermatitis herpetiformis. **Henoch-Schönlein purpura** is a systemic vasculitis that presents with the tetrad of palpable purpura (usually in the lower trunk or extremities), abdominal pain, joint inflammation, and renal failure due to IgA nephropathy.

1. **Pathology** is notable for increased mesangial cellularity and matrix. Immunofluorescence and electron microscopy reveal mesangial deposition of IgA and C3.
2. **Therapy** with glucocorticoids may be helpful in patients who have progressive disease. The use of omega-3 fatty acids, found in fish oil (6 g PO bid), may be beneficial in preventing the deterioration of renal function.

**III. Secondary glomerulopathies**

**A. Diabetic nephropathy** is the most common cause of ESRD in the United States (see Chap. 21, Diabetes Mellitus and Related Disorders). Two randomized trials, Irbesartan in Diabetic Nephropathy (IDNT) and Reduction of Endpoints in Non-Insulin Dependent Diabetes Mellitus with the Angiotensin II Antagonist Losartan (RENAAL), demonstrated a beneficial effect of ARBs over conventional antihypertensive medications on the progression of diabetic kidney disease. The ARB dose should be titrated to the maximal approved dose of these medications for optimal efficacy in reduction of proteinuria.

**B. SLE** may involve the kidney and can present as slowly progressive azotemia with urinary abnormalities, as nephrotic syndrome, or as rapidly progressive renal insufficiency. Renal biopsy is useful in SLE for evaluating disease activity and assessing irreversible changes such as glomerular sclerosis, tubular atrophy, and interstitial fibrosis.

1. A wide variety of **pathologic changes** may be seen on renal biopsy, including mesangial, membranous, focal or diffuse proliferative, and crescentic GN. A predominance of irreversible changes with little acute inflammation portends a poor response to therapy and should modify the aggressiveness of immunosuppressive treatment.
2. **Treatment** for patients with severe renal disease is methylprednisolone, 500 mg IV q12h for 3 days, followed by oral prednisone, 0.5–1.0 mg/kg PO qd. Prednisone should then be tapered over 6–8 weeks to the lowest dosage that controls disease activity, preferably using an alternate-day regimen. The addition of cyclophosphamide, 0.5–1.0 g/m$^2$ IV monthly for 6 months, then quarterly for up to 2 years, improves the likelihood of remission and appears to reduce the likelihood of progressive renal failure.

**C. Membranoproliferative glomerulonephropathy (MPGN)** exhibits a variety of clinical presentations, including acute GN, nephrotic syndrome, and asymptomatic hematuria and proteinuria. The diagnosis should be suspected if these clinical findings are associated with low complement levels. Hepatitis C accounts for most cases of MPGN and is often associated with **cryoglobulinemia** (see Chap. 23, Arthritis and Rheumatologic Diseases). MPGN progresses slowly to renal failure.

1. **Pathology** includes mesangial proliferation and alterations of the GBM with subendothelial (type I) or intramembranous (type II) electron-dense deposits.
2. **Therapy** for idiopathic MPGN has not been shown to improve disease-free survival.

**D. Dysproteinemias** include amyloidosis, light-chain and heavy-chain deposition diseases, and fibrillary/immunotactoid glomerulopathies and may be associated with multiple myeloma, Waldenström's macroglobulinemia, and other B-cell malignancies. The diagnosis is often suggested by an abnormal serum protein electrophoresis or urine protein electrophoresis. **Amyloidosis** is characterized by the extracellular deposition of 10-nm fibrils comprised of the variable region of monoclonal Ig light chains (typically lambda) in a beta-pleated configuration. **Light-chain deposition disease** is characterized by the extracellular deposition of the constant region of monoclonal Ig (kappa >80% of the time) light chains, whereas heavy and light chains are seen in **heavy-chain deposition disease.** Patients with dysproteinemias often have cardiac, hepatic, and neuropathic involvement in addition to kidney disease.

1. **Pathologic diagnosis of amyloidosis** can be made by Congo red–positive staining of the beta-pleated fibrils. In **light-chain deposition disease,** a granular pattern of deposition that is negative for Congo red staining is seen. Immunofluorescence staining for lambda and kappa light chains and heavy chains aids in making the appropriate diagnosis.
2. **Therapy** with melphalan and prednisone has proved to be beneficial for amyloidosis and light-chain deposition disease. For dysproteinemias associated with multiple myeloma, high-dose chemotherapy may be effective aggressive therapy in some patients.

**E. Infection-related GN** may occur in association with a variety of infectious processes, including **bacterial endocarditis, visceral abscesses, and infected shunts.** Treatment of the infection usually leads to the resolution of the active immune complex–mediated GN. **Poststreptococcal GN** is characterized by onset of edema, hypertension, and gross hematuria 7–28 days after a streptococcal pharyngeal or skin infection. It is associated with low complement levels and is usually self-limited with spontaneous resolution. **Hepatitis C** may cause MPGN, generally in association with **cryoglobulinemia.** Treatment with interferon-alpha can be attempted (see Chap. 17, Liver Diseases), but its effectiveness in resolving the renal manifestations of hepatitis C is unclear.

**F. Pulmonary-renal syndromes**

1. The most common cause of pulmonary-renal syndrome is **pneumonia with ATN.**
2. **Anti-GBM antibody disease** may present with pulmonary and renal involvement **(Goodpasture's syndrome)** or with renal disease alone. Anti-GBM disease often is rapidly progressive.
   a. **Diagnosis** is based either on the presence of anti-GBM antibodies in the serum or on linear deposition of IgG antibody along the basement membrane on renal biopsy. Of these patients, 10–30% may have a positive antineutrophil autoplasmic antibody (ANCA).
   b. **Standard therapy** is to clear anti-GBM antibodies from the serum while also suppressing formation of new antibodies. Daily total volume plasmapheresis for approximately 2 weeks, in combination with cyclophosphamide, 2 mg/kg PO qd for 8 weeks, and methylprednisolone, 7–15 mg/kg/day IV for 3 days, followed by prednisone, 60 mg PO qd tapered over 8 weeks, is usually effective. Frequent clinical evaluation and measurement of anti-GBM antibody titers monitor progress. Immunosuppression should be continued until the anti-GBM antibody is undetectable. Relapse is common and tends to occur within the first several months. Therapy may not be effective if the patient is already oliguric, is receiving dialysis, or has a Cr level of greater than 6.5 mg/dl.
3. **Wegener's granulomatosis** (see also Chap. 23, Arthritis and Rheumatologic Diseases)
   a. **Diagnosis** is made by tissue biopsy showing granulomatous inflammation. Immunofluorescence on kidney biopsy shows a paucity of immune deposits. Patients have a positive cytoplasmic ANCA directed against proteinase-3 in 90% of cases.
   b. **Therapy** includes a combination of cyclophosphamide, 2 mg/kg/day PO continued for at least 1 year beyond the induction of remission and subsequently tapered, plus prednisone, 1 mg/kg PO qd for 4 weeks followed by slow taper and conversion to alternate-day therapy over the next 6–9 months. Trimethoprim-sulfamethoxazole, 160 mg/800 mg (double strength) bid, has been shown to reduce extrarenal relapses in patients with Wegener's granulomatosis.
4. **Microscopic polyangiitis**
   a. **Diagnosis** can be confirmed on renal biopsy by the presence of focal necrotizing GN with crescent formation similar to that observed in Wegener's granulomatosis. Perinuclear ANCA serology with anti-

bodies to myeloperoxidase is often positive. **Churg-Strauss syndrome** can be distinguished from microscopic polyangiitis and Wegener's granulomatosis by the presence of asthma and eosinophilia (see also Chap. 10, Allergy and Immunology).

**b. Therapy** involves the combination of prednisone and cyclophosphamide similar to that used in the treatment of Wegener's granulomatosis.

**G. Sickle cell nephropathy** may present with microscopic or gross hematuria (which may be due to papillary necrosis), proteinuria, tubular dysfunction, and sclerosing glomerulopathy. Treatment may include maintenance of high urine output, alkalinization of urine, and correction of fluid and electrolyte derangements as needed. ACE-inhibitor therapy is beneficial in reducing proteinuria and possibly progression of sclerotic glomerular lesions.

**H. HIV-associated nephropathy** is characterized by proteinuria, edema, and hematuria with or without azotemia. The histologic appearance on biopsy is similar to that of collapsing focal segmental glomerulosclerosis. Antiretroviral therapy may stabilize renal function and reduce proteinuria. Prednisone, 60 mg/day for 3 months, may also improve renal function, and ACE inhibitors may be beneficial in reducing proteinuria. HIV infection has also been associated with other renal diseases, including membranous, membranoproliferative, proliferative, and crescentic GN; hemolytic-uremic syndrome/thrombotic thrombocytopenic purpura; and tubulointerstitial nephritis. Renal biopsy may be required to differentiate amongst these entities.

## Chronic Kidney Disease

CKD may result from many different etiologies and is often asymptomatic until severe renal insufficiency develops. The decline in GFR may be followed by plotting the reciprocal of serum Cr versus time. The resulting plot usually is linear, unless there is a superimposed renal insult, and is useful in end-stage planning and in predicting the time when dialysis is needed (typically, when GFR is $<10$ ml/minute in individuals without diabetes and $<15$ ml/minute in patients with diabetes). Avoidance of factors that are known to cause an acute decline in renal function and early referral to a nephrologist for implementation of conservative medical treatment of CKD may preserve renal function and postpone the need for dialysis.

**I. Acute deterioration in CKD** (i.e., a sudden decline in GFR that is more rapid than expected) should prompt a search for a superimposed, reversible process.

**A. Decreased renal perfusion** may be due to volume depletion or decreased cardiac output. Afterload reduction may be useful in volume-replete patients with cardiac dysfunction, but caution should be taken to avoid decreased renal perfusion pressure. Hypotension induced by antihypertensive agents can exacerbate CKD, as can poorly controlled hypertension. Thus, all significant fluctuations in BP control should be investigated, especially if they are associated with a reduction in renal function.

**B. Drugs** may cause direct toxicity to renal structures (e.g., aminoglycosides), decreased renal perfusion (e.g., nonsteroidal anti-inflammatory drugs, IV contrast), or allergic interstitial nephritis (e.g., allopurinol, antibiotics). Careful attention to drug dosing in patients with decreased GFR and avoidance of unnecessary use of nephrotoxic agents are appropriate.

**C. Urinary tract obstruction and infections** should be considered in any patient with an unexplained sudden decline in renal function.

**D. Progression of renal artery stenosis** may worsen preexisting renal failure.

**E. Cholesterol embolization** may worsen CKD and is seen most often in patients after procedures that require arterial catheterization (see Acute Renal Failure, sec. **III.I**).

**F. Renal vein thrombosis** may occur in nephrotic patients and exacerbate CKD and proteinuria.

**II. Conservative management** of CKD includes measures to correct and prevent metabolic derangements of renal failure and preserve remaining renal function.

**A. Dietary modification**

1. **Protein restriction** reduces accumulation of nitrogenous waste products and may slow the progression of renal failure. Intake should be reduced to 0.6–0.8 g/kg/day of high-biologic-value protein when the GFR falls below 30 ml/minute under supervision of a trained renal dietitian. Adequate caloric intake (35–50 kcal/kg/day) must be provided to avoid endogenous protein catabolism and malnutrition. In nephrotic patients, an amount of protein equal to that lost in the urine should be added to the daily allowance. The addition of an ACE inhibitor can reduce proteinuria and, hence, protein losses. ARBs may have similar efficacy in patients who are unable to tolerate ACE-inhibitor therapy.
2. **Potassium** should be restricted to 40 mEq/day when GFR falls below 20 ml/minute.
3. **Phosphorus and calcium** levels are altered in CKD due to (1) phosphorus retention, resulting in a rise in serum phosphorus levels and a reciprocal fall in calcium levels, with resultant stimulation of parathyroid hormone (PTH) secretion; (2) decreased generation of 1,25-dihydroxyvitamin $D_3$, further contributing to low serum calcium levels and decreasing suppression of PTH release; and (3) skeletal resistance to the action of PTH. Consequently, PTH secretion is increased (i.e., **secondary hyperparathyroidism**) and contributes to **renal osteodystrophy** (see sec. **III**). Hyperphosphatemia may also play a role in the progression of renal failure. The goal is to maintain predialysis serum phosphorus levels between 4.0 and 5.0 mg/dl. Dietary phosphorus should be restricted to 800–1000 mg/day when GFR is less than 50 ml/minute. As GFR falls further, phosphate restriction becomes less effective, and the addition of phosphate binders that prevent GI phosphate absorption is indicated. **Calcium carbonate** ($CaCO_3$), 500–1000 mg PO with meals, is effective in most patients. Serum calcium should be checked regularly. If the serum phosphate level cannot be reduced to 4–5 mg/dl with $CaCO_3$, or if the initial phosphate level is greater than 7 mg/dl, aluminum hydroxide antacids (e.g., Amphojel or Basaljel), 15–30 ml or one to three capsules PO with meals, may be used for a limited time. Chronic use of aluminum-containing antacids can lead to aluminum accumulation in CKD patients and can cause osteomalacia (see sec. **III**). **Sevelamer,** a phosphate binder that lacks aluminum and calcium, can be used in dialysis-dependent patients, although its use in CKD patients who are not yet on dialysis is limited by its propensity to worsen metabolic acidosis. Lack of dietary phosphate restriction is the most common reason that phosphate binders fail to control hyperphosphatemia. $CaCO_3$ should be stopped if the calcium phosphate product is consistently greater than 60, to avoid the possibility of metastatic calcification. If hypocalcemia (corrected for serum albumin) persists after phosphate has been controlled, nighttime $CaCO_3$ and supplementation of 1,25-dihydroxyvitamin $D_3$ may be indicated (see Chap. 3, Fluid and Electrolyte Management).
4. **Sodium and fluid restriction** must be determined on an individual basis. For most patients, a no-added-salt diet (NaCl, 8 g/day) is palatable and adequate. If necessary, 24-hour urinary sodium excretion can be determined to aid in sodium intake planning. Once a patient has reached an acceptable volume status, fluid intake should equal daily urine output plus an additional 500 ml for insensible losses. Additional fluid restriction is appropriate only in patients with dilutional hyponatremia. The presence of heart failure or refractory hypertension also may require greater restriction of

salt and water. In nephrotic patients with edema, salt restriction (2–3 g/day) and judicious use of diuretics should be implemented.

5. **Magnesium** is excreted by the kidney and accumulates in CKD. Extra dietary intake of magnesium (e.g., some antacids and cathartics) should be avoided.

**B. Hypertension** accelerates the rate of decline of renal function in patients with CKD and should be treated aggressively (see Chap. 4, Hypertension). Target BP in most forms of CKD should be 130/80 or less. ACE inhibitors appear to have renoprotective properties beyond their antihypertensive effect. ARBs may have similar efficacy with fewer side effects. Diuretic use must be carefully monitored to avoid volume depletion. Loop diuretics (e.g., furosemide) remain effective when the GFR is less than 25 ml/minute, although dose increases may be required to maintain adequate diuretic response.

**C. Metabolic acidosis** is treated with oral sodium bicarbonate, 650–1300 mg PO tid, when serum bicarbonate falls below 18–20 mEq/L. The additional sodium load from such therapy may require further dietary sodium restriction or administration of a diuretic. Although citrate is converted by the liver to bicarbonate, it should not be used in CKD because it dramatically enhances GI absorption of aluminum and can lead to acute aluminum neurotoxicity.

**D. Anemia** is responsible for many symptoms of CKD and can be corrected with the use of **recombinant human erythropoietin** after ensuring that iron stores are adequate. Treatment should be initiated in most patients with a hemoglobin of less than 10 mg/dl. The initial dose is 50–100 U/kg SC two to three times a week, with a target hematocrit of 31–36% (see Chap. 19, Anemia and Transfusion Therapy). A newer agent, **darbepoetin alfa,** has been approved for the anemia of CKD, which requires less frequent dosing (0.45 μg/kg SC once a week or once every 2 weeks). In patients who are receiving erythropoietin or darbepoetin, hematocrit should be checked at least monthly. Iron stores should also be assessed periodically, with evaluation of transferrin saturation and ferritin. If transferrin saturation is less than 20% or ferritin is less than 200 mg/dl, consideration should be given to iron repletion with IV preparations of iron dextran (1000 mg IV as a single dose, with an initial test dose of 25 mg), ferric gluconate (125 mg IV × 8 doses), or iron sucrose (100 mg IV × 10 doses).

**E.** Preparation for creation of a **permanent vascular access** should be initiated by protecting the veins of the nondominant forearm from peripheral IVs and blood draws. This increases the likelihood of successful future arteriovenous (AV) fistula or graft placement. Timely referral to an access surgeon can facilitate creation of a primary AV fistula, the preferred vascular access for hemodialysis (HD).

**F. Additional management of the nephrotic syndrome.** The nephrotic syndrome increases the risk of cardiac (e.g., atherosclerosis) and noncardiac (e.g., infection) comorbidities.

1. **Hyperlipidemia** in patients with long-standing nephrotic syndrome may increase the risk for atherosclerotic disease. Dietary restriction of cholesterol and saturated fat should be prescribed. HMG-CoA reductase inhibitors (see Chap. 5, Ischemic Heart Disease) are effective in improving the lipoprotein profile in these patients.
2. **Thromboembolic complications.** The nephrotic syndrome produces a hypercoagulable state, and the clinician should maintain a high index of suspicion for thromboemboli. Deep venous thrombosis of the upper and lower extremities, as well as renal vein thrombosis, may occur and should be treated with heparin anticoagulation, followed by long-term warfarin therapy (see Chap. 18, Disorders of Hemostasis).

**III. Renal osteodystrophy** refers to skeletal disorders seen in CKD and ESRD. It includes **high bone turnover diseases,** such as osteitis fibrosa, and **low bone**

**turnover diseases,** such as osteomalacia and adynamic bone disease. Therapy and prevention should be initiated early in the course of progressive renal failure. Goals include (1) maintenance of normal serum calcium and phosphorus levels, (2) halting the development of parathyroid gland hyperplasia with suppression of secondary hyperparathyroidism, (3) prevention of extraskeletal calcification, and (4) maintenance of normal bone histology.

A. **Osteitis fibrosa** is caused by **secondary hyperparathyroidism** (see sec. **II.A.3**). Clinical manifestations include bone pain, fractures, skeletal deformity, proximal muscle weakness, pruritus, and extraskeletal calcification. Serum PTH, measured by immunoassay for intact hormone, is markedly elevated. Radiographic studies typically show subperiosteal resorption and patchy osteosclerosis. Specific therapy includes the following:
   1. **Correction of hyperphosphatemia** (see sec. **II.A.3**)
   2. **Normalization of serum calcium levels and suppression of PTH** to 1–2 times the upper limit of normal in CKD patients and 1.5–4.0 times the upper limit of normal in dialysis-dependent patients
      a. **Vitamin D preparations** such as **calcitriol** (0.25–1.0 μg PO qd) can be used to suppress PTH and correct hypocalcemia. Serum calcium levels should be measured at least monthly and the dose adjusted accordingly at 1- to 2-month intervals to avoid hypercalcemia, which can reduce renal function. In HD patients, IV administration of **19-nor-1,25-dihydroxyvitamin $D_2$** (paricalcitol), a synthetic vitamin D analog that reduces the incidence of hypercalcemia, may suppress hyperparathyroidism more effectively than calcitriol.
      b. **Parathyroidectomy** may be required to control severe hyperparathyroidism. Indications include (1) **calciphylaxis** (ischemic necrosis of skin or soft tissue associated with metastatic calcification), (2) persistent severe hypercalcemia (after other causes of hypercalcemia are excluded), (3) progressive extraskeletal calcification, and (4) severe hyperparathyroidism (PTH >1000) despite maximal medical therapy.

B. **Mixed bone turnover disease** also occurs in the setting of hyperparathyroidism. It may be seen in patients with previously established osteitis fibrosa and with osteomalacia related to aluminum exposure.

C. **Low bone turnover disease** includes **osteomalacia** and **adynamic bone lesions** and occurs in the setting of relatively low PTH levels. Avoidance of vitamin D and use of sevelamer rather than calcium-based phosphate binders appears to increase PTH and presumably improves bone turnover. Aluminum as a cause of low bone turnover disease is now rare due to the decreased use of aluminum-based phosphate binders and prevention of aluminum contamination of dialysate.

## Renal Replacement Therapies

**Renal replacement therapy** in CKD is indicated when metabolic abnormalities can no longer be controlled with conservative management or when signs and symptoms of uremia develop; this generally occurs when $Cl_{Cr}$ falls below 10 ml/minute in nondiabetics and below 15 ml/min in diabetic patients. A variety of therapeutic options are available to the patient with ESRD.

I. **Hemodialysis (HD)** works by diffusion of small-molecular-weight solutes across a semipermeable membrane. Fluid removal occurs via ultrafiltration. Dialysis usually is performed three times a week. Because urea distributes through total body water, larger patients require longer treatment times; hence, the duration of each treatment is adjusted to achieve a urea reduction ratio (URR) of at least 65%, with most treatments lasting 3–4 hours. URR is calculated as follows:

$$\text{URR} = \frac{(\text{pre-HD BUN} - \text{post-HD BUN})}{\text{pre-HD BUN}} \times 100$$

When HD is instituted, dietary protein intake should be increased to 1.0–1.2 g/kg/day, and fluid intake should be adjusted to permit a weight gain of approximately 2 kg between dialysis sessions. Antihypertensive medication may have to be reduced, and short-acting antihypertensives may need to be withheld on dialysis days.

**A. Vascular access** for blood outflow and return is necessary. Permanent vascular access requires creation of a primary AV anastomosis or placement of a synthetic AV graft. **Primary AV fistulas** are considered the optimal form of permanent access; they have the lowest incidence of infection and thrombosis. Fistulas should be placed 3–6 months before anticipated dialysis because they take time to mature. In contrast, because **synthetic AV grafts** must merely heal and become incorporated, they usually are placed 1–3 months before anticipated dialysis. **Tunneled Silastic catheters** placed in the internal jugular vein are being increasingly used for long-term access; they have lower rates of infection than nontunneled catheters and fewer venous complications (stenosis, compromise of future arm grafts) than those placed in subclavian veins. Temporary access is usually via an internal jugular or femoral venous catheter.

1. **Infections** of vascular access sites are common and may produce local or systemic signs. Careful examination and ultrasonography of the access site may reveal a local abscess, which should be cultured and drained. Fevers, especially during an HD treatment, should be promptly evaluated. Blood cultures should be obtained, and empiric antibiotic coverage should be considered even in patients who lack an obvious source of infection. Initial therapy must include coverage for staphylococci and gram-negative organisms and should be continued for at least 3 weeks if bloodstream infection is documented. Removal of an infected access often is necessary.
2. **Thrombosis** of a vascular access site can be recanalized by balloon catheter embolectomy, thrombolysis, or thrombectomy. The access site usually can be used immediately after declotting.

**B. Hypotension during dialysis** is most commonly due to intravascular volume depletion and, less commonly, the use of antihypertensives or nitrates before dialysis, allergic reactions to the dialyzer, left ventricular dysfunction, or autonomic insufficiency. Acute treatment includes infusion of normal saline and reduction of the ultrafiltration rate. Other causes of hypotension, such as myocardial infarction, cardiac tamponade, sepsis, and bleeding, should be considered.

**C. Active bleeding and coagulopathies** may be exacerbated by the systemic anticoagulation used in HD. The heparin dosage used for HD can usually be minimized or even withheld in patients with such disorders, or a change to peritoneal dialysis (PD) should be considered. The platelet dysfunction seen in many uremic patients causes prolongation of the bleeding time and can be improved by the use of IV ddAVP (0.3 μg/kg in 50 ml saline q4–8h), IV conjugated estrogen (0.6 mg/kg/day for 5 days), or intranasal ddAVP (see Chap. 18, Disorders of Hemostasis).

**D. Dialysis-associated pericarditis** may occur in patients who are undergoing dialysis and appears to be different from uremic pericarditis. Treatment involves intensification of dialysis to six to seven times a week. If this therapy fails or if evidence of tamponade is found, pericardiectomy is indicated. Anticoagulation during HD should be minimized or discontinued until pericarditis resolves.

**E. Dialysis disequilibrium** is a syndrome that may occur during the first few treatments of profoundly uremic patients and is attributed to CNS edema from rapid osmolar shifts. Symptoms include nausea, emesis, and headache, with occasional progression to confusion and seizures. This complication can be prevented or ameliorated by using lower blood flows and shorter treatment duration during initial dialysis sessions.

**II. Peritoneal dialysis (PD)**

**A. Modalities.** PD can be used in ARF and ESRD. It uses the peritoneum as a dialysis membrane, with solutes removed by diffusion into the dialysate. Fluid removal is controlled by adjusting the dextrose concentration in the dialysate (1.5%, 2.5%, or 4.25% glucose) to create an osmotic gradient for water. Higher dextrose concentrations and more frequent exchanges increase the rate of fluid removal. A typical dialysis exchange is performed by infusion of 2 L fluid into the peritoneal cavity, followed by an equilibration period and dialysate drainage. In ARF, PD exchanges can be performed as often as every hour. **Continuous ambulatory PD** involves 2- to 3-L manual exchanges performed four to five times a day by the patient. **Continuous cycling PD** uses an automatic cycler to perform exchanges during sleep. It can be supplemented by daytime manual exchanges. PD should be avoided in patients with recent abdominal surgery or a history of multiple surgeries with adhesions. Strict sterile technique is mandatory when exchanges are being performed. Compared with HD, PD is less efficient and less useful in highly catabolic patients. PD usually is better tolerated by patients with dilated cardiomyopathies because it causes fewer abrupt changes in BP and electrolytes, and fluid removal is continuous. PD also offers greater independence to patients on chronic dialysis than does HD.

**B. Complications of PD**

1. **Infections** are the most significant problem in PD and include peritonitis, infection of the catheter tunnel, and infection of the catheter exit site. **Peritonitis** typically causes increasing abdominal pain and cloudy peritoneal fluid. It is usually secondary to a break in sterile technique. Patients are trained to save cloudy fluid for cell count and culture and then to initiate antibiotic therapy on an outpatient basis. A neutrophil count greater than 100 cells/μl in the dialysate is diagnostic of PD-associated peritonitis. Because of the concern for emerging vancomycin resistance, initial empiric therapy should consist of cefazolin plus ceftazidime (Table 11-3) added to the PD fluid, which then should dwell for 5–6 hours (*Perit Dial Int* 20:396, 2000). Further antibiotic therapy should be guided by Gram stain and cultures. Fluid balance must be closely monitored and dialysate concentration adjusted to avoid dehydration or volume overload. Hospitalization is indicated in patients with sepsis, resistant or recurrent infections, or suspicion of organ perforation or abscess formation. **Tunnel or exit site infections** involve skin organisms, frequently are difficult to treat, and may require catheter removal and temporary HD until the infection resolves.
2. **Hyperglycemia** may occur as a result of systemic absorption of glucose from PD fluid. Although regular insulin can be added to the dialysate, intraperitoneal insulin administration frequently results in unreliable dosing and an additional potential source of infectious contamination. Recent trends have favored traditional subcutaneous insulin administration for hyperglycemia in diabetic patients on PD.
3. **Protein loss** in PD can be excessive, and therefore dietary protein intake should be increased to 1.2–1.4 g/kg/day.

**III. Ultrafiltration and hemofiltration** remove large volumes of fluid with minimal removal of metabolic wastes. These filtration techniques are useful for removing fluid in patients with renal insufficiency and volume overload who do not need concomitant dialysis.

**A. Dry ultrafiltration** is performed in a manner similar to that of standard HD, except that no dialysate is used. Negative pressure applied across the dialyzer membrane causes an ultrafiltrate of plasma to form and be removed.

**Table 11-3.** Intraperitoneal antibiotics in peritoneal dialysis

| Antibiotic | Continuous dose (add to every exchange) | Intermittent dose (add to 1 exchange each day) |
|---|---|---|
| Cefazolin and cephalothin | Loading dose: 500 mg/L; maintenance dose: 125 mg/L | 500 mg/L (or 15 mg/kg); if UO >500 ml/d, increase by 0.6 mg/kg body weight |
| Ceftazidime | Loading dose: 250 mg/L; maintenance dose: 125 mg/L | 1000 mg/d in 1 exchange |
| Gentamicin, netilmicin, tobramycin | Loading dose: 8 mg/L; maintenance dose: 4 mg/L | If UO >500 ml/d, give 1.5 mg/kg loading dose, then 0.6 mg/kg/d[a]; if UO <500 ml/d, give 0.6 mg/kg/d without load |
| Imipenem | Loading dose: 500 mg/L; maintenance dose: 200 mg/L | 1000 mg intraperitoneally bid |

UO, urine output.
[a]Adjust dose based on blood levels (see Chap. 12, Antimicrobials).

Large volumes of fluid may be removed in a short period. The patient may experience hypotension, but fluid removal is usually better tolerated by isolated dry ultrafiltration than with concomitant HD.

**B. Slow, continuous renal replacement therapies** include **continuous venovenous hemofiltration** alone or with HD. These modalities were developed to treat critically ill patients in an ICU setting. Continuous treatment permits the slow removal of large amounts of volume and solutes while minimizing hemodynamic compromise. Continuous venovenous hemofiltration and continuous venovenous hemofiltration with HD use a blood pump that circulates blood though a double-lumen venous catheter, avoiding the need for an arterial line. Both modalities usually require systemic anticoagulation, and patients are bedbound during treatment. Fluid balance, electrolytes, and glucose must be closely monitored. Drug clearance may be higher than with HD or PD, and therefore drug levels should be monitored whenever possible.

**IV. Renal transplantation** offers patients a lifestyle that is closest to normal and may lead to improved survival over HD and PD. One-year graft survival rates are greater than 80% for cadaveric allografts and 90% for living-related donor grafts.

**A. Pretransplantation evaluation** of the recipient includes assessment of cardiovascular status and structural abnormalities of the urinary tract, correction of potential sources of infection, human lymphocyte antigen typing, and evaluation for preformed antibodies against potential donor antigens. The latter, along with blood group compatibility testing, should prevent hyperacute rejection in most cases. Contraindications to transplantation include most malignancies, active infections, and significant cardiac or pulmonary disease.

**B.** Immunosuppression, infectious complications, and long-term management of renal transplant recipients are discussed in Chap. 15, Solid Organ Transplant Medicine.

## Nephrolithiasis

**I. Clinical manifestations** of nephrolithiasis include hematuria, predisposition to urinary tract infection, and flank or costovertebral angle pain with passage of the stone. Renal stones may also be an incidental finding on radiographic studies. Oliguria and ARF may occur when both collecting systems are blocked by stones.

II. **Diagnostic evaluation** of an acute episode of flank pain and hematuria should include a plain abdominal radiogram, as most renal stones are radiopaque. Exceptions include cystine stones, which may be of intermediate opacity, and uric acid stones, which are radiolucent. **Noncontrast helical CT scanning** has largely supplanted IV pyelography for evaluation of renal colic and follow-up for patients with recurrent nephrolithiasis. Renal ultrasound may be useful to rule out obstruction of the collecting systems, particularly in the evaluation of pregnant patients with suspected nephrolithiasis. Urine should be cultured and examined for pH and crystals. Other initial studies include serum electrolytes, Cr, calcium, uric acid, and phosphorus levels. Urine should be strained and all passed stones should be saved for analysis. After resolution of the acute episode, further diagnostic evaluation can be guided by stone composition. The extent of the metabolic evaluation that should be undertaken for the patient with a single calcium stone has not been established, but recurrent calcium nephrolithiasis warrants complete investigation. Patients with noncalcium stones should undergo complete evaluation after the first episode. Additional studies may include PTH levels (if hypercalcemia is present) and 24-hour urine studies for measurement of calcium, phosphate, urate, oxalate, citrate, Cr, sodium, urea nitrogen, and cystine. Yearly follow-up examination of the patient with nephrolithiasis includes abdominal radiographs to check for new stone formation or growth of existing stones and repeat metabolic studies to assess the effects of specific therapies.

III. **Treatment** of acute episodes of nephrolithiasis includes narcotic analgesia and hydration. If the stone is obstructing outflow or is accompanied by infection, removal is indicated with urgent urologic intervention. After passage of a stone, treatment is directed at prevention of recurrent stone formation. In most patients, the foundation of therapy is maintenance of high urine output (>2.5 L/day) through oral hydration and avoidance of dietary excesses. Evaluation and management depend on the type of stone and are best performed in the outpatient setting.

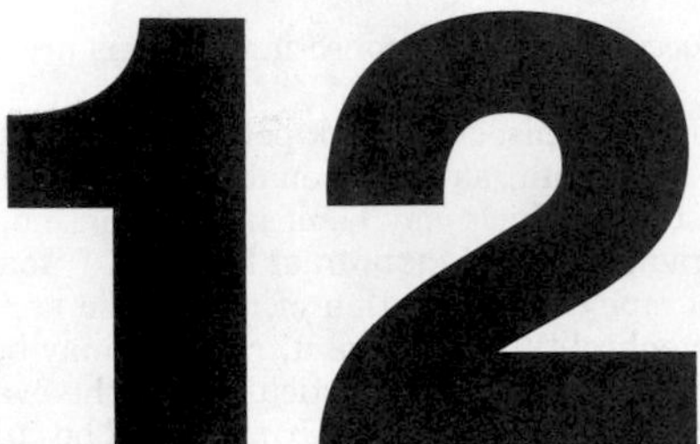

# Antimicrobials

David J. Ritchie and
Steven J. Lawrence

Empiric antimicrobial therapy should be initiated based on expected pathogens for a given infection. As microbial resistance is increasing in many pathogens, a review of institution antibiograms as well as local, regional, national, and global susceptibility trends also assists in the development of empiric therapy regimens. In addition, allergy history and pregnancy/lactation status should be evaluated, as several agents are contraindicated in these settings. Antimicrobial therapy should be modified, if possible, based on results of culture and sensitivity testing to agent(s) that have the narrowest spectrum possible. Attention should be paid to the possibility of switching from parenteral to oral therapy where possible, as many oral agents exhibit excellent oral bioavailability. Several antibiotics have major drug interactions (see Appendix C, Drug Interactions) or require alternate dosing in renal or hepatic insufficiency, or both (see Appendix E, Dosage Adjustments of Drugs in Renal Failure). For antiretroviral and antiparasitic agents, see Chap. 14, Human Immunodeficiency Virus Infection and Acquired Immunodeficiency Syndrome, and Chap. 13, Treatment of Infectious Diseases, respectively.

## Antibacterial Agents

**I. Penicillins (PCNs)** irreversibly bind PCN-binding proteins in the bacterial cell wall, causing osmotic rupture and death. Once the mainstay of antimicrobial therapy, these agents have a somewhat diminished role today because of acquired resistance in many bacterial species through alterations in PCN-binding proteins or expression of hydrolytic enzymes. However, PCNs remain among the drugs of choice for syphilis, group A streptococci, *Listeria monocytogenes*, *Pasteurella multocida*, *Actinomyces*, susceptible enterococcus species, and some anaerobic infections.

- **A. Aqueous penicillin G** [2–4 million U IV q4h or 18–24 million U qd by continuous infusion] is the IV preparation of PCN. This formulation is the therapy of choice for neurosyphilis (see Chap. 13, Treatment of Infectious Diseases). Although the potassium salt is more commonly used, the sodium salt is available and can be given in the setting of hyperkalemia or azotemia.
- **B. Procaine penicillin G** is an IM repository form of penicillin G that can be used as an alternate treatment for neurosyphilis at a dose of 2.4 million U IM qd in combination with probenecid, 500 mg PO qid for 10–14 days.
- **C. Benzathine PCN** is a long-acting IM repository form of penicillin G that is commonly used for treating early latent syphilis [<1 year duration (1 dose, 2.4 million U IM)] and late latent syphilis [unknown duration or >1 year (2.4 million U IM qwk for 3 doses)]. It is occasionally given for group A streptococcal pharyngitis and prophylaxis after acute rheumatic fever or poststreptococcal glomerulonephritis.
- **D. Penicillin V** (250–500 mg PO qid) is an oral formulation of PCN that is typically used to treat group A streptococcal pharyngitis.

E. **Ampicillin** (2–3 g IV q4–6h) is the drug of choice for treatment of infections caused by susceptible enterococcus species and *L. monocytogenes.* Oral ampicillin (250–500 mg PO qid) is commonly used for uncomplicated sinusitis, pharyngitis, otitis media, and urinary tract infections (UTIs). **Ampicillin/sulbactam** (1.5–3.0 g IV q6h) combines ampicillin with the beta-lactamase inhibitor sulbactam, thereby extending its spectrum to include oxacillin-sensitive *Staphylococcus aureus* (OSSA), anaerobes, and many Enterobacteriaceae. It is effective for the upper and lower respiratory tract, genitourinary tract, and abdominal, pelvic, and polymicrobial soft-tissue infections and is the IV antibiotic of choice for serious cellulitis due to human or animal bites.

F. **Amoxicillin** (250–500 mg PO tid) is an oral antibiotic similar to ampicillin that is commonly used for uncomplicated sinusitis, pharyngitis, otitis media, and UTIs. **Amoxicillin/clavulanic acid** [875 mg PO bid, or 500 mg PO tid, or 90 mg/kg/day divided q12h (Augmentin ES-600 suspension) or 2000 mg PO q12h (Augmentin XR)] is an oral antibiotic similar to ampicillin/sulbactam that combines amoxicillin with the beta-lactamase inhibitor clavulanate. It is useful for treating complicated sinusitis, otitis media, and skin infections and is the oral antibiotic of choice for prophylaxis in human or animal bites after appropriate local treatment. It is often used as a step-down therapy from IV ampicillin/sulbactam.

G. **Nafcillin and oxacillin** (2 g IV q4–6h) are penicillinase-resistant synthetic PCNs that are the drugs of choice for treating OSSA infections. These drugs have little activity against enterococci or gram-negative bacteria. Dose reduction by one-half should be considered in decompensated liver disease. **Dicloxacillin and cloxacillin** (250–500 mg PO qid) are oral antibiotics with a spectrum of activity similar to that of nafcillin and oxacillin. They are typically used to treat localized skin infections.

H. **Mezlocillin, ticarcillin, and piperacillin** (3 g IV q4h or 4 g IV q6h) are extended-spectrum PCN derivatives with enhanced gram-negative activity. These agents have reasonable antipseudomonal activity but generally require coadministration of an aminoglycoside for treatment of serious infections. Mezlocillin and piperacillin have significant enterococcal activity.

I. **Ticarcillin/clavulanic acid** (3.1 g IV q4–6h) combines ticarcillin with the beta-lactamase inhibitor clavulanic acid. This combination extends the spectrum to include most Enterobacteriaceae, OSSA, and anaerobes, making it a useful antibiotic for intra-abdominal and complicated soft-tissue infections. Ticarcillin/clavulanic acid also has a unique role in treatment of *Stenotrophomonas* infections. Alternative therapy with imipenem, meropenem, cefepime, or a fluoroquinolone should be used when bacteria with *AmpC*-inducible beta-lactamases (i.e., *Enterobacter*, *Citrobacter freundii*, *Serratia*, *Providencia*, and *Morganella* species) are identified as principal pathogens. Ticarcillin/clavulanic acid has a high sodium load and should be used cautiously in patients at risk for fluid overload.

J. **Piperacillin/tazobactam** (3.375 g IV q4–6h or 4.5 g IV q6h) combines piperacillin with the beta-lactamase inhibitor tazobactam. It has a similar spectrum and indications as ticarcillin/clavulanic acid but also has activity against ampicillin-sensitive enterococci. An aminoglycoside should generally be added to piperacillin/tazobactam for treatment of serious infections caused by *Pseudomonas aeruginosa* or for nosocomial pneumonia.

K. **Adverse effects.** All PCN derivatives have been associated with anaphylaxis, interstitial nephritis, anemia, and leukopenia. Oxacillin and nafcillin can cause hepatitis. Ticarcillin can aggravate bleeding by interfering with platelet adenosine diphosphate receptors. Prolonged high-dose therapy (>2 weeks) is typically monitored with weekly serum creatinine and blood counts [liver function tests (LFTs) are included with oxacillin/nafcillin]. **All patients should be asked about PCN or cephalosporin allergy.** These agents should not be used in patients with a reported serious PCN allergy without prior skin testing or desensitization, or both.

**II. Cephalosporins** kill bacteria by interfering with cell wall synthesis by the same mechanism as PCNs. These agents are clinically useful because of their low toxicity and broad spectrum of activity. However, all currently available cephalosporins are devoid of activity against enterococci and oxacillin-resistant *S. aureus* (ORSA).

**A. First-generation cephalosporins** have activity against staphylococci, streptococci, and community-acquired *Escherichia coli*, *Klebsiella*, and *Proteus* species. They have limited activity against other enteric gram-negative rods and anaerobes. These agents have similar spectra and indications and are commonly used for treating skin/soft-tissue infections, UTIs, and oxacillin-sensitive *S. aureus* infections. **Cefazolin** (1–2 g IV/IM q8h) is a parenteral formulation, and **cefadroxil** (500 mg–1 g PO bid), **cephalexin** (250–500 mg PO q6h), and **cephradine** (250–500 mg PO q6h) are oral preparations.

**B. Second-generation cephalosporins** have expanded coverage against enteric gram-negative rods and can be divided into above-the-diaphragm and below-the-diaphragm agents.

1. **Cefuroxime** (1.5 g IV/IM q8h) and **cefamandole** (1–2 g IV/IM q4–6h) are useful antibiotics for treatment of infections above the diaphragm. They have reasonable antistaphylococcal and antistreptococcal activity in addition to an extended spectrum against gram-negative aerobes and are typically used for skin/soft-tissue infections, complicated UTIs, and community-acquired pneumonia (cefuroxime). They do not cover *Bacteroides fragilis*.
2. **Cefoxitin** (1–2 g IV q4–8h), **cefotetan** (1–3 g IV/IM q12h), and **cefmetazole** (2 g IV q6–12h) are useful for treatment of infections below the diaphragm. They do not have dependable antistaphylococcal or antistreptococcal activity but have an extended spectrum against gram-negative aerobes and anaerobes, including *B. fragilis*. These antibiotics are typically used for intra-abdominal or gynecologic surgical prophylaxis and infections, including diverticulitis and pelvic inflammatory disease.
3. **Cefuroxime axetil** (250–500 mg PO bid), **cefprozil** (250–500 mg PO bid), and **cefaclor** (250–500 mg PO bid) are oral second-generation cephalosporins typically used for bronchitis, sinusitis, otitis media, UTIs, local soft-tissue infections, and step-down therapy for pneumonia or cellulitis responsive to parenteral cephalosporins. **Loracarbef** (200–400 mg PO q12–24h) is chemically classified as a carbacephem rather than a cephalosporin but is generally used for the same indications as the oral second-generation cephalosporins.

**C. Third-generation cephalosporins** have broad coverage against enteric, aerobic gram-negative rods and retain significant activity against streptococci other than enterococci. They have moderate anaerobic activity but do not reliably cover *B. fragilis*. Ceftazidime is the only third-generation cephalosporin that is useful for treating serious *P. aeruginosa* infections. Several of these agents have substantial CNS penetration and are useful in treating meningitis (see Chap. 13, Treatment of Infectious Diseases). Third-generation cephalosporins are not reliable for treatment of serious infections caused by organisms producing *AmpC*-inducible beta-lactamases regardless of the results of susceptibility testing. These microbes should be treated with cefepime, carbapenems, or quinolones.

1. **Ceftriaxone** (1–2 g IV/IM q12–24h), **cefotaxime** (1–2 g IV/IM q4–12h), **ceftizoxime** (1–4 g IV/IM q8–12h), and **cefoperazone** (2–4 g IV q12h) are very similar to one another in spectrum and efficacy. They can be used as empiric therapy for pyelonephritis, urosepsis, pneumonia (ceftriaxone or cefotaxime), intra-abdominal infections (combined with metronidazole), gonorrhea, and meningitis (ceftriaxone and cefotaxime). They can also be used for osteomyelitis, septic arthritis, endocarditis, and soft-tissue infections once an organism has been identified.
2. **Cefpodoxime proxetil** (100–400 mg PO bid), **cefdinir** (300 mg PO bid), **ceftibuten** (400 mg PO qd), and **cefditoren pivoxil** (200–400 mg PO bid)

are oral third-generation cephalosporins useful for the treatment of bronchitis and complicated sinusitis, otitis media, and UTIs. These agents can also be used as step-down therapy for pneumonia that is responsive to parenteral third-generation cephalosporins. Cefpodoxime can be used as single-dose therapy for uncomplicated gonorrhea.

3. **Ceftazidime** (1–2 g IV/IM q8h) is a drug of choice for infections caused by susceptible strains of *P. aeruginosa*.
4. **Cefepime** (500 mg–2 g IV/IM q8–12h) is a fourth-generation cephalosporin with excellent aerobic gram-negative rod coverage, including *P. aeruginosa* and other bacteria producing *AmpC* beta-lactamases. Its gram-positive spectrum is similar to that of third-generation cephalosporins (ceftriaxone, cefotaxime). Cefepime is routinely used for empiric therapy in febrile neutropenic patients (see Chap. 20, Medical Management of Malignant Disease). It has a role in treating antibiotic-resistant gram-negative bacteria and some polymicrobial infections (involving gram-negatives and gram-positives) in most sites, although clinical experience for treatment of meningitis is limited.
5. **Adverse effects.** All cephalosporins have been associated with anaphylaxis, interstitial nephritis, anemia, and leukopenia. **PCN-allergic patients have a 5–10% incidence of a cross-hypersensitivity reaction to cephalosporins.** These agents should not be used in a patient with a reported allergy without prior skin testing or desensitization, or both. Prolonged therapy (>2 weeks) is typically monitored with a weekly serum creatinine and CBC. Ceftriaxone (and possibly cefoperazone) can cause biliary sludging and symptomatic gallbladder disease, requiring discontinuation of the medication. Cefamandole, cefmetazole, cefoperazone, and cefotetan have an *N*-methylthiotetrazole side chain that interferes with vitamin K–dependent clotting factor metabolism and is associated with disulfiram-like reactions with ethanol intake. *N*-methylthiotetrazole–containing cephalosporins should be avoided when a prolonged course of therapy is likely, as a significant coagulopathy may develop.

III. **Aztreonam** (1–2 g IV/IM q6–12h) is a monobactam that is active only against aerobic gram-negative rods including *P. aeruginosa*. It has minimal gram-positive or anaerobic activity. Aztreonam is useful in patients with known PCN or cephalosporin allergies, as no apparent cross reactivity is present.

IV. **Carbapenems** kill bacteria by interfering with cell wall synthesis, similar to PCNs and cephalosporins. They are among the antibiotics of choice for infections caused by organisms producing *AmpC* beta-lactamases, including *P. aeruginosa*. Carbapenems are also active against most gram-positive and other gram-negative bacteria, including anaerobes. They are important agents for treatment of **antibiotic-resistant bacterial infections** at most body sites. These agents are commonly used for severe polymicrobial infections, including Fournier's gangrene, intra-abdominal catastrophes, and sepsis in compromised hosts. Notable bacteria that are resistant to carbapenems include ampicillin-resistant enterococci, ORSA, and *Stenotrophomonas* and *Burkholderia* species. In addition, ertapenem does not provide reliable coverage against *P. aeruginosa*, *Acinetobacter*, or enterococci; therefore, imipenem or meropenem would be preferred for empiric treatment of nosocomial infections. Meropenem is the preferred carbapenem for treatment of CNS infections.

A. **Imipenem** (500 mg–1 g IV/IM q6–8h), **meropenem** (1 g IV q8h), and **ertapenem** (1 g IV q24h) are the currently available carbapenems.

B. **Adverse effects.** Carbapenems can precipitate seizure activity, especially in older patients, individuals with renal insufficiency, and patients with preexisting seizure disorders or CNS pathology. Carbapenems should be avoided in these patients unless no reasonable alternative therapy is available. Like cephalosporins, carbapenems have been associated with anaphylaxis, interstitial nephritis, anemia, and leukopenia. **Patients who are allergic to PCNs/cephalosporins may have a cross-hypersensitivity reaction to carbapen-**

**ems,** and these agents should not be used in a patient with a reported severe PCN allergy without prior skin testing, desensitization, or both. Prolonged therapy (>2 weeks) is typically monitored with a weekly serum creatinine, LFTs, and CBC.

**V. Aminoglycosides** kill bacteria by binding to the bacterial ribosome, causing misreading during translation of bacterial messenger RNA into proteins. These drugs are commonly used as a component of combination therapy for severe infections caused by gram-positive and gram-negative aerobes. Prolonged low-dose therapy is indicated in combination therapy for patients with endovascular infections caused by enterococcus species, PCN/cephalosporin-resistant streptococci, or gram-negative endocarditis. Aminoglycosides tend to be synergistic with cell wall–active antibiotics such as PCNs, cephalosporins, and vancomycin. However, they do not have activity against anaerobes, and their activity is impaired in the low pH/low oxygen environment of abscesses. Resistance to one aminoglycoside is not routinely associated with resistance to all members of this class, and in cases of serious infections, susceptibility testing with each aminoglycoside is appropriate. Use of these antibiotics is limited by significant nephro- and ototoxicity.

**A. Traditional dosing** of aminoglycosides is q8h, with the upper end of the dose range reserved for life-threatening infections. Peak and trough levels should be obtained with the third or fourth dose and then every 3–4 days, along with regular serum creatinine monitoring. **Increasing serum creatinine or peak/troughs out of the acceptable range require immediate attention.** Traditional dosing, rather than extended-interval dosing, should be used for pregnant patients and for those with endocarditis, burns that cover more than 20% of the body, cystic fibrosis, anasarca, and creatinine clearance ($Cr_{Cl}$) of less than 20 ml/minute.

**B. Extended-interval dosing** of aminoglycosides is an alternative method of administration and is more convenient than traditional dosing for most indications. Extended-interval doses are given in the following sections with each drug. A drug level is obtained 6–14 hours after the first dose, and a nomogram (Fig. 12-1) is consulted to determine the subsequent dosing interval. Monitoring includes obtaining a drug level at 6–14 hours after the dosage at least every week and a serum creatinine three times a week. In patients who are not responding to therapy, a 12-hour level should be checked, and if that level is undetectable, extended-interval dosing should be abandoned in favor of traditional dosing. For obese patients (actual weight >20% above ideal body weight), an obese dosing weight should be used for determining doses for both traditional and extended-interval methods.

**C. Specific agents**

1. **Gentamicin** is the least expensive antibiotic in this class. Traditional dosing is an initial loading dose of 2 mg/kg IV (2–3 mg/kg in the critically ill) followed by 1.0–1.7 mg/kg IV q8h (peak, 4–10 μg/ml; trough, <2 μg/ml). Extended-interval dosing is an initial 5 mg/kg, with the subsequent dosing interval determined by a nomogram (Fig. 12-1).
2. **Tobramycin** traditional dosing is an initial loading dose of 2 mg/kg IV (2–3 mg/kg in the critically ill) followed by 1.0–1.7 mg/kg IV q8h (peak, 4–10 μg/ml; trough, <2 μg/ml). Extended-interval dosing is an initial 5 mg/kg, with the subsequent dosing interval determined by a nomogram (Fig. 12-1). Tobramycin is also available as an inhalational agent for adjunctive therapy for patients with cystic fibrosis or bronchiectasis complicated by *P. aeruginosa* infection (300 mg inhalation bid).
3. **Amikacin** has an additional unique role in mycobacterial and *Nocardia* infections. Traditional dosing is an initial loading dose of 5.0–7.5 mg/kg IV (7.5–9.0 mg/kg in the critically ill) followed by 5 mg/kg IV q8h or 7.5 mg/kg IV q12h (peak, 20–35 μg/ml; trough, <10 μg/ml). Extended-interval dosing is 15 mg/kg, with the subsequent dosing interval determined by a nomogram (Fig. 12-1).

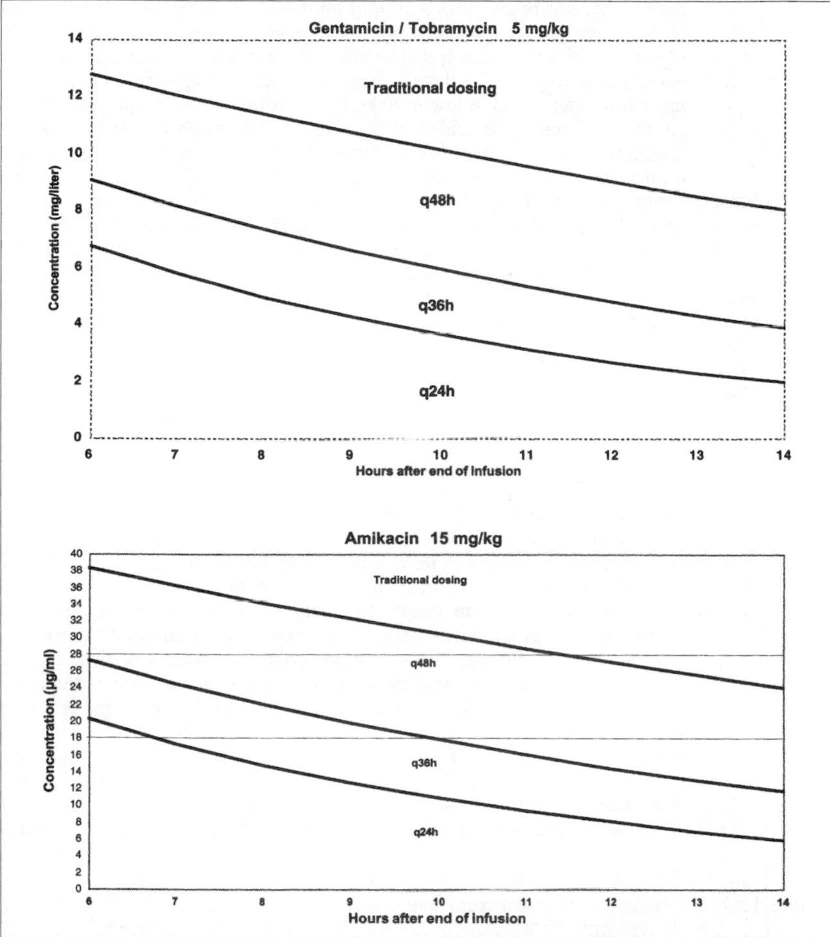


**Fig. 12-1.** Nomograms for extended-interval aminoglycoside dosing. (Adapted from RM Reichley, JR Little, TC Bailey, Barnes-Jewish Hospital and Washington University School of Medicine.)

4. **Streptomycin** is most commonly used for treating drug-resistant tuberculosis (TB; 15 mg/kg/day IM; the maximum dose per day is 1 g for daily dosing and 1.5 g for twice- or thrice-weekly dosing) and enterococcal endocarditis (7.5 mg/kg IM/IV q12h; maximum, 500 mg q12h). It generally has less gram-negative activity than the other aminoglycosides and no activity against *P. aeruginosa*. Other indications for streptomycin (tularemia, brucellosis, plague) have largely been supplanted by gentamicin or other antibiotics.
5. **Adverse effects. Nephrotoxicity** is the major adverse effect of aminoglycosides. If possible, prolonged therapy with aminoglycosides should be monitored by health care professionals who routinely administer home IV therapy and with systematic monitoring of laboratory studies. Nephrotoxicity is reversible when detected early but can be permanent, especially in patients with tenuous renal function due to other medical

conditions. Aminoglycosides should be used cautiously or avoided, if possible, in patients with decompensated liver disease. Ototoxicity (vestibular or cochlear) is also possible and requires weekly hearing tests with extended therapy (>14 days). Streptomycin is unique in that it causes more ototoxicity with a lower risk of nephrotoxicity. Concomitant administration of aminoglycosides with other known nephrotoxic agents (i.e., amphotericin B, foscarnet, nonsteroidal anti-inflammatory drugs, pentamidine, polymyxins, cidofovir, and cisplatin) should be avoided if possible.

**VI. Vancomycin** (15 mg/kg IV q12h; up to 30 mg/kg IV q12h for meningitis) is a glycopeptide antibiotic that kills gram-positive bacteria by interfering with cell wall synthesis. It binds a D-alanyl-D-alanine precursor that is critical for peptidoglycan cross-linking in most gram-positive (not gram-negative) bacterial cell walls. Vancomycin is bacteriostatic for enterococci. The **goal trough** is at least 5–15 μg/ml. Peak levels should generally only be measured in critically ill infected patients or in patients with endocarditis, osteomyelitis, meningitis, or other severe sequestered infections, with a goal of 30–45 μg/ml. **Patients with end-stage renal disease** should receive a single 15-mg/kg dose and then be redosed when the level drops below 10–15 μg/ml. Several factors, including the emergence of resistant nosocomial pathogens, low toxicity, and ease of administration, have led to an overuse of vancomycin and the evolution of vancomycin-resistant bacteria, most recently vancomycin-resistant *S. aureus* (VRSA).

**A. Indications for usage.** Today, most hospitals have serious problems with vancomycin-resistant *Enterococcus faecium* (VRE), and reports of vancomycin-intermediate *S. aureus* (VISA) and VRSA are increasing and will likely continue. See Table 12-1 for indications for vancomycin use.

**B. Vancomycin should not be used routinely** in the following circumstances: (1) routine surgical prophylaxis, (2) empiric therapy for nonseptic neutropenic fever, (3) treatment of single blood culture isolates of coagulase-negative staphylococcus or treatment of coagulase-negative staphylococcus blood cultures in cases in which the site of infection is inconsistent with the organism (e.g., community-acquired pneumonia or intra-abdominal infection), (4) routine treatment of *Clostridium difficile* colitis, (5) to complete a course of therapy in the absence of ORSA or ampicillin-resistant enterococci, (6) prophylaxis against catheter infections, and (7) use in topical application or irrigation. In dialysis patients, vancomycin use should be avoided in clinical situations in which

**Table 12-1.** Indications for vancomycin use

| |
|---|
| Treatment of serious infections caused by oxacillin-resistant *Staphylococcus aureus* (ORSA) |
| Treatment of serious infections caused by ampicillin-resistant enterococci |
| Treatment of serious infections caused by gram-positive bacteria in patients who are allergic to all other appropriate therapies |
| Oral treatment of *Clostridium difficile* colitis that has not responded to two courses of metronidazole or is failing metronidazole with a potentially life-threatening colitis |
| Surgical prophylaxis for placement of prosthetic devices at institutions with known high rates of ORSA or in patients who are known to be colonized with ORSA |
| Empiric use in suspected gram-positive meningitis until an organism has been identified and sensitivities confirmed |
| Life-threatening sepsis syndrome in a patient with known ORSA colonization or extended hospitalization until pathogen(s) are identified |
| Documented coagulase-negative staphylococcal endocarditis |
| Empiric use for serious dialysis catheter–related bloodstream infections until the results of blood culture data are available |

ORSA is unlikely. It should also be avoided in minor localized infections (e.g., cellulitis, carbuncles) well away from graft sites or catheters.

C. **Adverse effects.** Vancomycin is typically administered by slow IV infusion over at least 1 hour. More rapid infusion rates can cause the **red man syndrome,** which is a histamine-mediated reaction that is typically manifested by flushing and redness of the upper body (see Chap. 10, Allergy and Immunology).

VII. **Fluoroquinolones** kill bacteria by inhibiting bacterial DNA gyrase and topoisomerase, which are critical for DNA replication. In general, these antibiotics are well absorbed orally, with serum levels that approach those of parenteral therapy. These agents typically have poor activity against enterococci, although they may have some efficacy for enterococcal UTIs when other agents are inactive or contraindicated. Newer fluoroquinolones have activity against OSSA but should be considered only when oxacillin, nafcillin, and first-generation cephalosporins are contraindicated or inactive. Concomitant administration with aluminum- and magnesium-containing antacids, sucralfate, bismuth, oral iron, oral calcium, and oral zinc preparations can markedly impair absorption of all oral quinolones.

A. **Norfloxacin** (400 mg PO q12h) and **lomefloxacin** (400 mg PO qd) are useful for the treatment of UTIs caused by gram-negative rods; however, other fluoroquinolones are preferred in this setting. These agents are not used to treat systemic infections.

B. **Ciprofloxacin** [250–750 mg PO q12h or 500 mg PO qd (Cipro XR) or 200–400 mg IV q12h], **levofloxacin** (250–750 mg IV/PO q24h), and **ofloxacin** (200–400 mg IV or PO q12h) are active against gram-negative aerobes including many *AmpC* beta-lactamase–producing pathogens. These agents are commonly used for UTIs, pyelonephritis, infectious diarrhea, prostatitis, and intra-abdominal infections (with metronidazole). Ciprofloxacin is the most active quinolone against *P. aeruginosa* and is the quinolone of choice for serious infections with that pathogen. However, it has relatively poor activity against gram-positive cocci and anaerobes and should not be used as empiric monotherapy for community-acquired pneumonia, skin and soft-tissue infections, or intra-abdominal infections. Ciprofloxacin (500 mg), levofloxacin (250 mg), or ofloxacin (400 mg) can be used as single-dose therapy to treat gonorrhea. Oral and IV therapy with these agents give similar maximum serum levels; thus, oral therapy is appropriate unless contraindicated or coadministered with polyvalent metallic cations.

C. **Levofloxacin** (250–750 mg PO or IV q24h), **gatifloxacin** (400 mg PO/IV qd), and **moxifloxacin** (400 mg PO/IV qd) are newer fluoroquinolones with improved coverage of aerobic gram-positive bacteria (streptococci, staphylococci) and atypical respiratory pathogens (*Chlamydia pneumoniae, Mycoplasma, Legionella*) but less gram-negative activity (especially against *P. aeruginosa*) than ciprofloxacin. Moxifloxacin and gatifloxacin also have reasonable anaerobic activity, possibly expanding their role in mixed aerobic/anaerobic infections. These agents are useful for treatment of sinusitis, bronchitis, community-acquired pneumonia, and UTIs (except moxifloxacin, which is only minimally eliminated in the urine). They are reasonable therapy for soft-tissue infections if PCNs or cephalosporins are inactive or contraindicated. Some of these agents have activity against mycobacteria and have a potential role in treating drug-resistant TB and atypical mycobacterial infections.

D. **Adverse effects.** The principal adverse reactions with fluoroquinolones include nausea, CNS disturbances (drowsiness, headache, restlessness, and dizziness, especially in the elderly), rashes, and phototoxicity. Moxifloxacin, levofloxacin, and gatifloxacin can cause prolongation of the QTc interval and should not be used in patients who are receiving class I or class III antiarrhythmics, in patients with known electrolyte or conduction abnormalities, or in those who are taking other medications that prolong the QTc interval or induce bradycardia. These agents should also be used cautiously in the elderly, in whom asymptomatic conduction disturbances are more common. Fluoroquinolones should not be routinely used in patients younger than 18 years or in pregnant or lactating women due to the risk of arthropathy in pediatric patients. They may also cause an age-related arthropathy, particularly in elderly patients, and should be discontinued in individuals in whom joint pain or tendonitis (especially the Achilles tendon) develops. **This class of antibiotics has major drug interactions** (see Appendix C, Drug Interactions).

**VIII. Macrolide antibiotics** are bacteriostatic agents that block protein synthesis in bacteria by binding the 50S subunit of the bacterial ribosome. This class of antibiotics has activity against gram-positive cocci, including streptococci and staphylococci, and some upper respiratory gram-negative bacteria, with minimal activity against enteric gram-negative rods. They are commonly used to treat pharyngitis, otitis media, sinusitis, and bronchitis, especially in PCN-allergic patients, and are among the drugs of choice for treating *Legionella*, *Chlamydia*, and *Mycoplasma* infections. The newer macrolides can be used as monotherapy for nonbacteremic community-acquired pneumonia and have a unique role in the treatment and prophylaxis of *Mycobacterium avium* complex (MAC) infections in patients with HIV (see Chap. 14, Human Immunodeficiency Virus Infection and Acquired Immunodeficiency Syndrome). Many PCN-resistant strains of pneumococci are also resistant to macrolides.

**A. Erythromycin** (250–500 mg PO qid or 0.5–1.0 g IV q6h) possesses activity against gram-positive cocci (except enterococci) and can be used to treat bronchitis, pharyngitis, sinusitis, otitis media, and soft-tissue infections in PCN-allergic patients. It is effective for treatment of atypical respiratory tract infections due to *Legionella pneumophila* (1 g IV q6h), *C. pneumoniae*, and *Mycoplasma pneumoniae*. However, there is significant resistance to erythromycin among *Haemophilus influenzae* species, and therefore, efficacy of this drug for upper and lower respiratory tract infections is decreased. It can also be used for treatment of *Chlamydia trachomatis* infections (500 mg PO qid for 7 days) and as an alternate therapy for syphilis in PCN-allergic patients.

**B. Clarithromycin** (250–500 mg PO bid) has a spectrum of activity similar to that of erythromycin but with enhanced activity against some respiratory pathogens (especially *Haemophilus*). It is commonly used to treat bronchitis, sinusitis, otitis media, pharyngitis, soft-tissue infections, and community-acquired pneumonia. It has a prominent role in treating MAC infections in HIV patients and is an important component of regimens used to eradicate *Helicobacter pylori* (see Chap. 16, Gastrointestinal Diseases).

**C. Azithromycin** (500 mg PO × 1 day, then 250 mg PO qd × 4 days, 250–500 mg PO qd, 500 mg PO qd × 3 days, 500 mg IV qd) has a similar spectrum of activity to clarithromycin and is commonly used to treat bronchitis, sinusitis, otitis media, pharyngitis, soft-tissue infections, and community-acquired pneumonia. It has a prominent role in MAC prophylaxis (1200 mg PO qwk) and treatment (250–500 mg PO qd) in HIV patients. It is also commonly used to treat *C. trachomatis* infections (1 g PO single dose). An advantage of azithromycin is that it does not have the numerous drug interactions seen with erythromycin and clarithromycin.

**D. Dirithromycin** (500 mg PO qd) has a similar spectrum of activity and clinical application as erythromycin with the convenience of once-a-day dosing. Like azithromycin, it does not have the numerous drug interactions seen with erythromycin and clarithromycin.

**E. Clindamycin** (150–450 mg PO tid–qid or 600–900 mg IV q8h) is chemically classified as a lincosamide (related to macrolides), with a predominantly gram-positive spectrum similar to that of erythromycin and additional inclusion of activity against most anaerobes, including *B. fragilis*. It has excellent oral bioavailability (90%) and penetrates into bone and abscess cavities. In adults it is used for treatment of aspiration pneumonia and lung abscesses. A significant number of ORSA isolates remain susceptible to clindamycin, and the agent can be used as alternate chronic suppressive (not primary) therapy in this setting. It is typically used as a second agent in combination therapy for invasive streptococcal infections to decrease toxin production. It is also used for treatment of suspected anaerobic infections (peritonsillar/retropharyngeal abscesses, necrotizing fasciitis), except intra-abdominal infections, for which metronidazole is more commonly used (due to its more reliable activity against *B. fragilis*). Clindamycin has additional uses, including treatment of babesiosis (in combination with quinine), toxoplasmosis (in combination with pyrimethamine), and *Pneumocystis carinii* pneumonia (PCP; in combination with primaquine).

F. **Adverse effects.** Macrolides and clindamycin are associated with nausea, abdominal cramping, and LFT abnormalities (particularly erythromycin). Liver function profiles should be checked intermittently during extended therapy. Hypersensitivity reactions with prominent skin rash are more common with clindamycin, as is pseudomembranous colitis secondary to *C. difficile*. **Erythromycin and clarithromycin have major drug interactions** caused by inhibition of the cytochrome P-450 system (see Appendix C, Drug Interactions).

IX. **Sulfamethoxazole, sulfadiazine, sulfisoxazole, trimetrexate, and trimethoprim** slowly kill bacteria by inhibiting folic acid metabolism. This class of antibiotics is most commonly used for uncomplicated UTIs, sinusitis, and otitis media. They also have unique roles in treatment of PCP, *Nocardia*, *Toxoplasma*, and *Stenotrophomonas* infections.

A. **Sulfamethoxazole** (2 g PO, then 1 g PO q12h), **sulfisoxazole** (1 g PO q6h), and **trimethoprim** (100 mg PO bid) are occasionally used as monotherapy for treatment of UTIs. These drugs are more logically used in the combination preparations outlined in the following sections. Trimethoprim in combination with dapsone is an alternate therapy for mild PCP pneumonia (see Chap. 13, Treatment of Infectious Diseases).

B. **Trimethoprim/sulfamethoxazole** is a combination antibiotic (IV or PO) with a 1:5 ratio of trimethoprim to sulfamethoxazole. The IV preparation is dosed at 5 mg/kg IV q8h (based on the trimethoprim component) for serious infections. The oral preparations [160 mg trimethoprim/800 mg sulfamethoxazole per double-strength (DS) tablet] are extensively bioavailable, with similar drug levels obtained with IV and with PO formulations. Both components have excellent tissue penetration, including bone, prostate, and CNS. The combination has a broad spectrum of activity but typically does not inhibit *P. aeruginosa* or anaerobes. It is the therapy of choice for PCP (see Chap. 14, Human Immunodeficiency Virus Infection and Acquired Immunodeficiency Syndrome), *Stenotrophomonas maltophilia*, *Tropheryma whippelii*, and *Nocardia* infections. It is commonly used for treating sinusitis, otitis media, bronchitis, prostatitis, and UTIs (1 DS PO bid). Some strains of ORSA remain susceptible to trimethoprim/sulfamethoxazole, and the agent can be used as alternate chronic suppressive (not primary) therapy in this setting. It is used as PCP prophylaxis (1 DS PO twice a week, three times a week, or single strength or DS daily) in solid organ transplant patients, bone marrow transplant patients, patients receiving fludarabine, and HIV patients. IV therapy is routinely converted to the PO equivalent for patients who require prolonged therapy. For serious infections, such as *Nocardia* brain abscesses, it may be useful to monitor sulfamethoxazole peaks (100–150 μg/ml) and troughs (50–100 μg/ml) occasionally during the course of therapy and to adjust dosing accordingly. In patients with renal insufficiency, doses can be adjusted by following trimethoprim peaks (5–10 μg/ml). Prolonged therapy can cause bone marrow suppression, possibly requiring treatment with leucovorin (5–10 mg PO qd) until cell counts normalize.

C. **Sulfadiazine** (1.0–1.5 g PO q6h) in combination with pyrimethamine (200 mg PO followed by 50–75 mg PO qd) and leucovorin (10–20 mg PO qd) is the therapy of choice for toxoplasmosis. Sulfadiazine is also occasionally used to treat *Nocardia* infections.

D. **Trimetrexate** (45 mg/m$^2$ IV qd) combined with leucovorin (20 mg/m$^2$ PO or IV q6h continued for 3 days after the last dose of trimetrexate) is an alternate (salvage) therapy for PCP infections. Bone marrow suppression, renal insufficiency, and hepatotoxicity may occur.

**E. Adverse effects.** These drugs are associated with cholestatic jaundice, bone marrow suppression, interstitial nephritis, "false" elevations in serum creatinine, and severe hypersensitivity reactions (Stevens-Johnson syndrome/ erythema multiforme). Nausea is common with higher doses. **All patients should be asked whether they are allergic to "sulfa drugs,"** and specific commercial names should be mentioned (i.e., Bactrim or Septra).

**X. Chloramphenicol** (12.5–25.0 mg/kg IV q6h; maximum, 1 g IV q6h) is a bacteriostatic antibiotic that binds to the 50S ribosomal subunit, blocking protein synthesis in susceptible bacteria. It has broad activity against aerobic and anaerobic gram-positive and gram-negative bacteria, including *S. aureus*, enterococci, and enteric gram-negative rods. It also is active against spirochetes, *Rickettsia*, *Mycoplasma*, and *Chlamydia*. Today it is used almost exclusively for serious VRE infections. Because of its excellent CNS penetration, it also plays a role for treatment of meningitis caused by susceptible organisms in PCN-allergic patients and for meningitis caused by *Francisella tularensis* or *Yersinia pestis*. **Adverse effects** include idiosyncratic aplastic anemia (~1/30,000) and dose-related bone marrow suppression. Peak drug levels (1 hour postinfusion) should be checked every 3–4 days (goal peak <25 μg/ml) and doses adjusted accordingly. Dosage adjustment is necessary in the presence of significant liver disease. **This class of antibiotics has major drug interactions** (see Appendix C, Drug Interactions).

**XI. Metronidazole** (250–750 mg PO/IV q6–12h) kills anaerobic bacteria and some protozoa by accumulation of toxic metabolites that interfere with multiple biologic processes. It has excellent tissue penetration, including abscess cavities, bone, and CNS. Metronidazole has greater activity against gram-negative than gram-positive anaerobes but is active against *Clostridium perfringens* and *C. difficile*. It is the treatment of choice as monotherapy for *C. difficile* colitis and bacterial vaginosis, and it can be used in combination with other antibiotics to treat intra-abdominal infections and brain abscesses (see Chap. 13, Treatment of Infectious Diseases). Protozoal infections that are routinely treated with metronidazole include *Giardia*, *Entamoeba histolytica*, and *Trichomonas vaginalis*. A dose reduction may be warranted for patients with decompensated liver disease. **Adverse effects** include nausea, dysgeusia, disulfiram-like reactions to alcohol, and mild CNS disturbances (headache, restlessness). Rarely, this medication is associated with seizures and peripheral neuropathy.

**XII. Tetracyclines** are bacteriostatic antibiotics that bind the 30S ribosomal subunit, blocking protein synthesis. These agents have unique roles in the treatment of *Rickettsia*, *Ehrlichia*, *Chlamydia*, *Nocardia*, and *Mycoplasma* infections. They are used as therapy for Lyme disease–related arthritis and as alternate therapy for syphilis and *P. multocida* in PCN-allergic patients. Their general use is limited because of widespread resistance among more common bacterial pathogens.

**A. Tetracycline** (250–500 mg PO q6h) is commonly used for severe acne and in some *H. pylori* eradication regimens (see Chap. 16, Gastrointestinal Diseases). It can also be used for treatment of acute Lyme borreliosis, Rocky Mountain spotted fever, ehrlichiosis, psittacosis, *Mycoplasma* pneumonia, *Chlamydia* pneumonia, and chlamydial infections of the eye or genitourinary tract, but these infections are generally treated with doxycycline or other antibiotics. Aluminum- and magnesium-containing antacids and preparations that contain oral calcium, oral iron, or other cations can significantly impair oral absorption of tetracycline and should be avoided within 2 hours of the dose.

**B. Doxycycline** (100 mg PO/IV q12h) is the most commonly used tetracycline and is standard therapy for *C. trachomatis*, Rocky Mountain spotted fever, ehrlichiosis, and psittacosis. This agent also has a role for malaria prophylaxis and for treatment of community-acquired pneumonia.

**C. Minocycline** (200 mg IV/PO, then 100 mg IV/PO q12h) is similar to doxycycline in its spectrum of activity and clinical indications. It is second-line therapy for pulmonary nocardiosis and cervicofacial actinomycosis.

**D. Adverse effects.** Nausea and photosensitivity are common side effects. Patients should be warned about sun exposure. Rarely, these medications are associated with pseudotumor cerebri. **They should not routinely be given to children or to pregnant or lactating women** because they can cause tooth enamel discoloration in young children. Minocycline is associated with vestibular disturbances.

**XIII. Streptogramins** are a new class of antimicrobial agents that complex with bacterial ribosomes to inhibit protein synthesis.

**A. Quinupristin/dalfopristin** (7.5 mg/kg IV q8h) is the first U.S. Food and Drug Administration (FDA)–approved drug in this class. This antibiotic has activity against antibiotic-resistant gram-positive organisms, especially VRE, ORSA, VISA, and antibiotic-resistant strains of *Streptococcus pneumoniae*. It has some activity against gram-negative upper respiratory pathogens (*Haemophilus* and *Moraxella*) and anaerobes, but more appropriate antibiotics are available to treat these infections. Quinupristin/dalfopristin is bacteriostatic for enterococci and can be used for treatment of serious infections with VISA and VRE (however, it has little activity against *Enterococcus faecalis*). It can also be used for treatment of serious infections with ORSA and *S. pneumoniae* when vancomycin cannot be tolerated. This antibiotic may be an alternative for VRSA infections.

**B. Adverse effects** include arthralgias and myalgias, which occur frequently and can necessitate discontinuation of therapy. IV site pain and thrombophlebitis are common when the drug is administered through a peripheral vein. It has also been associated with elevated LFTs and, as it is primarily cleared by hepatic metabolism, patients with significant hepatic impairment require a dose adjustment. Quinupristin/dalfopristin is similar to erythromycin with regard to drug interactions (see Appendix C, Drug Interactions).

**XIV. Oxazolidinones** are a new class of antibiotics that block assembly of bacterial ribosomes to inhibit protein synthesis. **Linezolid** (600 mg IV/PO bid) is the first FDA-approved drug in this class, and IV and oral formulations produce equivalent serum levels. It has potent activity against gram-positive bacteria, including drug-resistant enterococci, staphylococci, and streptococci. Its activity against ORSA is comparable to that of vancomycin. However, it has no meaningful activity against Enterobacteriaceae and borderline activity against *Moraxella* and *H. influenzae*. **Use of linezolid should be restricted** to serious infections with VRE, for patients with an indication for vancomycin therapy who are intolerant of that medication, and possibly for oral therapy of ORSA infections when IV access is unavailable. Supporting data for treatment of osteomyelitis, endocarditis, and meningitis are minimal, and routine use for these infections cannot be recommended without additional clinical data. Resistance develops to this antibiotic, and it is imperative that abscesses be adequately drained to minimize this risk. Linezolid is well tolerated, and its principal **adverse effects** are diarrhea, nausea, and headaches. Thrombocytopenia occurs frequently in patients who receive greater than 2 weeks of therapy, and serial platelet count monitoring is indicated in this setting. A CBC, serum creatinine, and LFTs should be checked every 1–2 weeks during prolonged therapy with this new agent. **Linezolid has several important drug interactions.** It is a mild monoamine oxidase inhibitor, and patients should be advised not to take selective serotonin reuptake inhibitors while on the drug to avoid the serotonin syndrome. Over-the-counter cold remedies that contain pseudoephedrine or phenylpropanolamine should also be avoided, as coadministration with linezolid can elevate BP. Linezolid does not require dose adjustments for renal or hepatic dysfunction.

**XV. Daptomycin** (4 mg/kg IV q24h) belongs to a new class of antibiotics called the cyclic lipopeptides. The drug exhibits rapid bactericidal activity against a wide variety of gram-positive bacteria, including enterococci, staphylococci, and streptococci. Daptomycin also maintains activity against many of the bacteria that have become resistant to methicillin and vancomycin, and is currently FDA approved for treatment of complicated skin and skin structure infections.

**Adverse effects** include GI disturbances, injection site reactions, elevated liver function tests, and elevated creatine phosphokinase. Serum creatine phosphokinase should be monitored weekly, as daptomycin has been associated with skeletal muscle effects. Patients should also be monitored for signs of muscle weakness and pain, and the drug should be discontinued if these symptoms develop in conjunction with marked creatine phosphokinase elevations. Consideration should also be given to avoiding concomitant use of daptomycin and HMG-CoA reductase inhibitors due to the potential increased risk of myopathy.

**XVI. Fosfomycin** (3-g sachet dissolved in cold water PO once) is a bactericidal oral antibiotic that kills bacteria by inhibiting an early step in cell wall synthesis. It has a spectrum of activity that includes most urinary tract pathogens, including *P. aeruginosa*, *Enterobacter* species, and enterococci (including VRE). It is most useful for treating uncomplicated UTIs in women with susceptible strains of *E. coli* and *E. faecalis*. It should not be used to treat pyelonephritis or systemic infections. It should only be administered once, as therapeutic drug levels are maintained in the urine for approximately 48 hours. The most common **adverse effect** is diarrhea. Fosfomycin should not be taken with metoclopramide, as that drug interferes with fosfomycin absorption.

**XVII. Nitrofurantoin** (50–100 mg PO macrocrystals qid or 100 mg PO dual-release formulation bid for 5–7 days) is a bactericidal oral antibiotic that is useful for uncomplicated UTIs except those caused by *Proteus*, *P. aeruginosa*, or *Serratia*. The drug is metabolized by bacteria into toxic intermediates that inhibit multiple bacterial processes. It has had a modest resurgence in use, as it is frequently effective against uncomplicated VRE UTIs. Although it was commonly used in the past for UTI prophylaxis, this practice should be avoided, as prolonged therapy is associated with chronic pulmonary syndromes that can be fatal. Nitrofurantoin should not be used for pyelonephritis or any other systemic infections. Nausea is the most common **adverse effect,** and the drug should be taken with food to minimize this problem. Patients should be warned that their urine may become brown secondary to the medication. Furthermore, it should not be used in patients with an elevated serum creatinine, as the risk for development of treatment-associated neuropathy may be increased. Nitrofurantoin should not be given with probenecid, as this combination decreases the concentration of nitrofurantoin in the urine.

**XVIII. Methenamine** [methenamine hippurate or methenamine mandelate; 1 or 2 tablets (depending on the specific preparation) PO qid] is a urine/bladder antiseptic that is converted into formaldehyde in the urine when the pH is less than 6.0. Because the active drug is formaldehyde, most bacteria and fungi are potentially susceptible to therapy. The formaldehyde is generated while urine is retained in the bladder; therefore, methenamine is effective only in the lower urinary tract, and its efficacy is impaired in the setting of a draining Foley catheter. These drugs are rarely used because of the large number of alternative antibiotics that are available today. They do have a limited role in treating uncomplicated UTI caused by multiple drug–resistant bacteria or yeast. **Adverse effects** include bladder irritation, dysuria, and hematuria with prolonged use. Therapy should be limited to a maximum of 3 weeks at a time, and urine pH should be obtained once early during therapy to ensure an appropriately acidic pH. Vitamin C can be used to assist in urine acidification. **This drug is contraindicated** in the setting of glaucoma, significant renal insufficiency, and acidosis. It should not be given concomitantly with sulfonamides, as these drugs form an insoluble precipitate in the urine.

**XIX. Colistin** (colistimethate sodium; polymyxin E; IV therapy is 2.5–5.0 mg/kg/day divided into 2–4 doses; maximum dose, 5 mg/kg/day) and **polymyxin B** [12,000–15,000 U/kg/day by continuous infusion (500,000 U in 500 ml 5% dextrose in water; adjust rate to achieve desired daily dosing)] are bactericidal polypeptide antibiotics that kill by disrupting the cell membrane of gram-negative bacteria. These drugs have roles in the treatment of multiple drug–resistant gram-negative rods, predominantly *P. aeruginosa*, in patients with cystic fibrosis or bronchiectasis. **These medications should only be given under the guidance of an experienced cli-**

**nician,** as parenteral therapy has significant CNS side effects and potential nephrotoxicity. **Inhaled colistin** (75 mg given by standard nebulizer tid) is better tolerated, with only mild upper airway irritation, and has some efficacy as adjunctive therapy for *P. aeruginosa*. **Adverse effects** with parenteral therapy include paresthesias, slurred speech, peripheral numbness, tingling, and significant dose-dependent nephrotoxicity. The dosage should be carefully reduced in patients with renal insufficiency, as overdosage in this setting can result in neuromuscular blockade and apnea. If CNS side effects are significant with twice-daily dosing of colistin, four times daily dosing or continuous infusion (total daily dose in 500 ml 5% dextrose in water infused over 24 hours) should be arranged. Serum creatinine should be monitored daily early in therapy and then at a regular interval for the duration of therapy. **These antibiotics should not be coadministered with aminoglycosides, other known nephrotoxins, or neuromuscular blockers.**

## Antituberculous Agents

Effective therapy of *Mycobacterium tuberculosis* (MTB) infections requires combination chemotherapy designed to prevent the emergence of resistant organisms and maximize efficacy. Increased resistance to conventional antituberculous agents has led to the use of more complex regimens and has made susceptibility testing an integral part of TB management (see Chap. 13, Treatment of Infectious Diseases).

I. **Isoniazid** (INH, 300 mg PO qd) kills susceptible mycobacteria by interfering with the synthesis of the lipid components of the cell wall. It is well absorbed orally and has good penetration throughout the body including the CNS. INH is a component of nearly all treatment regimens and can be given twice a week in directly observed therapy (15 mg/kg/dose; 900 mg maximum). INH remains the drug of choice for recent purified protein derivative (PPD) conversions (300 mg PO qd for 9 months). **Adverse effects** include elevations in liver transaminases (20%). This effect can be idiosyncratic but is usually seen in the setting of underlying liver disease or concomitant consumption of alcohol and may be potentiated by rifampin. Transaminase elevations to greater than threefold the upper limit of the normal range necessitate holding therapy. Patients with known liver dysfunction should have weekly LFTs during the initial stage of therapy. INH also antagonizes vitamin $B_6$ and potentially can cause a peripheral neuropathy. This can be avoided or minimized by coadministration of pyridoxine, 25–50 mg PO qd, especially in the elderly, in pregnant women, and in patients with diabetes, renal failure, alcoholism, and seizure disorders.

II. **Rifamycins** kill susceptible mycobacteria by inhibiting DNA-dependent RNA polymerase, thereby halting transcription.

   A. **Rifampin** (600 mg PO qd or twice a week) is active against many gram-positive and gram-negative bacteria in addition to MTB. It is also used as adjunctive therapy in prosthetic valve endocarditis due to coagulase-negative staphylococci (300 mg PO q8h), for prophylaxis of close contacts of patients with infection caused by *Neisseria meningitidis* (600 mg PO q12h), and as adjunctive treatment of osteomyelitis associated with prosthetic material or devices. The drug is well absorbed orally and is widely distributed throughout the body including the cerebrospinal fluid (CSF).

   B. **Rifabutin** (300 mg PO qd) is principally used to treat TB and MAC infections in HIV-positive patients who are receiving highly active antiretroviral therapy, as it has less deleterious effects on protease inhibitor metabolism than does rifampin (see Chap. 14, Human Immunodeficiency Virus Infection and Acquired Immunodeficiency Syndrome).

   C. **Rifapentine** (600 mg PO twice a week for 2 months, then qwk to complete therapy) is a rifamycin that appears to be associated with more TB relapses than rifampin; therefore, it is typically not used as a first-line drug.

D. **Adverse effects.** Patients should be warned about reddish-orange discoloration of body fluids, and contact lenses should not be worn during treatment. Rash, GI disturbances, hepatitis, and interstitial nephritis can occur. Uveitis has been associated with rifabutin and hyperuricemia with rifapentine. **This class of antibiotics has major drug interactions** (see Appendix C, Drug Interactions).

III. **Pyrazinamide** (15–30 mg/kg PO qd; maximum, 2 g or 50–75 mg/kg PO twice a week; maximum, 4 g/dose) kills mycobacteria replicating in macrophages by an unknown mechanism. It is well absorbed orally and widely distributed throughout the body including the CSF. Pyrazinamide is typically used for the first 2 months of therapy. **Adverse effects** include hyperuricemia and hepatitis.

IV. **Ethambutol** (15–25 mg/kg PO qd or 50–75 mg/kg PO twice a week; maximum, 2.5 g/dose) is bacteriostatic with an unknown mechanism of action. It is included in initial TB regimens in areas where the prevalence of INH-resistant TB is greater than or equal to 4%. Doses should be reduced in the presence of renal dysfunction. **Adverse effects** include optic neuritis, which manifests as decreased red-green color perception, decreased visual acuity, or visual field deficits. Baseline and monthly visual examinations should be performed during therapy.

V. **Streptomycin** is an aminoglycoside that can be used as a substitute for ethambutol and for drug-resistant MTB. It does not adequately penetrate the CNS and should not be used for TB meningitis (see Antibacterial Agents, sec. **V.C.4**).

## Antiviral Agents

Current antiviral agents only suppress viral replication. Viral containment or elimination requires an intact host immune response.

I. **Anti-influenza drugs** include two recent drugs, zanamivir and oseltamivir, that block influenza A and B neuraminidases. This enzymatic activity is necessary for successful viral egress and release from infected cells. These drugs have shown modest activity in clinical trials, with a 1- to 2-day improvement in symptoms in patients who are symptomatic for no longer than 48 hours. However, annual influenza vaccination remains the intervention of choice for all high-risk patients and health care workers (see Appendix F, Immunizations and Post-Exposure Therapies).

A. **Amantadine and rimantadine** (100 mg PO bid for both; 100 mg PO qd in elderly patients, dialysis patients, or those with decompensated liver disease) prevent influenza A entry into cells by blocking endosomal acidification, which is necessary for fusion of the viral envelope with the host cell membrane. These agents have no activity against influenza B. They are effective when therapy is initiated within 48 hours of initial symptoms and continued for 7–10 days. Patients at high risk of complications (e.g., immunocompromised patients, the elderly, diabetics, dialysis patients, and patients with pulmonary or cardiac disease) should probably be treated even after 48 hours of symptoms in the absence of studies that specifically address the treatment of high-risk patients. These drugs can also be used for influenza prophylaxis in nonimmune individuals who have been exposed to the virus and in patients and staff members of nursing homes or hospitals during an epidemic. **Adverse effects** include GI disturbances and CNS dysfunction, including dizziness, nervousness, confusion, slurring of speech, blurred vision, and sleep disturbances. Rimantadine has fewer side effects than amantadine.

B. **Zanamivir** [10 mg (2 inhalations) q12h for 5 days, started within 48 hours of the onset of symptoms] is an inhaled neuraminidase inhibitor that is active against influenza A and B. Zanamivir is indicated for treatment of uncomplicated acute influenza infection in adults and adolescents older than 12 years of age who have been symptomatic for less than 48 hours. When used within

30 hours of the onset of influenza symptoms, zanamivir reduces the duration of symptoms by an average of 1–2 days. Limited evidence of its successful use for influenza prophylaxis has been shown, although it is currently not FDA approved for this use. **Adverse effects** of zanamivir include headache, GI disturbances, dizziness, and upper respiratory symptoms. Bronchospasm or declines in lung function, or both, may occur in patients with underlying respiratory disorders and may require a rapid-acting bronchodilator for control.

**C. Oseltamivir** (75 mg PO bid for 5 days) is an orally administered neuraminidase inhibitor that is active against influenza A and B. It is indicated for treatment of uncomplicated acute influenza in adults who have been symptomatic for less than 2 days and for prophylaxis of influenza after exposures. When used for treatment of influenza within 40 hours of the onset of influenza symptoms, oseltamivir was associated with a 1.3-day reduction in median time to clinical improvement. The most common **adverse effects** are nausea, vomiting, and diarrhea. Dizziness and headache may also occur.

**II. Antiherpetic agents** are nucleotide analogs that inhibit viral DNA synthesis.

**A. Acyclovir** [400 mg PO tid for herpes simplex virus (HSV), 800 mg PO 5 times a day for localized varicella-zoster virus (VZV) infections, 5 mg/kg IV q8h for severe HSV infections, and 10 mg/kg IV q8h for severe VZV infections and HSV encephalitis] is active against HSV and VZV. The drug has no effect on herpes viruses that are latent. Acyclovir is indicated for treatment of primary and recurrent genital herpes, severe herpetic stomatitis, and herpes simplex encephalitis. It is also used for herpes zoster ophthalmicus, disseminated primary VZV in adults (significant morbidity compared to the childhood illness), and severe disseminated primary VZV in children. It can be used as prophylaxis in patients who have frequent HSV recurrences (400 mg PO bid). **Adverse effects,** including a reversible crystalline nephropathy, may occur; preexisting renal failure, dehydration, and IV bolus dosing increase the risk of this effect. Rare cases of CNS disturbances, including delirium, tremors, and seizures, may also occur, particularly with high doses, in patients with renal failure and in the elderly.

**B. Valacyclovir** (1000 mg PO q8h for herpes zoster, 1000 mg PO q12h for initial episode of genital HSV infection, and 500 mg PO q12h or 1000 mg qd for recurrent episodes of HSV) is an orally administered prodrug of acyclovir used for the treatment of acute herpes zoster infections and for treatment or suppression of genital HSV infection. The most common **adverse effect** is nausea. Valacyclovir rarely can cause CNS disturbances, and high doses (8 g/day) have been associated with development of hemolytic-uremic syndrome/thrombotic thrombocytopenic purpura in immunocompromised patients, including those with HIV and bone marrow and solid organ transplants.

**C. Famciclovir** (500 mg PO q8h for herpes zoster, 250 mg PO q8h for the initial episode of genital HSV infection, and 125 mg PO q12h for recurrent episodes of genital HSV infection) is an orally administered antiviral agent used for the treatment of acute herpes zoster reactivation and for treatment or suppression of genital HSV infections. **Adverse effects** include headache, nausea, and diarrhea.

**D. Ganciclovir** [5 mg/kg IV q12h for 14–21 days for induction therapy of cytomegalovirus (CMV) retinitis, followed by 6 mg/kg IV for 5 days every week or 5 mg/kg IV qd; the oral dose is 1000 mg PO tid with food] is used to treat CMV. It has activity against HSV and VZV, but safer drugs are available to treat those infections. The drug is widely distributed in the body, including the CSF. It is indicated for treatment of CMV retinitis in immunocompromised patients and is also useful for other CMV diseases. Indefinite maintenance therapy generally is required to suppress CMV disease in patients with AIDS. **Valganciclovir** (900 mg PO qd–bid) is the oral prodrug of ganciclovir; it has excellent bioavailability and can be used for treatment of CMV retinitis and, thus, has supplanted the use of oral ganciclovir, which has poor oral bioavailability. The major **adverse effect** that limits ganciclovir therapy is neutropenia, which may require the addition of granulocyte colony-stimulating factor for management (300 mg SC qd–qwk). Thrombocytopenia, rash, confusion, headache, nephrotoxicity, and GI disturbances may also occur. Blood counts and electrolytes should be monitored weekly while the patient is receiving therapy. Other agents with nephrotoxic or bone marrow suppressive effects may enhance the adverse effects of ganciclovir.

E. **Foscarnet** (60 mg/kg IV q8h or 90 mg/kg IV q12h for 14–21 days as induction therapy, followed by 90–120 mg/kg IV qd as maintenance therapy for CMV; 40 mg/kg IV q8h for acyclovir-resistant HSV and VZV) is used to treat CMV retinitis in patients with AIDS. It is typically considered for use in patients who are not tolerating or responding to ganciclovir. Foscarnet is occasionally used for CMV disease in bone marrow transplant patients to avoid the bone marrow–suppressive effects of ganciclovir. It also has a role in treatment of acyclovir-resistant HSV/VZV infections or ganciclovir-resistant CMV infections. It has numerous **adverse effects,** the main one being nephrotoxicity. $Cr_{Cl}$ should be measured at baseline and repeated monthly during prolonged therapy. Electrolytes ($PO_4$, $Ca^{2+}$, $Mg^{2+}$, $K^+$) and serum creatinine should be checked twice a week. Normal saline (500–1000 ml) should be given before and during infusions to minimize nephrotoxicity. This drug should be avoided in patients with a serum creatinine of greater than 2.8 mg/dl or baseline $Cr_{Cl}$ of less than 50 ml/minute. Concomitant use of other nephrotoxins (e.g., amphotericin, aminoglycosides, pentamidine, nonsteroidal anti-inflammatory drugs, cisplatin, or cidofovir) also should be avoided. Foscarnet chelates divalent cations and can cause tetany even with normal serum calcium levels. Use of foscarnet with pentamidine can cause severe hypocalcemia. Other side effects include seizures, phlebitis, rash, and genital ulcers. **Prolonged therapy with foscarnet should be monitored by physicians who are experienced with administration of home IV therapy and can systematically monitor patients' laboratory results.**

F. **Cidofovir** (5 mg/kg IV qwk for 2 weeks as induction therapy, followed by 5 mg/kg IV q14d chronically as maintenance therapy) is used to treat CMV retinitis in patients with AIDS. Efficacy of the drug is not established for CMV in other organ systems or in patients without AIDS. It can be administered through a peripheral IV line. Nephrotoxicity is the most important adverse effect, and the drug should be avoided in patients with a $Cr_{Cl}$ of less than 55 ml/minute, a serum creatinine greater than 1.5 mg/dl, significant proteinuria, or a recent history of receipt of other nephrotoxic medications. **Each cidofovir dose should be administered with probenecid** (2 g PO 3 hours before the infusion and then 1 g at 2 and 8 hours after the infusion) along with 1 L normal saline IV 1–2 hours before the infusion to minimize nephrotoxicity. Patients should have a serum creatinine and urine protein checked before each dose of cidofovir is given. These patients should be followed by a physician regularly, as administration of this drug requires systematic monitoring of patients' laboratory studies.

## Antifungal Agents

I. **Amphotericin B** kills fungi by interacting with ergosterol to disrupt the fungal plasma membrane. Reformulation of this agent in various lipid complexes has decreased some of its adverse side effects.

A. **Amphotericin B deoxycholate** (standard; 0.3–1.25 mg/kg/day as a single infusion over 2–4 hours) is the mainstay of antifungal therapy for severely ill patients with fungal disease. A typical cumulative total dose for treatment of infection with noncandidal species is 1.0–1.5 g. It is not effective for *Pseudallescheria boydii* and some other uncommon fungal pathogens.

B. **Lipid complexed preparations** of amphotericin B, including amphotericin B lipid complex (5 mg/kg IV qd), liposomal amphotericin B (3–5 mg/kg IV qd), and amphotericin B colloidal dispersion (3–4 mg/kg IV qd), have decreased nephrotoxicity and are generally associated with fewer infusion-related reactions than amphotericin B deoxycholate. Despite these advantages, lipid complexed preparations have not yet been directly compared to standard amphotericin B therapy for most fungal infections. Based on currently available clinical data, no clear evidence exists for increased efficacy with the use of lipid complexed preparations, and minimal data are available that compare the lipid complexed preparations to each other. However, studies have shown lipid preparations to be at least equivalent and possibly slightly superior to standard amphotericin B for empiric therapy in neutropenic fevers.

C. The **major adverse effect** of all amphotericin B formulations, including the lipid formulations, is nephrotoxicity. Patients should receive 500–1000 ml normal saline before each infusion to minimize nephrotoxicity. Irreversible renal failure appears to be related to cumulative dosing. Therefore, concomitant administration of other known nephrotoxins should be avoided if possible. Common **infusion-related effects** include fever/chills, nausea, headache, and myalgias. Premedication with 500–1000 mg of acetaminophen and 50 mg of diphenhydramine may control many of these symptoms. More severe reactions may be prevented by premedication with hydrocortisone, 25–100 mg IV. Intolerable infusion-related chills can be managed with meperidine, 25–50 mg IV. Some advocate administration of a 1- to 5-mg test dose, but this is not routinely necessary. In addition, amphotericin B therapy is associated with **potassium and magnesium wasting** that generally requires supplementation. Serum creatinine and electrolytes (including $Mg^{2+}$ and $K^+$) should be monitored at least two to three times a week.

II. **Flucytosine** (25.0–37.5 mg/kg PO q6h) kills susceptible *Candida* and *Cryptococcus* species by interfering with DNA synthesis. Its main clinical uses are for treatment of cryptococcal meningitis and severe *Candida* infections in combination with amphotericin B. **Adverse effects** include dose-related bone marrow suppression and bloody diarrhea due to intestinal flora conversion of flucytosine to 5-fluorouracil. Peak drug levels should be monitored to keep peak levels between 50 and 100 μg/ml. Dose adjustment and close monitoring by levels are critical in the setting of renal insufficiency. LFTs should be obtained at least once a week.

III. **Azoles** are fungistatic agents that inhibit ergosterol synthesis.

A. **Itraconazole** (200–400 mg PO qd or 200 mg IV q12h for 4 doses, then 200 mg IV qd) is a triazole with broad-spectrum antifungal activity. It is commonly used to treat histoplasmosis, blastomycosis, and *Sporothrix* infections. Itraconazole is considered to be an alternative therapy for *Aspergillus* and is often used to consolidate a course of conventional amphotericin B. It can also be used to treat infections caused by dermatophytes, including onychomycosis of the toenails (200 mg PO qd for 12 weeks) and fingernails (200 mg PO bid for 1 week, with a 3-week interruption, and then a second course of 200 mg PO bid for 1 week). The capsules require adequate gastric acidity for absorption and, therefore, should be taken with food, whereas the liquid is not significantly affected by gastric acidity and is better absorbed on an empty stomach.

B. **Fluconazole** (100–400 mg PO/IV qd) is the drug of choice for localized candidal infections, such as UTIs, thrush, esophagitis, peritonitis, and hepatosplenic infection. It is also a viable agent for severe disseminated candidal infections and is a second-line agent for primary treatment of cryptococcal meningitis (400 mg PO qd for 10–12 weeks, then 200 mg PO qd). Fluconazole is also commonly used to suppress cryptococcal meningitis in immunocompromised patients (200 mg PO qd) after initial therapy with amphotericin B and flucytosine. Single-dose therapy is effective for vaginal yeast infections (150 mg PO once). Fluconazole does not, however, have activity against *Aspergillus* species and therefore should not be used for treatment of those infections. Its absorption is not dependent on gastric acid.

C. **Ketoconazole** (200–600 mg PO qd) is useful for treating histoplasmosis, blastomycosis, and chromomycosis infections outside of the CNS, but its use has been largely supplanted by the newer azole agents. It is also not effective for *Aspergillus* species. Its absorption is dependent on gastric acidity.

D. **Voriconazole** [loading dose of 6 mg/kg IV × 2 doses 12 hours apart followed by a maintenance dose of 4 mg/kg IV q12h or 200 mg PO bid (100 mg PO bid if <40 kg)] is a new triazole antifungal with a spectrum of activity against a wide range of pathogenic fungi. It has enhanced in vitro activity against all clinically important species of *Aspergillus*, as well as *Candida* (including non-*albicans*), *Scedosporium apiospermum*, *P. boydii*, and *Fusarium* species. Voriconazole is indicated for the treatment of invasive aspergillosis, for which it demonstrates typical response rates of 40–50% and superiority over conventional amphotericin B (*N Engl J Med* 347:408, 2002). One large trial showed fewer breakthrough fungal infections in febrile neutropenic patients who were empirically treated with voriconazole compared to liposomal amphotericin B but could not establish equivalence for overall response (*N Engl J Med* 346:225, 2002). Esophageal candidiasis and infections with *Scedosporium* and *Fusarium* species are also effectively treated with voriconazole.

An advantage of voriconazole is the easy transition from IV to PO therapy because of excellent bioavailability. For refractory diseases, a dose increase of 50% may be useful. The maintenance dose is cut in half for patients with moderate hepatic failure. Because of its metabolism through the cytochrome P-450 system (enzymes 2C19, 2C9, and 3A4), there are several **clinically significant drug interactions** that must be considered. Rifampin, rifabutin, carbamazepine (markedly reduce voriconazole levels), sirolimus (increased drug levels), and astemizole (prolonged QTc) are contraindicated while the patient is receiving voriconazole, and concomitantly administered cyclosporine, tacrolimus, and warfarin require more careful monitoring.

E. The most common **adverse effects** of azoles are nausea, diarrhea, and rash. Hepatitis is a rare but serious complication. Therapy must be monitored closely in the setting of compromised liver function (weekly LFTs) and should be monitored regularly with chronic use. Itraconazole levels should be checked after 1 week of therapy to confirm absorption. IV itraconazole should be avoided in patients with severe heart failure and in those with a $Cr_{Cl}$ of less than 30 ml/minute to avoid excessive accumulation of the hydroxyl-beta-cyclodextrin vehicle. Similarly, the IV formulation of voriconazole should not be used in patients with a $Cr_{Cl}$ of less than 50 ml/minute because of the potential for toxicity from the vehicle. Transient visual disturbance is a common adverse effect (30%) of voriconazole. Ketoconazole antagonizes testosterone metabolism, and antiandrogen side effects can occur with prolonged therapy. **This class of antibiotics has major drug interactions** (see Appendix C, Drug Interactions).

IV. **Caspofungin acetate** (70 mg IV loading dose, followed by 50 mg IV q24h) is the first available drug of the echinocandin class of antifungal agents, which act by inhibiting the synthesis of cell wall glucan. It has fungicidal activity against most *Aspergillus* and *Candida* species, including azole-resistant *Candida* strains. However, *Candida guilliermondi* and *Candida parapsilosis* may be relatively resistant. It also does not have appreciable activity against *Cryptococcus*, *Histoplasma*, or *Mucor* species. It is only available in an intravenous preparation, as it is not absorbed from the GI tract. Metabolism is mostly hepatic, although the cytochrome P-450 system is not significantly involved.

Caspofungin is FDA approved as salvage therapy for invasive aspergillosis based on limited clinical data showing favorable responses in a series of patients who failed or were intolerant of amphotericin B or itraconazole. Clinical studies that prove it to be at least as effective as, and better tolerated than, amphotericin B for the treatment of esophageal candidiasis, candidemia, and invasive candidiasis (*N Engl J Med* 347:2020, 2002) have led to approval for such indications. In addition, in vitro and limited clinical studies suggest a synergistic effect when caspofungin is given in conjunction with itraconazole, voriconazole, or amphotericin B for *Aspergillus* infections. Fever, rash, nausea, and phlebitis at the injection site are infrequent **adverse effects.** An increased dosage may be necessary with the use of drugs that induce hepatic metabolism (e.g., efavirenz, nelfinavir, phenytoin, rifampin, dexamethasone). The maintenance dose should be reduced to 35 mg for patients with moderate hepatic impairment; however, no dose adjustment is necessary for renal failure.

**V.** **Terbinafine** (250 mg PO qd for 6–12 weeks) is an allylamine antifungal agent that kills fungi by inhibiting ergosterol synthesis. It is approved for the treatment of onychomycosis of the fingernail (6 weeks of treatment) or toenail (12 weeks of treatment). It is not generally used for systemic infections. The main **adverse effects** are headache, GI disturbances, rash, LFT abnormalities, and taste disturbances. Terbinafine should not be used in patients with hepatic cirrhosis or a $Cr_{Cl}$ of less than 50 ml/minute because of inadequate data. It has only moderate affinity for cytochrome P-450 hepatic enzymes and does not significantly inhibit the metabolism of cyclosporine (15% decrease) or warfarin.

# 13 Treatment of Infectious Diseases

Steven J. Lawrence and
Linda M. Mundy

## Principles of Therapy

The decision to initiate, continue, and stop antimicrobial chemotherapy should be prudently determined. Aside from the irreversible decision to initiate therapy, indiscriminate use has been associated with adverse effects, the development of drug resistance, and excess costs. When antimicrobial therapy is indicated, a number of factors, reviewed in this chapter, must be considered. When antimicrobial agents are not readily available due to industry-related shortages, consultation with an infectious disease expert for alternative therapeutic options is prudent. For dosing of antimicrobial agents in patients with renal insufficiency, see Appendix E, Dosage Adjustments of Drugs in Renal Failure.

**I. Choice of initial antimicrobial therapy.** The infecting organism is often unknown when therapy is initiated. In these cases, empiric therapy should be directed against the most likely pathogens, using a regimen that possesses the narrowest spectrum that adequately covers the predicted organisms. Therapy should then be altered in accordance with the patient's course and laboratory results.

- **A. During the initial evaluation,** a Gram stain of potentially infected material often permits a rapid presumptive diagnosis and may be essential for interpretation of subsequent culture results.
- **B. Local susceptibility patterns** must be considered in selecting empiric therapy because patterns vary widely among communities and individual hospitals.
- **C. Cultures** are usually necessary for precise diagnosis and are required for susceptibility testing. Whenever organisms with special growth requirements are suspected, the microbiology laboratory should be consulted to ensure appropriate transport and processing of cultures.
- **D. Antimicrobial susceptibility testing** facilitates a rational selection of antimicrobial agents and should be performed on nearly all significant positive cultures.
- **E. Rapid diagnostic testing,** such as use of polymerase chain reaction (PCR) and antigen detection, may also provide early confirmation of an infectious etiologic agent.

**II. Status of the host.** The clinical status of the patient contributes to the speed with which therapy must be instituted, the route of administration, and the type of therapy (*Clin Infect Dis* 29:264, 1999). Patients should be evaluated promptly for hemodynamic stability, rapidly progressive or life-threatening infections, and immune defects.

- **A. Timing of the initiation of antimicrobial therapy.** In acute clinical scenarios, empiric therapy is usually begun immediately after appropriate cultures have been obtained. However, if the patient's condition is stable, delaying the empiric use of antimicrobials might permit specific therapy based on the results of initial diagnostic testing and avoid adverse effects from the use of unnecessary drugs. Urgent therapy is indicated in febrile patients who are neutropenic or asplenic. In other immunosuppressed patients, fever alone seldom warrants urgent therapy; rather, the overall clinical assessment determines the need for empiric antimicrobials. Sepsis, meningitis, and rapidly progressive anaerobic or necrotizing infections should also be treated promptly with antimicrobials.

B. **Route of administration.** Patients with serious infections should be given antimicrobial agents intravenously. In less urgent circumstances, IM or oral therapy often is sufficient. Oral therapy is acceptable when it is tolerated and able to achieve adequate drug concentrations at the site of infection.

C. **Type of therapy.** Bactericidal therapy is preferred over bacteriostatic regimens for patients with immunologic compromise or life-threatening infection. It is preferred also for infections characterized by impaired regional host defenses, such as endocarditis, meningitis, and osteomyelitis. Examples of bactericidal antibiotics include beta-lactams and fluoroquinolones.

D. **Pregnancy and the puerperium.** Although no antimicrobial agent is known to be completely safe in pregnancy, the penicillins and cephalosporins are used most often. **Tetracyclines and fluoroquinolones are among the agents specifically contraindicated,** and the sulfonamides and aminoglycosides should not be used if alternative agents are available (see Appendix B, Pregnancy and Medical Therapeutics). Most antibiotics that are administered in therapeutic dosages appear in breast milk and, therefore, should be used with caution in patients who are breast-feeding.

III. **Antimicrobial combinations.** The indiscriminate use of antimicrobial combinations should be avoided because of the potential for increased toxicity, pharmacologic antagonism, and the selection of resistant organisms. The empiric use of multiple antimicrobials to provide broader coverage is justified in seriously ill patients when (1) the identity of an infecting organism is not apparent, (2) the suspected pathogen has a variable antimicrobial susceptibility, or (3) failure to initiate effective antimicrobial therapy will likely increase morbidity or mortality. In addition, antimicrobial combinations are specifically indicated to produce synergism (e.g., in enterococcal endocarditis), to treat polymicrobial infections (e.g., peritonitis after rupture of a viscus), and to prevent the emergence of antimicrobial resistance [e.g., tuberculosis (TB)].

IV. **Assessment of antimicrobial therapy.** When therapy is initiated, continued, or discussed from the perspective of potential treatment failure, one should consider the following questions: Is the isolated organism the etiologic agent? Is adequate antimicrobial therapy being provided? Is the concentration of antimicrobial agent adequate at the site of infection? Have resistant pathogens emerged? Is a persistent fever due to underlying disease, an iatrogenic complication, a drug reaction, or another process?

V. **Duration of therapy.** The duration of therapy depends on the nature of the infection and the severity of the clinical presentation. Treatment of acute uncomplicated infections should be continued until the patient has been afebrile and clinically well, usually for a minimum of 72 hours. Infections at certain sites (e.g., endocarditis, septic arthritis, osteomyelitis) require prolonged therapy.

## Fever and Rash

Fever with rash is a common presentation of many infectious and noninfectious diseases that range from benign to life-threatening.

I. **Initial management.** Empiric antimicrobial therapy should be initiated immediately for those with severe illness or a rash suggesting a potentially life-threatening infection such as meningococcemia or **Rocky Mountain spotted fever (RMSF).** Ceftriaxone, 2 g IV q12h, with doxycycline, 100 mg IV or PO q12h, is a reasonable empiric regimen. If a pathogen is isolated, therapy should be tailored according to susceptibilities. Gloves should be worn while examining the rash, and respiratory isolation precautions should be considered if a transmissible pathogen is suspected (e.g., varicella, meningococcemia with meningitis, and certain bioterrorism agents).

II. **Diagnostic considerations.** The etiology of a febrile rash illness is often suggested by the type and distribution of the rash and historical data (travel; animal, insect, and drug exposures; immune status). Skin biopsy with Gram stain, culture, and microscopy is helpful and sometimes necessary. Rashes may be atypical, more severe, and caused by unusual organisms (including fungi) in immunocompromised hosts.

   A. **Maculopapular** rashes may suggest drug hypersensitivity, secondary syphilis, typhoid (rose spots), Lyme disease, acute HIV infection, or viral exanthems.

   B. **Vesicular** or **pustular** lesions can be seen with varicella, disseminated gonococcal infection, endocarditis, and smallpox (see the Bioterrorism section).

   C. **Diffuse erythematous** rashes, often with desquamation, should raise suspicion of toxin-mediated diseases (see the Toxin-Mediated Infections section) or toxic epidermal necrolysis.

   D. **Petechial** and **purpuric** lesions often herald life-threatening infections (meningococcemia, pneumococcemia, gram-negative bacterial sepsis, RMSF, malaria, viral hemorrhagic fevers) or autoimmune disorders.

III. **Specific pathogens**

   A. ***Neisseria meningitidis*** septicemia (meningococcemia) can occur with or without meningitis and presents with maculopapular lesions and petechiae, which may rapidly progress to extensive ecchymotic lesions (purpura fulminans) and death. Diagnostic tests include identification of gram-negative diplococci in a Gram-stained specimen or growth in culture from blood, cerebrospinal fluid (CSF), or lesion scrapings. Treatment of choice is a third-generation cephalosporin (e.g., ceftriaxone, 2 g IV q12h), particularly if penicillin is unavailable or if the strain is penicillin resistant. Chloramphenicol, 100 mg/kg/day IV (maximum, 4 g/day) divided q6h can be used in the severely beta-lactam–allergic patient. Duration of therapy is generally 10–14 days.

   B. **RMSF** is caused by *Rickettsia rickettsii* after a tick bite. Fever, headache, and myalgias are followed 1–5 days later with a petechial rash starting on the distal extremities that may be faint and difficult to detect. Death can occur when treatment is delayed. The antibiotic of choice is doxycycline, 100 mg q12h IV or PO for 7 days, or 2 days after becoming afebrile. Chloramphenicol is an alternative.

## Sepsis

I. **Sepsis,** a leading cause of death in the United States, involves a series of proinflammatory and procoagulant responses to invading pathogens. The mortality for patients with sepsis is 15%, and pathogens are bacteria more often than fungi and viruses. Sepsis is diagnosed when there is evidence of infection and criteria for the systemic inflammatory response syndrome are met.

   A. **Early use of appropriate antibiotics can reduce mortality from sepsis.** If a probable source of infection is evident, antimicrobials can be selected for the most likely pathogens and their anticipated antibiotic sensitivity pattern. If no obvious source is identified, empiric antimicrobial selection should be based on the clinical situation. Before therapy is initiated, specimens of potentially infected body fluids should be collected for Gram stain and culture. Two sets of blood cultures should be obtained from either separate venipuncture sites or one venipuncture and one central venous catheter (CVC) port. Empiric coverage usually includes a beta-lactam antimicrobial agent plus an aminoglycoside. Initial empiric coverage may also include vancomycin, particularly in a nosocomial setting or when a CVC is present.

B. **For community-acquired sepsis** with no obvious underlying disease, a third-generation cephalosporin plus an aminoglycoside covers most potential pathogens.

C. **Asplenic patients** are at particular risk for fulminant sepsis with encapsulated organisms such as *Streptococcus pneumoniae*, *Haemophilus influenzae*, and *N. meningitidis*. Penicillin G, 2 million units IV q2–4h, or vancomycin, 1 g IV q12h, plus a third-generation cephalosporin (e.g., ceftriaxone, 2 g IV q12h) should be administered promptly.

D. **Neutropenic hosts,** in whom *Pseudomonas aeruginosa* sepsis may be likely, should be initially treated with an antipseudomonal beta-lactam antimicrobial agent plus an aminoglycoside.

II. **Septic shock.** Beyond antimicrobial treatment, vasopressors, bolus IV fluids, physiologic doses of hydrocortisone, and activated protein C may play a role (see Chap. 8, Critical Care).

## Skin, Soft-Tissue, and Bone Infections

I. **General concepts.** Infections of intact skin are usually treated empirically; however, surgical sampling with culture is required for pathogen isolation in infections that are deep, severe, or will require prolonged antibiotics. For severe infections in which *Staphylococcus aureus* is the likely primary pathogen, empiric vancomycin, 1 g IV q12h, should be considered if the patient is at high risk of oxacillin-resistant *S. aureus* (ORSA; e.g., injection drug use, high local prevalence of ORSA, prior ORSA infection, recent prolonged hospitalization) until susceptibilities are available. Therapy should be switched to oxacillin or cefazolin if the strain proves susceptible.

II. **Skin infections. Erysipelas** is a painful, superficial, erythematous, sharply demarcated lesion that is usually found on lower extremities and is almost always caused by group A beta-hemolytic streptococci (GABHS) in the normal host. The **treatments of choice** are penicillin V, 250–1000 mg PO qid; procaine penicillin G, 600,000 units IM bid; or penicillin G, 0.6–2.0 million U IV q6h, depending on the severity of illness. In patients who are penicillin allergic, erythromycin, 500 mg PO qid, or other macrolides are alternatives.

III. **Soft-tissue infections**

A. **Cellulitis** involves the skin and underlying soft tissue superficial to fascia, with less distinct margins than erysipelas. GABHS and *S. aureus* are the usual pathogens and are clinically indistinguishable. **Initial therapy** is oxacillin, 1–2 g IV q4h; cefazolin, 1–2 g IV q8h; or vancomycin, 1 g IV q12h (see sec. **I**). Alternatives for the severely penicillin-allergic patient include macrolides or clindamycin. Mild disease can be treated with oral equivalents of the above. If present, coexisting **tinea pedis** should be treated with topical antifungals to prevent recurrence of lower extremity cellulitis.

1. **Diabetic patients** with cellulitis often require broader-spectrum coverage, including a beta-lactam/beta-lactamase inhibitor, third-generation cephalosporin, or carbapenem, depending on severity.
2. **Water-borne pathogens.** Severe cellulitis is sometimes seen after exposure to fresh (*Aeromonas hydrophila*) or salt water (*Vibrio vulnificus*). In these settings, initial therapy should include ceftazidime, 2 g IV q8h; cefepime, 2 g IV q8h; or ciprofloxacin, 400 mg IV q8h or 750 mg PO bid. Doxycycline, 100 mg IV/PO q12h should be added for *Vibrio* infections.

B. **Infected decubitus ulcers** and **limb-threatening diabetic foot ulcers** are usually polymicrobial; superficial swab cultures are unreliable. Osteomyelitis is a frequent complication and should be excluded (see sec. **IV**). **Treatment** consists of wound care and débridement. Moderately severe decubitus ulcers and most diabetic foot infections require systemic antibiotics covering *S. aureus*, anaerobes, and enteric gram-negative organisms. Options include clindamycin, 450–900 mg IV q8h with either a third-generation cephalosporin or ciprofloxacin, 500–750 mg PO bid, a beta-lactam/beta-lactamase inhibitor combination, or imipenem-cilastatin, 500 mg IV q6h, depending on the severity of illness. Less severe diabetic foot infections are usually due to *S. aureus* with or without *Streptococcus* species and can be managed with cephalexin, dicloxacillin, or clindamycin.

C. **Necrotizing fasciitis** is an infectious disease emergency with high mortality manifested by extensive soft-tissue infection and thrombosis of the microcirculation with resulting necrosis. It may present initially like simple cellulitis, with rapid progression to necrosis with dusky, hypoesthetic skin and bulla formation. Infection spreads quickly along fascial planes and may be associated with sepsis or streptococcal toxic shock syndrome (TSS). Fournier's gangrene is necrotizing fasciitis of the perineum. **Diagnosis** is mostly clinical. High suspicion should prompt **immediate surgical exploration** where lack of resistance to probing is diagnostic. Early in the disease process, CT scans and plain films may demonstrate gas and fascial edema. Bacterial etiology is either mixed anaerobic (*Bacteroides*, other anaerobes, aerobic gram-negative organisms, and *Streptococcus* species) or GABHS with or without *S. aureus*. Intraoperative Gram stain is used to differentiate among these. **Treatment** includes volume support, IV antibiotics, and aggressive surgical débridement, which are imperative. Initial antibiotic therapy should include penicillin G (or ampicillin), clindamycin, and gentamicin (or a third-generation cephalosporin). If the Gram stain and culture suggest mixed infection, imipenem or a beta-lactam/beta-lactamase inhibitor combination are alternatives. Penicillin and clindamycin should be continued if GABHS is the pathogen. Adjunctive hyperbaric oxygen may be useful.

D. **Anaerobic myonecrosis (gas gangrene)** usually is due to *Clostridium perfringens*, *Clostridium septicum*, *S. aureus*, GABHS, or other anaerobes. Distinguishing this condition from necrotizing fasciitis requires gross inspection of the involved muscle at the time of surgery. **Treatment** requires prompt surgical débridement and combination antimicrobial therapy with penicillin and clindamycin. Gentamicin, ciprofloxacin, or a third-generation cephalosporin should be added until the Gram stain excludes gram-negative involvement.

IV. **Osteomyelitis** should be considered when skin or soft-tissue infections overlie bone and when localized bone pain accompanies fever or sepsis. **Diagnosis** is made by detection of bone through a skin ulcer or by imaging with plain films, bone scintigraphy, or MRI. Biopsy of the affected bone should be performed (before initiation of antimicrobials, if possible) to determine the microbial etiology. If a causative organism is not identified, empiric therapy should be selected to cover *S. aureus* and any other likely pathogens. Cure typically requires at least 4–6 weeks of high-dose antimicrobial therapy. Parenteral therapy should be given initially; oral regimens can be considered after 2–3 weeks if the pathogen is susceptible and adequate bactericidal levels can be achieved. Erythrocyte sedimentation rate is usually markedly elevated and can be used to monitor the response to therapy.

A. **Acute hematogenous osteomyelitis** is caused most frequently by *S. aureus*. In the absence of vascular insufficiency or a foreign body, it can be treated with antimicrobial therapy alone. Vertebral osteomyelitis may be due to *S. aureus*, gram-negative bacilli, or *Mycobacterium tuberculosis*.

B. **Osteomyelitis associated with a contiguous focus of infection** may be due to *S. aureus*, gram-negative bacilli, coagulase-negative staphylococci (surgical site infections), or anaerobes (infected sacral decubitus ulcers).

C. **Osteomyelitis associated with vascular insufficiency** (e.g., in diabetic patients) seldom is cured by drug therapy alone; revascularization, débridement, or amputation often is required. Infections are generally polymicrobial, including anaerobes.

D. **Osteomyelitis in the presence of orthopedic devices** is most often caused by *S. aureus* or coagulase-negative *Staphylococcus* species. It is rarely eradicated by antimicrobials alone. Cure typically requires the removal of the device. When removal is impossible, the addition of rifampin (RIF), 600 mg PO qd, is recommended.

E. **Osteomyelitis associated with hemoglobinopathies** is caused most often by *S. aureus* or *Salmonella* species. *Salmonella* osteomyelitis may require surgical treatment and parenteral administration of high-dose ampicillin or chloramphenicol.

F. **Chronic osteomyelitis** usually is associated with a sequestrum of necrotic bone and frequently involves gram-negative pathogens as well as *S. aureus*. Eradication requires a combination of medical and surgical treatment to remove the persistent nidus of infection. Long-term, suppressive antimicrobial therapy can be used if surgery is not feasible. Hyperbaric oxygen may be a useful adjunctive therapy

## Toxin-Mediated Infections

I. **Clostridial infections**

A. **Botulism** (see the **Bioterrorism section**)

B. **Tetanus** (intoxication with *Clostridium tetani* toxin) is a rare disease in the United States but should be diagnosed when the classic presentation of generalized rigidity, trismus, risus sardonicus, and painful convulsive spasms of skeletal muscles is followed by autonomic dysfunction. A prior injury or wound has usually occurred. **Treatment** consists of human tetanus immunoglobulin, 3000–5000 U IM. Benzodiazepines, and occasionally paralytics, can be used to control spasms. Ventilatory support is often necessary. Antimicrobial therapy remains controversial; however, metronidazole is often used. Tetanus is best prevented by immunization and, for high-risk wounds, human tetanus immunoglobulin, 250 U IM is used.

C. ***Clostridium difficile*–associated diarrheal disease** is frequently seen after systemic antimicrobial therapy in hospitalized patients. Diagnosis is usually made by detection in the stool of the toxins that cause diarrhea and colitis.

1. **Treatment** is primarily targeted toward elimination of *C. difficile* from the gut. **First-line therapy** for initial episodes is metronidazole, 500 mg PO tid for 10–14 days, and discontinuation of the offending antibiotic, if possible. Antimotility agents should be avoided in severe disease. IV metronidazole is a less effective alternative when enteral therapy is not possible. Intracolonic vancomycin is sometimes used in severe cases in which gut motility is altered and surgical intervention is imminent (*Clin Infect Dis* 35:690, 2002).
2. **Recurrence** is common, and well-established effective regimens are lacking. A first recurrence is usually treated with metronidazole as for initial episodes. Multiply recurrent disease is often treated with metronidazole or vancomycin, 125–500 mg PO (IV is not effective) qid, in a regimen that is either of extended duration, tapered, or pulsed. Adjunctive therapy with oral rifampin (RIF), bacitracin, or a toxin-binding resin (cholestyramine) is sometime used, and adjunctive use of probiotics, such as *Saccharomyces boulardii* and *Lactobacillus* GG, may be useful.

II. **TSS** is a life-threatening disease caused by exotoxins produced by *S. aureus* or GABHS.

A. **Staphylococcal TSS** is most often associated with tampon use in young women, vaginitis, or colonization of surgical wounds. **Diagnosis** is made by the presence of fever, hypotension, macular desquamating erythroderma usually involving the palms and soles, and multisystem involvement, such as vomiting, diarrhea, and renal failure. Blood cultures are often negative. **Treatment is primarily supportive.** Tampons should be removed and avoided in the future. Oxacillin or cefazolin is administered for 10–14 days to decrease the rate of relapse.

B. **Streptococcal TSS** is associated with invasive GABHS infections, particularly necrotizing fasciitis. It is defined by isolation of GABHS, hypotension, and multiorgan failure with or without desquamating rash. **Treatment** is directed at the primary infection and should include penicillin G, 4 million U IV q4h, and clindamycin, 900 mg IV q8h. IV immunoglobulin also appears to be beneficial.

## Central Nervous System Infections

I. **Meningitis**

A. **Acute bacterial meningitis** is a medical emergency. Meningitis should be considered in any patient with fever and stiff neck or neurologic symptoms, especially if another concurrent infection or head trauma is present. Therapy should not be delayed for diagnostic measures because prognosis depends on rapid initiation of antimicrobial treatment.

1. **Diagnosis** requires lumbar puncture with measurement of opening pressure and examination of CSF protein, glucose, cell count with differential, and Gram stain with culture. Blood cultures should always be obtained. Depending on the clinical scenario, other potentially useful CSF studies include rapid plasma reagin (RPR), acid-fast stain, latex agglutination antigen detection, cryptococcal antigen, arbovirus antibodies, and PCR for herpes simplex virus (HSV) and enteroviruses. The performance of cranial CT scan before lumbar puncture is controversial but is generally not required for nonelderly, immunocompetent patients who present without focal neurologic abnormalities, seizures, or diminished level of consciousness (*N Engl J Med* 345:1727, 2001). Typical CSF findings include a neutrophilic pleocytosis, markedly elevated CSF protein, and decreased glucose level.

2. **Treatment consists of supportive measures and antimicrobial therapy.** Whenever acute bacterial meningitis is suspected, high-dose parenteral antimicrobial therapy should be started as soon as possible. Until the etiology of the meningitis is known, an **empiric regimen** should be based on the CSF Gram stain. If no organisms are seen, high-dose third-generation cephalosporins (ceftriaxone, 2 g IV q12h, or cefotaxime, 2 g IV q4h) and vancomycin, 500–750 mg IV q6h, are recommended while culture results are pending. Ampicillin, 2 g IV q4h, should be added for immunocompromised and older (>50 years of age) patients. In the postneurosurgical setting, or after head or spinal trauma, broad-spectrum coverage with high-dose vancomycin and ceftazidime, 2 g IV q8h, is indicated. Empiric regimens should be altered once culture and sensitivity data are known.

3. **Steroids.** Dexamethasone, 10 mg IV q6h, started just before or during initial antibiotics and given for 4 days, reduces the risk of a poor neurologic outcome. The benefit is greatest for meningitis caused by *S. pneumoniae* and *H. influenzae*; thus, it should be discontinued if a different pathogen is isolated (*N Engl J Med* 347:1549, 2002).

4. **Therapy for specific infections**

   a. **For *S. pneumoniae*,** IV penicillin G, 300,000 U/kg/day (maximum, 24 million U/day) divided into q2h or q4h doses for 10–14 days, is appropriate when the isolate is fully susceptible to penicillin. Options for severely penicillin-allergic patients are vancomycin plus RIF, 600 mg PO qd, or chloramphenicol, 1.0 g IV q6h. Penicillin-resistant pneumococci require ceftriaxone (or cefotaxime) and vancomycin. Vancomycin should not be used alone.

b. **For *N. meningitidis***, penicillin G or high-dose ceftriaxone or cefotaxime is continued for at least 5 days after the patient has become afebrile, usually a 7-day total course. Chloramphenicol is an option for the penicillin-allergic patient. Patients should be placed in a private room on respiratory isolation for at least the first 24 hours of treatment. Close contacts (e.g., persons living in the same household) should receive prophylaxis with RIF, 600 mg PO bid for 2 days, or single-dose therapy with either ciprofloxacin, 500 mg PO, or ceftriaxone, 250 mg IM. Terminal component complement deficiency (C6–C9) should be ruled out in patients with recurrent meningococcal infections.

c. ***Listeria monocytogenes*** meningitis is seen in immunosuppressed adults and the elderly. Treatment is with ampicillin, 2 g IV q4h, in combination with a systemically administered aminoglycoside for at least 3–4 weeks. Trimethoprim/sulfamethoxazole (TMP/SMX; TMP, 5 mg/kg IV q6h) is an alternative for the penicillin-allergic patient.

d. **Gram-negative bacillary meningitis** usually is a complication of head trauma and neurosurgical procedures. Third-generation cephalosporins, such as cefotaxime or ceftriaxone, are indicated for susceptible pathogens; however, ceftazidime, 2 g IV q8h, is used for *P. aeruginosa*. Alternatives include aztreonam, meropenem, and ciprofloxacin.

e. ***H. influenzae*** is now a rare cause of meningitis. Cefotaxime or ceftriaxone for 10 days is effective. Chloramphenicol is an alternative for patients allergic to penicillin and cephalosporins.

f. ***S. aureus*** meningitis is rare and usually a result of high-grade bacteremia, direct extension from a parameningeal focus, or neurosurgical procedures. Oxacillin or nafcillin, 2 g IV q4h, are the drugs of choice. First-generation cephalosporins do not reliably penetrate into the CSF. Vancomycin should be used for penicillin-allergic patients and when methicillin resistance is likely or confirmed. RIF may also be necessary.

g. **Ventriculitis and ventriculoperitoneal shunt infections** are typically caused by coagulase-negative staphylococci, *S. aureus*, and *Propionibacter* species. They are treated with IV vancomycin with or without RIF or intraventricular vancomycin, 10 mg qd–qod. Removal of an infected shunt is often necessary for cure.

**B. Aseptic meningitis** is usually milder than bacterial meningitis and is characterized by fever, headache, meningismus, and photophobia, often preceded by upper respiratory symptoms or pharyngitis. Viruses are common causes, as is drug-induced inflammation (e.g., nonsteroidal anti-inflammatory drugs, TMP/SMX). A lymphocytic CSF pleocytosis is common (although neutrophils may predominate very early in the disease course), and CSF PCR can detect enteroviruses, HSV-2, and HIV. For enteroviral meningitis, the treatment is supportive care. Pleconaril has been used on a compassionate basis for rare cases of severe disease. It is not clear how effective antiviral therapy is for mild HSV-2 meningitis, but acyclovir, 10 mg/kg IV q8h, is often used.

## II. Encephalitis

**A. HSV-1** is the most common and most important cause of sporadic infectious encephalitis. HSV encephalitis should be considered in any patient who presents with acute fever and neurologic abnormalities, particularly with personality change or seizures, and without meningeal signs. **Diagnosis** is confirmed by detection of HSV-1 in the CSF by PCR; however, a negative

PCR does not rule out HSV encephalitis. Temporal lobe enhancement is typically seen on brain MRI. **Treatment** is acyclovir, 10 mg/kg IV q8h infused over 1 hour with adequate hydration, which should be initiated at first suspicion and continued for 14–21 days. Delayed initiation of therapy greatly increases the risk of poor neurologic outcomes.

**B. West Nile virus** (WNV) (see the Arthropod-Borne Diseases, Zoonoses, and Bite Wounds section)

**III. Brain abscesses** in the immunocompetent host are usually bacterial in origin and are a result of spread from a contiguous focus or septic emboli from endocarditis. Infection is often mixed, with oral streptococci, *S. aureus*, and anaerobes being the most common pathogens. **Diagnosis** is radiographic, with ring-enhancing lesions seen on MRI or contrast CT scans. A microbiologic etiology must be determined by biopsy or at the time of surgery. **Therapy** is often surgical with the addition of systemic antimicrobials. Empiric therapy should be chosen to cover the most likely pathogens based on the primary infection site. When no preceding infection can be found, a third-generation cephalosporin combined with metronidazole and vancomycin is a reasonable regimen until culture data are available.

**IV. Neurocysticercosis** can present as new-onset seizures, hydrocephalus, or focal neurologic abnormalities. It is acquired from eating undercooked pork that contains the eggs of *Taenia solium*, which is endemic in Mexico and Central America. **Diagnosis** should be suspected in hosts with new-onset seizures of unknown etiology and exposure to endemic areas. Serologic tests are available at the Centers for Disease Control and Prevention (CDC). Brain imaging reveals multiple unilocular cysts that may or may not enhance. **Treatment** is controversial but may require surgery or high-dose albendazole or praziquantel, depending on the location of cysts and severity. Anticonvulsants and steroids are often necessary to control symptoms.

## Cardiovascular Infections

Cardiovascular infections occur from a variety of pathogens and may involve the endovascular system, cardiac valves, myocardium, or pericardium.

**I. Infective endocarditis (IE)** usually is caused by gram-positive cocci. Injection drug use and intravascular devices increase the risk for staphylococcal endovascular infection. Gram-negative and fungal IE occur infrequently and usually are associated with injection drug use or prosthetic valves. Patients may present within 3–10 days with critical illness **(acute bacterial endocarditis)** or subacutely **(subacute bacterial endocarditis)** with constitutional symptoms, immune complex disease (nephritis, arthralgias), and emboli (renal, splenic, and cerebral infarcts; petechiae; Osler's nodes; Janeway lesions). A deformed or previously damaged valve is the usual focus of infection in subacute bacterial endocarditis. Dental procedures and bacteremia from distant foci of infection are frequent seeding events; instrumentation of the genitourinary or GI tract is a less common cause.

**A. Diagnosis.** The most reliable diagnostic criterion is continuous bacteremia in a compatible clinical setting. **Blood cultures** are positive in at least 90% of patients. The yield is reduced if the patient has received antimicrobial therapy within 1–2 weeks. Three culture samples should be taken from separate sites over at least a 1-hour period before empiric therapy is begun. The diagnosis of IE remains essentially clinical and microbiologic, rather than echocardiographic. Patients with IE and vegetations seen by transthoracic echocardiography are at higher risk of embolism, heart failure, and valvular disruption; however, a negative transthoracic echocardiogram does not exclude the diagnosis of IE. When clinical evidence of IE exists, **transesophageal echocardiography** improves the sensitivity of the Duke criteria to diagnose and define IE, especially in hosts with prosthetic valves (*Am*

*Heart J* 139:945, 2000). The role of delayed echocardiography in IE is to define surgical disease. Presence of vegetations alone does not mandate surgical intervention. Vegetations seen on echocardiography may persist unchanged for at least 3 years after clinical cure.

**B. Treatment** of native valve IE requires high doses of antimicrobials for extended periods. Quantitative susceptibility testing of the responsible organism(s) to multiple antibiotics is more reliable than disk diffusion testing and is essential to ensure that optimal treatment is administered. **Baseline audiometry** is recommended for patients who will receive 7 or more days of aminoglycoside therapy, with follow-up audiometry contingent on the duration of treatment or development of symptoms.

**C. Acute bacterial endocarditis** requires empiric antimicrobial treatment before culture results become available. *S. aureus* and gram-negative bacilli are the most likely pathogens. Initial treatment for *S. aureus* should include oxacillin, 2 g IV q4h, plus gentamicin or tobramycin, 1.0–1.5 mg/kg IV q8h. If there is a high suspicion for ORSA, vancomycin should be used initially instead of oxacillin. Therapy should then be modified on the basis of culture and susceptibility data.

**D. Subacute bacterial endocarditis** is caused most often by streptococci. Penicillin therapy typically results in cure rates of more than 90%. *Streptococcus bovis* bacteremia and endocarditis are associated with lower GI disease, including neoplasms. Groups B and G streptococcal endocarditis may also be associated with lower intestinal pathology.

1. **For *viridans streptococci*,** penicillin G, 2 million units IV q4h for 4 weeks, is effective for penicillin-susceptible strains [minimal inhibitory concentration (MIC) <0.1 μg/ml]. Therapy with parenteral penicillin and an aminoglycoside for 2 weeks is an alternative, but extended aminoglycoside treatment should be avoided in the elderly and in patients who cannot tolerate the potential nephrotoxicity or ototoxicity. If the penicillin MIC equals or exceeds 0.1 μg/ml but is not more than 0.5 μg/ml, the addition of streptomycin or gentamicin may be appropriate for the first 2 weeks of therapy, followed by penicillin G alone for 2 more weeks. Patients with endocarditis caused by streptococci with penicillin MICs in excess of 0.5 μg/ml may require combination therapy similar to that given for enterococcal IE (see sec. **I.D.3**). Ampicillin, 2 g IV q4h, or ceftriaxone, 2 g IV q24h, can be substituted if penicillin G is unavailable. In patients who are allergic to penicillin, skin testing and desensitization should be considered. Vancomycin is an acceptable alternative, with maintenance of trough levels near 15 mg/L; peak levels generally do not need to be monitored regularly.
2. **GABHS and *S. pneumoniae*** should be treated with penicillin G, 2–4 million U IV q4h for 4–6 weeks. Penicillin-resistant pneumococci should be treated with ceftriaxone, 2 g IV q24h for 4–6 weeks.
3. ***Enterococcus* species** cause 10–20% of cases of subacute bacterial endocarditis. Isolates from patients with enterococcal endocarditis should be screened for beta-lactamase production and susceptibility to vancomycin, quinupristin/dalfopristin, and linezolid. Recommended treatment regimens for susceptible isolates are ampicillin, 2 g IV q4h, or penicillin G, 3–5 million units IV q4h, in combination with gentamicin, 1.0–1.5 mg/kg IV q8h, for 4–6 weeks. In susceptible strains, vancomycin in combination with an aminoglycoside is effective and should be used for penicillin-allergic patients or individuals with beta-lactamase–producing strains. Aminoglycoside and vancomycin levels should be monitored (see Appendix A, Barnes-Jewish Hospital Laboratory Reference Values). **Baseline and weekly audiometry is recommended for patients who receive aminoglycosides for more than 7 days.**
4. ***S. aureus*** should be treated with oxacillin, 2 g IV q4h for 6 weeks. An aminoglycoside can be added during the first 3–5 days of therapy or in

patients who do not respond to beta-lactam therapy alone. For young hosts with right-sided IE, treatment with oxacillin for 4 weeks may be sufficient. Older patients with aortic valve infection have a high mortality and often require surgical intervention. For IE caused by ORSA, vancomycin is the drug of choice.

5. ***Staphylococcus epidermidis*** IE primarily occurs in patients with valvular prostheses. These organisms often are resistant to beta-lactam agents; thus, the treatment of choice is vancomycin, 1 g IV q12h, in combination with RIF, 300 mg PO q8h, for at least 6–8 weeks, along with gentamicin, 1 mg/kg IV q8h for the first 2 weeks of therapy. Vancomycin and aminoglycoside levels should be monitored. Because detection of beta-lactam resistance in coagulase-negative staphylococci is potentially difficult, beta-lactam therapy for serious coagulase-negative staphylococcal infections is controversial.
6. **HACEK** is an acronym for a group of fastidious, slow-growing gram-negative bacteria (*Haemophilus*, *Actinobacillus*, *Cardiobacterium*, *Eikenella*, and *Kingella* species) that have a predilection for infecting heart valves. The treatment of choice is ceftriaxone, 2 g IV q24h for 4 weeks.
7. **Blood culture–negative IE** is usually encountered when antimicrobials are initiated before cultures are obtained or, rarely, with fastidious pathogens, such as nutritionally deficient streptococci, HACEK organisms (see section **I.D.6**), *Coxiella burnetii* (Q fever), *Bartonella*, *Tropheryma whippelii* (Whipple's disease), and fungi. Empiric therapy can be initiated despite negative cultures with penicillin G, 2–3 million U IV q4h, or ampicillin, 2 g IV q4h, plus oxacillin, 2 g IV q4h, and an aminoglycoside for 4–6 weeks. Vancomycin can be substituted for the beta-lactam agents in penicillin-allergic patients.

E. **Prosthetic valve endocarditis (PVE)** occurs in 1–4% of patients with prosthetic valves. Early infections (within 2 months of surgery) commonly are caused by *S. aureus*, *S. epidermidis*, gram-negative bacilli, *Candida* species, and other opportunistic organisms. PVE must be considered in any patient with sustained bacteremia after valve surgery. Treatment for oxocillin-sensitive *S. aureus* consists of combination therapy with oxacillin, 2 g IV q4h, plus RIF, 300 mg PO q8h, for at least 6 weeks. For ORSA, vancomycin, 1 g IV q12h, with RIF is used. Gentamicin, 1 mg/kg IV q8h, should be given for the initial 2 weeks of therapy in either case. Therapy should also be guided by the results of MIC testing. Late PVE (i.e., 2 or more months after surgery) usually is caused by organisms similar to those seen on native valves.

F. **Role of surgery.** Indications for urgent cardiac surgery include (1) uncontrolled infection as manifested by sustained bacteremia while on therapy, (2) refractory heart failure, (3) an unstable prosthetic valve, or (4) prosthetic valve obstruction. Surgical intervention might also be necessary when native valve endocarditis is complicated by recurrent systemic emboli, mycotic aneurysm, persistent conduction defects, chordae tendineae or papillary muscle rupture, or early closure of the mitral valve on echocardiography, or when PVE is complicated by a periprosthetic leak. In addition, fungal endocarditis is refractory to medical therapy and requires surgery for cure. Endocarditis due to gram-negative bacilli may be refractory to antimicrobials alone. Although a 10-day course of preoperative antimicrobials is desirable, surgery must not be delayed in patients whose condition is deteriorating.

G. **Response to antimicrobial therapy.** Frequently, clinical improvement is seen within 3–10 days. Daily blood cultures should be obtained until sterility is documented. Persistent or recurrent fever usually represents extensive cardiac infection but also might be due to septic emboli, drug hypersensitivity, or subsequent nosocomial infection. Such fever seldom represents the development of antimicrobial resistance.

H. **Prophylaxis** (*Ann Intern Med* 129:829, 1998). The American Heart Association recommends that prophylaxis for IE be provided to patients at moderate or high risk of infection (e.g., those with prosthetic cardiac valves or other intravascular prostheses, a history of IE, complex cyanotic heart disease, hypertrophic cardiomyopathy, or other valvular lesions including mitral valve prolapse with regurgitation and rheumatic valvular disease) before certain invasive procedures (see Table 13-1).

**II. Myocarditis.** When the heart is involved in an inflammatory process, the cause is often an infectious agent. Myocarditis may occur during and after viral, rickettsial, bacterial, and parasitic infection. It is also a rare complication following vaccination with vaccinia virus.

**A. Diagnostic considerations.** The clinical presentation varies greatly. Patients may be asymptomatic or may present with dysrhythmias, chest pain, or fulminant, fatal congestive heart failure. The workup can range from nasopharyngeal swab testing for viruses, serum titer and PCR studies, to tissue diagnoses via endomyocardial biopsies.

**B. Therapeutic considerations.** Given the range of infectious etiologies, the initial therapeutic regimens target the likely agents. Continued therapeutic regimens should be targeted to the identified agent. The role of IV immunoglobulin, pleconaril, and other antiviral agents in viral-mediated myocarditis remains anecdotal.

**III. Pericarditis.** Acute pericarditis is a syndrome caused by inflammation of the pericardium and characterized by chest pain, a pericardial friction rub, and diffuse ST-segment elevations on ECG (see Chaps. 5, Ischemic Heart Disease, and 6, Heart Failure, Cardiomyopathy, and Valvular Heart Disease). In most cases, viruses are implicated as the infectious etiologies of pericarditis. The role of antiviral therapies in viral pericarditis remains to be characterized. TB is another occasional cause (see the **Tuberculosis section**).

## Respiratory Tract Infections

**I. Upper respiratory tract infections**

A. Most cases of **pharyngitis** are caused by upper respiratory viruses, although distinction from streptococcal (GABHS) and gonococcal pharyngitis is difficult on clinical grounds.

1. **Diagnostic testing** in adults can be reserved for symptomatic patients who are exposed to streptococcal pharyngitis, individuals with signs of significant infection (i.e., fever, pharyngeal exudate, and cervical adenopathy), patients whose pharyngeal infection fails to clear despite symptomatic therapy, and those with a history of rheumatic fever. **Rapid antigen detection testing** (RADT) is useful to identify GABHS, which requires therapy to prevent acute pyogenic complications and rheumatic fever. A negative test does not reliably exclude GABHS, making a culture necessary when RADT is negative. Serology for Epstein-Barr virus (e.g., heterophil agglutinin or a monospot) and examination of a peripheral blood smear for atypical lymphocytes should be performed when infectious mononucleosis is suspected. Acute HIV infection should be considered in the differential diagnosis of pharyngitis with atypical lymphocytosis and negative streptococcus and Epstein-Barr virus testing.

2. **Treatment.** Most cases of pharyngitis are self-limited and do not require antimicrobial therapy. Treatment for GABHS should be initiated in the setting of a positive culture or RADT, if the patient is at high risk for development of rheumatic fever, or if the diagnosis is strongly suspected, pending the results of culture. Treatment schedules include penicillin V, 250 mg PO qid or 500 mg PO bid for 10 days, erythromycin, 250 mg PO qid for 10 days, or benzathine penicillin G, 1.2 million U IM as a one-time

**Table 13-1.** Endocarditis prophylaxis

| Clinical scenario | Drug and dosage |
|---|---|
| Standard prophylaxis | Amoxicillin, 2 g PO 1 hr before procedure |
| Unable to take PO | Ampicillin, 2 g IM or IV within 30 min before procedure |
| Penicillin-allergic patient | Clindamycin, 600 mg PO, or cephalexin or cefadroxil, 2 g PO,[a] or clarithromycin or azithromycin, 500 mg PO 1 hr before procedure |
| Penicillin-allergic and unable to take PO | Clindamycin, 600 mg IV, or cefazolin, 1 g IV within 30 min before procedure |
| Regimens for GI and genitourinary procedures | |
| High-risk patient | Ampicillin, 2 g IM or IV, plus gentamicin, 1.5 mg/kg (maximum, 120 mg) within 30 min before procedure; 6 hr later, ampicillin, 1 g IM or IV, or amoxicillin, 1 g PO |
| High-risk, penicillin-allergic patient | Vancomycin, 1 g IV, plus gentamicin, 1.5 mg/kg (maximum, 120 mg), timed to be completed within 30 min before procedure |
| Moderate-risk patient | Amoxicillin, 2 g PO 1 hr before procedure, or ampicillin, 2 g IM or IV within 30 min before procedure |
| Moderate-risk, penicillin-allergic patient | Vancomycin, 1 g IV timed to finish within 30 min before procedure |

*Note:* Regimens for dental, oral, respiratory tract, or esophageal procedures (including dental extractions, periodontal or endodontal procedures, professional teeth cleaning, esophageal sclerotherapy or dilatation, and endoscopic retrograde cholangiography; prophylaxis for transesophageal echocardiography, upper GI endoscopy, fiberoptic bronchoscopy, and vaginal delivery) are optional for high-risk patients.

[a]Cephalosporins should not be used in patients with anaphylactic or urticarial reactions to penicillin.

*Source*: Adapted from AS Dajani, KA Taubert, W Wilson, et al. Prevention of bacterial endocarditis: recommendations by the American Heart Association. *JAMA* 277:1794, 1997.

dose. Surgical intervention and parenteral therapy may be necessary for severe cases involving airway compromise or inability to take oral medications (*Clin Infect Dis* 35:113–125, 2002). For treatment of gonococcal pharyngitis, see the Sexually Transmitted Diseases section.

**B. Epiglottitis** should be considered in the febrile patient who complains of severe sore throat, odynophagia, new-onset drooling, and dysphagia but in whom minimal findings are noted on inspection of the pharynx.

1. **Diagnosis.** If epiglottitis is suspected, throat and blood cultures and a lateral soft-tissue radiograph of the neck should be obtained to assess airway occlusion.
2. **Treatment. Hospitalization and prompt otolaryngologic consultation for airway management are suggested in all suspected cases.** Antimicrobial therapy should include an agent that is active against *H. influenzae*, such as ceftriaxone, 1–2 g IV q24h, or cefotaxime, 1–2 g IV q6–8h.

**C. Sinusitis** is caused by blockage of the osteomeatal complex. The goals of medical therapy for acute and chronic sinusitis are to control infection, reduce tissue edema, facilitate drainage, maintain patency of the sinus ostia, and break the pathologic cycle that leads to chronic sinusitis.

1. **Acute sinusitis** in adults is a clinical diagnosis that presents with cough, purulent nasal discharge, and sinus tenderness with or without fever. It is most often caused by upper respiratory viruses. Bacterial pathogens, such as *S. pneumoniae*, *H. influenzae*, *Moraxella catarrhalis*, and anaerobes, should be considered if symptoms are severe or if they persist for

more than a week (*Ann Intern Med* 134:498, 2001). **Symptomatic treatment** is the mainstay of therapy, including systemic decongestants and analgesics with or without a short course of topical decongestant. Empiric antibiotic therapy is indicated when a bacterial etiology is suspected. First-line antibiotics include a 10-day regimen of amoxicillin, 500 mg PO tid, or, TMP/SMX, one double-strength (DS) tablet PO bid. Second-generation cephalosporins, amoxicillin/clavulanate, 875 mg PO bid, and macrolides are good second-line agents in case of primary treatment failure.

2. In **chronic sinusitis,** patients experience nasal congestion or obstruction. Secondary complaints include pain, pressure, postnasal discharge, and fatigue. Posttreatment coronal sinus CT with bone windows is the radiographic modality of choice; plain films are not recommended. Nasal endoscopy may complement CT scan by permitting direct inspection of the surface mucosa of the ethmoid air cells. The etiologic agents include those for acute sinusitis, as well as *S. aureus*, *Corynebacterium diphtheriae*, *Bacteroides* species, and *Veillonella* species. Antimicrobial therapy should include anaerobic antimicrobial coverage and, possibly, a nasal steroid spray. Some chronic cases require endoscopic surgery.

**D. Influenza virus infection.** Influenza virus causes an acute, self-limited febrile illness with myalgias, cough, and malaise. The virus is readily transmissible and associated with outbreaks of varying severity during the winter months. **Clinical sequelae** of influenza virus infection include viral pneumonia and secondary bacterial pneumonia. **Diagnosis** is made by nasopharyngeal swab. **Specific antiviral treatment** should be initiated within 48 hours of the onset of symptoms to be effective. Four antiviral treatment regimens are available. The neuraminidase inhibitors, oseltamavir and zanamivir, are used in treatment and prophylaxis of influenza A and B. Oseltamavir, 75 mg PO bid for 5 days, is well tolerated in capsule and elixir formulations. Zanamivir, 10 mg inhaled twice a day for 5 days, is an inhalational agent that may occasionally cause bronchospasm in patients with asthma. Amantadine and rimantadine, each 100 mg PO bid, are for the treatment and prophylaxis of influenza A only. These agents are inexpensive and have a high oral bioavailability but can be associated with adverse CNS effects in the elderly, in whom the dose should be reduced to 100 mg PO qd.

## II. Lower respiratory tract infections

### A. Acute bronchitis

1. **Diagnosis.** Acute bronchitis involves inflammation of the bronchi that causes the acute onset of cough, sputum production, and symptoms of upper respiratory tract infection. The usual causes are viral agents, such as coronavirus, rhinovirus, influenza, or parainfluenza. Uncommon causes include *Mycoplasma pneumoniae*, *Chlamydia pneumoniae*, and *Bordetella pertussis*. Pneumonia should be routinely ruled out either clinically or radiographically, and diagnostic tests for influenza should be performed if it is suspected. Cough that lasts for longer than 2 weeks in an adult should be evaluated for pertussis with a nasopharyngeal swab for culture or PCR, or both.
2. **Treatment.** Treatment is symptomatic and directed most often at controlling cough (dextromethorphan, 15 mg PO q6h). Routine antimicrobial use is not recommended (*Ann Intern Med* 134:521, 2001) unless influenza or pertussis is confirmed. Erythromycin is the drug of choice for pertussis, whereas azithromycin is a better-tolerated alternative. Pertussis cases should be reported to the local health department for contact tracing and administration of postexposure prophylaxis with erythromycin or azithromycin.

### B. Acute exacerbations of chronic bronchitis (AECB)

1. **Diagnosis.** AECB are characterized by an increase in volume or purulence of sputum with increased cough or dyspnea. *H. influenzae* is the major pathogen, followed by *S. pneumoniae* and *M. catarrhalis*. Many

episodes of AECB are incited by tobacco exposure, air pollution, occupational exposure, subclinical asthma, viral infection, or allergies.

2. **Treatment.** Uniformly active oral antibiotics include amoxicillin/clavulanate, third-generation cephalosporins, macrolides (azithromycin and clarithromycin), and doxycycline. For hosts with severe underlying disease and compromised respiratory status, broader treatment with a third-generation fluoroquinolone or cephalosporin is indicated. See Chap. 9, Pulmonary Disease, for further details.

C. **Pneumonia** occurs from inflammation of the pulmonary parenchyma caused by a microbial agent. The three routes of infection are inhalation, microaspiration, and large-volume aspiration. Traditionally, pneumonia is categorized as community-acquired pneumonia (CAP), hospital-acquired pneumonia, or ventilator-associated pneumonia (VAP) (see the Nosocomial Infections section).

1. **Diagnosis.** The diagnosis of CAP is made in patients whose chest radiograph reveals a new pulmonary infiltrate, usually combined with fever and respiratory symptoms (cough, sputum production, pleurisy, dyspnea). Physical examination reveals fever, tachypnea, crackles, or consolidation on auscultation. Most patients can be treated as outpatients, although all should be evaluated for severity of illness, comorbid factors, and oxygenation. Assessment of etiologic agents in all hospitalized patients should include **pretreatment expectorated sputum for Gram stain and culture, and blood cultures.** Fiberoptic bronchoscopy is used for detection of associated anatomic lesions, biopsy for histopathologic workup, or quantitative cultures of conventional bacteria. For patients with CAP, the predominant etiologic agent is *S. pneumoniae*, in which multidrug resistance is rapidly increasing. Pneumonia caused by atypical agents, such as *Legionella pneumophila*, *C. pneumoniae*, or *M. pneumoniae*, cannot be reliably determined clinically. If an atypical agent is suspected, urinary *Legionella* antigen and sputum culture should be sent. Rapid diagnostic tests such as throat-swab PCR are in transition from investigational to clinical use. Acute and convalescent serologic testing can retrospectively identify several atypical pathogens including *C. burnetii* (Q fever) and Hanta virus.

2. **Treatment of CAP.** The selection of antimicrobial agents should be pathogen-directed. Slight variations are found in treatment recommendations in currently published guidelines (CDC: *Arch Intern Med* 160:98, 2000; Infectious Diseases Society of America and Canadian Thoracic Society: *Clin Infect Dis* 31:347, 2000 and 31:383, 2000). Empiric therapy for immunocompetent outpatients who are younger than 40 years and who lack comorbidity should consist of doxycycline or a macrolide. Outpatients older than 60 years and those who have comorbidities should be treated with a second- or third-generation cephalosporin, amoxicillin, or amoxicillin/clavulanate with or without a macrolide. For hospitalized patients, ceftriaxone or cefotaxime with or without a macrolide or monotherapy with a fluoroquinolone that has antipneumococcal activity (e.g., moxifloxacin, gatifloxacin) is recommended. Consideration should be made to reserve fluoroquinolones for second-line therapy, as resistance to this class is also starting to appear. For all critically ill patients, the addition of a macrolide or fluoroquinolone to a beta-lactam regimen is necessary to provide coverage for *L. pneumophila*. Thoracentesis of pleural effusions should be performed, with analysis of pH, cell count, Gram stain and bacterial culture, protein, and lactate dehydrogenase (see Chap. 9, Pulmonary Disease), and empyemas should be drained.

D. **Lung abscess** typically results from macroaspiration of oral flora. Risk factors include periodontal disease and conditions which predispose patients to aspiration of oropharyngeal contents. Bacterial causes of lung abscess include oral anaerobes (*Bacteroides* spp., *Actinomyces* spp., and anaerobic and microaerophilic streptococcoi), enteric Gram-negative bacilli, *S. aureus*, and *S. pneumoniae* serotype III. Polymicrobial infection is common. The clinical presentation is typically indolent and reminiscent of pulmonary tuberculosis, with dyspnea, fever, chills, night sweats, weight loss, and cough productive of putrid or blood-streaked sputum. Chest radiography is very sensitive and typically reveals infiltrates with cavitation and air-fluid levels in dependent areas of the lung. **Therapy** involves postural drainage of the involved lung segment and antibiotic treatment with an antipneumococcal fluoroquinolone plus clindamycin or a beta-lactam-beta-lactamase inhibitor (*Clin Infect Dis* 26:811, 1998).

## Tuberculosis

TB is a systemic disease caused by *M. tuberculosis*. The most frequent clinical presentation is pulmonary disease. Extrapulmonary disease may present as lymphatic involvement, genitourinary disease, osteomyelitis, miliary dissemination, meningitis, peritonitis, or pericarditis. Most cases are the result of reactivation of prior infection, and persons at highest risk include those with HIV infection, silicosis, diabetes mellitus, chronic renal insufficiency, malignancy, malnutrition, and other forms of immunosuppression. The prevalence of TB, particularly multidrug-resistant forms, is increased among immigrants from Southeast Asia, China, the Indian subcontinent, and Central America.

I. **Diagnosis** is established by culture. Positive fluorochrome or acid-fast bacteria (AFB) smears of sputum are presumptive evidence of active TB, although nontuberculous mycobacteria and some *Nocardia* species may give positive results with these techniques. Use of radiometric culture systems and species-specific DNA probes can provide results faster than traditional methods. Drug susceptibility testing should be performed on all initial isolates as well as on follow-up isolates from patients who do not respond to standard therapy.

II. **Treatment** does not have to take place in a hospital setting, but hospitalization to initiate therapy provides an opportunity for intensive patient education. If a patient is hospitalized, proper isolation in a negative-pressure room is essential. The local health department should be notified of all cases of TB so that contacts can be identified and adherence to the regimen can be ensured by directly observed therapy (*Clin Infect Dis* 31:633–639, 2000).

   A. **Chemotherapy.** At least two drugs to which the organism is susceptible must be used because of the high frequency with which primary drug resistance to a single drug develops. Extended therapy is necessary because of the prolonged generation time of mycobacteria. Because adherence to multidrug regimens for prolonged periods is difficult, directly observed therapy should be used for all patients.

   B. **Initial therapy** of uncomplicated pulmonary TB should include four drugs unless the likelihood of drug resistance is very low [i.e., the rate of isoniazid (INH) resistance in the community is <4% or the patient has not received prior therapy for TB, has not been exposed to any contacts with drug-resistant TB, and is not from an area where drug-resistant TB is prevalent]. **INH** (5 mg/kg; maximum, 300 mg PO qd), **RIF** (10 mg/kg; maximum, 600 mg PO qd), **pyrazinamide** (PZA, 15–30 mg/kg PO qd), and either **ethambutol** (EMB, 15 mg/kg PO qd) or **streptomycin** (15 mg/kg; maximum, 1.5 g IM qd) should be administered initially. If the isolate proves to be fully susceptible to INH and RIF, EMB (or streptomycin) can be dropped and INH, RIF, and PZA continued to finish 8 weeks, followed by 16 weeks of INH and RIF. After at least 2 weeks of daily therapy, the drugs can be administered two or three times per week at adjusted doses. Pyridoxine (vitamin $B_6$), 25–50 mg PO qd, should be considered for all patients who take INH to prevent neuropathy.

**C. Organisms that are resistant** only to INH can be effectively treated with a 6-month regimen if a standard four-drug regimen consisting of INH, RIF, PZA, and EMB or streptomycin was started initially. When INH resistance is documented, the INH should be discontinued, and the remaining three drugs should be continued for the duration of therapy. Therapy for multidrug-resistant TB has been less well studied, and consultation with an expert in the treatment of TB should be considered.

**D. Extrapulmonary disease** in adults can be treated in the same manner as pulmonary disease, with 6- to 9-month regimens.

**E. Pregnant patients** with drug-sensitive TB should be treated with INH and RIF for 9 months, and pyridoxine, 50 mg PO qd. EMB should also be used initially until sensitivities are known. PZA and streptomycin should be avoided.

**F. Monitoring response to therapy.** Patients with pulmonary TB whose sputum AFB smears are positive before treatment should submit sputum for AFB smear and culture every 1–2 weeks until AFB smears become negative. Sputum should then be obtained monthly until negative cultures are documented. Conversion of cultures from positive to negative is the most reliable indicator of a response to treatment. Continued symptoms or persistently positive AFB smears or cultures after 3 months of treatment should raise the suspicion of drug resistance or nonadherence and prompt referral to an expert in the treatment of TB.

**G. Monitoring for adverse reactions.** Most patients should have a baseline laboratory evaluation at the start of therapy that includes hepatic enzymes, bilirubin, CBC, and serum creatinine. Routine laboratory monitoring for patients with normal baseline values is probably unnecessary, but some experts check transaminases monthly in patients older than 35 years of age. Monthly clinical evaluations with specific inquiries about symptoms of drug toxicity are essential. Patients who are taking EMB should be tested monthly for visual acuity and red-green color perception.

**H. Glucocorticoid administration.** In TB, the administration of glucocorticoids is controversial. Prednisone, 1 mg/kg PO qd initially, has been used in combination with antituberculous drugs for life-threatening complications such as meningitis and pericarditis.

**III. Latent tuberculosis infection (LTBI).** Untreated, approximately 5% of persons with LTBI develop active TB disease within 2 years of infection. TB disease develops in an additional 5% over the life span. Adequate prophylactic treatment can substantially reduce the risk of disease. LTBI is diagnosed by a positive tuberculin skin test (TST; 5TU administered by the Mantoux method).

**A. Criteria for a positive TST** vary depending on the host: (1) 5-mm induration in patients with HIV infection or another defect in cell-mediated immunity, close contacts of a known case of TB, patients with chest radiographs that are typical for TB, and individuals with organ transplantation or other immunosuppression; (2) 10-mm induration in immigrants from high-prevalence areas (Asia, Africa, Latin America, Eastern Europe), prisoners, the homeless, parenteral drug abusers, nursing home residents, low-income populations, patients with chronic medical illnesses or health and economic disparities, and those people who have frequent contact with these groups (e.g., health care workers, prison guards); and (3) 15-mm induration in individuals who are not in a high-prevalence group (*Am J Respir Crit Care Med* 161:S221 and 1376, 2000).

**B. Chemoprophylaxis for LTBI** should be administered only after active disease has been ruled out by a proper evaluation (chest radiography, sputum collection, or both). **INH,** 300 mg PO qd for 9 months, should be administered, regardless of age, to persons with LTBI who have risk factors for progression to active TB disease. Groups that are considered highest priority for treatment are (1) persons in whom a TST conversion develops within 2 years of a previously negative TST regardless of age; (2) persons with a history of untreated TB or chest radiographic evidence of previous infection; (3) persons with HIV infection, diabetes mellitus, end-stage renal disease, hematologic or lymphoreticular malignancy, conditions associated with rapid weight loss, chronic malnutrition, silicosis, or patients who are receiving immunosuppressive therapy; and (4) household members and other close contacts of patients with active disease who have a reactive TST. Persons with HIV infection who have had known contact with a patient with active TB should be treated for LTBI regardless of tuberculin status. Contacts with a nonreactive TST should undergo a repeat TST 3 months after the last exposure to the infectious person. A 9-month course of INH is adequate for all patients with LTBI even among those with HIV infection. Alternative regimens of shorter duration but higher toxicity can be considered in consultation with a TB expert. Referral to the health department for chemoprophylaxis is recommended to ensure adherence and to monitor for medication-related complications.

## Gastrointestinal and Abdominal Infections

I. **Infectious diarrhea** (see Chap. 16, Gastrointestinal Diseases)

II. **Peritonitis**

A. **Primary or spontaneous bacterial peritonitis** is a common complication of cirrhosis with ascites, which is discussed in Chap. 16, Gastrointestinal Diseases. *Escherichia coli*, other aerobic enteric gram-negatives, and *Streptococcus* species are the primary pathogens. A third-generation cephalosporin, such as ceftriaxone, 2 g IV q24h, or cefotaxime, 2 g IV q8h, is generally the treatment of choice. *M. tuberculosis* and *Neisseria gonorrhoeae* (Fitz-Hugh-Curtis syndrome in women) also occasionally cause peritonitis.

B. **Secondary peritonitis** is caused by spillage of bacteria from a perforated viscus in the GI or genitourinary tract, usually resulting in an acute surgical abdomen. Infections are virtually always mixed, with *E. coli*, *Bacteroides fragilis*, and other facultative and anaerobic gram-negatives predominating. Surgery and supportive care (particularly volume support) are the primary interventions, and **empiric antimicrobial therapy** must be broad in spectrum and should cover the likely pathogens from the presumed source. Optional regimens include monotherapy with a beta-lactam/beta-lactamase inhibitor combination, cefoxitin or cefotetan, or a carbapenem, depending on severity. Combination therapy options are an anaerobic agent with ampicillin and an aminoglycoside, or with a fluoroquinolone. **Intra-abdominal abscess** formation is a complication that usually requires drainage.

C. **Peritonitis related to peritoneal dialysis** (see Chap. 11, Renal Diseases)

III. **Hepatobiliary infections**

A. **Acute cholecystitis** is typically preceded by biliary colic associated with cholelithiasis and characteristically presents with fever, right upper quadrant tenderness with Murphy's sign, and vomiting. Acalculous cholecystitis occurs in 5–10% of patients. Ultrasonography or technetium-99m–hydroxy iminodiacetic acid scanning is the diagnostic imaging modality of choice. **Management** includes parenteral fluids, restricted PO intake, analgesia (meperidine causes less spasm of the sphincter of Oddi than morphine), and surgery. The **role of antimicrobials** for uncomplicated cholecystitis is unclear; however, perioperative antibiotics such as a beta-lactam/beta-lactamase inhibitor combination may reduce the risk of postsurgical infections. Advanced age; severe disease; or the presence of complications, such as gallbladder ischemia or perforation, peritonitis, or bacteremia, requires broad-spectrum antibiotics. Initial regimens include a beta-lactam/beta-lactamase inhibitor such as ampicillin/sulbactam, 3 g IV q6h; or piperacillin/tazobactam, 3.375 g IV q6h; or ampicillin, 2 g IV q6h; plus an aminoglycoside plus metronidazole, 500 mg IV q8h. Imipenem, 500 mg IV q6h, may be preferred for life-threatening disease or if the risk of *P. aeruginosa* is high. Immediate surgery is usually necessary for severe disease. The timing of cholecystectomy is controversial in uncomplicated cholecystitis and in many cases is delayed.

B. **Ascending cholangitis** is a sometimes fulminant infectious complication of an obstructed common bile duct. Charcot's triad of fever, right upper quadrant pain, and jaundice is the classic presentation. Bacteremia and shock are common. Dilated biliary ducts are seen on ultrasonography. The **mainstay of therapy** is aggressive supportive care and surgical or endoscopic decompression and drainage in all but the mildest cases. Broad-spectrum antibiotics as recommended for cholecystitis (see sec. **III.A**) are mandatory.

C. **Hepatitis** (see Chap. 17, Liver Diseases)

IV. **Appendicitis** requires surgical intervention, usually with adjuvant antimicrobial therapy as for secondary peritonitis.

V. **Diverticulitis** presents with left lower quadrant pain and fever and is diagnosed by abdominal/pelvic CT scan. Enteric gram-negative bacilli and gut anaerobes are the causative organisms. The standard regimen for mild disease is TMP/SMX, 160 mg/800 mg (DS) PO bid, or ciprofloxacin, 500 mg PO bid, and metronidazole, 500 mg PO bid, for 7–10 days. Broader antimicrobial coverage (as for secondary peritonitis) and surgical intervention are warranted for more severe disease.

## Genitourinary Infections

The diagnostic and therapeutic approach to adult genitourinary infections is determined by anatomic differences in sex, prior antimicrobial exposures, and the presence of medical devices.

I. **Lower urinary tract infections (UTIs)** in men and women are characterized by pyuria, often with dysuria, urgency, or frequency. A rapid presumptive diagnosis can be made by microscopic examination of a fresh, unspun, clean-voided urine specimen. A urine Gram stain can be helpful in guiding initial antimicrobial choices. Bacteriuria (>1 organism per oil-immersion field) or pyuria (>8 leukocytes per high-power field) correlates well with the presence of infection. Quantitative culture often yields more than $10^5$ bacteria/ml, but colony counts as low as $10^2$–$10^4$ bacteria/ml may indicate infection in women with acute dysuria.

A. **Acute uncomplicated cystitis in women** is caused primarily by *E. coli* (80%) and *Staphylococcus saprophyticus* (5–15%). If pyuria is present microscopically or by leukocyte esterase testing, empiric treatment with TMP/SMX, 160 mg/800 mg PO bid for 3 days, is recommended. In patients who are intolerant of sulfa, TMP, 100 mg PO bid, can be used. Second-generation fluoroquinolones (e.g., ciprofloxacin, 250 mg PO bid × 3 days) are more costly but should be considered in areas where *E. coli* resistance to TMP/SMX is high (*Clin Infect Dis* 34:1165, 2002). Nitrofurantoin is another alternative agent that is also effective for vancomycin-resistant enterococcus (VRE)–associated UTIs. A pretreatment urine culture is recommended for diabetics, patients who are symptomatic for more than 7 days, individuals with recurrent UTI, women who use a contraceptive diaphragm, and individuals older than 65 years. Therapy should be extended to 7 days in this subset of patients.

B. **Recurrent cystitis in women** is due to varying host-dependent risk factors, which vary for young women, healthy postmenopausal women, and older women who are institutionalized (*Clin Infect Dis* 30:152, 2000). Relapses with the original infecting organism that occur within 2 weeks of cessation of therapy should be treated for 2 weeks or more and may indicate a urologic abnormality. An alternative method of contraception might decrease the frequency of reinfection in women who use a diaphragm and spermicide. **Prophylactic therapy** can be beneficial for patients who experience frequent reinfection. Sterilization of the urine with a standard treatment regimen is necessary before prophylaxis is initiated. For women with relapses that correlate with sexual intercourse, TMP/SMX, 80 mg/400 mg (one single-strength tablet), or ciprofloxacin, 250 mg, after coitus may provide adequate prophylaxis. TMP/SMX, 40 mg/200 mg qd or qod, usually is sufficient to decrease recurrences that are unrelated to coitus.

C. **UTIs in men** are rare and do not necessarily indicate a urologic abnormality. In men, other risk factors for UTI include anal intercourse, lack of circumcision, and intercourse with a sex partner who has vaginal colonization with uropathogens. A pretreatment urine culture should be obtained routinely. If no complicating factors are present, a 7-day course of TMP/SMX, TMP alone, or a second-generation fluoroquinolone can be prescribed. If the response to therapy is prompt, a urologic evaluation is unlikely to be useful. Urologic studies are appropriate when treatment fails, in the event of recurrent infections, or when pyelonephritis occurs.

D. **Catheter-associated bacteriuria** is a common source of gram-negative bacteremia in hospitalized patients. **Prevention measures** include aseptic technique for urinary catheter insertion, use of a closed drainage system, and removal of the catheter as soon as possible. In patients with chronic indwelling catheters, the development of bacteriuria is inevitable, and long-term antimicrobial suppression simply selects for multidrug-resistant bacteria. Such patients should be treated with systemic antimicrobials only when symptomatic infection with pyuria is evident.

E. **Acute urethral syndrome** occurs in women who have lower UTI symptoms and pyuria with fewer than $10^5$ bacteria/ml urine. These patients may have bacterial cystitis or urethritis caused by *Chlamydia trachomatis*, *Ureaplasma urealyticum*, or, less frequently, *N. gonorrhoeae*. Specific cultures of the endocervix for sexually transmitted diseases should be performed (see the Sexually Transmitted Diseases section). If no specific etiology is found, doxycycline, 100 mg PO bid for 7 days, is recommended. Azithromycin, 1 g PO in a single dose, is an alternative.

F. Acute **prostatitis** is characterized by fever, chills, dysuria, and a boggy, tender prostate on examination. Patients with chronic prostatitis are usually asymptomatic, but some experience low back pain, perineal or testicular discomfort, mild dysuria, and recurrent bacteriuria. Quantitative urine cultures before and after prostatic massage may be necessary for diagnosis. Prostatitis often is associated with fewer than $10^3$ bacteria/ml of seminal fluid. Infections usually are caused by enteric gram-negative bacilli. TMP/SMX, 160 mg/800 mg (DS) PO bid for 14 days, is an effective, economical treatment for acute infections. Quinolones are useful alternatives. Patients with chronic bacterial prostatitis should receive prolonged therapy (for at least 1 month with the quinolones or 3 months with TMP/SMX).

G. **Epididymitis** usually is caused by *N. gonorrhoeae* or *C. trachomatis* in sexually active young men and by gram-negative enteric organisms in older men. Diagnosis and therapy should be directed accordingly, with ceftriaxone and doxycycline in young men and TMP/SMX or ciprofloxacin in men older than 40 years.

H. **When candiduria is present,** it is crucial to distinguish infection from colonization, which usually does not require treatment other than optimization of host status (glucose control in diabetics, removal or change of Foley catheter). Symptomatic candiduria with pyuria and asymptomatic candiduria in patients at high risk for development of candidemia (e.g., severely immunosuppressed) should receive fluconazole, 100–200 mg PO qd, for 5 days. Amphotericin continuous bladder irrigations have not been proven to be efficacious.

**II. Pyelonephritis**

**A. Acute uncomplicated pyelonephritis**

1. **Diagnosis.** Patients present with fever, flank pain, and lower UTI symptoms. Urine specimens characteristically demonstrate significant bacteriuria, pyuria, and occasional leukocyte casts. Urine cultures should be obtained in all suspect patients. Blood cultures should be obtained in those who are hospitalized, as bacteremia will be detected in 15–20%. The causative agent usually is *E. coli*.
2. **Treatment.** Patients with mild to moderate illness who are able to take oral medication can be safely treated as outpatients with TMP/SMX or fluoroquinolones for 10–14 days. Patients with more severe illness, those who are nauseated and vomiting, and pregnant patients should be treated initially with parenteral therapy. Appropriate empiric parenteral regimens include TMP/SMX, third-generation cephalosporins, second-generation fluoroquinolones, or aminoglycosides (with or without a beta-lactam agent). If enterococcal infection is suspected on the basis of a urine Gram stain, ampicillin, 1 g IV q6h, with or without gentamicin, 1 mg/kg IV q8h, is appropriate.

**B. Evaluation for anatomic abnormalities.** In patients who do not respond to initial empiric treatment within 48 hours, the presence of an anatomic abnormality such as intrarenal abscess or renal calculi should be evaluated by ultrasonography, CT scan, or IVP.

## Sexually Transmitted Diseases

**I. Ulcerative diseases**

**A. Genital herpes** is caused by human HSV, usually type 2, and is characterized by painful grouped vesicles in the genital and perianal regions that rapidly ulcerate and form shallow tender lesions. The initial episode may be associated with inguinal adenopathy, fever, headache, myalgias, and aseptic meningitis; recurrences usually are less severe.

1. **Diagnosis.** The confirmation of HSV infection requires culture or PCR; however, clinical presentation is often adequate for diagnosis.
2. **Treatment.** Acyclovir, 400 mg PO tid (or 200 mg PO 5 times a day) for 7–10 days, is recommended for all primary genital HSV infections if begun within 1 week of symptoms. Treatment is indicated for severe recurrences, and options include acyclovir, 400 mg PO tid (or 200 mg PO 5 times a day) for 5 days; valacyclovir, 500 mg PO bid for 5 days; or famciclovir, 125 mg PO bid for 5 days. Suppressive therapy with acyclovir, 400 mg PO bid, may be necessary for severe or frequent recurrences. Topical acyclovir has no proven benefit in the treatment or prophylaxis of HSV infection.

**B. Syphilis** is caused by the *Treponema pallidum* spirochete. Primary syphilis may develop within several weeks of exposure and involves one or more painless, indurated, superficial ulcerations (chancre). Secondary syphilis develops after the chancre resolves and involves a rash, mucocutaneous lesions, adenopathy, and constitutional symptoms. Tertiary syphilis includes cardiovascular, gummatous, and neurologic disease (general paresis, tabes dorsalis, or meningovascular syphilis).

1. **Diagnosis.** In **primary syphilis,** dark-field microscopy of the lesion exudate, a nontreponemal serologic test (e.g., RPR or VDRL), and a tre-

ponemal serologic test (e.g., fluorescent treponemal antibody absorption test, microhemagglutinin antigen–*T. pallidum*) are confirmatory. Diagnosis of **secondary syphilis** is made on the basis of positive serologic studies and the presence of compatible clinical illness. In the absence of symptoms, **latent syphilis** is a serologic diagnosis—early latent syphilis is defined as serologically positive for less than 1 year, and late latent syphilis is defined as serologically positive for more than 1 year. Diagnosis of **tertiary disease** requires clinical correlation with cardiovascular, neurologic, or systemic symptoms. Lumbar puncture should be performed in the presence of neurologic or ophthalmic signs or symptoms, evidence of tertiary disease, treatment failure, or serum RPR or VDRL of 1:32 or greater (unless the duration of infection is <1 year). Patients with HIV and syphilis of more than 1 year's duration also should undergo a lumbar puncture.

2. **Treatment.** To treat primary, secondary, and early latent disease, benzathine penicillin G, 2.4 million units IM in a single dose, is used. The alternative is doxycycline, 100 mg PO bid for 14 days. Treatment of late latent disease should include benzathine penicillin G, 2.4 million U IM, one dose per week for 3 weeks; an alternative is doxycycline, 100 mg PO bid for 4 weeks. Neurosyphilis treatment should include aqueous penicillin G, 12–24 million units IV qd in divided doses for 10–14 days; an alternative is procaine penicillin, 2.4 million units IM qd, plus probenecid, 500 mg PO qid for 10–14 days. Some practitioners follow this standard neurosyphilis regimen with an additional IM injection of benzathine penicillin G. An alternative, when penicillin is not available, is either IV or IM ceftriaxone.

## II. Vaginitis and vaginosis

**A. Trichomoniasis** is a parasitic infection caused by *Trichomonas vaginalis*. Clinical symptoms include malodorous purulent vaginal discharge; dysuria; and genital inflammation. Physical examination reveals profuse frothy discharge and cervical petechiae. The pH of vaginal fluid usually is 4.5 or higher. Diagnosis requires visualization of motile trichomonads on a saline wet mount of discharge. The **treatment** is metronidazole, 2.0 g PO in a single dose; intravaginal metronidazole gel is not effective. In the event of single-dose treatment failure, patients should receive metronidazole, 500 mg PO bid for 7 days. Because trichomoniasis is associated with adverse outcomes in pregnancy, it is recommended that pregnant women with symptoms of trichomoniasis be treated with a single dose of metronidazole, 2 g PO [*MMWR Morb Mortal Wkly Rep* 51(RR-6):45, 2002].

**B. Vulvovaginal candidiasis (VVC)** is caused by *Candida* species and commonly develops in relation to oral contraceptive use or antibiotic therapy. VVC, particularly if recurrent, may be a presenting manifestation of unrecognized HIV infection. It presents with thick, cottage cheese–like vaginal discharge in conjunction with intense vulvar inflammation, pruritus, and external dysuria. Definitive diagnosis requires visualization of fungal elements on a potassium hydroxide preparation of vaginal discharge fluid, but therapy often is initiated on the basis of the clinical presentation. **Treatment** is fluconazole, 100 mg PO qd for 3 days, or any of the intravaginal imidazole regimens (e.g., clotrimazole vaginal cream or suppository, 100 mg qhs for 7 days or 200 mg qhs for 3 days). For recurrent VVC, fluconazole, 100 mg PO, is usually effective. Duration of treatment is tailored to the individual case. Fluconazole failure could indicate the presence of a non–*albicans Candida* species.

**III. Cervicitis** is a frequent presentation of infection with ***N. gonorrhoeae*** **or** ***C. trachomatis*** and occasionally *Mycoplasma hominis*, *U. urealyticum*, and *T. vaginalis*. These infections frequently coexist, and the clinical presentations may be identical. Women with urethritis or cervicitis, or both, complain of mucopurulent vaginal discharge, dyspareunia, and dysuria. Men with urethritis complain of dysuria and a purulent penile discharge. A positive endocervical or urethral culture, endocervical DNA probe test, or urinary PCR is required for diagnosis. For gonorrhea, a Gram stain of endocervical or urethral discharge with gram-negative diplococci can also establish the diagnosis. Because of frequent coinfection, **simultaneous therapy for chlamydia** is recommended when gonorrhea is diagnosed. Single-dose antigonococcal therapies include ofloxacin, 400 mg PO, ciprofloxacin, 500 mg PO, ceftriaxone, 125 mg IM, or spectinomycin, 2 g IM. Effective antichlamydial therapy includes azithromycin, 1 g PO in a single dose; doxycycline, 100 mg PO bid for 7 days; or erythromycin stearate, 500 mg PO qid (or enteric-coated erythromycin base, 666 mg PO tid) for 7 days.

**IV. Pelvic inflammatory disease (PID)** is an upper genital tract infection in women, usually preceded by cervicitis that ranges from mild illness with lower abdominal pain and dyspareunia to peritonitis and tubo-ovarian abscess. Long-term consequences of untreated PID include chronic pain, infertility, and ectopic pregnancy. Cervical motion tenderness and the presence of at least ten WBCs per low-power field on endocervical smear Gram stain are consistent with PID. Endocervical cultures or probes for chlamydia and gonorrhea should be obtained. Severely ill, pregnant, HIV-infected, and severely nauseated patients should be hospitalized. **Treatment** for hospitalized patients should include either cefoxitin, 2 g IV q6h, or cefotetan, 2 g IV q12h, plus doxycycline, 100 mg IV or PO q12h. Clindamycin, 900 mg IV q8h, plus gentamicin is an alternative. Parenteral antibiotics are usually continued for at least 48 hours after the patient shows signs of improvement. Doxycycline, 100 mg PO bid for 14 days, can be used to complete the course of therapy. For outpatient therapy, several regimens are effective: (1) cefoxitin, 2 g IM, with probenecid, 1 g PO, plus doxycycline, 100 mg PO bid for 14 days; (2) ceftriaxone, 250 mg IM, plus doxycycline, 100 mg PO bid for 14 days, plus metronidazole, 500 mg PO bid for 7 days; or (3) ofloxacin, 400 mg PO bid for 14 days, plus metronidazole, 500 mg PO bid for 14 days. Intrauterine devices should be removed. Patients should abstain from sexual intercourse during therapy. All patients should receive follow-up within 72 hours to ensure adequate response to therapy.

## Systemic Mycoses

Fungal infections can often be identified by taking into account the clinical findings, site of infection, inflammatory response, and fungal appearance. Yeast-like fungi are typically round or oval and reproduce by budding, whereas molds are composed of tubular hyphae that grow by branching and longitudinal extension. The clinical presentations are protean and not pathogen specific.

**I. Candidiasis** is often associated with concurrent antibiotic use, contraceptive use, immunosuppressant and cytotoxic therapy, and indwelling foreign bodies. Candidiasis may present as mucocutaneous or invasive disease (e.g., candidemia with or without tissue dissemination). Mucocutaneous disease may resolve after elimination of the causative condition (e.g., antibiotic therapy) or may persist and progress in the setting of immunosuppressive conditions. Although isolated candidemia sometimes resolves spontaneously, particularly after catheter removal if disease is related to an infected catheter, serious complications, such as skin lesions, ocular disease, and osteomyelitis, can occur. Systemic antifungal therapy is recommended for all forms of invasive candidiasis.

**A. Diagnosis.** Mucocutaneous candidiasis is usually a clinical diagnosis, although a potassium hydroxide preparation of exudate provides confirmation. Cultures can be obtained in refractory cases to exclude the presence of non–*albicans Candida* species. Invasive candidiasis is diagnosed by positive cultures of blood or tissue.

**B. Treatment**

1. **Oral candidiasis,** or thrush, usually responds to topical therapy with clotrimazole troches, 10 mg dissolved in the mouth five times a day. Fluconazole, 100–200 mg PO qd, is very effective and preferred over topical therapy if the patient has esophageal involvement. Amphotericin B, 10–20 mg IV qd for 7–14 days; voriconazole; and caspofungin are effective alternatives for disease that is severe or failing fluconazole. The duration of therapy depends on clinical response and the reversibility of the underlying condition.
2. **Isolated catheter-related candidemia** (see the Nosocomial Infections section)
3. **Disseminated candidiasis** should be treated with more prolonged courses of either amphotericin B, 0.5 mg/kg/day IV for a total of 0.5–2.0 g, or a lipid formulation of amphotericin B. Fluconazole, 200–400 mg IV or PO qd, is an alternative for invasive disease caused by a sensitive organism. Most *C. albicans* and some non-*albicans* species including *Candida parapsilosis* and *Candida tropicalis* are generally sensitive to fluconazole (*Clin Infect Dis* 30:662, 2000). Voriconazole and caspofungin are alternatives if fluconazole fails and in patients who are intolerant of amphotericin B.

**II. Aspergillosis** is caused by *Aspergillus* species, which are ubiquitous environmental fungi.

**A. Allergic bronchopulmonary aspergillosis** has a natural history that includes remissions and exacerbations with eventual pulmonary bronchiectasis and fibrosis. **Diagnosis** generally requires the presence of asthma, eosinophilia, immunologic evidence of *Aspergillus* colonization, and radiographic abnormalities. **Treatment** consists of allergen avoidance and the intermittent use of corticosteroids.

**B. Pulmonary aspergilloma** has a variable natural history, ranging from spontaneous resolution to locally invasive disease. **Diagnosis** is made in the setting of a characteristic radiographic presentation ("fungus ball") and serum *Aspergillus* precipitins. **Treatment** is controversial because antifungal therapy has not been proven beneficial; however, surgical resection or bronchial artery embolization may be necessary for massive hemoptysis.

**C. Invasive aspergillosis** is a serious condition associated with vascular invasion, thrombosis, and ischemic infarction of involved tissues and progressive disease after hematogenous dissemination. **Diagnosis** requires characteristic histologic evidence of involved tissue and a positive culture. **Treatment** of serious invasive aspergillosis has traditionally required amphotericin B (1.0–1.5 mg/kg/day for 2.0–2.5 g total) or a lipid formulation of amphotericin B; however, newer agents are now available that exhibit similar or improved efficacy and less toxicity. Voriconazole, 6 mg/kg IV × two doses 12 hours apart followed by a maintenance dose of 4 mg/kg IV q12h or 200 mg PO bid, is a triazole antifungal that appears to be at least as efficacious, if not better than, conventional amphotericin B (*N Engl J Med* 347:408, 2002). Caspofungin, 70 mg IV loading dose followed by 50 mg IV q24h, is the first available drug of the echinocandin class of antifungal agents and is an alternative for salvage therapy. Itraconazole, 600 mg PO elixir qd for 4 days, then 200–400 mg PO elixir qd, may be effective in mild to moderate invasive aspergillosis.

**III. Cryptococcosis** is a mycosis that occurs worldwide and is caused by *Cryptococcus neoformans*, a yeast associated with soil and pigeon excrement. Definitive **diagnosis** requires detection of encapsulated yeast in tissue or body fluids with culture confirmation. The latex agglutination test for cryptococcal antigen in serum or CSF provides a supportive diagnosis. Lumbar puncture is necessary in persons with systemic disease to exclude coexistent CNS involvement. **Treatment** depends on the patient's immune function and the site of infection (*Clin Infect Dis* 30:710, 2000). In general, treatment is necessary for immunocompromised hosts, CNS or disseminated disease, and those with symptomatic infection. The treatment of choice for CNS disease is amphotericin B, 0.7–1.0 mg/kg IV qd, with flucytosine, 25 mg/kg PO q6h, for 2 weeks, followed by 3 months of fluconazole, 400 mg PO qd. Flucytosine dosage should be adjusted to achieve appropriate serum levels (peak, 70–80 mg/L, trough 30–40 mg/L) and to avoid serious adverse events. Immunocompetent hosts generally do not need prolonged maintenance therapy. For non-CNS disseminated disease, including cutaneous involvement or cryptococcemia, fluconazole, 200–400 mg PO qd for 6–12 months, is recommended. Isolated asymptomatic pulmonary cryptococcosis in an immunocompetent host can usually be followed without specific therapy.

IV. **Histoplasmosis,** a major endemic mycosis associated with bird and bat excrement primarily in the Ohio and Mississippi River Valleys, is caused by *Histoplasma capsulatum*. The **diagnosis** requires visualization of small yeasts in tissue or body fluids, or a positive culture, associated with positive complement fixation and immunodiffusion serology. Detection of *Histoplasma* antigen in urine, serum, or CSF is reliable in the diagnosis of disseminated infection of immunosuppressed hosts (*Clin Infect Dis* 30:688, 2000). Disease ranges from asymptomatic to mild pulmonary involvement to severe disseminated disease. **Standard therapy** for most symptomatic infections is itraconazole, 200 mg PO tid loading dose for 3 days, followed by 200–400 mg PO qd for 6–12 months; the elixir formulation is preferred given its more reliable absorption, and documentation of therapeutic levels is essential. More severe disease requires an initial course of amphotericin B, whereas mild pulmonary disease can be observed without specific therapy.

V. **Blastomycosis** is an endemic mycosis in North America caused by *Blastomyces dermatitidis*. The **diagnosis** of blastomycosis requires demonstration of large yeasts with broad-based buds or a positive culture from tissues or body fluids. Serologic studies are unreliable for diagnosis. Disease ranges from asymptomatic to chronic pulmonary involvement to severe disseminated disease. **Treatment** is usually itraconazole, 200–400 mg PO qd following a loading dose of 200 PO tid, for a minimum of 6 months. Amphotericin B, 0.7–1.0 mg/kg/day for a total dose of 1.5–2.5 g, should be used for life-threatening or CNS disease, often followed by a course of itraconazole (*Clin Infect Dis* 30:679, 2000).

VI. **Coccidioidomycosis,** a major endemic mycosis of the southwestern United States and Central America, is caused by *Coccidioides immitis*. The **diagnosis** of coccidioidomycosis requires visualization of an endosporulating spherule in tissue or body fluids, positive culture, or positive complement fixation serology. Lumbar puncture should be performed to rule out CNS involvement in persons with severe, rapidly progressive, or disseminated disease. **Treatment** is fluconazole, 400–600 mg PO qd, or itraconazole, 200 mg PO bid, for at least 6 months for mild or moderate nonmeningeal disease. High-dose fluconazole, 800 mg PO qd, with or without intrathecal amphotericin, is preferred for meningitis. Patients with disease that is severe, progressive, or disseminated may benefit from amphotericin B, 1.0–1.5 mg/kg IV q24h for a total of 1–3 g, depending on the clinical response. Some patients may require maintenance therapy with itraconazole (*Clin Infect Dis* 30:658, 2000).

VII. **Sporotrichosis** follows traumatic inoculation, generally of the extremities, after contact with soil or plant material, and lymphocutaneous disease is the usual manifestation. Untreated disease can persist and slowly progress over time; hematogenous dissemination occurs rarely in immunocompromised hosts, and pneumonia, arthritis, or meningitis can develop. The **diagnosis** requires demonstration of yeast in tissue or body fluids, a positive culture, or positive serologic studies. **Treatment** (*Clin Infect Dis* 30:684, 2000) for lymphocutaneous disease is itraconazole, 100–200 mg PO qd for 3–6 months, with documentation of therapeutic levels. A saturated solution of potassium iodide, 5 drops PO tid, increased to 40 drops tid as tolerated, for 3–6 months is an alternative. Severe and meningeal disease should be treated with amphotericin B, 0.5 mg/kg IV qd for 1–2 g total.

## Arthropod-Borne Diseases, Zoonoses, and Bite Wounds

**I. Arthropod-borne diseases**

**A. Tick-borne illnesses (TBIs)** are common during the summer months in many areas of the United States; prevalences for specific diseases depend on the local population of vector ticks and animal reservoirs. Coinfection with multiple TBIs is common and should be considered when patients present with overlapping syndromes. Risk for a TBI should be assessed by outdoor activity in endemic regions rather than known tick bite or attachment, as these are often unrecognized.

1. **Lyme borreliosis (Lyme disease)** is the most common vector-borne disease in the United States and is a systemic illness of variable severity caused by the spirochete *Borrelia burgdorferi*. Disease is seen in endemic regions, including northeastern coastal states, the upper Midwest, and northern California. The disease has three distinct stages, which start after an incubation period of 7–10 days. Stage 1 (**early local disease**) is characterized by erythema migrans, a slowly expanding macular rash greater than 5 cm in diameter, often with central clearing, and by mild constitutional symptoms. Manifestations of stage 2 (**early disseminated disease**) occur within several weeks to months and include multiple erythema migrans lesions, neurologic symptoms (e.g., seventh cranial nerve palsy, meningoencephalitis), cardiac symptoms (atrioventricular block, myopericarditis), and asymmetric oligoarticular arthritis. Stage 3 (**late disease**) occurs after months to years and includes chronic dermatitis, neurologic disease, and asymmetric monoarticular or oligoarticular arthritis. Chronic fatigue is not seen more frequently in patients with Lyme borreliosis than in control subjects. **Diagnosis** rests on clinical suspicion in the appropriate setting and is supported by two-tiered serologic testing (screening enzyme-linked immunosorbent assay followed by Western blot). Culture of *B. burgdorferi* from skin lesions provides a definitive diagnosis but is impractical. A substantial degree of coinfection occurs with babesiosis and ehrlichiosis. **Treatment** depends on stage and severity of disease. Oral therapy (doxycycline, 100 mg PO bid; amoxicillin, 500 mg PO tid; or cefuroxime axetil, 500 mg PO bid for 14–21 days) is used for early localized or disseminated disease without neurologic or cardiac involvement. Doxycycline has the added benefit of covering potential coinfection with ehrlichiosis. Parenteral therapy (ceftriaxone, 2 g IV qd; cefotaxime, 2 g IV q8h; penicillin G, 3–4 million U IV q4h) should be used for neurologic or cardiac disease. The routine use of prophylactic antimicrobials after a tick bite is not recommended (*Clin Infect Dis* 31:S1, 2000).
2. **RMSF** (see the Fever and Rash section)
3. **Ehrlichiosis** is a systemic TBI that is caused by intracellular pathogens of the *Ehrlichia* genus. Two similar syndromes are recognized: **human monocytic ehrlichiosis,** endemic in the south and south-central United States, and **human granulocytic ehrlichiosis,** found in the same regions as Lyme borreliosis due to a shared tick vector. Onset of illness usually occurs 1 week after exposure, with fever, headache, and myalgias. Unlike RMSF, a rash is only occasionally seen. Severe disease can result in respiratory failure, renal insufficiency, and neurologic decompensation. Leukopenia, thrombocytopenia, and elevated liver transaminases are the hallmark of moderately severe disease. **Identification of morulae** in circulating monocytes or granulocytes is uncommon but diagnostic in the appropriate clinical setting. Confirmation is by acute

and convalescent serology or PCR of blood or other fluids. Prompt initiation of **antimicrobial therapy** is likely to improve prognosis in severe disease. The drugs of choice are doxycycline, 100 mg PO or IV q12h, or tetracycline, 25 mg/kg/day PO divided qid, for 7–14 days.

4. **Tularemia** is a disease endemic to the south-central United States caused by the gram-negative *Francisella tularensis*. Disease onset with fever and malaise occurs 2–5 days after tick bite or exposure to infected animals (particularly rabbits). Infection can also occur from inhalation of an infectious aerosol. Presentation is one of several forms based on inoculation site and route of exposure. Painful regional lymphadenitis with a skin ulcer (ulceroglandular form), or without (glandular), is the most common finding. Systemic (typhoidal) and pneumonic disease are more likely to be severe, with high mortality if not treated promptly. **Diagnosis** can be confirmed by culture of blood, sputum, or pleural fluid, but it is insensitive. **The microbiology laboratory should be alerted promptly of culture specimens from patients with suspected tularemia to allow for advanced biohazard precautions.** Acute and convalescent serologic studies provide a retrospective diagnosis. Streptomycin, 1 g IM q12h for 10 days, has been the **treatment of choice;** however, gentamicin is nearly as effective and easier to administer. Doxycycline, 100 mg PO bid for 14–21 days, is an oral alternative but is more likely to result in relapse. Ciprofloxacin, 500 mg PO bid for 10–14 days, may also be effective.
5. **Babesiosis** is a malaria-like illness caused by the intraerythrocytic parasite *Babesia microti* after a tick bite. It is endemic in the same regions as Lyme borreliosis, with which patients may be coinfected. Disease ranges from subclinical to severe, with fever, chills, myalgias, headache, and dark urine due to hemolysis. Hemolytic anemia may also be present. **Diagnosis** is made by visualization of the parasite in erythrocytes on thick or thin blood smears. A serologic test is also available at the CDC. **Treatment** may be necessary for moderate or severe disease, especially in asplenic patients. Atovaquone, 750 mg PO bid, plus azithromycin, 500 mg PO $\times$ 1 followed by 250 mg PO qd, for 7 days is the first choice. Clindamycin, 600 mg PO/IV q8h, plus quinine, 650 mg PO tid, for 7 days should be considered for life-threatening disease.

**B. Mosquito-borne infections**

1. **Arboviral meningoencephalitis** is caused by multiple viral agents [**West Nile Virus (WNV),** Eastern and Western equine encephalitis, La Crosse encephalitis, St. Louis encephalitis]. Infections usually occur in the summer months, and most are subclinical. Symptomatic cases of WNV infection range from a mild febrile illness to aseptic meningitis, fulminant encephalitis, or a poliomyelitis-like presentation with flaccid paralysis. Long-term neurologic sequelae are common. In addition to mosquitoes, transmission can occur from blood transfusion, organ transplant, and possibly breast-feeding. **Diagnosis** is usually clinical or by acute and convalescent serologic studies. Specific IgM antibody detection in CSF is diagnostic for acute WNV. **Treatment** for all arboviral meningoencephalitides is supportive.
2. **Malaria** is a systemic parasitic disease that is endemic to most of the tropical and subtropical world. *Plasmodium falciparum* malaria, the most severe form of the disease, is a potential medical emergency. The onset of illness occurs within weeks or up to 6–12 months of infection with fever, headache, myalgias, and fatigue. Malaria is sometimes characterized by triphasic, periodic (every 48 hours for *Plasmodium ovale* and *Plasmodium vivax*) paroxysms of rigors followed by high fever with headache, cough, and nausea, then culminating in profuse sweating. Complicated, or severe, falciparum malaria is diagnosed in the setting of: hyperparasitemia (>5%), cerebral malaria, hypoglycemia, lactic acidosis, renal failure, acute respiratory distress syndrome, or coagulopathy.

a. **Diagnosis** is by visualization of parasites on examination of Giemsa-stained thin or thick blood smears. **Malaria should be suspected and excluded in all persons with fever who have been in an endemic area within the previous year.**

b. **Treatment** is dependent on the type of malaria, severity, and risk of chloroquine resistance where the infection occurred. Malaria remains chloroquine sensitive in most of Central America and the Caribbean and some of the Middle East. Updated information on geographic locations of chloroquine resistance can be found on the CDC web site, http://www.cdc.gov/travel/. **Usual treatment regimens** are

(1) **Uncomplicated *P. falciparum* from chloroquine-sensitive areas and *P. malariae*:** chloroquine, 600-mg base (1000 mg chloroquine phosphate) PO × 1, followed by 300-mg base PO 6, 24, and 48 hours later.

(2) ***P. ovale* and most *P. vivax*:** same as above, plus primaquine phosphate, 15.3-mg base (26.5 mg salt) PO qd, for 14 days to prevent relapse. Glucose 6-phosphate dehydrogenase deficiency must be ruled out before primaquine is initiated.

(3) **Uncomplicated *P. falciparum* from chloroquine-resistant areas and *P. vivax* from Australia or South America:** quinine sulfate, 650 mg PO tid for 3–7 days, plus doxycycline, 100 mg PO bid for 7 days. An alternative is atovaquone, 1 g PO qd, plus proguanil, 400 mg PO qd, both for 3 days.

(4) **Complicated or severe *P. falciparum*:** quinidine gluconate, 10 mg salt/kg (maximum, 600 mg) IV over 1–2 hours, followed by 0.02 mg/kg/minute as a continuous infusion for 72 hours or until parasitemia is less than 1%, at which time the 72-hour course can be completed with oral quinine sulfate as above. Exchange transfusion can be considered when *P. falciparum* parasitemia exceeds 15%, although the benefit has not been proven.

c. **Prophylaxis.** Pretravel advice and appropriate chemoprophylaxis regimens are available at the CDC web site, http://www.cdc.gov/travel/.

3. **Dengue fever** is an acute febrile illness that appears 4–7 days after transmission of dengue virus from a mosquito bite. Fever, chills, and prominent frontal headache lead to prostration and malaise. Hepatic involvement is common, and a hemorrhagic fever syndrome may occur. Diagnosis is serologic, and treatment is supportive.

## II. Zoonoses

A. **Cat-scratch disease**, or Bartonellosis, is a lymphadenitis syndrome caused by the bacterium *Bartonella henselae*. A single or a few papulopustular lesions appear 3–10 days after a cat bite or scratch, followed by regional lymphadenitis (usually cervical or axillary) and mild constitutional symptoms. Atypical presentations include oculoglandular disease, encephalopathy, arthritis, and severe systemic disease. **Diagnosis** is made by exclusion of other causes of lymphadenitis and by detection of antibodies to *B. henselae* or PCR of infected tissue, skin, or pus. **The role of routine antimicrobial therapy is not well established** because there is little evidence that therapy alters the natural course of disease, which usually resolves spontaneously over 2–4 months. If antimicrobial therapy is prescribed, azithromycin, 500 mg PO × 1 followed by 250 mg PO × 4 more days, seems to be the most likely to have an effect, although many other antibiotics are active against *B. henselae*. Needle aspiration of suppurative lymph nodes may provide symptomatic relief.

B. **Leptospirosis** is an acute febrile illness with varying presentations caused by *Leptospira interrogans*, a ubiquitous pathogen of wild and domestic mammals, reptiles, and amphibians. Onset of disease is 5–14 days after contact with infected animals or water contaminated with their urine. **Anic-**

**teric leptospirosis,** which accounts for most cases, is a biphasic illness that starts with influenza-like symptoms and proceeds to conjunctival suffusion and aseptic meningitis after a brief defervescent period. A minority progress directly to **Weil's disease (icteric leptospirosis),** with multiorgan failure manifested by severe jaundice, uremia, and hemorrhagic pneumonitis. **Diagnosis** is confirmed by specific cultures of urine or blood, PCR, or paired serologic studies. **Therapy** for anicteric disease, which can shorten the duration of illness, is doxycycline, 100 mg PO bid, or amoxicillin, 500 mg PO q6h. Penicillin G, 1.5 million U IV q4–6h, or ampicillin, 1 g IV q6h, is used for treatment of severe disease, during which a Jarisch-Herxheimer reaction is possible.

**C. Brucellosis** is a protean systemic infection caused by members of the *Brucella* genus of gram-negative coccobacilli. Infection usually is preceded by direct contact with body fluids of livestock animals or by eating unpasteurized dairy foods. Symptoms are initially nonspecific, but complications within every organ system can occur (diarrhea, arthritis, meningitis, endocarditis, pneumonia). Growth on blood or tissue culture confirms the **diagnosis. Antimicrobial therapy** with doxycycline, 100 mg PO bid, and gentamicin for 6 weeks reduces duration and complications of the disease. Audiometry should be performed weekly while gentamicin therapy is administered.

**D. Anthrax** (see the Bioterrorism section)

**E. Plague** (see the Bioterrorism section)

**III. Bite wounds**

**A. General considerations.** Bite wounds should be assessed for location and extent of injury, functional disability, evidence of infection, and need for rabies prophylaxis (see sec. **III.B**). Management includes obtaining cultures from visibly infected wounds, copious irrigation, and radiographic studies to exclude fracture, foreign body, or joint space involvement. Most wounds should not be sutured unless they are on the face and have been copiously irrigated. Wound elevation should be encouraged. Antimicrobial therapy is given to treat overt infection and as prophylaxis for high-risk bite wounds based on severity (moderate to severe), location (on hands, genitalia, or near joints), bite source (cats), immune status, and type of injury (puncture or crush). Tetanus booster should be given if none has been administered to the patient in the last 5 years.

**B.** The need for **rabies** vaccination and immunoglobulin prophylaxis (see Appendix F, Immunizations and Post-Exposure Therapies) should be determined after any animal bite. Rabies causes an invariably fatal, untreatable neurologic disease. Risk depends on the animal species and the geographic location. **Regardless of species, if the animal is rabid or suspected to be rabid, the human diploid vaccine and rabies immunoglobulin should be administered immediately.** Endemic rabies is present in some wild animals, particularly bats, mandating immediate prophylaxis following bites from these animals. Bites by domestic animals rarely require prophylaxis unless the animal's condition is unknown. Public health authorities should be consulted to determine if prophylaxis is recommended for most other animals. See Appendix F for further details.

**C. Human bites,** particularly clenched-fist injuries, are prone to infection and other complications. The normal oral flora of humans includes viridans streptococci, staphylococci, *Bacteroides* species, *Fusobacterium* species, peptostreptococci, and *Eikenella corrodens*. **Treatment** includes prophylaxis with amoxicillin/clavulanate, 875 mg/125 mg PO bid for 3–5 days for uninfected wounds. Infected wounds require parenteral therapy, such as ampicillin/sulbactam, 1.5 g IV q6h; cefoxitin, 2 g IV q8h; or ticarcillin/clavulanate, 3.1 g IV q6h, for 1–2 weeks. Therapy should be extended to 4–6 weeks if osteomyelitis is present.

**D. Dog bites.** For dogs, the normal oral flora includes *Pasteurella multocida*, streptococci, staphylococci, and *Capnocytophaga canimorsus*. Dog bites are responsible for 80% of animal bites, but only 20% become infected. **Prophy-**

**lactic antibiotic therapy** with amoxicillin/clavulanate, 875 mg/125 mg PO bid, for 3–5 days should usually be administered, unless the bite is trivial. For infected dog-bite wounds, amoxicillin/clavulanate, or clindamycin plus ciprofloxacin, is effective.

E. **Cat bites.** The normal oral flora of cats includes *P. multocida* and *S. aureus*. Because more than 80% of cat bites become infected, **prophylaxis** with amoxicillin/clavulanate should routinely be provided. For infected wounds, effective therapy includes amoxicillin/clavulanate, doxycycline, or cefuroxime axetil. Duration of therapy is 1–2 weeks for cellulitis and 4–6 weeks for osteomyelitis. Bartonellosis can also occur after bites (see sec. **II.A**).

F. **Wild animal bites.** The need for rabies vaccination should be determined (see sec. **III.B**). For most animals, amoxicillin/clavulanate is a good choice for prophylaxis and empiric treatment. Monkey bites should be treated with acyclovir because of the risk of *Herpesvirus simiae*.

## Nosocomial Infections

I. **General.** Hospital-acquired infections substantially contribute to morbidity, mortality, and excess health care costs. Efforts to control and prevent the spread of nosocomial infections require an institutional assessment of resources, priorities, and commitment to use of antimicrobial agents and infection control practices (see Appendix G, Infection Control and Isolation Recommendations).

II. **Catheter-related bloodstream infections (CR-BSIs).** CVCs are increasingly used in acute and chronic health care delivery today and contribute to more than 210,000 CR-BSIs annually, with associated increases in mortality, hospital stay, and medical costs.

A. **Diagnostic measures.** Clinical findings that increase the suspicion of CR-BSIs are local inflammation or phlebitis at the CVC insertion site, sepsis, endophthalmitis, lack of another source of bacteremia, and resolution of fever after catheter removal. Paired blood cultures should initially be drawn through the IV catheter and percutaneously.

B. **Therapy.** *S. aureus*, *S. epidermidis*, aerobic gram-negative species, and *Candida* species have most commonly been associated with CR-BSIs (*Clin Infect Dis* 32:1249–1272, 2001).

1. **Initial empiric antimicrobial therapy.** Host factors, such as comorbidities, severity of illness, multidrug-resistant colonization, prior infections, and current antimicrobial agents, are important considerations when selecting the initial antimicrobial regimen. Vancomycin, 1 g IV q12h, is usually appropriate for empiric therapy, as the majority of CR-BSI pathogens are gram-positive cocci.
2. **Pathogen-specific therapy.** Once the pathogen has been identified, antimicrobial therapy should be narrowed to the most effective regimen. Duration of treatment depends on whether the infection is complicated or uncomplicated. Duration of treatment should be longer if the CVC remains in situ.
3. **Isolated catheter-related candidemia** in hosts who are hemodynamically unstable or have had prolonged fluconazole therapy should be treated with amphotericin B, 0.5 mg/kg IV q24h. Patients who are hemodynamically stable, have had low fluconazole exposure, and have a *Candida* species that is usually sensitive to fluconazole can be treated with fluconazole, 200–400 mg IV or PO qd. Duration of antifungal treatment for candidemia should be for 14 days after the last positive blood culture result and when signs and symptoms of infection have resolved.
4. **CVC removal** may involve complex decision-making with consideration of host status, ongoing vascular access, and the identified pathogen.

CVCs should always be removed if local inflammation or phlebitis is present at the insertion site. Immunosuppressed patients with CVCs who have fever, neutropenia, and hemodynamic instability should also have CVCs removed. The majority of septic patients with short-term CVCs should have CVCs removed at the first signs of sepsis. Decisions for removal of long-term catheters are tailored to the clinical scenario.

**C. Prevention**

1. **Placement.** Aseptic insertion techniques are imperative with CVC placement. Tincture of iodine skin preparation can reduce the risk of pseudobacteremia from coagulase-negative staphylococci (*Am J Med* 107:119, 1999). Subclavian vein CVCs are associated with lower CR-BSI rates than internal jugular CVCs, whereas femoral CVCs have the highest rates of CR-BSIs and should be removed within 72 hours of placement. Subcutaneous tunneling and use of antiseptic-impregnated CVCs may further reduce the incidence of CR-BSIs (*JAMA* 281:261, 1999).
2. **Catheter care.** Strategies to decrease the incidence of CR-BSIs include the use of transparent dressings, strict adherence to aseptic technique and hand-washing, antiseptic-impregnated catheter cuffs, topical antiseptic solutions, and routine catheter changes by experienced health care workers. Topical antimicrobial ointment, inline membrane filters, and frequent dressing changes are interventions that have not been associated with reduced CR-BSIs. Exchange of CVCs over guidewires is not routinely recommended.

**III. Hospital and ventilator-associated pneumonia.** Hospital and ventilatory pneumonia occur in 0.3–0.7% of hospitalized patients. On clinical presentation there is a new pulmonary infiltrate in patients with fever, with or without cough, that occurs more than 48 hours after admission.

**A. Diagnosis.** Optimal specimens are uncontaminated sterile body fluids (pleural or blood), bronchoscopy aspirates (cultured quantitatively), or aspirates from endotracheal tubes. The most frequent pathogens are gram-negative bacilli and *S. aureus*. Fiberoptic bronchoscopy may be diagnostic (quantitative cultures) and therapeutic (re-expansion of lung segment) in these patients.

**B. Treatment.** Initial empiric antimicrobial therapy should target treatment of nosocomially acquired gram-negative pathogens, particularly *P. aeruginosa*. Targeted therapy should be based on culture results and in vitro sensitivity testing. Empyemas require drainage.

**IV. ORSA infections** should be distinguished from ORSA colonization. First-line therapy for most ORSA infections is vancomycin (dosed to therapeutic trough levels). Linezolid, 600 mg IV or PO q12h, is an alternative. Eradication of ORSA nasal carriage can be achieved with a 5-day course of twice-daily intranasal mupirocin.

**V. VRE infections.** A distinction exists between VRE colonization and infection. The majority of patients with VRE bloodstream infections are treated with linezolid, 600 mg IV or PO q12h, or chloramphenicol (dosed to therapeutic levels). Most VRE-related lower UTIs can be treated with nitrofurantoin, ampicillin, ciprofloxacin, or other agents that achieve high urinary concentrations, irrespective of the susceptibility profile of the clinical isolate. Eradication of enteric VRE colonization has been attempted without success.

## Bioterrorism

**I. General considerations.** Several highly fatal and easily produced micro-organisms have the potential to be used as agents of bioterrorism. Six diseases have been designated as the most likely to be used for such a purpose. All can produce substantial illness in large populations via an aerosol route of exposure. As most of the likely diseases are rare, a high index of suspicion is necessary to identify the first few cases. A bioterrorism-related outbreak should be considered if an unusually large number of patients present simultaneously with a respiratory, GI, or febrile rash syndrome; if several otherwise healthy patients present with unusually severe disease; or if an unusual pathogen for the region is isolated. Any suspected or confirmed cases of these diseases should be treated as an epidemiologic emergency and reported immediately to the local health department.

**II. Specific diseases**

**A. Anthrax** is caused by contact with spores from the gram-positive *Bacillus anthracis*. Spores germinate at the site of entry into the body, primarily the lung **(inhalational anthrax),** the skin **(cutaneous anthrax),** or the intestinal mucosa **(gastrointestinal anthrax).** The inhalational (45% mortality) and cutaneous forms are the most likely to be encountered in an intentional release.

1. **Clinical features.** Inhalational anthrax presents with an early prodrome of an influenza-like illness (fevers, malaise, myalgias but without nasal symptoms) or GI symptoms, or both, followed by fulminant respiratory distress, multiorgan failure, and death. Diagnosis is suggested by a **widened mediastinum** without infiltrates on chest radiography and confirmed by blood culture. Cutaneous anthrax is characterized by a painless black eschar with surrounding edema.
2. **Therapy.** Immediate antibiotic initiation on first suspicion of inhalational anthrax reduces mortality. **Empiric therapy** (*N Engl J Med* 287:2236, 2002) should be ciprofloxacin, 400 mg IV q12h, *or* doxycycline, 100 mg IV q12h, *and* one or two other antibiotics that are active against *B. anthracis* (RIF, clindamycin, penicillin, amoxicillin, vancomycin, imipenem, chloramphenicol). Patients with signs or symptoms of meningitis should receive at least one agent with good penetration into the CSF. On improvement, therapy can be switched to oral ciprofloxacin, 500 mg PO bid, *or* doxycycline, 100 mg PO bid, *and* one other active agent. The total course of therapy should be 60 days to reduce the risk of delayed spore germination. Uncomplicated cutaneous anthrax can be treated with oral ciprofloxacin, 500 mg bid, *or* doxycycline, 100 mg bid, for the same duration.
3. **Postexposure prophylaxis** consists of oral ciprofloxacin, 500 mg bid for 60 days after exposure. Doxycycline or amoxicillin is an alternative if the strain proves susceptible.

**B. Smallpox,** caused by variola virus, was declared eradicated as a naturally occurring disease in 1979; however, remaining viral stocks pose a potential bioterrorism threat to an unimmunized population. Smallpox is **transmitted person to person** through respiratory droplets and carries a **case-fatality rate of 25–30%.**

1. **Clinical features.** High fever, myalgias, low back pain, and headache appear 7–17 days after exposure, followed by the distinctive rash 3–5 days later. The rash starts on the face and distal extremities, including palms and soles, with relative sparing of the trunk, and all lesions in one area are in the same stage of development. These features help to distinguish smallpox from chickenpox (varicella). Lesions progress through stages of macules, deep vesicles, pustules, scabs, and permanent pitting scars. Diagnosis is primarily clinical but can be confirmed by electron microscopy, PCR, and culture at reference laboratories.
2. **Therapy** consists of supportive care, as **no specific antiviral treatment is available.** All suspected cases must be placed in contact and respiratory isolation until all scabs have separated to prevent secondary transmission.
3. **Postexposure prophylaxis** with live vaccinia virus vaccine within 3 days of exposure offers near complete protection for responders but is

associated with uncommon severe adverse reactions. Progressive vaccinia, eczema vaccinatum, and severe cases of generalized vaccinia can be treated with vaccinia immunoglobulin.

C. **Plague,** caused by the gram-negative bacillus *Yersinia pestis*, takes one of three forms: **bubonic,** with a local lymphadenitis (bubo) and 14% case-fatality rate; **septicemic,** with 30–50% case-fatality; and **pneumonic,** with 57% case fatality nearing 100% when treatment is delayed. Pneumonic disease can be transmitted from person to person and would be expected after inhalation of aerosolized *Y. pestis*. Naturally acquired plague occurs rarely in the southwestern United States after exposure to infected animals.
   1. **Clinical features.** An initial **influenza-like illness** precedes dyspnea, cough, and hemoptysis that rapidly progresses to **fulminant pneumonia** and gram-negative sepsis. Diagnosis is confirmed by isolation of *Y. pestis* from blood, sputum, or CSF.
   2. **Therapy** should be started at the first suspicion of plague, as rapid initiation of antibiotics improves survival. The agents of choice are streptomycin, 1 g IM q12h, or gentamicin, 5 mg/kg IV/IM q24h *or* a 2 mg/kg loading dose, then 1.7 mg/kg IV/IM q8h, with appropriate monitoring of drug levels. Alternatives include doxycycline, ciprofloxacin, and chloramphenicol. The switch to oral therapy can be made after clinical improvement, for a total course of 10–14 days. Respiratory droplet isolation precautions should be instituted on first suspicion.
   3. **Postexposure prophylaxis** is doxycycline, 100 mg PO bid, or ciprofloxacin, 500 mg PO bid, for 7 days after exposure.

D. **Tularemia** (see the Arthropod-Borne Diseases, Zoonoses, and Bite Wounds section)

E. **Botulism** is the result of intoxication with botulinum toxin, produced by the anaerobic gram-positive bacillus *Clostridium botulinum*. Rare sporadic outbreaks in the United States are due to ingestion of toxin from improperly canned foods **(food-borne botulism).** The toxin can also be inhaled directly from an aerosol source **(inhalational botulism).** Mortality is low when it is recognized early but may be very high in the setting of mass exposure if supportive care equipment supplies (i.e., ventilators) are exhausted.
   1. **Clinical features.** The classic symptom triad is lack of fever, a clear sensorium, and a **symmetric descending flaccid paralysis,** beginning with ptosis, diplopia, and dysarthria and progressing to loss of gag reflex and diaphragmatic function followed by diffuse skeletal muscle paralysis. Sensation remains intact. Paralysis lasts for weeks to months. Diagnosis is confirmed by detection of toxin in serum.
   2. **Therapy** is primarily supportive, particularly ventilatory support. Although the degree of paralysis that is evident at the time of presentation is not reversible, further progression can be halted by administration of **botulinum antitoxin,** which is available from the local health department (1 vial administered intravenously, with or without additional intramuscular administration, per package insert).
   3. **Postexposure prophylaxis** with antitoxin is not recommended because of the high incidence (10%) of hypersensitivity reactions and limited supply.

F. **Viral hemorrhagic fever** is a syndrome caused by many different RNA viruses, including filoviruses **(Ebola),** flaviviruses **(dengue),** bunyaviruses [**Hanta viruses, Congo-Crimean hemorrhagic fever** (CCHF), and arenaviruses **(South American hemorrhagic fevers)**]. All cause sporadic disease in endemic areas, and most can be transmitted as an aerosol or contact with infected body fluids. Lassa, CCHF, and Ebola may be transmissible through respiratory spread. Case-fatality rates are variable but can be as high as 90% for severe Ebola cases.
   1. **Clinical features.** Early symptoms are fevers, myalgias, and malaise. Severity ranges from mild to fulminant, and symptomatology varies depending on the specific virus. All can severely disrupt vascular perme-

ability and cause disseminated intravascular coagulation, manifested by edema, mucous membrane hemorrhage, petechiae, and shock. Thrombocytopenia, leukopenia, and hepatitis are common. Serologic tests can differentiate most viral agents of viral hemorrhagic fever from malaria, rickettsial diseases, meningococcemia, and other causes of disseminated intravascular coagulation.

2. **Therapy** is primarily supportive, particularly management of fluid and blood product status. IV ribavirin is an experimental treatment that has been used for CCHF, Lassa, and Rift Valley fevers. **All patients suspected of having viral hemorrhagic fever should be placed in respiratory and contact isolation** to prevent secondary transmission.
3. **Postexposure prophylaxis** with oral ribavirin has been studied for CCHF and Lassa fever.

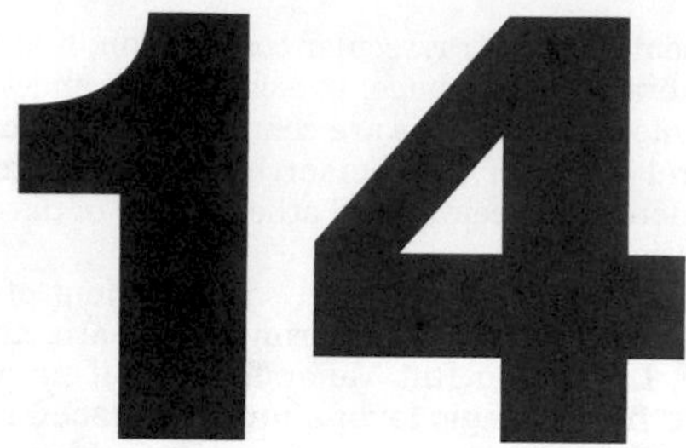

# 14 Human Immunodeficiency Virus Infection and Acquired Immunodeficiency Syndrome

Maria Ristig and
Pablo Tebas

## Screening and Evaluation of Patients with Human Immunodeficiency Virus

**I.** HIV type 1 is a human retrovirus that infects lymphocytes and other cells that bear the CD4 surface protein, as well as a coreceptor belonging to the chemokine receptor family. Infection usually leads to lymphopenia and CD4 T-cell depletion, impaired cell-mediated immunity, and polyclonal B-cell activation. Over time, this immune dysfunction gives rise to AIDS, which is characterized by opportunistic infections (OIs) and malignancies. The time from onset of HIV infection to development of AIDS varies from months to years (depending on host and viral factors), with a median incubation period of 10 years. The virus is transmitted sexually or parenterally. Therapy for HIV infection and AIDS includes antiretroviral therapy (ART), immunomodulation, prophylaxis for and treatment of opportunistic infections, and treatment of neoplasia.

**II. Before checking an individual's HIV serology,** informed consent should be obtained. Informed consent is required in most states and countries.

**A. Serology.** HIV serology should be checked in the following persons:

1. **Persons in high-risk categories,** including IV drug users, homosexual and bisexual men, hemophiliacs, sexual partners of the aforementioned patients, sexual partners of a known HIV patient, prostitutes and their sexual partners, persons with sexually transmitted diseases, persons who received blood products between 1977 and 1985, persons who have multiple sexual partners or who engage in unprotected intercourse, persons who consider themselves at risk, and patients with findings that are suggestive of HIV infection
2. **Pregnant women**
3. **Patients with active tuberculosis (TB)**
4. **Hospitalized patients** between the ages of 15 and 54 years if the community seroprevalence rate exceeds 1% or AIDS cases number more than 1 per 1000 discharges
5. **Donors of blood, semen, and organs**
6. **Health care workers** who perform invasive procedures (depending on the policy of the institution in which they work)
7. **Persons with occupational exposures** (e.g., needle-sticks) and source patients of the exposures

**B. Methods and results.** Screening is performed with an enzyme-linked immunosorbent assay (ELISA). The current HIV test used in the United States is a combination HIV-1/HIV-2 enzyme immunoassay test kit that is also sensitive to antibodies to HIV-2. The Centers for Disease Control and Prevention offer special tests for HIV-2 and HIV-1 non-B subtypes. A positive screening test is confirmed by a repeat positive ELISA and a positive

Western blot (presence of at least two of the following bands: p24, gp41, gp120/160). **An isolated positive ELISA result should not be reported to the patient until this result is confirmed by a Western blot.** An indeterminate test is one for which the ELISA is positive but the criteria for a positive Western blot are not fulfilled. A rapid HIV-1 antibody test has been approved by the U.S. Food and Drug Administration and can be considered for use outside of traditional laboratory and clinical settings.

**III. Initial evaluation** of persons with a positive HIV test should include the following measures:

**A. Complete history,** with emphasis on OIs, viral coinfections, and other complications

**B. Psychological and psychiatric history.** Depression and other psychological problems are common and should be identified and treated as necessary.

**C. Family and social support assessment**

**D. Contraception, safer sex practices,** educational issues, and detoxification for drug abusers

**E. Social worker referral** and open discussions about aggressiveness of care when the disease advances

**F. Complete physical examination**

**G. Laboratory tests**

1. **CBC, routine chemistry, and screening for other infections**
2. **CD4 cell count** (normal range, 600–1500 cells/μl) and CD4 percentage
3. **Virologic markers.** Several quantitative HIV type 1 RNA viral load assays are currently in use, but the polymerase chain reaction (PCR) assay is the only one approved by the U.S. Food and Drug Administration and is the most widely used. Regular PCR has a lower limit of detection of 400 viral copies/ml, whereas the ultrasensitive assay has a lower limit of detection of 40 copies/ml. The other two assays are a branched DNA assay and a nucleic acid sequence amplification assay.
4. **Tuberculin skin test**
5. **VDRL**
6. **Toxoplasma and cytomegalovirus (CMV) IgG and hepatitis A, B (HBsAg, HBsAb, HBcAb), and C serologies**
7. **Chlamydia/gonococcal urine probe**
8. **Cervical Papanicolaou smear** (most commonly using the thin prep method)
9. **HIV resistance testing** for individuals with recent infections and pregnant women

**H. Immunizations**

1. **Pneumococcal vaccine.** Efficacy has not been clearly established in this population. Antibody responses are better when CD4 cell counts are greater than 350 cells/μl. Revaccination after 5 years should be considered.
2. **Hepatitis A and B virus (HAV and HBV).** Vaccination for HAV is recommended for HIV-seropositive subjects who are negative for HAV antibodies, as hepatitis A superinfection can cause fulminant hepatitis in hepatitis C virus (HCV)–coinfected subjects who are not vaccinated or did not respond to immunization. HIV-positive patients are at higher risk of becoming chronic carriers of HBV after having an acute HBV infection. Therefore, if antibodies against hepatitis B core and hepatitis B surface antigens are negative, HBV vaccination is indicated. Coinfection with HCV is very prevalent in this population (especially among IV drug abusers); no vaccine for HCV currently exists.
3. **Influenza.** Influenza vaccination has been recommended in patients infected with HIV; however, vaccination may promote HIV replication and produce a transient increase in the viral load for up to 3 months after vaccination.

## Antiretroviral Therapy

**ART** should be individualized and closely monitored by measuring plasma HIV viral load. Reductions in plasma viremia correlate with increased CD4 cell counts and AIDS-free survival.

I. **Indications** for the initiation of ART include the following:
   A. **Therapy should be initiated in patients with a CD4 count of less than 200 cells/μl or in the symptomatic patient** (with AIDS, thrush, or unexplained fever) regardless of the CD4 count or viral load.
   B. **In the asymptomatic patient, if the CD4 count is between 200 and 350 cells/μl,** initiation of ART is recommended, although some controversy still exists. Initiation of ART depends on the patient's readiness, comorbidities, and drug toxicities.
   C. **In the asymptomatic patient, if the CD4 count is above 350 cells/μl,** there is no strong evidence of clinical benefit of early initiation of ART, and many experts would delay the initiation of treatment. Patients with viral loads greater than 55,000 copies/ml should be monitored closely.
   D. **General principles** for the treatment of HIV infection are outlined in Table 14-1.

II. **Antiretroviral drugs.** Specific drug information is summarized in Tables 14-2, 14-3, and 14-4. Approved antiretroviral drugs are grouped into four categories.
   A. **Nucleoside analog reverse transcriptase inhibitors (NRTIs)** constrain HIV replication by incorporating into the elongating strand of DNA, causing chain termination. All nucleoside analogs have been associated with **lactic acidosis,** presumably related to mitochondrial toxicity.

**Table 14-1.** General principles for treatment of human immunodeficiency virus infection

| |
|---|
| Ongoing HIV replication leads to immune system damage and progression to AIDS. |
| Plasma HIV RNA levels indicate the magnitude of HIV replication and its associated rate of CD4 cell destruction; CD4 counts indicate the extent of HIV-induced immune damage that has already been experienced. |
| Treatment decisions should be individualized by level of risk indicated by plasma HIV RNA levels and CD4 counts. |
| Complete suppression of HIV replications (measured by the ultrasensitive assay) should be the goal of therapy once it is initiated. |
| The most effective means of suppressing HIV replication is the simultaneous initiation of potent combination antiretroviral therapy. |
| Each drug should be used according to optimum schedules and dosages. |
| Any change in antiretroviral therapy increases future therapeutic constraints and potential drug resistance. |
| Women, especially if pregnant, should receive optimal antiretroviral therapy to reduce the risk of vertical transmission. |
| The same principles of antiretroviral therapy apply to HIV-infected children and adults. |
| Persons with acute primary HIV infections should be treated with potent antiretroviral therapy. |
| All HIV-infected persons, even those with viral loads below detectable limits, should be considered infectious. |

*Source:* From *2003 Guidelines for the use of antiretroviral agents in HIV-infected adults and adolescents;* http://aidsinfo.nih.gov.

**Table 14-2.** Nucleoside analog reverse transcriptase inhibitors (NRTIs)

| NRTIs | Dosage[a] | Food restrictions | Common side effects | Interactions with other antiretrovirals |
|---|---|---|---|---|
| Abacavir (ABC) | 300 mg PO bid or with combination tablet 3TC + AZT (Trizivir) | No | Hypersensitivity reaction[b] | If hypersensitivity reaction occurs, rechallenge can be fatal |
| Didanosine (ddI) | Preferred as an enteric-coated formula (Videx EC); >60 kg: 400 mg PO qd, <60 kg: 250 mg PO qd | On empty stomach | Pancreatitis, peripheral neuropathy, diarrhea | Increased incidence of lactic acidosis with d4T |
| Emtricitabine (FTC)[c] | Closely related to 3TC (cross resistance possible); 200 mg PO qd | No | Preliminary results show no common severe side effects, may have GI intolerance | Preliminary results show no significant interactions |
| Lamivudine (3TC) | 150 mg PO bid; <50 kg: 2 mg/kg bid; 300 mg qd | No | Rare | None |
| Stavudine (d4T) | >60 kg: 40 mg PO bid, <60 kg: 30 mg PO bid; extended-release form: >60 kg: 100 mg PO qd, <60 kg: 75 mg PO qd | No | Peripheral neuropathy | Antagonizes ZDV |
| Zidovudine (ZDV, AZT) | 300 mg PO bid or combination tablet with 3TC (Combivir) or 3TC + ABC (Trizivir) | No | Bone marrow suppression, GI intolerance | Antagonizes d4T |
| Tenofovir (TDF)[d] | 300 mg PO qd | With food | Rare | Dose adjustment of ddI if used together (Videx EC, 250 mg qd); decreases atazanavir levels |

[a]Dose adjustment required in patients with renal failure for most NRTIs.
[b]ABC-related hypersensitivity reaction: flu-like symptoms, fever, rash, upper respiratory symptoms, GI intolerance.
[c]Zalcitabine (ddC) belongs to this class of NRTIs; however, it is rarely used in clinical practice.
[d]Tenofovir (TDF) is a nucleotide that is available as tenofovir disoproxil fumarate.

**Table 14-3.** Nonnucleoside reverse transcriptase inhibitors (NNRTIs)

| NNRTIs | Dosage | Food restrictions | Side effects | Interactions[a] |
|---|---|---|---|---|
| Delavirdine (DLV) | 400 mg PO tid | No | Headaches | Inhibitor of the P-450 system |
| Efavirenz (EFV) | 600 mg PO qd | Avoid taking after high-fat meals because of ↑ peak concentration | CNS symptoms (dizziness, somnolence, insomnia, abnormal dreams), false-positive urine cannabinoid test[b] | Inducer/inhibitor of the P-450 system |
| Nevirapine (NVP) | 200 mg PO qd for 2 wk, then 200 mg PO bid or 400 mg qd | No | Hepatitis | Inducer of the P-450 system |

↑, increased.
[a]See Table 14-5 for interactions with other antiretrovirals.
[b]Use of gas chromatography or mass spectroscopy is recommended if screening for cannabis is desired.

**B. Protease inhibitors (PIs)** are a very potent group of drugs that block the action of the viral protease required for protein processing late in the viral cycle. They are used in combination regimens. All PIs can produce increased bleeding in hemophiliacs, GI intolerance, and increased liver function tests. These agents have also been associated with metabolic abnormalities such as glucose intolerance, increases in cholesterol and triglycerides, and body fat redistribution. **PIs have important drug interactions,** and concomitant medications should be reviewed carefully (see sec. **II.J**, Table 14-5, and Appendix C, Drug Interactions). Combinations of two PIs, especially with ritonavir, can decrease the dosage requirement of the other PIs.

**C. Nonnucleoside reverse transcriptase inhibitors (NNRTIs)** inhibit HIV by binding noncompetitively to the reverse transcriptase. A single dosage of nevirapine at the time of labor has been shown to decrease perinatal transmission of the virus. Side effects of NNRTIs include rash, increased AST and ALT, and Stevens-Johnson syndrome (more likely with nevirapine).

**D. HIV entry inhibitors** belong to a new class of antiretroviral agents that target different stages of the HIV entry process. **T-20 (enfuvirtide)** is a fusion inhibitor only available for use as an SC injection, 90 mg bid. The most frequent side effect is a local reaction at the injection site.

**E. Initial therapy.** ART is usually started in the outpatient setting by a physician with expertise in the management of patients with HIV infection. Adherence is the key factor for success of ART. Treatment should be individualized and adapted to the patient's lifestyle. Any treatment decision influences future therapeutic options because of the possibility of drug cross resistance. Potent ART generally consists of either a combination of two NRTIs plus one or two PIs or a nonnucleoside reverse transcriptase receptor. Alternatively, three NRTIs can be used.

**F. Monitoring of therapy.** Plasma HIV RNA load is used for monitoring of therapy. The goal is to reduce the viral load levels below the detection limits. CD4 cell counts should be checked periodically to assess the immune status

**Table 14-4.** Protease inhibitors (PIs)

| PIs | Dosage[a] | Food restrictions | Side effects |
|---|---|---|---|
| Fosamprenavir[b] (fAPV) | 1400 mg PO bid; combined with RTV(r): fAPV/r 700/100 mg bid or fAPV/r 1400/200 mg qd | Can be taken with or without food | Rash, diarrhea, nausea |
| Atazanavir (ATZ) | 400 mg PO qd; combined with RTV(r): ATZ/r, 300/100 qd | Take with food | Few metabolic effects; ↑ indirect bilirubin |
| Indinavir (IDV) | 800 mg PO tid usually with RTV(r): IDV/r, 800/100 mg bid; IDV/r 400/400 mg bid | No food if taken alone, can be taken with or without food if combined with RTV | Nephrolithiasis, ↑ indirect bilirubin, headache |
| Lopinavir (LPV) | Only available in fixed combination with RTV(r), 400/100 mg PO bid (Kaletra) or 533/133 mg (if used with EFV or NVP) | Take with food | Diarrhea, hyperlipidemia |
| Nelfinavir (NFV) | 750 mg PO tid or 1250 mg PO bid | Take with food | Diarrhea |
| Ritonavir (RTV)[c] | Usually added to achieve booster effect in combination with other PIs, in full dose, 600 mg PO bid (rarely used) | Take with food | Nausea and vomiting, paresthesia, hepatitis, taste perversion, asthenia |
| Saquinavir (SQV) | 1200 mg PO tid (soft gel, Fortovase) usually with RTV(r) SQV/r 1000/100 mg PO bid or SQV/r 400/400 mg bid or SQV/r 1600/100 mg qd | Take with food | Headache, diarrhea |

EFV, efavirenz; NVP, nevirapine; ↑, increased.
[a]See Table 14-5 for interactions with other antiretrovirals.
[b]fAPV is the prodrug of amprenavir; amprenavir is being phased out, and fAPV should be used instead.
[c]RTV is usually added using a lower dose to achieve a booster effect, especially with LPV, SQV, fAPV, and IDV.

of the patient and to define the start of prophylactic therapy. After starting or changing ART, the viral load should be checked after 4 weeks, and the regimen should be reassessed. When the ultrasensitive HIV RNA becomes undetectable and the patient is on a stable regimen, monitoring can be done every 3 months.

G. **Treatment failure** is defined as (1) less than a log (10-fold) reduction of the viral load 4–6 weeks after starting a new antiretroviral regimen; (2) failure to reach an undetectable viral load after 4–6 months of treatment; (3) detection of the virus after initial complete suppression of viral load, which suggests development of resistance; or (4) persistent decline of CD4 cells or clinical deterioration. Confirmed treatment failure should prompt changes in ART. In this situation, at least two of the drugs should be substituted with other drugs that have no expected cross resistance. **HIV resistance testing** at this stage may help determine a salvage regimen in the patients

**Table 14-5.** Interactions between antiretrovirals

| | Fosamprenavir (fAPV) | Atazanavir[a] (ATZ) | Delavirdine (DLV) | Efavirenz (EFV) |
|---|---|---|---|---|
| DLV | Insufficient data | Insufficient data | — | — |
| EFV | ↓ fAPV; use fAPV/r, 700/100 mg bid or 1400/300 mg qd | ↓ ATZ: use ATZ/r 300/100 or 400/100 qd | Insufficient data | — |
| IDV | ↑ fAPV but no change in dose | No data; avoid due to ↑ bilirubin | ↑ IDV: use IDV, 600 mg tid | ↓ IDV: use IDV, 1000 mg tid |
| LPV | ↓ LPV; should not be used together | No data | Insufficient data | ↓ LPV: use LPV/r, 533/133 mg bid = 4 caps bid |
| NFV | ↑ fAPV but no change in dose; insufficient data | No data | ↑ NFV ↓ DLV but no change in dose; monitor | ↑ NFV but no change in dose |
| NVP | ↓ fAPV; no data but probably dose as with EFV | No data | — | Should not be used together |
| SQV | ↓ fAPV; insufficient data | ↑ SQV: use ATZ/SQV, 400/1200 qd | ↑ SQV but no change in dose; insufficient data; monitor | ↓ SQV, ↓ EFV; avoid concomitant use |
| RTV | ↑ fAPV; for RTV boostering see Table 14-4 | ↑ ATZ; for boostering see Table 14-4 | Reduce RTV: 400 mg bid | ↑ RTV but no change in dose |

↑, increases level of; ↓, decreases level of; caps, capsules; r, short term for low-dose ritonavir used for boostering other protease inhibitors (PIs) (see also Table 14-4); RTV, ritonavir.
[a]When combined with tenofovir use ATZ/r 300/100 qd.
*Source:* From *2003 Guidelines for the use of antiretroviral agents in HIV-infected adults and adolescents*; see http://aidsinfo.nih.gov; all doses presented in this table are for PO use.

with prior antiretroviral therapy. The importance of adherence should be stressed. Referral to an HIV specialist is highly recommended in this situation.

H. **HIV resistance testing** is done using two different types of assays: genotypic, in which the reverse transcriptase and the polymerase genes are sequenced using different techniques, and phenotypic, in which the behavior of HIV in vitro in the presence of antiretroviral drugs is examined. Results of resistance testing can be used to guide ART.
I. **Therapeutic drug monitoring** is still considered experimental.
J. **Drug interactions.** Antiretroviral medications, especially PIs, have multiple drug interactions. **PIs and delavirdine both inhibit and induce the P-450 system,** and thus interactions are frequent with other inhibitors of the P-450 system, including macrolides (erythromycin, clarithromycin) and

| Indinavir (IDV) | Lopinavir (LPV) | Nelfinavir (NFV) | Nevirapine (NVP) | Saquinavir (SQV) |
|---|---|---|---|---|
| — | — | — | — | — |
| — | — | — | — | — |
| — | — | — | — | — |
| ↑ IDV: use IDV, 600 mg bid | — | — | — | — |
| ↑ IDV use: IDV, 1200 mg bid | Insufficient data | — | — | — |
| ↓ IDV: use IDV, 1000 mg tid | ↓ LPV: use LPV/r, 533/133 mg bid = 4 caps bid | ↓ NFV but no change in dose | — | — |
| ↑ SQV but no change in dose; insufficient data | ↑ SQV: use SQV, 800 mg bid | ↓ SQV, ↑ NFV: use SQV, 800 mg tid or 1200 mg bid | ↓ SQV but no change in dose; avoid use if SQV is only PI | — |
| ↑ IDV; for RTV boostering see Table 14-4 | For RTV boostering see Table 14-4 | ↑ NFV; NFV usually not boosted | No change in dose | For RTV boostering see Table 14-4 |

antifungals (ketoconazole, itraconazole), as well as other inducers, such as rifamycins (rifampin, rifabutin) and anticonvulsants (phenobarbital, phenytoin, carbamazepine). **Drugs with narrow therapeutic indexes that should be avoided or used with extreme caution** include antihistamines (although loratadine is safe), antiarrhythmics (flecainide, encainide, quinidine), long-acting opiates (fentanyl, meperidine), long-acting benzodiazepines (midazolam, triazolam), warfarin, 3-hydroxy-3-methylglutaryl coenzyme A (HMG-CoA) reductase inhibitors (pravastatin is the safest), and oral contraceptives. Sildenafil concentrations are increased, and methadone and theophylline concentrations are decreased with concomitant administration of certain PIs and NNRTIs. Grapefruit juice can increase levels of saquinavir and decrease levels of indinavir. See Table 14-5 for interactions between antiretroviral drugs.

**K. Complications of ART.** The long-term use of antiretrovirals has been associated with toxicity, the pathogenesis of which is only partially understood at this time.

1. **Lipodystrophy syndrome** is an alteration in body fat distribution and can be stigmatizing to individuals. Changes consist of the accumulation

of visceral fat in the abdomen, neck (buffalo hump), and pelvic areas, and/or the depletion of subcutaneous fat, causing facial or peripheral wasting. Lipodystrophy has been associated in particular with PIs and NRTIs, but other factors also may be important. Changes in the patient's ART regimen and lifestyle modifications such as exercise may improve morphologic changes. Other supplemental therapies such as rosiglitazone and cosmetic surgery are currently under investigation.

2. **Hyperlipidemia,** especially hypertriglyceridemia, is associated mainly with PIs (especially ritonavir). Improvement has been seen after treatment with atorvastatin, pravastatin, and/or gemfibrozil.
3. **Peripheral insulin resistance, impaired glucose tolerance, and hyperglycemia** have been associated with the use of PI-based regimens, mainly indinavir. Lifestyle changes or changing ART can be considered in these cases.
4. **Lactic acidosis** with liver steatosis is a rare but sometimes fatal complication associated with NRTIs. The mechanism appears to be mitochondrial toxicity. The clinical picture can range from asymptomatic hyperlactatemia to severe lactic acidosis with hepatomegaly and steatosis. Suspected drugs should be discontinued and supportive care given as needed.
5. **Osteopenia and osteoporosis** are described in HIV-infected individuals. The pathogenic mechanism of this problem is unknown.
6. **Osteonecrosis, particularly of the hip,** has been increasingly associated with HIV disease.

## Opportunistic Infections

I. **Impact of potent ART on OIs.** Potent ART has decreased the incidence, changed the manifestations, and improved the outcome of OIs. A new clinical syndrome associated with the immune enhancement induced by potent ART, **immune reconstitution syndrome,** has been described and generally presents as local inflammatory reactions. Examples include paradoxical reactions with TB reactivation, localized *Mycobacterium avium* complex adenitis, and CMV vitreitis immediately after the initiation of potent ART. Careful monitoring is important after starting ART. In this circumstance, ART is usually continued, and the addition of low-dose steroids might decrease the degree of inflammation.

II. **Prophylaxis for OIs** can be divided into primary and secondary prophylaxis.

A. **Primary prophylaxis** is established before an episode of OI occurs. Institution of primary prophylaxis depends on the level of immunosuppression as judged by the patient's CD4 cell count and percentage. The following interventions are considered standards of care and should be applied in every patient (*MMWR Morb Mortal Wkly Rep* 51:RR-8, 2001).

1. ***Pneumocystis carinii* pneumonia prophylaxis** should be initiated when the CD4 count is less than 200 cells/μl, if the CD4% has decreased to 15% or less, or if the patient has unexplained fever for more than 2 weeks or experiences an episode of oral candidiasis. Trimethoprim/sulfamethoxazole (TMP/SMX), 160 mg/800 mg [one double-strength (DS) tablet] PO once a day or three times a week, is the preferred regimen. If TMP/SMX is contraindicated, dapsone, 100 mg PO qd (after ruling out glucose 6-phosphate dehydrogenase deficiency); atovaquone, 1500 mg PO qd; or inhaled pentamidine, 300 mg once a month, are alternatives.
2. **TB prophylaxis** should be given to patients with a positive purified protein derivative (PPD) test (>5 mm of induration), a history of a previous untreated PPD test, or recent contact with an individual with active TB. Isoniazid (INH), 300 mg PO qd, plus pyridoxine, 50 mg PO qd, for 9

months is the regimen of choice. Rifampin, 600 mg PO qd, with pyrazinamide, 20 mg/kg qd, for 2 months is an alternative. In INH-resistant TB, rifampin for 4 months is indicated. Monitoring of liver toxicity is mandatory, especially in patients who are coinfected with hepatitis viruses.

3. ***Toxoplasma* prophylaxis** is indicated for seropositive patients with CD4 cell counts of less than 100 cells/μl. TMP/SMX DS, one tablet qd, is the preferred regimen. A combination of dapsone, 50 mg PO qd, plus pyrimethamine, 50 mg PO weekly, and leucovorin, 25 mg PO weekly, is an alternative.
4. ***M. avium* complex prophylaxis** is indicated if CD4 cell counts are less than 50 cells/μl and consists of azithromycin, 1200 mg PO weekly, or clarithromycin, 500 mg PO bid. Rifabutin, 300 mg PO qd, is an alternative, but its use may be limited by potential drug interactions.
5. **Varicella-zoster virus (VZV) prophylaxis** is indicated if a significant exposure to chickenpox or shingles occurs, the patient does not have a history of chickenpox, and the patient is VZV seronegative. VZV immunoglobulin (five vials of 1.25 ml each) should be given IM within 96 hours of exposure.
6. **Primary prophylaxis is not routinely recommended** for the following OIs: recurrent bacterial pneumonia, mucosal candidiasis, CMV retinitis, cryptococcosis, and endemic fungal infections such as histoplasmosis and coccidioidomycosis.

B. **Secondary prophylaxis** is instituted after an episode of infection has been adequately treated (see sec. **III**). Most OIs in AIDS are incurable, and the patient usually requires lifelong therapy.

C. **Withdrawal of prophylaxis.** Recommendations suggest withdrawing primary and secondary prophylaxis for most opportunistic infections if immune reconstitution has occurred (CD4 cell counts consistently above 150–200 cells/μl).

## III. Management of specific infectious complications

### A. Viral infections

1. **CMV infections.** CMV retinitis occurs very frequently and accounts for 85% of CMV disease in patients with AIDS. CMV also can affect the GI tract, the lungs, and the CNS.
   a. **Treatment of CMV retinitis** can be local or systemic and is administered in two phases, induction and maintenance.
      (1) **Valganciclovir,** a ganciclovir prodrug, has been approved for use in CMV retinitis. Drug levels are equivalent to those of IV ganciclovir. For induction, 900 mg PO bid for 21 days is given, followed by 900 mg once a day. **Treatment is indefinite unless immune reconstitution occurs.** Adverse effects are similar to those of ganciclovir.
      (2) **Ganciclovir** is given at an induction dosage of 5 mg/kg IV q12h for 14–21 days and a maintenance dosage of 5 mg/kg IV q24h indefinitely (unless immune reconstitution occurs). The most common side effect of ganciclovir is myelotoxicity resulting in neutropenia. The neutropenia may respond to granulocyte colony-stimulating factor therapy. An intraocular ganciclovir implant is effective but does not provide systemic CMV therapy.
      (3) **Foscarnet** is given at an induction dosage of 60 mg/kg IV q8h or 90 mg/kg IV q12h for 14–21 days, followed by a maintenance dosage of 90–120 mg/kg IV q24h indefinitely, unless immune reconstitution occurs. Nephrotoxicity is the major side effect; therefore, adequate hydration and electrolyte monitoring (including calcium) are required.
      (4) **Cidofovir** is effective at an induction dosage of 5 mg/kg IV weekly for 2 weeks, followed by a maintenance dosage of 5 mg/kg IV every 2 weeks. Probenecid (2 g PO 3 hours before and 1 g PO 2

and 8 hours after cidofovir is given) and saline hydration must be used to reduce the renal toxicity of cidofovir. Urinalysis and electrolytes should be monitored closely.

(5) **Fomivirsen** is an antisense oligonucleotide given intraocularly, 330 μg, on days 1 and 15 and then monthly. It does not provide systemic therapy.

(6) **Combination regimens** (ganciclovir and foscarnet) may be more effective than either drug alone, but together they are poorly tolerated.

b. **For other invasive CMV disease,** the optimal therapy is with IV ganciclovir, PO valganciclovir, IV foscarnet, or a combination of two drugs (in persons with prior anti-CMV therapy), for at least 3–6 weeks. Foscarnet has the best cerebrospinal fluid (CSF) penetration and is the drug of choice for CMV encephalitis and myelopathy. Maintenance therapy is indicated.

2. **Other herpesvirus infections**

a. **Herpes simplex virus infections** can be associated with large genital and perirectal lesions, esophagitis, proctitis, and pulmonary disease. Administration of acyclovir (400 mg PO tid), famciclovir (250 mg PO tid), or valacyclovir (500 mg PO tid) for 1 week is usually effective. For more severe disease, IV acyclovir, 5 mg/kg q8h, is recommended. Relapses are frequent, and acyclovir, 400 mg PO bid, may prevent their recurrence. Herpes simplex virus can become resistant to acyclovir, in which case foscarnet, 40 mg/kg IV q8h for 10–14 days, or one dose of cidofovir, 5 mg/kg IV, should be used.

b. **VZV** may cause typical dermatomal lesions or disseminated infection. Acyclovir, 10 mg/kg IV q8h for 7–14 days, is the recommended therapy. For milder cases, administration of acyclovir (800 mg PO five times a day), famciclovir (500 mg PO tid), or valacyclovir (1 g PO tid) for 1 week is usually effective.

c. **Epstein-Barr virus** (EBV) infection is common in AIDS patients. It causes oral hairy leukoplakia, for which no treatment is required. It is also associated with primary CNS lymphoma in patients with advanced AIDS.

d. **Human herpesvirus 8** is the causative agent of Kaposi's sarcoma (see sec. **IV.A**).

3. **JC virus** is a papovavirus associated with progressive multifocal leukoencephalopathy. Symptoms include mental status changes, weakness, and disorders of gait, and characteristic white matter lesions are seen on MRI. Potent ART has improved the survival of patients with progressive multifocal leukoencephalopathy.

4. **Parvovirus B19.** Chronic parvovirus infections can cause pure RBC aplasia. Treatment is with IV immunoglobulin, 0.4 g/kg IV qd for 10 days. Relapses are frequent.

5. **Hepatitis virus infections** can be aggravated with the immune reconstitution associated with ART.

a. **Hepatitis B** vaccination can prevent infection and is indicated in all seronegative subjects. Currently, there are three approved drugs for the treatment of hepatitis B: interferon alfa-2B (5 million U SC daily for 16 weeks), adefovir (10 mg PO qd), and lamivudine (150 mg PO bid or 300 mg PO qd). Tenofovir (300 mg PO qd), an antiretroviral drug approved for the treatment of HIV, is also active against hepatitis B. Patients who are coinfected with HBV should receive drugs that are active against both viruses to avoid the development of resistance. Pegylated interferon-alpha and new anti-HBV agents are currently being evaluated.

b. **Chronic hepatitis C** has a significant impact on morbidity and mortality in HIV-infected patients. Treatment using a combination of pegylated interferon-alpha and ribavirin is effective in HIV-positive patients, but sustained virologic response rates are much lower, specifically in genotype 1. New antiviral drugs against the hepatitis C virus are in development.

**B. Bacterial infections.** These are common in HIV-infected patients and often recur or follow atypical or aggressive courses. Intensive therapy generally is necessary, followed by chronic suppression.

1. **Bacillary angiomatosis** is caused by *Bartonella henselae* and is characterized by multiple nodular, purplish lesions in the skin and other organs. Erythromycin, 500 mg PO q6h, is the drug of choice. Doxycycline, 100 mg PO bid, is also effective. Other macrolides and ciprofloxacin, 500 mg PO bid, are alternatives.
2. ***Campylobacter jejuni*** can produce GI or disseminated infections in HIV-infected patients. Either erythromycin, 500 mg PO qid, or ciprofloxacin, 500 mg PO bid, can be used for treatment.
3. ***Rhodococcus equi*** can produce pulmonary infections, which should be treated with vancomycin, 1 g IV q12h, followed by chronic suppression with erythromycin, 500 mg PO qid, plus rifampin, 600 mg PO qd, or with ciprofloxacin, 500 mg PO bid.
4. ***Salmonella* species** produce recurrent bacteremia in AIDS patients. Antibacterial therapy should be based on susceptibility. Ceftriaxone (1 g IV qd), ampicillin (1 g IV q6h), TMP/SMX (1 DS tablet PO bid), and ciprofloxacin (500 mg PO bid) are options, depending on the sensitivities of the organism.
5. **Bacterial pneumonias** occur frequently in HIV-infected patients. If recurrent, they are considered AIDS defining. Usually, they are due to *Streptococcus pneumoniae* or *Haemophilus influenzae*. Gram-negative rods (especially *Pseudomonas aeruginosa*) may also produce pneumonia in advanced HIV disease.
6. **Syphilis** can have an atypical course in HIV-infected patients, and treatment failures are more frequent in this population. Benzathine penicillin, 2.4 million U IM one time for primary syphilis or weekly for 3 weeks for secondary or latent syphilis (of >1 year in duration), is the regimen of choice. Doxycycline, 100 mg PO bid for 14 days, is an alternative. A spinal tap is recommended in HIV-infected patients with latent syphilis to rule out neurosyphilis. If neurosyphilis is present, penicillin G, 12–24 million U IV qd for 14 days, is the treatment of choice. Patients who are allergic to penicillin should be desensitized. Data regarding the use of ceftriaxone, 1–2 g IV qd for 14 days, are limited. Close monitoring and follow-up using the VDRL test at 3, 6, and 12 months are necessary in all cases. Persons with a sustained positive VDRL should receive retreatment. (Sexually transmitted diseases treatment guidelines 2002. *MMWR Morb Mortal Wkly Rep* 51:RR-6, 2002.)
7. **Other sexually transmitted diseases** are treated as they would be in non–HIV-infected patients (see Chap. 13, Treatment of Infectious Diseases).

**C. Mycobacterial infections**

1. ***Mycobacterium tuberculosis*** [*MMWR Morb Mortal Wkly Rep* 49(9), 2000; 51:RR-8, 2002; 47:RR-20, 1998] is especially frequent among HIV-infected patients, particularly IV drug abusers. Primary as well as reactivated disease occurs. Clinical manifestations depend on the level of immunosuppression. Patients with higher CD4 cell counts tend to exhibit classic presentations with apical cavitary disease. More immunosuppressed patients may demonstrate atypical presentations that can resemble disseminated primary infection, with diffuse or localized pulmonary infiltrates and hilar lymphadenopathy. Extrapulmonary dissemination is very common. For treatment recommendations, see Chap. 13, Treatment of Infectious Diseases. Current recommendations suggest the substitu-

tion of rifabutin for rifampin in patients who are receiving concomitant ART, especially PIs. In subjects who are ART naïve, ART can be delayed for a few weeks after TB-specific therapy is started. The dosage for rifabutin should be reduced to 150 mg qd if the patient is receiving ritonavir, indinavir, nelfinavir, or fosamprenavir, whereas it should be increased to 450 mg qd when combined with nevirapine or efavirenz.

2. ***M. avium* complex** infection is the most commonly occurring mycobacterial infection in AIDS patients and is responsible for significant morbidity in patients with advanced disease (CD4 cell count <100 cells/μl). Disseminated infection with fever, weight loss, and night sweats is the most frequent presentation. Anemia and an elevated alkaline phosphatase level are the usual laboratory abnormalities. Initial therapy should include a macrolide (clarithromycin, 500 mg PO bid) and ethambutol (15 mg/kg PO qd). Rifabutin, 300 mg PO qd, or ciprofloxacin, 500 mg PO bid, can be added in severe cases.
3. ***Mycobacterium kansasii*** infection frequently occurs in HIV patients and should always be considered significant. Clinically, the infection appears similar to TB. A combination of rifampin (600 mg PO qd), ethambutol (15 mg/kg/day PO), and INH (300 mg PO qd) is the recommended therapy. Also recommended is consultation with an infectious disease specialist.
4. ***Mycobacterium haemophilum*** can produce ulcerative skin lesions in AIDS patients. It requires treatment with a macrolide, rifampin, and two other drugs active against the organism.

**D. Fungal infections**

1. **Candidiasis** (oral, esophageal, and vaginal infection) is common in the HIV-infected host. The severity of infection depends on the degree of the patient's immunosuppression. Oral and vaginal candidiasis usually respond to local therapy with troches or creams (nystatin or clotrimazole). For patients who do not respond or who have esophageal candidiasis, fluconazole, 100–200 mg PO qd, is the treatment of choice.
2. **Fluconazole-resistant candidiasis** is becoming increasingly frequent, especially in patients with advanced disease who have been receiving antifungal agents for prolonged periods. Itraconazole oral suspension (200 mg bid) is occasionally effective. Many patients require amphotericin B, either as an oral suspension (100 mg/ml swish and swallow qid) or parenterally. Caspofungin, an echinocandin, can be considered for refractory cases using an induction dose of 70 mg IV the first day and then 50 mg IV qd for maintenance. Voriconazole may also be useful.
3. ***Cryptococcus neoformans*** is the most frequent CNS fungal infection in AIDS patients, usually presenting with headaches, fever, and possibly mental status changes. Occasionally, the presentation is more subtle. Diagnosis is based on lumbar puncture results and on the determination of latex cryptococcal antigen, which is usually positive in the serum and in the CSF. CSF opening pressure should always be measured to assess the possibility of elevated intracranial pressure. Initial treatment is with amphotericin B, 0.7 mg/kg/day IV, and 5-flucytosine, 25 mg/kg PO q6h for 2–3 weeks, followed by fluconazole, 400 mg PO qd for 8–10 weeks and then 200 mg PO qd indefinitely. The 5-flucytosine level should be monitored during therapy to avoid toxicity. A lipid preparation of amphotericin can be used in patients with renal insufficiency. Repeat lumbar punctures (removing up to 30 ml CSF until the pressure is below 20–25 cm $H_2O$) may be required to relieve elevated intracranial pressure. In persons who have persistent elevation of intracranial pressure, a temporary lumbar drain is indicated.
4. ***Histoplasma capsulatum*** infections often occur in AIDS patients who live in endemic areas such as the Mississippi and Ohio River Valleys. Such infections are usually disseminated at the time of diagnosis. Patients present with fever, hepatosplenomegaly, and weight loss. Pan-

cytopenia is secondary to bone marrow involvement. Diagnosis is made by a positive culture, but the urine *Histoplasma* antigen can also be used for diagnosis and to monitor treatment. Amphotericin B, 0.5 mg/kg IV qd for a total dose of 0.5–1.0 g, followed by itraconazole, 400 mg PO qd indefinitely, is the therapy of choice. Itraconazole absorption should be documented by a serum drug level.

5. ***Coccidioides immitis*** is another frequent infection in AIDS patients in endemic areas of the southwestern United States. Extensive disease with extrapulmonary spread is common. Amphotericin B therapy is indicated initially, followed by lifelong suppression with fluconazole, 400 mg PO qd, or itraconazole, 400 mg PO qd. Coccidioidal meningitis requires intracisternal or intraventricular therapy with amphotericin B. Fluconazole may also be effective.
6. **Aspergillosis** is increasing among HIV-infected patients, especially those who are neutropenic and those with advanced disease (fewer than 50 CD4 cells/μl). This infection can involve the lungs, CNS, heart, kidneys, and sinuses. Diagnosis requires a biopsy of the tissue involved. Voriconazole is the treatment of choice. Alternatives include amphotericin B and itraconazole. Caspofungin can be used for refractory disease using an induction dose of 70 mg IV the first day and subsequently 50 mg IV qd for maintenance. Combination therapy is under study. Prognosis is poor for patients with invasive aspergillosis.

**E. *P. carinii* pneumonia** is the most common infection in patients with AIDS and is the leading cause of death in this population. Extrapulmonary disease has also been described, primarily in patients who are receiving inhaled pentamidine prophylaxis.

1. **TMP/SMX** is the treatment of choice. The dosage is 5 mg/kg of the TMP component IV q6–8h for severe cases, with a switch to oral therapy when the patient's condition improves. Total duration of therapy is 21 days. If no evidence of other infection is found, **prednisone** should be added if the patient has an arterial oxygen tension ($PaO_2$) of less than 70 mm Hg or an alveolar-arterial oxygen gradient [$P(A\text{-}a)O_2$] in excess of 35 mm Hg. The most frequently prescribed prednisone regimen is 40 mg PO bid on days 1–5 and 20 mg bid on days 6–10, followed by 20 mg qd on days 11–21.
2. **For patients who cannot receive TMP/SMX,** the following alternatives are available:
   - a. **For mild to moderately severe disease** [$PaO_2$ >70 mm Hg or $P(A\text{-}a)O_2$ < 35 mm Hg]
     - (1) **Trimethoprim,** 20 mg/kg/day PO, **and dapsone,** 100 mg PO qd. Glucose 6-phosphate dehydrogenase deficiency should be ruled out before dapsone is used.
     - (2) **Clindamycin,** 600 mg IV or PO tid, **plus primaquine,** 15 mg PO qd. Glucose 6-phosphate dehydrogenase deficiency should be ruled out before primaquine is used.
     - (3) **Atovaquone,** 750 mg PO tid. This drug should be administered with meals to increase absorption.
   - b. **For severe disease** [$PaO_2$ <70 mm Hg or $P(A\text{-}a)O_2$ >35 mm Hg]
     - (1) **Pentamidine,** 4 mg/kg IV qd, should be infused over 2 hours. Hypoglycemia or hyperglycemia is common, and monitoring of glucose and serum electrolytes (including calcium) is essential. Nephrotoxicity, hematologic toxicity, and hypotension also are frequent.
     - (2) **Trimetrexate,** 45 mg/$m^2$ IV qd over 90 minutes, and leucovorin, 20 mg/$m^2$ IV or PO q6h, can be given.
     - (3) **Prednisone** should be added (see sec. **III.E.1**).
3. **Prophylaxis** is indicated as described in sec. **II.A.1.**

**F. Protozoal infections**

1. ***Toxoplasma gondii*** typically causes multiple CNS lesions and presents with encephalopathy and focal neurologic findings. Disease represents

reactivation of a previous infection, and the serologic workup usually is positive. MRI of the brain is the best radiographic technique for diagnosis. Often, the diagnosis relies on response to empiric treatment, as seen by a reduction in the size of the mass lesions. Sulfadiazine, 25 mg/kg PO q6h, plus pyrimethamine, 100 mg PO on day 1 followed by 75 mg PO qd, is the therapy of choice. Leucovorin, 5–10 mg PO qd, should be added to prevent hematologic toxicity. For patients who are allergic to sulfonamides, clindamycin (600 mg IV or PO q8h) can be used instead of sulfadiazine. Doses are reduced after 3–6 weeks of therapy.

2. ***Cryptosporidium*** produces chronic diarrhea in HIV-infected patients. Diagnosis is based on the visualization of the parasite in an acid-fast stain of stool. Nitazoxanide, 500 mg PO bid, might be effective. Potent ART also has been reported to be effective.
3. ***Cyclospora*** is very similar to *Cryptosporidium* and produces chronic diarrhea. TMP/SMX, one DS tablet PO bid for 7 days, is usually effective.
4. ***Isospora belli*** also produces chronic diarrhea. Treatment with TMP/SMX, one DS tablet PO qid for 10 days, followed by chronic suppression with TMP/SMX, one DS tablet PO qd, is effective.
5. ***Microsporidia*** can produce diarrhea and biliary tree disease in patients with advanced infection. Diagnosis is difficult and requires special staining of the stool. *Enterocytozoon bieneusi* and *Encephalitozoon intestinalis* are most commonly found. *E. intestinalis* can cause disseminated disease. Conventional therapy is with albendazole, 400 mg PO bid, but this regimen has only modest success for *E. bieneusi* infections.
6. ***Strongyloides*** can produce disseminated infections in AIDS patients in endemic areas. Thiabendazole, 22 mg/kg (maximum, 1.5 g) PO qd for 2–3 days, is the drug of choice.

**IV. Neoplasms** associated with AIDS include Kaposi's sarcoma and Hodgkin's and non-Hodgkin's lymphoma. Patients should receive concomitant ART because it enhances the response to conventional therapy.

**A. Kaposi's sarcoma** is associated with human herpesvirus 8 infection. In AIDS patients, it commonly presents as skin lesions but can be disseminated. The GI tract and lung are the usual visceral organs involved. Potent ART can regress Kaposi's sarcoma lesions. Local therapy with liquid nitrogen or intralesional injection with alitretinoin or vinblastine has also been used. Cryotherapy or radiation may be useful as well. Systemic therapy involves chemotherapy (e.g., liposomal doxorubicin, paclitaxel, liposomal daunorubicin, thalidomide, retinoids), radiation, and interferon-alpha.

**B. Lymphoma** associated with AIDS is primarily non-Hodgkin's lymphoma. EBV appears to be the potential pathogen. Primary CNS lymphomas are common and can be multicentric; diagnosis is based on clinical symptoms, the presence of enhancing brain lesions, and a positive EBV-PCR of the CSF. Other OIs need to be ruled out. Other potential extranodal sites of involvement include bone marrow, GI tract, and liver. Treatment involves chemotherapy and radiation.

**C. Cervical and perianal neoplasias** are common. Certain oncogenic human papilloma virus subtypes such as 16 and 18 are oncogenic. Cancer can also arise from perianal condyloma acuminata. Yearly screening for vaginal dysplasia with a Papanicolaou smear is indicated. Screening for anal intraepithelial neoplasms is currently under evaluation.

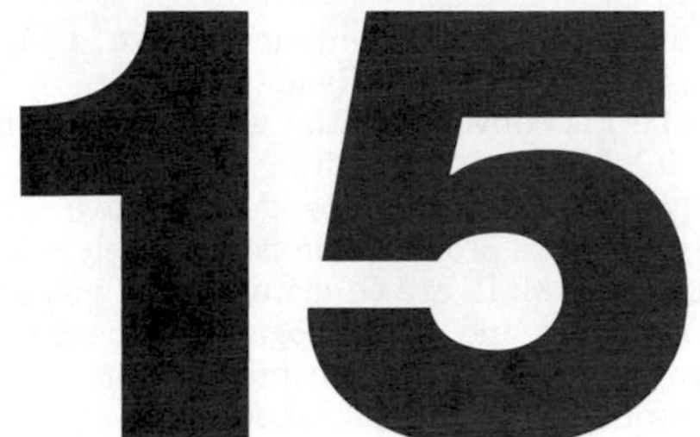

# Solid Organ Transplant Medicine

Brent W. Miller

Transplantation has become widely accepted as a treatment for end-stage organ failure. A continued increase in the number of patients awaiting solid organ transplant is anticipated. It is beyond the scope of this chapter to cover the entire field of transplantation; hence, this chapter should serve as an introduction to the subject with a selection of pertinent references. Immunosuppressive medications, graft rejection, and selected long-term complications are emphasized. For indications and contraindications of heart, lung, kidney, and liver transplantations, see Chaps. 6, Heart Failure, Cardiomyopathy, and Valvular Disease; 9, Pulmonary Disease; 11, Renal Diseases; and 17, Liver Diseases; respectively (*N Engl J Med* 331:365, 1994; *N Engl J Med* 340:1081, 1999; *Surg Clin North Am* 78:679, 1998; *J Hepatol* 32:198, 2000).

## Immunosuppressive Medications

**Immunosuppressive medications** are used to promote acceptance of a graft (induction therapy), to reverse episodes of acute rejection (rejection therapy), and to prevent rejection (maintenance therapy) (*JAMA* 278:1993, 1997; *Lancet* 353:1083, 1999). These agents are associated with immunosuppressive effects, immunodeficiency toxicity (e.g., infection and malignancy), and nonimmune toxicity (e.g., nephrotoxicity, diabetes mellitus, or neurotoxicity). Immunosuppressive medications should only be prescribed and administered by physicians and nurses who have appropriate knowledge and expertise. Many variables factor into the choice and dose of drug, and the guidelines for each specific organ are different.

I. **Glucocorticoids** are immunosuppressive and anti-inflammatory. Their mechanisms of action include inhibition of cytokine transcription, induction of lymphocyte apoptosis, down-regulation of adhesion molecule and major histocompatibility complex expression, and modification of leukocyte trafficking. The side effects of chronic glucocorticoid therapy are well known (see Chap. 23, Arthritis and Rheumatologic Diseases). As a result of the associated morbidity, steroids are tapered rapidly in the immediate posttransplant period to achieve maintenance doses of 0.1 mg/kg or less. Three further strategies are developing to minimize side effects: steroid-free immunosuppression, rapid steroid tapering, and steroid withdrawal.

II. **Antiproliferative agents**

A. **Azathioprine** is a purine analog that is metabolized by the liver to 6-mercaptopurine (active drug), which, in turn, is catabolized by xanthine oxidase. Azathioprine inhibits the synthesis of DNA and thereby suppresses the proliferation of activated lymphocytes. The major dose-limiting toxicity of this agent is myelosuppression, which is usually reversible after dose reduction or discontinuation of the drug. The usual maintenance dose is 1.5–2.5 mg/kg/day in a single dose. Drug levels are generally not obtained.

**B. Mycophenolate mofetil (MMF)** is converted to an active metabolite, mycophenolic acid (MPA). MPA inhibits the rate-limiting step in *de novo* purine synthesis. Because lymphocytes are relatively dependent on the *de novo* pathway for purine synthesis, lymphocyte proliferation is selectively inhibited by MPA. The major adverse effects of MMF are GI disturbances, including nausea, diarrhea, and abdominal pain, and hematologic disturbances, namely, leukopenia and thrombocytopenia. Antacids that contain magnesium and aluminum interfere with the absorption of MMF and should not be given concurrently. The usual dose is 1–2 g daily in divided doses. Additionally, the dosage of MMF should be reduced in the presence of renal impairment.

**C. Sirolimus (rapamycin)** is a macrocyclic antibiotic produced by *Streptomyces hygroscopics*. Sirolimus forms a complex with the same receptor-binding protein as tacrolimus; this complex inhibits the activation of a regulatory kinase, mammalian target of rapamycin, and thus prohibits T-cell progression from the G1 to the S phase of the cell cycle. Unlike the calcineurin inhibitors, sirolimus does not affect cytokine transcription but inhibits cytokine and growth factor–induced cell proliferation. The major adverse effects of this drug include hyperlipidemia, cytopenia, peripheral edema, oral ulcers, and gastrointestinal symptoms, although other less common side effects are present. Sirolimus is not nephrotoxic. The typical dose is 2–5 mg daily in a single dose. Therapeutic drug monitoring is being perfected, with current trough levels between 10 and 20 ng/ml most commonly being used.

**III. Calcineurin inhibitors** bind to immunophilins (intracellular binding proteins). The calcineurin inhibitor–immunophilin complex inhibits a key phosphatase that is involved in transducing the signal from the T-cell receptor to the nucleus. The net effect is blockade of interleukin-2 and other cytokine transcription, leading to inhibition of T-lymphocyte activation and proliferation. Current strategies are being developed for calcineurin withdrawal and avoidance in solid organ transplantation. Intravenous calcineurin inhibitors should be avoided because of their extreme toxicity and must never be given as a bolus under any circumstances.

**A. Cyclosporine (CsA)** is a cyclic 11–amino acid peptide derived from a fungus. Its major nonimmune side effect is nephrotoxicity due to afferent arteriolar vasoconstriction. This action leads to an immediate decline in glomerular filtration rate of up to 30% and a long-term vaso-occlusive fibrotic renal disease that often results in chronic renal failure. Angiotensin-converting enzyme inhibitors, volume depletion, and other nephrotoxins may potentiate this toxicity. Acute nephrotoxicity is reversible with dose reduction; chronic nephrotoxicity is generally irreversible. Other adverse effects include gingival hyperplasia, hirsutism, tremor, hypertension, glucose intolerance, hyperlipidemia, hyperkalemia, and, rarely, thrombotic microangiopathy. CsA has a narrow therapeutic window, and doses are adjusted based on blood levels (recommended maintenance trough levels of 100–300 ng/ml and 2-hour levels <800–1200 ng/ml). Usual doses are 6–8 mg/kg/day in divided doses, with careful attention to levels and toxicities.

**B. Tacrolimus (FK 506)** is a macrolide antibiotic and, like CsA, is nephrotoxic. Tacrolimus is more neurotoxic and diabetogenic than CsA, but it is associated with less hirsutism, hypertension, and gum hyperplasia. Tacrolimus dosing is based on trough blood levels (recommended maintenance levels of 5–15 ng/ml). Usual starting dose is 0.15 mg/kg/day in divided doses.

**IV. Biologic agents**

**A. Polyclonal antibodies**

**1. Antithymocyte globulin (ATGAM)** is a polyclonal, horse antihuman thymocyte antibody. ATGAM depletes circulating T lymphocytes as a result of complement-mediated lysis and clearance of antibody-coated cells by the reticuloendothelial system. ATGAM also interferes with lymphocyte function by blocking and modulating the expression of cell surface molecules. The drug is usually infused over 4–6 hours through a central vein to avoid thrombophlebitis. The most common side effects are fever, chills, and arthralgias. Other important adverse effects include myelosuppression, serum sickness, and, rarely, anaphylaxis.

2. **Thymoglobulin** is a polyclonal, rabbit antihuman thymocyte antibody. Its mode of administration and mechanism of action are similar to those of ATGAM, but the duration of lymphocyte depletion is more prolonged. Thymoglobulin has a side effect profile similar to that of ATGAM. Both drugs are used perioperatively for induction therapy and as needed postoperatively for the treatment of acute rejection.

**B. Monoclonal antibodies**

1. **Anti–interleukin-2 receptor monoclonal antibodies.** Daclizumab (humanized) and basiliximab (chimeric) are monoclonal antibodies that competitively inhibit the alpha subunit of the interleukin-2 receptor (CD25) and thereby inhibit activation of T cells. Humanization and chimerization reduce the murine sequences of these genetically engineered antibodies, respectively. This results in antibodies with an extended half-life and minimizes the chances of developing human antimurine antibodies. These drugs are administered by a peripheral vein perioperatively at the time of transplantation and are associated with few side effects.
2. **OKT3** is a murine monoclonal antibody directed against the CD3ε chain associated with the T-cell receptor. It is administered as a bolus injection via a peripheral vein. OKT3 depletes $CD3^+$ T cells and modulates CD3 expression. The most common side effect is cytokine release syndrome, characterized by fever, chills, nausea, vomiting, diarrhea, myalgia, and, occasionally, hypotension and noncardiogenic pulmonary edema. Other side effects include encephalopathy, seizures, and aseptic meningitis.

**V. Important drug interactions** are always a concern given the polypharmacy associated with transplant patients. The combination of allopurinol and azathioprine should be avoided or used cautiously due to the risk of profound myelosuppression. CsA is metabolized by cytochrome P-450 (3A4). Therefore, CsA levels are decreased by drugs that induce cytochrome P-450 activity, such as rifampin, isoniazid, barbiturates, phenytoin, and carbamazepine. Conversely, CsA levels are increased by drugs that compete for cytochrome P-450, such as verapamil, diltiazem, nicardipine, azole antifungals, erythromycin, and clarithromycin (see Appendix C, Drug Interactions). Similar effects are seen with tacrolimus and sirolimus. Tacrolimus and CsA should not be taken together because of the increased risk of severe nephrotoxicity. Lower doses of MMF should be used when either tacrolimus or sirolimus is taken concurrently. Concomitant administration of CsA and sirolimus may result in a twofold increase in sirolimus levels; to avoid this drug interaction, CsA and sirolimus should be dosed 4 hours apart.

## Rejection

**I. Acute rejection**

**A. Kidney** allograft rejection occurs in 10–30% of patients and is defined as an immunologically mediated, acute deterioration in renal function associated with specific pathologic changes on renal biopsy. Most episodes of acute rejection occur in the first 6 months after transplantation. Late acute rejection (>1 year after transplantation) usually results from inadequate immunosuppression or patient noncompliance.

1. **Manifestations** include an elevated serum creatinine, decreased urine output, increased edema, or worsening hypertension. Initial symptoms are often absent except for the rise in creatinine. Constitutional symp-

**Table 15-1.** Differential diagnosis of renal allograft dysfunction

| <1 wk posttransplant | <3 mo posttransplant | >3 mo posttransplant |
|---|---|---|
| Acute tubular necrosis | Acute rejection | Prerenal azotemia |
| Hyperacute rejection | Calcineurin toxicity | Calcineurin toxicity |
| Accelerated rejection | Prerenal azotemia | Acute rejection |
| Obstruction | Obstruction | Obstruction |
| Urine leak (ureteral necrosis) | Infection | Recurrent renal disease |
| Vascular thrombosis | Interstitial nephritis | *De novo* renal disease |
| Atheroemboli | Recurrent renal disease | Renal artery stenosis (anastomotic or atherosclerotic) |

toms (fever, malaise, arthralgia, painful or swollen allograft) are uncommon in the cyclosporine era.

2. **Differential diagnosis** varies with duration after transplantation (Table 15-1). Diagnosis of acute renal allograft rejection is made by renal biopsy after excluding prerenal azotemia via hydration and repeating laboratory tests, cyclosporine nephrotoxicity (trough and/or peak levels and associated signs), infection (urinalysis and culture), and obstruction (renal ultrasound). Rapid molecular diagnostic techniques for acute rejection using urine and blood are being developed.

B. **Lung** transplant rejection occurs frequently and most commonly in the first few months after transplantation. The majority of patients have at least one episode of acute rejection. Multiple episodes of acute rejection predispose to the development of chronic rejection (bronchiolitis obliterans syndrome).

1. **Manifestations** are nonspecific and include fever, dyspnea, and a nonproductive cough. The chest radiograph is usually unchanged, and, if it is abnormal in the early phase of rejection, the findings are generally nondiagnostic (perihilar infiltrates, interstitial edema, pleural effusions). Abnormal pulmonary function testing is not specific for rejection, but a 10% or greater decline in forced vital capacity or forced expiratory volume in 1 second, or both, is usually clinically significant.
2. **Differential diagnosis.** It is important to attempt to distinguish rejection from infection, because the treatments are markedly different.
3. **Diagnosis** is generally made by fiberoptic bronchoscopy with bronchoalveolar lavage and transbronchial biopsies.

C. **Heart** transplant recipients typically have two to three episodes of acute rejection in the first year after transplantation with a 50–80% chance of having at least one rejection episode, most commonly in the first 6 months.

1. **Manifestations** may include symptoms and signs of left ventricular dysfunction, such as dyspnea, paroxysmal nocturnal dyspnea, orthopnea, syncope, palpitations, new gallops, and elevated jugular venous pressure, but many patients are asymptomatic. Acute rejection may also be associated with a variety of tachyarrhythmias, atrial more often than ventricular.
2. **Diagnosis** is established by endomyocardial biopsy performed during routine surveillance or as prompted by symptoms. None of the noninvasive techniques has demonstrated sufficient sensitivity and specificity to replace the endomyocardial biopsy.

D. **Liver** transplant recipients commonly experience acute allograft rejection, with at least 60% having one episode. Acute rejection typically occurs within the first 3 months after transplant and often in the first 2 weeks after the operation. Acute rejection in the liver is generally reversible and does not portend a potentially serious adverse outcome as in other organs.

1. **Manifestations** may be absent, or the patients may have signs and symptoms of liver failure, including fever, malaise, anorexia, abdominal pain, ascites, decreased bile output, elevated bilirubin, and/or transaminases.
2. **Differential diagnosis** of early liver allograft dysfunction includes primary graft nonfunction, preservation injury, vascular thrombosis, biliary anastomotic leak, or stenosis. These should be excluded clinically or by Doppler ultrasonography. Late allograft dysfunction may be due to rejection, recurrent hepatitis B or C, cytomegalovirus (CMV) or Epstein-Barr virus (EBV) infection, cholestasis, or drug toxicity.
3. **Diagnosis** is made by liver biopsy after technical complications are excluded.

E. **Treatment of acute allograft rejection** depends on the histologic severity (grade). Mild rejection of heart and lung transplants is often left untreated. First-line therapy for acute rejection usually consists of either pulse methylprednisolone or high-dose prednisone, with a 60–80% response rate. Rejection that is more severe, recurrent, or refractory to glucocorticoid therapy is generally treated with antilymphocyte antibody preparations. Maintenance immunosuppressive agents are often added or substituted after an episode of acute rejection.

II. **Chronic rejection** is a slowly progressive, insidious decline in function of the allograft characterized by gradual vascular and ductal obliteration, parenchymal atrophy, and interstitial fibrosis. Diagnosis is often difficult and generally requires a biopsy. The process is mediated by immune and nonimmune factors. Chronic rejection or allograft dysfunction accounts for the vast majority of late graft losses and is the major obstacle to long-term graft survival. The manifestations of chronic rejection are unique to each organ system. To date, no effective therapy is available for established chronic rejection. Current investigational strategies are aimed at prevention.

## Infectious Complications

**Infectious complications** can occur in either the allograft (often causing allograft dysfunction and possibly enhancing rejection) or in other organs as a consequence of the immunosuppressed state (*N Engl J Med* 338:1741, 1998).

I. **Time course.** Infections follow a typical course depending on the organ transplanted, the time from transplantation, and the net state of immunosuppression. During the first month after transplantation, infections related directly to the surgery and hospitalization predominate (wound infections, pneumonia, catheter-related bacteremia, and urinary tract infections). Opportunistic viral, parasitic, and bacterial infections occur during the next 6 months and after aggressive treatment of acute rejection episodes. Signs or symptoms of infection should be pursued aggressively, as infection is the second leading cause of death in transplant recipients.

II. **Etiology.** Several opportunistic infections should be considered in the transplant recipient (Table 15-2).

III. **Prevention**

A. **Immunization.** Pneumococcal and hepatitis B vaccination should be given at the time of pretransplant evaluation. Influenza A vaccination should be administered yearly. Live vaccines should be avoided after transplantation.

B. **Prophylaxis**

1. Trimethoprim/sulfamethoxazole prevents urinary tract infections, *Pneumocystis carinii* pneumonia, and *Nocardia* infections. The optimal dose and duration of prophylaxis have not been determined.
2. Acyclovir prevents reactivation of herpes simplex virus but is ineffective in CMV prophylaxis. Lifetime acyclovir should also be used in EBV-seronegative patients who receive an EBV-positive organ.

**Table 15-2.** Timing and etiology of posttransplant infections

| Time period | Infectious complication | Etiology |
|---|---|---|
| <1 mo posttransplant | Nosocomial pneumonia, wound infection, urinary tract infection, catheter-related sepsis | Bacterial or fungal infections |
| 1–6 mo posttransplant | Opportunistic infections | Cytomegalovirus |
| | | *Pneumocystis carinii* |
| | | *Aspergillus* spp. |
| | | *Toxoplasma gondii* |
| | | *Listeria monocytogenes* |
| | | Varicella-zoster virus |
| | Reactivation of preexisting infections | *Mycobacteria* spp. |
| | | Endemic mycoses |
| >6 mo posttransplant | Community-acquired infections | Bacterial |
| | Chronic progressive infection | Hepatitis B |
| | | Hepatitis C |
| | | Cytomegalovirus |
| | | Epstein-Barr virus |
| | | Papillomavirus |
| | | Polyoma virus (BK) |
| | Opportunistic infections | *P. carinii* |
| | | *L. monocytogenes* |
| | | *Nocardia asteroides* |
| | | *Cryptococcus neoformans* |
| | | *Aspergillus* spp. |

3. Ganciclovir or valganciclovir prevents CMV infection when administered to patients who were previously CMV seropositive or receive a CMV-positive organ, or both. CMV hyperimmune globulin or IV ganciclovir can also be used for this purpose.
4. Fluconazole or ketoconazole can be given to patients with a high risk of systemic fungal infections or recurrent localized fungal infections. Both medications increase cyclosporine and tacrolimus levels (see Immunosuppressive Medications, sec. **V**). Nystatin suspension or clotrimazole troches are used to prevent oropharyngeal candidiasis (thrush).

## IV. Diagnosis and treatment

**A. CMV infection** from reactivation of CMV in a seropositive recipient or new infection from a CMV-positive organ can lead to a wide range of presentations from a mild viral syndrome to allograft dysfunction, invasive disease in multiple organ systems, and even death. CMV-seronegative patients who receive a CMV-seropositive organ are at substantial risk, particularly in the first year. Because of the potential progression and severity of untreated disease, treatment is usually indicated in the transplant patient without tissue diagnosis of invasive disease. Shell-vial culture of the buffy coat is accurate only when plated within 24 hours of sample collection. Seroconversion with a positive IgM titer or a fourfold increase in IgM or IgG titer suggests acute infection; however, many centers now use polymerase chain reaction–based diagnostic techniques. Treatment is with oral valganciclovir, 450–900 mg PO bid (adjusted for renal function) or IV ganciclovir, 2.5–5.0 mg/kg bid (adjusted for renal function), for 3–4 weeks. Hyperimmune globulin is often used in combination with ganciclovir for patients with organ involvement. Foscarnet is a more toxic alternative. Prophylaxis during the highest incidence of severe CMV infection episodes (e.g., 3–12 months after transplantation in patients who are either seropositive or receive a seropositive organ) with oral ganciclovir (1000 mg PO tid) or valganciclovir has markedly reduced the incidence of life-threatening CMV infections.

**B. Hepatitis B and C.** Patients with active hepatitis or cirrhosis are not considered for nonhepatic transplantation. Immunosuppression increases viral replication in organ transplant recipients with either hepatitis B or C. **Hepatitis B** can recur as fulminant hepatic failure even in patients with no evidence of viral DNA replication before transplantation. In liver transplantation, the risk of recurrent hepatitis B virus infection can be reduced by the administration of hepatitis B immunoglobulin during and after transplantation. Experience with lamivudine therapy initiated before transplantation to lower viral load has shown decreased likelihood of recurrent hepatitis B virus. **Hepatitis C** typically progresses slowly in nonhepatic transplants, and the effect of immunosuppression remains to be determined on mortality due to liver disease. Treatment protocols for hepatitis C in the nonhepatic transplant population are not yet established. Hepatitis C nearly always recurs in liver transplant recipients whose original disease was due to hepatitis C. Therapy for recurrent hepatitis C virus with a combination of ribavirin and interferon results in histopathologic improvement of disease, although dosage and duration of therapy remain controversial.

**C. EBV** plays a role in the development of posttransplant lymphoproliferative disease. This life-threatening lymphoma is treated by withdrawal or reduction in immunosuppression and often aggressive chemotherapy (see the section Long-Term Complications of Transplantation).

**D.** The role of newly discovered **viral agents** such as HHV-6, HHV-7, HHV-8, and polyoma (BK) virus after transplantation remains to be established, although BK virus is known to cause interstitial nephritis resulting in renal allograft loss.

**E. Fungal and parasitic infections,** such as *Cryptococcus*, *Mucor*, aspergillosis, and *Candida* species, result in increased mortality after transplantation and should be aggressively diagnosed and treated. The role of prophylaxis with oral fluconazole has not been established.

## Long-Term Complications of Transplantation

### I. Cardiovascular complications

**A. Hypertension** occurs in up to 80% of renal transplant patients and to a lesser degree in other solid organ transplant recipients. BP should be monitored and maintained below 130/80. Certain calcium channel blockers significantly increase CsA and tacrolimus levels (see Appendix C, Drug Interactions), and drug levels should be carefully monitored. Angiotensin-converting enzyme inhibitors should usually be avoided in the early posttransplant period because of the potential for increased nephrotoxicity when patients are receiving high doses of cyclosporine or tacrolimus. However, these agents may be renoprotective in the long term. When suspected, anastomotic or atherosclerotic renal artery stenosis should be excluded.

**B. Coronary heart disease.** Graft atherosclerosis in cardiac allografts is partially immunologic in nature. Cardiac disease is the leading cause of death in renal transplant recipients and should be screened aggressively before transplantation, with aggressive modification of risk factors after transplantation.

II. **Endocrine and metabolic complications**

A. **Obesity** is a common problem in the late posttransplant period, with average weight gains in excess of 40 lb by 1 year. The approach should be multidisciplinary and include dietary and exercise counseling. Most medications that promote weight loss, however, impair BP control.

B. **Hyperlipidemia** occurs in as many as 60% of solid organ transplant recipients. Elevated lipid levels may be related to medications (glucocorticoids, CsA, thiazides), comorbidity, and genetic factors. Hyperlipidemia is associated with cardiovascular disease and may also have a role in chronic allograft vasculopathy. Dietary intervention alone is often insufficient to achieve a therapeutic target, and treatment should follow the National Cholesterol Education Program guidelines.

C. **Diabetes mellitus.** Glucocorticoids, calcineurin inhibitors, and obesity all contribute to diabetes after transplantation. Tacrolimus may have a higher incidence of diabetes versus cyclosporine (approximately 20% vs. 5%, respectively). Patients should be screened with fasting plasma glucose levels as recommended by the American Diabetes Association.

D. **Bone disease.** Avascular necrosis and steroid-induced osteoporosis can be disabling, leading to multiple fractures and often requiring joint replacement. Bone densitometry at regular intervals monitors osteopenia, although cortical bone loss can occur rapidly within the first months of high-dose glucocorticoid therapy. Transplant recipients should be in positive calcium balance with calcium supplementation (calcium carbonate, 1000–1500 mg/day between meals or qhs). Vitamin D supplements, calcitonin, and bisphosphonates have been used in transplant recipients.

III. **Renal disease.** Chronic rejection is the leading cause of allograft loss in renal transplant recipients. Calcineurin inhibitor (CsA or tacrolimus) nephrotoxicity or recurrent native disease may also develop in these patients. Chronic calcineurin inhibitor nephrotoxicity may also lead to chronic renal insufficiency and end-stage renal disease (ESRD), requiring dialysis or transplantation in recipients of lung, heart, liver, or pancreas transplants. The incidence of ESRD secondary to calcineurin inhibitor toxicity in recipients of solid organ transplants is approximately 10%.

IV. **Malignancy** occurs in transplant patients with an overall incidence that is threefold to fourfold higher than that seen in the general population (age matched). Some cancers occur at the same rate, whereas other neoplasms have a much higher frequency than normal. The spontaneous malignancies that occur most frequently in transplant recipients include cancers of the skin and lips, lymphoproliferative disease, bronchogenic carcinoma, Kaposi's sarcoma, uterine/cervical carcinoma, renal cell carcinoma, and anogenital neoplasms (*N Engl J Med* 323:1767, 1990).

A. **Skin and lip cancers** are the most common malignancies (40–50%) seen in transplant recipients, with an incidence 10–250 times that of the general population. Risk factors include immunosuppression, ultraviolet radiation, and human papillomavirus infection. These cancers develop at a younger age, and they are more aggressive in transplant patients than in the general population. Using protective clothing and sunscreens and avoiding sun exposure are recommended. Examination of the skin is the principal screening test, and early diagnosis offers the best prognosis.

B. **Posttransplant lymphoproliferative disease** accounts for one-fifth of all malignancies after transplantation, with an incidence of approximately 1%. This is 30- to 50-fold higher than in the general population, and the risk increases with the use of antilymphocyte therapy for induction or rejection. The majority of these neoplasms are large-cell non-Hodgkin's lymphomas of the B-cell type. Posttransplant lymphoproliferative disease results from EBV-induced B-cell proliferation in the setting of chronic immunosuppression. The presentation is often atypical. Diagnosis requires a high index of suspicion followed by a tissue biopsy. Treatment includes reduction or withdrawal of immunosuppression and chemotherapy.

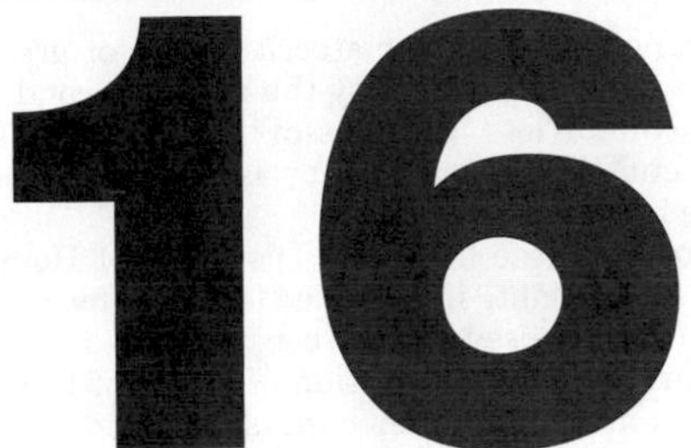

# Gastrointestinal Diseases

Chandra Prakash

## Gastrointestinal Bleeding

**Overt GI bleeding** presents with the passage of fresh or altered blood through the mouth [hematemesis, coffee-ground emesis, blood in nasogastric (NG) aspirate] or in the stool (melena, hematochezia, maroon stool). **Occult bleeding** refers to a positive fecal occult blood test (stool guaiac) or iron-deficiency anemia without visible blood in the stool. **Obscure bleeding** consists of GI blood loss of unknown origin that persists or recurs after negative initial endoscopic evaluation; obscure bleeding can be either overt or occult. The following sections refer primarily to overt bleeding.

I. **General considerations.** The initial evaluation is performed concurrently with resuscitative measures, regardless of the site of bleeding. History and physical examination are directed toward determining the anatomic level of bleeding, the quantity of blood lost, the etiology of bleeding, and precipitating factors.

A. **Initial evaluation**

1. **Intravascular volume and hemodynamic status.** Constant monitoring or frequent assessment of vital signs is necessary early in the evaluation, as a sudden increase in pulse rate or decrease in BP may be an early indicator of recurrent or ongoing blood loss. If the baseline BP and pulse are within normal limits, sitting the patient up or having the patient stand may result in **orthostatic hemodynamic changes** (drop in systolic BP of >10 mm Hg, rise in pulse rate of >15 beats/minute). Orthostatic changes in pulse and BP are seen with loss of 10–20% of the circulatory volume; supine hypotension suggests a greater than 20% loss. Hypotension with a systolic BP of <100 mm Hg or baseline tachycardia suggests significant hemodynamic compromise that requires urgent volume resuscitation.
2. **Laboratory evaluation.** A CBC, coagulation parameters (prothrombin time, partial thromboplastin time, platelet count), blood group, and cross-matching of 2–4 U of blood should be urgently performed. A chemistry profile including liver and renal function helps stratify risk when invasive intervention is required and may assist with differential diagnosis.

B. **Initial resuscitation**

1. **Restoration of intravascular volume.** Two large-bore IV lines with 14- to 18-gauge catheters or a central venous line should be urgently placed. Isotonic saline, lactated Ringer's solution, or 5% hetastarch can be initiated; patients in shock may require volume administration using pressure infusion devices or hand infused using large syringes and stopcocks. **Packed RBC transfusion** should be used for volume replacement whenever possible; O-negative blood or simultaneous multiple-unit transfusions may be indicated if bleeding is massive. Transfusion should be continued until hemodynamic stability is achieved and the hematocrit reaches 25% or greater; patients with cardiac or pulmonary

disease may require transfusion to a hematocrit of 30% or greater. The rate of volume infusion should be guided by the patient's condition and the rate and degree of volume loss. Vasopressors are generally not indicated, although transient IV pressor therapy is sometimes beneficial until enough volume is infused.

2. **Correction of coagulopathy** (see Chap. 18, Disorders of Hemostasis). Discontinuation of anticoagulant, if possible, followed by infusion of fresh frozen plasma can be used to correct prolonged coagulation parameters from warfarin. An initial infusion of 2–4 U of **fresh frozen plasma** can be supplemented with further infusion based on reassessment of the coagulation parameters. Parenteral **vitamin K** (10 mg SC or IM) may be indicated for prolonged prothrombin time from warfarin therapy or hepatobiliary disease but takes several hours to days for adequate reversal; it should be repeated daily for a total of three doses in hepatobiliary disease. Protamine infusion (1 mg antagonizes ~100 U of heparin) can be used for immediate reversal of anticoagulation from heparin infusion. Platelet infusion may be indicated when the platelet count is less than 50,000/mm$^3$.
3. **Airway protection.** Endotracheal intubation to prevent aspiration should be considered when altered mental status (shock, hepatic encephalopathy), massive hematemesis, or active variceal hemorrhage is present (see Airway Management and Tracheal Intubation in Chap. 8, Critical Care).

## II. History

A. **Degree of volume loss.** Estimation of the amount of blood lost can be attempted but is often inaccurate. If the baseline hematocrit is known, the drop in hematocrit provides a rough estimate of blood loss. In general, patients with lower GI bleeding have less hemodynamic compromise than those with upper GI bleeding.

B. **Level of bleeding.** Hematemesis, coffee-ground emesis, and aspiration of blood or coffee grounds from an NG tube suggest an upper GI source of blood loss. **Melena,** black sticky stool with a characteristic odor, indicates an upper GI source of blood loss, although small-bowel and sometimes right colonic bleeds can result in melena. Various shades of red blood are seen in the stool with distal small-bowel or colonic bleeding, depending on the rate of blood loss and colonic transit. Although patients with upper GI bleeding can also present with red blood in their stool, this is almost invariably associated with hemodynamic compromise and circulatory shock. Bleeding from the anorectal area typically results in bright blood coating the exterior of formed stool, sometimes associated with distal colonic symptoms (e.g., rectal urgency, straining, or pain with defecation).

C. **Etiology of bleeding.** Important points in the medical history include prior bleeding episodes, alcohol use, liver disease, coagulation disorders, and bleeding tendencies. A history of emesis preceding upper GI bleeding may suggest a Mallory-Weiss tear. Nonsteroidal anti-inflammatory drugs (NSAIDs) and aspirin can result in mucosal damage anywhere in the GI tract. Hypotension and hypovolemic shock preceding the bleeding episode may suggest ischemic colitis. Radiation therapy to the prostate or pelvis suggests radiation proctopathy, and prior aortic graft surgery raises suspicion of an aortoenteric or aortocolonic fistula. Chronic constipation may suggest bleeding from stercoral (stool-induced) ulceration of the rectum. A history of recent polypectomy may indicate postpolypectomy bleeding. GI angiodysplasia can develop in patients with chronic renal disease, and patients with hereditary hemorrhagic telangiectasia can have GI telangiectasia as a source for blood loss.

D. **Precipitating factors.** Coagulation abnormalities can propagate bleeding from a preexisting lesion in the GI tract. Bleeding cannot be attributed to coagulation abnormalities alone, and workup to identify the etiology of blood loss is recommended, usually after coagulopathy has been corrected. Usual medications that are known to affect the coagulation process include warfarin, heparin, aspirin, NSAIDs, clopidogrel (Plavix), and thrombolytic agents. Newer antithrombotic agents can also propagate bleeding and include glycoprotein IIb/IIIa receptor antagonists [abciximab (ReoPro), eptifibatide (Integrelin), tirofiban (Aggrastat)] and direct thrombin inhibitors (argatroban, bivalirudin) (see Chap. 5, Ischemic Heart Disease, and Chap. 18, Disorders of Hemostasis). Disorders of coagulation, such as liver disease, von Willebrand's disease, vitamin K deficiency, and disseminated intravascular coagulation, can also influence the course of GI bleeding (see Chap. 18, Disorders of Hemostasis).

**III. Physical examination**

**A. Color of stool.** Direct examination of spontaneously passed stool or stool obtained during a digital rectal examination can provide important clues as to the level of bleeding (see sec. **II.B**).

**B. NG aspiration.** An NG aspirate is useful in the diagnosis of upper GI bleeding. In a small fraction of patients, a bleeding source in the duodenum can result in a negative NG aspirate. Hemoccult testing of a normal-appearing NG aspirate is of no clinical utility; the aspirate should be considered positive only if blood or dark particulate matter ("coffee grounds") is seen. Gastric lavage with water or saline may be useful in assessing the activity and severity of upper GI bleeding and in clearing the stomach of blood and clots before endoscopic examination. After a diagnosis of upper GI bleeding is made, the NG tube is not required further in a stable patient, especially if endoscopy is to follow.

**C. Anoscopy/sigmoidoscopy.** A digital rectal examination helps assess the color of stool and may identify a potential source of bleeding in the anorectum. Anal fissures, typically seen in the posterior midline, can result in extreme pain during a rectal examination (see Other Gastrointestinal Disorders, sec. **VII.C**). Anoscopy may be useful in the detection of internal hemorrhoids and anal fissures. In an outpatient or emergency room setting, anoscopy and sigmoidoscopy may be useful in rapid diagnosis of the level of bleeding before patient triage but is usually followed by colonoscopy after bowel preparation.

**IV. Further evaluation and therapy.** The level of bleeding, acuity of blood loss, and general comorbid illnesses of the patient should be considered in test selection.

**A. Esophagogastroduodenoscopy (EGD)** is the preferred method of investigation and therapy of upper GI bleeding and is associated with high diagnostic accuracy, therapeutic capability, and low morbidity. Volume resuscitation or blood transfusion should precede endoscopy in hemodynamically unstable patients. Although early diagnostic endoscopy does not reduce mortality, therapeutic endoscopy reduces transfusion requirements, need for surgery, and length of hospital stay (*N Engl J Med* 325:1142, 1991). Patients with ongoing bleeding benefit most from urgent EGD, whereas stable patients with minimal bleeding (e.g., coffee-ground emesis with stable hematocrit) can have the procedure performed electively during the hospitalization.

**B.** Early **colonoscopy** can be performed after a rapid bowel purge in patients whose condition has clinically stabilized and who can tolerate an adequate bowel purge. The yield of finding a potential bleeding source in the colon is greatest if colonoscopy is performed within the initial 24 hours of presentation. Patients who are unable to drink adequate amounts of the balanced electrolyte solution can have an NG tube placed for infusion of the bowel purge. All patients with acute lower GI bleeding from an unknown source should eventually undergo endoscopic evaluation of the colon during the initial hospitalization, regardless of the initial mode of investigation.

**C. Tagged red blood cell (TRBC) scanning.** RBCs that are labeled with technetium-99m remain in circulation for as long as 48 hours and extravasate into the bowel lumen with active bleeding. This extravasation can be detected as pooling of the radioactive tracer on gamma camera scanning. The pattern of peristaltic movement of the pooled tracer can help identify the potential site of bleeding. Bleeding rates as low as **0.1 ml/minute** can be detected in research settings. A positive TRBC scan identifies patients who are likely to require invasive intervention and have high in-hospital morbidity, in contrast to a negative test, which may imply a better short-term prognosis. However, the scan is only positive 45% of the time. When positive, it is accurate in identification of the location of the bleeding source in 80% of cases. The false localization rate of approximately 20% precludes use of this test alone in directing surgical resection of the bleeding bowel segment. Therefore, the clinical utility of this test is for screening before arteriography, a more invasive test that requires a higher rate of bleeding.

D. **Arteriography** allows rapid localization and potential therapy of GI bleeding by demonstrating extravasation of the dye into the intestine when bleeding rates exceed **0.5 ml/minute.** Arteriography may also identify the bleeding lesion, especially bleeding diverticula or angiodysplasia. A tumor blush or a late draining vein of angiodysplasia may be seen even in the absence of active bleeding. In upper GI bleeding, arteriography is reserved for situations in which brisk bleeding makes endoscopy difficult. In small-bowel or lower GI bleeding, arteriography is used for diagnosis and for therapy of the bleeding lesion, typically after initial localization with TRBC scanning. Immediate or early extravasation on TRBC scanning carries the greatest likelihood of a positive arteriogram. In stable patients with recurrent, difficult-to-localize GI bleeding, infusion of anticoagulants (e.g., heparin), thrombolytic agents (e.g., streptokinase), or intra-arterial vasodilators in a controlled fashion may increase the diagnostic yield of angiography. These provocative measures can be associated with excessive bleeding and should only be used in specialized centers in stable patients without comorbid illnesses. When an actively bleeding lesion is found during angiography, intra-arterial infusion of vasopressin can cause vasoconstriction and stop bleeding. **Embolization** of the bleeding artery can also be performed but carries a small risk of bowel infarction.

E. **Advanced procedures.** When radiologic evaluation suggests a jejunal bleeding source, or in recurrent (obscure) GI bleeding, **enteroscopy** to the jejunum can be performed using dedicated small-bowel enteroscopes. The distal ileum can be examined during colonoscopy after intubation of the ileocecal valve. **Capsule endoscopy** is a novel diagnostic procedure that has high diagnostic yield in obscure GI bleeding of suspected small-bowel origin; this procedure is typically performed after push-enteroscopy and colonoscopy exclude a bleeding source within reach of conventional endoscopy. When capsule endoscopy diagnoses a potential bleeding lesion in the small bowel, or when the risk of recurrent bleeding outweighs the risks of laparotomy, the entire small bowel can be examined endoscopically during exploratory laparotomy, with a surgeon manually threading bowel over an orally or rectally inserted endoscope; a potential bleeding source can be resected at the same operation, if found.

F. **Surgery.** Emergent total colectomy may be required as a lifesaving maneuver for massive, unlocalized, colonic bleeding; this should be preceded by emergent EGD to rule out a rapidly bleeding upper source whenever possible. Certain lesions (e.g., neoplasia, Meckel's diverticulum) require surgical resection for a cure. Splenectomy is curative in bleeding gastric varices from splenic vein thrombosis. Ongoing bleeding with transfusion requirements exceeding 4–6 U over 24 hours or 10 U overall or greater than 2–3 recurrent bleeding episodes from the same source have been considered indications for surgery.

V. **Therapy of specific lesions**

A. **Peptic ulcer disease (PUD).** The use of high-dose **proton pump inhibitors** (PPIs; e.g., omeprazole, 40 mg PO bid) reduces the rate of recurrent bleeding and the need for surgery in patients with upper GI bleeding who are awaiting endoscopic treatment or if endoscopy is contraindicated or postponed (*N Engl J Med* 336:1054, 1997). Conventional oral doses of PPIs (Table 16-1) may suffice after endoscopic therapy has been administered. PPI therapy, oral or IV, is

**Table 16-1.** Dosage of acid-suppressive agents

| Medication | Peptic ulcer disease | GERD | Parenteral therapy |
|---|---|---|---|
| Cimetidine[a] | 300 mg qid<br>400 mg bid<br>800 mg qhs | 400 mg qid<br>800 mg bid | 300 mg q6h |
| Ranitidine[a] | 150 mg bid<br>300 mg qhs | 150–300 mg bid–qid | 50 mg q8h |
| Famotidine[a] | 20 mg bid<br>40 mg qhs | 20–40 mg bid | 20 mg q12h |
| Nizatidine[a] | 150 mg bid<br>300 mg qhs | 150 mg bid | — |
| Omeprazole | 20 mg qd | 20–40 mg qd–bid | — |
| Esomeprazole | 40 mg qd | 20–40 mg qd | — |
| Lansoprazole | 15–30 mg qd | 15–30 mg qd–bid | — |
| Rabeprazole | 20 mg qd | 20 mg qd–bid | — |
| Pantoprazole | 20 mg qd | 20–40 mg qd–bid | 40 mg q12–24h *or* 80 mg IV followed by 8-mg/hr infusion |

GERD, gastroesophageal reflux disease.
[a]Dosage adjustment required in renal insufficiency (see Appendix E, Dose Adjustments of Drugs in Renal Failure).

better than IV histamine$_2$-receptor antagonist ($H_2$RA) therapy in bleeding peptic ulcers. Therapeutic endoscopy offers the advantage of immediate treatment and should be implemented in all patients early in the hospital course (within 24 hours). Fluid resuscitation and hemodynamic stability are essential before endoscopy. Surgery may be required for intractable or recurrent bleeding. **Surgical consultation** should be obtained early in severe bleeding with significant transfusion requirements or in recurrent bleeding after nonsurgical management. Angiography and embolization of the bleeding artery can be considered in poor surgical candidates. **Risk factors** for increased morbidity and mortality include age older than 60 years, more than one comorbid illness, blood loss of greater than 5 U, shock on admission, bright-red hematemesis with hypotension, coagulopathy, large (>2 cm) ulcers, recurrent hemorrhage (within 72 hours), and requirement for emergency surgery (see the section Peptic Ulcer Disease).

**B. Variceal hemorrhage**

1. **General measures. ICU admission** and **endotracheal intubation** for airway protection should be considered when active bleeding from varices is suspected. **Octreotide** infusion should be initiated immediately (50- to 100-μg bolus, followed by infusion at 25–50 μg/hour). Octreotide infusion acutely reduces portal pressures and controls variceal bleeding with very few side effects, improving the diagnostic yield and therapeutic success of subsequent endoscopy. **Vasopressin** (0.3 U/minute IV, followed by increments of 0.3 U/minute q30min until hemostasis is achieved, side effects develop, or the maximum dose of 0.9 U/minute is reached) is an alternate agent, rarely used because of significant cardiovascular complications including cardiac arrest and myocardial infarction. If used, vasopressin should be administered in an

ICU setting with cardiac monitoring and the infusion reduced or terminated if significant side effects develop. Concomitant infusion of **nitroglycerin** may reduce undesirable cardiovascular side effects and provide more effective control of bleeding. Nitroglycerin is administered only if the systolic BP is greater than 100 mm Hg, at a dose of 10 μg/minute IV, increased by 10 μg/minute q10–15min until the systolic BP falls to 100 mm Hg or a maximum dose of 400 μg/minute is reached.

2. **Esophageal varices**
   a. **Variceal ligation** or **banding** is the endoscopic therapy of choice. It is effective in controlling active hemorrhage and achieves variceal eradication rapidly, with lower rates of rebleeding and fewer complications compared to sclerotherapy. Complications of banding include superficial ulceration, dysphagia, transient chest discomfort, and, rarely, esophageal strictures.
   b. **Sclerotherapy** is also effective but is used less frequently because of complications (ulcerations, strictures, perforation, pleural effusions, adult respiratory distress syndrome, sepsis). Recurrent bleeding may be seen in up to 50% of patients but usually responds to repeat sclerotherapy. Fever may be seen in 40% of patients within the first 2 days of therapy; fever that lasts longer than 2 days should prompt investigation for bacteremia.
   c. **Transjugular intrahepatic portosystemic shunt** (TIPS) is a radiologic procedure wherein an expandable metal stent is deployed between the hepatic veins and the portal vein to decompress the portal system and reduce portal venous pressure. **Indications** include refractory variceal bleeding that is unresponsive to variceal ligation or sclerotherapy and bleeding from gastric varices in the setting of portal hypertension. **Hepatic encephalopathy** may occur in up to 25% of patients but is usually controlled with medical therapy (see Complications of Hepatic Insufficiency, sec. **II,** in Chap. 17, Liver Diseases). Shunt stenosis is another significant complication that may respond to balloon dilation. Screening for shunt stenosis with duplex Doppler ultrasound is recommended if variceal bleeding redevelops or the patient has recurrence of esophageal or gastric varices on endoscopy.
   d. **Shunt surgery** (portacaval or distal splenorenal shunt) should be considered in patients with good hepatic reserve if the patient (1) fails endoscopic or pharmacologic therapy, (2) is unable to return for follow-up visits, (3) is at high risk of death from recurrent bleeding because of cardiac disease or difficulty in obtaining blood products, or (4) lives far from medical care. Although bleeding may be controlled in 95% of cases, hospital death rates are high, and there is a significant incidence of postoperative encephalopathy, especially among patients with higher grades of Child-Turcotte-Pugh classification (see Table 17-5 in Chap. 17, Liver Diseases).
   e. **Balloon tamponade** has a very limited role in the therapy of variceal hemorrhage. It should only be used to temporize bleeding in situations in which definitive therapy is subsequently available. Octreotide infusion and endoscopic therapy should have been attempted before balloon placement in all instances. The Sengstaken-Blakemore tube and the Minnesota tube have a gastric and esophageal balloon, whereas the Linton tube has a large-volume gastric balloon without an esophageal balloon. These tubes should be used according to the manufacturer's specific directions for placement, traction, and balloon volume. The following are general guidelines for the use of balloon tamponade: (1) **ICU admission** is mandatory, as is **endotracheal intubation.** (2) Modification of the Sengstaken-Blakemore tube by the placement of an NG tube above

the esophageal balloon should be completed before insertion. This NG tube should be connected to intermittent suction to prevent aspiration of oropharyngeal secretions. The tube should be clearly labeled and not used for lavage. (3) Gastric balloon position should be confirmed by radiography before it is inflated. Inflating the gastric balloon in the esophagus can result in esophageal rupture. (4) **Complications** including mucosal ulceration and necrosis may occur, especially if large balloon volumes, high pressure, or traction are necessary to control bleeding. Balloon tamponade is associated with a high rate of major complications and mortality from tube displacement. Balloon pressure should be reduced intermittently, as stated in the manufacturer's instructions, and when bleeding has been controlled. The tube, with its balloon deflated, can be left in place so that pressure can be applied again if bleeding resumes. (5) Scissors must be kept at the patient's bedside to transect and withdraw the tube immediately, if necessary.

3. **Gastric varices.** Octreotide infusion or other pharmacologic therapy should be initiated early as for esophageal variceal bleeding (see sec. **V.B.1**). Variceal ligation or banding is usually unsuccessful in controlling gastric variceal bleeding. Sclerotherapy can be attempted, but larger volumes of sclerosant solution are generally required. When bleeding gastric varices are due to portal hypertension, **TIPS** needs to be considered early in the clinical course. Assessment of the portal circulation with duplex Doppler ultrasound or portal venography is essential, as isolated gastric varices from splenic vein thrombosis can be effectively treated with splenectomy. If balloon tamponade is necessary, the Linton tube offers better control of bleeding than does the Sengstaken-Blakemore tube (see sec. **V.B.2.e**).
4. **Pharmacologic prophylaxis** with β-adrenergic antagonists has been shown to reduce portal pressure and lower the risk of recurrent bleeding. **Propranolol** and **nadolol** in doses sufficient to reduce the resting heart rate by 25% are effective prophylactic therapy for recurrent bleeding as well as for primary prophylaxis, although no benefit in overall survival has been shown. Contraindications or side effects may limit their use. The addition of oral nitrates improves the therapeutic benefit of β-adrenergic antagonists.
5. **Liver transplantation** in selected patients can reverse portal hypertension, thereby eliminating the risk of variceal bleeding.

C. **Angiodysplasia** can occur anywhere in the GI tract and cause occult or overt GI bleeding. Renal failure and hereditary hemorrhagic telangiectasias are important predisposing factors. Iron therapy and intermittent blood transfusions should be continued for several months as an initial approach to persistent anemia from angiodysplasia. **Endoscopic ablation** is recommended even for nonbleeding angiodysplasias in patients with iron deficiency, especially if no other bleeding source is identified. Actively bleeding angiodysplasias are best treated by endoscopic therapy (heater probe, laser or argon plasma coagulator), intra-arterial vasopressin, embolization during angiography, or surgical resection. Capsule endoscopy may be useful in identification of small-bowel angiodysplasia beyond the reach of push enteroscopy; intraoperative enteroscopy for ablation or limited resection of isolated lesions can be considered in good surgical candidates. In patients with refractory life-threatening anemia despite ablation, intermittent transfusions and iron therapy and combination hormone therapy with estrogen and progesterone can be attempted (estradiol, 0.035–0.05 mg; norethisterone, 1 mg administered bid). Side effects are particularly troublesome for men and include sexual dysfunction, feminization, loss of libido, and gynecomastia; breast tenderness and vaginal bleeding can develop in women. A higher incidence of vascular thrombosis may be found in either sex.

D. **Stress ulcer** is encountered in the ICU setting, especially in patients who require mechanical ventilation for longer than 48 hours, with coagulopathy, sepsis, burns, renal failure, or CNS processes. **Prophylactic therapy** should be administered in patients who are considered to be at increased risk. IV infusions of $H_2$RAs in standard doses (Table 16-1) or oral sucralfate (4–6 g/day) are effective in preventing severe bleeding. PPIs can also be used in standard doses (Table 16-1). IV PPIs may also be effective for stress ulcer prophylaxis, although it is unclear whether this adds any advantage over $H_2$RA and sucralfate.

E. **Mallory-Weiss tear** is a mucosal tear at the gastroesophageal junction. The classic history of retching or emesis followed by hematemesis is obtained in some but not all patients. Bleeding ceases spontaneously in most instances, and few patients require endoscopic or angiographic therapy. Acid suppression should be initiated for 1–2 weeks to promote healing.

F. **Diverticulosis** is a common finding at routine endoscopy, but bleeding develops in only approximately 5% of patients with diverticula. Spontaneous cessation of bleeding is seen in 80%, but recurrent bleeding may occur. Persistent or brisk bleeding may require intra-arterial vasopressin at angiography or even surgical resection (see Other Gastrointestinal Disorders, sec. **V**).

G. **Aortoenteric fistula** is an uncommon but lethal cause of GI bleeding. Most patients have a history of aortic graft surgery and present with bleeding months to years after surgery. The fistula is generally aortoduodenal but can be anywhere in the small bowel or colon. The classic presentation is a herald bleed hours to weeks before massive GI bleeding. Recognition of this condition is essential, as undiagnosed aortoenteric fistulas are uniformly fatal. Endoscopy with examination of the fourth portion of the duodenum should be performed immediately. Angiography or CT scanning may demonstrate leakage at the graft site, but a negative study does not exclude an aortoenteric fistula; surgery should not be delayed to perform such procedures if the index of suspicion is high.

H. **Radiation proctopathy/colopathy** can result months to years after exposure to radiation therapy. Typically, intermittent hematochezia results from aberrant superficial mucosal vasculature in the distal colon. Treatment consists of supportive measures and endoscopic ablation of the mucosal telangiectasias. Recurrence is common, and repeat sessions may be required. Use of aspirin and NSAIDs should be avoided, if possible.

I. **Hemorrhoids** are the most common outpatient cause of hematochezia. Bleeding typically ceases spontaneously. Dietary fiber supplements and avoidance of constipation form the mainstay of supportive management (see Constipation, sec. **II.A** and **II.B**). Hemorrhoids that result in recurrent or constant bleeding can be surgically ligated or treated with band ligation.

## Esophageal Disorders

I. **Gastroesophageal reflux disease (GERD).** The predominant symptom of GERD is heartburn, and response to a therapeutic trial of a PPI can be diagnostic (*Aliment Pharmacol Ther* 13:59, 1999). Early endoscopic evaluation is recommended for patients with **warning symptoms** of dysphagia, odynophagia, early satiety, weight loss, or bleeding, and **atypical symptoms** (cough, asthma, hoarseness, chest pain, aphthous ulcers, hiccups, dental erosions). Patients with symptoms that are refractory to empiric acid suppression or require continuous medication for prolonged periods should also undergo endoscopy. **Ambulatory pH monitoring** is used to establish the diagnosis of GERD in patients with ongoing symptoms despite acid suppression (especially if endoscopy is negative) or those with atypical symptoms. **Complications** of GERD include ulceration, stricture formation, iron-deficiency anemia, and Barrett's esophagus. Endoscopic surveillance for Barrett's esophagus should be considered in patients with a symptom history that exceeds 5 years.

**A.** The basics of **lifestyle modification** include eating small meals; refraining from eating for 2–3 hours before lying down; elevating the head of the bed 6 in.; decreasing intake of fatty foods, chocolate, coffee, cola, and alcohol; and smoking cessation. Medications such as calcium channel blockers, theophylline, sedatives/tranquilizers, anticholinergics, and oral bisphosphonates may potentiate reflux and should be avoided if possible. Over-the-counter antacids and $H_2$RAs can be used prophylactically if necessary.

**B. Medical therapy**

1. **$H_2$RAs.** Standard doses of $H_2$RAs (Table 16-1) can result in symptomatic benefit in up to 60% of patients and endoscopic healing in 50%. Higher doses of $H_2$RAs (equivalent to ranitidine, 600 mg qd) improve the healing rate to 75% at a higher cost. Dosage adjustments are required in renal insufficiency.
2. **PPIs** have been demonstrated to be more effective than placebo or standard-dose $H_2$RA in symptomatic relief as well as endoscopic healing of GERD. Higher doses (omeprazole, 20–40 mg PO bid or equivalent) may be required in severe esophagitis. Continuous long-term PPI therapy is safe and effective in maintaining remission of GERD symptoms and is recommended for patients with erosive esophagitis, Barrett's esophagus, and severe symptoms. An attempt to step down treatment using $H_2$RA can be considered after initial response in patients with mild symptoms. Breakthrough nocturnal symptoms can sometimes be treated by adding an $H_2$RA (ranitidine, 150–300 mg or equivalent) at bedtime.
3. **Prokinetic agents** are not in common use in the management of GERD.

**C. Surgery.** Indications for fundoplication include the need for continuous or increasing doses of medication in patients who are good surgical candidates. All patients who require aggressive long-term medical therapy should be offered the surgical option. Other indications include patient preference for surgery and noncompliance with medical therapy. Patients with medical treatment failures need careful evaluation to determine whether symptoms are indeed related to acid reflux before surgical options are considered; these patients often have other diagnoses, including visceral hypersensitivity and functional heartburn. The success rate of **laparoscopic fundoplication** in controlling GERD symptoms exceeds 90%, with fewer complications compared to the open technique.

**II. Infectious esophagitis** usually presents with odynophagia or dysphagia. Major pathogens include *Candida albicans*, herpes simplex virus (HSV), and cytomegalovirus (CMV). Infectious esophagitis is seen most often in immunocompromised states (AIDS, organ transplant recipients), disorders of esophageal emptying (e.g., achalasia), malignancy, diabetes mellitus, and antibiotic use. However, HSV and varicella esophagitis can occur in the normal healthy host. The presence of typical oral lesions (thrush, herpetic vesicles) may suggest an etiologic agent. Endoscopy with biopsy and brush cytology is often diagnostic. Symptomatic relief can be achieved with 2% viscous lidocaine swish and swallow (15 ml PO q3–4h prn) or sucralfate slurry (1 g PO qid). Concomitant acid suppression should also be administered.

**A. *Candida* esophagitis.** Topical therapy is usually ineffective, and systemic therapy with triazoles is the current standard. **Fluconazole,** 100 mg/day, or **itraconazole,** 200 mg/day, for 14–21 days is recommended as initial therapy. For infections that are refractory to azoles, a short course of parenteral amphotericin B (0.3–0.5 mg/kg/day) should be considered (see Opportunistic Infections, sec. **III.D.1** and **III.D.2**, in Chap. 14, Human Immunodeficiency Virus Infection and Acquired Immunodeficiency Syndrome). When new-onset dysphagia or odynophagia occurs in the immunocompromised host, and typical oropharyngeal lesions of *Candida* infection are visualized, empiric therapy for *Candida* esophagitis can be initiated and endoscopy reserved for patients who do not respond.

B. **HSV esophagitis.** No treatment may be necessary in immunocompetent hosts, although quicker symptom resolution may result with antiviral therapy when esophageal symptoms are severe. In immunocompromised patients, HSV esophagitis can be treated with acyclovir, 400–800 mg PO five times a day for 14–21 days or 5 mg/kg IV q8h for 7–14 days. Famciclovir and valacyclovir are alternate agents.

C. **CMV esophagitis.** IV therapy with ganciclovir, foscarnet, or cidofovir is effective for a variety of GI CMV infections in immunocompromised hosts (see Opportunistic Infections, sec. **III.A.1**, in Chap. 14, Human Immunodeficiency Virus Infection and Acquired Immunodeficiency Syndrome). Ganciclovir, 5 mg/kg IV q12h, or foscarnet, 90 mg/kg IV q12h, for 3–6 weeks can be used as initial therapy. Oral valganciclovir may also be effective.

III. **Chemical esophagitis.** Ingestion of caustic agents or medications such as oral potassium, doxycycline, quinidine, iron, NSAIDs, and aspirin can result in mucosal irritation and damage. Cautious early endoscopy is recommended to evaluate the extent and degree of mucosal damage in caustic ingestion; the procedure may have to be terminated if extensive damage is encountered. A second caustic agent to neutralize the first is contraindicated.

IV. **Nonspecific ulceration.** Nonspecific ulceration can be seen with medication, malignancy, or AIDS (idiopathic ulcer). Multiple biopsies, brushings, and culture specimens should be obtained at endoscopy. Idiopathic ulcer of AIDS may respond to oral steroid or thalidomide therapy. Concomitant acid suppression should always be administered.

V. **Other esophageal disorders**

A. **Achalasia** is the most frequently recognized motor disorder of the esophagus, characterized by failure of the lower esophageal sphincter (LES) to relax completely with swallowing and aperistalsis of the esophageal body. **Presenting symptoms** can include dysphagia, regurgitation, chest pain, weight loss, and aspiration pneumonia. Barium radiographs may demonstrate a typical appearance of a dilated intrathoracic esophagus with impaired emptying, an air-fluid level, absence of gastric air bubble, and tapering of the distal esophagus with the appearance of a bird's beak. Endoscopy may help exclude a stricture or neoplasia of the distal esophagus; the esophageal body may be dilated and contain food debris, whereas the LES, although pinpoint, typically allows passage of the endoscope into the stomach with minimal resistance. Achalasia is associated with a 0.15% risk of squamous cell cancer of the distal esophagus, a 33-fold higher risk relative to the nonachalasic population.

1. **Pharmacologic therapy** consists of smooth-muscle relaxants such as nitrates or calcium channel blockers administered immediately before meals. Overall, medications are not very effective and are only indicated as temporizing measures.
2. **Botulinum toxin** injection into the LES at endoscopy can result in relief of achalasia symptoms that can last for several weeks to months. This approach may be useful in elderly and frail patients who are poor surgical risks or as a bridge to more definitive therapy. Botulinum toxin injection may induce fibrosis in the region of the LES, making subsequent surgery more cumbersome.
3. Disruption of the circular muscle of the LES using **pneumatic dilation** can result in lasting reduction of LES pressure and symptomatic relief. Gastroesophageal reflux can result, treated with lifelong acid suppression. Esophageal perforation occurs in 3–5% of cases, requiring prompt surgical repair.
4. A **surgical (Heller) myotomy** offers good efficacy and lasting symptom relief. It can be performed laparoscopically with minimal complications.

Laparoscopic myotomy is typically combined with an antireflux procedure to prevent symptoms from acid reflux.

**B. Diffuse esophageal spasm** is a spastic disorder characterized by simultaneous, nonperistaltic contractions in the esophageal body. Concomitant incomplete LES relaxation may be present. The major symptoms are dysphagia and chest pain. Diagnosis is made after esophageal manometry; barium studies may show a beaded or "corkscrew" esophagus, sometimes with pseudodiverticula. Smooth-muscle relaxants, such as nitrates and calcium channel blockers, are commonly used. Low-dose tricyclic antidepressants (TCAs) can be effective for symptom relief not only in diffuse esophageal spasm but also in other nonspecific spastic motor disorders of the esophagus. Resistant cases may require empiric esophageal dilation, botulinum toxin injection, or even surgical myotomy; these treatments are typically reserved for patients with severe symptoms.

**C. Esophageal hypomotility** is typically idiopathic but can be associated with connective tissue diseases, Barrett's esophagus, and diabetes mellitus. Scleroderma can cause fibrosis that results in aperistalsis and atony of the distal esophagus and LES; the esophagus is involved in 75–85% of cases, with dysphagia and heartburn being the predominant symptoms. No specific therapy exists for esophageal hypomotility from connective tissue diseases. Acid suppression with a PPI is recommended for acid reflux; periodic dilation may be necessary for strictures.

## Peptic Ulcer Disease

**I. General considerations.** The presence of **alarm symptoms** (weight loss, early satiety, bleeding, anemia, and lack of appropriate response to acid suppression) indicates the need for an aggressive approach to exclude neoplasia or a bleeding lesion. Endoscopy is the gold standard for diagnosis; although barium studies also have good sensitivity for peptic ulcers, they may miss lesions that are less than 5 mm. The goals of therapy in PUD include relief of symptoms and prevention of recurrence and complications.

**A. *Helicobacter pylori*,** a spiral, gram-negative urease-producing bacillus, is thought to be responsible for approximately 80% of ulcers that are not due to NSAIDs. **Serum *H. pylori* antibody** assessment is the cheapest noninvasive test for diagnosis; the antibody remains detectable as long as 18 months after successful eradication, and therefore this test cannot be used to document successful therapy of the organism. **Rapid urease assay (CLO test)** and histopathologic examination of endoscopic biopsy specimens are commonly used for diagnosis in patients undergoing endoscopy; these tests may be falsely negative in patients who are receiving PPI therapy. **Carbon-labeled urea breath testing** is the most accurate noninvasive test for diagnosis. This test is often used to document successful eradication after therapy in patients with ongoing dyspeptic symptoms or complicated ulcer disease. The current standard of care is to eradicate *H. pylori* in all patients with new-onset or recurrent peptic ulcers who test positive for this organism. Eradication requires antimicrobial therapy in addition to antisecretory medication (Table 16-2).

**B. NSAIDs and aspirin** can result in mucosal damage anywhere in the GI tract and are associated with an increased incidence of gastritis and PUD. **Risk factors** for NSAID-related peptic ulcers include past history of PUD, age older than 60 years, concomitant corticosteroid or anticoagulant therapy, high-dose or multiple NSAID therapy, and the presence of serious comorbid medical illnesses. Patients with these risk factors may benefit from *H. pylori* testing and eradication before initiation of long-term NSAID therapy, as the

**Table 16-2.** Regimens used for eradication of *Helicobacter pylori*[a]

| Regimen | Dosage | Duration (days) | Eradication rate (%) |
|---|---|---|---|
| Bismuth subsalicylate | 524 mg PO qid | 14 | >85 |
| Metronidazole | 250 mg PO qid | | |
| Tetracycline | 500 mg PO qid | | |
| Acid-suppressive agent | Standard dose | | |
| Ranitidine bismuth subcitrate (Tritec)[b] | 400 mg PO bid (14 d), then 1000 mg PO bid | 28 | 77–82 |
| Clarithromycin | 500 mg PO tid | 14 | |
| Clarithromycin[b] | 500 mg PO bid | 10–14 | 86–92 |
| Amoxicillin | 1 g PO bid | | |
| PPI | bid | | |
| Metronidazole | 500 mg PO bid | 10–14 | 87–91 |
| Clarithromycin | 500 mg PO bid | | |
| PPI | bid | | |
| Metronidazole | bid | 10–14 | 77–83 |
| Amoxicillin | bid | | |
| PPI | bid | | |
| Clarithromycin[b] | 500 mg PO tid | 14 | 70–80 |
| PPI | Standard dose | | |
| Amoxicillin[b] | 1 g PO tid | 14 | 20–70 |
| PPI | Standard dose | | |

PPI, proton pump inhibitor, standard dose (see Table 16-1).
[a]These doses are for patients with normal renal function (see Appendix E).
[b]U.S. FDA approved.

coexistence of *H. pylori* and NSAID use may amplify the risk for PUD. Continuous **PPI therapy** may ameliorate dyspeptic symptoms in patients who have strong indications for long-term NSAID therapy. PPI therapy is superior to $H_2$RAs in preventing and healing NSAID-related ulcers. **Misoprostol,** a synthetic prostaglandin E derivative (200 μg PO qid), can prevent and heal NSAID-related mucosal damage when given in full doses, but side effects (abdominal pain, diarrhea) can be limiting, especially in the elderly. **Pregnancy should be excluded in women of reproductive age before administration. Cyclooxygenase-2 (COX-2) inhibitors** cause less GI toxicity than traditional NSAIDs; patients with risk factors for PUD who require continuous NSAID therapy may benefit from the use of COX-2 inhibitors instead of traditional NSAIDs. Use of concomitant aspirin may negate the advantage of COX-2 inhibitors.

C. **Malignant ulcers.** Gastric ulcers can be malignant in fewer than 5% of cases. The likelihood of malignancy is higher in solitary ulcers, ulcers located in the greater curvature, chronic atrophic gastritis, pernicious anemia, gastric adenomatous polyps, and prior surgery for PUD. Endoscopic biopsy should be performed in all suspicious gastric ulcers. Follow-up EGD or upper GI series should be performed 8–12 weeks after initial diagnosis of all gastric ulcers to document healing; repeat endoscopic biopsy or surgical management should be considered for nonhealing ulcers. Duodenal ulcers are almost never malignant, and therefore documentation of healing is unnecessary in the absence of symptoms.

**D. Zollinger-Ellison syndrome** is caused by a gastrin-secreting, non-beta islet cell tumor of the pancreas or duodenum. Multiple endocrine neoplasia type I is associated with this syndrome in 25% of patients. The resultant hypersecretion of gastric acid can cause multiple peptic ulcers in unusual locations, ulcers that fail to respond to standard medical therapy, or recurrent ulceration after surgical therapy. Diarrhea and gastroesophageal reflux symptoms are common. Gastric acid output is typically greater than 15 mEq/L, and gastric pH is less than 1.0. A fasting **serum gastrin level** while off acid suppression for at least 5 days serves as a screening test; a value greater than 1000 pg/ml is seen in 90% of patients. When serum gastrin is elevated but less than 1000 pg/ml, a **secretin stimulation test** may demonstrate a paradoxical 200-pg increment in serum gastrin level after IV secretin in patients with gastrinomas. PPIs are generally required in higher doses than those used for PUD. Specialized nuclear medicine scans (octreotide scans) can be useful in localizing the neoplastic lesion for curative resection (*Ann Intern Med* 125:26, 1996).

## II. Treatment

**A. Acid suppression.** Regardless of etiology, acid suppression is the main aspect of therapy of PUD. Oral agents suffice in most instances; parenteral administration of $H_2$RAs or PPIs may be necessary when oral administration is not tolerated or not possible (Table 16-1). Dosage intervals should be prolonged for $H_2$RAs in the presence of renal insufficiency. Side effects are uncommon, but headache and mental status abnormalities (lethargy, confusion, depression, hallucinations) can result from $H_2$RA therapy; abdominal pain and diarrhea are common side effects of PPI therapy. Rare hepatotoxicity, thrombocytopenia, and leukopenia have been observed with $H_2$RA use. Cimetidine can impair metabolism of many drugs, including warfarin anticoagulants, theophylline, and phenytoin (see Appendix C, Drug Interactions).

**B. Other agents. Sucralfate** acts by coating the mucosal surface without blocking acid secretion and can be as effective as $H_2$RAs or high-dose antacids in healing duodenal ulcers. Side effects include constipation and reduction of bioavailability of certain drugs [e.g., cimetidine, digoxin, fluoroquinolones, phenytoin, and tetracycline (see Appendix C, Drug Interactions)] when administered concomitantly. **Antacids** are rarely used as primary therapy for PUD but can be useful as supplemental therapy for pain relief. The choice of antacid is determined by buffering capacity, formulation, and side effects. A typical dose is 30 ml of a high-potency liquid antacid, administered four to six times a day. Magnesium-containing antacids should be avoided in renal failure.

**C. *H. pylori* eradication.** Eradication of *H. pylori* promotes healing and markedly reduces recurrence of gastric and duodenal ulcers. Several antimicrobial and antisecretory agent regimens are available (Table 16-2), and eradication is recommended in all *H. pylori*–infected patients with PUD. Metronidazole resistance (predominantly in females and patients of Asian descent) and poor compliance with therapy may affect eradication rates.

**D. Nonpharmacologic measures.** Dietary modification should only include the avoidance of foods that are reproducibly associated with dyspeptic symptoms. Cigarette smoking doubles the risk of peptic ulcer development, delays healing, and promotes recurrence; therefore, cessation of cigarette smoking should be encouraged in all instances. Alcohol in high concentrations can damage the gastric mucosal barrier, but no evidence exists to link alcohol with ulcer recurrence. NSAIDs and aspirin should be avoided, if possible (see sec. **I.B**).

**E. Surgery.** Since the advent of improved medical therapies, the requirement for surgical therapy of PUD has declined dramatically. However, surgery is still occasionally required for intractable symptoms, GI bleeding, Zollinger-Ellison syndrome, and other complications of PUD. Surgical options vary depending on the location of the ulcer and the presence of associated complications. Significant morbidity can occur after surgical therapy of PUD, and adequate therapy requires a thorough understanding of the postsurgical complications.

1. **Abdominal symptoms.** Postoperative abdominal discomfort or vomiting after meals can be secondary to recurrent ulcer, afferent loop obstruction, bile reflux gastritis, gastric outlet obstruction, or stump carcinoma (a late complication). The **dumping syndrome** is caused by rapid gastric emptying of a large osmotic load into the small intestine and occurs after gastroenteric anastomosis with or without subtotal gastrectomy, vagotomy, and pyloroplasty. **Early dumping syndrome** occurs 15–30 minutes after eating and is due to osmotic fluid shifts into the gut lumen. Symptoms can be abdominal (nausea, vomiting, abdominal pain) or vasomotor (palpitations, sweating, dizziness). **Late dumping syndrome** consists of similar symptoms 2–4 hours after meals due to excessive serum insulin response to rapid delivery and absorption of sugars from the small intestine. Dietary modification to multiple small meals high in protein and low in refined carbohydrates can be beneficial; liquids with meals should be avoided. Anticholinergics, fiber supplements, and ephedrine may relieve the vasomotor symptoms. In refractory situations, SC administration of octreotide may be necessary. Mild diarrhea can be a common problem after vagotomy. Symptomatic measures are usually adequate (see Diarrhea, sec. **V**).
2. **Malabsorption.** Mild steatorrhea can occur as a result of decreased intestinal transit time and inadequate mixing of food with bile and pancreatic secretions. Bacterial overgrowth due to afferent loop stasis can also lead to steatorrhea (see Other Gastrointestinal Disorders, sec. **IV**).
3. **Anemia.** Deficiencies of folate, vitamin $B_{12}$, and iron can lead to anemia. Postoperative iron-deficiency anemia is usually a result of dietary iron malabsorption, but blood loss from gastritis or recurrent ulcers may contribute.

## III. Complications of PUD

**A. GI bleeding** (see the section Gastrointestinal Bleeding)

**B. Gastric outlet obstruction** is more likely to occur with ulcers that are close to the pyloric channel. Nausea and vomiting, sometimes several hours after meals, may occur. Plain abdominal radiographs often show a dilated stomach with an air-fluid level. NG suction should be maintained for 2–3 days to decompress the stomach, while repleting fluids and electrolytes intravenously. Although medical management may be temporarily effective, recurrence is common, and endoscopic balloon dilation or surgery is often necessary for definitive correction.

**C. Perforation** occurs in a small number of PUD patients and usually necessitates emergency surgery. Perforation may occur in the absence of previous symptoms of PUD and may be asymptomatic in patients who are receiving glucocorticoids. A plain upright radiograph of the abdomen may demonstrate free air under the diaphragm.

**D. Pancreatitis** can result from penetration into the pancreas, most commonly seen with ulcers in the posterior wall of the duodenal bulb. The pain becomes severe and continuous, radiates to the back, and is no longer relieved by antisecretory therapy. Serum amylase may be elevated. CT scanning may be diagnostic. These patients frequently require surgery (see Pancreaticobiliary Disorders).

# Inflammatory Bowel Disease

**Ulcerative colitis (UC)** is an idiopathic chronic inflammatory disease of the colon and rectum, characterized by mucosal inflammation and typically presenting with bloody diarrhea. Rectal involvement is almost universal. Patients with disease refractory to medical therapy or with complications (toxic megacolon, neoplasia) often require surgery; total proctocolectomy can be curative. In contrast to UC, **Crohn's disease** can affect any part of the tubular GI tract and is characterized by transmural inflammation of the gut wall. Common presenting symptoms include nonbloody diarrhea, abdominal pain, and weight loss. Fistulas, strictures, and abscesses can occur as complications. Bowel resection may be required for obstruction or refractory disease but does not afford a cure.

## I. Anti-inflammatory agents

**A. 5-Aminosalicylate (ASA) compounds.** Drugs that deliver 5-ASA to the bowel mucosa constitute first-line therapy in inflammatory bowel disease (IBD). The choice of agent depends on the site of disease activity.

1. **Sulfasalazine** reaches the colon intact, where it is metabolized to 5-ASA and a sulfapyridine moiety. It is therefore used for colonic disease (UC and Crohn's disease limited to the colon), either as initial therapy (0.5 g PO bid, increased as tolerated to 0.5–1.5 g PO qid) or to maintain remission (1 g PO bid–qid). **Adverse effects** are mainly caused by the sulfapyridine moiety and include headache, nausea, vomiting, and abdominal pain; a reduction in dose may be beneficial. Hypersensitivity reactions are less common and include skin rash, fever, agranulocytosis, hepatotoxicity, and aplastic anemia. Reversible reduction in sperm counts can be seen in males. Paradoxical exacerbation of colitis is a rare adverse effect. Folic acid supplementation is recommended, as sulfasalazine impairs folate absorption.
2. **Newer 5-ASA preparations** lack the sulfa moiety of sulfasalazine and are associated with fewer side effects. **Mesalamine** (5-ASA) is available in several formulations. An oral preparation released at pH greater than 7 (Asacol, 800–1600 mg PO tid) is useful in UC as well as ileocecal/colonic Crohn's disease. A second preparation, balsalazide (Colazal, 2.25 g PO tid for active disease, 1.5 g PO bid for maintenance), is cleaved by colonic bacteria to mesalamine and an inert carrier molecule and is useful for colonic inflammation. A third preparation with time- and pH-dependent release of the active ingredient throughout the GI tract (Pentasa, 0.5–1.0 g PO qid) is useful in diffuse Crohn's disease that also affects the small bowel; it can be used in UC as well. Rare hypersensitivity reactions occur and include pneumonitis, pancreatitis, hepatitis, and nephritis. Mesalamine preparations can be used for initiation and maintenance therapy. **Olsalazine** is a 5-ASA dimer that is cleaved by bacteria in the colon and can be used in UC and Crohn's colitis. Diarrhea is a major side effect and can limit its use.

**B. Glucocorticoids** are beneficial in inducing remission of active UC and Crohn's disease. They are not recommended for mild disease; they can be used concurrently with other anti-inflammatory agents in moderate to severe disease, especially with flare-ups of disease activity. Extracolonic manifestations of IBD (ocular lesions, skin disease, and peripheral arthritis) also respond to glucocorticoids. A typical starting oral dose of prednisone is 40–60 mg given once a day in the morning. Depending on response, the dose can be reduced by 10 mg every 5–10 days and tapered off in 3–6 weeks. In severe disease or in patients who cannot tolerate oral medication, IV administration (methylprednisolone, 20–40 mg qd–bid, or equivalent) may be necessary for brief periods; higher doses may be necessary in refractory disease.

Glucocorticoids are not recommended for maintenance therapy, and alternatives should be sought for the patient who appears dependent on these medications. **Glucocorticoids should not be prescribed before ruling out an infectious process and should not be initiated for the first time over the telephone.**

C. **Immunosuppressive agents** (see Chap. 15, Solid Organ Transplant Medicine, and Chap. 23, Arthritis and Rheumatologic Diseases). **6-Mercaptopurine,** a purine analog, and **azathioprine,** its S-imidazole precursor, cause preferential suppression of T-cell activation and antigen recognition. They are used orally in doses of 1.0–1.5 mg/kg body weight qd. Both agents have more favorable side effect profiles than glucocorticoids and are used as steroid-sparing agents in severe or refractory IBD. Response may be delayed for up to 1–2 months. Side effects include reversible bone marrow suppression, pancreatitis, and allergic reactions. **Methotrexate** (15–25 mg IM or PO weekly) has also been used as a steroid-sparing agent in Crohn's disease. Side effects include hepatic fibrosis, bone marrow suppression, alopecia, pneumonitis, allergic reactions, and teratogenicity. IV **cyclosporine** has been used in refractory cases of UC; however, the benefit is temporary. Side effects include nephrotoxicity, hepatotoxicity, hypertrichosis, seizures, and lymphoproliferative disorders.

D. **Antibiotics.** Metronidazole (250–500 mg PO tid) can be used as an alternate first-line agent or adjunctive therapy in mild to moderate Crohn's disease. Peripheral neuropathy is a concern with long-term use. Ciprofloxacin (500 mg PO bid) has also been used in Crohn's disease. The two agents can be used concurrently in perianal Crohn's disease for prolonged periods with good results. An alternative agent that is sometimes used is sulfamethoxazole/trimethoprim.

E. **Infliximab** (Remicade) is a monoclonal antibody against tumor necrosis factor-α that induces inflammatory cell lysis by binding to tumor necrosis factor receptors on the cell surface. Infliximab (IV infusions of 5 mg/kg) is approved for therapy of fistulous Crohn's disease as well as refractory inflammatory-type Crohn's disease that is unresponsive to conventional therapy. Induction regimens typically consist of doses at 0, 2, and 6 weeks, with maintenance doses every 8 weeks. CHF may worsen after therapy with infliximab. Sepsis and reactivation of latent tuberculosis or histoplasmosis may occur; a tuberculin test may be indicated to evaluate for latent tuberculosis before treatment. Serious infusion reactions may occur, and constant monitoring is essential during infusion.

F. **Local therapy.** UC that is limited to the rectum or distal left colon can be treated effectively with 5-ASA or glucocorticoid enemas or suppositories, or both, administered once to twice a day; concurrent systemic therapy may be required in severe cases. Symptomatic benefit may be achieved in perianal Crohn's disease with sitz baths, analgesics, hydrocortisone creams, and local heat, in addition to systemic anti-inflammatory agents and antibiotics.

II. **Supportive therapy**

A. **Antidiarrheal agents** may be useful as adjunctive therapy in selected patients with mild exacerbations or postresection diarrhea. They are contraindicated in severe exacerbations and toxic megacolon.

B. **Diet and nutrition.** For patients whose disease is in remission, no specific dietary restrictions are necessary. A low-roughage diet often provides symptomatic relief in patients with mild to moderate disease or in individuals with strictures. Elemental diets (see Chap. 2, Nutritional Support, sec. **III.B.2**) have been used in acute phases of the diseases, especially Crohn's disease, but are unpalatable and disliked by patients. Total parenteral nutrition (see Chap. 2, Nutritional Support, sec. **IV**) and bowel rest may be required in severe disease, for nutritional maintenance and symptom relief while waiting for the effects of medical treatment, or as a bridge to surgery. Patients with Crohn's ileitis or ileocolonic resection may need vitamin $B_{12}$ supplementation. Specific oral replacement of calcium, magnesium, folate, iron, vitamins A and D, and other micronutrients may be necessary in patients with small-bowel Crohn's disease (see Chap. 2, Nutritional Support). Extensive small-bowel Crohn's disease and ileal resection may also predispose to calcium oxalate nephrolithiasis; this is treated with a low-fat, low-oxalate, high-calcium diet.

C. **Surgery** in IBD is generally reserved for patients with fistulas, obstruction, abscess, perforation, or bleeding; rarely, it is performed on those with medically refractory disease and neoplastic transformation. Surgery in IBD should be performed by experienced surgeons who are well versed in the diseases.

III. **Special considerations**

A. **UC.** In patients with colitis that lasts longer than 8–10 years, annual colonoscopic surveillance for neoplasia with four quadrant mucosal biopsies every 5–10 cm is recommended. Histopathologic evidence of any grade of dysplasia is an indication for total colectomy.

B. **Crohn's disease.** The most common indications for surgery in Crohn's disease are bowel obstruction, strictures, fistulas, and inflammatory masses. Recurrence close to the resected margins is common after bowel resection. Efforts should be made to avoid multiple resections in Crohn's disease because of the risk of short-bowel syndrome. Immunosuppressive agents should be discontinued before surgery and reinstituted if necessary during the postoperative period. Metronidazole, ciprofloxacin, oral immunosuppressive agents, and infliximab are useful in the medical management of fistulous and perianal disease.

C. **Fulminant colitis and toxic megacolon.** Acute fulminant colitis presents as severe diarrhea with abdominal pain, bleeding, fever, sepsis, electrolyte disturbances, and dehydration. Toxic megacolon occurs in 1–2% of patients with UC; the colon becomes atonic and modestly dilates, but systemic toxicity is the dominant feature. Patients should be given nothing by mouth (NPO), with NG suction if there is evidence of small-bowel ileus. Dehydration and electrolyte disturbances should be treated vigorously. Anticholinergic and opioid medication should be discontinued. Intensive medical therapy with IV corticosteroids (hydrocortisone, 100 mg IV q6h or equivalent) and broad-spectrum antimicrobials should be initiated. Deterioration or lack of improvement despite 7–10 days of intensive medical management, evidence of bowel perforation, or peritoneal signs are indications for urgent total colectomy.

D. **Intestinal obstruction.** Stricture formation can result in intestinal obstruction in Crohn's disease. Presentation may resemble a flare, and a careful history, physical examination, and imaging studies are essential for diagnosis. NG tube decompression, parenteral hydration, and bowel rest may resolve minor episodes, but surgery may be necessary. Stricturoplasty is an accepted procedure for focal tight strictures; biopsies should be obtained to rule out cancer at stricture sites. Patients with intermittent obstructive symptoms should avoid highly indigestible foods such as nuts, pits, hulls, skins, seeds, and pulps that may precipitate obstruction.

## Functional Gastrointestinal Disorders

I. **General considerations.** Functional GI disorders are characterized by the presence of abdominal symptoms in the absence of a demonstrable organic disease process. Symptoms can arise from any part of the luminal gut. Irritable bowel syndrome (IBS), primarily characterized by abdominal pain linked to altered bowel habits, is the best-recognized functional bowel disease and the most commonly diagnosed GI illness. Clinical evaluation and investigation should be directed toward prudently excluding organic processes in the involved area of the gut while initiating therapeutic trials when functional symptoms are suspected.

**II. Therapy** is dependent on the nature and severity of symptoms and the degree of functional impairment.

**A. Nonspecific measures.** Patient education, reassurance, and help with diet and lifestyle modification are key to an effective physician-patient relationship. The psychosocial contribution to symptom exacerbation should be determined, as its management may be sufficient for many patients. Low-dose TCAs (e.g., amitriptyline, nortriptyline, imipramine, doxepin: 25–100 mg PO qhs) have neuromodulatory and analgesic properties that are independent of their psychotropic effects and can be beneficial, especially in pain-predominant functional GI disorders. Selective serotonin reuptake inhibitors (e.g., fluoxetine, 20 mg PO qd; paroxetine, 20 mg PO qd; sertraline, 50 mg PO qd) are less effective but have better side effect profiles.

**B. Functional esophageal symptoms** can coexist with GERD as well as disorders of affect, including anxiety and depression. Patients with functional chest pain and heartburn may have symptomatic relief from standard-dose PPI therapy with or without concomitant low-dose TCAs.

**C. Nonulcer dyspepsia.** In young individuals with short-lived symptoms and no other explanation for dyspepsia, noninvasive testing for *H. pylori* (serology or urea breath test) is recommended. If the organism is found, eradication (Table 16-2) may result in symptom improvement or resolution in up to half the patients over 1 year follow-up (*BMJ* 324:1012, 2002). When testing for the organism is negative, acid suppression and low-dose TCA therapy may be beneficial. Older patients with new-onset dyspepsia, individuals with long-standing symptoms or symptoms that are not responsive to empiric therapy, and patients with alarm symptoms (GI bleeding, anemia, weight loss, early satiety) need further workup with endoscopy and imaging studies.

**D. Functional nausea and vomiting** consist of intermittent or persistent symptoms in the absence of a structural or organic etiology. Antiemetic agents, acid suppression, and low-dose TCAs form the mainstay of therapy. Anecdotal evidence suggests that patients with cyclic vomiting syndrome (stereotypic episodes of vigorous vomiting with asymptomatic intervals between episodes) may also benefit from sumatriptan (25–50 mg PO, 5–10 mg transnasally, or 6 mg SC at the beginning of an episode), especially if it is administered during a prodrome or early in the episode.

**E. Irritable bowel syndrome (IBS).** When pain and bloating are the predominant symptoms, antispasmodic or anticholinergic medications (hyoscyamine, 0.125–0.25 mg PO/SL up to qid; dicyclomine, 10–20 mg PO qid) or low-dose TCAs (see sec. **II.A**) are recommended. **Constipation-predominant IBS** may benefit from increased dietary fiber (25 g/day) supplemented with laxatives prn. Newer 5-$HT_4$–receptor agonists such as tegaserod (Zelnorm, 6 mg bid) may be useful in women with constipation-predominant IBS, but studies in men are inconclusive. Alosetron (Lotronex, 1 mg qd–bid), a 5-$HT_3$ antagonist, is useful in women with **diarrhea-predominant IBS**; its use is restricted to women with symptoms that are refractory to other measures because of the potential for ischemic colitis in a small proportion of patients. Loperamide (2–4 mg, up to qid/prn) can reduce stool frequency, urgency, and fecal incontinence.

## Acute Intestinal Pseudo-Obstruction (Ileus)

**I. General considerations.** Acute intestinal pseudo-obstruction or ileus consists of obstructive symptoms (nausea, vomiting, abdominal distention, lack of bowel movements) and intestinal dilatation on imaging studies without a mechanical explanation. Predisposing causes include virtually any medical insult, particularly life-threatening systemic diseases, infection, vascular insufficiency, surgery, and electrolyte abnormalities. **Ogilvie's syndrome** or acute colonic pseudo-obstruction describes colonic dilation without a mechanical obstruction in the presence of a competent ileocecal valve, which may be complicated by cecal rupture when dilation is rapid or massive. A careful history and physical examination and conventional laboratory studies (blood count, complete metabolic profile) are important initial steps in assessing for a primary intra-abdominal inflammatory process or mechanical obstruction that may require surgical attention and to exclude electrolyte abnormalities. An **obstructive series** (supine and upright abdominal x-rays with a chest x-ray) determines the distribution of intestinal gas and assesses for the presence of free intraperitoneal air. Additional imaging studies, including CT scanning, contrast enema, or small-bowel series, may be required.

**II. Therapy**

**A. General measures.** Basic supportive measures consist of NPO, fluid replacement, and correction of electrolyte imbalances. Prompt antimicrobial therapy is indicated if an infectious process is suspected. Medications that slow GI motility (adrenergic agonists, TCAs, sedatives, narcotic analgesics) should be withdrawn or doses reduced. The ambulatory patient is encouraged to remain active and to undertake short walks. Temporary total parenteral nutrition may be required in protracted cases.

**B. Decompression.** Intermittent NG suction prevents swallowed air from passing distally. In protracted cases, gastric decompression, either using an NG tube or a percutaneous endoscopic gastrotomy tube, eliminates upper GI secretions and decreases vomiting and gastric distention. Rectal tubes help decompress the distal colon; more proximal colonic distention may necessitate **colonoscopic decompression,** especially when the cecal diameter approaches 9–10 cm. A flexible decompression tube can be left in the proximal colon during colonoscopy. Turning the patient from side to side may potentiate the benefit of colonoscopic decompression.

**C. Surgery.** Surgical consultation is required when the clinical picture is suggestive of mechanical obstruction or if peritoneal signs are present. Cecostomy is rarely required when colonoscopic decompression fails in acute colonic distention. Surgical exploration is reserved for acute cases with peritoneal signs, ischemic bowel changes, or other evidence for perforation.

**D. Medications. Neostigmine** (2 mg IV administered slowly over 3–5 minutes) is beneficial in selected patients with acute colonic distention (*N Engl J Med* 341:137, 1999). The drug can induce rapid re-establishment of colonic tone and is **contraindicated** if mechanical obstruction remains in the differential diagnosis. Side effects include abdominal pain, excessive salivation, symptomatic bradycardia, and syncope. A trial of neostigmine may be warranted before colonoscopic decompression in patients without contraindications. Erythromycin (200 mg IV) acts as a motilin agonist and stimulates upper gut motility; it has been used with some success in refractory postoperative ileus. Guanethidine, bethanechol, and metoclopramide have all been used, with mixed results.

## Pancreaticobiliary Disorders

**I. Acute pancreatitis.** The most common causes are alcohol and gallstone disease. Less common causes include abdominal trauma, hypercalcemia, hypertriglyceridemia, and a variety of drugs; post–endoscopic retrograde cholangiopancreatography (ERCP) pancreatitis occurs in 5–10% of patients undergoing ERCP. The morbidity and mortality associated with acute pancreatitis are higher when necrosis is present, especially if the necrotic area is also infected; therefore, dual-

**Table 16-3.** Ranson criteria for severity assessment in acute pancreatitis[a]

| | Alcoholic pancreatitis | Nonalcoholic pancreatitis |
|---|---|---|
| **On admission** | | |
| Age | >55 yr | >70 yr |
| WBC count | >16,000/μl | >18,000/μl |
| Blood glucose | >200 mg/dl | >220 mg/dl |
| LDH | >350 IU/L | >400 IU/L |
| AST | >250 U/L | >440 U/L |
| **During the first 48 hr of admission** | | |
| Fall in hematocrit | >10% | >10% |
| Serum calcium | <8 mg/dl | <8 mg/dl |
| Base deficit | >4.0 mEq/L | >5.0 mEq/L |
| Increase in blood urea | >5 mg/dl | >2 mg/dl |
| Fluid sequestration | >6 L | >6 L |
| Arterial $PO_2$ | <60 mm Hg | <60 mm Hg |

LDH, lactic dehydrogenase; $PO_2$, oxygen tension.
[a]The presence of three or more criteria indicates severe pancreatitis.

phase CT scanning is useful in the initial evaluation of severe acute pancreatitis. The Ranson criteria (Table 16-3) provide helpful prognostic information.

**A. Therapy** is largely supportive. Specific therapy is reserved for complications.

1. Aggressive **volume repletion** with IV fluids must be undertaken, with careful monitoring of fluid balance and awareness of the potential for significant fluid sequestration within the abdomen. Serum electrolytes, calcium, and glucose levels should be monitored and supplemented as necessary. Urine output, hemodynamics, and laboratory parameters help assess adequacy of volume repletion.
2. **Narcotic analgesics** are usually necessary for pain relief. Meperidine is the most commonly used agent. Although morphine is frequently avoided, there is no conclusive evidence that morphine has deleterious effects on sphincter of Oddi pressure. Patient-controlled analgesia is frequently necessary for adequate relief of pain.
3. Patients should be **NPO** until they are free of pain and nausea. NG suction is reserved for patients with ileus or protracted emesis. Total parenteral nutrition may be necessary when inflammation is slow to resolve. Enteral nutrition through a tube placed distal to the ligament of Treitz is usually tolerated and may be safer than total parenteral nutrition.
4. Urgent **ERCP and biliary sphincterotomy** within 72 hours of presentation can improve the outcome of severe gallstone pancreatitis. This is thought to result from reduced biliary sepsis rather than true improvement of pancreatic inflammation.
5. **Acid suppression** may be necessary in severely ill patients with risk factors for stress ulcer bleeding (see Gastrointestinal Bleeding, sec. **V.D**).

**B. Complications**

1. **Necrotizing pancreatitis** represents a severe form of acute pancreatitis, usually identified on dynamic dual-phase CT scanning with IV contrast. The presence of radiologically identified pancreatic necrosis increases the morbidity and mortality of acute pancreatitis. Increasing abdominal pain, fever, marked leukocytosis, and bacteremia suggest infected pancreatic necrosis that requires broad-spectrum antibiotics and often sur-

gical débridement. CT-guided percutaneous aspiration for Gram stain and culture can confirm the diagnosis of infected necrosis.

2. The presence of **pseudocysts** is suggested by persistent pain or hyperamylasemia. Complications include infection, hemorrhage, rupture (pancreatic ascites), and obstruction of adjacent structures. Generally, asymptomatic nonenlarging pseudocysts can be followed clinically with serial imaging studies. Decompression of symptomatic, rapidly enlarging, or complicated pseudocysts can be performed by percutaneous, endoscopic, or surgical techniques.
3. **Infection.** Potential sources of fever include pancreatic necrosis, abscess, infected pseudocyst, cholangitis, and aspiration pneumonia. Cultures should be obtained, and broad-spectrum antimicrobials that are appropriate for bowel flora should be administered (see Chap. 13, Treatment of Infectious Diseases). In the absence of fever or other clinical evidence for infection, prophylactic antimicrobial therapy has no clear role in acute pancreatitis.
4. **Pulmonary complications.** Atelectasis, pleural effusion, pneumonia, and acute respiratory distress syndrome (ARDS) can develop in severely ill patients (see Chap. 8, Critical Care).
5. **Renal failure.** Severe intravascular volume depletion or acute tubular necrosis can cause renal failure (see Chap. 11, Renal Diseases).
6. **Other complications.** Metabolic complications include hypocalcemia, hypomagnesemia, and hyperglycemia. GI bleeding can result from stress gastritis, pseudoaneurysm rupture, or gastric varices from splenic vein thrombosis.

## II. Gallstone disease

**A. Asymptomatic cholelithiasis** is a common incidental finding for which no specific therapy is generally necessary. **Symptomatic cholelithiasis** may present as biliary colic, a constant pain lasting for hours, located in the right upper quadrant, radiating to the back or right shoulder, and sometimes associated with nausea or vomiting. Other complications of gallstones include acute cholecystitis, acute pancreatitis, cholangitis, and gallbladder cancer.

1. **Cholecystectomy** is the therapy of choice for symptomatic gallstone disease. Laparoscopic cholecystectomy compares favorably with the open procedure, with lower morbidity, shorter hospital stay, and better cosmetic results.
2. **Medical therapy** with ursodeoxycholic acid (8–10 mg/kg/day PO in 2–3 divided doses for prolonged periods) might be prudent in a small select group of patients with small cholesterol stones in normally functioning gallbladders who are at high risk of complications from surgical therapy. Side effects include diarrhea and reversible elevation in serum transaminase levels.
3. **Other nonsurgical therapies** include percutaneous instillation of contact solvents such as methyl-tertiary-butyl ether into the gallbladder and extracorporeal shock-wave lithotripsy combined with oral bile acid dissolution therapy. Experience with these therapies is limited, and neither is definitive as the gallbladder remains in place.

**B. Acute cholecystitis** is caused most often by obstruction of the cystic duct by gallstones, but acalculous cholecystitis can occur in severely ill, hospitalized patients. Ultrasound scans have a high degree of accuracy in diagnosis; a hydroxy iminodiacetic acid (HIDA) scan can demonstrate nonfilling of the gallbladder in difficult cases. Cholecystectomy is the mainstay of treatment. Supportive measures include IV fluid resuscitation and broad-spectrum antimicrobial agents, especially in the event of complications such as sepsis, perforation, peritonitis, abscess, or empyema formation. Percutaneous cholecystotomy and decompression of the gallbladder can be performed under fluoroscopy in severely ill patients who are not surgical candidates.

C. **Choledocholithiasis.** In patients who have undergone cholecystectomy, retained common bile duct stones can complicate the postoperative course. Common bile duct obstruction, jaundice, biliary colic, cholangitis, or pancreatitis can result. The diagnosis can be made on ultrasonography, CT scanning, or MR cholangiography. ERCP with sphincterotomy and stone extraction is curative.

D. Patients with **acute ascending cholangitis** present with right upper quadrant pain, fever with chills, and jaundice (Charcot's triad), usually in the setting of biliary obstruction (choledocholithiasis, neoplasia, sclerosing cholangitis, biliary stent occlusion). Elderly patients may lack abdominal symptoms. Cholangitis represents a medical emergency with high morbidity and mortality if biliary decompression is not performed urgently. The patient's condition should be stabilized with IV fluids and broad-spectrum antibiotics (see Chap. 13, Treatment of Infectious Diseases). Drainage of the biliary tree can be performed through the endoscopic (ERCP with sphincterotomy) or percutaneous approach under fluoroscopic guidance.

III. **Chronic pancreatitis** is commonly seen with chronic alcohol abuse. A plain abdominal radiograph may demonstrate a calcified pancreas.

A. **Pain management** is critical in chronic pancreatitis. Alcohol cessation may improve pain in alcoholics. Narcotic analgesics are frequently required, and narcotic dependence is common. In patients with mild to moderate exocrine insufficiency, the addition of oral pancreatic enzyme supplements may be beneficial for pain control. Patients with pancreatic duct obstruction from stones, strictures, or papillary stenosis may benefit from ERCP and sphincterotomy. Intractable pain may necessitate celiac ganglion block or even surgery.

B. **Exocrine insufficiency** typically manifests as **weight loss** and **steatorrhea.** In the presence of steatorrhea, a serum trypsinogen level of less than 10 ng/ml is diagnostic of chronic pancreatitis. Most patients can be managed with a low-fat diet (<50 g/day) and pancreatic enzyme supplements. Non–enteric-coated pancrelipase preparations (Viokase or Cotazym, 2–4 tablets with each meal) are administered with acid suppression to prevent degradation by gastric acid. Enteric-coated preparations (Pancrease or Creon, 1–2 capsules with meals) are stable at acid pH and should not be given with concomitant acid suppression. Fat-soluble vitamin supplementation may be necessary (see Table 2-3).

C. **Endocrine insufficiency** may result from destruction of islet cells. The resultant diabetes mellitus is characteristically brittle, as glucagon-producing islet cells are also destroyed. Insulin therapy is generally required (see Chap. 21, Diabetes Mellitus and Related Disorders).

IV. **Sphincter of Oddi dysfunction.** Patients with biliary-type pain in association with at least two of the following benefit from sphincterotomy: (1) a dilated common bile duct, (2) slow drainage (>45 minutes) of contrast from the biliary tree during ERCP, and (3) abnormal liver function tests on two separate occasions. If only one of the three features is present in addition to biliary-type pain, sphincter of Oddi **manometry** is indicated, with sphincterotomy only if basal sphincter pressures are greater than 40 mm Hg. Medical therapy with anticholinergic agents, calcium channel blockers, or low-dose TCAs is recommended for patients with only biliary-type pain without objective evidence of biliary pathology. Pancreatic duct correlates of sphincter of Oddi dysfunction have also been identified.

## Other Gastrointestinal Disorders

I. **Gastroparesis** can result from chronic disorders (diabetes mellitus, scleroderma, intestinal pseudo-obstruction, previous gastric surgery) or, less frequently, from acute metabolic derangements (hypokalemia, hypercalcemia, hypocalcemia, hyperglycemia) or medications (narcotic analgesics, anticholinergic agents, chemotherapeutic agents). Mechanical obstruction should always be excluded. Symptoms include nausea, bloating, and vomiting, often hours after a meal. A gastric-emptying study consisting of gamma camera scanning after a radiolabeled meal can confirm the diagnosis. Patients should avoid high-fat, high-fiber meals; high-calorie liquid iso-osmotic meals may be beneficial in refractory situations. Underlying metabolic derangements should be corrected. **Prokinetic agents** have been used with varying degrees of success. Metoclopramide (10 mg PO qid half an hour before meals) has variable efficacy, and side effects (drowsiness, tardive dyskinesia, parkinsonism) may be limiting. Erythromycin (250 mg PO tid or 200 mg IV) also stimulates gastric motility. Tegaserod, a 5-$HT_4$ agonist with prokinetic properties, is being studied for use in gastroparesis. Intermittent nausea and vomiting in patients with gastroparesis may also respond to treatment for functional nausea and vomiting (see Functional Gastrointestinal Disorders, sec. **II.D**).

**II.** Patients with **celiac sprue** are sensitive to gluten, a group of proteins that are present in wheat, barley, and rye. The resulting inflammation in the small-bowel mucosa causes malabsorption of dietary nutrients. Noninvasive tests include antiendomysial and antitissue transglutaminase antibodies, but endoscopic biopsy revealing severe blunting or complete absence of villi is the gold standard for diagnosis. Secondary lactase deficiency may coexist. Prompt improvement in symptoms results from a **gluten-free diet.** Patients may require iron, folate, calcium, and vitamin supplements. Corticosteroids (prednisone, 10–20 mg/day) may be required in refractory cases, although the most common cause of refractory disease is dietary indiscretion. If symptoms persist despite a strict gluten-free diet, radiologic and endoscopic evaluation of the small bowel should be performed to rule out **small-bowel lymphoma.**

**III.** **Lactose intolerance** results from selective deficiency of lactase in the intestinal brush border. Undigested lactose in the intestinal lumen results in osmotic diarrhea, abdominal cramps, and flatulence. Symptoms are associated with ingestion of dairy products. Temporary lactase deficiency may result from bacterial or viral enteritis. Avoidance of dairy products is usually sufficient for diagnosis and treatment. Lactose tolerance and hydrogen breath tests can be used for diagnosis in difficult cases. Lactase supplements (2–4 tablets or capsules with each lactose meal) can be used for treatment.

**IV.** **Bacterial overgrowth** of the small intestine can result from any condition that causes intestinal stasis (small-bowel diverticulosis, afferent loop obstruction, scleroderma, intestinal pseudo-obstruction, strictures, adhesions). Hypochlorhydria and immunodeficiency are other predisposing conditions. Deconjugation of bile salts by the bacteria causes **fat malabsorption.** The bacteria also may compete for dietary vitamin $B_{12}$, causing anemia. Diagnosis is suspected by history and radiography and can be confirmed using breath tests and culture of small-bowel aspirate obtained at endoscopy. Broad-spectrum antimicrobials (tetracycline, 250 mg PO qid; amoxicillin/clavulanate, 250–500 mg PO tid; ciprofloxacin, 250 mg PO bid) can be used in 2-week courses intermittently. Vitamin supplementation may be necessary (see Tables 2-3 and 2-4). Surgical correction of the predisposing disorder may be indicated.

**V.** **Diverticulosis** is asymptomatic and does not require any specific treatment other than increased dietary fiber. **Diverticular bleeding** can be profuse and may require invasive measures, including angiography, intra-arterial vasopressin infusion, or surgery for control (see Gastrointestinal Bleeding, sec. **V.F**). **Diverticulitis** results from microperforation of a diverticulum and resultant extracolonic or intramural inflammation. Typical presenting symptoms include left lower quadrant abdominal pain, fevers and chills, and alteration of bowel habits, usually associated with an elevated WBC count. Imaging studies [CT scanning, sodium diatrizoate (Hypaque) enema] are useful in confirming the diagnosis; colonoscopy is contraindicated for 4–6 weeks after acute diverticulitis. Mild cases can be managed in the outpatient setting with a low-residue diet and oral antibiotics (e.g., ciprofloxacin, 500 mg PO bid, and metronidazole, 500 mg PO tid for 10–14 days). Hospital admission, bowel rest, IV fluids, and broad-spectrum IV antimicrobial agents are typically required in moderate to severe cases. Surgical consultation should be obtained early, as operative intervention may be necessary should complications arise.

VI. **Acute mesenteric ischemia** results from arterial (or, rarely, venous) compromise to the superior mesenteric circulation. Emboli are the most common cause, although **nonocclusive mesenteric ischemia** from vasoconstriction can also give rise to the disorder. Patients present during the ischemic episode with abdominal pain, but physical examination and imaging studies may be unremarkable until infarction has occurred. As a result, diagnosis is late and mortality is high. Angiography should be urgently performed if the diagnosis is suspected. Treatment is essentially surgical. **Ischemic colitis** is more common, resulting from mucosal ischemia in the inferior mesenteric circulation during a low flow state (hypotension, arrhythmias, sepsis, aortic vascular surgery) in patients with atherosclerotic disease. Vasculitis, sickle cell disease, vasospasm, and marathon running can also predispose to ischemic colitis. Ischemic colitis may manifest as transient bleeding or diarrhea; severe insults can lead to stricture formation, gangrene, and perforation. Symptoms may follow a hypotensive event. Characteristic "thumbprinting" may be seen on plain x-rays of the abdomen. Colonoscopy may reveal mucosal erythema, edema, and ulceration, sometimes in a linear configuration; evidence of gangrene or necrosis is an indication for surgical intervention. In the absence of peritoneal signs or evidence of gangrene or perforation, expectant management with fluid and electrolyte repletion, broad-spectrum antimicrobials, and maintenance of an adequate BP usually suffices.

VII. **Anorectal disorders**

A. **Thrombosed external hemorrhoids** present as acutely painful, tense, bluish lumps covered with skin in the anal area. The thrombosed hemorrhoid can be surgically excised under local anesthesia for relief of severe pain. In less severe cases, oral analgesics, sitz baths (sitting in a tub of warm water), stool softeners, and topical ointments (see sec. **VII.B**) may provide symptomatic relief.

B. **Internal hemorrhoids** commonly present with either bleeding or a prolapsing mass with straining. Bulk-forming agents such as fiber supplements are useful in preventing straining at defecation. Sitz baths and Tucks pads (cotton soaked in witch hazel) may provide symptomatic relief. Ointments and suppositories that contain topical analgesics, emollients, astringents, and hydrocortisone [e.g., Anusol-HC Suppositories, 1 per rectum (PR) bid for 7–10 days] can also be used to decrease edema. Hemorrhoidectomy or band ligation can be curative and is indicated in patients with recurrent or constant bleeding.

C. **Anal fissures** present with acute onset of pain during defecation and are often caused by passage of hard stool. Anoscopy reveals an elliptical tear in the skin of the anus, usually in the posterior midline. Acute fissures generally heal in 2–3 weeks with the use of stool softeners, oral or topical analgesics, and sitz baths. Topical nitroglycerin ointment, 0.2%, applied three times a day may be beneficial (*Dis Colon Rectum* 42:1000, 1999). Chronic fissures often require surgical therapy.

D. **Perirectal abscess** commonly presents as a painful induration in the perianal area. Patients with IBD and immunocompromised states are particularly susceptible. Prompt drainage is essential to avoid the serious morbidity associated with delayed treatment. Antimicrobials directed against bowel flora (metronidazole, 500 mg PO tid, and ciprofloxacin, 500 mg PO bid) should be administered in patients with significant inflammation, systemic toxicity, or immunocompromised states.

## Dysphagia and Odynophagia

**Oropharyngeal dysphagia** (difficulty in transferring food from the mouth to the esophagus, often associated with symptoms of nasopharyngeal regurgitation and pulmonary aspiration) needs to be distinguished from **esophageal dysphagia,** characterized by the sensation of difficulty in passage of food down the esophagus. Dysphagia usually necessitates a search for an esophageal obstructive process or a motility disorder (e.g., achalasia, diffuse esophageal spasm). Progressive symptoms are typically seen with neoplasia or a motility disorder; webs and rings result in intermittent symptoms. Acute onset of dysphagia, usually in temporal relationship to a meal, suggests food impaction. **Odynophagia** refers to painful swallowing and indicates the presence of esophagitis, particularly infectious esophagitis and pill esophagitis.

I. **General considerations. Oropharyngeal dysphagia** is typically caused by neuromuscular or structural disorders involving the oropharynx and proximal esophagus. Assessment is initiated with barium videofluoroscopy (usually a modified barium swallow) and may include detailed ear, nose, and throat examination; CT scanning; and laboratory tests (for polymyositis, myasthenia gravis, and other neuromuscular disorders). **Esophageal dysphagia** of insidious onset is characteristically investigated with upper endoscopy; however, subtle rings and webs may not be visualized unless a barium swallow is performed using a solid bolus. Barium swallow is also a suitable initial test for esophageal dysphagia, although biopsies and esophageal dilation require endoscopy. Esophageal manometry can characterize esophageal motor disorders when other studies are normal or suggest a motility disorder. **Acute esophageal obstruction** is best investigated with endoscopy. Nutrition needs to be addressed in patients with prolonged dysphagia that causes weight loss; patients with dysphagia are typically advised to chew their food well and eat foods of soft consistencies.

II. **Therapy**

A. **Dysphagia.** Modification of diet and swallowing maneuvers may benefit patients with oropharyngeal dysphagia. Enteral feeding through a gastrostomy tube may be indicated in patients with frank tracheal aspiration on attempted swallowing. Patients with drooling of saliva can be treated with anticholinergic medication (e.g., transdermal scopolamine). Inflammatory myopathies and myasthenia may respond to medical therapy, whereas benign or early-stage tumors and Zenker's diverticulum can be treated surgically. Benign structural lesions including webs and rings can be dilated using rigid dilators. Recurrence of dysphagia can occur but usually responds to repeat dilation. Esophageal stent placement can alleviate dysphagia in inoperable neoplasia. Endoscopic retrieval of an obstructing food bolus can result in dramatic resolution of acute dysphagia from food impaction. Glucagon (2- to 4-mg IV bolus) can be attempted but is frequently unsuccessful; sublingual nitroglycerin can also be given, but meat tenderizer should not be administered. Subsequent esophageal dilation or manometry, or both, should be scheduled and acid suppression prescribed. (See the section Esophageal Disorders for management of esophageal motility disorders and esophagitis.)

B. **Odynophagia** generally responds to specific therapy of the lesion that is causing the esophagitis (see the section Esophageal Disorders). Concomitant acid suppression and viscous lidocaine swish-and-swallow solutions may afford additional symptomatic relief.

## Nausea and Vomiting

Nausea and vomiting may result from systemic illnesses, CNS disorders, and primary GI disorders, and as side effects of medications. Vomiting that occurs during or immediately after a meal can result from a pyloric channel ulcer or from functional disorders. Vomiting within 30–60 minutes after a meal suggests gastric or duodenal pathology, whereas delayed vomiting after a meal with undigested food from a previous meal can suggest gastric outlet obstruction or gastroparesis. **Bowel obstruction and pregnancy should be ruled out.** The patient's medication list should be scrutinized.

I. **Nonspecific measures.** Oral intake should be withheld or limited to clear liquids. Many patients with self-limited illnesses require no further therapy. NG decompression may be required for patients with bowel obstruction or protracted nausea and vomiting of any etiology. Correction of fluid and electrolyte imbalances is an important supportive measure. Patients with protracted nausea and vomiting may sometimes require enteral feeding through jejunal tubes, or rarely even total parenteral nutrition.

II. **Pharmacotherapy.** Empiric pharmacotherapy is often initiated while investigation is in progress or when the etiology is thought to be self-limited.

   A. **Phenothiazines and related agents.** Prochlorperazine (Compazine), 5–10 mg PO tid–qid, 10 mg IM or IV q6h, or 25 mg PR bid; promethazine (Phenergan), 12.5–25.0 mg PO, IM, or PR q4–6h; and trimethobenzamide (Tigan), 250 mg PO tid–qid, 200 mg IM tid–qid, or 200 mg PR tid–qid are effective. Drowsiness is a common side effect, and acute dystonic reactions or other extrapyramidal effects may occur.

   B. **Dopamine antagonists** include metoclopramide (10 mg PO 30 minutes before meals and at bedtime), a prokinetic agent that also has central antiemetic effects. IV metoclopramide can be used in nausea and vomiting associated with chemotherapy (see Chap. 20, Medical Management of Malignant Disease). Metoclopramide can also be tried in chronic cases in which dysmotility of the upper GI tract is thought to play a significant role in symptoms. Drowsiness and extrapyramidal reactions may occur. Domperidone is an alternate agent that does not readily cross the blood–brain barrier and therefore has no CNS side effects; however, it is not uniformly available.

   C. **Antihistaminic agents** are most helpful for nausea and vomiting related to motion sickness but may also be useful for other causes. Agents used include diphenhydramine (Benadryl, 25–50 mg PO q6–8h or 10–50 mg IV q2–4h), dimenhydrinate (Dramamine, 50–100 mg PO or IV q4–6h), and meclizine (Antivert, 12.5–25.0 mg 1 hour before travel).

   D. **Serotonin 5-HT$_3$–receptor antagonists. Ondansetron** (Zofran, 0.15 mg/kg IV q4h for 3 doses, or 32 mg IV infused over 15 minutes beginning 30 minutes before chemotherapy) is effective in chemotherapy-associated emesis. It can also be used in emesis that is refractory to other medications (4–8 mg PO or IV up to q8h). Constipation may occur (see Chap. 20, Medical Management of Malignant Disease). **Granisetron** (Kytril, 10 μg/kg IV for 1–3 doses 10 minutes apart, or 1 mg PO bid) is an alternate agent.

## Diarrhea

I. **General considerations.** Empiric therapy of diarrhea is used as a temporizing measure while diagnostic testing is being conducted, when specific therapy of the etiology fails to provide symptomatic benefit, and when diagnostic testing fails to identify a cause.

**II. Acute diarrhea.** Infectious agents, toxins, and drugs are the major causes of acute diarrhea. IBD may also present with acute diarrhea. In hospitalized patients, pseudomembranous colitis, antibiotic- or drug-associated diarrhea, and fecal impaction should be considered. Stool cultures, *Clostridium difficile* toxin assay, fecal leukocytes, stool ova and parasite examination, and flexible sigmoidoscopy may be warranted in patients with severe, prolonged, or atypical symptoms. Patients in whom diarrhea develops after bone marrow transplantation should be investigated for graft-versus-host disease (see Hematopoietic Stem Cell Transplantation, sec. **III.B,** in Chap. 20, Medical Management of Malignant Disease).

**A. Bacterial and viral infections.** Viral enteritis and bacterial infections with *Escherichia coli*, *Shigella*, *Salmonella*, *Campylobacter*, and *Yersinia* species constitute the most common causes of acute diarrhea. Most cases are self-limiting and do not require antimicrobial therapy. Empiric antibiotic therapy is only recommended in patients with moderate to severe disease and associated systemic symptoms, while awaiting stool cultures. Fluoroquinolones (ciprofloxacin, 500 mg PO bid for 3 days, or norfloxacin, 400 mg PO bid for 3 days) and trimethoprim/sulfamethoxazole (160 mg/800 mg PO bid for 5 days) can be used. **Pseudomembranous colitis** is usually seen in the setting of antimicrobial therapy and is caused by toxins produced by *C. difficile.* Oral metronidazole is the treatment of choice; oral vancomycin is reserved for resistant cases or intolerance to metronidazole (see Toxin-Mediated Infections, sec. **I.C,** in Chap. 13, Treatment of Infectious Diseases, for further details).

**B. Parasitic infections. Amebiasis** may cause acute diarrhea, especially in travelers to areas with poor sanitation and in homosexual men. Demonstration of trophozoites or cysts of *Entamoeba histolytica* in the stool, or a serum antibody test, confirms the diagnosis. Treatment of symptomatic disease is with metronidazole, 750 mg PO tid or 500 mg IV q8h for 5–10 days. This should be followed by paromomycin, 500 mg PO tid for 7 days, or iodoquinol, 650 mg PO tid for 20 days, to eliminate cysts. **Giardiasis** is confirmed by identification of *Giardia lamblia* trophozoites in the stool, in duodenal aspirate, or in small-bowel biopsy specimens. A stool immunofluorescence assay is also available for rapid diagnosis. Therapy consists of metronidazole, 250 mg PO tid for 5–7 days, or tinidazole, 2-g single dose. Quinacrine, 100 mg PO tid for 7 days, is an alternative agent. More prolonged therapy may be necessary in the immunocompromised patient.

**C. Diarrhea related to medication use.** Common offending agents include laxatives, antacids, cardiac medications (e.g., digitalis, quinidine), colchicine, and antimicrobial agents. Symptoms usually respond to discontinuation of the offending agent.

**III. Chronic diarrhea** is defined as the passage of loose stools with or without increased stool frequency for more than 4 weeks. A careful history and thorough physical examination can complement routine laboratory tests. Stool should be tested for ova and parasites in the appropriate clinical setting. Further investigation is performed to classify diarrhea into one of the following categories: watery diarrhea (secretory or osmotic), inflammatory diarrhea, or fatty diarrhea (steatorrhea). The **fecal osmotic gap** is calculated as $290 - 2([Na^+] + [K^+])$ in watery stools. Secretory processes typically have stool osmotic gaps of less than 50 mOsm/kg, whereas osmotic diarrheas have gaps of greater than 125 mOsm/kg. A positive fecal occult blood test or fecal leukocyte test suggests inflammatory diarrhea. Steatorrhea is traditionally diagnosed by demonstration of fat excretion in stool of greater than 7 g/day in a 72-hour stool collection while the patient is on a 100 g/day fat diet. Sudan staining of a stool specimen is an alternate test; greater than 100 fat globules per high-power field is suggestive of steatorrhea. Laxative screening should be considered in any patient with chronic diarrhea that remains undiagnosed.

**IV. Diarrhea in HIV disease.** Opportunistic agents, including *Cryptosporidium*, *Microsporidium*, CMV, *Mycobacterium avium* complex, and *Mycobacterium tuberculosis*, may cause diarrhea in patients with advanced HIV and should be looked for specifically (see Opportunistic Infections in Chap. 14, Human Immunodeficiency Virus Infection and Acquired Immunodeficiency Syndrome). Venereal infections (syphilis, gonorrhea, chlamydiosis, HSV infection), as well as other nonvenereal infections (amebiasis, giardiasis, salmonellosis, shigellosis), may also cause diarrhea. Other causes of diarrhea in this population include intestinal lymphoma and Kaposi's sarcoma. Stool studies (ova and parasites, culture), endoscopic biopsies, and serologic testing may assist diagnosis. The most likely cause of undiagnosed diarrhea is missed pathogens; however, drugs, antibiotics, HIV acting as a pathogen, autonomic disturbance, and abnormal intestinal motility may also contribute to diarrhea. Management consists of specific therapy if pathogens are identified; symptomatic measures may be of benefit in idiopathic cases.

**V. Symptomatic therapy.** Adequate hydration is an essential part of the therapy of diarrheal disease (see Chap. 3, Fluid and Electrolyte Management). IV hydration is required in severe cases. Long-term IV fluids or parenteral nutrition are sometimes necessary in refractory diarrhea. Symptomatic therapy is recommended in simple self-limiting GI infections in which diarrhea is frequent or troublesome, while diagnostic workup is in progress, when specific management fails to improve symptoms, or when a specific etiology is not identified. Opiates (loperamide, 2–4 mg up to four times a day; tincture of opium; belladonna; and opium capsules) and anticholinergic agents [diphenoxylate and atropine (Lomotil), 15–20 mg/day diphenoxylate in divided doses] are the most effective nonspecific antidiarrheal agents. Pectin and kaolin preparations (bind toxins) and bismuth subsalicylate (antibacterial properties) are also useful in symptomatic therapy of acute diarrhea. Bile acid–binding resins (e.g., cholestyramine, 1 g up to qid) are beneficial in bile acid–induced diarrhea. Octreotide (100–200 $\mu$g bid–qid prn) is useful in hormone-mediated secretory diarrhea but can be of benefit in refractory diarrhea.

## Constipation

**I. General considerations.** The acuity of onset of constipation is critical in the initial assessment. A recent change in bowel habits may indicate an organic cause, whereas constipation of several years' duration is more likely due to a functional disorder. Medication (e.g., calcium blockers, opiates, anticholinergics, iron supplements, barium sulfate) and systemic disease (e.g., diabetes mellitus, hypothyroidism, systemic sclerosis, myotonic dystrophy) may contribute. Other predisposing factors include lack of exercise, disorders that cause pain on defecation (e.g., anal fissures, thrombosed external hemorrhoids), and prolonged immobilization. Colonoscopy and barium studies help rule out structural disease, particularly in older individuals. Colonic transit studies, anorectal manometry, and defecography are reserved for resistant cases without an organic explanation.

**II. Therapy.** Treatment of underlying disease and correction of predisposing conditions are important initial steps. Regular exercise and adequate fluid intake are other nonspecific measures that may be of benefit.

**A. Fiber supplementation.** An increase in dietary fiber intake to 20–30 g/day may be beneficial in many adults with constipation. Fecal impactions should be resolved before fiber supplementation is initiated. A fiber supplement such as wheat bran or psyllium with water two to four times a day can be initiated; fluid intake should be increased with these preparations. Transient bloating often occurs.

**B. Laxatives**

1. **Emollient laxatives** consist of docusate salts and mineral oil. Docusate sodium, 50–200 mg PO qd, and docusate calcium, 240 mg PO qd, allow water and fat to penetrate the fecal mass. Mineral oil (15–45 ml PO q6–8h) can be given orally or by enema. Tracheobronchial aspiration of mineral oil can result in lipoid pneumonia.
2. **Stimulant cathartics** such as castor oil, 15 ml PO, stimulate intestinal secretion and increase intestinal motility. Anthraquinones (cascara, 5 ml PO qd; senna, 1 tablet PO qd–qid) stimulate the colon by increasing fluid and water accumulation in the proximal colon. Chronic use can result in benign staining of the colonic mucosa (melanosis coli) and colonic atony from smooth-muscle atrophy and damage to the myenteric plexus. Bisacodyl (10–15 mg PO qhs, 10-mg rectal suppositories) is structurally similar to phenolphthalein and stimulates colonic peristalsis.
3. **Osmotic cathartics** include nonabsorbable salts or carbohydrates that cause water retention in the lumen of the colon. Magnesium salts include milk of magnesia (15–30 ml q8–12h) and magnesium citrate (200 ml PO); they should be avoided in renal failure. Lactulose (15–30 ml PO bid–qid) can cause bloating as a side effect.

**C. Enemas.** Sodium biphosphate (Fleet) enemas (1–2 rectally prn) can be used for mild to moderate constipation and for bowel cleansing before sigmoidoscopy. However, these should be avoided in patients with renal failure because of the risk of developing hyperphosphatemia and subsequent hypocalcemia. Tap water enemas (1 L) are also useful for bowel cleansing. Oil-based enemas (cottonseed Colace, Hypaque) are reserved for refractory constipation.

**D. Bowel-cleansing agents.** Patients should be placed on a clear liquid diet the previous day and kept NPO for 6–8 hours or overnight before the bowel examination (colonoscopy or barium enema). An iso-osmotic **polyethylene glycol solution** (GoLYTELY or NuLYTELY, 1 gal, administered at a rate of 8 oz every 10 minutes) is commonly used as a bowel-cleansing agent before colonoscopy. This agent has a mildly salty taste and can be more palatable if chilled; it can also be administered through an NG tube, if necessary. Flavored preparations are available as well. **Nonabsorbable phosphate** (Fleet Phospho-Soda, 20–45 ml with 10–24 oz liquid, taken the day before and morning of the procedure) produces bowel movements in 0.5–6.0 hours. The dose can be taken with 4 oz liquid and followed with at least 8 oz more of liquid, or 15 ml each can be mixed with three 8-oz glasses of liquid and taken within 30 minutes. Phospho-Soda can result in severe dehydration, hyperphosphatemia, hypocalcemia, hypokalemia, hypernatremia, and acidosis. It should be avoided in the elderly and in patients with electrolyte imbalances, CHF, and ascites; it is contraindicated in renal failure and hepatic dysfunction. **Two-day bowel preparation** is sometimes indicated in elderly or debilitated individuals when the above agents are contraindicated. This consists of magnesium citrate (120–300 ml PO) administered on 2 consecutive days while the patient remains on a clear liquid diet; bisacodyl (30 mg PO or 10-mg suppository) can also be administered on both days. Oral bowel-cleansing agents should be avoided in patients with suspected bowel obstruction, ileus, bowel perforation, toxic colitis, or toxic megacolon. **Tap water enemas** (1 L volume, repeated one to two times) can cleanse the distal colon when colonoscopy is indicated in patients with proximal bowel obstruction.

**E. Other agents.** Polyethylene glycol in powder form (MiraLax, 17 g PO qd–bid) can be used regularly or intermittently for the treatment of constipation. Serotonin 5-$HT_4$–receptor agonists (tegaserod, 6 mg bid) may be of benefit for some women with constipation-predominant IBS.

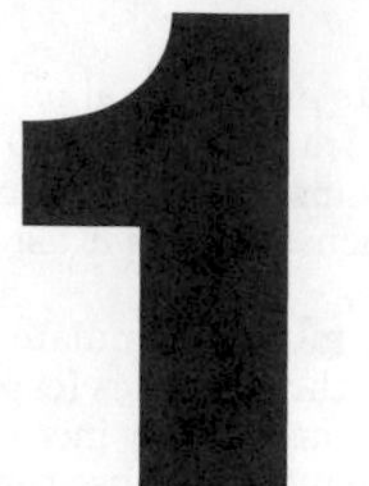
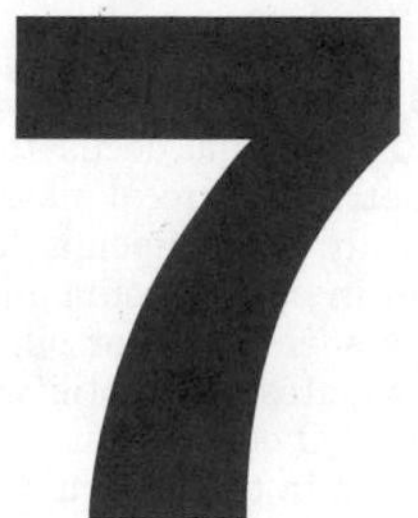

# Liver Diseases

Mauricio Lisker-Melman
and Marc A. Fallah

## Evaluation of Liver Function

Liver disease is classified according to the duration of abnormalities as either acute (<6 months) or chronic (>6 months).

I. **Laboratory evaluation**

A. **Serum enzymes.** Hepatic disorders associated predominantly with elevation in aminotransferases are referred to as **hepatocellular;** hepatic disorders with predominant elevation in alkaline phosphatase (AP) are referred to as **cholestatic.**

1. Elevation of **serum aminotransferases (AST and ALT)** indicates hepatocellular injury and necrosis. Markedly elevated levels (>1000 U/L) typically occur with acute hepatocellular injury (e.g., viral, drug-induced, or ischemic), whereas mild to moderate elevations may be seen in a variety of conditions (e.g., acute or chronic hepatocellular injury, infiltrative diseases, biliary obstruction). The ratio of serum AST to ALT is typically greater than 2 in alcoholic liver disease. In viral hepatitis, this ratio is characteristically less than 1.
2. **Alkaline phosphatase (AP)** is an enzyme that is present in a variety of body tissues (bone, intestine, kidney, leukocytes, liver, and placenta). The concomitant elevation of other hepatic enzymes (e.g., gamma-glutamyl transpeptidase or 5'-nucleotidase) assists in establishing the hepatic origin of AP. Serum AP level is often elevated in biliary obstruction, space-occupying lesions, infiltrative disorders, and conditions that cause intrahepatic cholestasis [primary biliary cirrhosis, primary sclerosing cholangitis, drug-induced cholestasis]. The degree of elevation of AP does not differentiate the site or cause of cholestasis.
3. **5'-Nucleotidase** is comparable to AP in sensitivity in detecting biliary obstruction, cholestasis, and infiltrative hepatobiliary diseases.
4. **Gamma-glutamyl transpeptidase (GGT)** is an enzyme that is present in a variety of tissues. Increases in GGT and AP tend to occur in similar hepatic diseases. GGT may be elevated in individuals who ingest barbiturates, phenytoin, or alcohol even when other liver enzyme and bilirubin levels are normal.

B. **Excretory products**

1. **Bilirubin** is a degradation product of hemoglobin and nonerythroid hemoproteins (e.g., cytochrome, catalase). Total serum bilirubin is composed of conjugated (direct) and unconjugated (indirect) fractions. Unconjugated hyperbilirubinemia occurs as a result of **excessive bilirubin production** (neonatal or physiologic jaundice, hemolysis and hemolytic anemias, ineffective erythropoiesis, and resorption of hematomas), **reduced hepatic bilirubin uptake** (Gilbert's syndrome and drugs such as rifampin and probenecid), or **impaired bilirubin conjugation** (Gilbert's or Crigler-Najjar

syndromes). Elevation of conjugated and unconjugated fractions occurs in Dubin-Johnson and Rotor syndromes and in conditions associated with **intrahepatic** (from hepatocellular, canalicular, or ductular damage) and **extrahepatic** (from mechanical obstruction) **cholestasis.**

2. **Bile acids** are produced in the liver and are secreted into bile, where they are required for lipid digestion and absorption. Elevated levels of serum bile acids are specific but not sensitive markers of hepatobiliary disease. Levels of individual bile acids are not useful in the differential diagnosis of liver disorders.
3. **Serum ammonia** levels are often elevated in hepatic encephalopathy. However, absolute levels do not correlate with clinical findings or grade of encephalopathy.

**C. Synthetic products**

1. **Serum albumin** concentration is frequently decreased in chronic liver disease. However, chronic inflammation, expanded plasma volume, and gastrointestinal or renal losses may also lead to hypoalbuminemia. Because the half-life of albumin is relatively long (20 days), serum levels may be normal in acute liver disease.
2. Several important proteins involved in **hemostasis** and **fibrinolysis** [coagulation factors (except factor VIII, which is produced by the liver and endothelium), $\alpha_2$-antiplasmin, antithrombin, heparin cofactor II, high-molecular-weight kininogen, prekallikrein, protein C, and protein S] are synthesized by the liver. The synthesis of factors II, VII, IX, and X and proteins C and S depends on the presence of vitamin K. The adequacy of hepatic synthetic function can be estimated by the **prothrombin time (PT)** (see Chap. 18, Disorders of Hemostasis, sec. **I.B.2**). PT prolongation may result from impaired coagulation factor synthesis or vitamin K deficiency. Normalization of PT after administration of vitamin K indicates vitamin K deficiency. In **fulminant hepatic failure (FHF)** (see the section Complications of Hepatic Insufficiency, sec. **I**), the level of factor V (half-life, 2 hours) predicts outcome.
3. Other synthetic products whose levels can be measured in specific liver diseases are **$\alpha_1$-antitrypsin, alpha-fetoprotein, and ceruloplasmin.**
4. **Cholesterol** is synthesized in the liver. Patients with advanced liver disease may have very low cholesterol levels. However, in primary biliary cirrhosis, levels of serum cholesterol may be markedly elevated.

## II. Radiographic evaluation

**A. Ultrasonography** is used to screen for dilation of the biliary tree and to detect gallstones and cholecystitis in patients with right-sided abdominal pain associated with abnormal liver blood tests. It can detect and characterize liver masses, abscesses, and cysts. Color-flow Doppler ultrasonography can assess patency and direction of blood flow in the portal and hepatic veins. Ultrasonography is the diagnostic modality of choice for hepatocellular carcinoma screening.

**B. Helical CT** scan with IV contrast is useful in the evaluation of parenchymal liver disease. It has the added feature of contrast enhancement to define space-occupying lesions (e.g., abscess and tumor) and allows for the calculation of liver volume.

**C. MRI** offers information similar to that provided by CT scan and also visualizes vessels without the use of IV contrast. IV gadolinium is used to help differentiate between malignant lesions such as hepatocellular carcinoma and benign masses such as focal nodular hyperplasia and hemangioma.

**D. Percutaneous transhepatic cholangiography and endoscopic retrograde cholangiopancreatography (ERCP)** involve the instillation of contrast into the biliary tree. They are most useful after the preliminary determination of biliary tree abnormalities detected by ultrasonography, CT, or MRI. The risk of acute pancreatitis following ERCP is approximately 5%. **Magnetic reso-**

**nance cholangiopancreatography (MRCP)** provides an alternative noninvasive diagnostic modality for visualizing the bile ducts. However, therapeutic intervention is not possible with MRCP.

E. **Technetium-99m RBC scan** is helpful in confirming the diagnosis of hepatic hemangioma.

F. **Positron emission tomography (PET)** is an emerging modality that uses differences in metabolism among normal, inflammatory, and malignant tissues. PET scans are helpful in assessing the presence of hepatic metastasis in colorectal cancer. PET scans may also be helpful in diagnosing cholangiocarcinoma.

III. **Pathologic evaluation.** Percutaneous liver biopsy can be performed with or without radiographic (ultrasound or CT) guidance. In the presence of coagulopathy, thrombocytopenia, and/or ascites, a biopsy can be obtained by the transjugular route. Biopsy of masses that are suspicious for carcinoma is usually performed with ultrasonographic or CT guidance. Laparoscopy is an alternative method for obtaining liver tissue. Liver biopsy is generally safe and can be performed as an outpatient procedure with observation for 4–6 hours after biopsy. Bleeding, pain, infection, and injury to neighboring organs are possible complications.

## Viral Hepatitis

I. The hepatotropic viruses include **hepatitis A (HAV), hepatitis B (HBV), hepatitis C (HCV), hepatitis D (HDV),** and **hepatitis E (HEV)** (Tables 17-1 and 17-2). Hepatitis G and TT virus are both hepatotropic RNA viruses, but they have failed to show a pathogenic role in acute or chronic liver disease. **Acute viral hepatitis** is a major public health problem, with approximately 300,000 cases reported annually in the United States. HAV and HEV (fecal-oral route of transmission) infections have no chronic form. In contrast, HBV, HCV, and HDV (parenteral route of transmission) infections may progress to chronic hepatitis, cirrhosis, and hepatocellular carcinoma. **Chronic viral hepatitis** is defined as the presence of persistent (at least 6 months) necroinflammatory injury that can lead to cirrhosis. Histopathologic classification of chronic viral hepatitis is based on etiology, grade, and stage. Grading and staging are measures of the severity of the necroinflammatory process and fibrosis, respectively.

II. **Clinical presentation** in acute and chronic (HBV, HCV, HDV) hepatitis tends to be similar for the hepatotropic viruses. **Acute hepatitis** can be silent (subclinical), especially in children and young adults. Symptoms vary from mild illness to FHF. Malaise, fatigue, pruritus, headache, abdominal pain, myalgias, arthralgias, nausea, vomiting, anorexia, and fever are common but nonspecific symptoms. Jaundice, dark urine, and acholic stools are associated findings. **Extrahepatic manifestations** (believed to be mediated by circulating immune-complexes), such as arthritis, skin rash, vasculitis, cryoglobulinemia, glomerulonephritis, and aplastic anemia, are infrequent. **Chronic hepatitis** runs an indolent course, sometimes for decades. Fatigue is a common symptom. The disease may only become clinically apparent late in the natural course, when symptoms typically seen in end-stage liver disease (ESLD) appear. Physical examination can be unrevealing.

A. **HAV** infection is usually transmitted via the fecal-oral route; large-scale outbreaks due to contamination of food and drinking water can occur. Sexual transmission and parenteral transmission may occur, although the period of viremia is brief. The period of greatest infectivity is the 2 weeks before the onset of clinical illness; however, fecal shedding continues for 2–3 weeks after the onset of symptoms. The diagnosis of HAV is made by detection of

**Table 17-1.** Clinical and epidemiologic features of hepatotropic viruses

| Organism | Hepatitis A | Hepatitis B | Hepatitis C | Hepatitis D | Hepatitis E |
|---|---|---|---|---|---|
| Incubation | 15–45 d | 30–180 d | 15–150 d | 30–150 d | 30–60 d |
| Transmission | Fecal-oral | Blood<br>Sexual<br>Perinatal | Blood<br>Sexual (rare)<br>Perinatal (rare) | Blood<br>Sexual (rare) | Fecal-oral |
| Risk groups | Residents of and travelers to endemic regions<br>Children and caregivers in day care centers | Injection drug users<br>Multiple sexual partners<br>Men having sex with men<br>Infants born to infected mothers<br>Health care workers<br>Transfusion recipients | Injection drug users<br>Transfusion recipients | Any person with hepatitis B virus<br>Injection drug users | Residents of and travelers to endemic regions |
| Sequelae | | | | | |
| Fatality rate | 1.0% | 1.0% | <0.1% | 2–10% | 1% |
| Carrier state | No | Yes | Yes | Yes | No |
| Chronic hepatitis | None | 2–10% in adults; 90% in children <5 yr | 70–85% | Variable | None |
| Cirrhosis | No | Yes | Yes | Yes | No |

**Table 17-2.** Viral hepatitis serologies

| Hepatitis | Acute | Chronic | Recovered/ latent | Vaccinated |
|---|---|---|---|---|
| HAV | IgM anti-HAV+ | NA | IgG anti-HAV+ | IgG anti-HAV+ |
| HBV | IgM anti-HBc+<br>HBeAg+<br>HBsAg+<br>HBV DNA+ | IgG anti-HBc+<br>HBeAg±<br>Anti-HBe±[a]<br>HBsAg+<br>HBV DNA±[a] | IgG anti-HBc+<br>HBV DNA–<br>HBeAg–<br>Anti-HBe±[a]<br>HBsAg–<br>Anti-HBs+ | Anti-HBs+ only |
| HCV | All tests possibly negative<br>HCV RNA+<br>Anti-HCV Ab+ in 8–10 wk | Anti-HCV Ab+<br>HCV RNA+ | Anti-HCV Ab+<br>HCV RNA[b]– | NA |
| HDV | IgM anti-HDV+[c]<br>HDV Ag+[c] | IgG anti-HDV+[c] | IgG anti-HDV+[c] | NA[d] |
| HEV | Available from CDC and research specialty laboratories | NA | Available from CDC and research specialty laboratories | NA |

Ab, antibody; CDC, Centers for Disease Control and Prevention; HAV, hepatitis A virus; HBc, hepatitis B core antigen; HBeAg, hepatitis B e antigen; HBsAg, hepatitis B surface antigen; HBV, hepatitis B virus; HCV, hepatitis C virus; HDV, hepatitis D virus; HEV, hepatitis E virus; NA, not applicable.

[a]HBeAg is present during periods of high replication along with HBV DNA. Anti-HBe is present during periods of low replication when HBeAg and HBV DNA may be undetectable.

[b]Negative HCV RNA results should be interpreted with caution. Differences are found in thresholds for detection among assays and among laboratories.

[c]Markers of HBV infection are also present, because HDV cannot replicate in the absence of HBV.

[d]Although no vaccine is available for HDV, immunity to HBV protects against HDV infection (see text, Viral Hepatitis sec. **II.D** and **III.A.4**).

**IgM anti-HAV antibody.** Liver biopsy is usually not necessary for diagnosis. **IgG anti-HAV antibody** develops after recovery or immunization and provides lifelong immunity.

**B. HBV** infection is transmitted by parenteral routes (e.g., needle-stick injury, injection drug use, transfusion, sexual contact, and from mother to infant). Although blood is the most effective vehicle for transmission, HBV is present in other body fluids (e.g., saliva and semen). Therefore, patients with HBV infection should avoid intimate contact (e.g., sharing razors and toothbrushes, unprotected sex) with nonimmune individuals. Immunity may develop after recovery from infection or immunization with **HBV vaccine, hepatitis B Ig (HBIg), or both.** HBV is a DNA virus that contains a number of antigens that elicit a corresponding antibody response. **Hepatitis B surface antigen (HBsAg)** is detectable in serum in acute and chronic HBV infection and disappears after clearance of the virus. **Hepatitis B core**

**antigen (HBcAg)** is not found in serum but can be detected within liver cells by immunoperoxidase staining during active viral replication. **Hepatitis B e antigen (HBeAg)** appears shortly after HBsAg in the serum, and its persistence is indicative of active viral replication and a high degree of infectivity. The presence of HBeAg is usually associated with the detection of serum **HBV viral DNA (HBV DNA).** The presence of HBV DNA also provides a measure of active replication. **Antibody against HBsAg (anti-HBs)** appears after the disappearance of HBsAg and after vaccination. Anti-HBs confers immunity (except in rare cases of chronic HBV infection with very low titers of heterotypic anti-HBs). **IgM antibody against HBcAg (IgM anti-HBc)** usually is present in acute infection and occasionally can be detected during periods of high viral replication in chronic disease. **IgG anti-HBc** is detectable in chronic infection and, in association with anti-HBs, after recovery. Rarely, patients with isolated IgG anti-HBc can reactivate HBV in the setting of immunosuppression (e.g., transplantation). **Antibody against HBeAg (anti-HBe)** usually indicates low-level replication and a lower degree of infectivity. Some patients harbor HBV mutants (e.g., precore, core promoter), in which case the conventional serologic markers may vary.

**C. HCV** is transmitted parenterally (e.g., transfusion, injection drug use, needlestick injury). It can be transmitted sexually and from mother to offspring, although at a much lower frequency than HBV. The screening test that is most widely used to detect antibody to HCV virus is performed by the **enzyme-linked immunosorbent assay (ELISA)** technique. The antibody may be undetectable for the first 8 weeks after infection, although acute HCV infection is usually subclinical. The antibody does not confer immunity. The ELISA has a sensitivity of 97%; however, the positive predictive value in a low-risk population is only 25%. The **recombinant immunoblot assay (RIBA)** is a supplementary test in low-risk individuals, but it has been replaced by **polymerase chain reaction (PCR)** tests that detect HCV RNA in serum as early as 1–2 weeks after infection. **Qualitative** (reported as positive or negative) and **quantitative** (estimate of viral load) PCR assays use different techniques for amplification and have different thresholds for detection. Tests to detect **HCV genotypes, subtypes, or serotypes** are commercially available. HCV genotype influences the duration, dosage, and response to treatment (see sec. **III.B.2**). A new test that detects HCV antigen is currently under investigation.

**D. HDV** is found throughout the world. It is endemic to the Mediterranean basin, the Middle East, and portions of South America. Outside these areas, infections occur primarily in individuals who have received transfusions or in injection drug users. HDV requires the presence of HBV for infection and replication. Clinical forms of presentation are **coinfection** (simultaneous acquisition with HBV infection) and **superinfection** (acute HDV infection in chronic HBV infection). Chronic hepatitis occurs more often after superinfection. Diagnosis is made by finding HDV RNA or HDV antigen in serum or liver and by detecting antibody to HDV antigen.

**E. HEV** has been implicated in epidemics in India, Southeast Asia, Africa, and Mexico. Reported cases in the United States have been in travelers to endemic areas. Transmission closely resembles that of HAV. The diagnosis of HEV infection is made by the detection of **IgM anti-HEV antibody. IgG anti-HEV antibody** develops after recovery from an acute infection. HEV is associated with a high fatality rate in pregnant women.

**F. Non A-E hepatitis** is the exclusionary category of hepatotropic viruses that remains when serologic tests for other viruses are negative.

## III. Prophylaxis

### A. Pre-exposure prophylaxis (see Appendix F, Immunizations and Post-Exposure Therapies)

#### 1. HAV

**a. Pre-exposure prophylaxis** with **HAV vaccine** should be given to travelers to endemic areas, men who have sex with men, illegal drug users, persons with high occupational risk for infection (research personnel working with HAV or HAV-infected primates), persons who have clotting factor disorders, and persons with chronic liver disease. In the United States, children residing in areas where the incidence of hepatitis A is twice the national average and people living in communities with local outbreaks of HAV should be vaccinated. Vaccinations should be administered at 0 and 6 months.

- **b.** Vaccination should be initiated at least 4 weeks before travel to an endemic area. For individuals who require immediate protection, the first dose of HAV vaccine can be administered concomitantly with **Ig** 0.02 ml/kg, at different anatomic injection sites.
- **c.** Travelers who are allergic to a vaccine component or who elect not to undergo vaccination should receive a single dose of Ig (0.02 ml/kg if the desired duration of protection is <2 months or 0.06 ml/kg if the desired duration is 2–5 months). The dose should be repeated if the travel period exceeds 5 months.

**2. HBV**

- **a. Pre-exposure prophylaxis** with **HBV vaccine** should be considered for everyone, particularly in individuals with multiple anticipated transfusions (e.g., transplant recipients, clotting factor deficiencies), patients with chronic renal failure (who are receiving or are likely to receive hemodialysis), health care workers, injection drug users, household and heterosexual contacts of HBsAg carriers, men having sex with men, residents and employees of residential care facilities, travelers (>6 months) to hyperendemic regions, and natives of Alaska, Asia, and the Pacific Islands.
- **b.** Many countries have included HBV vaccination (0, 1, and 6 months) in their infant or adult immunization programs. The Centers for Disease Control and Prevention has recommended a universal vaccination program for infants and sexually active adolescents in the United States.
- **c.** Prevaccination screening for previous exposure or infection is recommended in high-risk groups to avoid vaccinating recovered individuals or those with chronic infection.
- **d.** For patients who require rapid immunity, the dosage schedule can be escalated to 0, 1, and 2 months, but a follow-up booster at 6 months is required for long-lasting immunity.
- **e.** Additional doses, higher doses, or revaccination can be considered in nonresponders and hyporesponders (anti-HBs <10 mIU/ml) to elicit protective levels of immunity. Booster doses may be needed in immunosuppressed individuals in whom anti-HBs levels fall below 10 mIU/ml on annual testing.

**3.** A combined HAV and HBV vaccine is currently available and is highly immunogenic. The combined vaccine has very low rates of adverse effects, and it is given in three doses to persons older than 18 years of age.

**4.** Pre-exposure prophylaxis for HCV and HEV is not available. Individuals who are successfully vaccinated against HBV are protected against HDV.

**B. Postexposure prophylaxis** (see Appendix F, Immunizations and Post-Exposure Therapies)

**1. HAV**

- **a. Postexposure prophylaxis** for HAV with Ig (0.02 ml/kg) should be given within 2 weeks of the last exposure to unvaccinated individuals.
- **b.** Household and sexual contacts and persons who have shared illegal drugs with a person who has serologically confirmed acute HAV should receive Ig and the first dose of vaccine at different anatomic sites.
- **c.** Ig should be administered to all previously unvaccinated staff and attendees of day care centers if one or more cases of HAV are recognized in children or employees or if cases are recognized in two or

more households of center attendees. HAV vaccine can be administered at the same time as Ig at different anatomic sites.

**d.** If a food handler is diagnosed with HAV, Ig should be administered to other food handlers at the same establishment and to patrons who can be identified and treated within 2 weeks of exposure.

**2. HBV**

**a.** Infants born to HBsAg-positive mothers should receive **HBV vaccine** and **HBIg,** 0.5 ml, within 12 hours of birth. Immunized infants should be tested at approximately 12 months of age for HBsAg, anti-HBs, and anti-HBc. The presence of HBsAg indicates that the infant is actively infected. The presence of both anti-HBs and anti-HBc suggests that infection occurred but was probably modified by immunoprophylaxis and that immunity is likely to be prolonged. The presence of anti-HBs alone is indicative of vaccine-induced immunity.

**b.** Susceptible sexual partners of individuals with HBV and victims of needle-stick injury (with HBV contamination) should receive HBIg (0.04–0.07 ml/kg) and the first dose of HBV vaccine at different sites on the body as soon as possible (preferably within 48 hours but no more than 7 days after exposure). A second dose of HBIg can be administered 30 days after exposure, and the vaccination schedule should be completed.

**c.** Postexposure prophylaxis with HBIg and lamivudine should be used after liver transplantation for ESLD that results from HBV (see sec. **III.B.1** and the section Liver Transplantation). The use of adefovir dipivoxil is under investigation for this indication.

## IV. Management of viral hepatitis

**A. Acute viral hepatitis.** Management is supportive and generally occurs in the ambulatory clinic setting. Serum liver enzymes (AST and ALT), hepatic synthetic function (albumin and PT), bilirubin, and the appropriate serologic tests (see sec. **I** and Table 17-2) should be monitored to assess recovery. **Symptomatic treatment** of nausea and vomiting is recommended. Rarely, patients require hospitalization for dehydration. Alcohol should be avoided. In a small group of patients (Table 17-1), FHF ensues, as reflected by alteration in mental status (hepatic encephalopathy) and prolongation of PT (unresponsive to vitamin K supplementation). Such patients should be monitored in an ICU and urgently referred for liver transplantation (see the section Liver Transplantation). **Treatment of acute HCV** with interferon (IFN)-alpha (standard or pegylated) for 6 months has been associated with a high rate of sustained HCV-RNA clearance. The role of ribavirin in addition is under investigation.

**B. Chronic viral hepatitis** is associated with HBV, HCV, and HDV infections (Table 17-1).

**1. Treatment for chronic HBV** involves either the use of **IFN-alfa-2b, lamivudine, or adefovir dipivoxil.** The use of IFN for chronic HBV is restricted to patients with active viral replication and elevated serum ALT who have no evidence of decompensated liver disease (i.e., no history of variceal bleeding, ascites, or encephalopathy). IFN-alfa-2b (5 million units SC qd or 10 million units SC 3 times/week) is administered for 16 weeks. This results in a sustained loss of viral replication (disappearance of HBV DNA and HBeAg and appearance of anti-HBe) and biochemical and histologic remission in approximately one-third of patients. Loss of HBsAg occurs in about 10%. **Side effects of IFN** include flu-like symptoms (fatigue, fever, chills, nausea, vomiting, myalgias, and headaches), bone marrow suppression (leukopenia, neutropenia, and thrombocytopenia), neuropsychiatric alterations (emotional lability, mood disorders, and depression), and thyroid dysfunction (hypo- or hyperthyroidism). Rarely, patients may have suicidal ideation that mandates cessation of therapy and psychiatric consultation. **Lamivudine** (100 mg PO qd) is similarly effective and is better tolerated than IFN. Unresolved issues with lamivudine include duration of therapy and emergence of resistant polymerase mutants (10–15% per year). **Adefovir dipivoxil** (10 mg PO qd) appears to be safe, well tolerated, and effective. Its use has been associated with a very low rate of emergence of resistant strains. Other nucleoside analogs, such as tenofovir, clevudine, and emtricitabine, have been evaluated in clinical trials, but final recommendations are pending. Combination therapy using IFN and a nucleoside analog has no proven benefit. HDV coinfection makes successful treatment less likely.

2. **Treatment of chronic HCV** consists of a combination of **pegylated-interferon (PEG-IFN)** and **ribavirin** (10.6–13.0 mg/kg/day, PO in 2 divided doses) administered for 6–12 months. The addition of polyethylene glycol to the standard IFN molecule results in prolonged half-life with improved bioavailability. Pegylation allows for weekly dosing with improved therapeutic effect. PEG-IFN alpha-2a (180 μg SC/week) and PEG-IFN alpha-2b (1.5 μg/kg SC/week) are similar in efficacy. Sustained response (defined as normalization of serum ALT and clearance of HCV RNA from serum 6 months after completion of treatment) is observed in approximately 55% of all patients. **HCV genotype** and **viral load** determination are important in patient management. Genotype 1 represents two-thirds of the HCV genotypes in the United States and requires 12 months of full-dose therapy with a 30–50% sustained response rate. Genotypes 2 and 3 are "favorable" genotypes, as they require only 6 months of lower-dose therapy and have a 75–80% sustained response rate. Additional toxicity from ribavirin includes reversible hemolysis, cough, skin rash, insomnia, and teratogenicity. Contraindications to treatment with ribavirin include pregnancy or unwillingness to practice birth control, chronic renal insufficiency, and the inability to tolerate anemia (15–30%). Selected patients may receive monotherapy with PEG-IFN with a 20–30% sustained response rate.
3. **Liver transplantation** may be indicated in advanced viral disease, but disease recurrence is frequent (see Chap. 15, Solid Organ Transplant Medicine).

## Drug-Related Hepatotoxicity and Alcoholic Liver Disease

Chemical agents that damage the liver include **intrinsic hepatotoxins** (e.g., carbon tetrachloride and elemental phosphorus) and **idiosyncratic hepatotoxins** (e.g., isoniazid).

I. **Intrinsic hepatotoxicity** results from the direct hepatotoxic effects of the drug or its metabolite. This mechanism is predictable and dose dependent.

II. **Idiosyncratic hepatotoxicity** can be mediated by immunologic (hypersensitivity) or metabolic mechanisms and is unpredictable.

A. **Hypersensitivity reactions** are characterized by clinical (fever, rash, and/or eosinophilia) and histologic (eosinophilic or granulomatous inflammation) features of hypersensitivity and occur after a sensitization period of 1–5 weeks in susceptible individuals. Repeat challenge with the same agent leads to prompt recurrence of the reaction. Examples include sulfonamides, dapsone, and sulindac.

B. **Metabolic hepatotoxicity** occurs in susceptible patients as a result of altered drug clearance or accelerated production of hepatotoxic metabolites (e.g., isoniazid and methyldopa).

III. **Management of hepatotoxicity** includes cessation of exposure to the offending drug and institution of supportive measures. An attempt to remove the agent from the GI tract should be made in most cases of acute toxic ingestion using lavage or cathartics (see Chap. 25, Medical Emergencies, the section Overdosage). No specific therapy is available in most cases.

**IV. Acetaminophen** may cause significant hepatocellular injury in accidental or intentional overdose. Toxic potentiation of alcohol in combination with even therapeutic doses of acetaminophen has been demonstrated to cause significant hepatocellular injury. Management of acetaminophen overdose is a medical emergency (see Chap. 25, Medical Emergencies, the section Overdosage, sec. **VII**). Observation for signs of **FHF** is necessary (see the section Complications of Hepatic Insufficiency, sec. **I**).

**V. Alcoholic liver disease** is a significant medical and socioeconomic problem. Although ethyl alcohol exerts a direct toxic effect on the liver, significant liver damage develops in only 10–20% of chronic alcoholics. Thus, additional factors (e.g., genetic, nutritional, environmental) may be important in the pathogenesis of alcoholic liver disease. The spectrum of alcoholic liver disease is broad, and a single patient may be affected by more than one of the following conditions. Potentially dangerous interactions may occur between alcohol and a variety of medications, including sedative-hypnotics, anticoagulants, and acetaminophen, even in the absence of alcoholic liver disease, because of shared metabolic pathways.

**A. Fatty liver** is the most commonly observed abnormality in alcoholics. Patients are usually asymptomatic. Clinical findings include hepatomegaly and mild liver enzyme abnormalities. The disorder may be reversible if alcohol intake is stopped and an adequate diet is consumed.

**B. Alcoholic hepatitis** may be clinically silent or severe enough to lead to the rapid development of hepatic failure and death. Clinical features include fever, upper abdominal pain, anorexia, nausea, vomiting, and weight loss. Laboratory tests typically demonstrate elevation in serum aminotransferases (AST higher than ALT) and AP. Hyperbilirubinemia and prolongation of PT may be seen. Although clinical presentation is helpful, liver biopsy confirms the diagnosis. Features associated with a poor prognosis include renal failure, leukocytosis, a markedly elevated total bilirubin, and prolongation of the PT that does not normalize with vitamin K. A **discriminatory factor (DF) = 4.6 × (PT patient – PT control) + serum bilirubin** can be determined to assess in-hospital mortality. A DF of greater than 32 indicates a 50% in-hospital mortality.

**C. Alcoholic cirrhosis** is a common cause of cirrhosis and hepatocellular carcinoma worldwide.

**D. Therapy for alcoholic liver disease** includes abstinence from alcohol and nutritional support. Treatment of acute alcoholic hepatitis with corticosteroids is controversial. However, there is some evidence that patients with a DF greater than 32 who have hepatic encephalopathy may benefit from steroid therapy. Oral prednisone can be started at 40–60 mg/day and subsequently tapered as clinically indicated. Pentoxifylline (400 mg PO tid) is a nonselective phosphodiesterase inhibitor with anti-inflammatory properties and an excellent safety profile that has shown improved survival in severe (DF >32) alcoholic hepatitis. *S*-Adenosylmethionine, antioxidants, tumor necrosis factor inhibitors, and glutathione prodrugs are under investigation in alcoholic liver disease.

## Immune-Mediated Liver Disease

**I. Autoimmune hepatitis (AIH)** is an unresolving inflammation of the liver of unknown cause. It is characterized by the presence of elevated levels of serum aminotransferases, **circulating autoantibodies** (antinuclear antibody, smooth-muscle antibody, and liver-kidney microsomal antibody), and hypergammaglobulinemia. It occurs most often in women (10–30 years and late middle age) and frequently presents with cirrhosis. In approximately 30% of cases, the presentation is acute and similar to viral hepatitis. Patients may present in FHF or with asymptomatic elevation of serum ALT. Extrahepatic manifestations (arthritis, skin rashes, thyroiditis) are common. **Diagnosis** requires the presence of characteristic histology (plasmacytic inflammation of the portal triads with interface hepatitis), autoimmune markers, and the absence of viral, toxic, or alcoholic injury. **Therapy** is initiated with either (1) prednisone alone (40–60 mg/day) or (2) a combination of prednisone (40–60 mg/day) and azathioprine (1–2 mg/kg/day). Prednisone is tapered with biochemical and clinical improvement to a maintenance dose of 5 mg/day. Remission (normalization of serum bilirubin, immunoglobulin levels, AST, ALT; disappearance of symptoms; resolution of histologic changes) is achieved in 65% and 80% of patients within 1.5 and 3 years, respectively. Relapses occur in at least 50% after cessation of therapy, and some patients require lifelong low-dose therapy. Liver transplantation should be considered in patients with end-stage disease. After transplantation, recurrent AIH or de novo AIH (in patients transplanted for non-autoimmune diseases) has been described.

**II. Primary biliary cirrhosis (PBC)** is a cholestatic hepatic disorder of unknown etiology that most often affects middle-aged women and progresses along a path of increasingly severe histologic damage (florid bile duct lesion, ductular proliferation, fibrosis, and cirrhosis). The course is highly variable, and patients may be asymptomatic for many years. Fatigue, jaundice, and pruritus are often the most troublesome symptoms. Typical features include elevated levels of AP, cholesterol, IgM, and bile acids; **antimitochondrial antibodies** are present in more than 90% of patients. Treatment includes control of pruritus, management of steatorrhea and malabsorption, and symptom-specific therapy. No curative therapy is available. **Ursodeoxycholic acid** (13–15 mg/kg/day PO) improves liver function test abnormalities and appears to delay progression of disease when given long term (>4 years). Liver transplantation may be necessary in advanced disease, and recurrent PBC after transplantation has been documented.

**III. Primary sclerosing cholangitis (PSC)** is an idiopathic cholestatic liver disorder characterized by inflammation, fibrosis, and eventual obliteration of the extrahepatic and intrahepatic bile ducts. Most patients are middle-aged men, and the disorder is frequently associated with **inflammatory bowel disease** (70% with ulcerative colitis). PSC should be considered in individuals with inflammatory bowel disease who have increased levels of AP even in the absence of symptoms of hepatobiliary disease. Clinical manifestations typically include intermittent episodes of jaundice, hepatomegaly, pruritus, weight loss, and fatigue. It is confirmed by demonstration of strictures or irregularity of the intrahepatic and extrahepatic bile ducts by ERCP or MRCP. Liver biopsy is helpful in the diagnosis of small-duct PSC, in the exclusion of other diseases, and in the staging of disease. Patients are at risk for development of **ascending bacterial cholangitis** and **cholangiocarcinoma.** No specific therapy has proven to be successful. Colectomy does not affect the course of PSC associated with ulcerative colitis. Episodes of cholangitis should be managed with IV antibiotics and with dilatation and stent placement across dominant strictures. Patients with advanced disease or recurrent cholangitis should be referred for liver transplantation. Cholangiocarcinoma is a contraindication to liver transplantation. Recurrent PSC after liver transplantation has been documented.

**IV. Complications of cholestasis**

**A. Nutritional deficiencies** result from fat malabsorption (see Chap. 2, Nutritional Support, and Table 2-4). In patients with steatorrhea, a low-fat diet (40–60 g/day) helps to decrease symptoms but may compromise total energy intake. **Fat-soluble vitamin deficiency** (vitamins A, D, E, K) is often present in advanced disease and is particularly common in patients with steatorrhea. Fat-soluble vitamin replacement can be accomplished by water-soluble preparations of **vitamin A,** 5000–10,000 IU PO qd; **vitamin K,** 5–10 mg PO qd; and **vitamin E,** 100 IU PO qd. Vitamin D deficiency can be corrected by **25-hydroxyvitamin D3 (25-cholecalciferol),** 20–50 mg PO three to five times a week. Serum levels of vitamin A and 25-cholecalciferol should be monitored to assess the adequacy of replacement therapy and avoid toxicity. Zinc deficiency may occur in some patients and is corrected with **zinc sulfate,** 220 mg PO daily (50 mg elemental zinc) for 4 weeks.

B. **Osteoporosis and osteomalacia** can occur in patients with cholestatic liver disease. Bone mineral density should be measured in all patients at the time of diagnosis. Treatment of bone disease includes exercise, oral calcium supplementation (1.0–1.5 g/day), bisphosphonate therapy, and vitamin D supplementation.

C. **Pruritus** is best treated with **cholestyramine,** a basic anion exchange resin. It binds bile acids and other anionic compounds in the intestine and inhibits their absorption. The dose is 4 g mixed with water before and after the morning meal, with additional doses before lunch and dinner to control symptoms. The maximum recommended dose is 16 g/day. Cholestyramine should not be given concurrently with vitamins or other medications, as it may impair absorption. **Colestipol,** another similar resin, is also available. **Antihistamines** (diphenhydramine or doxepin, 25 mg PO qhs) and petrolatum may provide symptomatic relief. **Rifampin** (300–600 mg/day) and **naltrexone** (25–50 mg/day) are reserved for intractable pruritus. Plasmapheresis, charcoal hemoperfusion, and partial external biliary diversion are invasive therapeutic procedures that can also be administered when medical therapy has failed.

## Metabolic Liver Disease

A number of treatable metabolic disorders present with hepatocellular dysfunction, including Wilson's disease and hereditary hemochromatosis. Other rare disorders include glycogen storage disease, phospholipidosis, and $\alpha_1$-antitrypsin deficiency.

I. **Wilson's disease (WD)** (incidence, 1 in 30,000) is an autosomal-recessive disorder (ATP7B gene on chromosome 13) that results in progressive copper overload. The average age at presentation of liver dysfunction is 10–15 years; neuropsychiatric disorders can manifest later. The diagnosis of WD should be considered in patients with unexplained liver disease with or without neuropsychiatric symptoms, first-degree relatives with WD, or individuals with FHF (with or without hemolysis). Prompt recognition of WD is crucial in patients with FHF (5% in the United States). The diagnosis is suggested by Kayser-Fleischer rings on slit lamp examination of the eyes (50% and 98% of patients with hepatic and neurologic presentations, respectively), elevated serum free copper level (>25 μg/dl), low serum **ceruloplasmin** level (<20 mg/dl), and elevated 24-hour urinary copper level (>100 μg). The liver histology (steatosis, glycogenated nuclei, chronic hepatitis, fibrosis, cirrhosis) and brain imaging (basal ganglia changes) findings are nonspecific. Elevated **hepatic copper levels** of greater than 250 μg/g dry weight (normal <40 μg/g) on biopsy are highly suggestive of WD. Treatment is with copper-chelating agents (penicillamine or trientine and zinc salts). Liver transplantation is the only therapeutic option in FHF or in progressive dysfunction despite chelation therapy. Liver transplantation is curative.

II. **Hereditary hemochromatosis** (incidence, 1 in 200 to 1 in 800) is an autosomal-recessive disorder of iron overload, usually not diagnosed until middle age (40–60 years). The disorder is related to abnormal iron absorption in the duodenum that leads to excessive and damaging iron deposition in various organs.

Affected persons may present with slate-colored skin, diabetes, cardiomyopathy, arthritis, hypogonadism, or hepatic dysfunction. The diagnosis is suggested by high fasting transferrin saturation (>55% in men, >45% in women). The diagnosis is subsequently confirmed by the presence of specific mutations in the **hemochromatosis gene (HFE).** The presence of the **abnormal HFE genotypes** C282Y homozygous (95%), C282Y/H63D compound heterozygous (4%), or H63D homozygous (1%) in the setting of iron overload is diagnostic of hereditary hemochromatosis. HFE genotype determination has replaced the role of liver biopsy in making the diagnosis. Presently, a liver biopsy is most helpful in staging the disease, especially in individuals who are at increased risk of having advanced fibrosis or cirrhosis. In cases in which the abnormal HFE genotypes are not present but the index of suspicion is very high, a liver biopsy allows for the measurement of the **hepatic iron concentration** and the calculation of the **hepatic iron index.** A hepatic iron concentration of greater than 4000 µg/g dry weight and a hepatic iron index of greater than 1.9 are both diagnostic of hemochromatosis. Genetic counseling is important. First-degree relatives should be screened if the HFE mutation is detected in the proband or if they have a high serum transferrin saturation. Therapy consists of **phlebotomy** (500 ml blood/week) until iron depletion is confirmed by either mild anemia (hemoglobin <10 g/dl) or ferritin levels below 50 ng/ml. Thereafter, maintenance phlebotomy of 1–2 U of blood three to four times a year is continued for life. Patients with cirrhosis are at increased risk for the development of hepatocellular carcinoma despite therapy. The survival rate in appropriately treated noncirrhotic patients is identical to that of the general population. Patients who undergo liver transplantation for hemochromatosis tend to have poorer 1- and 5-year survivals when compared to other liver transplant recipients.

**III.** **$\alpha_1$-Antitrypsin deficiency** (incidence, 1 in 1600) is an autosomal-recessive disease that may present with pulmonary, hepatic, or pancreatic manifestations. Chronic hepatitis, cirrhosis, or hepatocellular carcinoma may develop in 10–15% of patients with the PiZZ phenotype during the first 20 years of life. Controversy exists as to whether liver disease develops in heterozygotes (PiMZ). The presence of significant pulmonary and hepatic disease in the same patient is very rare (1–2%). The diagnosis is suggested by a low serum $\alpha_1$-antitrypsin level (10–15% of normal). The liver biopsy shows characteristic periodic acid-Schiff–positive, diastase-resistant globules in the periportal hepatocytes. No specific medical therapy for the hepatic disease is available, but transplantation is curative, with survival rates of 90% at 1 year and 80% at 5 years.

## Miscellaneous Disorders

**I. Vascular diseases** of the liver can be due to impaired arterial or venous blood flow. The portal vein and the hepatic artery provide two-thirds and one-third of hepatic blood flow, respectively.

**A. Ischemic hepatitis** results from liver hypoperfusion. Clinical circumstances include severe blood loss, severe burns, cardiac failure, heat stroke, and sepsis. Characteristic features include the rapid rise and fall in levels of serum AST, ALT, and lactic dehydrogenase accompanied by midzonal and centrilobular necrosis on liver biopsy. Prognosis is determined by the rapid and effective treatment of the underlying cause.

**B. Budd-Chiari syndrome** results from hepatic venous outflow obstruction. Etiologies include webs in the suprahepatic inferior vena cava, tumors, and thrombosis (often related to hypercoagulable states such as myeloproliferative disorders, estrogen use, and paroxysmal nocturnal hemoglobinuria). Approximately 20% of cases are idiopathic. Patients may present with an acute, subacute, or chronic illness characterized by **ascites, hepatomegaly,**

and **right upper quadrant abdominal pain.** Serum to ascites albumin gradient is greater than 1.1 g/dl, and serum albumin, bilirubin, AST, ALT, and PT are mildly abnormal. Hepatic venography or MRI establishes the diagnosis. Nonsurgical management [anticoagulants, thrombolytics, diuretics, angioplasty, stents, transjugular intrahepatic portosystemic shunt (TIPS)], surgical decompressive procedures, and liver transplantation are the main therapeutic options.

C. **Veno-occlusive disease (VOD)** refers to obliteration of terminal hepatic venules within the liver and consequent sinusoidal engorgement and necrosis of hepatocytes in the centrilobular region of the hepatic acinus. It is seen in bone marrow transplant recipients who have received total body irradiation and high-dose chemotherapy, in renal transplant recipients who are immunosuppressed with azathioprine, and in association with ingestion of Jamaican bush teas. Diagnosis is based on the triad of **hepatomegaly, weight gain** (2–5% of baseline body weight), **and hyperbilirubinemia** (>2 mg/dl), generally occurring within 3 weeks after transplantation. The severity of VOD varies from mild, reversible disease to multiorgan failure. Chemotherapeutic drugs and radiation therapy affect the incidence and severity of VOD. Reported mortality ranges from 0 to 67%. Treatment is supportive, as the disease is self-limited in the majority of patients.

D. **Portal vein thrombosis** in adults is seen in a variety of clinical settings, including abdominal trauma, cirrhosis, malignancy, hypercoagulable states, intra-abdominal infections, and pancreatitis, and after portocaval shunt surgery or splenectomy. It can manifest with variceal hemorrhage or ascites. **Ultrasonographic Doppler** examination is sensitive and specific for establishing the diagnosis. Angiography or magnetic resonance angiography can also be used when portosystemic shunt surgery is being considered. Portosystemic shunts are primarily indicated in patients with variceal bleeding in whom endoscopic management fails or when endoscopic management is not indicated (portal hypertensive gastropathy or extraesophageal varices) (see Chap. 16, Gastrointestinal Diseases, the section Gastrointestinal Bleeding, sec. **V.B**).

II. **Hepatic abscess** may be either pyogenic or amebic.

A. **Pyogenic abscess** can result from hematogenous infection, spread from intra-abdominal infection or ascending infection from the biliary tract. Approximately 20% of cases are cryptogenic in origin. Clinical features include fever, chills, weight loss, jaundice, and abdominal pain from tender hepatomegaly. Laboratory studies may demonstrate leukocytosis and elevated AP. Diagnosis is confirmed by CT, MRI, or ultrasonography. More than half the patients have positive blood cultures at the time of presentation. Treatment includes a prolonged course of antibiotic therapy, and, in select cases, imaging-guided percutaneous or surgical drainage. Repeat imaging is recommended to document resolution.

B. **Amebic abscess** should be considered in patients from endemic areas. Diagnosis requires a high index of clinical suspicion. Specific serologic tests for *Entamoeba histolytica* such as the indirect hemagglutination determination are helpful in establishing the diagnosis in low-prevalence areas. Amebic abscesses are treated with metronidazole.

III. **Granulomatous hepatitis** presents primarily as a cholestatic disorder. Patients typically have fever and elevated liver enzyme levels (particularly AP) and may have hepatosplenomegaly. The differential diagnosis includes infections (e.g., syphilis and mycobacterial, fungal, and rickettsial diseases), sarcoidosis, drug-induced injury, and idiopathic causes. Specific therapy is directed at the underlying cause. If the clinical suspicion for tuberculosis is high, an empiric trial of antituberculous therapy may be warranted despite negative mycobacterial cultures.

IV. **Nonalcoholic fatty liver disease (NAFLD)** is the most common liver disease in the United States (5% of general population, 25–75% in patients with obesity and type II diabetes mellitus). The spectrum of histologic forms includes hepatic steatosis (benign clinical course), steatosis with nonspecific inflammation, and nonalcoholic steatohepatitis (NASH). NASH is characterized by steatosis, inflammation, necrosis, and fibrosis. Approximately 25% of patients with NASH progress to cirrhosis over a 10- to 15-year period. Up to 70% of cases of **cryptogenic cirrhosis** have NASH as the underlying etiology. Conditions associated with NAFLD include diabetes mellitus (type II), insulin resistance syndrome, obesity, and dyslipidemia. Secondary causes include hepatotoxic drugs (amiodarone, nifedipine, estrogens), surgical procedures (jejunoileal bypass, extensive small-bowel resection, biliary and pancreatic diversions) and miscellaneous conditions (total parenteral nutrition, hypobetalipoproteinemia, environmental toxins). A liver biopsy remains the gold standard by which the diagnosis is made. However, the decision to perform a liver biopsy should take into account the specific clinical questions that are relevant to each case. No established treatment is available for NAFLD. Therapies to correct or control associated conditions are warranted. Liver transplantation should be considered in patients with ESLD, although recurrence can develop.

## Complications of Hepatic Insufficiency

I. **Fulminant hepatic failure (FHF)** is defined as the onset of hepatic encephalopathy within 8 weeks of initial symptoms of liver disease in an otherwise healthy individual. Acetaminophen hepatotoxicity and viral hepatitis are the most common causes of FHF. Other causes are AIH, drug and toxin exposure, ischemia, acute fatty liver of pregnancy, WD, and Reye's syndrome. Manifestations of FHF include encephalopathy, worsening jaundice, GI bleeding, sepsis, coagulopathy, hypoglycemia, renal failure, and electrolyte abnormalities. Supportive therapy in the ICU setting (in cooperation with a hepatology-liver transplant team) is essential. Blood glucose, electrolytes, and fluid status should be monitored carefully. Vitamin K should be administered to attempt to correct underlying coagulopathy, and stress ulcer prophylaxis should be given. Fresh frozen plasma and blood should be administered when evidence of active hemorrhage is found. In patients with signs that are suggestive of elevated intracranial pressure (see Chap. 24, Neurologic Disorders, the section Alterations in Consciousness, sec. **III.F.1**) or grade III or IV hepatic encephalopathy (Table 17-3), an intracranial pressure monitor can be placed. Transplantation should be urgently considered in cases of FHF. Mortality exceeds 80% in patients with grade IV encephalopathy who do not receive a transplant. Death often results from progressive liver failure, GI bleeding, cerebral edema, sepsis, or arrhythmia.

II. **Hepatic encephalopathy** is the syndrome of disordered consciousness and altered neuromuscular activity that is seen in patients with acute or chronic hepatocellular failure or portosystemic shunting. The pathogenesis of hepatic encephalopathy is controversial, and numerous mediators have been implicated.

  A. **Precipitating factors** include azotemia; use of a tranquilizer, opioid, or sedative-hypnotic medication; GI hemorrhage; hypokalemia and alkalosis (diuretics and diarrhea); constipation; infection; high-protein diet; progressive hepatocellular dysfunction; and portosystemic shunts (surgical or TIPS).

  B. **Grading** of hepatic encephalopathy is outlined in Table 17-3.

  C. **Treatment** should be initiated promptly.

    1. Precipitating factors should be identified and corrected if possible.
    2. The rationale and benefit of dietary protein restriction are controversial. Once the patient is able to eat, a diet containing 30–40 g protein per day is initiated. Special diets (vegetable protein or branched-chain amino acid enriched) may be beneficial in patients with encephalopathy that is refractory to the usual measures.
    3. **Medical therapies** include **nonabsorbable disaccharides** (lactulose, lactitol, and lactose in lactase-deficient patients), neomycin, and metro-

**Table 17-3.** Grading system for hepatic encephalopathy

| Grade | Level of consciousness | Personality and intellect | Neurologic abnormalities | EEG abnormalities |
|---|---|---|---|---|
| 0 | Normal | Normal | Normal | Normal |
| 1 | Inverted sleep pattern, restless | Forgetful, mild confusion, agitation, irritable | Tremor, apraxia, incoordination, impaired handwriting | Slowing triphasic waves |
| 2 | Lethargic, slow responses | Disorientation for time, amnesia, decreased inhibitions, inappropriate behavior | Asterixis, dysarthria, hypoactive reflexes | Slowing triphasic waves |
| 3 | Somnolent but can be aroused, confused | Disorientation for place, aggressive | Asterixis, hyperactive reflexes, Babinski's sign, muscle rigidity | Slowing triphasic waves |
| 4 | Coma | Nil | Decerebrate | Slow delta activity |

*Source:* From NC Gitlin. Hepatic encephalopathy. In: D Zakim, TD Boyer (eds). *Hepatology* (3rd ed). Philadelphia: WB Saunders, 1996:611, with permission.

nidazole. The initial dose of lactulose is 15–45 ml PO bid–qid. Maintenance dose should be adjusted to produce three to five soft stools per day. Oral lactulose should not be given to patients with an ileus or possible bowel obstruction. **Lactulose enemas** (prepared by the addition of 300 ml lactulose to 700 ml distilled water) can be administered. **Neomycin** can be given by mouth (500–1000 mg q6h) or as a retention enema (1% solution in 100–200 ml isotonic saline). Approximately 1–3% of the administered dose of neomycin is absorbed, with the attendant risk of ototoxicity and nephrotoxicity. The risk of toxicity is increased in patients with renal insufficiency. Because lactulose is as effective as neomycin, it is preferred for initial and maintenance therapy. Combination therapy with lactulose and neomycin should be considered in cases that are refractory to either agent alone. **Metronidazole** (250 mg PO q8h) is useful for short-term therapy when neomycin is unavailable or poorly tolerated. Long-term metronidazole is not recommended due to its associated toxicities.

**III. Portal hypertension** frequently complicates cirrhosis and presents with ascites, GI bleeding, and splenomegaly. The presence of portal hypertension is established by determining the pressure difference between the hepatic vein and the portal vein. A pressure gradient of greater than 10 mm Hg is seen in portal hypertension, and complications can occur when the pressure gradient is greater than 12 mm Hg. GI bleeding from portal hypertension most often results from varices (esophageal and gastric). Other sources of bleeding include duodenal and rectal varices, hemorrhoids, and portal hypertensive gastropathy and colopathy. The cause of bleeding is generally determined by endoscopy (see Chap. 16, Gastrointestinal Diseases, for diagnosis and treatment). Causes of portal hypertension in patients without cirrhosis include idiopathic portal hypertension, schistosomiasis, congenital hepatic fibrosis, sarcoidosis, cystic fibrosis, arteriovenous fistulas, splenic and portal vein thrombosis, myeloproliferative diseases, nodular regenerative hyperplasia, and focal nodular hyperplasia.

**IV. Ascites** is the abnormal (>25 ml) accumulation of fluid within the peritoneal cavity. It is a common manifestation of decompensation in cirrhosis. It is a consequence of portal hypertension, decreased plasma oncotic pressure, and avid sodium retention by the kidneys. In cirrhosis, the ascitic fluid has a low albumin concentration and low opsonic activity.

**A.** A **serum to ascites albumin gradient** that is greater than 1.1 g/dl indicates portal hypertension–related ascites (97% specificity). A serum to ascites albumin gradient of less than 1.1 g/dl is found in nephrotic syndrome, peritoneal carcinomatosis, serositis, tuberculosis, and biliary and pancreatic ascites.

**B. Management**

1. **Dietary salt restriction** (2 g salt or 88 mmol $Na^+$/day) should be initiated and continued thereafter unless the renal ability to excrete sodium spontaneously improves. In selected cases, it may be necessary to restrict sodium intake further. The use of potassium-containing salt substitutes can lead to serious hyperkalemia. Routine water restriction is not necessary. If dilutional hyponatremia (serum $Na^+$ <120 mmol/L) occurs, fluid restriction to 1000–1500 ml/day usually suffices.
2. **Diuretic therapy** can be initiated along with salt restriction. The goal of diuretic therapy should be a daily weight loss of no more than 1.0 kg in patients with edema and approximately 0.5 kg in those without edema until ascites is adequately controlled. Diuretics should not be administered to individuals with an increasing serum creatinine level. **Spironolactone** (100 mg PO in a single daily dose with food) is the diuretic of choice. The daily dose can be increased by 50–100 mg every 7–10 days until satisfactory weight loss, a maximum dose of 400 mg, or side effects occur. Hyperkalemia and gynecomastia are common side effects. Amiloride or triamterene (potassium-sparing diuretics) are substitutes that can be used in patients in whom painful gynecomastia develops from spironolactone. **Loop diuretics,** such as furosemide (20–40 mg, increasing to a maximum dose of 160 mg PO qd) or bumetanide (0.5–2.0 mg PO qd), can be added when a 200-mg dose of spironolactone fails to initiate a diuresis. Patients should be observed closely for signs of dehydration, electrolyte disturbances, encephalopathy, muscle cramps, and renal insufficiency. Nonsteroidal anti-inflammatory agents may blunt the effect of diuretics and increase the risk of renal dysfunction.
3. **Paracentesis** should be performed for diagnosis [e.g., new-onset ascites, suspicion of malignant ascites, or spontaneous bacterial peritonitis (SBP)] or as a therapeutic maneuver when tense ascites causes significant discomfort or respiratory compromise. Routine diagnostic testing should include fluid cell and differential counts, albumin, total protein, and culture. Amylase and triglyceride measurement, cytology, and mycobacterial smear/culture should be performed to confirm specific diagnoses. **Bleeding** and **intestinal perforation** are possible complications. Rarely, rapid large-volume paracentesis may lead to circulatory collapse, encephalopathy, and renal failure. Concomitant administration of IV colloid (5–8 g albumin/L ascites removed) can be used to minimize these complications, especially in the setting of renal insufficiency or the absence of peripheral edema.
4. **TIPS** has proved effective in the management of refractory ascites (fluid overload that is nonresponsive to a sodium-restricted diet and high-dose diuretic therapy). Complications include shunt occlusion, bleeding, infection, cardiopulmonary compromise, and hepatic encephalopathy.

**V. SBP** is an infectious complication of portal hypertension–related ascites. Its occurrence is related to low protein level and impaired opsonic activity in ascitic fluid.

**A. Clinical manifestations** include abdominal pain and distention, fever, decreased bowel sounds, and worsening of hepatic encephalopathy; however, the disease may be present in the absence of specific clinical signs. Therefore, cirrhotic patients with ascites and evidence of any clinical deterioration should undergo diagnostic paracentesis to exclude SBP.

B. **The diagnosis is likely when the ascitic fluid contains more than 250 neutrophils/µl.** Gram stain reveals the organism in only 10–20% of samples. A positive culture confirms the diagnosis. **Cultures are more likely to be positive when 10 ml ascitic fluid is inoculated into two blood culture bottles at the bedside.** The most common organisms are *Escherichia coli*, *Klebsiella*, and *Streptococcus pneumoniae*. Blood cultures are positive in approximately one-half of cases with SBP. Polymicrobial infection is uncommon and should lead to the suspicion of secondary bacterial peritonitis.

C. In suspected cases (fever, abdominal pain, or tenderness) without more than 250 neutrophils/µl, empiric **antibiotic therapy** with a third-generation cephalosporin (e.g., ceftriaxone, 1 g IV qd, or cefotaxime, 1–2 g IV q6–8h, depending on renal function; see Appendix E) or a quinolone (ciprofloxacin, 500 mg IV q12h) is appropriate for 5 days. Paracentesis should be repeated if no clinical improvement occurs in 48–72 hours, especially if the initial ascitic fluid culture was negative.

D. **Norfloxacin** (400 mg PO qd) can be used as secondary prophylaxis by reducing the frequency of recurrent episodes of SBP. However, the use of antibiotic prophylaxis has not been clearly shown to improve survival and does select resistant gut flora.

VI. **Coagulopathy** occurs as a result of impaired hepatic synthesis of coagulation factors and thrombocytopenia. Vitamin K deficiency can be corrected by parenteral administration of 10 mg/day for 3 consecutive days. Transfusion of fresh frozen plasma and platelets should be reserved for patients with active bleeding or for those who are undergoing invasive procedures (see Chap. 18, Disorders of Hemostasis).

VII. **Hepatorenal syndrome (HRS)** is characterized by impairment in renal function in the setting of acute or, more commonly, chronic liver disease. Major and minor diagnostic criteria are summarized in Table 17-4. **Type I** HRS is characterized by the acute onset of rapidly progressive, oliguric renal failure unresponsive to volume expansion. **Type II** HRS progresses more slowly but relentlessly and often clinically manifests as diuretic-resistant ascites. No clear or established treatments are available for HRS. Although transplantation may be curative, prognosis without transplantation is grave.

VIII. **Hepatocellular carcinoma** (hepatoma) frequently occurs in patients with cirrhosis, especially in association with viral hepatitis (HBV or HCV), alcoholic cirrhosis, $\alpha_1$-antitrypsin deficiency, and hemochromatosis. It can be multifocal. Early diagnosis is essential, as surgical resection and liver transplantation can improve long-term survival. Alternative therapy for unresectable tumors includes percutaneous alcohol or acetic acid injection, arterial chemoembolization, microwave coagulation therapy, or radiofrequency ablation. Patients with cirrhosis should therefore be monitored for hepatocellular carcinoma by periodic measurement of **serum alpha-fetoprotein level** and radiologic imaging (MRI, CT, or ultrasonography).

## Liver Transplantation

The severity of chronic liver disease is often graded on the basis of **Child-Turcotte-Pugh** classification (Table 17-5). The prioritization for liver transplantation in chronic liver disease is determined by the **Model for End Staged Liver Disease (MELD)** score.

**Table 17-4.** Diagnostic criteria of hepatorenal syndrome

| |
|---|
| **Major criteria** |
| Low glomerular filtration rate, as indicated by serum creatinine >1.5 mg/dl or 24-hr creatinine clearance <40 ml/min |
| Absence of shock, ongoing bacterial infection, fluid losses, and current treatment with nephrotoxic drugs |
| No sustained improvement in renal function (decrease in serum creatinine to 1.5 mg/dl or increase in creatinine clearance to 40 ml/min) after diuretic withdrawal and expansion of plasma volume with 1.5 L of a plasma expander |
| Proteinuria <500 mg/dl and no ultrasonographic evidence of obstructive uropathy or parenchymal renal disease |
| **Additional criteria** |
| Urine volume < 500 ml/d |
| Urine sodium < 10 mEq/L |
| Urine osmolality greater than plasma osmolality |
| Urine RBCs <50/high-power field |
| Serum sodium concentration <130 mEq/L |

*Note*: All major criteria must be present for the diagnosis of hepatorenal syndrome. Additional criteria are not necessary for the diagnosis but provide supportive evidence.
*Source:* From V Arroyo, P Gines, AL Gerbes, et al. Definition and diagnostic criteria of refractory ascites and hepatorenal syndrome in cirrhosis. International Ascites Club. *Hepatology* 23:164, 1996, with permission.

**I. Indications**

**A.** In patients with **FHF** and signs of advanced encephalopathy (grade III or IV; Table 17-3), marked coagulopathy (PT >20 seconds), or hypoglycemia, liver transplantation is the accepted therapy.

**B.** Timing of liver transplantation in patients with **chronic liver disease** is a complex issue. Patients should be evaluated for transplantation when they have a decline in hepatic synthetic or excretory functions, ascites, hepatic encephalopathy (Child-Turcotte-Pugh class B or C), or other complications, such as SBP, HRS, hepatocellular carcinoma, and recurrent SBP or variceal bleeding. Patients with cholestatic liver disease can be transplanted for disabling, intractable pruritus.

**C.** The MELD score has been used to estimate the probability of 3-month survival and helps determine the need for transplantation in patients with chronic liver disease. The MELD score is determined by the use of an algorithm that takes into account serum bilirubin, serum creatinine, and international normalized ratio (INR).

**II. Contraindications.** Contraindications to liver transplantation include severe and uncontrolled extrahepatic infection, advanced cardiac or pulmonary disease, extrahepatic malignancy, multiorgan failure, and unresolved psychosocial and medical noncompliance issues.

**III. Recurrent disease.** Certain forms of liver disease (especially viral hepatitis) recur after transplantation (see Chap. 15, Solid Organ Transplant Medicine, the section Infectious Complications, sec. **IV.B**).

**A. Recurrent HBV** can be prevented by the coadministration of HBIg and lamivudine after transplantation. Lamivudine (100 mg PO qd) or adefovir dipivoxil (10 mg PO qd) initiated before transplantation lowers viral load and reduces the likelihood of recurrent HBV.

**B. Recurrent HCV** cannot be prevented. Treatment of recurrent infection with combination PEG-IFN and ribavirin is feasible in selected cases.

**Table 17-5.** Child-Turcotte-Pugh scoring system to assess severity of liver disease

| | Points scored for increasing abnormality | | |
|---|---|---|---|
| Clinical and biochemical measurements | 1 | 2 | 3 |
| Albumin | >3.5 | 2.8–3.5 | <2.8 |
| Bilirubin (mg/dl) | <2 | 2–3 | >3 |
| For cholestatic diseases: bilirubin (mg/dl) | <4 | 4–10 | >10 |
| PT (secs prolonged)[a] *or* | <4 | 4–6 | >6 |
| INR[a] | <1.7 | 1.7–2.3 | >2.3 |
| Ascites | Absent | Mild | Moderate |
| Encephalopathy (grade) | 0 | 1 and 2 | 3 and 4 |

[a]Either the prothrombin time (PT) or international normalized ratio (INR) can be used for scoring.

| Class | Total points |
|---|---|
| A | 5–6 |
| B | 7–9 |
| C | 10–15 |

**IV.** The number of transplants performed is limited by the availability of organs. Improvements in surgical technique have resulted in successful **split liver and live donor (partial liver) transplants.** Immunosuppressive, infectious, and long-term complications are discussed in Chap. 15, Solid Organ Transplant Medicine.

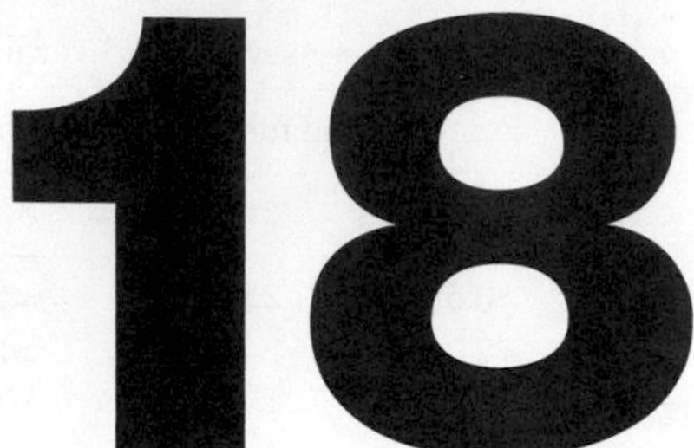

# Disorders of Hemostasis

Leslie Andritsos,
Roger D. Yusen, and
Charles Eby

## Evaluation of Patients with Hemostatic Disorders

I. **Normal hemostasis** involves a complex sequence of interrelated reactions, leading to platelet aggregation (primary hemostasis) and activation of the coagulation cascade (secondary hemostasis) to produce a durable vascular seal.

A. **Primary hemostasis** is an immediate (seconds to minutes) but temporary response to vessel injury. Platelets and von Willebrand factor (vWF) interact to form a primary plug, after which platelet activation occurs and blood vessels constrict, limiting flow.

B. **Secondary hemostasis (coagulation)** is a slower process (minutes to hours) that results in the formation of a fibrin clot (Fig. 18-1). Coagulation is initiated when vascular damage exposes extravascular tissue factor to factor VII, with subsequent activation of factors V, VIII, and XI, leading to accelerated and sustained generation of thrombin, conversion of fibrinogen to fibrin, and formation of a durable clot (*Annu Rev Med* 46:103, 1995).

C. **History and physical examination.** A detailed history is crucial for determining whether a bleeding disorder is present and whether it is likely to be congenital or acquired, mild or severe, and involving primary or secondary hemostasis. Prolonged bleeding after challenges such as dental extractions, circumcision, menstruation, labor and delivery, trauma, or surgery may suggest an underlying bleeding disorder, especially if blood transfusion or hospital admission for hemostasis is required. Self-reporting of easy bruising and prolonged bleeding with minor cuts is often noninformative unless accompanied by objective abnormal bleeding events. A detailed family history may reveal evidence to support an inherited bleeding disorder. Acquired bleeding disorders may be suggested by comorbid conditions (liver disease, alcohol consumption, autoimmune disease) or commonly implicated medications. On **physical examination,** primary hemostasis defects are suggested by mucosal bleeding and bruising. The latter may manifest as focal areas (<2 mm) of subcutaneous bleeding that do not blanch with pressure, called **petechiae;** larger patches (<1 cm), designated **purpura;** or extensive areas of bruising (>1 cm), called **ecchymoses.** Petechiae typically present in areas that are subjected to increased hydrostatic force (lower legs) or the periorbital area after coughing or vomiting. Disorders of secondary hemostasis usually produce deep ecchymoses, hematomas, hemarthroses, or delayed bleeding after trauma or surgery.

II. **Laboratory evaluation** of patients with suspected hemostatic disorders is guided by the history and physical examination. Initial studies should include a platelet count, prothrombin time (PT), activated partial thromboplastin time (aPTT), and peripheral blood smear review.

A. **Tests of primary hemostasis**

1. A low **platelet count** on a CBC report requires a manual slide review to rule out a platelet clumping artifact due to the anticoagulant ethylene

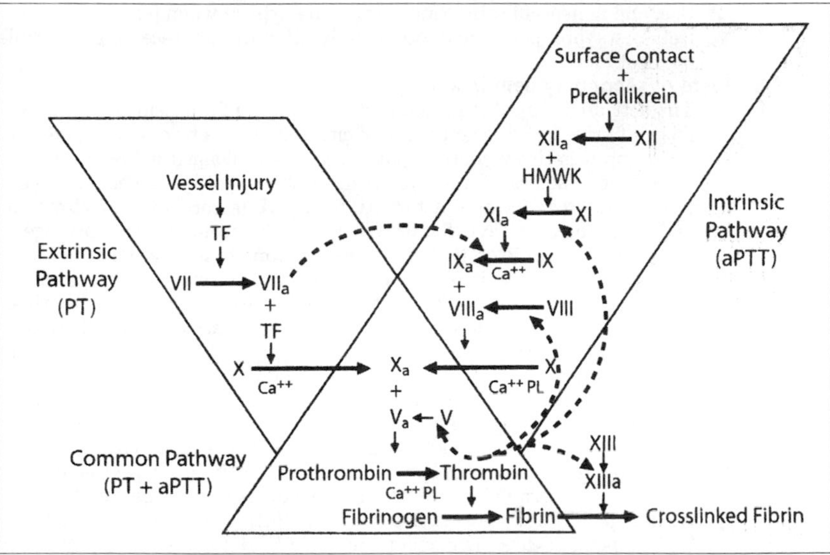


**Fig. 18-1.** Coagulation cascade. *Solid arrows* indicate activation, and *dashed lines* indicate additional substrates activated by factor VIIa or thrombin. aPTT, activated partial thromboplastin time; HMWK, high-molecular-weight kininogen; PL, phospholipase; PT, prothrombin time; TF, tissue factor. (Modified from GJ Broze Jr. Tissue factor pathway inhibitor and the revised theory of coagulation. *Annu Rev Med* 46:103, 1995.)

diamine tetra-acetic acid (EDTA) or unusually large platelets that are misclassified by the automated hematology instrument.

2. A prolonged **bleeding time (BT)** may be due to qualitative or quantitative disorders of platelets or vWF, or abnormalities of capillary integrity. It is generally not prolonged by disorders of secondary hemostasis. The BT is not useful for predicting the risk of bleeding complications before invasive procedures in unselected patients and may be prolonged after ingestion of medications that interfere with platelet function, such as aspirin. Other variables that can artificially prolong the BT include differences in technician performance, subcutaneous edema, thinning of the skin, and anemia. Therefore, when platelet dysfunction is suspected and the BT is prolonged, additional platelet function assays may be appropriate.
3. The **PFA-100** (Dade Behring, Deerfield, IL) instrument simulates primary hemostasis. It is used to screen for von Willebrand's disease and to detect acquired platelet dysfunction due to medications. However, this test currently cannot be used to predict bleeding risk, as adequate clinical investigations have not been performed (*Thromb Haemost* 82:35–39, 1999).
4. **von Willebrand factor antigen (vWF:Ag)** is a measure of circulating vWF protein by immunoassay.
5. **von Willebrand factor activity, Ristocetin cofactor (vWF:RCo)** is a functional assay of vWF-mediated agglutination of platelets in the presence of the antibiotic ristocetin.
6. **In vitro platelet aggregation** studies measure platelet secretion and aggregation in response to purified platelet agonists and are used to evaluate patients who are suspected of having an inherited qualitative platelet disorder. Performance requires considerable technical exper-

tise, and nonspecific abnormal results are typical when platelet aggregation tests are performed on acutely ill patients receiving multiple medications.

**B. Tests of secondary hemostasis**

1. The activated partial thromboplastin time **(aPTT)** measures the time to form a fibrin clot after activation of citrated plasma by calcium, phospholipid, and negatively charged particles. It is prolonged by deficiencies of coagulation factors of the "intrinsic pathway" (high-molecular-weight kininogen, prekallikrein, factor XII, factor XI, factor IX, and factor VIII) and "common pathway" (factor V, factor X, prothrombin, and fibrinogen).
2. The **prothrombin time (PT)** measures the time to form a fibrin clot after the addition of thromboplastin (tissue factor and phospholipid) and calcium to citrated plasma. This test is sensitive to deficiencies of "extrinsic pathway" factor VII and common pathway coagulation factors. Thromboplastins vary in sensitivity to factor deficiencies, which complicates monitoring of oral anticoagulation therapy (OAT) when PTs are obtained from different laboratories. Reporting PT ratios as an international normalized ratio (INR) reduces interlaboratory variation. Manufacturers compare the sensitivity to OAT of each lot of thromboplastin to a World Health Organization reference thromboplastin and assign an international sensitivity index (ISI). Laboratories convert PT ratios to INR using the equation $INR = (\text{patient PT}/\text{mean normal PT})^{ISI}$ (*Thromb Haemost* 49:238–244, 1983). Several point-of-care instruments measure PT/INR from a drop of whole blood for use in coagulation clinics or home monitoring.
3. The **thrombin time (TT)** measures time to clot formation after the addition of thrombin to citrated plasma. It is sensitive to quantitative and qualitative deficiencies of fibrinogen, fibrin degradation products, some monoclonal antibodies, heparin, and direct thrombin inhibitor drugs. The presence of heparin is confirmed if a prolonged TT corrects after adding protamine, which neutralizes heparin.
4. **Fibrinogen concentration (Clauss method)** is inversely proportional to the prolongation of the TT performed on diluted plasma.
5. **Mixing studies** are performed to determine if a prolonged PT or aPTT is due to a factor deficiency(ies) or an inhibitor. When patient plasma is mixed 1:1 with normal pooled plasma (all factor activities = 100%), deficient factors are restored to at least 50%, sufficient to normalize or nearly normalize the PT or aPTT. Most inhibitors are still detected after a 1:1 mix, and the prolonged PT or aPTT does not correct. The next step is to perform selected factor activity assays (Table 18-1) to identify the deficiency(ies).
6. **Clot urea stability** is a qualitative functional test used to screen for severe (<5%) congenital deficiency of factor XIII in patients who have a clinical bleeding disorder but no evidence of a primary hemostasis defect and normal PT, aPTT, and TT. After activation by thrombin, FXIIIa forms covalent cross links between fibrin molecules to produce a durable clot.

**Table 18-1.** Factor deficiencies that cause prolonged prothrombin time (PT) or activated partial thromboplastin time (aPPT)

| Abnormal assay | Suspected factor deficiency |
|---|---|
| aPTT | XI, IX, XII, or VIII |
| PT | VII vs. multiple factors |
| PT and aPTT | II, V, X, or fibrinogen vs. multiple factors |

**C.** Evaluation for **thrombophilia risk factors** may be appropriate in some patients with venous thromboembolic events (see Thromboembolic Disorders, secs. **V** and **VI**).

## Platelet Disorders

**I. Thrombocytopenia** is defined as a platelet count of less than 140,000/μl at Barnes-Jewish Hospital. Usually, increased bleeding is not attributable to thrombocytopenia until the count drops below 50,000/μl. The risk of spontaneous life-threatening (e.g., CNS, GI) bleeding increases at counts below 20,000/ml and substantially at counts below 10,000/μl. A helpful diagnostic strategy is to differentiate disorders of marrow production from conditions that result in increased platelet destruction or sequestration. A bone marrow examination, which can be performed safely at platelet counts above 10,000/ml, may be helpful in making this distinction. Agents such as aspirin, nonsteroidal anti-inflammatory drugs (NSAIDs), and anticoagulants that further impair hemostasis are relatively contraindicated in patients with thrombocytopenia.

**A. Drug-induced** thrombocytopenia may be idiosyncratic or dose dependent. Of the several mechanisms of drug-induced thrombocytopenia, the two most common are antibody mediated. Antibodies may be directed against drugs that are covalently bound to platelet membrane glycoproteins, so-called hapten-dependent antibodies. Drugs may also stimulate formation of antibodies that bind platelet membrane proteins only when the drug is circulating (*Semin Hematol* 36[1 Suppl 1]:2–6, 1999 [review]). The most common medications that are reported to cause thrombocytopenia include quinidine, quinine, rifampin, trimethoprim/sulfamethoxazole, and methyldopa (*Ann Intern Med* 129:886–890, 1998). Some drugs, such as ethanol, directly inhibit thrombopoiesis. Drug-induced thrombocytopenia is a diagnosis of exclusion and is confirmed only after normalization of platelet counts with discontinuation of the drug. Intravenous immunoglobulin (IVIg) can be administered if thrombocytopenia is life-threatening.

**B. Marrow infiltration (myelophthisis)** by tumors, storage diseases, chronic myeloproliferative disorders, or granulomatous disease may interfere with normal platelet production. The diagnosis is confirmed by examination of a bone marrow biopsy and aspirate. The presence of nucleated RBCs, teardrop cells, and immature myeloid forms on a peripheral smear may indicate a myelophthisic process. Treatment is directed toward the underlying cause of the marrow infiltration.

**C. Infections** can cause thrombocytopenia in a variety of ways. Some organisms, such as fungi and mycobacteria, infiltrate the bone marrow. HIV is commonly associated with thrombocytopenia, either through direct infection of megakaryocytes or by accelerated peripheral destruction secondary to an immune thrombocytopenia (*Blood Rev* 16:73–76, 2002). HIV is known to be associated with thrombotic thrombocytopenic purpura (TTP), and thrombocytopenia may arise as a result of opportunistic infections or as a complication of antiretroviral therapy. HHV-6 causes thrombocytopenia in immunosuppressed patients by suppressing production of megakaryocyte progenitor cells (*J Gen Virol* 81:663–673, 2000).

**D. Prolonged vitamin $B_{12}$ or folate deficiency** usually cause pancytopenia but may result in thrombocytopenia, which resolves with appropriate supplementation.

**E. Immune thrombocytopenia** is caused by the binding of antibodies (usually IgG) to platelet surface antigens, resulting in premature clearance by the reticuloendothelial system.

**1.** The diagnosis of **immune thrombocytopenic purpura (ITP)** is suggested by isolated thrombocytopenia in the absence of a likely underlying caus-

**Table 18-2.** Indications for therapy in pregnancy and immune thrombocytopenic purpura

| Platelet count | Trimester | Bleeding | Therapy |
|---|---|---|---|
| Any | Any | Present | IVIg or steroids |
| >50,000 | Any | Absent | Observation |
| 30,000–50,000 | First or second | Absent | Observation |
| 10,000–30,000 | Second or third | Present or absent | IVIg or steroids |
| <10,000 | Any | Present or absent | IVIg or steroids |

IVIg, intravenous immunoglobulin.
Adapted from Hoffman et al. *Hematology* (3rd ed). Philadelphia: Harcourt, Inc., 2000.

ative disease or medication. In adults, ITP typically presents as mild mucocutaneous bleeding that develops over several weeks. Immune thrombocytopenia may arise as a result of other underlying diseases, such as systemic lupus erythematosus (SLE), antiphospholipid antibody (APA) syndrome, HIV, hepatitis C virus, or lymphoproliferative disorders, and testing for these diseases is performed based on history, physical examination, and laboratory findings (*N Engl J Med* 346:995–1008, 2002). Serologic tests for antiplatelet antibodies generally are not helpful due to poor sensitivity. Bone marrow biopsy may be useful in selected patients to exclude a primary bone marrow disorder, especially in individuals over the age of 60, patients with persistent thrombocytopenia, or those who do not respond to therapy (*Blood* 88:398–403, 1996).

2. Not all patients with immune thrombocytopenia require **treatment** (Table 18-2). Initial therapy, when indicated, consists of glucocorticoids with the addition of IVIg if the patient is bleeding. Most patients who are treated respond to therapy within 1–3 weeks. Patients who fail initial therapy are treated either with splenectomy or immunosuppressive therapy. Splenectomy is the treatment of choice, as it can salvage approximately two-thirds of refractory ITP patients. Of patients who respond to glucocorticoid therapy, 30–40% relapse during steroid taper, and these individuals are considered to have chronic ITP. As is the case for primary refractory ITP, splenectomy is the treatment of choice. Pneumococcal, meningococcal, and *Haemophilus influenzae* type B vaccines should be administered at least 2 weeks before splenectomy. If a patient is a poor surgical candidate or unwilling to undergo splenectomy, medical salvage therapy may include prednisone, anti-D immunoglobulin (WinRho) in Rh-positive patients, androgen therapy with danazol, or immunosuppressive agents, such as vincristine, cyclophosphamide (Cytoxan), rituximab, or azathioprine (*Blood* 88:398–403, 1996; 98:952–957, 2001). The minority of patients who fail splenectomy are managed similarly to those with primary refractory ITP, with the exception of the use of WinRho, which is ineffective in the absence of a spleen.
3. **ITP during pregnancy** may be difficult to distinguish from gestational thrombocytopenia, preeclampsia, and HELLP (**h**emolysis, **e**levated **l**iver enzymes, **l**ow **p**latelets) syndrome and is a diagnosis of exclusion (Table 18-2). IVIg is recommended for initial therapy, but glucocorticoids can also be used if an appropriate response to IVIg does not occur. Patients who fail initial therapy with IVIg and glucocorticoids and who have a platelet count of less than 10,000 or are bleeding can be considered for splenectomy. Pregnant patients with ITP can safely undergo vaginal delivery or cesarean section if the platelet count is greater than 50,000. Platelet transfusion before delivery is recommended in patients for

whom a cesarean section is planned, if the platelet count is less than 10,000, or if the patient is bleeding. Because most antiplatelet antibodies are IgG and are able to cross the placenta, some neonates who are born to affected mothers have severe thrombocytopenia and may be at risk for intracranial hemorrhage during vaginal delivery. Centers with high-risk obstetric services can perform fetal blood sampling either by percutaneous umbilical vein sampling or fetal scalp vein sampling to determine the fetal platelet count before delivery. Cesarean section is recommended when the fetal platelet count is less than 20,000 (*Blood* 88:398–403, 1996).

**F. Posttransfusion purpura (PTP)** is a rare syndrome characterized by the formation of alloantibodies against platelet surface antigens, most commonly the antigen $PL^{A1}$, resulting in severe thrombocytopenia. The syndrome occurs in a minority of $PL^{A1}$-negative patients who receive blood or platelet transfusions from $PL^{A1}$-positive donors, and it is most common in multiparous women who are transfused for the first time. Thrombocytopenia occurs within approximately 7–10 days of transfusion. Effective treatment options are IVIg or plasmapheresis. Platelet transfusions from random donors are not helpful because they are rapidly destroyed, as more than 99% of the population is $PL^{A1}$ positive. $PL^{A1}$-negative blood products can be used but are difficult to procure. The diagnosis of PTP is confirmed by detecting platelet-specific antibodies in the patient's serum. If PTP is clinically suspected but $PL^{A1}$ antibodies are not detected, further testing should be done for other uncommon platelet alloantibodies.

**G. Heparin-induced thrombocytopenia (HIT)** is an acquired hypercoagulable disorder caused by antibodies that target heparin and platelet factor 4 (PF4) complexes, which leads to platelet activation and clot formation (*Blood* 101:31–37, 2003). HIT usually develops between 5 and 14 days after heparin exposure, but it may develop in patients with recent exposure to heparin and circulating antibodies as early as 10 hours after initiation of heparin therapy (*N Engl J Med* 344:1286–1292, 2001). It rarely develops after 2 weeks of heparin use. Typically, HIT produces modest reductions in platelet counts to 50,000–100,000/$\mu$l. The incidence of HIT is approximately 2% with adjusted-dose unfractionated heparin and even lower with prophylactic-dose unfractionated heparin (*Blood* 101:2955, 2003) and low-molecular-weight heparin (LMWH). Thrombosis develops in approximately 50% of patients with HIT, and the risk of thrombosis persists for up to 6 weeks after discontinuation of heparin.

1. The **diagnosis** of HIT is suggested by the development of thrombocytopenia during heparin therapy by any route (including heparin flushes) and a prompt recovery of platelet count after cessation of heparin, in the absence of other causes of thrombocytopenia. The diagnosis is suspected when thrombocytopenia (<140,000) or a decrease in the platelet count of 50% or more from baseline develops in patients who are receiving heparin. When the clinical evidence for HIT is not compelling, laboratory testing for HIT antibodies is recommended. Two types of assays are available: **functional** (platelet aggregometry or serotonin release assay to detect activation of donor platelets in the presence of patient serum and heparin) and **antigenic** (enzyme-linked immunosorbent assay to detect antibodies against heparin-PF4 complexes). Functional assays are generally considered to be more specific and enzyme-linked immunosorbent assay more sensitive. Results for both types of HIT tests are rarely immediately available, and initial management decisions must be made based on clinical judgment.
2. **Therapy** begins with the discontinuation of heparin, including heparin flushes. Patients with thromboses require alternative anticoagulation with a direct thrombin inhibitor, either recombinant **hirudin (lepirudin)** or **argatroban** (see Anticoagulants, secs. **V–VI**). LMWH should be

avoided due to high rates of cross reactivity with HIT antibodies. Thrombocytopenia is generally not regarded as a contraindication to anticoagulation, unless the patient is bleeding. In one series, 50% of patients with thrombocytopenia and documented HIT were found to have subclinical lower extremity deep venous thromboses (DVTs). Therefore, screening lower extremity Doppler ultrasound in such patients is reasonable, as the finding of a DVT mandates anticoagulation for 3–6 months (*Blood* 101:31–37, 2003). Oral anticoagulation therapy with warfarin should not be initiated until the platelet count normalizes because of the risk of limb gangrene.

**H. TTP** is a systemic disorder that results from decreased circulating levels of vWF-cleaving protease, leading to elevated levels of the high-molecular-weight multimers of vWF (*N Engl J Med* 339:22, 1998). This often occurs as a result of autoantibodies inhibiting the von Willebrand–cleaving protease. The presence of high-molecular-weight vWF multimers leads to platelet aggregation in the microcirculation and subsequent microangiopathy. The complete clinical pentad, which is present in fewer than 30% of cases, includes consumptive thrombocytopenia, microangiopathic hemolytic anemia, fever, renal dysfunction, and fluctuating neurologic deficits. Thrombocytopenia and microangiopathic hemolytic anemia are sufficient to raise suspicion for TTP in the absence of other identifiable causes. The **hemolytic-uremic syndrome** may share a common pathogenesis with TTP but usually arises in the setting of GI bacterial infection (*Shigella*, *Escherichia coli* O157:H7) and is associated with more pronounced renal dysfunction. TTP may occur postpartum and in pregnancy, has been associated with HIV, and can be drug induced (e.g., cyclosporine, ticlopidine, quinine). Rare autosomal-recessive inherited deficiencies of vWF-cleaving protease with chronic relapsing TTP also exist. The differential diagnosis of thrombotic microangiopathy includes disseminated intravascular coagulation (DIC), malignant hypertension, preeclampsia, HELLP syndrome, and vasculitis.

1. **Laboratory evaluation** shows evidence of intravascular hemolysis (anemia, low haptoglobin, elevated lactate dehydrogenase), thrombocytopenia, normal coagulation studies, and renal insufficiency. The peripheral smear is significant for evidence of mechanical red cell damage (schistocytes) and thrombocytopenia. Assays for vWF-cleaving protease activity are offered by some reference laboratories, although protease levels have not been shown to correlate directly with response to treatment or risk for relapse (*Blood* 102:60–68, 2003).
2. **Treatment** of TTP is critical, as it is a medical emergency that requires immediate hospitalization. **Plasma exchange** of 1.0–1.5 plasma volumes daily is the mainstay of therapy. Remission rates are as high as 90% when plasma exchange is initiated without delay. If plasma exchange is not available or will be delayed, therapy with fresh frozen plasma (FFP) should be instituted immediately. The addition of **glucocorticoids** has become standard practice, ranging from methylprednisolone, 1.0 g IV qd, to prednisone, 1 mg/kg PO qd. RBC transfusion can be given as needed. Platelet transfusion in the absence of significant bleeding is relatively contraindicated because of the potential risk of clinical deterioration. The end point of therapy is not well defined, but plasma exchange is usually continued for at least 5 days or for 2 days after normalization of the platelet count and lactate dehydrogenase, resolution of neurologic signs, and improvement in microangiopathy. Schistocytes may persist for several weeks into a durable remission. Renal failure may be slower to improve, and persistent azotemia does not necessarily indicate treatment failure. Patients who do not respond initially to plasma exchange usually receive a trial of plasma exchange with cryosupernatant (depleted of vWF) in place

of FFP. Relapse occurs most commonly within 1 month after discontinuing plasma exchange. Patients with relapsing TTP may experience long remissions with intermittent plasma exchange. **Splenectomy** may salvage some patients with TTP that is refractory to plasma exchange or may reduce the frequency of relapses in patients who experience recurrent episodes (*Blood* 96:1223–1229, 2000). **Immunosuppression** with vincristine may be beneficial for relapsed TTP (*Ann Hematol* 81:7–10, 2002). **Rituximab,** an anti-CD20 monoclonal antibody, has proved effective in achieving durable remissions, according to several case reports (*Ann Intern Med* 138:105, 2003).

I. **Gestational thrombocytopenia** is a common (5–10%) finding in the third trimester. Platelet counts typically range between 100,000/L and 150,000/L [Hoffman, et al. *Hematology* (3rd ed). Philadelphia: Harcourt, Inc., 2000]. However, thrombocytopenia can be seen in **preeclampsia** (in 15–20% of cases), **eclampsia** (in 40–50% of cases), **HELLP** syndrome, **TTP,** and **DIC,** and a thorough evaluation for evidence of hemolysis, infection, hypertension, and liver dysfunction is required to distinguish between these syndromes. Gestational thrombocytopenia, preeclampsia, and eclampsia usually resolve promptly after delivery; the management of TTP is similar to that of the nonpregnant patient (*Semin Hematol* 34:159, 1997). The neonate is unaffected in gestational thrombocytopenia, and at platelet counts greater than 100,000/μL there is no contraindication to vaginal delivery [Hoffman, et al. *Hematology* (3rd ed). Philadelphia: Harcourt, Inc., 2000].

J. **Hypersplenism** is a syndrome characterized by splenomegaly and sequestration of up to 90% of circulating platelets. A variety of disorders may result in splenomegaly, such as portal hypertension, but most produce only a modest decrease in the platelet count. Treatment is directed toward the underlying condition. Splenectomy is a consideration if the cause of splenomegaly is not remediable or the splenomegaly is symptomatic, or as a diagnostic procedure in idiopathic splenomegaly.

## II. Thrombocytosis

A. **Reactive thrombocytosis,** typically less than 1,000,000/μl, may occur in response to splenectomy or conditions such as iron deficiency, chronic infectious or inflammatory conditions, and malignancy. Patients with this condition apparently do not have an increased risk of bleeding or thrombosis. No specific therapy is required except for correction of the underlying disorder.

B. **Essential thrombocythemia (ET)** is a chronic myeloproliferative disorder characterized by persistent thrombocytosis and an increased susceptibility to thrombosis and hemorrhage. Like the other myeloproliferative disorders (e.g., chronic myelogenous leukemia, polycythemia vera, and myelofibrosis), ET is a clonal disorder of hematopoietic stem cells (*Blood* 58:916–919, 1981).

1. **Diagnosis and clinical features.** Diagnostic criteria for ET have been defined by the Polycythemia Vera Study Group and include a platelet count of greater than 600,000, a normal hematocrit, adequate iron stores, absence of Philadelphia chromosome on karyotype analysis, no evidence of myelofibrosis or myelodysplastic syndrome, and no cause for reactive thrombocytosis (*Semin Hematol* 34:29–39, 1997). Megakaryocyte hyperplasia is usually identified on bone marrow biopsy. Median age at diagnosis is 60 years, and 3–5% of patients ultimately progress to acute myeloid leukemia. Thromboses may be arterial or venous, and the risk of thrombosis increases with age, prior thrombosis, duration of disease, and comorbidities (*Blood* 93:417–424, 1999). Hemorrhage is typically associated with platelet counts greater than 1,000,000 and is secondary to an acquired deficiency of large vWF multimers (*Blood* 82:1749–1757, 1993).

2. **Management** of ET must be individualized. Younger asymptomatic patients without excess risk of thrombosis can be observed. Erythromelalgia, distal burning and redness due to platelet microaggregates, usually responds to low-dose aspirin. In older patients with a high risk of throm-

bosis, particularly a prior thrombosis, the majority of thrombotic complications occur at modest elevations of platelets. Therefore, a reasonable treatment goal is a platelet count of 400,000 or less. This can be accomplished with the use of platelet-lowering agents such as anagrelide or hydroxyurea, or with interferon-alpha during pregnancy and childbearing years (*Blood* 97:863–866, 2001). Low-dose aspirin can be prescribed, but its additional benefit to cytoreduction is unclear, and its use may lead to worsening platelet dysfunction. Acute arterial thrombosis is managed best with platelet pheresis in combination with aspirin. Platelet transfusion is appropriate for life-threatening hemorrhage.

III. **Qualitative platelet disorders** are suggested by a prolonged BT or PFA-100 closure time despite a normal platelet count. Acquired defects are more prevalent than hereditary disorders.

A. **Acquired defects** in platelet function generally cause milder disorders of hemostasis than do the inherited disorders. Patients with isolated platelet dysfunction may not bleed abnormally unless superimposed coagulation defects are present.

1. **Drug-induced** platelet dysfunction is an effect of a wide variety of drugs, including aspirin, high-dose penicillin, bismuth subsalicylate (Pepto-Bismol), and ethanol. Numerous other drugs, such as beta-lactam antibiotics, beta-blockers, calcium channel blockers, and selective serotonin reuptake inhibitors, cause platelet dysfunction in vitro but rarely are associated with bleeding complications.
2. **Antiplatelet agents** are useful for their anti-inflammatory and antithrombotic effects. **Aspirin** is an irreversible cyclooxygenase-1 and -2 inhibitor. After aspirin is discontinued, its effects gradually diminish over approximately 7 days as new platelets are produced. Patients receiving aspirin who are scheduled to undergo elective procedures are advised to stop the medication 5–7 days before surgery. However, the risk of significant bleeding in most patients on aspirin who require urgent surgery is probably too low to warrant a delay, excluding ophthalmologic and neurosurgery (*N Engl J Med* 324:27, 1991). All other **NSAIDs** reversibly inhibit cyclooxygenase-1, and their effect lasts only as long as they remain in plasma. **Cyclooxygenase-2 inhibitors** have antiplatelet activity in large doses but at therapeutic doses have a minimal effect on platelets. **Clopidogrel** inhibits platelet aggregation by blocking the platelet adenosine diphosphate receptor. Because of its prolonged half-life, clopidogrel should be withheld beginning 10 days before elective invasive procedures. **Dipyridamole** is a platelet adhesion inhibitor that is available either alone or in combination with aspirin (Aggrenox). The antiplatelet agents **abciximab, eptifibatide,** and **tirofiban** block platelet IIb/IIIa–dependent aggregation and are approved for use in acute coronary syndromes (see Chap. 5, Ischemic Heart Disease). Platelet transfusion compensates for drug-induced platelet dysfunction described above, except that caused by tirofiban and eptifibatide, and is thus effective therapy for patients with significant bleeding.
3. **Uremia.** BTs can be increased in patients with uremia; however, the associated risk of bleeding is variable. Moreover, the BT is independently prolonged by anemia, which is itself a result of renal failure. Treatment is generally reserved for individuals with bleeding complications. **Dialysis** rapidly improves uremia and may be appropriate for bleeding patients. Increasing the hematocrit to at least 30%, either with the use of RBC transfusion or erythropoietin, shortens bleeding time. **Desmopressin** [diamino-8-D-arginine vasopressin (DDAVP)] can shorten a prolonged BT in uremic patients and is commonly administered before renal biopsy or during a bleeding episode. Conjugated **estrogens** (0.6 mg/kg IV qd for 5 days) may improve platelet function for up to 2 weeks. Transfused platelets acquire the uremic defect rapidly but can have transient utility in actively bleeding patients.

**B. Inherited disorders** of platelet function are rare and are categorized as either secretory (e.g., storage pool disease) or adhesive (e.g., Glanzmann's thrombasthenia, Bernard-Soulier syndrome). Patients with these disorders are managed conservatively, with platelet transfusions reserved for significant bleeding.

**IV. Platelet transfusion guidelines**

**A. Platelet products.** Platelets can be separated from a unit of donated whole blood (random-donor platelets) or collected by apheresis (single-donor platelets). In patients with thrombocytopenia resulting from a platelet production defect, transfusion of either one single-donor apheresis unit or six random-donor units results in an immediate increment of approximately 30,000/μl. Removing WBC by filtration of whole blood after collection or of pooled random-donor platelets during infusion can reduce the risk of alloimmunization and refractoriness to platelet transfusion in patients who are likely to require chronic platelet support. Single-donor apheresis platelet products are free of significant WBC contamination. Platelets are infused over 30 minutes, and premedication with acetaminophen and diphenhydramine (Benadryl) is indicated if the patient has had a prior platelet transfusion reaction. Many of the risks and complications of RBC transfusion (see Chap. 19, Anemia and Transfusion Therapy) apply to platelet transfusion as well.

**B. Transfusion threshold.** Platelet transfusion is appropriate for asymptomatic outpatients with platelet counts of less than 20,000/μl and asymptomatic inpatients with platelet counts of less than 10,000/μl. Prophylactic transfusion is reasonable for patients with counts of 10,000–20,000/μl if a minor invasive procedure is performed or if a coagulopathy is also present. If a major invasive procedure is performed, a 50,000/μl threshold is generally used. High-risk surgery (e.g., neurosurgery, ophthalmic surgery, cardiopulmonary bypass) may warrant prophylactic transfusion to keep the platelet count greater than 100,000/μl. Platelet transfusion thresholds change if there is evidence of bleeding. For minor mucosal bleeding (minor epistaxis, occult GI bleeding, petechiae), the goal for platelet transfusion is a platelet count greater than 20,000/μl. In the event of major bleeding (postoperative, CNS bleeding), the goal is a level of approximately 100,000/μl. Unless the platelet half-life is shortened severely, as in sepsis, fever, or alloimmunization, there is no rationale for monitoring counts and transfusing more frequently than every 24 hours.

**C. Platelet refractoriness** can be due to alloantibody development in multiply transfused patients and is documented by measuring the platelet count before and 60 minutes after transfusion. An increment of less than 5000/μl after one apheresis unit or six random-donor units indicates refractoriness. Using HLA-matched single-donor platelets, ABO-compatible platelets, or IVIg before transfusion may improve platelet increments.

## Inherited Bleeding Disorders

**I. Hemophilia.** Hemophilia A and B are X-linked coagulation disorders caused by defects in the genes encoding factors VIII and IX, respectively. Deficiencies of these coagulation factors lead to impaired intrinsic pathway coagulation.

**A. Hemophilia A** affects approximately 1 in 5000 live male births. Approximately 30% of cases occur in families with no prior history of hemophilia, reflecting the high rate of spontaneous germ line mutations in the factor VIII gene (*N Engl J Med* 344:662–667, 2001). The clinical phenotype is determined by the factor VIII activity level: severe (<1% activity), moderate (1–5% activity), and mild (>5% activity). Patients with hemophilia have normal primary hemostasis but experience delayed bleeding after trauma or surgery. Patients with severe hemophilia (<1% activity) experience frequent spontaneous hemorrhages, including hemarthroses, hematomas, hematuria, and delayed posttraumatic and postoperative bleeding. Repeated bleeding into a "target" joint can cause chronic synovitis and hemophilic arthropathy. Moderate hemophiliacs have fewer spontaneous bleeding episodes, and mild hemophiliacs may only bleed excessively after trauma or surgery.

1. **Primary therapy** is determined by the severity of the patient's disease and the type of hemorrhage. Patients with mild to moderate hemophilia A and a minor bleeding episode can be treated with **DDAVP,** which increases plasma factor VIII levels by three- to fivefold within 30 minutes, with a half-life of 5–8 hours. The usual dose is 0.3 μg/kg IV (in 50–100 ml normal saline infused over 30 minutes) or SC or 300 μg intranasally (Stimate, 1.5 mg/ml) dosed every 12 hours. Tachyphylaxis may occur after several doses (*Blood* 90:2515–2521, 1997).
2. Patients with mild to moderate hemophilia with major bleeding episodes or those with severe hemophilia with any prolonged source of hemorrhage require **FVIII replacement** for bleeding challenges. This treatment may consist of either purified FVIII concentrate from pooled plasma or recombinant FVIII (rFVIII). The choice of replacement is determined by the availability of product, the patient's history of viral exposure, and patient preference. Testing for viral pathogens combined with viral inactivation procedures has dramatically improved the safety of plasma-derived coagulation factor concentrates. In general, previously untreated patients and those who are HIV and hepatitis B and C negative receive the more expensive rFVIII to minimize the risk of viral transmission. Typically, FVIII levels increase 2% for every 1 U/kg factor VIII concentrate infused with a half-life of 8–12 hours, regardless of type of product. Thus, 50 U/kg IV bolus would be expected to raise factor VIII levels to approximately 100% over baseline. This dosage can be followed by 25 U/kg IV bolus q12h. To stop most mild hemorrhages, infusion of FVIII to achieve peak activities of 30–50% of normal is necessary. Home therapy with factor replacement allows outpatient therapy of minor hemorrhages. One to three doses of factor usually suffice. Moderate to severe hemorrhages require infusions of FVIII to achieve peak activities of 50–100% for adequate hemostasis. Inpatient treatment and dose adjustments guided by daily monitoring of peak and trough FVIII activity may be necessary to ensure adequate hemostasis without wasting expensive concentrates, which are occasionally in short supply (*Hematol Oncol Clin North Am* 12:1315–1344, 1998).
3. **Inhibitors.** Alloantibodies to FVIII and FIX develop in approximately 20% and 12% of severe hemophilia A and B patients, respectively, in response to replacement therapy. These alloantibodies bind to and neutralize the activity of infused FVIII or FIX and prevent correction of the coagulopathy. Determining the titer of a FVIII inhibitor, using a laboratory assay that reports inhibitor strength in Bethesda units (BU), is useful for predicting inhibitor behavior and for guiding therapy. Patients with high inhibitor titers (>5 BU) frequently have rapid anamnestic responses to repeat exposures and are defined as "high responders." Low responders have low inhibitor titers (<5 BU) and usually have minimal anamnesis on repeat exposure to FVIII or FIX. Several treatment options are available for hemophiliacs with potent FVIII or FIX inhibitors.
   a. **Recombinant factor VIIa (rFVIIa, NovoSeven)** is currently approved for use in patients with hemophilia A and B in whom inhibitors to factor replacement have developed. rFVIIa promotes hemostasis by activating the tissue factor/extrinsic pathway. It is available in 1.2-,

2.4-, or 4.8-mg vials and is dosed at 90 μg/kg every 2 hours until hemostasis is achieved (*Semin Hematol* 38[4 Suppl 12]:43–47, 2001).

**b.** Alternative replacement products include **porcine factor VIII (Hyate-C)** and activated prothrombin complex concentrate (Autoplex). Large doses of human FVIII may be effective in hemophiliacs with weak inhibitors (BU <5–10).

**c.** **Gene therapy** for hemophilia A and B is an area of active investigation; however, no therapy has yet been able to increase factor levels sufficiently to eliminate dependence on factor replacement.

**B.** **Hemophilia B** is clinically indistinguishable from hemophilia A, but the distinction is important, as the therapy consists of FIX replacement with either FIX concentrate from pooled plasma or recombinant FIX (BeneFIX). Postinfusion peak and trough targets and duration of replacement for treatment of hemophilia B–related bleeding episodes are similar to the guidelines provided for hemophilia A. Each unit of FIX replacement per kilogram of body weight typically effects a 1% increase in factor IX levels, with a half-life of approximately 24 hours. For moderate to severe bleeding events, a loading dose of 100 U/kg is administered followed by 50 U/kg every 18–24 hours until hemostasis is achieved or 10–14 days postoperatively.

**C.** **von Willebrand's disease,** which represents qualitative or quantitative disorders of vWF, is the most common inherited bleeding disorder, affecting an estimated 0.1% of the population. The spectrum of bleeding is broad, and the inheritance of most forms is autosomal dominant, although autosomal-recessive forms exist. vWF has two important functions: to facilitate adherence of platelets to injured vessel walls and to stabilize factor VIII in plasma. The characteristic clinical findings are mucocutaneous bleeding (epistaxis, menorrhagia, GI bleeding) and easy bruising. Trauma, surgery, or dental extractions may result in life-threatening bleeding in severely affected individuals. Patients with mild disease may remain undiagnosed into adulthood (*Blood* 97:1915–1919, 2001).

**1.** **Classification** follows a revised nomenclature for vWD that recognizes three main types: type 1 vWD, partial quantitative deficiency; type 2 vWD, qualitative deficiency; and type 3 vWD, severe quantitative deficiency. Type 1 accounts for 70–80% of cases, and vWF:Ag and activity are proportionately low. In most subtypes of type 2 vWD, FVIII activity is normal, whereas vWF:RCo is decreased out of proportion to vWF:Ag levels. In type 3 vWD, levels of vWF:Ag are extremely low or undetectable (*Blood* 97:1915–1919, 2001).

**2.** **Diagnosis.** vWF:Ag tests measure circulating vWF protein by immunoassay. A deficiency of vWF is sensitive for type 1 and 3 vWD and may be low normal for type 2 forms. vWF:RCo is a functional test of vWF-mediated agglutination of platelets in the presence of the antibiotic ristocetin. Decreased agglutination is due either to a deficiency of vWF (type 1 and 3) or vWF mutations that cause a selective loss of large multimers (type 2A and B). Factor VIII activity may be low due to a quantitative deficiency of vWF (type 1 and 3) or due to a vWF mutation that reduces FVIII binding to vWF (type 2N vWD). If a qualitative defect in vWF is suspected due to a vWF:Ag greater than vWF:RCo, obtain vWF multimer analysis by gel electrophoresis to determine if large vWF multimers are absent (type 2A and 2B) and a ristocetin-induced platelet aggregation test to distinguish type 2A (attenuated) from type 2B (exaggerated) responses.

**3.** **Management** consists of raising vWF:RCo and factor VIII to levels that ensure adequate hemostasis.

**a.** **Minor bleeding** in type 1 vWD usually responds to DDAVP. A test dose should be administered, and FVIII increase confirmed, to determine each patient's responsiveness. DDAVP usually is not effective in type 2A vWD and is contraindicated in type 2B due to the risk of postinfusion thrombocytopenia, and it is not useful in type 3 vWD (for dosing, see sec. **I.A.1**). Oral contraceptives may be useful for management of menorrhagia. vWF:RCo levels of greater than 50% are sufficient to correct most minor hemorrhages.

**b. Severe bleeding** and **major surgery** require vWF replacement provided by infusion of vWF as intermediate purity FVIII concentrates (Alphanate or Humate-P) or cryoprecipitate q12–24h to raise vWF:RCo levels to 100% initially and maintain them between 50% and 100% until healing is complete (typically 5–10 days). Factor VIII activity is usually used as a surrogate marker because STAT in vitro measurement of vWF:RCo is rarely available. In general, 50 IU vWF:RCo/kg raises the vWF:RCo level to 100%. High-purity (monoclonal) plasma-derived and recombinant FVIII concentrates do not contain vWF and should not be used for vWD. Cryoprecipitate contains significant amounts of vWF and FVIII and is an alternative replacement product; however, it does not undergo viral inactivation. Type 1 vWD patients who are undergoing minor invasive procedures can receive DDAVP 1 hour before surgery and q12–24h for 2–3 days postoperatively, with or without the oral antifibrinolytic drug aminocaproic acid (Amicar), but for more extensive surgery vWF should be administered. In type 3 vWD, platelet transfusions may complement infusions of vWF to control bleeding by releasing vWF stored in alpha granules at the site of vascular injury (*Blood* 97:1915–1919, 2001).

## Acquired Coagulation Disorders

**I. Vitamin K deficiency** is usually caused by malabsorption states or poor dietary intake combined with antibiotic-associated loss of intestinal bacterial colonization. Hepatocytes require vitamin K to complete the synthesis (gamma-carboxylation) of clotting factors (II, VII, IX, X) and the natural anticoagulant proteins C and S. Vitamin K deficiency is suspected when an at-risk patient has a prolonged PT that corrects after a 1:1 mix with normal pooled plasma.

**A. Vitamin K replacement** can be given orally, subcutaneously, or intravenously. Vitamin K absorption is variable when administered subcutaneously, especially in edematous patients, and intravenous vitamin K is effective but carries the risk of anaphylaxis. Oral administration is superior to subcutaneous vitamin K for reversing the effects of warfarin in outpatients (*Ann Intern Med* 137:251–254, 2002). With adequate replacement therapy, the PT should begin to normalize within 12 hours and should normalize completely in 24–48 hours.

**B. FFP** rapidly but temporarily corrects acquired coagulopathies secondary to vitamin K deficiency and is indicated in patients who are actively bleeding or who require immediate invasive procedures. The usual starting dose is 2 U (400–450 ml), with measurement of the PT and aPTT after the infusion to determine the need for additional therapy. Up to 10–15 ml/kg may be needed for severe bleeding with significant PT prolongation. Because factor VII has a half-life of only 6 hours, the PT may again become prolonged and require additional FFP. Vitamin K replacement is initiated concomitantly with FFP.

**II. Liver disease** can seriously impair hemostasis because coagulation factors, with the exception of vWF, are produced in the liver. Hemostatic abnormalities associated with liver disease are usually stable unless liver synthetic function is rapidly worsening, as in fulminant hepatic failure (*N Engl J Med* 305:242–248, 1981). Other complications of end-stage liver disease that may lead to abnormal hemostasis include portal hypertension, leading to hypersplenism with splenic sequestration of platelets, and cholestasis, which impairs vitamin K absorption. **Vitamin K** replacement may be helpful in correcting mild prolongation of the PT in liver dysfunction; however, this is not effective if hepatic synthetic dysfunction is the underlying etiology. **FFP** is indicated for patients who are bleeding or require an invasive procedure and have abnormal coagulation parameters (PT or aPTT >1½ times control). **Cryoprecipitate,** a concentrated source of fibrinogen, can be given at a dose of 1.5 U/10 kg body weight to correct severe hypofibrinogenemia (<100 mg/dl) if there is bleeding or the need for invasive procedures. This should be followed by periodic measurement of the fibrinogen level. **Platelet transfusion** is indicated for bleeding in the setting of thrombocytopenia, especially for counts of less than 20,000/ml.

**III. Disseminated intravascular coagulation (DIC)** is seen in a variety of systemic illnesses, including sepsis, trauma, burns, shock, obstetric complications, and malignancies (notably, acute promyelocytic leukemia). The underlying cause is exposure of tissue factor to the circulation, which leads to the generation of tissue factor/FVIIa complexes followed by excessive and uncontrolled generation of thrombin and fibrin, generalized microthrombi, and consumption of platelets, coagulation factors and regulators (protein C, protein S, antithrombin). **Clinical consequences** include diffuse bleeding, global organ dysfunction secondary to microvascular thrombi and ischemia, and, less often, large arterial and venous thrombosis (*N Engl J Med* 341:586–592, 1999). Although no one test confirms a diagnosis of DIC, affected patients commonly have prolonged PT and aPTT, thrombocytopenia, low fibrinogen levels, elevated fibrin degradation products, and a positive D-dimer. **Treatment** consists of supportive care, correction of the underlying disorder if possible, and administration of FFP, cryoprecipitate, and platelets (see secs. **I** and **II**), as needed. The use of heparin to prevent thrombosis in DIC is controversial, but adjusted-dose **heparin** (see Anticoagulants, sec. **I**) is appropriate therapy for large-vessel thrombosis in DIC.

**IV. Acquired inhibitors of coagulation factors** may arise de novo or may develop in hemophiliacs who have been exposed to factor replacement. The most common acquired specific inhibitor is directed against factor VIII. Patients present with an abrupt onset of bleeding, prolonged aPTT that does not correct after 1:1 mixing, and a normal PT. Bleeding complications in patients with acquired factor VIII inhibitors are managed in the same manner as for hemophiliacs with acquired alloantibodies to factor VIII (see the section Inherited Bleeding Disorders). Long-term therapy consists of immunosuppression with cyclophosphamide, prednisone, rituximab, or vincristine to reduce production of the autoantibody (*Blood* 100:3426–3428, 2002).

**V. Disorders of fibrinogen** may be acquired or, rarely, inherited. Fibrinogen is an acute-phase reactant whose synthesis in the liver is increased by inflammatory states or malignancy. Hyperfibrinogenemia is associated with an increased risk for arterial and venous thrombotic events. Hypofibrinogenemia secondary to decreased liver synthesis and dysfibrinogenemia secondary to production of abnormal fibrinogen molecules leading to delayed fibrin polymerization can cause impaired coagulation (*J Clin Invest* 60:89–95, 1977). Characteristic laboratory findings consist of prolonged thrombin and reptilase times.

**VI. Use of anticoagulants.** Hospitalized patients often receive heparin during peripheral IV or central venous catheter flushes or may have blood drawn through heparinized lines. Coagulation studies consistent with warfarin effect and an otherwise negative evaluation may indicate accidental or surreptitious ingestion of warfarin. Detection of warfarin metabolites in serum is a confirmatory test. Ingestion of anticoagulant rodenticides containing "superwarfarin" (brodifacoum) causes prolonged elevation of the PT lasting up to 1 year. FFP and vitamin K are indicated for patients with associated bleeding. Standard doses of vitamin K are usually not sufficient to correct this coagulopathy, and high doses (100–150 mg/day orally) are required until the PT normalizes (*Arch Intern Med* 158:1929–1932, 1998).

## Thromboembolic Disorders

**Venous thromboembolism (VTE)** consists of **deep venous thrombosis (DVT)** and **pulmonary embolism (PE)**. VTE is often unsuspected, leading to diagnostic and therapeutic delays that can increase morbidity and mortality. DVTs most commonly develop in the lower limbs, and half cause pulmonary emboli in the absence of treatment. Venous thromboemboli arise under conditions of stasis, hypercoagulability, and acute trauma to venous endothelial surfaces. Hypercoagulable states may be inherited or acquired, such as those seen in cancer patients (see secs. **V**. and **VI**).

**I. Diagnosis of DVT.** Venous thrombosis is typically described by anatomic location. Thrombosis in the lower extremity can be classified as *deep* or *superficial* and as *proximal* or *distal*. The *superficial femoral vein* is actually a deep vein, and its preferred term is *femoral vein*. A lower extremity DVT found in or superior to the popliteal vein is considered **proximal,** whereas a DVT that is found inferior to the popliteal vein is considered **distal.** DVTs that arise from the proximal veins of the lower extremities and pelvis primarily produce PE. Calf vein DVTs uncommonly cause significant emboli, unless they propagate proximally. Up to 30% of untreated calf vein DVTs extend into the proximal lower extremity, and some cause PE. DVTs that occur in upper extremity veins, often secondary to an indwelling catheter, may also cause PE.

**A. History and physical examination** are neither sensitive nor specific for DVT. Thus, the presence of symptoms or signs such as pain or edema implies the need for objective diagnostic testing. However, pretest assessment of the probability of a DVT is still useful, when combined with the results of compression ultrasound or a D-dimer test, or both, in determining whether to exclude or accept the diagnosis of DVT or perform additional imaging studies (*Lancet* 350:1795–1798, 1997). Clinical suspicion may dictate the speed and type of evaluation.

**B.** The **differential diagnosis** for unilateral lower extremity **swelling** includes Baker's cysts, hematoma, venous insufficiency, lymphedema, sarcoma, arterial aneurysm, myositis, cellulitis, rupture of the medial head of the gastrocnemius, and abscess. Additional diseases to consider in association with lower extremity **pain** include musculoskeletal and arteriovascular disorders. Compression ultrasound, MRI, and CT are useful for detecting pathology other than DVT.

**C. Diagnostic testing**

**1.** The initial diagnostic test for symptomatic acute DVT should be a **noninvasive test,** typically **compression ultrasound** (called *duplex examination* when performed with Doppler testing) (*Am J Respir Crit Care Med* 160:1043, 1999). Compression ultrasound is not sensitive at detecting calf DVT and may fail to visualize other veins as well, especially parts of the deep femoral vein, part of the upper extremity venous system, and the pelvic veins. Noninvasive testing is also difficult to interpret in the setting of an old DVT, unless the original thrombus is known to have resolved. Noninvasive testing has a low sensitivity in asymptomatic patients.

**a. Serial noninvasive testing** can improve the diagnostic yield. If the initial noninvasive test is negative in a patient with a clinically suspected lower extremity DVT, anticoagulant therapy may be withheld provided that testing is repeated at least once 3–14 days later.

**b. Simplified compression ultrasound** limited to the common femoral vein in the groin and the popliteal vein down to the trifurcation of the calf veins is not as sensitive as a complete examination; however, repeating simplified noninvasive tests within a few weeks improves sensitivity. When noninvasive testing or patient follow-up is unreliable, complete noninvasive testing or venography should be used.

2. **Venography** is the gold standard technique for diagnosing DVT, although it requires placement of a pedal IV catheter, administration of iodinated contrast, and exposure to radiation. Thus, noninvasive tests are preferred in symptomatic patients with suspected DVT. Contraindications to venography include renal dysfunction and dye allergy.
3. **D-Dimer** is a cross-linked fibrin degradation product. Various assays are available, and each differs in accuracy (see Table H-2 in Appendix H, Clinical Epidemiology). D-dimer testing has a low positive predictive value, and thus, **patients with a positive test require further evaluation.** In contrast, the negative predictive value of a negative D-dimer is high enough to exclude a DVT when a noninvasive test is negative (*Arch Intern Med* 157:1077, 1997) and/or the clinical probability is low (http://med.mssm.edu/ebm/cpr/dvt2.html). In settings in which the pretest probability is moderate or high, including patients with cancer, a negative D-dimer test is not useful because it does not have a sufficient negative predictive value to rule out DVT (*Ann Intern Med* 131:17, 1999).
4. **MRI** is noninvasive and has demonstrated good sensitivity for acute, symptomatic proximal DVT in small studies.
5. **CT venography** is being used to diagnose DVT in conjunction with a contrast-enhanced spiral CT for diagnosis of PE (see sec. **II.C.2** and Table H-2 in Appendix H, Clinical Epidemiology). CT venography allows for visualization of the veins in the abdomen, pelvis, and proximal lower extremities. Use of spiral CT for DVT evaluation appears to be less accurate than CT for PE diagnosis (*Ann Intern Med* 132:227, 2000).

**II. Diagnosis of PE** involves performance of a careful history and physical examination to establish clinical suspicion, followed by judicious use of diagnostic testing to confirm the diagnosis and rapidly initiate appropriate therapies.

**A. History and physical examination.** Symptoms and signs of PE are neither sensitive nor specific. Predictors of PE include shortness of breath, chest pain (pleuritic), hypoxemia, hemoptysis, pleural rub, new right-sided heart failure, and tachycardia (*Ann Intern Med* 129:997, 1998). Validated **clinical risk factors** for a PE in outpatients who present to an emergency department include signs and symptoms of DVT, high suspicion of PE by the clinician, tachycardia, immobility in the past 4 weeks, history of VTE, active cancer, and hemoptysis (*Ann Intern Med* 129:997, 1998). **Clinical suspicion of PE should lead to objective diagnostic evaluation.** Nondiagnostic tests such as electrocardiography, blood gases, and chest radiography may help determine the pretest probability, focus the differential diagnosis, and assess the cardiopulmonary reserve.

**B.** The **differential diagnosis** of PE includes dissecting aortic aneurysm, pneumonia, acute bronchitis, bronchocarcinoma, pericardial or **pleural disease, heart failure, costochondritis, and myocardial ischemia.**

**C. Diagnostic testing** (*Am J Respir Crit Care Med* 160:1043–1066, 1999).

1. **Ventilation-perfusion ($\dot{V}/\dot{Q}$) scanning** requires administration of radioactive material (via both inhaled and IV routes). $\dot{V}/\dot{Q}$ scanning is most useful in a patient with a normal chest radiograph, because nondiagnostic scans are extremely common in the setting of an abnormal chest radiograph. $\dot{V}/\dot{Q}$ scans may be classified as normal, nondiagnostic (i.e., very low probability, low probability, intermediate probability), or high probability for pulmonary embolism. Clinical suspicion improves the accuracy of $\dot{V}/\dot{Q}$ scanning: In patients with normal or high probability $\dot{V}/\dot{Q}$ scans and matching pretest clinical suspicion, the accuracy is 96% (*JAMA* 263:2753, 1990). When the $\dot{V}/\dot{Q}$ findings and the pretest probability conflict, further testing should be performed. See Table H-2 in Appendix H, Clinical Epidemiology, for sensitivity and specificity data.

2. **Contrast-enhanced spiral (helical) chest CT** requires IV administration of iodinated contrast and exposure to radiation. Used according to standardized protocols in conjunction with expert interpretation, spiral CT appears accurate for large (proximal) pulmonary emboli, but the sensitivity is lower for small (distal) emboli (see Table H-2 in Appendix H, Clinical Epidemiology). In contrast to $\dot{V}/\dot{Q}$ scans, most spiral CT scans produce a diagnostic result (positive or negative), with fewer indeterminate or inadequate studies. CT has the benefit of suggesting alternative diagnoses, such as dissecting aortic aneurysm, pneumonia, malignancy, pleural disease, and so forth. Contraindications to spiral CT include renal dysfunction and dye allergy.
3. **MRI** appears to be sensitive for diagnosing acute PE. Similar to spiral CT, MRI may provide alternative diagnoses. The role of MRI in the diagnosis of PE is not clearly defined.
4. **D-Dimer** testing is sensitive but not specific for diagnosing PE. Consequently, **patients with a positive test require further evaluation.** However, a negative D-dimer in combination with low pretest probability can exclude almost all PE (*Ann Intern Med* 129:1006, 1998). Thus, some experts reserve the use of D-dimer for patients who have a low pretest probability for PE (*Arch Intern Med* 161:567, 2001).
5. **Pulmonary angiography** is the gold standard for diagnosing PE, although noninvasive tests are preferred for the initial evaluation. Even though angiography is the gold standard, it can be inadequate or inaccurate in some situations. Angiography requires placement of a pulmonary artery catheter, infusion of IV contrast, and exposure to radiation. Contraindications to angiography include renal dysfunction and dye allergy.
6. **Noninvasive testing of the legs** (see sec. **I.C.1**) is useful for a patient with a suspected PE who has a nondiagnostic $\dot{V}/\dot{Q}$ scan and in a patient with a nondiagnostic or negative CT scan without an alternative explanation for symptoms, serving as an alternative means to diagnose venous thromboembolic disease. However, further evaluation is required if the noninvasive test is negative.

**III. Treatment and management of PE and proximal DVT.** The ideal strategy for management of DVT and PE is to identify patients at high risk of thromboembolism and to institute prophylactic measures (see Chap. 1, Patient Care in Internal Medicine, sec. **I.D**). The goals of VTE therapy are to reduce the immediate risk of PE and long-term complications of the postphlebitic syndrome (pain, edema, and possibly ulceration after DVT), pulmonary hypertension, and recurrent VTE.

**Initial treatment** of VTE should consist of parenteral anticoagulation, either with IV **UFH** or SC **LMWH.** A CBC and PT/aPTT should be obtained before starting UFH/LMWH to detect preexisting cytopenias, coagulopathies, or lupus anticoagulant (LA) and to serve as baselines to monitor UFH infusion, development of HIT, and bleeding. A platelet count should be monitored during days 4–10 in patients treated with UFH or LMWH, and earlier if the patient has been exposed to UFH within the past 100 days (*Arch Pathol Lab Med* 126:1415–1423, 2002). If the clinical presentation is highly suspicious for inherited hypercoagulable risk factors, testing ideally should be delayed until some future time when the patient is in stable health and off anticoagulation therapy for at least 2 weeks. If there is a compelling reason to screen for hypercoagulable risk factors immediately, specimens for measuring protein C, protein S, and antithrombin should be collected before starting anticoagulation therapy. Although normal levels rule out congenital deficiencies, an abnormal, low result requires repeat testing to confirm or screening first-degree relatives to rule out a temporary deficiency related to the acute thrombosis.

**A. UFH** therapy is initiated with a 60 U/kg IV bolus followed by a continuous infusion at 14 U/kg/hour (Table 18-3). aPTT should be measured every 6 hours thereafter. For a complete discussion of UFH therapy, see Anticoagulants, sec. **I.**

**Table 18-3.** Weight-based heparin dosing[a]

| | |
|---|---|
| Initial therapy | |
| Bolus | 60 U/kg[b] |
| Infusion | 14 U/kg/hr |
| Adjustments[c] | |
| aPTT <40 | 3000 U IV bolus; increase infusion by 3 U/kg/hr |
| aPTT 40–50 | 2000 U IV bolus; increase infusion by 2 U/kg/hr |
| aPTT 45–70 | No change |
| aPTT 71–80 | Decrease infusion by 1 U/kg/hr |
| aPTT 81–90 | Hold for 0.5 h; decrease infusion by 2 U/kg/hr |
| aPTT >90 | Hold for 1 h; decrease infusion by 3 U/kg/hr |

*Note:* Target activated partial thromboplastin time (aPTT) can vary among hospitals depending on reagents and instruments used.
[a]Round all doses to nearest 100 U.
[b]Maximum, 5000 U.
[c]Draw aPTT 6 hours after any bolus or change in infusion rate.
*Source:* Barnes-Jewish Hospital Pharmacy, St. Louis, MO.

**B. LMWH** can be administered on an inpatient or outpatient basis. Patients selected for outpatient therapy should be ambulatory, have adequate cardiopulmonary reserve, have received instruction in the warning signs of abnormal bleeding, have access to a telephone and transportation, be able to inject the drug or have a responsible caretaker, and have adequate outpatient follow-up with a physician who can manage daily INRs or complications (*Chest* 115:972, 1999). Long-term anticoagulation with LMWH is the first choice in **pregnant** women with thromboses, and it is an alternative for patients who have clearly **failed oral anticoagulation** (objectively confirmed new DVT/PE despite consistently therapeutic INRs) or have unacceptable INR lability. For a complete discussion of LMWH therapy, see Anticoagulants, sec. **II.**

**C. Thrombolytic therapy** may be appropriate for patients with PE and systemic hypotension (*Chest* 119:1768, 2001). Compared to heparin alone, thrombolytic therapy for DVT causes more bleeding complications and produces more rapid and complete vein patency rates. However, there is no definitive evidence that thrombolytic therapy reduces the incidence and severity of the postphlebitic syndrome. Thrombolytic therapy could be considered for patients with massive iliofemoral DVT causing venous congestion that compromises the arterial supply to the limb. Currently, no consensus has been reached regarding the use of systemic versus catheter-directed thrombolysis. Systemic therapy is more effective than catheter delivery but is associated with an increased risk of major bleeding, including intracranial hemorrhage, and PE (*J Am Coll Cardiol* 36:1336–1343, 2000).

**D. Inferior vena cava (IVC) filters** should be reserved for acute DVT situations in which there are absolute contraindications to anticoagulation: active bleeding, severe thrombocytopenia, urgent surgery, or recurrent thromboemboli despite therapeutic anticoagulation. Relative indications for IVC filters that require individualized decision making include primary or metastatic CNS cancer, free-floating proximal iliac vein thrombi, or patients with limited cardiopulmonary reserve. Anticoagulation therapy should be resumed when it is safe to do so to reduce the risk of filter-related thromboses. Prophylactic IVC filters in patients with acute DVT/PE do not reduce overall mortality and increase DVT recurrences (*N Engl J Med* 338:409–415, 1993).

**E. Warfarin** (typically 5 mg) can be started on the first day of heparin therapy, with daily INR monitoring and dose adjustments as indicated. UFH/LMWH

**Table 18-4.** Warfarin nomogram

| Day | INR | Dosage (mg) |
|---|---|---|
| 2 | <1.5 | 5.0 |
| | 1.5–1.9 | 2.5 |
| | 2.0–2.5 | 1.0–2.5 |
| | >2.5 | 0 |
| 3 | <1.5 | 5.0–10.0 |
| | 1.5–1.9 | 2.5–5.0 |
| | 2.0–3.0 | 0.0–2.5 |
| | <3.0 | 0 |
| 4 | <1.5 | 10.0 |
| | 1.5–1.9 | 5.0–7.5 |
| | 2.0–3.0 | 0.0–5.0 |
| | >3.0 | 0 |
| 5 | <1.5 | 10.0 |
| | 1.5–1.9 | 7.5–10.0 |
| | 2.0–3.0 | 0.0–5.0 |
| | >3.0 | 0 |

INR, international normalized ratio.
*Source:* Adapted from *Ann Intern Med* 127:333, 1997.

is continued for at least 5 days, as the initial INR rise primarily reflects depletion of factor VII with relatively little depletion of factor II, while the anticoagulant effects of proteins C and S are reduced by warfarin (*Arch Intern Med* 159:1005, 1998). In addition, UFH/LMWH should be continued until INRs of greater than 2.0 are achieved on 2 consecutive days. After an initial 5-mg dose, warfarin induction can be guided by an algorithm (Table 18-4). Because it often takes several weeks to determine a patient's stable warfarin dose, INRs should be monitored frequently during the first month. Thereafter, monitoring should be performed at least every 4 weeks in patients with a high percentage of therapeutic INRs and stable warfarin doses and more often in those with labile INRs. More frequent monitoring is required when medications are added or discontinued, especially antibiotics, due to potential interactions with warfarin metabolism. For further information on warfarin therapy, see Anticoagulants, sec. **IV.**

**F. Duration of anticoagulation** must be individualized for each patient based on an assessment of his or her risk of recurrent DVT off therapy versus the risk of bleeding complications with continued anticoagulation. In addition, the patient's level of concern regarding these potential complications should be considered.

1. **DVTs due to reversible risk factors** (surgery, major trauma) are at very low risk of recurrence, and anticoagulation can be stopped after 3 months.
2. **Idiopathic DVT/PE** and VTE associated with less compelling risk factors, such as prolonged travel, oral contraceptive pills/hormone replacement therapy, or minor injuries, typically benefit from 6 months of OAT. No definite guidelines have been established for the duration of anticoagulant therapy for most patients with spontaneous DVTs, regardless of whether inherited hypercoagulable risk factors are present. After 6–12 months of oral anticoagulation (INR 2–3), options include stopping OAT, long-term OAT (ELATE study, *N Engl J Med* 349:631–639, 2003), or

long-term OAT at a lower target INR (1.5–2.0) (PREVENT study, *N Engl J Med* 348:1425–1434, 2003). If treatment is discontinued, temporary prophylactic anticoagulation is required during periods of increased VTE risk, including surgery, trauma, immobilization, hospitalization for medical illnesses, and postpartum. Infusion of ATIII concentrate should be considered in congenitally deficient patients during an acute thrombosis, perioperatively, and during pregnancy (*Br J Haemotol* 50:531–535, 1982).

3. **Isolated calf vein DVT** is treated with anticoagulation if it is symptomatic. If not treated with anticoagulation, patients with calf vein DVTs should undergo serial compression ultrasonography to assess for proximal extension, which would mandate anticoagulant therapy. Duration of treatment is determined in the manner outlined above.
4. Patients with **recurrent idiopathic VTE** should receive anticoagulation for life or until a contraindication develops.

**G. Special circumstances**

1. **Perioperative management of VTE** requires close coordination with the surgical service (see Perioperative Medicine in Chap. 1, Patient Care in Internal Medicine). The benefit of treatment should be weighed against the risk of hemorrhage by individual case. If an absolute contraindication to anticoagulation exists, IVC filter placement should be considered for patients with acute VTE. **Holding warfarin** for 4–5 days before surgery allows the INR to drift below 1.5 (*Ann Intern Med* 122:40, 1995). If anticoagulation is needed until just before surgery, LMWH or UFH can be given, with discontinuation of LMWH 24 hours before surgery and discontinuation of UFH at least 6 hours before surgery.
2. **VTE in pregnancy.** Elevated estrogen levels, decreased mobility, and pressure on the IVC and iliac veins predispose to the development of DVT in the peripartum period. The recommendations for DVT prophylaxis and postpartum anticoagulation vary depending on the patient's history of DVT and/or thrombophilia. In general, postpartum anticoagulation for 4–6 weeks is recommended for all women with a history of DVT or thrombophilia. DVT prophylaxis during pregnancy with UFH or LMWH is recommended for women with a history of DVT and thrombophilia, especially antithrombin deficiency. In patients with APA syndrome and recurrent fetal loss, the addition of low-dose aspirin to this regimen may help to reduce complications in pregnancy. Women with a history of DVT associated with transient risk factors or idiopathic DVT, or thrombophilia without a history of DVT, may be followed with surveillance compression venous ultrasounds or may be treated prophylactically as clinically indicated. A first DVT occurring during pregnancy is treated with LMWH or UFH, with treatment held for 24 hours before the induction of labor. Because warfarin is teratogenic, pregnant patients with mechanical heart valves are managed as inpatients with UFH or as outpatients with adjusted SC UFH to maintain the aPTT at twice normal or anti-Xa heparin level of 0.35–0.70 (*Chest* 119[Suppl]:122s–131s, 2001). Caution is advised when considering the use of LMWH for thromboprophylaxis in pregnant patients with mechanical heart valves because enoxaparin in this setting has been associated with valve thrombosis and sudden death. Heparin does not cross the placenta and is not excreted in breast milk.
3. **Upper extremity DVTs** should be diagnosed and managed like lower extremity DVTs. Some do occur spontaneously; however, most are associated with indwelling venous catheters used for chemotherapy, total parenteral nutrition, or antibiotic therapy. Catheter-associated DVT rates are highest in cancer patients, ranging from 12–38%, and many are asymptomatic. Pulmonary emboli can occur, but the incidence and significance of this complication are disputed. No consensus has been reached on management of symptomatic catheter-associated thrombosis. Treatment options include elevation of the affected arm, catheter

removal, anticoagulation with heparin followed by warfarin, and thrombolytic therapy. Prophylactic anticoagulation with warfarin 1.0 mg/day (*Ann Int Med* 112:423–428, 1990) or dalteparin (Fragmin) 2500 IU/day (*Thromb Haemost* 74:251–253, 1996) has been studied and is beneficial in selected patients with central venous catheters.

IV. **Superficial thrombophlebitis** is associated with varicose veins, trauma, infection, and hypercoagulable disorders. **It presents as a tender, warm, erythematous, and often palpable thrombosed vein.** Initial treatment consists of elevation, heat, NSAIDs, and compression stockings. Because superficial venous thrombosis can be a sign of DVT, compression ultrasound is recommended to rule out DVT. Most resolve within a few weeks with symptomatic therapy. Recurrent superficial thrombophlebitis may be treated with anticoagulation or vein stripping (*Angiology* 50:523, 1999).

V. **Inherited thrombophilic disorders** are suggested by a history of spontaneous VTE at a young age (<50 years), recurrent VTE, documented VTE in first-degree relatives, thrombosis in unusual anatomic locations, and recurrent fetal loss. The established inherited risk factors for VTE include two gene polymorphisms that are common in whites (factor V Leiden and prothrombin gene G20210A), and deficiencies of the natural anticoagulants protein C, protein S, and antithrombin. Hyperhomocystinemia is an uncommon inborn error of metabolism associated with extremely high plasma homocysteine and arterial and venous thromboembolic events in childhood. More commonly, milder homocysteine elevations arise from an interaction between genetic mutations that affect enzymes involved in homocysteine metabolism and acquired factors such as inadequate folate consumption (*N Engl J Med* 344:1222–1231, 2001). Although elevated factor VIII activity and factor XI and IX antigen concentrations are also associated with a mildly increased risk for VTE, expert opinions remain divided regarding the utility of these tests for guiding individual patient management. No compelling evidence has been found that inherited deficiencies of protein C, protein S or antithrombin, or factor V Leiden and prothrombin G20210A mutations are important risk factors for arterial disease, and routine ordering of these tests is not recommended in patients with myocardial infarction, ischemic stroke, or peripheral vascular disease.

VI. **Acquired hypercoagulable states** may arise secondary to malignancy, nephrotic syndrome, estrogen use, pregnancy, and central venous catheters. Any condition leading to prolonged immobilization (trauma, surgery, and other major medical illnesses) predisposes to development of thromboemboli. Both heparin-induced thrombocytopenia and the APA syndrome can cause arterial or venous thrombi. Unusual spontaneous thromboses, such as cavernous sinus thrombosis, mesenteric vein thrombosis, or portal vein thrombosis, may be the initial presentation of paroxysmal nocturnal hemoglobinuria (PNH), and flow cytometry for PNH markers on red cells or leukocytes is indicated under these circumstances. Patients with a history of spontaneous thrombosis even in the absence of an inherited thrombophilia are predisposed to the development of future thromboses (*N Engl J Med* 344:1222–1231, 2001). (See Table 18-5 for guidelines to the laboratory evaluation of thrombophilic states.)

**Antiphospholipid antibody (APA) syndrome** is defined by the occurrence of arterial or venous thrombosis, thrombocytopenia, or recurrent fetal loss in the presence of autoantibodies that react with negatively charged phospholipids. APAs are a heterogeneous group of autoantibodies that are detected with serologic tests (anticardiolipin antibodies, IgG and IgM) or clotting assays [lupus anticoagulant (LA)], which are prolonged in their presence. Performing both assays improves sensitivity. The aPTT may be elevated in LA patients but does not predispose to bleeding. At least 10% of patients with SLE have evidence of LAs; however, most patients with LAs do not have SLE. **Therapy** for isolated asymptomatic APAs is not warranted. Acute thrombosis is treated with heparin, although monitoring in an LA patient with an elevated baseline aPTT is problematic. Options include measuring heparin activity (anti-Xa) or treating with LMWH without monitoring. The duration and intensity of oral anticoagulation depend on patient-

**Table 18-5.** Laboratory evaluation of thrombophilic states

| **Inherited thrombophilia** | **Laboratory assessment** |
|---|---|
| Prothrombin gene mutation | G20210A mutation |
| Protein C deficiency | Protein C activity |
| Protein S deficiency | Free protein S antigen |
| Antithrombin deficiency | Antithrombin heparin cofactor activity |
| Factor V Leiden | Activated protein C resistance, if positive factor V Leiden PCR confirmation |
| Hyperhomocystinemia | Fasting plasma homocysteine level |
| **Acquired thrombophilias** | **Laboratory assessment** |
| Antiphospholipid antibody syndrome | Anticardiolipin antibody, lupus anticoagulant |
| PNH | RBC or WBC flow cytometry for CD55, CD59, CD24 |

PCR, polymerase chain reaction; PNH, paroxysmal nocturnal hemoglobinuria.

specific assessment of risk for recurrent thrombosis versus risk of bleeding complications. Typically, indefinite warfarin therapy (target INR, 2.5; range, 2–3) is recommended for patients with thrombotic complications associated with antiphospholipid syndrome. Women with APA and recurrent fetal loss have been managed successfully through pregnancy with aspirin, prednisone, and heparin, alone or in combination [*N Engl J Med* 346(10):752–763, 2002].

## Anticoagulants

**Anticoagulants** are used to treat or prevent thromboses and generally have narrow therapeutic windows. Bleeding is the major complication of anticoagulation, occurring in 1.2–2.0% of patients who receive unfractionated heparin and 0.5–2.0% of patients receiving LMWH (*N Engl J Med* 334:677–681, 1996). Concomitant use of antiplatelet agents increases the risk of bleeding and should be avoided if possible. Occult GI bleeding is a relative contraindication to anticoagulation and warrants investigation for an underlying anatomic abnormality. Concurrent use of heparin or LMWH with spinal punctures and epidurals should be avoided because of the risk of development of **spinal hematomas.** If mild bleeding occurs during heparin use, discontinuation is usually sufficient to restore normal hemostasis. For major bleeding episodes, heparin can be completely reversed by infusion of **protamine sulfate.** Approximately 1 mg protamine sulfate IV neutralizes 100 U of circulating heparin, up to a maximum dose of 250 mg. Because of the risk of anaphylaxis with rapid infusion, protamine is administered IV over 10 minutes. Protamine sulfate is less effective for reversal of LMWH, neutralizing only approximately 60% (*Br J Haematol* 116:178–186, 2002).

I. **Unfractionated heparin** is derived from porcine intestinal mucosa or bovine lung tissue and is administered IV or SC. It catalyzes the inactivation of thrombin and factor Xa by antithrombin. Factor VIIa is unaffected. Therefore, heparin administration at usual doses prolongs the TT and aPTT, but generally not the PT. Because the anticoagulant effects of heparin administration normalize within hours of discontinuation and heparin is reversible with protamine sulfate, it is the therapy of choice for patients with increased

**Table 18-6.** Low-molecular-weight heparin dosages for treatment of deep venous thrombosis

| Drug | Dosage |
|---|---|
| Enoxaparin | Outpatient: 1.0 mg/kg SC q12h |
| | Inpatient: 1.0 mg/kg SC q12h *or* 1.5 mg/kg SC q24h |
| Tinzaparin | 175 IU/kg SC qd[a] |
| Dalteparin | 200 IU/kg SC qd[b] |

IU, anti-Xa units; for enoxaparin, 1.0 mg = 100 anti-Xa units.
[a]U.S. Food and Drug Administration (FDA) approved for treatment of pulmonary embolism in absence of deep venous thrombosis.
[b]Not an FDA-approved indication.

risk of bleeding. For **DVT prophylaxis,** the dosage is 5000 U SC q8–12h, and aPTT monitoring is not necessary. For **therapeutic anticoagulation,** heparin is administered IV by weight-based dosing, with a bolus followed by continuous infusion. This method provides the most rapid and reliable prolongation of the aPTT into the therapeutic range (*Ann Intern Med* 119:874, 1993). Clearance is prolonged in hepatic and renal dysfunction. Table 18-5 provides an example of a weight-based dosing algorithm; however, the therapeutic aPTT range can vary among hospitals, depending on reagents and instruments used. It is possible to measure plasma heparin activity directly and adjust the heparin infusion rate to obtain a therapeutic concentration; however, few hospital laboratories currently offer STAT heparin activities. Consultation with your hospital pharmacy and clinical laboratory is recommended to determine how each hospital-specific therapeutic range is determined. Because of the risk of HIT (see the section Platelet Disorders), frequent platelet counts are recommended when heparin is administered by any route. Osteoporosis is a potential complication of long-term heparin use.

II. **LMWH** preparations (Table 18-6) are comprised of smaller fractions of the heparin molecule and are administered subcutaneously. LMWH inactivates factor Xa to a greater extent than it does thrombin; therefore, the aPTT is minimally prolonged at therapeutic plasma concentrations. Extensive clinical trials confirm that weight-based dosing of LMWH without laboratory monitoring of anticoagulant effect is safe and efficacious. However, LMWH pharmacokinetics may not be as reliable in patients with a creatinine clearance of less than 30 ml/minute, in patients whose weight is greater than 100 kg, or in women who are pregnant (*N Engl J Med* 337:688–699, 1997). To ensure therapeutic anticoagulation with LMWH for such patients, peak plasma LMWH activity (anti-Xa activity), measured 4 hours after a subcutaneous dose, should be 0.6–1.0 IU/ml for q12h dosing and 1.0–2.0 IU/ml for q24h dosing (*Blood* 99:3102–3110, 2002). The incidence of osteoporosis appears to be lower than that of unfractionated heparin. Although LMWH is less likely to induce HIT, most antibodies to the PF4/heparin complex cross-react with LMWH, and therefore LMWH should not be substituted for heparin in thrombocytopenic patients with suspected HIT (*Blood* 101:31–37, 2003).

III. **Fondaparinux** is a synthetic pentasaccharide that is a selective inhibitor of factor Xa. It is structurally similar to the region of the heparin molecule that binds antithrombin and is currently approved for DVT prophylaxis in patients undergoing total hip replacement (*N Engl J Med* 345:18, 2001). Unlike other LMWH, it does not appear to cross react with HIT antibodies (*Blood* 101:31–37, 2003). The recommended dose is 2.5 mg SC qd.

IV. **Warfarin** is an oral anticoagulant that inhibits reduction of vitamin K to its active form. Consequently, administration of warfarin leads to depletion of the vitamin K–dependent clotting factors II, VII, IX, and X and proteins C and S.

**Table 18-7.** Lepirudin infusion rates in renal impairment per manufacturer's guidelines[a]

| Creatinine clearance (ml/min) | Serum creatinine (mg/dl) | Adjusted infusion rate (mg/kg/hr) |
|---|---|---|
| 45–60 | 1.6–2.0 | 0.075 |
| 30–44 | 2.1–3.0 | 0.045 |
| 15–29 | 3.1–6.0 | 0.0225 |
| <15 | >6.0 | Avoid or stop infusion |

[a]Dose adjustment is required for patients on hemodialysis or continuous venovenous hemodialysis.

**A. Administration.** Warfarin is well absorbed orally but requires 4–5 days before the full anticoagulant effect is achieved. For this reason, parenteral anticoagulation is continued until the INR is in the therapeutic range in two samples measured 24 hours apart. The recommended starting dose of warfarin is 5 mg PO qd followed by dose adjustments for the target INR. For most indications, an INR in the 2.0–3.0 range is adequate. Patients with mechanical valves require a higher level of anticoagulation (INR, 2.5–3.5). If invasive procedures are planned, warfarin therapy should be discontinued 4–5 days before elective surgery, allowing the INR to drift below 1.5 (*Ann Intern Med* 122:40, 1995), then resumed at the previous dose postoperatively as soon as adequate hemostasis is assured, typically within 24 hours. If a temporary interruption of anticoagulation is unacceptable, IV heparin or SC LMWH can be substituted until a few hours or 24 hours (respectively) before surgery.

**B. Possible complications and reversal of warfarin.** Major bleeding occurs in approximately 3% of patients who receive chronic OAT. Minor bleeding or asymptomatic, minor INR elevations should be managed by holding or reducing warfarin therapy until the INR returns to the appropriate range. Marked elevation of the INR (>5) in asymptomatic patients can be corrected partially with low-dose vitamin K (1.0–2.5 mg PO) without jeopardizing anticoagulant control. Higher doses of vitamin K (3–5 mg PO) can be given if the INR is greater than 9.0 in asymptomatic patients. Serious hemorrhages should be treated with IV vitamin K (10 mg) by slow IV infusion and FFP. Recombinant FVIIa may be beneficial for life-threatening bleeding (*Semin Hematol* 38[4 Suppl 12]:43–47, 2001). **Coumadin-induced skin necrosis** is a rare complication that can occur during initiation of warfarin therapy because of rapid depletion of the anticoagulant factor protein C. Necrosis occurs most often in areas with a high percentage of adipose tissue, such as breast tissue, and can be life-threatening. This complication can be prevented by first achieving therapeutic anticoagulation with a parenteral agent and avoiding "loading doses" of warfarin. **Warfarin is contraindicated in pregnancy because of teratogenicity** but is safe for infants of nursing mothers (*Chest* 119[Suppl]:1S–370S, 2001). Important drug interactions for warfarin exist (see Appendix C).

**V. Lepirudin (Refludan, recombinant hirudin)** is a direct thrombin inhibitor that is currently approved for use in the treatment of **HIT.** It has a half-life of 1.5 hours and is renally cleared; it requires dose adjustment in renal insufficiency (Table 18-7). No reversal agent is available for lepirudin. The treatment dose for patients with HIT and associated thrombosis is a bolus of 0.4 mg/kg (up to 110 kg body weight) followed by 0.15 mg/kg body weight/hour (up to 110 kg body weight) as a continuous IV infusion. See Figure 18-2 for a dose adjustment algorithm. Because lepirudin can also increase the PT, this must be taken into account when interpreting INRs of patients who are receiving warfarin (*Blood* 101:31–37, 2003).

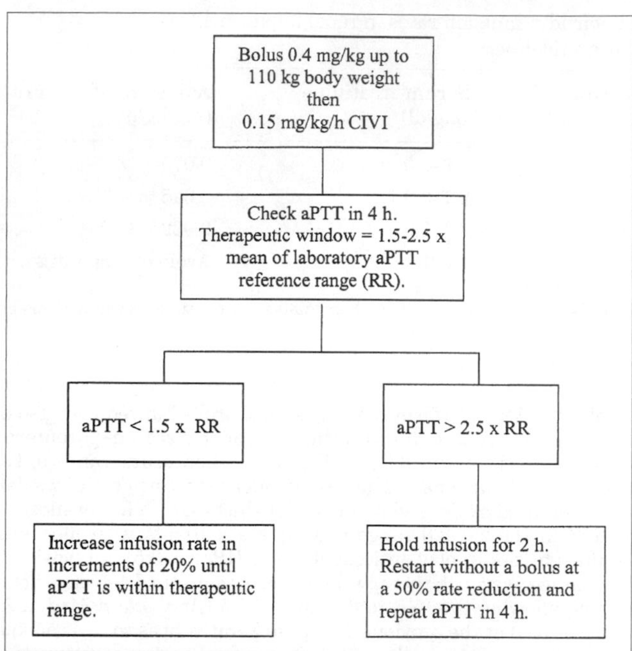


**Fig. 18-2.** Lepirudin dosing algorithm. aPTT, activated partial thromboplastin time; CIVI, continuous intravenous infusion. (Adapted from BM Alving. How I treat heparin-induced thrombocytopenia and thrombosis. *Blood* 101:31–37, 2003.)

**VI. Argatroban** is a synthetic direct thrombin inhibitor that is approved for prevention and treatment of thrombosis in PTCA and HIT patients. The recommended dosage in individuals with HIT is an intravenous infusion (without a bolus) of 2.0 μg/kg/minute, not to exceed 10.0 μg/kg/minute. An aPTT is obtained 2 hours after beginning the infusion, and the infusion rate is adjusted to achieve a steady-state aPTT of 1.5–3.0 times the patient's normal baseline aPTT. No reversal agent is available for argatroban; however, the half-life is less than 1 hour. Argatroban is hepatically cleared, and dose adjustment is necessary in patients with hepatic dysfunction. The PT is prolonged by argatroban; therefore, when warfarin is coadministered, argatroban should be discontinued when the INR is greater than 4. After discontinuation of argatroban, the INR is measured again within 4–6 hours, and if it is subtherapeutic, argatroban should be resumed and the warfarin dose adjusted daily until a therapeutic INR is achieved off argatroban. If the argatroban dose is greater than 2.0 μg/kg/minute during warfarin coadministration, the effect of warfarin on the INR is less predictable. Therefore, the argatroban infusion should be temporarily reduced to 2.0 μg/kg/minute and the INR is checked 4–6 hours later and adjusted accordingly (*Blood* 101:31–37, 2003).

**VII. Ximelogatran** is an oral direct thrombin inhibitor that is currently being evaluated in clinical trials for prophylaxis and therapeutic anticoagulation. Unlike warfarin, it does not require monitoring of coagulation studies (*N Engl J Med* 349:1703–1712, 1713–1721, 2003).

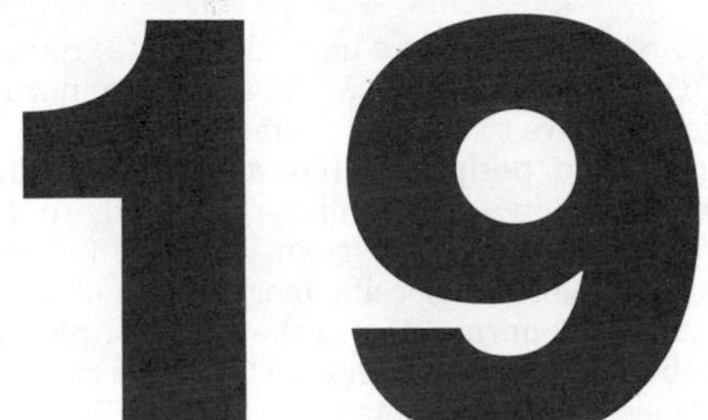

# Anemia and Transfusion Therapy

Morey A. Blinder and
Leslie Andritsos

## Approach to the Patient with Anemia

Anemia is a commonly encountered clinical condition caused by acquired or hereditary abnormalities of the RBC or its precursors, or may be a manifestation of an underlying nonhematologic disorder. Anemia is defined as a decrease in the circulating RBC mass; the usual criteria are a hemoglobin (Hb) of less than 12 g/dl [hematocrit (Hct) <36%] in women and less than 14 g/dl (Hct <41%) in men.

I. **Clinical manifestations** of anemia vary depending on the etiology, magnitude, and rapidity of onset. Other underlying disorders such as cardiopulmonary disease may contribute to the severity of symptoms. Severe anemia may be well tolerated if it develops gradually, but generally patients with a Hb of less than 7 g/dl generally have symptoms of tissue hypoxia (fatigue, headache, dyspnea, lightheadedness, angina). Pallor, visual impairment, syncope, and tachycardia may signal anemic hypovolemia, which requires immediate attention.

II. **History and physical examination.** The acuity or chronicity of the anemia should be assessed, and clues to any underlying systemic process should be sought. One must look for a family history of anemia, drug exposure (including ethanol), or blood loss. Physical findings that aid in diagnosis include lymphadenopathy, hepatic or splenic enlargement, jaundice, bone tenderness, neurologic symptoms, and evidence of blood in the feces.

III. **Laboratory evaluation** should always include the Hb and Hct, reticulocyte count, mean cellular volume (MCV), and an examination of the peripheral blood smear.

A. **The Hb and Hct** serve as an estimate of the RBC mass, but their interpretation must take into consideration the volume status of the patient. Immediately after acute blood loss, the Hb is unchanged because compensatory mechanisms have not had time to restore normal plasma volume.

B. **The reticulocyte count** reflects the rate of production of RBCs and is an indicator of the bone marrow response to the anemia. The reticulocyte count is usually reported as reticulocytes/100 RBCs (% reticulocytes), but newer methods in determining the reticulocyte count may also report an absolute number:

**Absolute reticulocyte count** = % reticulocytes × RBC count (per $mm^3$)

An increase of reticulocytes to greater than 100,000/$mm^3$ suggests a hyperproliferative bone marrow associated with loss or destruction of RBCs. Anemia with a low reticulocyte count suggests impaired RBC production.

C. **The MCV** is often used in classifying anemia (microcytic, normocytic, and macrocytic for anemia with low, normal, and high MCV, respectively). Proper use of the MCV in establishing a diagnosis depends on examination of the peripheral smear for the following reasons: (1) Small and large cells may be present simultaneously, resulting in a normal MCV; (2) reticulocytes are larger than mature RBCs and raise the MCV; and (3) abnormal cells may be present in numbers that are too small to affect the MCV.

D. **Examination of a well-prepared peripheral blood smear** is mandatory. RBC morphology is best evaluated in a portion of the smear where the RBCs are nearly touching one another. Heterogeneity in RBC size (anisocytosis) and shape (poikilocytosis) may be seen. Specific morphologic abnormalities should be sought, as well as any abnormalities in the WBCs or platelets.

E. **Additional testing** to establish an exact diagnosis should be guided by the initial findings, and, whenever possible, some tests should be performed before blood transfusions [peripheral smear, glucose-6-phosphate dehydrogenase (G6PD) level, Hb analysis, iron studies].

IV. **Classification of anemias.** Typically, anemia is characterized by the MCV and reticulocyte count. Determination of the MCV and an examination of the peripheral smear often suggest a single diagnosis or a limited number of diagnoses that can be investigated with specific tests. Anemia may be multifactorial in origin (e.g., alcoholism with GI bleeding, nutritional deficiencies, and liver disease). Evaluation of anemia also requires consideration of the WBC and platelet count, because bicytopenia or pancytopenia often suggests other causes.

## Anemias Associated with Decreased Red Blood Cell Production

I. **Iron-deficiency anemia** is a common disorder worldwide. In the United States, most cases are caused by menstrual blood loss and increased iron requirements of pregnancy. In the absence of menstrual bleeding, GI blood loss is the presumed etiology in most patients; appropriate radiographic and endoscopic procedures should be performed to identify a source and to exclude occult malignancy. Decreased iron absorption (celiac disease, postgastrectomy) or increased iron requirements (lactation) may also lead to iron deficiency. Complete evaluation of iron deficiency requires identification of the cause.

A. **History and physical examination.** Evidence for a source of blood loss (melena, menorrhagia) should be sought. In severe iron-deficiency anemia, a history of **pica** (consumption of substances such as ice, starch, or clay) can be obtained. Splenomegaly, koilonychia ("spoon nail"), and the Plummer-Vinson syndrome (glossitis, dysphagia, and esophageal webs) are rare findings.

B. **Laboratory results.** The MCV is usually normal in early iron deficiency. As the Hct falls below 30%, anisocytosis increases and hypochromic microcytic cells appear, followed by a decrease in the MCV. Other findings on the peripheral smear include "pencil cells" and occasional target cells. The platelet count may be increased. Diagnosis requires the documentation of low iron stores, which can usually be accomplished indirectly by measuring serum ferritin.

1. **A serum ferritin level** of less than 10 ng/ml in women or 20 ng/ml in men is indicative of low iron stores. Ferritin is an acute-phase reactant, so that normal levels may be seen in inflammatory states, liver disease, or malignancy despite low iron stores. A serum ferritin level of greater than 200 ng/ml generally indicates adequate iron stores regardless of other underlying conditions. **Serum iron** is usually low (<50 μg/dl), and **total iron-binding capacity** is increased (>420 μg/dl) in iron deficiency, but these values may fluctuate in a number of common clinical conditions and hence are less reliable indicators of iron stores than the serum ferritin.

2. **A bone marrow aspirate** should be stained for iron and, if absent, is definitive for establishing iron deficiency. Alternatively, a **therapeutic challenge** with supplemental iron can help identify anemias that are iron responsive. Either approach is useful when the ferritin level is not diagnostic.

C. **Therapy** of iron-deficiency anemia requires repleting iron stores with supplemental oral or parenteral iron; normal dietary intake only meets daily losses. With therapy, the reticulocyte count peaks in 5–10 days, and the Hb rises over 1–2 months. The most common cause of a poor response to therapy is noncompliance; other causes, such as poor absorption, continued blood loss, or a multifactorial anemia, must also be considered.

1. **Oral therapy** with ferrous sulfate, 325 mg (65 mg elemental iron) PO tid taken between meals to maximize absorption, usually corrects the anemia and repletes iron stores (as determined by normalization of the serum ferritin) over approximately 6 months. Concomitant use of acid-neutralizing medications is an underappreciated cause of an impaired response to oral iron. **GI side effects,** such as constipation, cramping, diarrhea, or nausea, develop in approximately 25% of patients. These side effects can be decreased by initially administering the drug with meals or once a day and increasing the dose as tolerated. Ferrous gluconate and fumarate at a similar dose may be better tolerated alternative therapies. One capsule of iron polysaccharide complex (Niferex) contains 150 mg elemental iron and, given twice daily, is as effective as other preparations at a similar cost and seems to have fewer GI side effects. Sustained-release or enteric-coated preparations dissolve poorly and generally should not be recommended.

2. **Parenteral iron therapy** may be useful in patients with (1) poor absorption (e.g., inflammatory bowel disease, malabsorption), (2) very high iron requirements that cannot be met with oral supplementation (e.g., ongoing bleeding), or (3) intolerance of oral preparations. **Iron dextran** (INFeD), sodium ferric gluconate (Ferrlecit), and iron sucrose (Venofer) are the currently available parenteral agents. A formula is available in the package insert for iron dextran to approximate the amount of iron that is required to restore the Hb to normal levels and replenish the iron stores. Patients can be treated with 1000–2000 mg iron dextran in a single IV dose to correct the deficit. A single dose of IV iron dextran (diluted in 500–1000 ml normal saline and infused at 6 mg/minute) has been used with few complications and is the generally preferred route (*J Lab Clin Med* 111:566, 1988). Iron dextran may rarely be complicated by **anaphylaxis**, and therefore a 0.5-ml (25 mg) IV test dose should be administered 1 hour before therapy is initiated. Epinephrine should be available to treat any anaphylactic reaction. Delayed reactions to IV iron, such as arthralgia, myalgia, fever, pruritus, and lymphadenopathy, may be seen within 3 days of therapy and usually resolve spontaneously or after treatment with nonsteroidal anti-inflammatory agents. **Sodium ferric gluconate** is an alternative to iron dextran can be used in patients who have an adverse reaction to iron dextran. It is not given as a single dose because of adverse reactions including hypotension. The recommended dosage is 125 mg diluted in 100 ml normal saline infused IV over 1 hour, repeated as needed to achieve the target dose. Because of the low risk of acute adverse reactions, a test dose is not needed. Doses greater than 250 mg/day are not recommended due to the risk of complications. **Iron sucrose** given at 100 mg in 100 ml normal saline IV over 15–30 minutes and repeated one to three times/week is another alternative.

II. **The thalassemias** are a heterogeneous group of inherited disorders characterized by underproduction of either the alpha- or beta-globin chains of the Hb molecule. Thalassemia occurs in persons of Mediterranean, African, Middle

Eastern, Indian, and Asian descent. In beta-thalassemia, there is a reduced production of beta-globin chains with normal amounts of alpha-globin production. The excess alpha-globin chains form insoluble tetramers in the RBCs, resulting in membrane damage, ineffective erythropoiesis, and hemolytic anemia. In alpha-thalassemia, the beta-tetramers that form are more soluble, and thus the clinical severity is milder. A family history of microcytosis or microcytic anemia may aid in the diagnosis. Splenomegaly and bone abnormalities caused by the expanded marrow are common in more severe forms of thalassemia. Microcytic, hypochromic cells with poikilocytosis, target cells, and nucleated RBCs may be present on the peripheral smear. Hb analysis may aid in the diagnosis.

**A. Alpha-thalassemia.** Clinically apparent alpha-thalassemia occurs with a deletion or mutation of three alpha-globin genes, resulting in hemoglobin H (HbH) disease, which is characterized by splenomegaly, chronic hemolytic anemia, and the presence of beta-globin tetramers. A loss of all four alpha-globin genes causes hydrops fetalis. HbH disease rarely requires transfusion or splenectomy, but oxidant drugs similar to those that exacerbate G6PD deficiency should be avoided because increased hemolysis may occur (see Table 19-2).

**B. Beta-thalassemia.** Production of beta-globin chains may be reduced or absent from each allele; they are described as beta$^{+}$-thalassemia or beta$^{o}$-thalassemia, respectively. Beta-thalassemia is commonly classified phenotypically by the severity of anemia; many genotypes exist for each phenotype. **Thalassemia minor (trait)** is caused by diminished or absent beta-globin chain synthesis from one gene. Patients are asymptomatic with a hypochromic microcytic anemia (Hb >10 g/dl). **Thalassemia intermedia** is usually associated with dysfunction of both beta-globin genes. Clinical severity is intermediate (Hb, 7–10 g/dl), and patients are usually not transfusion dependent. **Thalassemia major (Cooley's anemia)** is caused by severe dysfunction of both beta-globin genes. Anemia is severe, and RBC transfusions are required to sustain life. In severe forms of thalassemia, the transfusions result in tissue iron overload, which may cause CHF, hepatic dysfunction, glucose intolerance, and secondary hypogonadism. Iron chelation therapy with deferoxamine mesylate (Desferal) delays or prevents these complications (see sec. **II.B.3**).

1. **Transfusions.** A Hb of greater than 9 g/dl improves exercise tolerance and prevents skeletal deformities and can usually be achieved with 1 U of RBCs every 2–3 weeks or 2 U every month.
2. **Splenectomy** removes the primary site of extravascular hemolysis and should be considered if RBC transfusion requirements increase and exceed one and a half times the previous levels. It should not be performed if the patient is younger than 5–6 years because of the risk of sepsis. To decrease the risk of postsplenectomy sepsis, immunization against *Pneumococcus*, *Haemophilus influenzae*, and *Neisseria meningitidis* should be administered at least 2 weeks before surgery if not previously vaccinated (see Appendix F, Immunizations and Post-Exposure Therapies).
3. **Iron chelation therapy** with deferoxamine mesylate, 40 mg/kg/day, is usually administered by continuous SC infusion for 8–12 hours/day beginning in childhood when the iron burden has reached approximately 50 U of RBCs. Once clinical organ deterioration has begun, it may not be reversible. Therapy may be complicated by local irritation at the injection site, and pruritus and hypotension may occur if the drug is infused too rapidly. Continuous IV infusion of deferoxamine through an indwelling venous catheter at the same dosage and schedule can also be used (*Am J Hematol* 41:61, 1992). Although iron chelation therapy is generally safe, long-term side effects, particularly with high-dose therapy, include optic neuropathy, sensorineural hearing loss, and increased

risk of infection. Patients who are receiving deferoxamine should have baseline and yearly vision and hearing examinations.

4. **Stem cell transplant (SCT)** should be considered in young patients with thalassemia major who have HLA-identical related donors.

III. **Refractory anemias** are a heterogeneous group of acquired or hereditary disorders characterized by a hypoproliferative normocytic anemia. Presentations range from mild asymptomatic anemia to severe pancytopenia.

IV. **Myelodysplastic syndrome (MDS)** is an acquired clonal disorder of hematopoietic stem cells that has recently been reclassified according to morphologic findings on the blood and the bone marrow along with cytogenetic analysis. MDS is often idiopathic but may be secondary to prior radiation, chemotherapy, or toxin exposure and is almost always characterized by anemia. Associated findings include ringed sideroblasts, multilinear dysplasia, excess blasts, or an isolated chromosome deletion [del (5q)] (*Blood* 100:2292, 2002).

A. **Therapy** of MDS is supportive and rarely curative. Myelosuppressive drugs should be stopped, and nutritional deficiencies should be corrected. **Deferoxamine mesylate** (see sec. **II.B.3**) should be considered in patients with a good prognosis after 50–100 U of RBCs have been transfused.

1. **Pyridoxine,** 50–200 mg PO qd, can be tried empirically, although the response rate is low and usually occurs in patients with refractory anemia with ringed sideroblasts.
2. **Erythroid-stimulating factors** may be useful in decreasing RBC transfusion requirements in approximately 20% of patients and is more likely to be effective when the serum erythropoietin (Epo) level is below 200 mU/ml (Table 19-1). **Granulocyte colony-stimulating factor,** 1–5 μg/kg SC qd, is likely to result in improved neutrophil counts in patients with neutropenia.
3. **Chemotherapy** is not usually of benefit for MDS but is frequently attempted in patients in reasonable health; a variety of chemotherapeutic regimens have been used, often administered in the setting of a research protocol. **SCT** should be considered in patients younger than 50 years of age who have an HLA-identical sibling.

**Table 19.1.** Guidelines for the use of erythroid-stimulating factors

| | Agent and initial dose (SC or IV) | |
|---|---|---|
| Indication | Erythropoietin[a] | Darbepoetin[b] |
| Chemotherapy-induced anemia from nonmyeloid malignancy, multiple myeloma, lymphoma; anemia secondary to malignancy or MDS | 40,000 U/wk *or*<br>150 U/kg tiw | 2.25 μg/kg/wk *or*<br>100 μg/wk *or*<br>200 μg/2 wk |
| Anemia associated with renal failure | 50–150 U/kg tiw | 0.45 μg/kg/wk |
| Anemia associated with HIV infection | 100–200 U/kg tiw | Not approved |
| Anemia of chronic disease | 150–300 U/kg tiw | Not approved |
| Anemia in patients unwilling or unable to receive RBC; anemic patients undergoing major surgery | 600 U/kg/wk × 3 *or*<br>300 U/kg/d × 1–2 wk | Not recommended |

MDS, myelodysplastic syndrome; tiw, thrice weekly.
[a]Dose increase after 4–8 wk up to 900 U/kg/wk or 60,000 U/wk; discontinue if hematocrit (Hct) is greater than 40%; resume when Hct is less than 36% at 75% of previous dose.
[b]Dose increase after 6 wk up to 4.5 μg/kg/wk or 150 μg/wk or 300 μg/2 wk; hold dose if Hct is greater than 36%; then resume when Hct is less than 36% at 75% of previous dose.

4. **Immunosuppressive therapy** with antithymocyte globulin, cyclosporine, and glucocorticoids can also be considered in patients with refractory anemia.

V. **Sideroblastic anemias** are a group of RBC disorders characterized by abnormal iron metabolism. Causes of acquired sideroblastic anemia include drugs (Table 19-2), lead toxicity, or chronic ethanol use, and treatment includes withdrawing the offending agent.

VI. **The megaloblastic anemias** are a group of disorders associated with altered morphology of hematopoietic cells and other rapidly dividing cells because of abnormalities in DNA synthesis. Almost all cases are because of folic acid or vitamin $B_{12}$ deficiency. **Folic acid deficiency** may develop within a few months, and common causes include (1) decreased intake often associated with alcoholism, (2) malabsorption, and (3) increased utilization (hemolytic anemia, pregnancy). In addition, some drugs (ethanol, trimethoprim, pyrimethamine, methotrexate, sulfasalazine, oral contraceptives, and anticonvulsants) may lead to perturbed folate metabolism. **Vitamin $B_{12}$ deficiency** takes years to develop because very little of the body's store is used each day. Causes of vitamin $B_{12}$ deficiency include (1) pernicious anemia, (2) gastrectomy, (3) pancreatic insufficiency, (4) GI bacterial overgrowth, (5) ileitis or ileal resection, and (6) intestinal parasites.

A. **History and physical examination.** Symptoms are primarily attributable to anemia, although glossitis, jaundice, and splenomegaly may be present. Vitamin $B_{12}$ deficiency may cause decreased vibratory and positional sense, ataxia, paresthesias, confusion, and dementia. Neurologic complications may occur in the absence of anemia and may not resolve completely despite adequate treatment. Folic acid deficiency does not directly result in neurologic disease.

B. **Laboratory results.** A macrocytic anemia is usually present, and leukopenia and thrombocytopenia may occur. The peripheral smear is characterized by RBC macro-ovalocytes and hypersegmented neutrophils (containing ≥ 5 nuclear lobes). Lactate dehydrogenase (LDH) and indirect bilirubin are typically elevated, reflecting ineffective erythropoiesis and premature destruction of RBCs.

1. **Serum vitamin $B_{12}$ and RBC folate levels** should be measured. RBC folate is a more accurate indicator of body folate stores than serum folate, particularly if measured after folate therapy or improved nutrition has been initiated.
2. **Serum methylmalonic acid (MMA) and homocysteine (HC)** may be useful when the vitamin $B_{12}$ or folate level is equivocal. MMA and HC are elevated in vitamin $B_{12}$ deficiency; only HC is elevated in folic acid deficiency.
3. **A Schilling test** may be useful in the diagnosis of pernicious anemia due to vitamin $B_{12}$ deficiency but rarely affects the therapeutic approach. The presence of **antibodies to intrinsic factor** is specific for the diagnosis of pernicious anemia.
4. **Bone marrow biopsy** may be necessary to rule out MDS and hematologic malignancy; these disorders may present with findings similar to those of megaloblastic anemia on peripheral smear.

C. **Therapy** is directed toward replacing the deficient factor. Symptomatic hypokalemia may occur within 48 hours of initiating therapy, and supplemental potassium may be needed. Blood transfusions are rarely required and may be associated with volume overload when used for these disorders. With therapy, reticulocytosis should begin within 1 week, followed by a rising Hb over 6–8 weeks. Coexisting iron deficiency is present in one-third of patients with vitamin $B_{12}$ deficiency and is a common cause for an incomplete response to therapy. Because pernicious anemia is associated with hypothyroidism, thyroid studies should be checked.

1. **Folic acid** can be administered at 1 mg PO qd until the deficiency is corrected. High doses of folic acid (5 mg PO qd) may be needed in patients with malabsorption syndromes.

**Table 19-2.** Drugs that can induce red blood cell disorders

| | | | Immune hemolytic anemia | | |
|---|---|---|---|---|---|
| Sideroblastic anemia | Aplastic anemia[a] | Hemolytic episode in G6PD deficiency | Autoantibody | Hapten | Immune complex[b] |
| Chloramphenicol | Acetazolamide | Dapsone | α-Methyldopa | AK-Fluor 25% | Amphotericin B |
| Cycloserine | Antineoplastic agents | Furazolidone | Cephalosporins | Cephalosporins | Antazoline |
| Ethanol | Carbamazepine | Methylene blue | Diclofenac | Penicillins | Cephalosporins |
| Isoniazid | Chloramphenicol | Nalidixic acid | Ibuprofen | Tetracycline | Chlorpropamide |
| Pyrazinamide | Gold salts | Nitrofurantoin | Interferon-alpha | Tolbutamide | Diclofenac |
| | Hydantoins | Phenazopyridine | L-Dopa | | Diethylstilbestrol |
| | Penicillamine | Primaquine | Mefenamic acid | | Doxepin |
| | Phenylbutazone | Sulfacetamide | Procainamide | | Hydrochlorothiazide |
| | Quinacrine | Sulfamethoxazole | Teniposide | | Isoniazid |
| | | Sulfanilamide | Thioridazine | | *p*-Aminosalicylic acid |
| | | Sulfapyridine | Tolmetin | | Probenecid |
| | | | | | Quinidine |
| | | | | | Quinine |
| | | | | | Rifampin |
| | | | | | Sulfonamides |
| | | | | | Thiopental |
| | | | | | Tolmetin |

G6PD, glucose-6-phosphate dehydrogenase.
[a]Drugs with more than 30 cases reported; many other drugs rarely are associated with aplastic anemia and are considered low risk.
[b]Some sources list the mechanism for many of these drugs as unknown.
*Source*: Data compiled from multiple sources. Agents listed are available in the United States.

2. **Vitamin $B_{12}$** deficiency is corrected by administering cyanocobalamin. A typical schedule is 1 mg IM qd for 7 days, then weekly for 1–2 months or until normalization of the Hb occurs. Long-term therapy is 1 mg IM monthly.

VII. **Anemia of chronic renal insufficiency** is attributed primarily to decreased endogenous Epo production and may occur as the creatinine clearance declines below approximately 50 ml/minute (see also Chap. 11, Renal Diseases, the section Chronic Kidney Disease, sec. **II.D.**

A. **Laboratory results.** The Hct is usually 20–30%, and the MCV is normal. On peripheral smear the RBCs are often hypochromic, with the occasional presence of echinocytes (burr cells).

B. **Treatment** of anemia of chronic renal insufficiency has been revolutionized by the availability of recombinant human Epo (Procrit, Epogen, Aranesp). Therapy is indicated in predialysis and dialysis patients who are symptomatic. Objective benefits of reversing the anemia include enhanced exercise capacity, improved cognitive function, elimination of RBC transfusions, and reduction of iron overload. Subjective benefits include increased energy, enhanced appetite, better sleep patterns, and improved sexual activity.

1. **Administration of Epo** can be IV (hemodialysis patients) or SC (predialysis or peritoneal dialysis patients). More than 97% of patients increase their Hct by ten points or to a level greater than 32% within 12 weeks of therapy. A long-acting form of Epo has been developed [darbepoetin (Aranesp)], and a typical dosing schedule is shown in Table 19-1.
2. **Adverse reactions** to Epo or darbepoetin therapy are uncommon. Hypertension may develop or worsen in some patients while the Hct is increasing. Seizures may occur, although the etiology is not well characterized.
3. **Suboptimal responses** may occur with coexisting iron deficiency or iron-restricted erythropoiesis; thus, many patients benefit from IV iron supplementation despite normal serum ferritin. Sodium ferric gluconate or iron sucrose, 100–125 mg one to three times/week IV, is typically used in this setting. Chronic inflammatory conditions and acute or chronic bleeding affect the response to erythroid-stimulating factors as well. Hemodialysis patients may also suffer from aluminum intoxication, which blunts the response to erythroid-stimulating factors. Secondary hyperparathyroidism may cause bone marrow fibrosis and relative resistance to the action of Epo.

VIII. **Anemia of chronic disease** often develops in patients with long-standing inflammatory diseases, malignancy, autoimmune disorders, and chronic infection. Abnormalities in iron metabolism and Epo production, as well as humoral inhibition of erythropoiesis, have all been implicated in the pathogenesis.

A. **Laboratory results.** A normocytic normochromic anemia is typical. The peripheral smear is usually normal, although microcytes may be present. Ferritin is generally normal but may be elevated because it is an acute-phase reactant. No laboratory test is diagnostic for the anemia of chronic disease. However, when anemia of chronic disease is difficult to distinguish from iron-deficiency anemia, determining the level of serum transferrin receptor may help in the diagnosis (elevated in iron deficiency, normal in anemia of chronic disease).

B. **Treatment** is directed at the underlying cause and at eliminating exacerbating factors such as nutritional deficiencies and marrow-suppressive drugs. Doses of Epo that are effective are higher than those reported in anemia from renal insufficiency (Table 19-1). If no response has been observed at 900 U/kg/week, further escalation is unlikely to be effective. Whether the use of supplemental iron is of benefit is uncertain. Treatment should only be considered in patients with symptoms of severe anemia or a Hb of less than 10 g/dl.

C. **Anemia in cancer patients** may be successfully prevented and treated with erythroid-stimulating factors (Table 19-1) (see Chap. 20, Medical Management of Malignant Disease, the section Complications of Treatment, sec. **I.B.4.c.**

**IX. Anemia associated with HIV infection** is common. In many cases dysplasia similar to that seen in MDS is found on bone marrow examination. Treatment with an erythroid-stimulating factor should be considered in symptomatic anemic patients with a serum Epo level of less than 500 mU/ml. Certain situations warrant specific mention.

**A. Mycobacterium avium complex** infections are frequently associated with severe anemia, and this may occur in the absence of other cytopenias. This diagnosis should be considered in patients in whom new-onset or worsening anemia develops. The treatment of *M. avium* complex is described in Chap. 14, Human Immunodeficiency Virus and Acquired Immunodeficiency Syndrome, the section Opportunistic Infection, sec. **III.C.2.**

**B. Parvovirus B19** should be considered in HIV-infected patients with transfusion-dependent anemia and a low reticulocyte count. The diagnosis is established by finding parvovirus in the serum by **polymerase chain reaction (PCR).** Antiparvovirus antibodies, which develop in immunocompetent patients and provide long-term immunity, are typically not elevated in HIV-infected patients. Treatment with IV immunoglobulin (0.4 g/kg IV qd for 5–10 days) results in erythropoietic recovery. Relapses have occurred between 2 and 6 months and can be successfully managed with intermittent IV immunoglobulin at an empiric maintenance dose of 0.4 g/kg IV for 1 day given every 4 weeks (*Ann Intern Med* 113:926, 1990).

**C. Zidovudine** induces a macrocytic anemia in all treated patients and can be used to assess compliance with therapy. Erythroid-stimulating factor (Table 19-1) improves the Hct in patients with an endogenous Epo level of less than or equal to 500 mU/ml. RBC transfusion requirements are decreased by approximately one-half, and up to 40% of patients become transfusion independent. No hematologic benefit occurs if the serum Epo level is greater than or equal to 500 mU/ml. Stavudine (d4T) has also been reported to cause macrocytic anemia.

**X. Pancytopenia** may occur in a variety of situations, including MDS, acute leukemia, HIV infection, and infiltration of the marrow with tumor or granuloma. In immunocompromised patients, pancytopenia is frequently due to immunosuppressive agents or viral infection. A bone marrow examination is frequently required to establish the diagnosis.

**Aplastic anemia** is an acquired abnormality of hematopoietic stem cells that usually presents with pancytopenia. Most cases are idiopathic, although approximately 20% are associated with drug or chemical exposure (Table 19-2) and another 10% are associated with viral illnesses [e.g., viral hepatitis, Epstein-Barr virus, cytomegalovirus (CMV)]. Presenting symptoms are usually due to anemia or thrombocytopenia, although some patients present with fever and leukopenia. The diagnosis may be difficult to distinguish from hypocellular MDS and may also be associated with paroxysmal nocturnal hemoglobinuria. **Therapy** for aplastic anemia is potentially curative. Any suspected offending drugs should be discontinued and exacerbating factors corrected.

**A. Early referral** to a center that is experienced in managing aplastic anemia is recommended. When feasible, **SCT** from an HLA-identical sibling is generally recommended and has achieved a long-term survival of 60–70%. **Immunosuppressive treatment** with cyclosporine, glucocorticoids, and antithymocyte globulin should be considered in patients who do not undergo an SCT (*Ann Intern Med* 136:534, 2002).

**B. Transfusions** with RBCs should be kept to a minimum. Prophylactic platelet transfusions are generally recommended if the platelet count is below 10,000/µl. Transfusion with blood products from family members should be avoided while SCT is being considered.

**C. Infection.** Patients should be instructed to seek medical attention immediately in the event of fever over 38.5°C. Fevers with neutropenia require a diagnostic and empiric antimicrobial regimen similar to that used in patients with chemotherapy-induced myelosuppression (see Chap. 20, Medical Management of Malignant Disease, the section Complications of Treatment, sec. **I.B**).

## Anemias Associated with Increased Red Blood Cell Loss or Destruction

Anemias associated with increased erythropoiesis (i.e., an elevated reticulocyte count) are caused by bleeding or destruction of RBCs (hemolysis) and may exceed the capacity of normal bone marrow to correct the Hct. Typically, the bilirubin and LDH are normal in the bleeding patient and elevated in the patient with hemolysis.

**I. Bleeding is much more common than hemolysis.** Occult sites of bleeding (retroperitoneum, fractured hip) may result in laboratory findings that are similar to those seen with a hemolytic process. All patients with suspected hemolysis should have a direct antiglobulin test (DAT, or direct Coombs' test). This test detects the presence of IgG and the third component of complement (C3) on the surface of RBCs and usually differentiates between immune and nonimmune causes of hemolysis.

**II. Hemolytic anemias** are characterized by the predominant site of hemolysis.

- **A. Intravascular hemolysis** may present with fever, chills, tachycardia, and backache. Serum haptoglobin levels are invariably decreased, as this protein binds and removes Hb from the plasma. If hemolysis is severe, free Hb can be measured in the plasma and urine. Renal failure may develop with hemoglobinuria (see Chap. 11, Renal Diseases, the section Acute Renal Failure, sec. **III.D**).
- **B. Extravascular hemolysis** is characterized by RBC destruction in the reticuloendothelial system, primarily the spleen. Jaundice and splenomegaly may be present. Haptoglobin levels are normal or slightly reduced.

**III. Sickle cell disease** includes homozygous sickle cell anemia (HbSS) and other sickling syndromes with double-heterozygous conditions (HbS–beta-thalassemia, HbSC). These disorders are associated with structurally abnormal Hb molecules that polymerize under reduced oxygen conditions. The clinical features are a consequence of a chronic hemolytic anemia and vaso-occlusive ischemic tissue injury. A monograph on sickle cell disease is available and provides useful guidelines (National Institutes of Health publication No. 02-2117 at http://www.nhlbi.nih.gov/health/prof/blood/sickle). **Sickle cell trait** occurs in individuals who are heterozygous for HbS. Individuals with sickle cell trait are healthy but are at increased risk of sudden death with rigorous exercise, which may be precipitated by dehydration.

- **A. Laboratory results.** The Hb ranges from 5 to 10 g/dl in HbSS, and the MCV may be slightly elevated due to the increased reticulocyte count. Chronic neutrophilia (10,000–20,000/$mm^3$) is often present, and the platelet count may be increased. The peripheral smear shows the classic distorted sickle-shaped erythrocytes. Target cells may be present, particularly in HbS–beta-thalassemia and HbSC. Hb analysis by electrophoresis or high-pressure liquid chromatography distinguishes HbSS from sickle cell trait and other abnormal HbS.
- **B. Routine care and health maintenance**
  1. **Dehydration and hypoxia** should be avoided because they may precipitate or exacerbate sickling. Intense exercise, activities at high altitude, and flying in unpressurized aircraft should be strongly discouraged.
  2. **Folic acid,** 1 mg PO qd, should be administered to patients with sickle cell disease because of chronic hemolysis.

3. **Antimicrobial prophylaxis** with penicillin VK, 125 mg PO bid up to age 3 years, then 250 mg PO bid until 5 years, is effective in reducing the risk of infection. Patients who are allergic to penicillin should receive erythromycin, 10 mg/kg PO bid. In most patients, antimicrobial prophylaxis should be discontinued after 5 years of age (*J Pediatr* 127:685, 1995).
4. **Immunizations** in adults should include a polyvalent pneumococcal vaccine. Hepatitis B vaccine is recommended for hepatitis B surface antibody–negative patients. Yearly influenza vaccine is recommended (see Appendix F, Immunizations and Post-Exposure Therapies).
5. **Regular yearly ophthalmologic examinations** are recommended in adults because of a high incidence of proliferative retinopathy leading to vitreous hemorrhage and retinal detachment. Laser photocoagulation is effective in preventing these complications.
6. **Surgery and anesthesia.** Local and regional anesthesia can be used without special precautions. With general anesthesia, measures to avoid volume depletion, hypoxia, and hypernatremia are crucial. For major surgery, RBC transfusions to increase the Hb concentration to 10 g/dl seem to be as effective as more aggressive transfusion regimens in most circumstances (*N Engl J Med* 333:206, 1995).

C. **Infections in adults** are often related to indwelling venous access devices, and therefore infections with *Staphylococcus* are common. Tissues that are susceptible to vaso-occlusive infarcts (bone, kidney, lung) and the urinary tract are also at risk of infection, and treatment should be directed by culture data. Pneumonia is most likely to be caused by *Mycoplasma*, *Staphylococcus aureus*, or *H. influenzae* and must be distinguished from acute chest syndrome (see sec. **III.E.2**).

D. **Complications of chronic hemolysis**

1. **Aplastic crisis** is characterized by a sudden decrease in Hb and reticulocyte count. This crisis is usually a complication of infection with parvovirus B19. Transfusion with RBCs is the mainstay of therapy, and most patients recover in 10–14 days. Individuals who are suspected of having a parvovirus infection should be in respiratory isolation to prevent exposure to other susceptible patients and pregnant women.
2. **Cholelithiasis,** primarily with bilirubin stones, is present in most adult patients, and biliary pain is common. Elective laparoscopic cholecystectomy is generally effective and should be considered in most patients. Acute cholecystitis should be treated medically, and cholecystectomy should be performed when the attack subsides (see Chap. 16, Gastrointestinal Diseases, the section Pancreatobiliary Disorders, sec. **II**).

E. **Clinical features of sickle cell disease**

1. **Vaso-occlusive pain crises** are the most common manifestation of sickle cell disease. Pain typically occurs in the back, ribs, and limbs and lasts for 5–7 days. The pattern of pain is usually consistent in any one patient from crisis to crisis. A deviation from the pattern may suggest another diagnosis such as cholecystitis. Precipitating factors such as an infection should be excluded. Many painful episodes are managed on an outpatient basis with PO fluids (3–4 L/day) and analgesia. Patients who require parenteral opioids, who cannot consume adequate PO fluids, or in whom another complication is suspected (infection, acute chest syndrome) require hospital admission. **Opioids** (see Chap. 1, Patient Care in Internal Medicine, the section Acute Inpatient Care, sec. **V.E**) are typically used and are effectively administered by a patient-controlled analgesia pump, allowing for the patient to self-administer medication within a set limit of infusions (lockout interval) and basal rate. Morphine (2 mg/hour basal rate with boluses of 2–10 mg every 6–10 minutes) is the drug of choice for moderate or severe pain. If patient-controlled analgesia is not used, morphine (0.1–0.2 mg/kg IV q2–3h) or hydromorphone (0.02–0.04 mg/kg IV q2–3h) is recommended. Careful recording of dosing facili-

tates appropriate care during subsequent episodes of pain. The use of a pain scale [analog scale 0 (absent) to 10 (worst)] is helpful in guiding efficacy and dosing. Supplemental oxygen does not benefit acute pain crisis unless hypoxia is present. **RBC transfusions do not change the immediate course of an acute pain crisis.** Some patients do not require significant amounts of analgesic therapy between crises, although opioids may be required by others. Patients who experience severe recurrent pain crisis that requires frequent medical intervention may benefit from chronic partial exchange transfusions or treatment with hydroxyurea (see sec. **III.F.2**).

2. **Acute chest syndrome** is associated with chest pain, pulmonary infiltrates, leukocytosis, and hypoxia and is indistinguishable from pneumonia. The most frequently identified pathogens are *Chlamydia pneumoniae*, *Mycoplasma* species, respiratory syncytial virus, and *S. aureus*. Initial management should include hospitalization, administration of supplemental oxygen to correct hypoxia, adequate analgesia, and empiric coverage with antimicrobials such as a cephalosporin or macrolide is recommended. Transfusion of RBCs is recommended in most cases, and exchange transfusion should be considered in patients with multiple-lobe involvement, worsening disease, or hypoxemia (arterial oxygen tension <60 mm Hg) (*N Engl J Med* 342:1859, 2000).
3. **Splenic sequestration crisis** is associated with rapid onset of splenomegaly due to pooling of blood into the spleen causing severe anemia. Hemodynamic support and RBC transfusions are usually required. Splenic infarction, causing severe left upper quadrant pain, may also result. Splenectomy should be considered for recurrent events. In adults, this complication generally occurs in patients with an intact spleen, such as those with HbSC or HbS–beta$^+$-thalassemia.
4. **Priapism** refers to painful erection from vaso-occlusion, which may respond to hydration and analgesics. Transfusions and surgical drainage should be considered for acute events that last longer than 24 hours. Permanent impotence can occur.
5. **Osteonecrosis** of the femoral and humeral heads causes considerable morbidity in approximately one-third of patients. Treatment consists of local heat, analgesics, and avoidance of weight bearing. Hip and shoulder arthroplasty are often effective in decreasing symptoms and improving function and should be considered.
6. **Stroke** occurs most commonly in children younger than 10 years and is usually caused by cerebral infarction. Without treatment approximately two-thirds of patients experience recurrent stroke. Long-term transfusions to maintain the HbS concentration at less than 50% for a minimum of 5 years reduce the incidence of recurrence.
7. **Leg ulcers** should be treated with rest, leg elevation, and intensive local care. Wet-to-dry dressings should be applied every 4–6 hours to débride the ulcer. Local care with moist occlusive dressings and control of edema with leg elevation, Ace wraps, and careful diuresis are usually helpful. An Unna's boot (zinc oxide–impregnated bandage), changed weekly for 3–4 weeks, can be used for nonhealing or more extensive ulcers. Otherwise, long-term transfusions, split-thickness skin grafts, and free-flap grafts may be necessary.
8. **Renal tubular defects** caused by sickling in the anoxic hyperosmolar environment of the renal medulla may lead to isosthenuria (inability to concentrate urine) and hematuria in sickle cell disease and sickle cell trait. These conditions predispose patients to dehydration, which increases the risk of vaso-occlusive events. Renal insufficiency occurs in 10–20% of patients.

**F. Treatment**

1. **RBC transfusions** are indicated for patients with strokes, transient ischemic attacks, acute chest syndrome, aplastic crisis, priapism that is unresponsive to supportive care, and in preparation for general anes-

thesia. Guidelines for chronic transfusions should be followed (see the section Transfusion Therapy).

2. **Hydroxyurea** (15–35 mg/kg PO qd) has been shown to increase levels of fetal Hb and decrease the incidence of vaso-occlusive pain episodes by approximately 50% and acute chest syndrome by approximately 70% in adults with sickle cell anemia (*N Engl J Med* 332:1317, 1995).

IV. **G6PD deficiency** is the most common of the hereditary RBC enzyme deficiencies. It is a sex-linked disorder that typically affects men. The enzyme deficiency results in RBCs that are more susceptible to oxidant stress than normal RBCs, leading to chronic or episodic hemolysis.

A. **Classification.** A mild form of the deficiency occurs in approximately 10% of men of African heritage and is characterized by hemolytic episodes that are triggered by infections or drug exposure (Table 19-2). A more severe enzyme deficiency, such as the Mediterranean variety, results in hemolysis when susceptible individuals are exposed to fava beans. The most severe type causes a chronic, hereditary, nonspherocytic hemolytic anemia in the absence of an inciting cause.

B. **Laboratory results.** The peripheral smear shows "bite cells"; denatured Hb inclusions **(Heinz bodies)** are seen with special stains. Measurement of enzyme levels usually establishes the diagnosis. However, senescent RBCs contain less G6PD and are more easily destroyed than younger cells so that after a hemolytic episode, the G6PD level may be normal, reflecting the younger population of cells in the circulation.

C. **Treatment** consists of adequate hydration to protect renal function during hemolysis, avoidance of precipitating factors, and, if necessary, RBC transfusion.

V. **Autoimmune hemolytic anemia (AIHA)** is caused by antibodies to RBCs. In warm AIHA, antibodies interact best with RBCs at 37°C, whereas in cold AIHA, antibodies are most active at lower temperatures. The DAT is often positive in both forms of AIHA.

A. **Warm antibody AIHA** is usually caused by an IgG autoantibody. It may be idiopathic or associated with an underlying malignancy (lymphoma, chronic lymphocytic leukemia), collagen vascular disorder, or drugs (Table 19-2).

1. **Clinical presentation** may include weakness, jaundice, and splenomegaly. Severe hemolysis may be associated with fever, chest pain, syncope, CHF, and hemoglobinuria.
2. **Laboratory findings** include a decrease in haptoglobin, an increase in LDH, and a positive DAT for IgG. The peripheral smear shows spherocytes.
3. **Therapy** should be directed at identifying and treating any underlying cause. In most cases the hemolysis should be treated with glucocorticoids. The approach to treatment is similar to that of immune thrombocytopenic purpura (see Chap. 18, Disorders of Hemostasis, the section Platelet Disorders, sec. **I.E**). **RBC transfusions** are occasionally necessary in severe cases and pose a special problem. The conventional cross-matching procedure is difficult because autoantibodies are commonly present in the serum so that alloantibodies may escape detection, posing a risk of hemolysis. Treatment with folic acid is also recommended.

B. **Cold antibody AIHA** is associated with episodic cold-induced intravascular hemolysis and vaso-occlusive events resulting in cyanosis of the ears, nose, fingers, and toes. **Cold agglutinin disease** is the most common syndrome. The chronic form is caused by a paraprotein (lymphoma, Waldenström's macroglobulinemia) in approximately one-half of cases and is usually idiopathic in the others. Acute cold agglutinin syndrome, secondary to an infection (*Mycoplasma*, Epstein-Barr virus), is usually transient. IgM and C3 are found on the RBCs (the DAT identifies only the presence of C3). **Treatment** is directed at the underlying disease; the acute form usually requires only supportive measures. When transfusions are indicated, the blood should be warmed to 37°C before infusion to prevent exacerbation of hemolysis.

VI. **Drug-induced hemolytic anemia** may be caused by any of three distinct mechanisms. In all cases, treatment consists of discontinuing the offending agent. Medications that are known to cause these effects are listed in Table 19-2.

A. **Drug-induced autoantibodies** present similarly to warm antibody AIHA. The DAT is positive for IgG, and the anemia gradually resolves after discontinuation of the drug.

B. **Haptens** form when a drug (usually an antimicrobial) coats RBC membranes, forming a new antigenic determinant. If antibodies against the drug are present and the patient receives the drug (particularly at high doses), a DAT-positive (IgG) hemolytic anemia may result.

C. **Immune complexes.** IgM (occasionally IgG) antibodies may develop against a drug and form a drug-antibody complex that adheres to RBCs. Because the antibody involved is usually an IgM, the DAT is positive only for C3.

VII. **Microangiopathic hemolytic anemia** is a syndrome of traumatic intravascular hemolysis that is thought to be caused by deposition of fibrin strands in the lumen of small blood vessels. It may be seen in disseminated intravascular coagulation (DIC), thrombotic thrombocytopenic purpura, hemolytic-uremic syndrome, severe hypertension, vasculitis, eclampsia, and some disseminated malignancies. The peripheral smear shows schistocytes (fragmented RBCs) and frequently thrombocytopenia. Management of DIC, thrombotic thrombocytopenic purpura, and hemolytic-uremic syndrome is described in Chap. 18, Disorders of Hemostasis. **Traumatic (macroangiopathic) hemolytic anemia** refers to intravascular hemolysis that is most commonly associated with a malfunctioning prosthetic aortic valve. Porcine valves or valves in the mitral position are not as likely to cause significant hemolysis. The peripheral smear shows schistocytes, and therapy involves correction of the mechanical abnormality.

## Transfusion Therapy

Advances in collection, preparation, and administration have allowed transfusion of blood components to become useful in a wide variety of clinical situations. However, blood products are a limited resource, and their administration exposes the patient to the risk of a number of adverse effects, some of which may be life-threatening. **The benefits and risks of transfusion therapy must be carefully weighed in each situation.** In each case, the indications for transfusion should be recorded in the medical record. It is generally agreed that, if possible, informed consent should be obtained for the administration of all blood products. In elective surgery, this may require informing the patient several weeks in advance of the procedure so that the options of autologous donation and directed donation can be explored.

I. **RBC transfusion** is indicated to increase the oxygen-carrying capacity of blood in anemic patients when the anemia is responsible for poor tissue oxygenation. Adequate tissue oxygenation can usually be attained with a Hb of 7–8 g/dl in a normovolemic patient. One unit of RBCs increases the Hb by 1 g/dl in the average adult. Patient age, cause and severity of anemia, and coexisting disorders such as cardiopulmonary disease must be considered when determining the need for transfusion. If the cause of anemia is easily treatable (e.g., iron or folic acid deficiency) and no cerebrovascular or cardiopulmonary compromise is present, it is preferable to avoid transfusions. Many options are available to the responsible physician regarding the preparation and administration of blood (e.g., types of filter, flow rates), and these should be detailed in the medical orders.

II. **Preparation and administration of RBCs**

A. **The type and screen procedure** tests the recipient's RBCs for the A, B, and D (Rh) antigen and also screens the recipient's serum for antibodies against other RBC antigens. **Cross-matching** tests the patient's serum for antibodies against antigens on the donor's RBCs and is performed before a specific unit of blood is dispensed for a patient.

B. **Leukocyte-depleting (Leuko-poor) filters** remove 99.9% of WBCs from blood products and are recommended in the following circumstances: (1) in patients who have had one or more nonhemolytic febrile transfusion reactions that were not responsive to acetaminophen and diphenhydramine, (2) in patients who are undergoing RBC exchange transfusions, (3) in patients in whom cross-match incompatibilities are identified, and (4) to prevent CMV infection in patients who require CMV-negative blood products that are not available. Red blood cell products are often leukocyte depleted in the blood bank as a routine procedure in the absence of a specific indication.

C. **Irradiation of blood products** eliminates immunologically competent lymphocytes and is recommended for immunocompromised bone marrow or organ transplant recipients or for any patient who is receiving directed donations from HLA-matched donors or first-degree relatives.

D. **Washed RBCs** are rarely indicated but should be considered in patients in whom plasma proteins may cause a serious reaction (e.g., IgA-deficient recipients or patients with paroxysmal nocturnal hemoglobinuria).

E. **CMV-negative blood products** are indicated in immunocompromised bone marrow or organ transplant recipients who are CMV antibody negative.

F. **Premedication** with acetaminophen and diphenhydramine, 25–50 mg PO or IV, is recommended in all patients who are receiving RBC transfusion (except older patients at risk of delirium from diphenhydramine). Occasionally, glucocorticoids (e.g., hydrocortisone, 50–100 mg IV) are also of benefit in patients with previous nonhemolytic reactions.

G. **Administration.** Patient and blood product identification procedures must be carefully followed to avoid mishandling errors. The IV catheter should be at least 18 gauge to allow adequate flow. All blood products that are not leukocyte depleted should be administered through a 170- to 260-µm "standard" filter to prevent infusion of macroaggregates, fibrin, and debris. Only 0.9% NaCl should be used with blood components to prevent cell lysis. Patients should be observed for the first 5–10 minutes of each transfusion for adverse side effects and at regular intervals thereafter. Each unit of blood should be administered within 4 hours.

III. **Risks are incurred with all blood component therapy.** Patient concerns are primarily focused on transfusion-associated viral infections.

A. **Transfusion-transmitted infections.** Current testing for viral infections includes HIV-1, HIV-2, human T-lymphotropic virus type 1, hepatitis B virus, and hepatitis C virus. The risk of transfusion-associated transmission of HIV-1, HIV-2, human T-lymphotropic virus type 1, and hepatitis C from screened blood is estimated to be 1 in 2,000,000–3,000,000. The estimated risk of hepatitis B virus transmission is approximately 1 in 500,000. Viral infections occur when donors are in the seronegative window period, allowing the infection to escape detection. CMV transmission from RBC and platelet transfusion is an important risk in immunocompromised patients. CMV-negative blood products are recommended, but leukocyte-depleting filters seem to be effective in decreasing the risk. Infection with parvovirus B19 may occur and is a threat to specific patients. Risks from other viruses including West Nile Virus are not defined. Bacterial transmission may occur from either a donor infection or a contaminant at the time of collection; *Yersinia* is most frequently described with RBC transfusions. Parasitic infections, including *Plasmodium*, *Babesia*, or *Trypanosoma*, have occurred. Transfusion-transmitted prion disease appears possible but has not yet been identified.

B. **Noninfectious hazards of transfusion**

1. **Hemolytic transfusion reactions**

a. **Acute hemolytic reactions** are usually caused by preformed antibodies in the recipient and are characterized by intravascular hemolysis of the transfused RBCs soon after administration of ABO incompatible blood. Fever, chills, back pain, chest pain, nausea, vomiting, and symptoms related to hypotension may develop. Acute renal failure with hemoglobinuria may occur. In the unconscious patient, hypotension or hemoglobinuria may be the only manifestation. If a hemolytic transfusion reaction is suspected, the transfusion should be stopped immediately and all IV tubing should be replaced. Clotted and EDTA–treated samples of the patient's blood should be delivered to the blood bank along with the remainder of the suspected unit for repeat of the cross-match. Serum bilirubin and tests for DIC should be obtained, and the plasma and freshly voided urine should be examined for free Hb. **Management** includes preservation of intravascular volume and protection of renal function. Urine output should be maintained at 100 ml/hour or greater with the use of IV fluids and diuretics or mannitol, if necessary. The excretion of free Hb can be aided by alkalinization of the urine. Sodium bicarbonate can be added to IV fluids to increase the urinary pH to 7.5 or greater (see Chap. 11, Renal Diseases, the section Acute Renal Diseases, sec. **III.D**).

b. **Delayed hemolytic transfusion reactions** may occur within 3–4 weeks after transfusion and are caused by either a primary or an amnestic antibody response to specific RBC antigens. Usually the Hb and Hct fall and the bilirubin increases. While hemolysis is ongoing, the DAT may be positive, resulting in confusion with AIHA. Delayed hemolytic transfusion reaction may at times be severe; these cases should be treated similarly to acute hemolytic reactions.

2. **Nonhemolytic febrile transfusion reactions** are characterized by fevers, chills, urticaria, pruritus, and respiratory distress and are usually seen in previously transfused patients or multiparous women. Antibodies against donor plasma proteins or leukocyte antigens are thought to be the cause. Treatment of symptoms with acetaminophen for fever and diphenhydramine, 25–50 mg PO or IV, is usually sufficient. Rarely, epinephrine or glucocorticoids are required. Meperidine, 25–50 mg IV, is effective in preventing shaking chills. Some patients require premedication with acetaminophen and diphenhydramine, or leukocyte-depleting filters to prevent recurrence with subsequent transfusions. **Anaphylactic reactions** may be seen in patients with IgA deficiency who receive IgA-containing blood products and develop anti-IgA antibodies.

C. **Volume overload** with signs of CHF may be seen when patients with cardiovascular compromise are transfused with RBCs. Slowing the rate of transfusion and judicious use of diuretics help prevent this complication.

D. **Transfusion-related acute lung injury (TRALI)** is indistinguishable from acute respiratory distress syndrome and occurs within 4 hours of a transfusion. A number of patients require ventilatory assistance. Antileukocyte antibodies are frequently identified in the donor's serum, causing dyspnea, hypotension, fever, chills, and hypoxemia. Despite clinical or radiographic findings that suggest edema, available data indicate that diuretics have no role and may be detrimental.

E. **Transfusion-associated graft-versus-host disease** is usually seen in immunocompromised patients and is thought to result from the infusion of immunocompetent T lymphocytes. This entity has been reported in immunocompetent patients who share an HLA haplotype with HLA-homozygous blood donors (usually a relative or members of inbred populations). Rash, elevated liver function tests, and severe pancytopenia are seen. The mortality is greater than 80%. Irradiation of blood products prevents this disease (see sec. **II.C**). Because the chances of shared HLA haplotypes with a random blood donor are extremely low, irradiation of nonrelated blood products is not indicated for the immunocompetent patient.

F. **Posttransfusion purpura** is a rare syndrome of severe thrombocytopenia and purpura or bleeding that starts 7–10 days after exposure to blood products that contain platelets. The disorder is described in Chap. 18, Disorders of Hemostasis, the section Platelet Disorders, sec. **I.F.**

IV. **Adverse effects due to massive transfusion.** Administration of blood products greater than the normal blood volume of the patient in a 24-hour period **(massive transfusion)** may be associated with several additional complications.

A. **Hypothermia** caused by rapid infusion of chilled blood may cause cardiac dysrhythmias. A blood-warming device can prevent this problem.

B. **Citrate intoxication** occurs in patients with hepatic dysfunction and can cause hypocalcemia, resulting in paresthesias, tetany, hypotension, and decreased cardiac output. On rare occasions the patient may require calcium gluconate, 10 ml of a 10% solution IV. Calcium should never be added directly to the transfusion product because it may cause the blood to clot.

C. **Acidemia and hyperkalemia** may occur. Hyperkalemia is not usually significant unless the patient was hyperkalemic before transfusion (e.g., because of renal failure or muscle injury). Twenty-four hours after massive transfusion, hypokalemia may occur as RBCs become more metabolically active and take up potassium from the plasma.

D. **Bleeding complications** from dilution of platelets and plasma coagulation factors may be seen during massive transfusion. Correction of platelet and coagulation factor deficiencies should be based on clinical findings and laboratory monitoring rather than an empiric formula.

V. **Long-term RBC transfusion therapy** is indicated in a variety of diseases. These patients likely require either premedication or leukocyte-depleting filters to prevent nonhemolytic febrile reactions. Transfusion burdens in excess of approximately 50 U of RBCs require consideration of iron chelation therapy (see the section Anemias Associated with Decreased Red Blood Cell Production, sec. **II.B.3**). Consideration should also be given to performing an expanded RBC antigen panel to determine RBC phenotypic matches and decrease the risk of RBC alloimmunization and delayed hemolytic transfusion reactions.

VI. **Emergency RBC transfusions** should be used only in situations in which massive blood loss has resulted in cardiovascular compromise. Volume expansion with normal saline should be attempted initially. Blood typing can be performed in 10 minutes and cross-matching within 30 minutes in emergency situations. If unmatched blood must be used, it should be group O/Rh-negative type that has been previously screened for reactive antibodies. At the first sign of a transfusion reaction, the infusion should be stopped.

VII. **Approach to patients who are unwilling or unable to receive RBC transfusions.** The treatment of acute or severe anemia in which transfusions are not an option (i.e., patient refusal) raises difficult issues for the health care team. Understanding and documentation of any ethical or religious preferences and the patient's beliefs (e.g., Jehovah's Witness) along with early consultation with any liaison groups help to avoid confrontation and delay in therapy. Management includes reducing blood loss by phlebotomy and obtaining necessary testing in pediatric tubes. The use of Epo is often of benefit (Table 19-1). In most cases, concurrent use of oral or parenteral iron is also recommended (see Anemias Associated with Decreased Red Blood Cell Production, sec. **I.C.2**). An increase in Hb of 1–2 g/dl over approximately a week is generally observed.

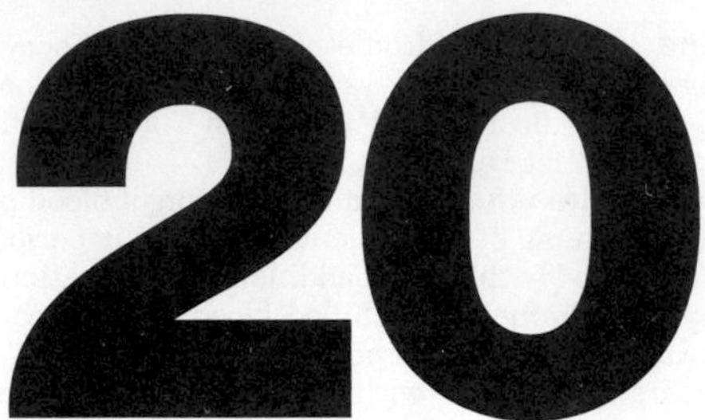

# Medical Management of Malignant Disease

Michael Naughton

## Approach to the Cancer Patient

**I. General.** Before treatment of a cancer patient is initiated, all patients should have a diagnosis of cancer based on tissue pathology, and, if possible, a clinical, biochemical, or radiographic marker of disease should be identified to assess the results of therapy.

**A. Stage and grade of tumor. Stage** is a clinical or pathologic assessment of tumor spread. The major role of staging is to define the optimal therapy and prognosis in subsets of patients. **Treatment plans are generally determined by the stage of the tumor.** The role of local therapies, surgery, and radiation are determined by regional spread of disease. The role of systemic therapy, or chemotherapy, is also dependent on the stage of the tumor. In general, the probability of survival correlates well with tumor stage. The **grade** of a tumor defines its retention of characteristics compared to the cell of origin. It is designated as low, moderate, or high as the tissue loses its normal appearance. Although grade is important in determining prognosis for many tumors, it is not used as commonly as stage in defining treatment plans.

**B. Performance status.** Performance status is a gauge of a patient's overall functional status. Two scales are commonly used: the Karnofsky performance status scale and the Eastern Cooperative Oncology Group scale (Table 20-1). Performance status is an essential component of the evaluation of cancer patients, as it helps predict response to treatment, duration of response, and survival. For most solid tumors, patients with poor performance status are unlikely to derive significant benefit from systemic chemotherapy. However, patients with tumors that respond dramatically to chemotherapy may benefit from this treatment, even if they have poor performance status.

**C. Therapy.** Cancer is in general treated with surgery, radiation, chemotherapy, or a combination of these modalities. Cancers are generally characterized as "liquid" or "solid" malignancies. Leukemias and lymphomas comprise the liquid group; the solid tumors include tumors that arise in any solid organ or tissue. The treatment of liquid tumors is usually chemotherapy or radiation therapy, or both. Solid tumors are treated with surgery, radiation therapy, chemotherapy, or some combination of these modalities.

**D. Chemotherapy** is administered in several different settings. **Induction chemotherapy** is used to achieve a complete remission. **Consolidation chemotherapy** is administered to patients who initially respond to treatment. **Maintenance therapy** refers to low-dose, outpatient treatment used to prolong remissions; its use has proved effective in a few malignancies. **Adjuvant chemotherapy** is given after complete surgical or radiologic eradication of a primary malignancy to eliminate any presumed but unmeasurable metastatic disease. **Neoadjuvant chemotherapy** is given in the presence of local disease, before planned local therapy.

**Table 20-1.** Performance status

| Karnofsky performance status scale | | ECOG performance status scale | |
|---|---|---|---|
| % | Definition | Grade | Definition |
| 100 | Normal; no complaints; no symptoms of disease | 0 | Fully active, able to carry on all predisease activity without restriction |
| 90 | Able to carry on normal activity; minor signs or symptoms of disease | 1 | Restricted in physically strenuous activity but ambulatory and able to carry out work of a light or sedentary nature |
| 80 | Normal activity with effort; some signs or symptoms of disease | | |
| 70 | Able to care for self; unable to carry on normal activity or to do active work | 2 | Ambulatory and capable of all self-care but unable to carry out any work activities; up and about >50% of waking hours |
| 60 | Requires occasional care for most needs | 3 | Capable of only limited self-care; confined to bed or chair >50% of waking hours |
| 50 | Requires considerable assistance and frequent medical care | | |
| 40 | Disabled; requires special care and assistance | 4 | Completely disabled; cannot carry on any self-care; totally confined to bed or chair |
| 30 | Severely disabled; hospitalization is indicated, although death is not imminent | | |
| 20 | Very sick; hospitalization necessary; active supportive treatment necessary | | |
| 10 | Moribund; fatal process progressing rapidly | | |
| 0 | Dead | | |

ECOG, Eastern Cooperative Oncology Group.

**E. Response to treatment** can be defined either by clinical or pathologic criteria. A **complete response** (or remission) is achieved when all evidence of malignancy is eradicated. A **partial response** is defined as a decrease in tumor mass by more than 50%.

**F. Palliative care and pain management.** Patients with cancer experience a multitude of symptoms. Studies have revealed that individuals with advanced cancer often experience ten or more symptoms, including pain, nausea, fatigue, weakness, constipation, and dyspnea. In addition to physical symptoms, patients also suffer emotionally and spiritually. Individuals with early-stage cancer experience similar symptoms, but with less frequency. The optimal management of cancer patients includes a careful assessment of symptomatology and appropriate management of these symptoms. **Palliative care** focuses on the relief of symptoms and coping with the implications of advanced cancer, as most patients with advanced cancer die from their disease. Defining appropriate treatment plans must include realistic assessments of prognosis and relative benefits of planned therapy.

1. **Pain** is present at diagnosis in 5–10% of patients with localized cancer and 60–90% of individuals with metastases. Improved oral analgesics, use of indwelling venous access devices, development of home nursing care agencies, and public acceptance of the hospice philosophy now allow patients to receive a large portion of their palliative treatment out of the hospital. Successful treatment of the underlying disease usually provides relief of pain. Painful foci of disease that are refractory to systemic intervention can be controlled with local radiation therapy, regional nerve block, or an ablative surgical procedure. In many situations, however, analgesics are necessary (see Chap. 1, Patient Care in Internal Medicine).
   a. **Mild or moderate cancer pain** may respond to nonopioid analgesics such as acetaminophen or nonsteroidal anti-inflammatory drugs. **Moderate to severe pain** almost always requires an opioid analgesic to attain significant relief. Medication administered on a prescribed schedule is more effective in maintaining analgesia than that taken intermittently once pain has developed. Several potent opioids are available in sustained-release formulations, including morphine, oxycodone hydrochloride, and fentanyl. Methadone has a long half-life and can be used as a long-lasting pain medication. Most patients with cancer pain have some combination of chronic and intermittent pain.
   b. **Optimal pain management** includes a long-lasting pain medication with prn dosing for breakthrough pain. Occasionally, infusions of morphine, 3–5 mg/hour IV, increased by 2–4 mg/hour as needed, are necessary. Under supervision, morphine drips can be used in the home setting. Morphine, as well as most other parenteral opioids, can also be administered subcutaneously. This reduces the difficulty of delivering these medications, especially in the home setting. Although tolerance and physical dependency can develop with long-term narcotic administration, **drug abuse and psychological dependency seldom occur** in the setting of chronic pain from cancer. These concerns should not compromise the patient's ability to achieve adequate analgesia.
   c. **Nonopioid adjuvant pain medications.** Acetaminophen and nonsteroidal anti-inflammatory drugs may offer some relief even in the setting of severe pain, allowing a lower dose of opioid to be used. Other adjuvant pain medications include tricyclic antidepressants and antiseizure medications, which may be especially useful for neuropathic pain. The bisphosphonates may improve the treatment of bone pain.
2. **Palliative care** is defined by the World Health Organization as "the active total care of the patient whose disease is not responsive to curative intent." Control of pain and other symptoms, as well as addressing psychological, social, and spiritual problems, is paramount (World Health Organization, Technical Report 804, 1990). A detailed overview of palliative care is beyond the scope of this chapter. The basic principles include a multidisciplinary approach to patient assessment and management. A careful and detailed assessment of symptoms, physical as well as psychological, is essential to this process, as is an assessment of the disease and patient status. This allows for realistic expectations regarding the disease process and prognosis to be determined, which in turn allow for informed decision making to formulate a plan of care.

**II. Therapy of selected solid tumors.** Guidelines for treatment of selected tumors are provided below; however, consultation with an oncologist should be obtained for recommendations regarding specific chemotherapeutic regimens.

**A. Breast cancer**

1. **Approach to an undiagnosed lump in the breast.** Breast cancer develops in approximately 11% of women during their lifetime in the United States. A breast lump in a premenopausal woman is less likely to be cancerous than a breast lump in a postmenopausal woman. In a younger woman, a mass should be observed for 1 month to identify any cyclic changes that suggest benign disease. If the mass is still present, bilateral mammography should be performed. The accuracy of mammography to diagnose cancer in pre- and postmenopausal women is approximately 90%. Nevertheless, a woman with a clinically suspicious lump and negative mammograms should undergo biopsy.
2. **Surgical options.** Treatment is focused on local control and the risk of systemic spread. Local control with **tylectomy** (lumpectomy and axillary lymph node dissection) is as effective as a modified radical mastectomy. An axillary lymph node dissection should be included because it provides prognostic information and is of therapeutic value. **Sentinel lymph node mapping** and dissection allow many women to be spared full axillary dissection. In this procedure, blue dye, a radiotracer, or both are injected around the tumor bed. The lymph node(s) that pick up the dye/tracer are excised. If no cancer cells are seen in these lymph nodes, further axillary dissection can be avoided.
3. **Adjuvant therapy.** The presence or absence of axillary lymph node metastases is the most important prognostic factor in breast cancer. All women with axillary nodal involvement should receive adjuvant therapy. Women with node-negative breast cancer should also be considered for adjuvant therapy if the tumor is greater than 1 cm, is estrogen receptor (ER) negative, or has overexpression of her-2. Chemotherapy should be considered in patients who are premenopausal, have cancers that are ER negative, or overexpress her-2. **Tamoxifen,** 20 mg PO qd for 5 years, is recommended for all ER-positive breast cancers (*J Natl Cancer Inst* 90:1601, 1998). **Anastrozole,** an aromatase inhibitor, has been compared to tamoxifen in the adjuvant setting in postmenopausal women and appears likely to be equivalent or slightly more effective than tamoxifen (*Lancet* 359:2131, 2002).
4. **Metastatic disease.** Menopausal status, hormone receptor status, her-2 expression, and sites of metastatic disease dictate initial treatment. ER-negative breast cancer, lymphangitic lung disease, and liver metastasis seldom respond to hormonal manipulation and should be treated with chemotherapy. In other metastatic sites, ER-positive disease is treated with hormonal manipulation. Premenopausal women are initially treated with tamoxifen and a luteinizing hormone–releasing hormone (LHRH) agonist; postmenopausal women should receive a hormonal agent such as tamoxifen or an aromatase inhibitor. If the disease responds to hormonal therapy, subsequent disease progression may respond to other hormonal agents. Chemotherapy should be considered if there is no response to initial hormonal therapy or if progression occurs during subsequent hormonal manipulations. In her-2 overexpressing cancers, the addition of the humanized antibody **trastuzumab** (see Chemotherapy, sec. **III.H.1.a**) to first-line chemotherapy produced an improvement in survival compared to chemotherapy alone (*N Engl J Med* 344:783, 2001). In women with more than one osteolytic metastasis, the monthly administration of **zoledronic acid,** 4 mg IV, produces an improvement in quality of life, greater response to therapy, fewer extravertebral fractures, and possibly a prolongation in survival (*Cancer J* 7:377, 2001).

5. **Inflammatory and unresectable cancers.** Inflammatory breast cancer manifests as "peau d'orange" changes or erythema involving more than one-third of the chest wall. Because of the high likelihood of metastases at diagnosis, these patients and those with inoperable primary breast cancers are initially treated with chemotherapy. Subsequently, surgery and radiation therapies are used for maximal local control.
6. **Radiation therapy** is indicated for patients treated with tylectomy and for some individuals with axillary lymph node involvement. It can also be used for palliation of painful or obstructing metastatic lesions.

B. **GI malignancies** commonly present with vague symptoms and are often advanced at the time of diagnosis.

1. **Esophageal cancers** are either squamous cell (associated with cigarette smoking and alcohol use) or adenocarcinoma (arising in Barrett's esophagus). Surgical resection of the esophagus is recommended in small primary tumors and in selected patients after chemoradiation. Local control of unresectable cancers can be achieved with combined chemotherapy and radiation therapy (*N Engl J Med* 335:462, 1996). Palliation of obstructive symptoms can be accomplished by radiation therapy, dilatation, prosthetic tube placement, or laser therapy.
2. **Gastric cancer** is usually adenocarcinoma and can be cured with surgery in the rare patient with localized disease. Adjuvant chemotherapy and concurrent radiation have been shown to improve outcomes in surgically resected gastric cancer (*N Engl J Med* 345:725, 2001). Locally advanced but unresectable cancers may benefit from concomitant chemotherapy and radiation therapy. Chemotherapy may offer palliation for metastatic disease.
3. **Colon and rectal adenocarcinomas** are primarily treated by surgical resection. A prolonged survival in patients with colon cancer and regional lymph node involvement is seen with administration of postoperative 5-fluorouracil (FU) and levamisole for 12 months or FU and leucovorin (LV) for 6 months (*Ann Intern Med* 122:321, 1995). Rectal cancer that arises below the peritoneal reflection commonly recurs locally after surgery alone; postoperative radiation therapy and FU are recommended. A number of chemotherapy agents are available for the treatment of metastatic colorectal cancer. These include FU, irinotecan, capecitabine, and oxaliplatin. In metastatic disease, the addition of irinotecan to FU/LV produces a higher likelihood of response and possible survival advantage (*N Engl J Med* 343:905, 2000). Selected patients with metastases confined to the liver may be candidates for liver resection (*J Clin Oncol* 15:938, 1997). In all patients who are undergoing surgical resection of colon or rectal cancer, a preoperative **carcinoembryonic antigen** level should be measured and followed. A persistently elevated or increasing level may indicate residual or recurrent tumor.
4. **Anal cancer.** Chemotherapy with concurrent radiation therapy appears to result in a higher cure rate than surgical resection and usually preserves the anal sphincter and fecal continence (*Cancer* 76:1731, 1995). Surgical resection should be used only as salvage therapy.

C. **Genitourinary malignancies**

1. **Bladder cancer** in the United States is usually a transitional cell carcinoma. A variety of chemical carcinogens, including those in cigarette smoke, have been implicated. Unifocal tumors confined to the mucosa should be managed with cystoscopy and transurethral resection or fulguration, repeated at approximately 3-month intervals; multifocal mucosal disease is treated with intravesicular bacillus Calmette-Guérin, thiotepa, or mitomycin-C. Locally invasive cancers should be resected. Adjuvant chemotherapy improves survival when regional lymph node

involvement is confirmed in the cystectomy specimen. In metastatic or recurrent disease, the highest response rates are seen with cisplatin-containing regimens.

2. **Prostate cancer.** Local control of the primary lesion can be achieved with either prostatectomy or radiation therapy. **Prostate-specific antigen** is useful as a marker for recurrence, bulk of disease, and response to therapy and may detect asymptomatic early-stage disease. In patients with metastatic disease, bilateral orchiectomy and LHRH analogs with or without an antiandrogen produce tumor regression in approximately 85% of patients for a median of 18–24 months. Disease that has relapsed after hormonal therapy may respond to withdrawal of that antiandrogen (*Urol Clin North Am* 24:421, 1997). Anthracyclines, taxanes, vinblastine, and estramustine may be of palliative value in hormone-refractory disease. Anemia and bone pain dominate the advanced phases of this disease and are best relieved with transfusions, growth factors, and palliative radiation therapy.
3. **Renal cell cancer** is treated by surgical resection, which may be curative if disease is localized; no effective adjuvant therapy is available. Chemotherapy, interferon-alpha, and interleukin-2 have reported response rates of 15–30%.
4. **Testicular cancer** is considered one of the most curable malignancies and should be treated aggressively. A patient suspected of having cancer of the testis should only have tissue obtained through an inguinal orchiectomy because a transscrotal incision facilitates tumor spread to the inguinal lymph nodes. The initial evaluation should also include **serum alpha-fetoprotein and β–human chorionic gonadotropin levels** and a CT scan of the abdomen and pelvis. Most patients with **seminoma** should be treated with radiation therapy. In **nonseminomatous germ cell cancer,** a retroperitoneal lymph node dissection should be performed for staging, except in the instance of bulky abdominal disease or pulmonary metastasis. If microscopic disease is identified at surgery, two alternatives are acceptable: two cycles of postoperative chemotherapy or observation until relapse occurs followed by institution of chemotherapy. With gross metastatic disease, cisplatin-based chemotherapy is curative for most germ cell cancers. If tumor markers normalize after chemotherapy but a radiographic mass persists, exploratory surgery should be performed. The lesion proves to be residual cancer in approximately one-third of the patients. Patients with residual cancer should receive additional chemotherapy (*J Clin Oncol* 8:1777, 1990).

**D. Gynecologic malignancies**

1. **Cervical cancer.** The recognized **risk factors** are multiparity, multiple sexual partners, and infection with human papillomavirus. Carcinoma in situ and superficial disease can be treated by endocervical cone biopsy. Microinvasive disease is treated with an abdominal hysterectomy. Advanced local disease (invasion of the cervix or local extension) is initially treated with surgery or radiation therapy, or both. The addition of chemotherapy to radiation therapy postoperatively is associated with improved survival (*N Engl J Med* 340:1154, 1999). Inoperable cancer can be controlled with radiation therapy; metastatic disease is treated with cisplatin-based chemotherapy.
2. **Ovarian cancer** is primarily a disease of postmenopausal women. Because symptoms are uncommon with localized disease, most patients present with advanced local disease, malignant ascites, or peritoneal metastases. Surgical staging and treatment include an abdominal hysterectomy, bilateral oophorectomy, lymph node sampling, omentectomy, peritoneal cytology, and removal of all gross tumor. If the tumor is localized to the ovary, the surgery may be curative and further treatment is not routinely recommended. However, if microscopic foci of cancer are

identified, chemotherapy is administered postoperatively. The serum marker **CA-125,** although not specific, is elevated in more than 80% of women with epithelial ovarian cancer and is a sensitive indicator of response. After a response is achieved, a "second-look laparotomy" is performed to restage and remove residual tumor. Approximately one-third of the patients who are in pathologic complete remission after a second-look laparotomy are cured. Those patients who have residual cancer should receive additional chemotherapy.

**E. Endometrial cancer** risks include obesity, nulliparity, polycystic ovaries, and the use of unopposed estrogens (including tamoxifen). Patients generally present with vaginal bleeding. Surgery and radiation therapy are often curative.

**F. Head and neck cancer** is usually a squamous cell cancer. It may arise in a variety of sites, each of which has a different natural history. Early lesions can be cured with surgery, radiation therapy, or both. Despite aggressive surgical and radiation therapy, approximately 65% of patients with head and neck cancer have uncontrolled local disease. The addition of chemotherapy to radiation therapy improves the survival in patients with nasopharyngeal cancers and selected patients with other primary disease sites (*J Natl Cancer Inst* 91:2081, 1999).

**G. Lung cancer** is the most common cause of cancer death in the United States and is the most preventable given its relationship to cigarette smoking. Treatment is based on the histology and stage of the disease. Whenever possible, surgical resection should be attempted for non–small-cell lung cancer because it affords the best chance of cure. Small-cell and non–small-cell lung cancers are treated according to whether disease is limited (confined to one hemithorax and ipsilateral regional lymph nodes) or extensive stage.

1. **Small-cell lung cancer** is often responsible for a variety of paraneoplastic syndromes in addition to local symptoms (see Complications of Cancer, sec. **II**). For **limited disease,** combination chemotherapy and radiation therapy result in an 85–90% response rate, a median survival of 12–18 months, and a cure in 5–15% of patients. With **extensive disease,** the median survival is 8–9 months, and cures are rare. For patients who achieve a complete remission with chemotherapy, **prophylactic whole-brain radiation therapy** has been shown to decrease the risk of CNS metastases (*N Engl J Med* 341:476, 1999). Radiation therapy to the chest as consolidation therapy may improve survival in limited disease but is not recommended in extensive disease except for palliation of local symptoms.
2. **Non–small-cell lung cancer** survival rates after resection are not improved with adjuvant chemotherapy or radiation therapy. For unresectable disease confined to the lung and regional lymph nodes, radiation therapy is the conventional treatment. The use of chemotherapy before or concurrent with radiation may improve survival in patients with a good performance status. In patients with metastatic disease, cisplatin-based combination chemotherapy may modestly improve survival.

**H. Malignant melanoma** should be considered in any changing or enlarging nevus, and suspicious lesions should be removed by **excisional biopsy.** Subsequently, a wide local excision is performed to remove possible vertical and radial spread of tumor. Deeper invasion is associated with a worse prognosis. **High-dose interferon** prolongs the survival of selected high-risk resected patients (*J Clin Oncol* 14:7, 1996). Systemic disease may respond to dacarbazine, interferon-alpha, or interleukin-2 in 10–30% of patients.

**I. Sarcomas** are tumors arising from mesenchymal tissue and occur most commonly in soft tissue or bone. Initial evaluation should include a CT scan of the chest, as hematogenous spread to the lungs is common.

1. The prognosis for **soft-tissue sarcoma** is primarily determined by tumor grade and not by the cell of origin. Surgical resection should be

performed when feasible and may be curative. In low-grade tumors, local and regional recurrence is most common, and adjuvant radiation therapy may be of benefit. High-grade tumors often recur systemically, but no advantage to the routine use of adjuvant chemotherapy has been demonstrated. In metastatic disease, doxorubicin, ifosfamide, and dacarbazine produce responses in 40–55% of patients.

2. **Osteogenic sarcomas** are treated with surgical resection followed by adjuvant chemotherapy for 1 year. Treatment of isolated pulmonary metastasis by surgical resection is associated with long-term survival.
3. **Kaposi's sarcoma** in an immunocompetent patient is generally a low-grade lesion of the lower extremities that is readily treated with local radiation therapy or vinblastine. When Kaposi's sarcoma complicates organ transplantation or AIDS, it is more aggressive and may arise in visceral sites. Liposomal doxorubicin alone is as effective as combination chemotherapy for palliation (*J Clin Oncol* 14:2353, 1996).

J. **Cancer with an unknown primary site.** Approximately 5% of cancer patients present with symptoms of metastatic disease, but no primary tumor site is identifiable on physical examination, routine laboratory studies, or chest radiography. The histopathologic cell type and the site of the metastasis should direct a search for the primary lesion. Immunohistochemical stains may identify specific tissue antigens that help to define the origin of the tumor and guide subsequent therapy. Two potentially curative circumstances are described below.

1. **Cervical adenopathy** suggests cancer of the lung, breast, head and neck, or lymphoma. In this case, initial evaluation usually includes panendoscopy (nasendoscopy, laryngopharyngoscopy, bronchoscopy, and esophagoscopy) and biopsy of any suspicious lesion before excision of the lymph node. If squamous cell carcinoma is identified, the patient is presumed to have primary head and neck cancer, and radiation therapy may be curative.
2. **Midline mass in the mediastinum or retroperitoneum.** In both sexes, a midline mass in the mediastinum or retroperitoneum may be an extragonadal germ cell cancer. Elevations in alpha-fetoprotein or β–human chorionic gonadotropin further suggest this diagnosis. This neoplasm is potentially curable (see sec. **II.C.4**).

## III. Therapy of hematologic tumors

A. **Lymphoma** is usually diagnosed by biopsy of an enlarged lymph node.

1. **Staging** of Hodgkin's disease and non-Hodgkin's lymphoma is organized into four categories.
   a. **Stage I** is disease localized to a single lymph node or group.
   b. **Stage II** is disease involving more than one lymph node group but confined to one side of the diaphragm.
   c. **Stage III** is disease in the lymph nodes or the spleen and occurs on both sides of the diaphragm.
   d. **Stage IV** is disease involving the liver, lung, skin, or bone marrow.
   e. **B symptoms** include fever above 38.5°C, night sweats that require a change in clothes, or a 10% weight loss over 6 months. These symptoms suggest bulky disease and a worse prognosis.
2. **Hodgkin's disease** usually presents with cervical adenopathy and spreads in a predictable manner along lymph node groups. Treatment is based on the presenting stage of the disease; the cell type is relatively unimportant in the natural history and prognosis. **Initial evaluation** includes a CT scan of the chest, abdomen, and pelvis, and bilateral bone marrow biopsies to determine the clinical stage of the disease. Exploratory laparotomy with splenectomy and liver biopsy is performed if the findings will change the disease stage and treatment. **Stage IA and IIA** disease are treated with radiation therapy or a combination of chemotherapy and radiation. **Stage IIIA** disease can be treated either by radia-

tion therapy or chemotherapy, whereas all **stage IV** patients should receive combination chemotherapy. When **B symptoms** are present, chemotherapy is recommended regardless of the stage.

3. **Non-Hodgkin's lymphoma** is classified as low, intermediate, or high grade based on the histologic type. Staging evaluation is the same as for Hodgkin's disease, but non-Hodgkin's lymphoma has a less predictable pattern of spread. Advanced-stage disease (stage III or IV) is very common and can usually be diagnosed by CT scan or bone marrow biopsy; exploratory laparotomy and lymphangiography are rarely necessary.
   a. **Low-grade lymphoma** often involves the bone marrow at diagnosis, but the disease has an indolent course. Because this tumor is not curable with standard chemotherapy, treatment can be delayed until the patient is symptomatic ("watch and wait"). Radiation therapy or an alkylating agent (e.g., cyclophosphamide) can be used to ameliorate symptoms. Radiation therapy may produce a long-term complete remission in stage I or II disease. **Rituximab** is a humanized monoclonal antibody that recognizes the CD20 antigen expressed by most indolent lymphomas (see Chemotherapy, sec. **III.H.1.b**). This agent produces an objective response in approximately 50% of patients with follicular lymphoma without the usual toxicities of chemotherapy.
   b. **Intermediate-grade lymphoma** has a more aggressive course, usually does not involve the bone marrow at diagnosis, and can be cured with chemotherapy. Complete response rates exceed 80%. Features associated with a lower likelihood of cure include an elevated lactate dehydrogenase level, stage III/IV disease, age older than 60 years, more than one extranodal site, and poor performance status.
   c. **High-grade lymphoma** (Burkitt's, lymphoblastic) includes the most aggressive subtypes and has a high frequency of CNS and bone marrow involvement. **Cerebrospinal fluid (CSF) cytology** should be included as part of the initial evaluation. Combination chemotherapy is the mainstay of treatment and should include CNS prophylaxis if the CSF is cytologically free of tumor. If tumor cells are seen in the CSF, additional therapy may be indicated (see Complications of Cancer, sec. **I.B**). Prophylaxis to prevent **tumor lysis syndrome** (see Complications of Treatment, sec. **I.F**) should be initiated before induction chemotherapy.

B. **Acute leukemias** may present with manifestations of cytopenias, including fatigue and dyspnea (anemia), cutaneous or mucosal hemorrhage (thrombocytopenia), and fever/infection (neutropenia). Patients may also present with leukemic infiltration of organs, manifested as lymphadenopathy, splenomegaly (more common in acute lymphocytic leukemia), gingival hyperplasia, and skin nodules (more common in acute myeloid leukemia). Leukemic blasts are usually present in the blood. Bone marrow aspiration/biopsy is performed to establish the diagnosis and often shows nearly complete replacement by blasts. **Flow cytometry and cytogenetics** must be performed on the bone marrow aspirate for classification and to provide prognostic information.

1. **Acute myeloid leukemia** constitutes approximately 80% of adult acute leukemia. Approximately 50–80% of patients achieve complete remission with induction chemotherapy that includes cytarabine [cytosine arabinoside (ara-C)] and daunorubicin. Consolidation is given with at least one additional cycle of chemotherapy, which is typically ara-C at a dose of 10–30 times that used for induction (high-dose ara-C). High-dose ara-C consolidation results in cure in approximately 30–40% of patients younger than 60 years. Pretreatment factors associated with a low (<10%) chance for cure include preceding myelodysplastic syndrome; prior exposure to radiation, benzene, or chemotherapy; and

adverse cytogenetic abnormalities. For these high-risk patients, allogeneic stem cell transplant in first remission increases the likelihood of cure. **Acute promyelocytic leukemia** is characterized by a chromosomal translocation [t(15;17)] that results in a hybrid protein (pml-rar). Treatment with oral tretinoin (*all-trans* retinoic acid) results in complete remission in greater than 90% of patients. After consolidation chemotherapy, approximately 75% of patients are cured.

2. **Acute lymphocytic leukemia** is predominantly a disease of childhood, with only 25% of all cases occurring in patients older than the age of 15 years. For adults, induction and consolidation involve treatment with multiple chemotherapeutic agents over a period of approximately 6 months followed by at least 18 months of lower-dose maintenance chemotherapy. To prevent CNS relapse, patients receive intrathecal (IT) chemotherapy and either cranial radiation or CNS penetrating chemotherapy. Approximately 60–80% of adults achieve complete remission, with about 30–40% being cured; increasing age, higher WBC, and longer time to remission are associated with reduced survival. Cytogenetics are crucial in determining prognosis, and allogeneic stem cell transplantation during the first remission should be considered in patients with a poor prognosis.

C. **Chronic lymphocytic leukemia (CLL)** usually presents with lymphocytosis, lymphadenopathy, and splenomegaly. Malignant cells resemble mature lymphocytes. Treatment is similar to that for **low-grade lymphoma** (see sec. **III.A.3.a**) except that fludarabine appears to be more active than alkylating agents. Median survival is approximately 6–8 years; anemia and thrombocytopenia are associated with shortened survival. As in low-grade lymphoma, patients are treated for control of symptoms or cytopenias. Because CLL is accompanied by immunodeficiency, **life-threatening infections may occur.** Therefore, febrile patients must be evaluated carefully. Immune hemolytic anemia or immune thrombocytopenia may develop as complications of CLL. Treatment of these conditions is with glucocorticoids (e.g., prednisone, 1 mg/kg PO qd) or chemotherapy, or both. CLL may transform to an intermediate- or high-grade lymphoma (Richter's transformation).

D. **Chronic myelogenous leukemia (CML)** presents with leukocytosis and a left shift, as well as splenomegaly. Thrombocytosis, basophilia, and eosinophilia are also common. The diagnosis is confirmed by demonstration of the **Philadelphia chromosome** (t9:22), which results in production of a hybrid protein (bcr-abl). During the **stable phase** of the disease, leukocytosis, thrombocytosis, and splenomegaly can be controlled for several years with oral hydroxyurea, and most patients are asymptomatic. However, **acute leukemic transformation (blast phase)** is inevitable and unpredictable, with a median time to transformation of 5–7 years. Blast phase is highly resistant to treatment and is usually fatal. For younger patients (40–50 years old) with HLA-identical siblings, allogeneic stem cell transplantation performed in stable phase within 1 year of diagnosis is the treatment of choice, resulting in a 50–70% likelihood of cure. For older patients and for those without an HLA-identical sibling, options include unrelated donor transplant or therapy with interferon-alpha. The latter agent delays blast phase in some patients. **STI571** (Gleevec) is an orally administered medication designed specifically to inhibit the bcr-abl tyrosine kinase. Because STI571 is more active and has far fewer toxicities than interferon, it is currently the first-line therapy for this disease. Even blast phase CML or Philadelphia chromosome–positive acute leukemia may respond to Gleevec. Responses in this setting are generally of relatively short duration.

E. **Hairy-cell leukemia** represents 2–3% of all adult leukemias. Clinical presentation includes splenomegaly, pancytopenia, and infection. Patients are at increased risk for bacterial, viral, and fungal infections and have a unique susceptibility to atypical mycobacterial infections. Bone marrow biopsy reveals infiltration by cells that have prominent cytoplasmic projections. A single 7-day course of **chlorodeoxyadenosine** produces remission in more than 90% of patients. Although this drug is not curative, 5-year progression-free survival exceeds 50%.

F. **Multiple myeloma** is a malignant plasma cell disorder that is usually accompanied by a serum or urine paraprotein, or both. Presenting manifestations may include hypercalcemia, anemia, lytic bone lesions with bone pain, and acute renal failure. The **initial evaluation** should include a radiographic bone survey, bone marrow aspiration and biopsy, serum and urine protein electrophoresis, $\beta_2$-microglobulin, and quantitative immunoglobulins. Treatment generally includes a combination of an oral alkylating agent (i.e., melphalan) and prednisone or vincristine/doxorubicin/dexamethasone. Local radiation therapy can be used to relieve painful bone lesions, and **zoledronic acid,** 4 mg IV q month, decreases skeletal complications. After induction chemotherapy, consolidation with high-dose therapy and autologous stem cell transplant improves survival (see the section Hematopoietic Stem Cell Transplantation). **Thalidomide,** an immunomodulatory agent, has been shown to be effective in multiple myeloma. Because thalidomide can cause severe fetal malformations, prescribing this medication requires participation in a prescriber program. Combinations of dexamethasone and thalidomide are also active in the treatment of multiple myeloma. **Bortezomib** (Velcade), a proteasome inhibitor that degrades ubiquitinated proteins, has recently been approved for the treatment of multiple myeloma that has progressed despite two previous treatments. Toxicities of bortezomib are primarily thrombocytopenia and neuropathy.

## Complications of Cancer

### I. Complications related to tumor mass

A. **Brain metastasis.** Patients with parenchymal brain metastasis may present with headache, mental status changes, weakness, or focal neurologic deficits. Papilledema is observed in only 25% of patients. In individuals with malignancy, a CT scan of the head showing one or more round, contrast-enhancing lesions surrounded by edema is usually sufficient for the diagnosis. If cancer has not been diagnosed previously, tissue should be obtained from the brain lesion or a more accessible site before radiation therapy is initiated. Therapy with **dexamethasone,** 10 mg IV or PO, should be initiated to decrease cerebral edema and should be continued at a dosage of 4–6 mg PO q6h throughout the course of radiation therapy, or longer if symptoms related to edema persist. Subsequent therapy depends on the number and location of the brain lesions as well as the prognosis of the underlying cancer. Patients with a chemotherapy-responsive neoplasm and a solitary accessible lesion should be considered for surgical resection. **All patients who have not received prior radiation therapy should be given whole-brain radiation therapy.**

B. **Meningeal carcinomatosis** should be suspected in a cancer patient with headache or cranial neuropathies. This pattern of spread is most often seen with lung or breast cancer, melanoma, or lymphoma; the diagnosis is confirmed by cytology of the CSF. A CT scan of the head should be performed to rule out parenchymal metastases or hydrocephalus before a lumbar puncture is performed. Local radiation therapy or IT chemotherapy may provide temporary relief of symptoms (see Chemotherapy, sec. **II.C**). Meningeal lymphoma may respond to IV ara-C.

C. **Spinal cord compression** is most commonly caused by hematogenous spread of cancer to the vertebral bodies followed by expansion into the spinal canal or ischemia of the spinal cord. The most common malignancies causing spinal cord compression are breast, lung, and prostate cancer, but **the diagnosis should be considered in any patient with cancer who complains of back pain.** Evaluation and therapy are discussed in Chap. 24, Neurologic Disorders.

D. **Superior vena cava obstruction** is most commonly caused by cancers, such as lymphoma or lung cancer, that arise in or spread to the mediastinum. The compressed superior vena cava leads to swelling of the face or trunk, chest pain, cough, and shortness of breath. Dilated superficial veins of the chest, neck, or sublingual area suggest an engorged collateral circulation. The presence of a mass on chest radiograph or CT scan usually confirms the diagnosis. Because collateral veins develop, the cerebral circulation is not significantly affected, but a **mediastinal mass may compromise the airway.** If the histologic origin of the obstruction is unknown, tissue can be obtained for diagnosis via bronchoscopy or mediastinoscopy. Therapy is directed at the underlying disease. Chemotherapy should be administered through a vein that is not obstructed by the lesion. Neoplasms that are not responsive to chemotherapy are treated with radiation therapy (*J Clin Oncol* 2:961, 1984).

E. **Malignant effusions**

1. **Malignant pericardial effusions** commonly result from cancer of the breast or lung. Initial presentation ranges from dyspnea to acute cardiovascular collapse from cardiac tamponade requiring emergency pericardiocentesis. After cardiovascular stabilization, some patients may improve with treatment if the tumor is chemotherapy sensitive. When the pericardial effusion is a complication of uncontrolled disease, palliation can be achieved by pericardiocentesis with sclerosis; the effusion should be completely drained, followed by instillation of 30–60 mg bleomycin through the drainage catheter, which is subsequently clamped for 10 minutes and then withdrawn (*Int J Cardiol* 16:155, 1987). Subxiphoid pericardiotomy can be performed in patients whose effusions do not respond to other treatment (*JAMA* 257:1088, 1987).
2. **Malignant pleural effusions** develop as a result of pleural invasion by tumor or obstruction of lymphatic drainage. When systemic control is not feasible and reaccumulation of fluid occurs rapidly after drainage, removal of the fluid followed by instillation of a sclerosing agent into the pleural space is recommended. Resistant effusions can be controlled with pleurectomy.
3. **Malignant ascites** is most commonly caused by peritoneal carcinomatosis and is best controlled by systemic chemotherapy. Therapeutic paracenteses can provide symptomatic relief. Intraperitoneal instillation of chemotherapy has been used but is not routinely recommended.

F. **Bone metastases** may result in spontaneous fracture. Prophylactic surgical pinning and radiation therapy may be indicated. Bisphosphonates may also protect against skeletal complications from myeloma and breast cancer (*N Engl J Med* 334:488, 1996).

II. **Paraneoplastic syndromes** are complications of malignancy that are not directly caused by a tumor mass effect and are presumed to be mediated by either secreted tumor products or the development of autoantibodies. Paraneoplastic syndromes can affect virtually every organ system, and in most cases, successful treatment of the underlying malignancy eliminates these effects.

A. **Metabolic complications**

1. **Hypercalcemia** is the most common metabolic complication in malignancy and can cause mental status changes, GI discomfort, and constipation. Acute and chronic management of hypercalcemia is discussed in Chap. 3, Fluid and Electrolyte Management.
2. **Syndrome of inappropriate antidiuretic hormone (SIADH)** should be considered in a euvolemic cancer patient with unexplained hyponatremia

(see Chap. 3, Fluid and Electrolyte Management). Although a variety of neoplasms have been described in association with SIADH, small-cell lung cancer is most often responsible. If chemotherapy is ineffective, radiation therapy may decrease the tumor mass and relieve symptoms.

3. **Cancer anorexia and cachexia** refers to the clinical syndrome of anorexia, distortion of taste perception, and loss of muscle mass. The asthenic appearance of patients is more often related to tumor type than to tumor burden. **Megestrol acetate,** 160 mg PO qd, has been used as an appetite stimulant and results in weight gain in some patients (*J Natl Cancer Inst* 89:1763, 1997). Other appetite stimulants include steroids, cannabinoids, and promotility agents such as metoclopramide.

**B. Neuromuscular complications**

1. **Polymyositis and dermatomyositis.** Dermatomyositis, more often than polymyositis, has been associated with a variety of malignancies, including non–small-cell lung cancer and colon, ovarian, and prostate cancers. In some patients, successful treatment of the underlying malignancy has resulted in resolution of the symptoms. An exhaustive search for a malignancy is not recommended because a primary malignancy is found in fewer than 20% of patients (*N Engl J Med* 326:363, 1992) (see Chap. 23, Arthritis and Rheumatologic Diseases).
2. **Lambert-Eaton myasthenic syndrome** is characterized by proximal muscle weakness, decreased or absent deep tendon reflexes, and autonomic dysfunction. Electromyography using high-frequency nerve stimulation may show posttetanic potentiation. Small-cell lung cancer is most often associated with this syndrome, and effective chemotherapy may result in improvement. Worsening symptoms have been reported with the use of calcium channel antagonists; these agents are contraindicated in this syndrome (*N Engl J Med* 321:1567, 1989).

**C. Hematologic complications.** Although cytopenias occur more often as a complication of treatment (see Complications of Treatment, sec. **I.B**) or marrow involvement with cancer, elevated counts may be explained by paraneoplastic syndromes.

1. **Erythrocytosis** is a rare complication of hepatoma, renal cell cancer, and benign tumors of the kidney, uterus, and cerebellum. Debulking the tumor with surgery or radiation therapy generally results in resolution of the erythrocytosis. Occasionally, therapeutic phlebotomy is indicated.
2. **Granulocytosis** (leukemoid reaction), in the absence of infection, occurs in cancer that arises in the stomach, lung, pancreas, brain, and lymphoma. Because the neutrophils are mature and seldom exceed 100,000/mm$^3$, complications are rare and intervention is generally unnecessary.
3. **Thrombocytosis** in patients with cancer may be caused by splenectomy, iron deficiency, acute hemorrhage, or inflammation; treatment is usually not necessary.
4. **Thromboembolic complications.** Mucin-secreting adenocarcinomas of the GI tract and lung cancer have been associated with a "hypercoagulable state," resulting in recurrent venous and arterial thromboembolism. Nonbacterial thrombotic (marantic) endocarditis, usually involving the mitral valve, may also occur. Heparin anticoagulation or low-molecular-weight heparin should be instituted, as well as treatment of the underlying cancer. Long-term warfarin with a target international normalized ratio of 2–3 or daily low-molecular-weight heparin is recommended to prevent subsequent thrombi (*Ann Intern Med* 130:800, 1999). In many patients, biochemical evidence of disseminated intravascular coagulation coexists with thromboemboli (see Chap. 18, Disorders of Hemostasis).

**D. Glomerular injury** resulting in renal failure has been observed as a paraneoplastic syndrome. Minimal change disease is often associated with lymphoma, especially Hodgkin's disease; membranous glomerulonephritis is more often seen with solid tumors. The process can be reversed with treatment of the underlying cancer (see Chap. 11, Renal Diseases).

E. **Clubbing of the fingers** and **hypertrophic osteoarthropathy** (polyarthritis and periostitis of long bones) are most often observed in non–small-cell lung cancer but are also seen with lesions that are metastatic to the mediastinum. Some improvement in the osteoarthropathy can be achieved with nonsteroidal anti-inflammatory drugs, but definitive therapy requires treatment of the underlying malignancy.

F. **Fever** may accompany lymphoma, renal cell cancer, and hepatic metastasis. Once an infectious etiology for the fever has been excluded, nonsteroidal anti-inflammatory drugs (e.g., ibuprofen, 400 mg PO qid, or indomethacin, 25–50 mg PO tid) may provide symptomatic relief.

## Chemotherapy

I. **Administration of chemotherapeutic drugs.** The dosage of chemotherapy is usually based on body surface area (Table 20-2); for some agents, dosage is determined by body weight and should be adjusted when changes in body weight occur. An assessment of the patient disease status, determination of side effects from the previous treatment, and a CBC should be obtained before each cycle of chemotherapy. Drug dosages usually must be adjusted for the following conditions: (1) neutropenia, (2) thrombocytopenia, (3) stomatitis, (4) diarrhea, or (5) limited metabolic capacity for the drug. **The advice of an oncologist and precise adherence to a treatment plan are mandatory because of the low therapeutic index of chemotherapeutic agents.**

II. **Route of administration**

A. **Oral drug administration** may be accompanied by nausea and vomiting and may require antiemetic therapy. For some agents, oral absorption is erratic and parenteral administration is preferred.

B. **IV drug administration** should be performed by experienced personnel. Care should be taken to ensure free flow of fluid to the vein, and adequate blood return should be verified before instillation of chemotherapy. Infusions should be through a large-caliber, upper extremity vein. When possible, veins of the antecubital fossa, wrist, dorsum of the hand, and arm ipsilateral to an axillary lymph node dissection should be avoided. In patients with poor peripheral venous access or those who require many doses of chemotherapy, **indwelling venous catheter devices** should be considered (*JAMA* 253:1590, 1985).

C. **Intrathecal chemotherapy** is administered for the treatment of meningeal carcinomatosis or as CNS prophylaxis. Side effects include acute arachnoiditis, subacute motor dysfunction, and progressive neurologic deterioration (leukoencephalopathy). Decreased cognitive function has been found in children. Impaired cognitive function and leukoencephalopathy occur more often when IT chemotherapy is combined with whole-brain radiation. **Methotrexate,** 10–12 mg, is diluted in 5 ml preservative-free nonbacteriostatic isotonic solution. Before administration, 5–10 ml CSF should be allowed to drain; methotrexate is then injected into the spinal canal over 5–10 minutes. To decrease the risk of arachnoiditis, patients should remain in a supine position for 15 minutes after the infusion is completed. Slow-release cytarabine, 50 mg, or ara-C, 50–100 mg in 5–10 ml diluent, can be administered in a similar manner (*J Clin Oncol* 17:3110, 1999).

D. **Intracavitary instillation** of chemotherapy may be useful in some circumstances. **Thiotepa,** 30–60 mg, is commonly instilled in the bladder for the treatment of bladder carcinoma. Doxorubicin and cisplatin have been given

**Table 20-2.** Doses and common toxicities of antineoplastic agents

| Agent | Dose range–schedule | N & V | Mucositis | Diarrhea | Days to nadir | Myelosuppression | Other toxicity or cautions |
|---|---|---|---|---|---|---|---|
| **Antimetabolites** | | | | | | | |
| Capecitabine | 1250 mg/m² PO q12h × 14 d/off 7 d | + | + | ++ | 7–14 | + | Hand-foot syndrome |
| Cytarabine (cytosine arabinoside) | 20 mg/m² IV infusion × 14–21 d | 0 | 0 | + | 10–14 | +++ | — |
| | 100–200 mg/m² IV qd × 5–7 d | ++ | + | ++ | 10–14 | +++ | — |
| | 1.5–3 g/m² IV q12h × 3–6 d | +++ | + | ++ | 10–14 | +++ | Cerebellar dysfunction, conjunctivitis |
| Fludarabine | 15–30 mg/m² qd × 5 d | + | 0 | 0 | 7–14 | +++ | Neurotoxicity |
| 5-Fluorouracil | 250–450 mg/m² IV × 5 d | 0 | + | + | 7–14 | ++ | — |
| | 200–1000 mg/m² infusion × 5 d | 0 | +++ | +++ | 7–14 | + | Phlebitis, cerebellar symptoms |
| | Often with leucovorin 20 mg/m² qd | 0 | + | +++ | 7–14 | + | Hand-foot syndrome |
| Gemcitabine | 1 g/m² q1wk × 3 doses every 4 wk | + | 0 | 0 | | ++ | Peripheral edema |
| Methotrexate | 10–60 mg/m² IV every 1–3 wk | + | ++ | ++ | 7–14 | ++ | Dermatitis, interstitial nephritis, pneumonitis; modify dose for renal dysfunction |
| | If >1.5 g IV qd × 1 wk, then requires leucovorin rescue | +++ | +++ | +++ | 7–14 | +++ | Modify dose with effusions |
| Pentostatin (2-deoxycoformycin) | 4 mg/m² IV every 2 wk | + | 0 | 0 | 7 | + | Erythema, lethargy, renal failure |

| | | | | | | | |
|---|---|---|---|---|---|---|---|
| 6-Mercaptopurine | 75–100 mg/m² PO qd | + | 0 | 0 | 7–14 | ++ | Hepatotoxicity; modify dose for renal dysfunction, allopurinol |
| Thioguanine | 100 mg/m² PO qd × 1–4 d | + | + | 0 | 10–30 | ++ | Modify dose for renal dysfunction |
| Cladribine (2-chlorodeoxyadenosine) | 0.09 mg/kg/d IV × 7 d | + | 0 | 0 | 7–14 | +++ | — |
| **Alkylating agents** | | | | | | | |
| Busulfan | 2–4 mg/m² PO qd | 0 | + | 0 | 14–28 | ++ | Hyperpigmentation Addison-like syndrome, pulmonary fibrosis |
| Chlorambucil | 6–14 mg PO qd | 0 | 0 | 0 | 10–14 | ++ | — |
| Cyclophosphamide | 60–150 mg/m² PO qd × 14 d | + | 0 | 0 | 10–12 | ++ | Interstitial pneumonitis, hemorrhagic cystitis |
| | 500–1500 mg/m² IV every 21 d | ++ | + | 0 | 7–14 | ++ | Hemorrhagic cystitis |
| | 120–200 mg/kg IV × 2–4 doses for BMT | +++ | +++ | +++ | 7–14 | +++ | Cardiomyopathy |
| Dacarbazine (DTIC) | 150–250 mg/m² IV qd × 5 d every 21–28 d | +++ | 0 | 0 | — | — | Flu-like symptoms; modify dose for renal dysfunction |
| Altretamine (hexamethylmelamine) | 260 mg/m²/d PO × 14–21 d | ++ | 0 | 0 | 21–28 | + | Peripheral neuropathy |
| Ifosfamide | 800–1500 mg/m² IV qd × 3–5 d every 21–28 d | +++ | 0 | 0 | 7–10 | +++ | Encephalopathy, hemorrhagic cystitis, administer with mesna (bladder protection) |

*(continued)*

**Table 20-2.** Continued

| Agent | Dose range–schedule | N & V | Mucositis | Diarrhea | Days to nadir | Myelosuppression | Other toxicity or cautions |
|---|---|---|---|---|---|---|---|
| Mechlorethamine | 8 $mg/m^2$ IV every 28 d | +++ | + | + | 7–14 | ++ | Rash; vesicant |
| Melphalan | 4–8 $mg/m^2$ PO qd × 4 d | 0 | 0 | 0 | 10–14 | ++ | — |
| Thiotepa | Up to 1.25 $g/m^2$ IV with BMT | ++ | +++ | +++ | 7–14 | +++ | Rash |
| **Nitrosoureas** | | | | | | | |
| Carmustine (BCNU) | 60–100 $mg/m^2$ IV qd × 3 d | +++ | 0 | 0 | 28–35 | ++ | Interstitial pneumonitis |
| Lomustine (CCNU) | 130 $mg/m^2$ PO × 1 d | + | 0 | 0 | 21–42 | ++ | — |
| **Tumor antimicrobials** | | | | | | | |
| Bleomycin | 10–20 $mg/m^2$ SC qwk | 0 | 0 | 0 | — | — | Erythroderma, interstitial pneumonitis, modify dose for renal dysfunction, requires test dose |
| Dactinomycin | 0.4–1.0 $mg/m^2$ IV qwk | ++ | ++ | 0 | 14–21 | ++ | Rash |
| Daunorubicin | 45–60 $mg/m^2$ IV qd × 3 d | ++ | + | + | 7–14 | +++ | Vesicant; cardiotoxicity; modify dose for renal and hepatic dysfunction |
| Doxorubicin | 10–60 $mg/m^2$ IV every 7–28 d | ++ | + | + | 7–14 | +++ | Vesicant; cardiotoxicity; modify dose for renal and hepatic dysfunction |

| | | | | | | | |
|---|---|---|---|---|---|---|---|
| Idarubicin | 12 mg/m² IV qd × 3 d | ++ | + | + | 7–14 | +++ | Vesicant; cardiotoxicity; modify dose for renal and hepatic dysfunction |
| Mitomycin-C | 10–20 mg/m² IV every 4–6 wk | + | + | 0 | 21–28 | ++ | Vesicant; hemolytic-uremic syndrome |
| Mitoxantrone | 10–30 mg/m² IV every 21–28 d | + | + | + | 7–14 | ++ | Cardiotoxicity |
| Streptozocin | 500 mg/m² IV qd × 5 d or 1000–1500 mg/m² IV qwk | +++ | 0 | 0 | — | — | Glycosuria, nephrotoxicity |
| **Plant alkaloids** | | | | | | | |
| Etoposide | 50–200 mg/m² PO or IV qd × 3–5 d | 0 | 0 | 0 | 10–14 | ++ | — |
| Vinblastine | 5–10 mg/m² IV every 1–4 wk | + | + | 0 | 4–10 | ++ | Vesicant; neuropathy (especially obstipation); modify dose for hepatic dysfunction |
| Vincristine | 1–2 mg IV every 1–4 wk | 0 | 0 | 0 | — | — | Vesicant; neuropathy (especially sensory); modify dose for hepatic dysfunction |
| Vinorelbine | 30 mg/m² IV qwk | + | 0 | 0 | — | — | Pain at infusion site; neuropathy |
| Paclitaxel (Taxol) | 135–250 mg/m² every 21 d | + | 0 | 0 | 10–14 | ++ | Premedicate with steroids to avoid anaphylactoid reaction; neuropathy; dose modification for hepatic dysfunction |

(*continued*)

**Table 20-2.** Continued

| Agent | Dose range–schedule | N & V | Mucositis | Diarrhea | Days to nadir | Myelosuppression | Other toxicity or cautions |
|---|---|---|---|---|---|---|---|
| Docetaxel (Taxotere) | 60–100 mg/m$^2$ every 21 d | + | 0 | 0 | 10–14 | ++ | Decadron starting 1 d pretreatment qd × 5 d to avoid third spacing of fluids; modify dose in hepatic dysfunction |
| **Other agents** | | | | | | | |
| Carboplatin | 200–360 mg/m$^2$ IV every 21–28 d | ++ | 0 | 0 | 14–28 | ++ | Modify dose with renal failure |
| Cisplatin | 20–120 mg/m$^2$ IV qd × 1–5 d | +++ | 0 | 0 | — | — | Peripheral neuropathy; nephropathy; ototoxicity |
| Oxaliplatin | 60–130 mg/m$^2$ every 14–21 d | + | 0 | 0 | 7–10 | ++ | Peripheral neuropathy |
| Hydroxyurea | 500–2000 mg PO qd | 0 | 0 | 0 | 7–10 | ++ | Atrophic skin |
| L-Asparaginase | 1000–10,000 IU SC qd × 3 d | 0 | 0 | 0 | — | — | Coagulopathy, pancreatitis, hypersensitivity reactions |
| Procarbazine | 100–200 mg/m$^2$ PO qd × 7–14 d | + | 0 | 0 | 7–10 | ++ | Rash, encephalopathy |
| Topotecan | 1.5 mg/m$^2$ IV qd × 5 d every 21 d | ++ | 0 | + | 10–14 | +++ | Modify dose for renal dysfunction |
| Irinotecan | 125 mg/m$^2$ qwk × 4 wk | ++ | + | +++ | 7–10 | +++ | Diarrhea controlled with atropine in first 24 hr, then with loperamide; asthenia, fever, abdominal pain common |

0, none; +, mild; ++, moderate; +++, severe; BMT, bone marrow transplant; N & V, nausea and vomiting.

through an implanted peritoneal catheter for the treatment of peritoneal metastasis.

E. **Intra-arterial chemotherapy** is advocated as a method of achieving high drug concentrations at specific tumor sites. Although it is of theoretical advantage, there are no absolute indications for chemotherapy administered by this route.

III. **Chemotherapeutic agents.** A summary of commonly used chemotherapeutic agents, dosages, and toxicities is given in Table 20-2. Class-specific or unique side effects are described here.

A. **Antimetabolites** exert antitumor activity by acting as pseudosubstrates for essential enzymatic reactions. Their greatest toxicity occurs in tissues that are actively replicating (e.g., GI mucosa, hematopoietic cells).

1. **Ara-C** is an analog of deoxycytidine that is most useful in hematologic neoplasms. In standard doses, myelosuppression and GI toxicity are dose limiting. In high doses, conjunctivitis is common, and prophylaxis with dexamethasone eye drops, two drops in each eye tid, should be administered. Cerebellar ataxia, pancreatitis, and hepatitis may also develop. If cerebellar dysfunction occurs during treatment, ara-C must be discontinued.
2. **FU** is a pyrimidine analog that is administered as an injection or as a continuous infusion. When it is administered as a bolus injection, myelosuppression is dose limiting; with a 4- to 5-day infusion, stomatitis and diarrhea are dose limiting. Cerebellar ataxia has been reported with both schedules and requires discontinuation of the drug. Chest pain ascribed to coronary artery vasospasm may occur with infusions and, if suspected, should be treated with a calcium channel antagonist (e.g., nifedipine) or by discontinuing the chemotherapy (*Cancer* 61:36, 1988). FU can be administered over 6–8 weeks and is limited by the development of a palmar-plantar dermatologic toxicity (the hand-foot syndrome can be palliated with vitamin $B_6$, 150 mg/day). **LV** can be coadministered with FU to potentiate cytotoxicity; diarrhea is dose limiting (*J Clin Oncol* 7:1419, 1989).
3. **Methotrexate** is an inhibitor of dihydrofolate reductase and has numerous toxicities. Mucositis is dose limiting.
   a. **Prolonged reabsorption.** Methotrexate is polyglutamated, and these metabolites accumulate in effusions to produce substantial toxicity. Patients with effusions should either have the fluid drained before receiving methotrexate or have the dosage drastically reduced.
   b. **Interstitial pneumonitis,** unrelated to cumulative dose and associated with a peripheral eosinophilia, may occur. It should be treated with glucocorticoids (e.g., prednisone, 1 mg/kg PO qd or equivalent) and precludes additional use of methotrexate.
   c. **Hepatitis** may occur with long-term oral administration but may also occur after a single high dose.
   d. **High-dose methotrexate** may be associated with crystalline nephropathy and renal failure. Urine alkalinization with sodium bicarbonate should be maintained to minimize this risk. **LV** is used to "rescue" normal tissue after high-dose methotrexate. The dose depends on the amount of methotrexate used, but the usual dosage is 5–25 mg IV or PO q6h for 8–12 doses, or until the serum methotrexate concentration is less than 50 nM.
4. **6-Mercaptopurine** is a purine analog that is partially metabolized by xanthine oxidase. To avoid increased toxicity, the dose of 6-mercaptopurine should be decreased by 75% in patients taking allopurinol. Hepatic cholestasis has also been observed.
5. **Fludarabine** is an adenosine monophosphate analog that produces myelosuppression (*J Clin Oncol* 9:175, 1991).

6. **Cladribine (2-chlorodeoxyadenosine)** is a purine substrate analog that is resistant to degradation by adenosine deaminase. Myelosuppression is predictable (*Lancet* 340:952, 1994).
7. **Gemcitabine** is a nucleoside analog that may produce fever, edema, flu-like symptoms, and rash. Pneumonitis is an uncommon complication.

B. **Alkylating agents** are useful in a wide variety of malignancies. These drugs cause DNA cross-linking and strand breaks. Most alkylating agents are cytotoxic to resting and dividing cells. Patients should be counseled that irreversible sterility may develop after treatment with alkylating agents. Chlorambucil, cyclophosphamide, melphalan, and mechlorethamine have been implicated in the development of acute myeloid leukemia and myelodysplasia 3–10 years after treatment.
1. **Busulfan** can cause interstitial pneumonitis and gynecomastia. A reversible syndrome resembling Addison's disease may develop with long-term daily oral administration.
2. **Chlorambucil** is a well-tolerated orally administered drug. Myelosuppression is dose limiting and usually readily reversible.
3. **Cyclophosphamide** can cause hemorrhagic cystitis (see Complications of Treatment, sec. **I.E**); therefore, adequate hydration to maintain urine output is required during treatment. Oral cyclophosphamide should be given early in the day to ensure adequate hydration. High-dose cyclophosphamide is used as a preparative agent before stem cell transplantation; at these doses a hemorrhagic myocarditis can occur.
4. **Dacarbazine** can produce a flu-like syndrome consisting of fever, myalgias, facial flushing, malaise, and marked elevations of hepatic enzymes.
5. **Ifosfamide** is chemically similar to cyclophosphamide, but the incidence of hemorrhagic cystitis is much higher (occurring in 20–30% of treated patients). Administration of 2-mercaptoethanesulfonate (mesna) is recommended to lower the incidence of cystitis (see Complications of Treatment, sec. **I.E**). Ifosfamide can also cause neurologic toxicity, including seizures.
6. **Mechlorethamine (nitrogen mustard)** is a skin irritant; protective gloves and eyewear must be used during drug preparation and administration. Development of a drug rash does not prevent further use of this agent.
7. **Melphalan** is available in oral and injectable forms. An idiosyncratic interstitial pneumonitis may occur, and, although usually reversible, it precludes further use of the drug.
8. **Nitrosoureas [carmustine (BCNU) and lomustine (CCNU)]** are lipid soluble and penetrate the blood-brain barrier. BCNU is usually administered in an ethanol solution, and toxicity from the vehicle, including giddiness, flushing, and phlebitis, may occur. Because delayed myelosuppression occurs 6–8 weeks after treatment and may be cumulative, these agents are commonly given at 8-week intervals.
9. **Thiotepa** can be administered IV with bone marrow rescue. When used intravesically, 60–90 mg is administered in 60–100 ml water and instilled over 2 hours.

C. **Antitumor antibiotics** intercalate adjacent DNA nucleotides, interrupting replication and transcription to cause strand breaks; they are cell cycle nonspecific.
1. **Anthracycline antibiotics are associated with a cardiomyopathy** consisting of intractable CHF and dysrhythmias. With doxorubicin, this complication is seen in approximately 2% of patients who receive a **cumulative lifetime dose of 550 mg/m²**. The incidence increases dramatically at higher cumulative doses. Concomitant cyclophosphamide or previous chest irradiation may potentiate this toxicity. As the cumulative dose approaches 450–550 $mg/m^2$, serial radionuclide ventriculography should be performed, and the anthracycline should be discontinued if LV function is compromised. Myocardial damage is related to peak serum concentrations and cumulative dosage; longer

(96-hour) infusions have allowed for higher cumulative dosages. These agents may also produce a radiation recall effect that consists of acute toxicity to previous radiation fields, usually to the heart, GI region, or lungs. The cardioprotectant **dexrazoxane** has been shown to decrease the incidence and severity of the cardiomyopathy associated with doxorubicin (*Ann Intern Med* 125:47, 1996).

a. **Daunorubicin** is used in the treatment of acute leukemia. Bone marrow suppression is expected, and the dose-limiting toxicity is usually mucositis. Red urine may be caused by the drug and its metabolites.

b. **Doxorubicin** toxicity is similar to that of daunorubicin, although this drug has a broader spectrum of activity. **Liposomal doxorubicin** is indicated for Kaposi's sarcoma and has similar toxicities.

c. **Mitoxantrone** is structurally similar to doxorubicin and daunorubicin but is associated with less cardiac toxicity. Mucositis and myelosuppression are dose limiting; a bluish discoloration of the urine and sclera may occur.

d. **Idarubicin** is more rapidly taken up in cells than other anthracyclines. Toxicity is similar to that of daunorubicin.

2. **Bleomycin** is useful in combination chemotherapy because it is rarely myelosuppressive. **A test dose, 1–2 mg SC, should be administered before full doses are instituted** because severe allergic reactions with hypotension may occur, especially in patients with lymphoma. Interstitial pneumonitis, which occasionally results in irreversible pulmonary fibrosis, is more common in patients with underlying pulmonary disease or previous lung irradiation or those who received a cumulative dose of 200 mg/$m^2$. Pulmonary symptoms and chest radiographs should be monitored.
3. **Mitomycin-C** is associated with delayed myelosuppression that worsens with repeated use of the drug. Interstitial pneumonitis has also been observed. The **hemolytic-uremic syndrome** has been reported, is exacerbated by RBC transfusions, and should be suspected in patients with sudden onset of a microangiopathic hemolytic anemia and renal failure.
4. **2-Deoxycoformycin** (Pentostatin) is isolated from *Streptomyces* and acts as an inhibitor of adenosine deaminase. Myelosuppression is the chief toxicity.

D. **Plant alkaloids** are naturally occurring nitrogenous bases. Most inhibit cell division through inhibition of mitotic spindle formation.

1. **Vincristine** often causes a dose-limiting neuropathy. Paresthesias followed by loss of deep tendon reflexes are the usual manifestations. Neuritic pain, jaw pain, diplopia, constipation, abdominal pain, and an adynamic ileus occur less often. Other adverse effects include SIADH and Raynaud's phenomenon.
2. **Vinblastine** is less neurotoxic than vincristine; dosage is usually limited by myelosuppression. At high doses, myalgias, obstipation, and transient hepatitis may occur.
3. **Etoposide (VP-16).** The major dose-limiting toxicity is myelosuppression.
4. **Teniposide (VM-26)** is a semisynthetic derivative of podophyllotoxin. Toxicities include myelosuppression, hypersensitivity reactions, alopecia, and hypotension.
5. **Paclitaxel (Taxol)** has a unique antitubulin mechanism that disrupts microtubule assembly. Because paclitaxel is dissolved in cremophor, anaphylactoid reactions may occur and are partially related to the rate of infusion. All patients should be premedicated with dexamethasone and $H_1$ and $H_2$ blockers. In addition, myelosuppression, arthralgias, neuropathy, and arrhythmias may occur.
6. **Docetaxel (Taxotere)** can be administered more rapidly than paclitaxel without anaphylactoid reactions. Dexamethasone, 8 mg bid for 3 days beginning the day before chemotherapy, is administered to prevent third-space fluid collections.

**Table 20-3.** Recommendations for antiemetic therapy

| |
|---|
| Phenothiazines[a] |
| Prochlorperazine, 5–10 mg PO or IV q4–6h (maximum IV dose, 40 mg/d) |
| Prochlorperazine, 25 mg per rectum q4–6h |
| Chlorpromazine, 10 mg PO q4–6h |
| Trimethobenzamide, 100 mg PO or IM q4–6h |
| Serotonin-receptor antagonists |
| Granisetron, 1 mg IV or 2 mg PO 15 min before chemotherapy |
| Ondansetron, 8–32 mg IV 15–30 min before chemotherapy or 24 mg PO or 8 mg PO tid |
| Dolasetron, 100 mg IV or PO 30 min before chemotherapy |
| Butyrophenone |
| Droperidol, 1–5 mg IV q4–6h |
| Metoclopramide,[a] 2–3 mg/kg IV before chemotherapy and q2h × 3 doses |
| Antihistamine |
| Diphenhydramine, 50 mg PO or IV q4–6h |
| Anxiolytic |
| Lorazepam, 1–2 mg PO or IV tid–qid |
| Glucocorticoid |
| Dexamethasone, 10–30 mg IV before chemotherapy |

[a]May cause extrapyramidal side effects that can be treated with either diphenhydramine, 25–50 mg PO or IV q4–6h, or benztropine mesylate, 1–2 mg IV or PO q4–6h.

7. **Navelbine** may produce pain in the IV injection site.

**E. Platinum-containing agents** act as intercalators, causing single- and double-strand breaks in DNA.

1. **Cisplatin** produces severe nausea and vomiting; aggressive antiemetic therapy is mandatory (Table 20-3). The patient should be aggressively volume expanded with 1 L isotonic saline administered over 4–6 hours before and after chemotherapy to prevent renal toxicity. The dosage of cisplatin should be reduced for patients with renal insufficiency and should be withheld if the serum creatinine is greater than 3 mg/dl. Other toxicities include hypomagnesemia and ototoxicity. Pretreatment with **amifostine** may reduce the cumulative hematologic, renal, and neurologic toxicities (*J Clin Oncol* 14:2101, 1996).
2. **Carboplatin** is a cisplatin analog with less neurotoxicity, ototoxicity, and nephrotoxicity than cisplatin; myelosuppression is the dose-limiting toxicity.
3. **Oxaliplatin** is a recently approved platinum-containing agent with activity in colorectal cancer. It is associated with a sensory neuropathy.

**F. Other agents**

1. **Hydroxyurea,** an oral agent that inhibits ribonucleotide reductase, is used in the management of the chronic phase of CML and other myeloproliferative diseases. The dosage is adjusted according to the peripheral blood neutrophil and platelet count.
2. **L-Asparaginase** hydrolyzes asparagine, depleting cells of an essential substrate in protein synthesis. Allergic or anaphylactic reactions may occur. Other toxicities include hemorrhagic pancreatitis, hepatic failure with depression of clotting factors, and encephalopathy.
3. **Procarbazine** is an oral agent that inhibits DNA, RNA, and protein synthesis. It is a monoamine oxidase inhibitor, and therefore tricyclic antide-

pressants, sympathomimetic agents, and tyramine-containing foods should be avoided. Procarbazine has a disulfiram-like effect, and therefore ethanol should not be ingested while this medication is being administered.

4. **Topotecan** is a topoisomerase I inhibitor. Myelosuppression is dose limiting.
5. **Irinotecan** has a similar mechanism of action to topotecan. It can produce severe diarrhea, which can be treated with atropine and loperamide.

G. **Hormonal agents** lack direct cytotoxicity. In general, they have few serious adverse effects. In disseminated disease, eventual resistance to hormonal agents should be anticipated.

1. **Tamoxifen** is a selective ER modulator. It acts as an ER antagonist in some tissues including breast and as an ER agonist on others. The usual dosage is 10 mg PO bid. After 7–14 days of treatment, a **hormone flare** (increasing bone pain, erythema, and hypercalcemia) occurs in approximately 5% of women with ER-positive breast cancer and bone metastases. The symptoms abate over 7–10 days, and 75% of these patients respond to tamoxifen; therefore, palliation of pain, control of hypercalcemia, and continuation of the drug are recommended. Long-term administration of tamoxifen is not associated with a systemic antiestrogen effect (vaginal atrophy, osteoporosis, or increased risk of heart disease) but is related to some estrogen effects (endometrial cancer and deep vein thrombosis).
2. **Aromatase inhibitors.** Third-generation aromatase inhibitors have become available for the treatment of postmenopausal women with hormone-responsive breast cancer. Two nonsteroidal agents, **anastrazole** (Arimidex, 1 mg/day) and **letrozole** (Femara, 2.5 mg/day), and one steroidal agent, **exemestane** (Aromasin, 25 mg/day), are available. All three agents have been found to be active in hormone-sensitive breast cancer (*J Clin Oncol* 19:881, 2001). The most common side effects of aromatase inhibitors are hot flashes and night sweats.
3. **Gonadotropin agonists.** Two LHRH agonists are used in the treatment of metastatic prostate cancer. **Leuprolide acetate** and **goserelin acetate** can be given as monthly SC depot injections, and leuprolide acetate is also available in a daily injection form. The first weeks of treatment may be associated with an initial flare in tumor symptoms, bone pain, fluid retention, hot flashes, sweats, and impotence. One should monitor for signs of neurologic dysfunction or urinary obstruction.
4. **Progestational agents. Megestrol acetate,** 40 mg PO qid, and **medroxyprogesterone,** 10 mg PO qd, have been used in the treatment of a variety of neoplasms. Principal toxicities include weight gain, fluid retention, hot flashes, and vaginal bleeding with discontinuation of therapy. Both agents also have been used in the treatment of cachexia associated with cancer and AIDS (see Complications of Cancer, sec. **II.A.3**).
5. **Antiandrogens. Flutamide** and **bicalutamide** may produce nausea, vomiting, gynecomastia, and breast tenderness (*Cancer* 71:1083, 1993). In advanced prostate cancer, withdrawal of flutamide results in tumor regression in 25% of patients (*J Clin Oncol* 11:1566, 1993).

H. **Immunotherapy.** Immunotherapeutic agents may be selective or nonspecific.

1. **Selective agents** include monoclonal antibodies, most of which are partially humanized.
   a. **Trastuzumab** (4 mg/kg over 90 minutes week 1, then 2 mg/kg over 30 minutes weekly) should be added to the first-line chemotherapy in patients with metastatic breast cancer whose cancers overexpress her-2 as measured by gene amplification or protein expression. Its use is associated with an improved survival. As a single agent, it has modest activity and a different mechanism of action than chemotherapy (*N Engl J Med* 17:2639, 1999).
   b. **Rituximab,** an unconjugated antibody targeted to CD20, is administered weekly for 1 month for treatment of low-grade non-Hodgkin's

lymphomas that are CD20 positive. Toxicities include chills and fevers during administration and rare hypersensitivity reactions (*J Clin Oncol* 16:2825, 1998).

c. **Campath** is a humanized antibody to CD52 (present on normal B and T cells) and has been used to treat CLL. Because of a high incidence of opportunistic infections from resulting immunodeficiency, prophylactic antifungals and antivirals are recommended (*Br J Haematol* 93:151, 1996).

2. **Nonspecific immunotherapy**
   a. **Interferon-alpha** is used for hairy-cell leukemia, CML, and melanoma. Toxicity includes nausea and vomiting, flu-like symptoms, and headaches. Acute toxicity may respond to acetaminophen; with continued administration these symptoms subside.
   b. **Aldesleukin (interleukin-2)** can produce responses in melanoma or renal cell carcinoma; some of these remissions are durable. At high doses this agent is toxic, producing increased vascular permeability with fluid overload, hypotension, prerenal azotemia, and elevation of liver enzymes.

I. **Chemopreventive agents**
   1. **Retinoids** have been used as therapeutic and chemopreventive agents. Isotretinoin (13-cis-retinoic acid), 50–100 mg/m$^2$ PO qd for 12 months, has been shown to lower the incidence of second primary tumors in patients who were previously treated for head and neck cancer (*N Engl J Med* 323:795, 1990). Common toxicities include dry skin, cheilitis, hyperlipidemia, and elevation of transaminases (*Cancer* 76:602, 1995).
   2. **Tamoxifen,** 20 mg PO qd administered for 5 years, has been shown to decrease the incidence of breast cancer in women with a high risk of developing breast cancer (*JNCI* 90:1371, 1998).

## Complications of Treatment

I. **Chemotherapy** often causes serious or life-threatening toxicity. The most common and predictable toxicities are to the rapidly proliferating cells of hematopoietic and mucosal tissue. Because repair of these tissues cannot be accelerated, palliation during the healing process is the primary goal.
   A. **Extravasation** of certain chemotherapeutic agents from venous infusion sites may lead to severe local tissue injury. Offending agents are identified as **vesicants** in Table 20-2. Initial symptoms of pain or erythema may appear within hours or may be delayed for up to 1–2 weeks. When extravasation occurs, the steps described below should be taken.
      1. **Stop the chemotherapy infusion.** With the venous catheter still in place, approximately 5 ml blood should be aspirated to remove any residual drug.
      2. **Certain drugs require hot or cold compresses** and may be neutralized by instillation of agents locally through the catheter and subcutaneously into the nearby tissue (Table 20-4).
      3. **Observe the area closely** for signs of tissue breakdown; surgical intervention for débridement or skin grafting may be necessary. Because extravasation injuries usually result in severe pain, adequate analgesia should be supplied (*J Clin Oncol* 5:1116, 1987).
   B. **Myelosuppression** from most agents reaches its peak 7–14 days after treatment (Table 20-2).
      1. **The risk of infection** increases dramatically with neutropenia (defined as an absolute neutrophil count of less than 500/mm$^3$) and is directly related to the duration of the neutropenia. In the absence of neutrophils, signs of

**Table 20-4.** Treatment of extravasation of selected chemotherapeutic agents

| Drug | Compress | Antidote |
|---|---|---|
| Dacarbazine | Hot | Isotonic thiosulfate IV and SC |
| Daunorubicin | Cold | DMSO applied topically to vein |
| Doxorubicin | Cold | DMSO applied topically to vein |
| Etoposide | Hot | Hyaluronidase (150 U/ml), 16 ml SC × 1 |
| Mechlorethamine | — | Isotonic thiosulfate IV and SC |
| Mitomycin-C | — | Isotonic thiosulfate IV and SC |
| Vinblastine | Hot | Hyaluronidase (150 U/ml), 16 ml SC × 1 |
| Vincristine | Hot | Hyaluronidase (150 U/ml), 16 ml SC × 1 |

DMSO, dimethyl sulfoxide.

infection or inflammation may be muted. **A febrile neutropenic patient should be presumed to be infected and must be evaluated and treated promptly.** A complete physical examination should be performed to locate potential sites of infection, with particular attention to indwelling catheter sites, sinuses, and the oral and rectal areas. **Cultures** of blood, urine, stool, sputum, and other foci that are susceptible to bacterial infections (e.g., fluid collections) should be collected, and a chest radiograph should be obtained. **Empiric antimicrobial treatment should be initiated immediately** after cultures are obtained. In the absence of any obvious source, the antimicrobials should provide broad coverage for gram-negative bacilli (including *Pseudomonas aeruginosa*) and gram-positive cocci (including alpha-hemolytic *Streptococcus* species). In choosing a regimen, local susceptibility patterns should also be considered. Empiric therapy may consist of an aminoglycoside and semisynthetic penicillin or a single agent such as cefepime. Vancomycin should not be included in initial empiric regimens unless the patient is clinically unstable or has had a recent oxacillin-resistant *Staphylococcus aureus* infection. Low-risk patients (afebrile after institution of antibiotics, negative cultures, and anticipated to recover from myelosuppression in <1 week) can be discharged on an oral broad-spectrum agent such as a fluoroquinolone or trimethoprim/sulfamethoxazole. **Modification of the antimicrobial regimen** according to the culture data or clinical picture may become necessary. Additional agents to treat *Staphylococcus epidermidis*, *Clostridium difficile*, or anaerobic infections are commonly necessary based on physical examination findings and suspected foci of infection. Persistent fever, in the absence of other data, usually does not warrant an empiric change in the antibacterial therapy. However, **empiric antifungal therapy** with amphotericin B (starting at 0.5 mg/kg and advanced to 1.0 mg/kg qd) should be added if the fever continues for longer than 72 hours (see Chap. 13, Treatment of Infectious Diseases). Antimicrobials are continued until the neutrophil count is greater than 500/mm$^3$. Neutropenic patients should be maintained in modified reverse isolation. Those who enter the room should wash their hands thoroughly with antiseptic soap or an alcohol-based hand-cleaning solution. Visitors with colds should wear a mask, and those with fevers should not enter. Due to the risk of fungal infection, live plants should not be allowed in the room.

2. **Thrombocytopenia** below 10,000/mm$^3$ that is the result of chemotherapy should be treated with platelet transfusions to minimize the risk of spontaneous hemorrhage (see Chap. 18, Disorders of Hemostasis).

When prolonged thrombocytopenia is anticipated, histocompatibility testing should be performed before therapy so that HLA-matched single-donor platelets can be provided when alloimmunization makes the patient refractory to random-donor platelets.

3. **RBC transfusions** are indicated for patients who have symptoms of anemia, active bleeding, or a hemoglobin concentration below 7–8 g/dl (see Chap. 18, Disorders of Hemostasis). Because of anecdotal reports of graft-versus-host disease (GVHD) associated with transfusions, radiation of all blood products is generally recommended for immunosuppressed marrow transplant patients.
4. **Growth factors** include many cytokines that may ameliorate the myelosuppression associated with cytotoxic chemotherapy. They act on hematopoietic cells, stimulating proliferation, differentiation, commitment, and some functional activation. Because they can increase myelosuppression, they **should not be given within 24 hours of chemotherapy or radiation.**
   a. **Granulocyte colony-stimulating factor (G-CSF),** given at an initial dose of 5 μg/kg SC or IV beginning the day after the last dose of cytotoxic chemotherapy, may reduce the incidence of febrile neutropenic events. Blood counts should be monitored twice a week during therapy. Bone pain is a common toxicity that can be managed with nonnarcotic analgesics.
   b. **Granulocyte-macrophage colony-stimulating factor (GM-CSF),** given subcutaneously at a dose of 250 μg/m$^2$/day beginning the day after the last dose of cytotoxic chemotherapy, shortens the period of neutropenia after stem cell transplant.
   c. **Recombinant erythropoietin** given at a starting dose of 150 U/kg SC three times a week has been shown to improve anemia and decrease transfusion requirements in cancer patients, particularly those in whom the anemia is predominantly caused by cytotoxic chemotherapy (*Oncology* 16[9 Suppl 10]:41, 2002). Hematocrit should be monitored weekly during therapy, and the dosage should be adjusted accordingly. Darbepoetin alfa has also become available. This agent represents a modified formulation of recombinant erythropoietin with a longer half-life. It is indicated for the treatment of chemotherapy-induced anemia in patients with solid tumors and can be dosed every 2 weeks (*Oncology* 16[9 Suppl 11]:31).
   d. **Interleukin-11** was approved to reduce the duration and severity of thrombocytopenia after chemotherapy. However, limited efficacy and significant toxicity (fluid retention and atrial arrhythmias) have limited its use.

C. **GI toxicity**

1. **Stomatitis** is an unpleasant consequence of many chemotherapeutic agents (Table 20-2) and is commonly the dose-limiting toxicity of methotrexate and FU. With simultaneous administration of radiation therapy, the toxicity is more severe. Healing generally occurs within 7–10 days of the development of symptoms. The severity of stomatitis ranges from mild (oral discomfort) to severe (ulceration, impaired oral intake, and hemorrhage). In mild cases, **oral rinses** (chlorhexidine, 15–30 ml swish and spit tid, or the combination of equal parts diphenhydramine elixir, saline, and 3% hydrogen peroxide) may provide relief. In severe cases, IV morphine is appropriate. **IV fluids** should be used to supplement oral intake as needed. Aspiration may develop in patients with moderate or severe stomatitis; precautions should include elevation of the head of the bed and availability of a hand-held suction apparatus. In severe or prolonged episodes, superinfection with *Candida* or herpes simplex is possible and requires appropriate diagnosis and antimicrobial intervention.

2. **Diarrhea** is the result of cytotoxicity to proliferating cells of the intestinal mucosa. In some cases, IV fluids are necessary to avoid intravascular volume depletion. The use of oral opioid agents as antidiarrheals is commonly limited by abdominal cramping. Severe diarrhea associated with FU and LV has been reported to respond to octreotide, 150–500 µg SC tid. Diarrhea secondary to irinotecan can be treated with loperamide, 4 mg PO then 2 mg q2h while awake, and 4 mg q4h during the night.
3. **Nausea and vomiting** may develop in varying degrees and frequency (see Table 20-2). Suggestions for antiemetic agent(s) are listed in Table 20-3.

D. **Interstitial pneumonitis** may develop as a dose-related, cumulative toxicity or as an idiosyncratic reaction. The implicated agent should be discontinued, and institution of glucocorticoids (e.g., prednisone, 1 mg/kg PO qd or equivalent) may be of some benefit. The long-term outcome is unpredictable.

E. **Hemorrhagic cystitis** may develop with either cyclophosphamide or ifosfamide. It is best anticipated and treated with prophylactic mesna at a dosage of at least 0.6 mg mesna to 1 mg ifosfamide. Treatment consists of continuous bladder irrigation with isotonic saline and should continue until the hematuria resolves.

F. **Tumor lysis syndrome** occurs in patients with rapidly proliferating neoplasms that are highly sensitive to chemotherapy. Rapid tumor cell death releases intracellular contents and causes **hyperkalemia, hyperphosphatemia,** and **hyperuricemia.** Although reported in the treatment of a variety of malignancies, it is usually associated with **high-grade non-Hodgkin's lymphoma** and **acute leukemia.** During induction chemotherapy, prophylactic measures should include **allopurinol,** 300–600 mg PO qd, and aggressive IV volume expansion (e.g., 3000 ml/m$^2$/day). The addition of **sodium bicarbonate,** 50 mEq/1000 ml IV fluid, to alkalinize the urine above a pH of 7 may prevent uric acid nephropathy and acute renal failure. When hyperphosphatemia accompanies hyperuricemia, urine alkalinization should be avoided because calcium phosphate precipitation may result in renal failure. Despite these preventive measures, hemodialysis may be needed for hyperkalemia, hyperphosphatemia, acute renal failure, or fluid overload.

II. **Radiation therapy** toxicity is related to the location of the therapy, total dose delivered, and rates of delivery. Large dose fractions of radiation are associated with greater toxicity to the normal tissues encompassed in the radiation field.

A. **Acute toxicity** develops within the first 3 months of therapy and is characterized by an inflammatory reaction in the tissue receiving radiation. Such toxicity may respond to anti-inflammatory agents such as glucocorticoids. Local irritations or burns in the treatment field generally resolve with time. Close observation and treatment of any infections and palliation of symptoms such as pain, dysphagia, dysuria, or diarrhea (depending on the site of treatment) are the mainstays of supportive care until healing has occurred.

B. **Subacute toxicities** between 3 and 6 months of therapy and chronic toxicity after 6 months are less amenable to therapy, as fibrosis and scarring are present. Daily **amifostine** before head and neck radiation therapy decreases the incidence of xerostomia (*J Clin Oncol* 13:490, 1996).

## Hematopoietic Stem Cell Transplantation

Hematopoietic stem cell transplantation involves IV infusion of either hematopoietic progenitors (collected from the bone marrow by aspiration from the iliac crests) or peripheral blood stem cells (collected by apheresis after treatment of the donor with G-CSF or GM-CSF). **Allogeneic** stem cells are collected from another person (the donor), whereas **autologous** stem cells are collected from the patient. For autologous transplant, peripheral blood stem cells have largely replaced bone marrow as the source of progenitors because hematologic recovery is more rapid.

I. **Allogeneic stem cell transplant.** HLA-matched siblings are the most common donors, but matched unrelated donors can be identified for many patients through the National Bone Marrow Donor Registry. Allogeneic transplants can be performed to restore normal hematopoiesis or immune function in patients with aplastic anemia, immunodeficiency, or hemoglobinopathies and are also used to treat resistant leukemia and lymphoma. For patients with resistant acute leukemia, allogeneic transplant is generally favored, whereas for those with resistant lymphoma, autologous transplant is usually preferred. The **"preparative regimen"** is given immediately before transplant and includes chemotherapy with or without total body irradiation. For patients with nonmalignant conditions, the preparative regimen provides immunosuppression, which is needed for engraftment. For patients with resistant malignancy, the preparative regimen is designed to promote engraftment and to kill tumor cells. Unlike autologous transplant, allogeneic transplants may be accompanied by a **graft-versus-tumor effect,** which appears to be a very important part of curing leukemia or lymphoma (see sec. **III.B**).

II. **Autologous stem cell transplantation.** Eradication of malignancy is entirely the result of the preparative regimen, because no graft-versus-tumor effect can occur. The major advantage of autologous transplant is that GVHD (see sec. **III.B**) does not occur; therefore, the risk of death from transplant-related complications is less than 5%. Most autologous transplants are performed for relapsed lymphoma. In patients with relapsed large-cell lymphoma who achieve at least a partial response to salvage chemotherapy, cure can be achieved in 30–50%. Autologous transplant also prolongs the survival of patients with multiple myeloma and is a viable option for individuals with acute leukemia in first remission who lack a compatible sibling donor.

III. **Complications of transplantation** may be the result of high-dose therapy, pancytopenia, immunodeficiency, or GVHD.

A. **Infections.** After the preparative regimen, 7–10 days of profound pancytopenia (absolute neutrophil count <100, platelets <10,000) develops in all patients. During this time nearly all patients experience fever and require empiric broad-spectrum antibiotic therapy. Patients who are seropositive for herpes simplex virus should also receive acyclovir prophylaxis until neutrophil recovery. G-CSF or GM-CSF is usually given starting on the day after transplant until neutrophil recovery. Patients who have undergone autologous transplant recover immune function within 3–6 months. However, patients who undergo allogeneic transplant have profound and prolonged impairment of humoral and cell-mediated immunity that persists until GVHD resolves. Therefore, **patients who are febrile after allogeneic transplant should be cultured and immediately receive IV broad-spectrum antibiotics** even if they are not neutropenic. After allogeneic transplant, patients receive long-term prophylaxis for varicella-zoster virus with acyclovir and for *Pneumocystis* with trimethoprim/sulfamethoxazole. Patients are also at risk for reactivation and systemic infection with cytomegalovirus (CMV). One strategy for preventing overt infection is to perform shell vial cultures or polymerase chain reaction assays on blood weekly or biweekly during the period of maximal risk (1–6 months posttransplant). Ganciclovir or foscarnet is given if testing is positive for CMV. Patients who have undergone allogeneic transplant require reimmunization.

B. **GVHD** is an immunologic response by the donor to recipient antigens and is the major complication of allogeneic transplantation. GVHD within the first 100 days of transplant (**acute GVHD**) produces a skin rash, diarrhea, and liver dysfunction. Despite prophylaxis with cyclosporine and methotrexate, significant acute GVHD occurs in 30–50% of transplants from matched sibling donors. **Chronic GVHD** occurs more than 100 days after transplant and resembles an autoimmune disorder with protean manifestations, including keratoconjunctivitis sicca, lichenoid changes of the buccal mucosa, and sclerodermatous skin changes. Overall, GVHD accounts for most of the 20–30% mortality that accompanies matched sibling transplant, with death usually resulting from infection. After allogeneic transplant, donor T cells can mediate immunologic destruction of residual tumor cells. This "graft-versus-tumor effect" is unique to allogeneic transplant and plays a key role in eradicating residual malignancy.

C. **Veno-occlusive disease** occurs in 1–5% of patients, usually within 21 days of treatment. Risk factors include extensive prior therapy and elevated transaminase values before transplant. Manifestations include hyperbilirubinemia, ascites, tender hepatomegaly, and fluid retention.

D. **Pulmonary complications.** CMV pneumonia usually occurs within 6 months of allogeneic transplant in patients who are seropositive or who receive transplants from seropositive donors. It is uncommon after autologous transplant. Treatment is with ganciclovir or foscarnet. Interstitial pneumonitis may complicate total body radiation or high-dose chemotherapy and is manifested by cough, dyspnea, and interstitial infiltrates that present 1–3 months after transplant. Prior chest radiotherapy is a risk factor; treatment with prednisone usually results in rapid and long-term improvement.

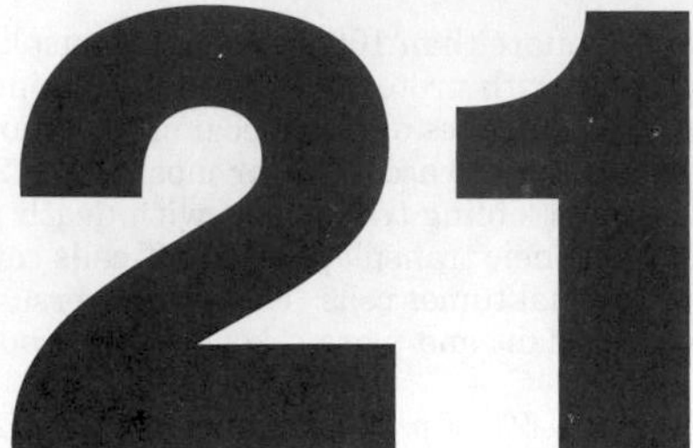

# Diabetes Mellitus and Related Disorders

Ernesto Bernal-Mizrachi and Carlos Bernal-Mizrachi

## Diabetes Mellitus

**Diabetes mellitus (DM)** is a group of metabolic diseases characterized by hyperglycemia resulting from defects in insulin secretion, insulin action, or both.

I. **Classification of diabetes and related disorders** (*Diabetes Care* 26[Suppl 1]:S5, 2003)
   A. **DM** is classified into two broad types and a third, miscellaneous category.
      1. **Type 1 diabetes** accounts for fewer than 10% of all cases of DM and results from a cellular-mediated autoimmune destruction of the β cells of the pancreas. The rate of destruction is rapid in some individuals (mainly infants and children) and slow in others (mainly adults and known as late-onset autoimmune diabetes). This form of diabetes is characterized by severe insulin deficiency. Exogenous insulin is required to control blood glucose, prevent diabetic ketoacidosis (DKA), and preserve life. A transient period of insulin independence ("honeymoon phase") or reduced insulin requirement may occur early in the course of type 1 DM.
      2. **Type 2 diabetes** accounts for more than 90% of all cases of DM. Usually a disease of adults, type 2 DM is being increasingly diagnosed in younger age groups. Obesity, insulin resistance, and relative insulin deficiency are characteristic findings. Insulin secretion is usually sufficient to prevent ketosis under basal conditions, but DKA can develop during severe stress.
      3. **Other specific types of DM** include those that result from genetic defects in insulin secretion or action, exocrine pancreatic disease, pancreatectomy, endocrinopathies (e.g., Cushing's syndrome, acromegaly), drugs, and other syndromes.
   B. **Gestational DM** complicates approximately 4% of all pregnancies and usually resolves after delivery, although affected women remain at an increased risk for development of type 2 DM later in life.
   C. **Impaired glucose tolerance (IGT) and impaired fasting glucose (IFG)** refer to intermediate states between normal glucose tolerance and DM. IFG and IGT are associated with insulin resistance and appear to be risk factors for type 2 DM and micro- and macrovascular complications.

II. **Diagnosis**
   A. **The diagnosis of DM** can be established using any of the following criteria:
      1. **Plasma glucose of 126 mg/dl or greater** after an overnight fast. This should be confirmed with a repeat test.
      2. **Symptoms of diabetes** and a random plasma glucose of **200 mg/dl** or greater.
      3. **Oral glucose tolerance test** that shows a plasma glucose of **200 mg/dl** or greater at 2 hours after a 75-g glucose load.

The authors express gratitude to Matilde Mizrachi for careful review of the manuscript.

**B. IGT** is defined by a 2-hour oral glucose tolerance test plasma glucose greater than 140 mg/dl but less than 200 mg/dl.

**C. IFG** is defined by fasting plasma glucose of 110 mg/dl or greater but less than 126 mg/dl. Both lifestyle changes and treatment with metformin reduced the incidence of diabetes in persons at risk. The lifestyle interventions were more effective than metformin (*N Engl J Med* 346:393, 2002).

**III. Principles of management.** The therapeutic goals are alleviation of symptoms, achievement of metabolic control, and prevention of acute and long-term complications of diabetes. **Glycemic control** is set at the same goal for type 1 and type 2 diabetes: average preprandial blood glucose values of 90–130 mg/dl, bedtime blood glucose of 100–140 mg/dl, and hemoglobin $A_{1c}$ ($HbA_{1c}$) of 7% or lower (*Diabetes Care* 26[Suppl 1]:S33, 2003). This degree of glycemic control has been associated with the lowest risk for long-term complications in patients with type 1 (*N Engl J Med* 329:978, 1993) as well as type 2 DM (*Lancet* 352:837, 1998). An individualized, comprehensive diabetes care plan is necessary to accomplish these goals. The mnemonic **MEDEM** (**m**onitoring, **e**ducation, **d**iet, **e**xercise, **m**edications) can be used to recall the modalities of diabetes care.

**A. Monitoring** of diabetes control consists of the following:

1. **$HbA_{1c}$** provides an integrated measure of blood glucose profile over the preceding 2–3 months; it should be obtained approximately every 3 months or at least twice a year in well-controlled patients.
2. **Self-monitoring of blood glucose** is an important tool for diabetes management and is recommended for all the patients.
3. **Urine glucose** correlates poorly with blood glucose, is dependent on renal glucose threshold (150–300 mg/dl), and should only be used for monitoring DM therapy if self-monitoring of blood glucose is impractical.
4. **Ketonuria** grossly reflects ketonemia. All DM patients should monitor urine ketones using Ketostix or Acetest tablets during febrile illness or persistent elevated glucose (>300 mg/dl) or if signs of impending DKA (e.g., nausea, vomiting, abdominal pain) develop.

**B. Patient education** is integral to successful management of diabetes. Diabetes education should be reinforced at every opportunity, particularly during hospitalization for diabetes-related complications.

**C. Dietary modification.** A balanced diet that provides adequate nutrition and maintains an ideal body weight is desirable. Caloric restriction is recommended for overweight persons. An allowance of 10–20% of total caloric intake as protein, less than 30% as total fat (<10% saturated fat), and less than 300 mg/day cholesterol is appropriate. Patients with diabetic nephropathy usually are allowed a protein intake of 0.8 g/kg/day. With deterioration in renal function, further restriction in protein intake (0.6 g/kg) can be considered in selected patients. Carbohydrate allowance should be individualized based on glycemic control, plasma lipids, and weight goals.

**D. Exercise** improves insulin sensitivity, reduces fasting and postprandial blood glucose, and offers numerous metabolic, cardiovascular, and psychological benefits in diabetic patients.

**E. Medications** for diabetes are most effective if instituted as part of a comprehensive management approach that includes dietary and exercise counseling. Therapy for diabetes includes insulin and oral agents, which are described in Tables 21-1 and 21-2.

## Diabetes Mellitus in Hospitalized Patients

**I. Indications for hospitalization.** Hospital admission can be considered for stabilization of newly diagnosed diabetes, newly recognized diabetes of pregnancy, and management of complications of diabetes. Inpatient care is particularly appropriate in the following situations:

A. **DKA,** as indicated by a plasma glucose of greater than 250 mg/dl in association with an arterial pH of less than 7.30 or serum bicarbonate level of less than 15 mEq/L and moderate ketonuria or ketonemia
B. **Hyperosmolar nonketotic state,** usually suggested by marked hyperglycemia (≥400 mg/dl) and elevated serum osmolality (>315 mOsm/kg), often accompanied by impaired mental status
C. **Hypoglycemia** (<50 mg/dl), especially if induced by a sulfonylurea drug or resulting in coma, seizures, or altered mental status

II. **Management of diabetes in hospitalized patients** (*Diabetes Care* 18:870, 1995; *Am J Med* 113:317, 2002). Glycemic control seldom receives priority attention when diabetic patients are hospitalized for reasons other than diabetes, despite evidence linking hyperglycemia to (1) decreased cerebral blood flow, (2) impaired wound healing, (3) infections, and (4) delayed drug clearance (especially narcotic analgesics). Even in previously stable patients, glycemic control tends to deteriorate during hospitalization because of the stress of illness, erratic insulin absorption, inappropriate dietary practices, and effects of medications (corticosteroids, sympathomimetic agents, beta-blockers, cyclosporine, thiazide diuretics). Hospital admission also provides an opportunity to reinforce the elements of diabetes management and optimize glycemic control.

A. **Patients hospitalized for reasons other than diabetes who are eating normally** should continue their usual diabetes treatment, unless specifically contraindicated. The common practice of **sliding-scale** administration of regular insulin alone, q6h, based on bedside capillary blood glucose levels, seldom gives satisfactory results; regimens that include intermediate-acting insulin give superior glycemic control (*Arch Intern Med* 157:545, 1997).

1. **Monitoring.** Blood glucose should be monitored at least two to four times a day, especially in patients treated with insulin. Extreme values (>300 mg/dl or <60 mg/dl) from bedside capillary blood glucose meters should be confirmed using laboratory measurements. If persistent hyperglycemia is observed in febrile or sick patients, urine ketone reaction should be determined using dipstick (Ketostix) or Acetest tablets. $HbA_{1c}$ should be measured if no recent result is available.
2. **Education** regarding optimal diabetes care should be reinforced at every opportunity.
3. **Dietary intervention.** Restriction of total and saturated fat intake, with increased complex carbohydrates and dietary fiber, is appropriate.
4. **Exercise.** Physical activity should be encouraged, as appropriate.
5. **Medications** for diabetes should be reviewed with regard to potential toxicities.
   a. **Metformin** should be withheld 1 day before any diagnostic evaluation that involves the use of iodinated radiocontrast dyes. It can be restarted 48 hours after radiocontrast exposure and documentation of normal renal function. Metformin therapy should also be discontinued in the presence of sepsis, CHF, renal dysfunction, or other conditions that predispose to lactic acidosis.
   b. **Thiazolidinediones (TZDs)** should not be administered to patients with hepatic dysfunction, as indicated by elevated serum transaminases or CHF.
   c. **Glucosidase inhibitors** should be continued unless the patient has a GI illness.

B. **Patients hospitalized for reasons other than diabetes who are required to fast** should discontinue oral antidiabetic medications. In patients who require insulin, IV insulin infusion is recommended (see Chap. 1, Patient Care in Internal Medicine, the section Perioperative Medicine, sec. **V**). Another alternative is to give one-half to two-thirds of the patient's long or intermediate insulin dose along with a short-acting insulin by sliding scale.

An IV infusion of 5% dextrose in water ($D_5W$) or dextrose in saline at 75–125 ml/hour should be provided to maintain plasma glucose between 100 and 200 mg/dl. Additional SC doses of short-acting insulin (1–4 U) are indicated when blood glucose levels are greater than 200 mg/dl.

**C. Enteral nutrition** (*Mayo Clin Proc* 71:587, 1996). Short-acting insulin by sliding scale should be used initially until the patient is tolerating tube feedings. When infusion rates are greater than 30 ml/hour, one should start neutral protamine hagedorn (NPH) or lente at one-half of the patient's morning preadmission dose, adjusting the dose daily to keep glucose levels between 100 and 200 mg/dl.

**D. Total parenteral nutrition** (TPN). Individuals with type 2 diabetes who require TPN are likely to require large amounts of insulin. See Chap. 2, Nutrition Support, sec. **IV.B.3** for insulin management of patients on TPN.

**E. Newly diagnosed type 1 DM** and **newly recognized gestational DM** may be indications for hospitalization, even in the absence of ketoacidosis (see the section Type 1 Diabetes and Diabetic Ketoacidosis).

**F.** Patients with **newly diagnosed type 2 DM** who meet the criteria for hospitalization often have severe hyperglycemia and may require insulin therapy for initial stabilization, even in the absence of ketoacidosis or hyperosmolar syndrome (see the section Type 2 Diabetes and Nonketotic Hyperosmolar Syndrome, sec. **I**).

## Type 1 Diabetes and Diabetic Ketoacidosis

A comprehensive approach, including monitoring, education, dietary and exercise counseling, and insulin therapy, is necessary for successful management of type 1 DM (see Diabetes Mellitus, sec. **III**). Glycemic goals include average preprandial blood glucose values of 90–130 mg/dl, bedtime blood glucose of 100–140 mg/dl, and $HbA_{1c}$ of 7% or lower. A team approach, tailored to the individual patient's needs, that uses the expertise of diabetes educators, dietitians, and other members of the diabetes care team offers the best chance of success.

**I. Treatment of type 1 DM** requires lifelong insulin replacement.

**A. Insulin preparations.** After SC injection, there is individual variability in the duration and peak activity of insulin preparations and day-to-day variability in the same subject (Table 21-1).

1. **Rapid-acting insulins** include regular insulin, lispro, and insulin aspart. Regular insulin can be administered IV, IM, or by the more familiar SC route. Absorption of IM injection is variable and undependable, especially in hypovolemic patients. IV regular insulin is given as a bolus, usually followed by continuous infusion, for the treatment of hyperglycemic crises. An IV bolus of regular insulin exerts maximum effect in 10–30 minutes and is quickly dissipated.
2. **Intermediate-acting insulins** include NPH (isophane) and lente (zinc). These insulins are released slowly from SC sites and reach peak activity after 6–12 hours, followed by gradual decline.
3. **Long-acting insulins** are absorbed more slowly than the intermediate-acting preparations. Long-acting insulins provide a steady "basal" supply of circulating insulin when administered once or twice a day. **Glargine** is a "peakless" bioengineered human insulin analog with an extended duration of activity. Insulin glargine is generally administered once a day as a subcutaneous injection at bedtime, in a regimen that also includes premeal regular insulin or insulin lispro. In some patients with type 1 DM, two injections are required for 24-hour coverage.

**Table 21-1.** Approximate kinetics of human insulin preparations after subcutaneous injection[a]

| Insulin type | Onset of action (hr) | Peak effect (hr) | Duration of activity (hr) |
|---|---|---|---|
| **Rapid acting** | | | |
| Lispro, Aspart | 0.25–0.50 | 0.50–1.50 | 3–5 |
| Regular | 0.50–1.00 | 2–4 | 6–8 |
| **Intermediate acting** | | | |
| NPH | 1–2 | 6–12 | 18–24 |
| Lente | 1–3 | 6–12 | 18–26 |
| **Long acting** | | | |
| Ultralente | 4–6 | 10–16 | 24–48 |
| PZI | 3–8 | 14–24 | 24–40 |
| Glargine | 4–6 | None[b] | 18 |

NPH, neutral protamine hagedorn; PZI, protamine zinc insulin.
[a]Insulin dosage and individual variability in absorption and clearance rates affect pharmacokinetic data. Human insulins may peak earlier and be dissipated faster than porcine or bovine insulins. Duration of insulin activity is prolonged in renal failure.
[b]After a lag time of approximately 5 hours, insulin glargine has a flat peakless effect over a 24-hour period.

4. **Concentration.** Most insulins now contain 100 U/ml (U-100). A U-500 preparation is available for the rare patient with severe insulin resistance.
5. **Mixed insulin therapy.** Rapid-acting insulins (regular, lispro, and aspart) can be mixed with intermediate-acting (NPH and lente) or long-acting (ultralente) insulins in the same syringe for convenience. The rapid-acting insulin should be drawn first, cross contamination should be avoided, and the mixed insulin should be injected immediately. **Insulin glargine and protamine zinc insulin should not be mixed with other forms of insulin.** Commercial premixed insulin preparations do not allow dose adjustment of individual components but are convenient for patients who are unable or unwilling to do the mixing themselves.
6. **SC insulin delivery** is accomplished using disposable syringes with fine hypodermic needles, insulin pens, and pumps. The anterior abdominal wall, thighs, buttocks, and arms are the preferred sites for SC insulin injection. Absorption is fastest from the abdomen, followed by the arm, buttocks, and thigh, probably as a result of differences in blood flow. Injection sites should be rotated within the regions rather than randomly across separate regions, to minimize erratic absorption. Clean techniques should be adopted, and areas of scarring, ulceration, or infection should be avoided. Exercise, or massage over the injection site may accelerate insulin absorption.

B. **Initial insulin dosage** for optimal glycemic control is approximately 0.5–1.0 U/kg/day for the average nonobese patient. A conservative total daily dose is given initially; the dose is then adjusted, using blood glucose values.
   1. A regimen of **multiple daily insulin injections** is preferred to obtain optimal control. This regimen provides approximately 40–50% of the total daily dose of insulin as basal insulin supply, using one or two injections of long-acting or intermediate-acting insulin. The remainder is given as three doses of rapid-acting insulin divided across the main meals, empirically or in proportion to the carbohydrate content. An allowance of 1.0 U/10–15 g carbohydrate consumed is typical.

2. **The conventional insulin regimen** uses a mixture of short- and intermediate-acting (so-called split-mixed) insulins administered before breakfast and before the evening meal. Approximately two-thirds of the total daily dose is injected in the morning and one-third in the evening. Approximately two-thirds of each injection comprises intermediate-acting insulin and one-third is rapid-acting insulin ("rule of thirds"). These proportions should be modified for patients with unusual work schedules or eating patterns. The units of individual insulin components of each injection are then adjusted using data from preprandial and bedtime blood glucose monitoring.
3. **Continuous SC insulin infusion** is a tool for intensive diabetes control in selected patients. It provides 50% of total daily insulin as basal insulin and the remainder as multiple preprandial boluses of insulin, using a programmable insulin pump. As with the multiple daily insulin injections regimen, the premeal insulin doses are estimated from the carbohydrate content of each meal.
4. **Sliding-scale** administration of regular insulin alone to hospitalized patients, based on bedside capillary blood glucose levels, rarely achieves satisfactory glycemic control; regimens that include intermediate-acting insulin give superior results (*Arch Intern Med* 157:545, 1997).
5. **Monitoring.** Blood glucose should be monitored at least four times a day (preprandially and at bedtime) in hospitalized patients with type 1 DM. The $HbA_{1c}$ should be obtained if no recent result is available. Urine should be tested for ketones whenever hyperglycemia (>300 mg/dl) persists.

**II. DKA,** a potentially fatal complication, occurs in up to 5% of patients with type 1 DM annually; it is seen less frequently in type 2 DM. It is a manifestation of severe insulin deficiency, often in association with stress and activation of counterregulatory hormones (e.g., catecholamines, glucagon).

**A. Precipitating factors** for DKA include inadvertent or deliberate interruption of insulin therapy, sepsis, trauma, myocardial infarction, and pregnancy. DKA may be the first presentation of type 1 and, rarely, type 2, diabetes.

**B. Diagnosis.** A high index of suspicion is warranted, because clinical presentation may be nonspecific.

1. **Clinical features** include nausea, vomiting, and vaguely localized abdominal pain. Prominent GI symptoms may give rise to suspicion for intra-abdominal pathology. Dehydration is invariable, and respiratory distress, shock, and coma can occur.
2. **Laboratory evaluation** shows an anion gap metabolic acidosis and positive serum ketones. Plasma glucose usually is elevated, but the degree of hyperglycemia may be moderate (≤ 300 mg/dl) in 10–15% of patients in DKA. Pregnancy and alcohol ingestion are associated with "euglycemic DKA." The urine ketone reaction correlates poorly with ketonemia but is usually positive in DKA. Hyponatremia, hyperkalemia, azotemia, and hyperosmolality are other findings. Serum amylase and transaminases may be elevated. A focused search for a precipitating infection is always prudent. An ECG should be performed to evaluate electrolyte abnormalities and for unsuspected myocardial ischemia.

**C. Management of DKA** should preferably be conducted in an ICU. If treatment is conducted in a non-ICU setting, close monitoring by a physician is mandatory until ketoacidosis resolves and the patient's condition has stabilized. The therapeutic priorities are fluid replacement, adequate insulin administration, and potassium repletion. Administration of bicarbonate, phosphate, magnesium, or other therapies may be advantageous in selected patients but is not a first-line consideration.

1. **IV access and supportive measures** should be instituted without delay.

2. **Fluid** deficits of several liters are common in DKA patients and can be estimated by subtracting the current weight from a recently known dry weight. Hypotension indicates a loss of 10% or more of body fluids.
   a. Initially, **restoration of circulating volume** using isotonic (0.9%) saline should be accomplished. The first liter should be infused rapidly (if cardiac function is normal) and should be followed by additional fluids at a rate of 1 L/hour until the volume deficit is corrected. Hypotonic saline (0.45%) can be used in patients with severe hypernatremia (>155 mEq/L).
   b. The next goal is to **replenish total body water deficits;** this can be accomplished using a 0.45% saline infusion at 150–500 ml/hour, depending on degree of dehydration and cardiac and renal status.
   c. **Maintenance fluid replacement** is continued at a tapered rate until the fluid intake/output records indicate an overall positive balance of approximately 6 L. Complete fluid replacement in a typical DKA patient may require 12–24 hours to accomplish.
3. **Insulin therapy.** Sufficient insulin must be administered to turn off ketogenesis and correct hyperglycemia.
   a. **An IV bolus of regular insulin,** 10–15 U (0.15 U/kg), can be administered. This should be followed by a continuous infusion of regular insulin at an initial rate of 5–10 U/hour (or 0.1 U/kg/hour). A solution of regular insulin, 100 U in 500 ml 0.9% saline, infused at a rate of 50 ml/hour, delivers 10 U/hour of insulin. It is not necessary to add albumin routinely to the solution to prevent adsorption of insulin to the glass bottle and infusion tubing. Instead, running the initial 50–100 ml of the solution down the sink should saturate adsorption sites in the infusion apparatus and ensure proper delivery of insulin to the patient.
   b. **IM injection of regular insulin,** 5–10 U q1h, is an alternative to IV infusion, but absorption from this route is unreliable, particularly in hypotensive patients.
   c. **A decrease in blood glucose of 50–75 mg/dl/hour** is an appropriate response; lesser decrements suggest insulin resistance, inadequate volume repletion, or a problem with insulin delivery. If insulin resistance is suspected, the hourly dose of regular insulin should be increased progressively by 50–100% until an appropriate glycemic response is observed.
   d. **Excessively rapid correction of hyperglycemia** at rates greater than 100 mg/dl/hour should be avoided to reduce the risk of osmotic encephalopathy.
   e. **Maintenance insulin infusion rates of 1–2 U/hour** are appropriate when serum bicarbonate rises to 15 mEq/L or higher and the anion gap has closed. Once oral intake resumes, insulin can be administered SC and the intravenous route can be discontinued. It is prudent to give the first SC injection of insulin approximately 30 minutes before stopping the IV route.
4. **Dextrose (5%)** in saline should be infused once plasma glucose decreases to 250 mg/dl, and the insulin infusion rate should be decreased to 0.05 U/kg/hour to prevent dangerous hypoglycemia.
5. A **potassium deficit** should always be assumed or anticipated, regardless of plasma levels on admission. Insulin therapy results in a rapid shift of potassium into the intracellular compartment.
   a. The goal is to maintain plasma potassium in the normal range and thereby prevent the potentially fatal cardiac effects of hypokalemia. Potassium status should be documented from the outset; this includes an ECG to rule out life-threatening hyperkalemia.
   b. Potassium should be added routinely to the IV fluids at a rate of 10–20 mEq/hour except in patients with hyperkalemia (>6.0 mmol/L

and/or ECG evidence), renal failure, or oliguria confirmed by bladder catheterization.

c. Patients who present with hypokalemia should receive higher doses of potassium, 40 mEq/hour or greater, depending on severity.

d. Potassium chloride is an appropriate initial choice, but this can later be changed to potassium phosphate to reduce chloride load.

6. **Monitoring of therapy.** Blood glucose should be monitored hourly, serum electrolytes every 1–2 hours, and arterial blood gases as often as necessary. Serum sodium tends to rise as hyperglycemia is corrected; failure to observe this trend suggests that the patient is being overhydrated with free water. Serial serum ketone assays are not necessary, because ketonemia lags behind clinical recovery; closure of the anion gap is a more reliable index of metabolic recovery. Use of a flowchart is an efficient method of tracking clinical data (e.g., weight, fluid balance, mental status) and laboratory results during the management of DKA. Continuous ECG monitoring may be required for proper management of dyskalemia in patients with oliguria or renal failure.

7. **Bicarbonate therapy** is not routinely necessary and may be deleterious in certain situations. However, bicarbonate therapy may be appropriate and should be considered for DKA patients who develop (1) shock or coma, (2) severe acidosis (pH, 6.9–7.1), (3) severe depletion of buffering reserve (plasma bicarbonate <5 mEq/L), (4) acidosis-induced cardiac or respiratory dysfunction, or (5) severe hyperkalemia. Sodium bicarbonate, 50–100 mEq in 1 L 0.45% saline infused over 30–60 minutes, can be given in these situations. Bicarbonate treatment should be guided by arterial pH measurement and continued until the indications are no longer present. Care should be taken to avoid hypokalemia; an additional dose of potassium, 10 mEq, should be included with each infusion of bicarbonate unless hyperkalemia is present.

8. **Phosphate and magnesium** stores are subnormal in DKA patients, and plasma levels (particularly phosphate) decline further during insulin therapy. The clinical significance of these changes is unclear, and routine replacement of phosphate or magnesium is not necessary. In hypophosphatemic patients with compromised oral intake, the use of potassium phosphate in maintenance IV fluids can be considered (see Chap. 3, Fluid and Electrolyte Management). Magnesium therapy is indicated in patients with ventricular arrhythmia and can be administered as magnesium sulfate 1–2 g IV over 30–60 minutes.

9. **IV antimicrobial therapy** should be started promptly for documented bacterial, fungal, and other treatable infections. Empiric broad-spectrum antibiotics can be started in septic patients, pending results of blood cultures (see Chap. 13, Treatment of Infectious Diseases).

D. **Complications of DKA** include life-threatening conditions that must be recognized and treated promptly.

1. **Lactic acidosis** may result from prolonged dehydration, shock, infection, and tissue hypoxia in DKA patients. Lactic acidosis should be suspected in patients with refractory metabolic acidosis and a persistent anion gap despite optimal therapy for DKA. Adequate volume replacement, control of sepsis, and judicious use of bicarbonate constitute the approach to management.

2. **Arterial thrombosis** manifesting as stroke, myocardial infarction, or an ischemic limb occurs with increased frequency in DKA. However, routine anticoagulation is not indicated except as part of the specific therapy for a thrombotic event.

3. **Cerebral edema,** a dire complication of DKA, is observed more frequently in children than adults. Symptoms of increased intracranial pressure (e.g., headache, altered mental status, papilledema) or a sud-

den deterioration in mental status after initial improvement in a patient with DKA should raise suspicion for cerebral edema. Overhydration with free water and excessively rapid correction of hyperglycemia are known risk factors. A fall in serum sodium or failure to rise during therapy of DKA is a clue to imminent or established overhydration with free water. Neuroimaging with a CT scan can establish the diagnosis. Prompt recognition and treatment with IV mannitol is essential and may prevent neurologic sequelae in patients who survive cerebral edema.

4. **Rebound ketoacidosis** can occur as a result of premature cessation of insulin therapy.

E. **Prevention of DKA.** Every episode of DKA suggests a breakdown in clinical communication. Diabetes education should therefore be reinforced at every opportunity, with special emphasis on (1) self-management skills during prodromal sick days; (2) the body's need for more, rather than less, insulin during such illnesses; (3) testing of urine for ketones; and (4) procedures for obtaining timely and preventive medical advice.

## Type 2 Diabetes and Nonketotic Hyperosmolar Syndrome

The glycemic goals for patients with type 2 DM are the same as for type 1 DM: average preprandial blood glucose values of 90–130 mg/dl, bedtime blood glucose of 100–140 mg/dl, and $HbA_{1c}$ of 7% or lower (*Diabetes Care* 26[Suppl 1]:S33, 2003).

I. **Treatment of type 2 diabetes** requires a comprehensive approach that incorporates lifestyle and pharmacologic interventions (see Diabetes Mellitus, sec. **III**). The choice of **oral antidiabetic agents** (Table 21-2) for control of hyperglycemia in patients with type 2 DM is a matter of clinical judgment, as **monotherapy with maximum doses of insulin secretagogues, metformin, or TZDs yields comparable glucose-lowering effects.** Glycemic control with monotherapy is less likely to occur in patients with very high glucose readings (>240 mg/dl) at the time of diagnosis (*Ann Intern Med* 131:281, 1999). Insulin secretagogues exert their glucose-lowering effects within days, but approximately 20% of patients do not respond to these agents ("primary failure"). In contrast, the maximum effects of metformin or TZDs may not be observed for several weeks. Because residual pancreatic β-cell function is required for the glucose-lowering effects of sulfonylureas, repaglinide, metformin, and TZDs, many patients with advanced type 2 DM do not respond satisfactorily to these agents. Insulin therapy may thus be an early choice for such patients. Moreover, the toxicity profile of some oral agents may preclude their use in patients with preexisting illnesses.

A. **Insulin secretagogues**

1. **Sulfonylureas** lower blood glucose by augmenting insulin secretion. Similar glucose-lowering effects are obtained with equivalent doses of different sulfonylureas, and the mean decrease in fasting glucose is approximately 60 mg/dl. Sulfonylureas should be taken 30–60 minutes before food and should never be administered to patients who are observing a voluntary or imposed fast. Chlorpropamide and glyburide are metabolized to an active metabolite with significant renal excretion and should be avoided in the setting of impaired renal function and used with caution in elderly patients. Therapy should be initiated with the lowest effective dose and increased gradually over several days or

**Table 21-2.** Characteristics of oral antidiabetic agents

| Drug | Daily dosage range | Dose(s)/d | Duration of action (hr) | Main adverse effects |
|---|---|---|---|---|
| **Insulin secretagogues** | | | | |
| Sulfonylureas | | | | |
| First generation | | | | Hypoglycemia, weight gain |
| Tolbutamide | 0.5–2.0 g | 2–3 | 12 | |
| Acetohexamide | 0.25–1.5 g | 1–2 | 12–24 | |
| Tolazamide | 0.1–1.0 g | 1–2 | 12–24 | |
| Chlorpropamide | 100–500 mg | 1 | 36–72 | |
| Second generation | | | | |
| Glyburide | 1.25–20 mg | 1–2 | 16–24 | |
| Glipizide | 5–40 mg | 1–2 | 12 | |
| Glimepiride | 1–8 mg | 1 | 24 | |
| Rapid acting | | | | Hypoglycemia, weight gain |
| Nateglinide | 180–360 mg | 2–4 | 1–2 | |
| Repaglinide | 1–16 mg | 2–4 | | |
| **Biguanide** | | | | GI intolerance, lactic acidosis |
| Metformin | 1.0–2.5 g | 2–3 | 6–12 | |
| **Alpha-glucosidase inhibitors** | | | | GI intolerance, flatulence |
| Acarbose | 75–300 mg | 3 | N/A | |
| Miglitol | 75–300 mg | 3 | N/A | |
| **Thiazolidinediones** | | | | Fluid retention, CHF, hepatotoxicity, weight gain |
| Rosiglitazone | 2–8 mg | 1–2 | 12–24 | |
| Pioglitazone | 15–45 mg | 1 | 24 | |

N/A, not applicable because agents do not act systemically.

weeks to the optimal dose. Hypoglycemia and weight gain are notable adverse effects of sulfonylureas.

2. **Repaglinide** is a meglitinide analog that augments food-stimulated insulin secretion with a similar glucose-lowering effect as sulfonylureas. Unlike sulfonylureas, however, the meglitinides have a very short onset of action and a short half-life. Repaglinide can be used as a single agent or in combination with metformin in patients with type 2 DM. The dose range is 0.5–4.0 mg PO with two to four meals daily; the drug should be taken within 30 minutes before meals and skipped if no meal is planned. Adverse effects include hypoglycemia and weight gain.
3. **Nateglinide,** a D-phenylalanine derivative that is chemically distinct from other insulin secretagogues, acts directly on the pancreatic β cells to stimulate early insulin secretion (*Diabetes Care* 23:202, 2000). It is taken 10 minutes before breakfast, lunch, and dinner and leads to significant insulin secretion within 15 minutes with a return to baseline in 3–4 hours, effectively controlling postprandial hyperglycemia. The maximum effective dose is 120 mg with each meal. The potential exists for

**drug interactions** between nateglinide and medications that are affected by the cytochrome P-450 system. The drug is well tolerated, and the risk of hypoglycemia appears minimal.

B. **Metformin,** the only biguanide in current clinical use, inhibits hepatic glucose output and stimulates glucose uptake by peripheral tissues. It is the preferred agent for patients in whom weight gain is not desirable. Metformin is taken with food and, beginning with a single 500-mg or 850-mg tablet, the dose is increased slowly every 1–2 weeks until optimal glycemic effect is achieved or 2000 mg/day is reached. GI symptoms occur frequently but are seldom serious. **Lactic acidosis,** the most serious adverse effect, has an incidence of approximately three cases per 100,000 patient-years and a significant mortality. Risk factors for lactic acidosis include renal dysfunction, hypovolemia, tissue hypoxia, infection, alcoholism, and cardiopulmonary disease. **A serum creatinine level of 1.5 mg/dl or greater in men (≥1.4 mg/dl in women) or a glomerular filtration rate of less than 70 ml/minute is a contraindication to metformin use.** Metformin should be discontinued at the time of the radiographic contrast procedure and not restarted for 48 hours. Other situations in which metformin therapy should be avoided include cardiogenic or septic shock, CHF that requires pharmacologic therapy, severe liver disease, pulmonary insufficiency with hypoxemia, or severe tissue hypoperfusion (*N Engl J Med* 334:574, 1996).

C. **Alpha-glucosidase inhibitors** block carbohydrate digestion and decrease postprandial hyperglycemia when administered with food. Two members of this class, acarbose and miglitol, exert maximal effects at a dosage of approximately 150 mg/day. Each drug should be initiated at low dosages (25 mg PO qd–tid, with food) and increased slowly in weekly steps of 25 mg to minimize GI intolerance. Monotherapy with these agents seldom gives satisfactory results, but their addition to other drugs can improve glycemic control. Dose-related adverse effects are symptoms of carbohydrate malabsorption (e.g., diarrhea, bloating, abdominal cramping). Acarbose has been associated with elevation in liver enzymes, and therefore periodic monitoring of transaminases is recommended. **Hypoglycemia in patients who are receiving regimens that include alpha-glucosidase inhibitors should be treated with glucose, not sucrose.**

D. **TZDs** increase insulin sensitivity in muscle, adipose tissue, and liver. The risk of drug-induced hepatotoxicity with this class mandates close monitoring of liver function, particularly during the initial 12 months of drug exposure. Edema and cytopenia, from increased plasma volume, also occur with these agents. **TZDs can precipitate CHF** in patients who have cardiovascular disease and are in borderline compensation; therefore, therapy with these agents is not recommended in patients with significant heart disease (New York Heart Association class III and IV cardiac status). The risk of CHF is increased when TZDs are used in combination with insulin. Resumption of ovulation may occur in some premenopausal women with anovulatory cycles after TZD therapy. Therefore, contraceptive practice should be reviewed to prevent unintended pregnancy. The two TZDs that are currently available, rosiglitazone and pioglitazone, appear to have similar efficacy on glycemia.

   1. **Rosiglitazone** can be used alone as an adjunct to diet and exercise or in combination with metformin or a sulfonylurea. The usual starting dosage is 4 mg PO qd (or 2 mg PO bid) taken with or without food. This can be advanced to 8 mg PO qd (or 4 mg PO bid) after 12 weeks if glycemic response is inadequate. Although data from clinical trials suggest a low propensity for hepatotoxicity, regular monitoring of hepatic transaminases is required in patients treated with rosiglitazone.
   2. **Pioglitazone** can also be used as a single agent (as an adjunct to diet and exercise) or in combination with a sulfonylurea, metformin, or insulin. The initial dosage is 15 mg or 30 mg PO qd, taken with or with-

out food; this dosage can be increased after several weeks to 45 mg PO qd for optimal effect. Regular monitoring of hepatic transaminases is required during pioglitazone therapy.

**E. Insulin therapy in type 2 DM** is indicated for refractory hyperglycemia, DKA, nonketotic hyperosmolar crisis, and during pregnancy and other situations in which oral antidiabetic agents are contraindicated. The success of insulin therapy depends on the use of a sufficiently large dose of insulin (typical range, 0.6 to >1.0 U/kg/day) to achieve normoglycemia, rather than any specific pattern of insulin administration. Once-daily injections of intermediate-acting or long-acting insulin at bedtime or before breakfast, daily or twice-daily combinations of intermediate- and short-acting insulins, and more complex regimens have all been used with good results. Large doses of insulin (>100 U/day) usually are required for optimal glycemic control due to insulin resistance. The risk of insulin-induced hypoglycemia is low in this population, but weight gain can be considerable.

**F. Drug combinations.** Patients who are receiving monotherapy may have worsening of metabolic control during the first 5 years of therapy, and concurrent use of two or more medications with a different mechanism of action may be necessary. Widely used regimens include a sulfonylurea plus metformin or a TZD plus a sulfonylurea. Triple combination therapy has not been studied extensively and is considered somewhat controversial. The combination of a TZD plus insulin is less accepted because of a higher incidence of CHF exacerbations.

**II. Nonketotic hyperosmolar syndrome (NKHS)** results from severe dehydration and hyperglycemia in patients with type 2 DM. Ketoacidosis is absent because residual insulin secretion, although inadequate for glycemic control, effectively inhibits lipolysis and ketogenesis. Precipitating factors include stress, infection, stroke, noncompliance with medications, dietary indiscretion, alcohol, and cocaine abuse. Impaired glucose excretion is a contributory factor in patients with renal insufficiency or prerenal azotemia.

**A. Clinical manifestations.** In contrast to DKA, the onset of NKHS is usually insidious. Several days of deteriorating glycemic control are followed by increasing lethargy. Clinical evidence of severe dehydration is the rule. Focal neurologic deficits may be found at presentation or may develop during therapy. Therefore, repeated neurologic assessment is recommended.

**B. Laboratory** findings include (1) hyperglycemia, often greater than 600 mg/dl; (2) plasma osmolality greater than 320 mOsm/L; (3) absence of ketonemia; and (4) pH greater than 7.3 and serum bicarbonate greater than 20 mEq/L. Prerenal azotemia and lactic acidosis can develop. Although some patients have detectable urine ketones, most patients do not have a metabolic acidosis. Lactic acidosis may develop from an underlying infection or other cause.

**C. Management** of NKHS consists of (1) fluid replacement, (2) insulin therapy, (3) correction of electrolyte deficits, and (4) detection and treatment of precipitating causes. An IV access line should be secured promptly, and supportive measures should be provided. A focused search for precipitating factors (e.g., infection) is appropriate, but such efforts should not delay fluid replacement and insulin therapy.

**1. Fluid replacement** initially should aim to restore intravascular volume and later correct total body water deficit.

**a. Initial fluid therapy** can be given as isotonic (0.9%) saline. In the absence of cardiac or renal compromise, a rapid infusion rate of 1–2 L/hour in the first 1–2 hours can be administered, followed by 1 L/hour until intravascular volume is restored.

**b. Free water deficits** can be corrected using infusion of 0.45% saline to replace one-half of the water deficit over the first 12 hours and the remainder in the next 24 hours at a rate guided by serum sodium level and osmolarity, after repletion of intravascular volume (see

Chap. 3, Fluid and Electrolyte Management). Caution should be exercised when replacing fluids in the elderly and in patients with cardiac or renal dysfunction.

c. **Dextrose (5%)** should be added to the 0.45% saline infusion once plasma glucose decreases to 250–300 mg/dl. If plasma sodium is greater than 150 mmol/L, $D_5W$ can be infused instead.

d. **Maintenance fluids** should be infused at a rate guided by clinical status, especially urine output and evidence of volume repletion or overload. Patients with NKHS may require as much as 10–12 L positive fluid balance over 24–36 hours to restore total deficits.

2. **Insulin therapy** is indicated for all patients with NKHS. In individuals with marked hyperglycemia (>600 mg/dl), regular insulin, 5–10 U IV, should be given immediately, followed by continuous infusion of 0.1–0.15 U/kg/hour. Lower doses of a regular insulin bolus can be used for less severe hyperglycemia. Once plasma glucose decreases to 250–300 mg/dl, insulin infusion can be decreased to 1–2 U/hour and 5% dextrose should be added to the intravenous fluids. After full rehydration and clinical recovery, regular insulin can be given SC and patients can thereafter resume their usual diabetes therapy.

3. **Electrolyte management.** Hypokalemia after initiation of IV insulin therapy should be anticipated and corrected (see Type I Diabetes and Diabetic Ketoacidosis, sec. **II.C.5**). Lactic acidosis requiring bicarbonate therapy may develop as a complication of NKHS or metformin therapy (see Diabetes and Diabetic Ketoacidosis, sec. **II.C.7**).

4. **Monitoring of therapy.** Use of a flowchart is helpful for tracking clinical data and laboratory results. Initially, blood glucose should be monitored every 30–60 minutes and serum electrolytes every 1–2 hours; frequency of monitoring can be decreased during recovery. Neurologic status must be reassessed frequently; persistent lethargy or altered mentation indicates inadequate therapy. On the other hand, relapse after initial improvement in mental status suggests too-rapid correction of serum osmolarity.

5. **Other considerations.** The clinician should be alert to predisposing factors and possible complications of NKHS.

   a. **Diabetes education and weight loss** should be reinforced, with emphasis on self-management skills during intercurrent illness.

   b. **IV antimicrobial therapy** should be started promptly for documented bacterial, fungal, and other treatable infections. Empiric broad-spectrum antibiotics can be started in septic patients, pending results of blood cultures.

   c. **Acute renal failure** may result from severe and prolonged hypovolemia. Evaluation by a nephrologist may be required if oliguria persists despite correction of volume deficit.

   d. **Coagulopathy** that presents either with thrombotic or bleeding episodes requires specialist evaluation and management.

## Chronic Complications of Diabetes Mellitus

Prevention of long-term complications is one of the main goals of diabetes management. Appropriate treatment of established complications may delay their progression and improve quality of life.

I. **Microvascular complications** include diabetic retinopathy, nephropathy, and neuropathy. These complications are directly related to hyperglycemia and can be prevented by maintaining scrupulous glycemic control.

A. **Diabetic retinopathy** is the most frequent cause of new cases of blindness among adults aged 20–74 years and includes background retinopathy (microaneurysms, retinal infarcts) and proliferative retinopathy.

1. Background retinopathy usually is not associated with loss of vision. However, the development of macular edema or proliferative retinopathy (particularly new vessels near the optic disk) requires elective laser photocoagulation therapy to preserve vision. Vitrectomy is indicated for patients with vitreous hemorrhage or retinal detachment.
2. **Annual examination by an ophthalmologist** is recommended from the outset for all patients with type 2 DM and beginning at puberty or 3–5 years after diagnosis for those with type 1 DM.
3. **Other ocular abnormalities** associated with diabetes include cataract formation, dyskinetic pupils, glaucoma, optic neuropathy, extraocular muscle paresis, floaters, and fluctuating visual acuity. The latter is related to changes in blood glucose. The presence of floaters may be indicative of preretinal or vitreous hemorrhage; immediate referral for ophthalmologic evaluation is warranted.

B. **Diabetic nephropathy** is the leading cause of end-stage renal disease and is preceded by microalbuminuria (30–300 mg albumin/24 hours), a potentially reversible state.

1. **Microalbuminuria** precedes overt proteinuria (>300 mg albumin/day) by several years in type 1 and type 2 DM. The mean duration from diagnosis of type 1 diabetes to development of overt proteinuria is 17 years, and the time from the occurrence of proteinuria to end-stage renal disease averages 5 years. In type 2 DM, microalbuminuria can be present at the time of diagnosis.
2. **Annual screening for microalbuminuria** should be performed in type 1 patients who have had diabetes for longer than 5 years and all type 2 diabetic patients starting at diagnosis. Measurement of microalbumin-creatinine ratio (normal, <30 mg albumin/g creatinine) in a random urine sample is recommended for screening. At least two to three measurements within a 6-month period should be performed to make the diagnosis (*Diabetes Care* 26:S94, 2003).
3. **Intensive control of diabetes and hypertension** is an effective intervention for incipient or established diabetic nephropathy. In type 1 and type 2 patients with microalbuminuria and with or without hypertension, **angiotensin-converting enzyme inhibitors** delay the progression of nephropathy. In type 2 patients with hypertension, creatinine greater than 1.5 mg/dl, and microalbuminuria, **angiotensin II–receptor blockers** delay progression of nephropathy. Nondihydropyridine calcium channel blockers or beta-blockers can be used in patients who are unable to tolerate angiotensin-converting enzyme inhibitors or angiotensin II–receptor blockers (*Diabetes Care* 26:S94, 2003). Dietary protein restriction may be beneficial in some patients.

C. **Diabetic neuropathy** may result in sensory, motor, autonomic, or combined deficits. Sensorimotor diabetic peripheral polyneuropathy is a major risk factor for foot trauma, ulceration, Charcot's arthropathy, and limb amputation. Sensation in the lower extremities should be documented at least annually, using either a light-touch monofilament or a tuning fork.

1. **Painful peripheral neuropathy** responds variably to treatment with tricyclic antidepressants (e.g., amitriptyline, 10–150 mg PO qhs), topical capsaicin (0.075% cream), or anticonvulsants (e.g., carbamazepine, 100–400 mg PO bid). Patients should be warned about adverse effects: sedation and anticholinergic symptoms (tricyclics), burning sensation (capsaicin), and blood dyscrasias (carbamazepine).
2. **Orthostatic hypotension** is a manifestation of autonomic neuropathy, but common etiologies (e.g., dehydration, anemia, medications) should be excluded. Treatment is symptomatic: postural maneuvers, use of

compressive garments (e.g., Jobst stockings), and intravascular expansion using sodium chloride, 1–4 g PO qid, and fludrocortisone, 0.1–0.3 mg PO qd. Hypokalemia, supine hypertension, and CHF are some adverse effects of fludrocortisone.

3. **Intractable nausea and vomiting** in diabetes are manifestations of impaired GI motility from autonomic neuropathy. **Surveillance for DKA** is warranted in insulin-treated patients with nausea and vomiting because interruption of insulin therapy is widespread among such patients. Other causes of nausea and vomiting also should be excluded.
   a. **Management of diabetic gastroenteropathy** can be challenging. Frequent, small meals (6–8/day) of soft consistency that are low in fat and fiber provide relief for some patients. Parenteral nutrition may become necessary in some individuals. Improvement in glycemic control also is beneficial, because hyperglycemia delays gastric emptying.
   b. **Pharmacologic therapy** includes the prokinetic agent metoclopramide, 10–20 mg PO (or as a suppository) before meals and qhs, and erythromycin, 125–500 mg PO qid. Extrapyramidal side effects (tremor and tardive dyskinesia) from the antidopaminergic actions of metoclopramide may limit therapy.
   c. **Cyclical vomiting** that is unrelated to a GI motility disorder or other clear etiology may also occur in diabetic patients and appears to respond to amitriptyline, 25–50 mg PO qhs.
4. **Diabetic cystopathy,** or bladder dysfunction, results from impaired autonomic control of detrusor muscle and sphincteric function. Manifestations include urgency, dribbling, incomplete emptying, overflow incontinence, and urinary retention. Recurrent urinary tract infections are common in patients with residual urine. Treatment with bethanechol, 10 mg PO tid, or intermittent self-catheterization may be required to relieve retention.
5. **Diabetic diarrhea** should only be diagnosed after exclusion of other causes of diarrhea. Because the pathogenesis of diabetic diarrhea is unclear, treatment is empiric. Repeated courses of broad-spectrum antibiotics (e.g., azithromycin, tetracycline, cephalosporins) may be beneficial; loperamide or octreotide, 50–75 μg SC bid, can be effective in patients with intractable diarrhea.

II. **Macrovascular complications of DM** include coronary artery disease, stroke, and peripheral vascular disease. **Risk factors** for macrovascular disease include insulin resistance, hyperglycemia, microalbuminuria, hypertension, hyperlipidemia, cigarette smoking, and obesity. Glycemic control should be optimized; hypertension should be controlled to a target blood pressure of less than 130/80 mm Hg (or <125/75 mm Hg in patients with proteinuria), and hyperlipidemia should be treated appropriately, with a target low-density lipoprotein cholesterol level of less than 100 mg/dl, high-density lipoprotein cholesterol levels of greater than 40 mg/dl, and triglyceride levels of less than 150 mg/dl. Cigarette smoking should be actively discouraged, and weight loss should be promoted in obese patients. Aspirin, 81–325 mg/day, is of proven benefit in secondary prevention of myocardial infarction or stroke in diabetic patients.

A. **Coronary artery disease** occurs at a younger age and may have atypical clinical presentations in patients with diabetes. Myocardial infarction carries a worse prognosis, and angioplasty gives less satisfactory results in diabetic patients. ECG should be obtained yearly, and there should be a low threshold for ordering stress tests.

B. **Management of diabetes after acute myocardial infarction.** Optimization of glycemic control during and after admission for acute myocardial infarction improves survival. Routine IV infusion of regular insulin and glucose to improve glycemic control in the hospital, followed by intensive insulin therapy at home, significantly reduces acute and long-term mortality (*BMJ* 314:1512, 1997; *J Am Coll Cardiol* 26:57, 1995).

1. **Initial insulin infusion** rates of 1–4 U/hour and dextrose infusion of 5 g/hour (100 ml/hour $D_5W$) can be used and adjusted, as necessary, to maintain plasma glucose in the 100- to 150-mg/dl range.
2. **Potassium chloride,** 10–20 mEq, can be added to each liter of insulin-glucose infusion to prevent hypokalemia in patients with normal renal function.
3. **Close supervision of therapy** is mandatory, because hypoglycemia triggers release of counterregulatory hormones, some of which (e.g., catecholamines) may be arrhythmogenic.

**III. Miscellaneous complications,** such as erectile dysfunction and diabetic foot ulcers, have multiple etiologies.

**A. Erectile dysfunction** may result from diabetic neuropathy, vascular insufficiency, adverse drug effects, endocrinopathy, psychological factors, or a combination of these etiologies. Glycemic control should be intensified, and specialist referral should be considered if the problem persists. If endocrinologic evaluation proves negative and other treatable causes have been excluded, a trial of the phosphodiesterase V inhibitor, sildenafil, 50–100 mg PO precoitally, may be appropriate. **Sildenafil should not be used concurrently with nitrates** to prevent severe and potentially fatal hypotensive reactions.

**B. Diabetic foot ulcers** result from chronic neuropathy, vascular insufficiency, and polymicrobial infection. Poorly managed foot ulcers may result in limb loss from amputation. Patient education should emphasize prevention: daily foot examination, application of moisturizing lotion, use of proper footwear, and caution with self-pedicure. The exposed feet should be inspected and palpated at every patient encounter; significant findings, such as calluses, hammertoes or other deformities, and soft-tissue lesions, should be evaluated. Screening for peripheral vascular disease clinically or by noninvasive methods is a mandatory part of diabetic foot care. **Diabetic foot infections** should be treated aggressively. Proper management includes a multidisciplinary approach that includes orthopedic surgeons, specialized nursing care, and close monitoring. The presence of deep infection with abscess, cellulitis, gangrene, or osteomyelitis is an indication for hospitalization and prompt surgical drainage. Treatment of foot infections is dependent on severity, as outlined below.

1. **Mild to moderate cellulitis.** Rest, elevation of the affected foot, and relief of pressure are essential components of treatment and should be initiated at first presentation. In localized cellulitis and new ulcers, *Staphylococcus aureus* and streptococci are the most frequent pathogens. Therapy with oral dicloxacillin, first-generation cephalosporin, amoxicillin/clavulanate, or clindamycin is recommended.
2. **Moderate to severe cellulitis.** This type of involvement requires intravenous therapy and admission to the hospital. Consultation for débridement and aerobic and anaerobic cultures are necessary when necrotic tissue is present. Intravenous oxacillin or nafcillin, a first-generation IV cephalosporin, ampicillin/sulbactam, clindamycin, or vancomycin are options for therapy. Antibiotic coverage should subsequently be tailored according to the clinical response of the patient, culture results, and sensitivity testing.
3. **Moderate to severe cellulitis with ischemia or significant local necrosis.** It is important to determine the presence of bone involvement and peripheral vascular disease because failure to diagnose osteomyelitis and ischemia often results in failure of wound healing. **Bone involvement** is present if bone is seen at the base of the ulcer or is easily detected by gentle probing with a blunt sterile probe. Radiographs are not very sensitive for diagnosis, and leukocyte scanning or magnetic resonance imaging offers better specificity. Presence of **peripheral vascular disease** is suspected by absence of pedal pulses or decreased capillary filling. An ankle-to-brachial index of less than 0.9 by Doppler

ultrasound has a 95% sensitivity for detecting angiogram-positive peripheral vascular disease (*Int J Epidemiol* 17:248, 1988). Intravenous antibiotics, bed rest, surgical débridement, culture obtained from the base of the ulcer, and bone culture help direct antibiotic therapy. Ampicillin/sulbactam and ticarcillin/clavulanate are first-line agents; piperacillin/tazobactam, clindamycin plus ciprofloxacin, ceftazidime, cefepime, cefotaxime, or ceftriaxone plus metronidazole are good alternatives for initial therapy. In the presence of osteomyelitis, 10–12 weeks of intravenous antibiotic therapy is recommended. Ulcers with localized or generalized gangrene require surgical amputation.

## Hypoglycemia

Hypoglycemia is uncommon in the general population but is a significant problem among patients with diabetes. Iatrogenic factors usually account for hypoglycemia in the setting of diabetes, whereas spontaneous hypoglycemia in the nondiabetic population has multiple etiologies.

I. **Iatrogenic hypoglycemia** complicates therapy with insulin or sulfonylureas and is a limiting factor to achieve glycemic control during intensive therapy in patients with DM. Diabetic patients should be familiar with the warning symptoms of hypoglycemia and be taught to respond appropriately to such episodes.
   A. **Risk factors** for iatrogenic hypoglycemia include skipped or insufficient meals, unaccustomed physical exertion, misguided therapy, alcohol ingestion, and drug overdose. Recurrent episodes of hypoglycemia impair recognition of hypoglycemic symptoms, thereby increasing the risk for severe hypoglycemia.
   B. **Symptoms**
      1. **Autonomic (or neurogenic) symptoms** include tremulousness, sweating, palpitations, and hunger. Increased secretion of counterregulatory hormones (e.g., epinephrine) accounts for these symptoms.
      2. **Neuroglycopenic symptoms** develop as glucose decreases further. These symptoms include impaired concentration, irritability, blurred vision, lethargy, and development of seizure or coma.
      3. **Patients with hypoglycemia unawareness** and defective glucose counterregulation have a blunting of autonomic symptoms and counterregulatory hormone secretion during hypoglycemia. Seizures or coma may develop in such patients without the usual warning symptoms of hypoglycemia.
      4. **Plasma or capillary blood glucose** should be obtained, whenever feasible, to confirm hypoglycemia.
   C. **Treatment of hypoglycemia.** Isolated episodes of mild hypoglycemia may not require specific intervention. Recurrent episodes require a review of lifestyle factors; adjustments may be indicated in the content, timing, and distribution of meals, as well as medication dosage and timing. Severe hypoglycemia is an indication for supervised treatment.
      1. **Readily absorbable carbohydrates** (e.g., glucose and sugar-containing beverages) can be administered orally to conscious patients for rapid effect. Alternatively, milk, candy bars, fruit, cheese, and crackers may be adequate in some patients with mild hypoglycemia. Hypoglycemia associated with acarbose or miglitol therapy should preferentially be treated with glucose. Glucose tablets and carbohydrate supplies should be readily available to patients with DM at all times.
      2. **IV dextrose** is indicated for severe hypoglycemia, in patients with altered consciousness, and during restriction of oral intake. An initial bolus, 20–50 ml 50% dextrose, should be given immediately, followed by

infusion of $D_5W$ (or 10% dextrose in water) to maintain blood glucose above 100 mg/dl. Prolonged IV dextrose infusion and close observation are warranted in sulfonylurea overdose, in the elderly, and in patients with defective counterregulation.

3. **Glucagon,** 1 mg IM (or SC), is an effective initial therapy for severe hypoglycemia in patients who are unable to receive oral intake or in whom IV access cannot be secured immediately. Vomiting is a frequent side effect, and therefore care should be taken to prevent the risk of aspiration. A glucagon kit should be available to patients with a history of severe hypoglycemia; family members and roommates should be instructed in its proper use.
4. **Education** regarding etiologies of hypoglycemia, preventive measures, and appropriate adjustments to medication, diet, and exercise regimens are essential tasks to be addressed during hospitalization for severe hypoglycemia.
5. **Hypoglycemia unawareness** can develop in patients who are undergoing intensive diabetes therapy. These patients should be encouraged to monitor their blood glucose frequently and take timely measures to correct low values (<60 mg/dl). In patients with very tightly controlled diabetes, slight relaxation in glycemic control and scrupulous avoidance of hypoglycemia can restore the lost warning symptoms.

II. **Spontaneous hypoglycemia,** unrelated to diabetes therapy, is an infrequent problem in general medical practice. Major categories include fasting and postprandial hypoglycemia.

A. **Fasting hypoglycemia** can be caused by inappropriate insulin secretion (e.g., insulinoma), alcohol abuse, severe hepatic or renal insufficiency, hypopituitarism, glucocorticoid deficiency, or surreptitious injection of insulin or ingestion of a sulfonylurea.

1. **Episodic autonomic symptoms** suggestive of hypoglycemia may be present, but, more commonly, neuroglycopenic symptoms predominate.
2. **Recurrent seizures, dementia, and bizarre behavior** may occasion referral for neuropsychiatric evaluation, which may delay timely diagnosis of hypoglycemia.
3. **Definitive diagnosis** of fasting hypoglycemia requires hourly blood glucose monitoring during a supervised fast lasting up to 72 hours and measurement of plasma insulin, C-peptide, and sulfonylurea metabolites if hypoglycemia (<50 mg/dl) is documented.
4. **Patients who develop hypoglycemia** and have measurable plasma insulin and C-peptide levels without sulfonylurea metabolites require further evaluation for an insulinoma.

B. **Postprandial hypoglycemia** often is suspected, but seldom proven, in patients with vague symptoms that occur 1 or more hours after meals.

1. **Alimentary hypoglycemia** is a tenable consideration in a patient with a history of partial gastrectomy or intestinal resection in whom recurrent symptoms develop 1–2 hours after eating. The mechanism is thought to be related to too-rapid glucose absorption, resulting in a robust insulin response. Thus, frequent small meals with reduced carbohydrate content may ameliorate symptoms.
2. **Functional hypoglycemia.** Symptoms that are possibly suggestive of hypoglycemia, which may or may not be confirmed by plasma glucose measurement, occur in some patients who have not undergone GI surgery. This condition is referred to as *functional hypoglycemia*. The symptoms tend to develop 3–5 hours after meals. Current evaluation and management of functional hypoglycemia are imprecise; some patients show evidence of IGT and may respond to dietary therapy.

# 22 Endocrine Diseases

William E. Clutter

## Evaluation of Suspected Thyroid Disease

The major hormone secreted by the thyroid is **thyroxine ($T_4$)**, which is converted in many tissues to the more potent **triiodothyronine ($T_3$).** Both are bound reversibly to plasma proteins, primarily **thyroxine-binding globulin (TBG).** Only the free (unbound) fraction enters cells and produces biologic effects. $T_4$ secretion is stimulated by **thyroid-stimulating hormone (TSH).** In turn, TSH secretion is inhibited by $T_4$, forming a negative feedback loop that keeps free $T_4$ levels within a narrow normal range. Diagnosis of thyroid disease is based on clinical findings, palpation of the thyroid, and measurement of plasma TSH and thyroid hormones (*Arch Intern Med* 160:1573, 2000).

**I. Thyroid palpation** determines the size and consistency of the thyroid and the presence of nodules, tenderness, or a thrill.

**II. Plasma TSH is the initial test of choice in most patients with suspected thyroid disease,** except when thyroid function is not in a steady state (*Endocrinol Metab Clin North Am* 30:245, 2001). TSH levels are elevated even in mild primary hypothyroidism and are suppressed to less than 0.1 μU/ml even in mild hyperthyroidism. Thus, **a normal plasma TSH level excludes hyperthyroidism and primary hypothyroidism.** Because even slight changes in thyroid hormone levels affect TSH secretion, **abnormal TSH levels are not specific for clinically important thyroid disease.** Changes in plasma TSH lag behind changes in plasma $T_4$, and TSH levels may be misleading when plasma $T_4$ levels are rapidly changing, as during treatment of hyperthyroidism.

- **A. Plasma TSH is mildly elevated** (up to 20 μU/ml) in some euthyroid patients with **nonthyroidal illnesses** and in mild (also known as subclinical) hypothyroidism.
- **B. TSH levels may be suppressed to less than 0.1 μU/ml** in **severe nonthyroidal illness,** in mild (also known as subclinical) hyperthyroidism, and during treatment with dopamine or high doses of glucocorticoids. Also, TSH levels remain less than 0.1 μU/ml for some time after hyperthyroidism is corrected.
- **C. TSH levels are usually within the reference range in secondary hypothyroidism and are not useful for detection of this rare form of hypothyroidism.**

**III. Plasma free $T_4$** confirms the diagnosis and assesses the severity of hyperthyroidism when plasma TSH is less than 0.1 μU/ml. It is also used to diagnose secondary hypothyroidism and adjust $T_4$ therapy in patients with pituitary disease. Most laboratories measure free $T_4$ by analog immunoassays. Older tests, such as total $T_4$ assays or $T_4$ index, are less reliable and should no longer be used.

**IV. Free $T_4$ measured by equilibrium dialysis** is the most reliable measure of thyroid status, but results seldom are rapidly available. It is needed only in rare cases in which the diagnosis is not clear from measurement of plasma TSH and free $T_4$ by analog immunoassay.

**V. Effect of nonthyroidal illness on thyroid function tests** (*Endocrinol Metab Clin North Am* 31:159, 2002). Many illnesses alter thyroid tests without causing true thyroid dysfunction (the nonthyroidal illness or euthyroid sick syndrome). These changes must be recognized to avoid mistaken diagnosis and therapy.

- **A. The low $T_3$ syndrome** occurs in many illnesses, during starvation, and after trauma or surgery. Conversion of $T_4$ to $T_3$ is decreased, and plasma $T_3$ levels are low. Plasma free $T_4$ and TSH levels are normal. This may be an adaptive response to illness, and thyroid hormone therapy is not beneficial.
- **B. The low $T_4$ syndrome** occurs in severe illness. Plasma total $T_4$ levels fall as a result of decreased levels of TBG and perhaps inhibition of $T_4$ binding to TBG. When measured by commonly available analog immunoassays, free $T_4$ may be low. **However, plasma free $T_4$ measured by equilibrium dialysis usually remains normal. TSH levels decrease early in severe illness,** sometimes to less than 0.1 μU/ml. **During recovery they rise, sometimes to levels higher than the normal range** (although rarely >20 μU/ml).

**VI. A number of drugs affect thyroid function tests** (Table 22-1). Iodine-containing drugs (**amiodarone** and radiographic contrast media) may cause hyperthyroidism or hypothyroidism in susceptible patients. Other drugs alter thyroid function tests, especially plasma total $T_4$, without causing true thyroid dysfunction. In general, plasma TSH levels are a reliable guide to determining whether true hyperthyroidism or hypothyroidism is present.

**Table 22-1.** Effects of drugs on thyroid function tests

| Effect | Drug |
|---|---|
| **Decreased free and total $T_4$** | |
| True hypothyroidism (TSH elevated) | Iodine (amiodarone, radiographic contrast) |
| | Lithium |
| Inhibition of TSH secretion | Glucocorticoids |
| | Dopamine |
| Multiple mechanisms (TSH normal) | Phenytoin |
| **Decreased total $T_4$ only** | |
| Decreased TBG (TSH normal) | Androgens |
| Inhibition of $T_4$ binding to TBG (TSH normal) | Furosemide (high doses) |
| | Salicylates |
| **Increased free and total $T_4$** | |
| True hyperthyroidism (TSH <0.1 μU/ml) | Iodine (amiodarone, radiographic contrast) |
| Inhibited $T_4$ to $T_3$ conversion (TSH normal) | Amiodarone |
| **Increased free $T_4$ only** | |
| Displacement of $T_4$ from TBG in vitro (TSH normal) | Heparin, low-molecular-weight heparin |
| **Increased total $T_4$ only** | |
| Increased TBG (TSH normal) | Estrogens, tamoxifen |

$T_3$, triiodothyronine; $T_4$, thyroxine; TBG, thyroxine-binding globulin; TSH, thyroid-stimulating hormone.

## Hypothyroidism

I. **Etiology. Primary hypothyroidism** (due to disease of the thyroid itself) accounts for more than 90% of cases. **Chronic lymphocytic thyroiditis (Hashimoto's disease)** (*N Engl J Med* 348:2646, 2003) is the most common cause and may be associated with Addison's disease and other endocrine deficits. Its prevalence is greatest in women and increases with age. **Iatrogenic hypothyroidism** due to thyroidectomy or radioactive iodine (RAI, $^{131}$I) therapy is also common. Transient hypothyroidism occurs in postpartum thyroiditis and subacute thyroiditis, usually after a period of hyperthyroidism. **Drugs that may cause hypothyroidism** include iodine, lithium, interferon-alpha, interleukin-2, and thalidomide. **Secondary hypothyroidism** due to TSH deficiency is uncommon but may occur in any disorder of the pituitary or hypothalamus. However, it rarely occurs without other evidence of pituitary disease.

II. **Clinical findings.** Most symptoms of hypothyroidism are nonspecific and develop gradually. They include cold intolerance, fatigue, somnolence, poor memory, constipation, menorrhagia, myalgias, and hoarseness. Signs include slow tendon-reflex relaxation, bradycardia, facial and periorbital edema, dry skin, and nonpitting edema (myxedema). Mild weight gain may occur, but hypothyroidism does not cause marked obesity. Rare manifestations include hypoventilation, pericardial or pleural effusions, deafness, and carpal tunnel syndrome. Laboratory findings may include hyponatremia and elevated plasma levels of cholesterol, triglycerides, and creatine kinase. The ECG may show low-voltage and T-wave abnormalities.

III. **Diagnosis.** Hypothyroidism is readily treatable and should be suspected in any patient with compatible symptoms, especially in the presence of a diffuse goiter or a history of RAI therapy or thyroid surgery.

A. **In suspected primary hypothyroidism, plasma TSH is the best initial diagnostic test.** A normal value excludes primary hypothyroidism, and a markedly elevated value (>20 μU/ml) confirms the diagnosis. Mild elevation of plasma TSH (<20 μU/ml) may be due to nonthyroidal illness but usually indicates **mild (or subclinical) primary hypothyroidism,** in which thyroid function is impaired but increased secretion of TSH maintains plasma free $T_4$ levels within the reference range (see sec. **IV.D**). These patients may have nonspecific symptoms that are compatible with hypothyroidism and a mild increase in serum cholesterol and low-density lipoprotein cholesterol. They develop more severe hypothyroidism at a rate of 2.5%/year.

B. **If secondary hypothyroidism is suspected because of evidence of pituitary disease, plasma free $T_4$ should be measured.** Plasma TSH levels are usually within the reference range in secondary hypothyroidism and cannot be used alone to make this diagnosis. Patients with secondary hypothyroidism should be evaluated for other pituitary hormone deficits and for a mass lesion of the pituitary or hypothalamus (see the Anterior Pituitary Gland Dysfunction section).

C. **In severe nonthyroidal illness,** the diagnosis of hypothyroidism may be difficult (*Endocrinol Metab Clin North Am* 31:1159–1172, 2002). Plasma total $T_4$ and free $T_4$ measured by routine assays may be low.

1. **Plasma TSH is the best initial diagnostic test.** A normal TSH value is strong evidence that the patient is euthyroid, except when there is evidence of pituitary or hypothalamic disease or in patients treated with dopamine or high doses of glucocorticoids. Marked elevation of plasma TSH (>20 μU/ml) establishes the diagnosis of primary hypothyroidism.

2. **Moderate elevations of plasma TSH (<20 μU/ml) may occur in euthyroid patients with nonthyroidal illness and are not specific for hypothyroidism.** Plasma free $T_4$ by analog immunoassay should be measured if TSH is moderately elevated, or if secondary hypothyroidism is suspected, and patients should be treated for hypothyroidism if

plasma free $T_4$ is low. Thyroid function in these patients should be reevaluated after recovery from illness.

**IV. Therapy.** $T_4$ (levothyroxine) is the drug of choice. The usual replacement dose is 100–125 μg PO qd, and most patients require doses between 75 and 150 μg qd. In elderly patients, the average replacement dose is somewhat lower. The need for lifelong treatment should be emphasized. $T_4$ should be taken 30 minutes before a meal, because dietary fiber may interfere with its absorption, and should not be taken with medications that affect its absorption (see sec. **IV.C**).

**A. Initiation of therapy.** Young, otherwise healthy adults should be started on 100 μg qd. This regimen gradually corrects hypothyroidism, as several weeks are required to reach steady-state plasma levels of $T_4$. Symptoms begin to improve within a few weeks. In otherwise healthy elderly patients, the initial dose should be 50 μg qd. Patients with cardiac disease should be started on 25–50 μg qd and monitored carefully for exacerbation of cardiac symptoms.

**B. Dose adjustment and follow-up**

1. **In primary hypothyroidism, the goal of therapy is to maintain plasma TSH within the normal range.** Plasma TSH should be measured 2–3 months after initiation of therapy. The dose of $T_4$ then should be adjusted in 12- to 25-μg increments at intervals of 6–8 weeks until plasma TSH is normal. Thereafter, annual TSH measurement is adequate to monitor therapy and to ensure compliance. TSH should also be measured in the first trimester of pregnancy, because the $T_4$ dose requirement increases at this time. Overtreatment, indicated by a subnormal TSH, should be avoided because it increases the risk of osteoporosis and atrial fibrillation.
2. **In secondary hypothyroidism, plasma TSH cannot be used to adjust therapy.** The goal of therapy is to maintain the **plasma free $T_4$** near the middle of the reference range. The dose of $T_4$ should be adjusted at 6- to 8-week intervals until this goal is achieved. Thereafter, annual measurement of plasma free $T_4$ is adequate to monitor therapy.
3. **Coronary artery disease** may be exacerbated by treatment of hypothyroidism. The dose of $T_4$ should be increased slowly in patients with coronary artery disease, with careful attention to worsening angina, heart failure, or arrhythmias.

**C. Situations in which $T_4$ dose requirements change.** Difficulty in controlling hypothyroidism is most often due to **poor compliance** with therapy. Observed therapy may be necessary in some cases. Other causes of increasing $T_4$ requirement include (1) **malabsorption** due to intestinal disease or **drugs that interfere with $T_4$ absorption** (e.g., **calcium carbonate, ferrous sulfate,** cholestyramine, sucralfate, aluminum hydroxide); (2) **drug interactions that increase $T_4$ clearance** (e.g., estrogen, rifampin, carbamazepine, phenytoin) or block conversion of $T_4$ to $T_3$ (**amiodarone**); (3) **pregnancy,** in which $T_4$ requirement increases in the first trimester; and (4) gradual failure of remaining endogenous thyroid function after RAI treatment of hyperthyroidism.

**D. Mild (or subclinical) hypothyroidism** (see sec. **III.A**) should be treated with $T_4$ if any of the following are present: (1) **nonspecific symptoms compatible with hypothyroidism,** (2) a **goiter,** (3) **hypercholesterolemia** that warrants treatment, or (4) a **plasma TSH that is greater than 10 μU/ml** (*N Engl J Med* 345:260, 2001). Untreated patients should be monitored annually, and $T_4$ should be started if symptoms develop or serum TSH increases to greater than 10 μU/ml.

**E. Urgent therapy** is rarely necessary for hypothyroidism. Most patients with hypothyroidism and concomitant illness can be treated in the usual manner (see secs. **IV.A** and **IV.B**). However, hypothyroidism may impair survival in critical illness by contributing to hypoventilation, hypotension, hypothermia, bradycardia, or hyponatremia. Little evidence supports the contention that severe hypothyroidism alone causes coma or shock; most reports of alleged "myxedema coma" predate recognition that nonthyroidal illness itself lowers thyroid hormone levels.

1. Hypoventilation and hypotension should be treated intensively, along with any concomitant diseases. Confirmatory tests (plasma TSH and free $T_4$) should be obtained before thyroid hormone therapy is started in a severely ill patient.
2. **$T_4$, 50–100 μg IV, can be given q6–8h for 24 hours,** followed by 75–100 μg IV qd until oral intake is possible. Replacement therapy should be continued in the usual manner if the diagnosis of hypothyroidism is confirmed. No clinical trials have determined the optimum method of thyroid hormone replacement, but this method rapidly alleviates $T_4$ deficiency while minimizing the risk of exacerbating underlying coronary disease or heart failure. **Such rapid correction is warranted only in extremely ill patients. Vital signs and cardiac rhythm should be monitored carefully to detect early signs of exacerbation of heart disease. Hydrocortisone,** 50 mg IV q8h, is usually recommended during rapid replacement of thyroid hormone.

## Hyperthyroidism

I. **Etiology. Graves' disease** (*N Engl J Med* 343:1236, 2000) causes most cases of hyperthyroidism, especially in young patients. This autoimmune disorder may also cause **proptosis** (exophthalmos) and pretibial myxedema, neither of which is found in other causes of hyperthyroidism. **Toxic multinodular goiter** (MNG) is a common cause of hyperthyroidism in older patients. Unusual causes include **iodine-induced hyperthyroidism** (usually precipitated by drugs such as **amiodarone** or radiographic contrast media), thyroid adenomas, subacute thyroiditis (painful tender goiter with transient hyperthyroidism), painless thyroiditis (nontender goiter with transient hyperthyroidism, most often seen in the postpartum period), and surreptitious ingestion of thyroid hormone. TSH-induced hyperthyroidism is extremely rare.

II. **Clinical findings.** Symptoms include heat intolerance, weight loss, weakness, palpitations, oligomenorrhea, and anxiety. Signs include brisk tendon reflexes, fine tremor, proximal weakness, stare, and eyelid lag. Cardiac abnormalities may be prominent, including sinus tachycardia, atrial fibrillation, and exacerbation of coronary artery disease or heart failure. **In the elderly,** hyperthyroidism may present with only atrial fibrillation, heart failure, weakness, or weight loss, and a high index of suspicion is needed to make the diagnosis.

III. **Diagnosis.** Hyperthyroidism should be suspected in any patient with compatible symptoms, as it is a readily treatable disorder that may become very debilitating.

A. **Plasma TSH is the best initial diagnostic test, as a TSH level greater than 0.1 μU/ml excludes clinical hyperthyroidism.** If plasma TSH is less than 0.1 μU/ml, **plasma free $T_4$** should be measured to determine the severity of hyperthyroidism and as a baseline for therapy. If plasma free $T_4$ is elevated, the diagnosis of clinical hyperthyroidism is established.

B. **If plasma TSH is less than 0.1 μU/ml but free $T_4$ is normal,** the patient may have clinical hyperthyroidism due to **elevation of plasma $T_3$ alone;** therefore, plasma $T_3$ should be measured in this case. Very **mild (or subclinical) hyperthyroidism** may lower TSH to less than 0.1 μU/ml, and therefore suppression of TSH alone does not confirm that symptoms are due to hyperthyroidism. TSH may also be suppressed by **severe nonthyroidal illness** (see Evaluation of Suspected Thyroid Disease, sec. **V**). A **third-generation TSH assay** with a detection limit of 0.02 μU/ml may be helpful in patients with suppressed TSH and nonthyroidal illness. Most patients with clinical hyper-

**Table 22-2.** Differential diagnosis of hyperthyroidism

| Signs | Diagnosis |
|---|---|
| Diffuse, nontender goiter | Graves' disease or painless thyroiditis |
| Multiple thyroid nodules | Toxic multinodular goiter |
| Single thyroid nodule | Thyroid adenoma |
| Tender painful goiter | Subacute thyroiditis |
| Normal thyroid gland | Graves' disease, painless thyroiditis, or factitious hyperthyroidism |

thyroidism have plasma TSH levels that are less than 0.02 μU/ml in such assays, whereas nonthyroidal illness rarely suppresses TSH to this degree (*Endocrinol Metab Clin North Am* 30:245, 2001).

**C. Differential diagnosis** (Table 22-2). The etiology of hyperthyroidism affects the choice of therapy. Differentiating features include (1) the presence of **proptosis** or pretibial myxedema, seen in Graves' disease (although many patients with Graves' disease lack these signs); (2) a **diffuse nontender goiter** on palpation of the thyroid, consistent with Graves' disease or painless thyroiditis; or (3) a history of recent **pregnancy, neck pain, or iodine administration,** suggesting causes other than Graves' disease. In rare cases, **24-hour radioactive iodine uptake (RAIU)** is needed to distinguish Graves' disease or toxic MNG (in which RAIU is elevated) from postpartum thyroiditis, iodine-induced hyperthyroidism, or factitious hyperthyroidism (in which RAIU is very low). **Thyroid imaging with ultrasound or radionuclide scan is not useful in diagnosing hyperthyroidism.**

**IV. Therapy.** Some forms of hyperthyroidism (subacute or postpartum thyroiditis) are transient and require only symptomatic therapy. Three methods are available for definitive therapy (none of which controls hyperthyroidism rapidly): RAI, thionamides, and subtotal thyroidectomy. **During treatment, patients are followed by clinical evaluation and measurement of plasma free $T_4$.** Plasma TSH is useless in assessing the initial response to therapy, as it remains suppressed until after the patient becomes euthyroid. Regardless of the therapy used, all patients with Graves' disease require lifelong follow-up for recurrent hyperthyroidism or development of hypothyroidism. Patients with symptomatic Graves' eye disease should be managed in consultation with an ophthalmologist.

**A. Symptomatic therapy.** A **β-adrenergic antagonist** (such as **atenolol,** 25–100 mg qd) is used to relieve symptoms of hyperthyroidism, such as palpitations, tremor, and anxiety, until hyperthyroidism is controlled by definitive therapy or until transient forms of hyperthyroidism subside. The dose is adjusted to alleviate symptoms and tachycardia, then reduced gradually as hyperthyroidism is controlled. Verapamil at an initial dose of 40–80 mg PO tid can be used to control tachycardia in patients with contraindications to β-adrenergic antagonists.

**B. Choice of definitive therapy**

1. **In Graves' disease, RAI therapy is the treatment of choice for almost all patients.** It is simple and highly effective, but **cannot be used in pregnancy. Propylthiouracil (PTU) should be used to treat hyperthyroidism in pregnancy.** Long-term control of Graves' disease with thionamides is achieved in fewer than one-half of patients, and they carry a small risk of life-threatening side effects (see sec. **IV.D.3**). Thyroidectomy should be used only in patients who refuse RAI therapy and who relapse or develop side effects with thionamide therapy.
2. **Other causes of hyperthyroidism.** Toxic MNG and toxic adenoma should be treated with RAI (except in pregnancy). Transient forms of

hyperthyroidism due to thyroiditis should be treated symptomatically with atenolol. Iodine-induced hyperthyroidism is treated with thionamides and atenolol until the patient is euthyroid. Although treatment of some patients with amiodarone-induced hyperthyroidism with glucocorticoids has been advocated, **nearly all patients with amiodarone-induced hyperthyroidism respond well to thionamide therapy** (*Circulation* 105:1275, 2002).

**C. RAI therapy.** A single dose permanently controls hyperthyroidism in 90% of patients, and further doses can be given if necessary. A **pregnancy test** is done immediately before therapy in potentially fertile women. A 24-hour RAIU is usually measured and used to calculate the dose. Thionamides interfere with RAI therapy and should be stopped at least 3 days before treatment. If iodine treatment has been given, it should be stopped at least 2 weeks before RAI therapy. Most patients with Graves' disease are treated with 8–10 mCi, although treatment for toxic MNG requires higher doses.

1. **Follow-up.** Usually, several months are needed to restore euthyroidism. Patients are evaluated at 4- to 6-week intervals, with assessment of clinical findings and plasma free $T_4$.
   a. **If thyroid function stabilizes within the normal range,** the interval between follow-up visits is increased gradually to annual intervals.
   b. **If symptomatic hypothyroidism develops,** $T_4$ therapy is started (see Hypothyroidism, sec. **IV**). Mild hypothyroidism after RAI therapy may be transient, and asymptomatic patients can be observed for a further 4–6 weeks to determine whether hypothyroidism will resolve spontaneously.
   c. **If symptomatic hyperthyroidism persists after 6 months, RAI treatment is repeated.**
2. **Side effects. Hypothyroidism** occurs in more than half of patients within the first year and continues to develop at a rate of approximately 3%/year thereafter. Because of the release of stored hormone, a slight rise in plasma $T_4$ may occur in the first 2 weeks after therapy. This development is important only in **patients with severe cardiac disease,** which may worsen as a result. Such patients should be treated with thionamides to restore euthyroidism and to deplete stored hormone before treatment with RAI. No convincing evidence has been found that RAI has a clinically important effect on the course of Graves' eye disease. It does not increase the risk of malignancy. No increase in congenital abnormalities has been found in the offspring of women who conceive after RAI therapy, and the radiation exposure to the ovaries is low, comparable to that from common diagnostic radiographs. Concern for potential teratogenic effects should not influence physicians' advice to patients.

**D. Thionamides.** Methimazole and PTU inhibit thyroid hormone synthesis. PTU also inhibits extrathyroidal conversion of $T_4$ to $T_3$. Once thyroid hormone stores are depleted (after several weeks to months), $T_4$ levels decrease. These drugs have no permanent effect on thyroid function. **In the majority of patients with Graves' disease, hyperthyroidism recurs within 6 months after therapy is stopped.** Spontaneous remission of Graves' disease occurs in approximately one-third of patients during thionamide therapy and, in this minority, no other treatment may be needed. Remission is more likely in mild, recent-onset hyperthyroidism and if the goiter is small.

1. **Initiation of therapy.** Before starting therapy, patients must be warned of side effects and precautions. Usual starting doses are PTU, 100–200 mg PO tid, or methimazole, 10–40 mg PO qd; higher initial doses can be used in severe hyperthyroidism.
2. **Follow-up.** Restoration of euthyroidism takes up to several months. Patients are evaluated at 4-week intervals with assessment of clinical findings and plasma free $T_4$. If plasma free $T_4$ levels do not fall after 4–8

weeks, the dose should be increased. Doses as high as PTU, 300 mg PO qid, or methimazole, 60 mg PO qd, may be required. Once the plasma free $T_4$ level falls to normal, the dose is adjusted to maintain plasma free $T_4$ within the normal range. No consensus exists on the optimal duration of therapy, but periods of 6 months to 2 years are used most commonly. Patients must be monitored carefully for recurrence of hyperthyroidism after the drug is stopped.

3. **Side effects** are most likely to occur within the first few months of therapy. Minor side effects include rash, urticaria, fever, arthralgias, and transient leukopenia. **Agranulocytosis** occurs in 0.3% of patients treated with thionamides. Other life-threatening side effects include **hepatitis,** vasculitis, and drug-induced lupus erythematosus. These complications usually resolve if the drug is stopped promptly. **Patients must be warned to stop the drug immediately if jaundice or symptoms suggestive of agranulocytosis develop (e.g., fever, chills, sore throat)** and to contact their physician promptly for evaluation. Routine monitoring of the WBC is not useful for detecting agranulocytosis, which develops suddenly.

E. **Subtotal thyroidectomy.** This procedure provides long-term control of hyperthyroidism in most patients.
   1. Surgery may trigger a perioperative exacerbation of hyperthyroidism, and patients should be prepared for surgery by one of two methods:
      a. **A thionamide** is given until the patient is nearly euthyroid (see sec. **IV.D**). **Supersaturated potassium iodide (SSKI),** 40–80 mg (1–2 drops) PO bid, is then added 1–2 weeks before surgery. Both drugs are stopped postoperatively.
      b. **Atenolol** (50–100 mg qd) is started 1–2 weeks before surgery. The dose of atenolol is increased, if necessary, to reduce the resting heart rate below 90 beats/minute and is continued for 5–7 days postoperatively. SSKI is dosed as above.
   2. **Follow-up.** Clinical findings and plasma free $T_4$ and TSH should be assessed 4–6 weeks after surgery. If thyroid function is normal, the patient is seen at 3 and 6 months, then annually. If symptomatic hypothyroidism develops, $T_4$ therapy is started (see Hypothyroidism, sec. **IV**). Mild hypothyroidism after subtotal thyroidectomy may be transient, and asymptomatic patients can be observed for a further 4–6 weeks to determine whether hypothyroidism will resolve spontaneously. Hyperthyroidism persists or recurs in 3–7% of patients.
   3. **Complications** of thyroidectomy include **hypothyroidism** in 30–50% of patients and **hypoparathyroidism** in 3%. Rare complications include permanent vocal cord paralysis, due to recurrent laryngeal nerve injury, and perioperative death. The complication rate appears to depend on the experience of the surgeon.

F. **Mild (or subclinical) hyperthyroidism** is present when the plasma TSH is suppressed to less than 0.1 μU/ml but the patient has no symptoms that are definitely caused by hyperthyroidism, and plasma levels of free $T_4$ and $T_3$ are normal (*N Engl J Med* 345:512, 2001). Subclinical hyperthyroidism increases the risk of **atrial fibrillation** in the elderly and those with heart disease and predisposes to **osteoporosis** in postmenopausal women; it should be treated in these groups of patients (see sec. **IV.C**). Asymptomatic young patients with mild Graves' disease can be observed for spontaneous resolution of hyperthyroidism or the development of symptoms or increasing free $T_4$ levels that warrant treatment.

G. **Urgent therapy** is warranted when hyperthyroidism exacerbates heart failure or coronary artery disease and in rare patients with severe hyperthyroidism complicated by fever and delirium. Concomitant diseases should be treated intensively, and confirmatory tests should be obtained before therapy is started, including serum TSH and free $T_4$.
   1. **PTU, 300 mg PO q6h,** should be started immediately.

2. **Iodide (SSKI, 1–2 drops PO q12h)** should be started approximately 2 hours after the first dose of PTU, to inhibit thyroid hormone secretion rapidly.
3. **Propranolol,** 40 mg PO q6h (or an equivalent dose IV), should be given to patients with angina or myocardial infarction, and the dose should be adjusted to prevent tachycardia. Propranolol may benefit some patients with heart failure and marked tachycardia but can further impair left ventricular systolic function. In patients with clinical heart failure, it should be given only with careful monitoring of left ventricular function.
4. Plasma free $T_4$ is measured every 3–7 days, and the doses of PTU and iodine gradually are decreased when free $T_4$ approaches the normal range. RAI therapy should be scheduled 2 weeks after iodine is stopped (see sec. **IV.C**).

**H. Hyperthyroidism in pregnancy.** If hyperthyroidism is suspected, plasma TSH should be measured. Plasma TSH declines in early pregnancy, but rarely to less than 0.1 μU/ml. If TSH is less than 0.1 μU/ml, the diagnosis should be confirmed by measurement of plasma free $T_4$. RAI is contraindicated in pregnancy, and therefore patients should be treated with PTU (see sec. **IV.D**). The dose should be adjusted at 4-week intervals to maintain the plasma free $T_4$ near the upper limit of the normal range. The dose required often decreases in the later stages of pregnancy. Atenolol, 25–50 mg PO qd, can be used to relieve symptoms while awaiting the effects of PTU. The fetus and neonate should be monitored carefully for hyperthyroidism.

## Euthyroid Goiter

The diagnosis of euthyroid goiter is based on palpation of the thyroid and evaluation of thyroid function. If the thyroid is enlarged, the examiner should determine whether the enlargement is diffuse, multinodular, or whether a single palpable nodule is present. All three forms of euthyroid goiter are common, especially in women. Imaging studies, such as thyroid scans or ultrasonography, provide no useful additional information about goiters that are diffuse or multinodular by palpation and should not be performed in these patients. Furthermore, 20–50% of people have nonpalpable thyroid nodules that are detectable by ultrasound. These nodules rarely have any clinical importance, and their incidental discovery may lead to unnecessary diagnostic testing and treatment (*Endocrinol Metab Clin North Am* 29:187, 2000).

**I. Diffuse goiter.** Almost all euthyroid diffuse goiters in the United States are due to **chronic lymphocytic thyroiditis (Hashimoto's thyroiditis)** (*N Engl J Med* 348:2646, 2003). Because Hashimoto's thyroiditis may also cause hypothyroidism, plasma TSH should be measured even in patients who are clinically euthyroid. Small diffuse goiters usually are asymptomatic, and therapy is seldom required. Symptomatic diffuse goiters may shrink with suppression of plasma TSH to the lower part of the normal range by $T_4$ therapy. If $T_4$ is not given, the patient should be monitored regularly for the development of hypothyroidism.

**II. MNG** is common in older patients, especially women. Most patients are asymptomatic and require no treatment. In a few individuals, **hyperthyroidism** (toxic MNG) develops (see Hyperthyroidism, sec. **I**). In rare patients, the gland compresses the trachea or esophagus, causing dyspnea or dysphagia, and treatment is required. $T_4$ treatment has little, if any, effect on the size of MNGs. RAI therapy reduces gland size and relieves symptoms in most patients. Subtotal thyroidectomy can also be used to relieve compressive symptoms. The risk of malignancy in MNG is low, comparable to the frequency of incidental thyroid carcinoma in clinically normal glands. Evaluation for thyroid carcinoma with needle biopsy is warranted only if one nodule is disproportionately enlarged.

**III. Single thyroid nodules** are usually benign, but a small number are thyroid carcinomas (*Lancet* 361:501, 2003). Clinical findings that increase the likelihood of carcinoma include the presence of cervical lymphadenopathy, a history of radiation to the head or neck in childhood, and a family history of medullary thyroid carcinoma or multiple endocrine neoplasia syndromes type 2A or 2B. A hard fixed nodule, recent nodule growth, or hoarseness due to vocal cord paralysis also suggests malignancy. However, most patients with thyroid carcinomas have none of these risk factors, and nearly all **palpable single thyroid nodules should be evaluated with needle aspiration biopsy** (*Endocrinol Metab Clin North Am* 30:361, 2001). Patients with thyroid carcinoma should be managed in consultation with an endocrinologist. Nodules with benign cytology should be re-evaluated periodically by palpation. $T_4$ therapy has little or no effect on the size of single thyroid nodules and is not indicated (*Endocrinol Metab Clin North Am* 31:699, 2002). Radionuclide thyroid scans cannot distinguish benign from malignant nodules and should not be performed. The management of nonpalpable thyroid nodules discovered incidentally by ultrasound is controversial (*J Clin Endocrinol Metab* 87:1938, 2002).

## Adrenal Failure

**I. Etiology.** Adrenal failure may be due to disease of the adrenal glands (**primary adrenal failure, Addison's disease**), with deficiency of cortisol and aldosterone and elevated plasma adrenocorticotropic hormone (ACTH), or to ACTH deficiency caused by disorders of the pituitary or hypothalamus (**secondary adrenal failure**), with deficiency of cortisol alone.

**A. Primary adrenal failure** (*J Clin Endocrinol Metab* 86:2909, 2001) is most often due to **autoimmune adrenalitis,** which may be associated with other endocrine deficits (e.g., hypothyroidism). Infections of the adrenal gland such as **tuberculosis** and **histoplasmosis** also may cause adrenal failure. **Hemorrhagic adrenal infarction** may occur in the postoperative period, in coagulation disorders and hypercoagulable states, and in sepsis. Adrenal hemorrhage often causes abdominal or flank pain and fever; CT scan of the abdomen reveals high-density bilateral adrenal masses. Adrenoleukodystrophy causes adrenal failure in young males. Adrenal failure may develop in patients with AIDS, caused by disseminated cytomegalovirus, mycobacterial or fungal infection, or adrenal lymphoma. The drugs ketoconazole and etomidate inhibit steroid hormone synthesis and can cause adrenal failure.

**B. Secondary adrenal failure** is due most often to **glucocorticoid therapy;** ACTH suppression may persist for a year after therapy is stopped. Any disorder of the pituitary or hypothalamus can cause ACTH deficiency, but other evidence of these disorders is usually obvious.

**II. Clinical findings** in adrenal failure are nonspecific, and without a high index of suspicion, the diagnosis of this potentially lethal but readily treatable disease is easily missed. Symptoms include **anorexia, nausea, vomiting, weight loss, weakness, and fatigue. Orthostatic hypotension** and **hyponatremia** are common. Usually, symptoms are chronic, but **shock** may develop suddenly and is fatal unless promptly treated. Often, this adrenal crisis is triggered by illness, injury, or surgery. All these symptoms are due to cortisol deficiency and occur in primary and in secondary adrenal failure. **Hyperpigmentation** (due to marked ACTH excess) and **hyperkalemia** and **volume depletion** (due to aldosterone deficiency) occur only in primary adrenal failure.

**III. Diagnosis** (*Ann Intern Med* 139:194, 2003). Adrenal failure should be suspected in patients with hypotension, weight loss, hyponatremia, or hyperkalemia.

**A. The short cosyntropin (Cortrosyn) stimulation test** is used for diagnosis. Cosyntropin, 250 μg, is given IV or IM, and **plasma cortisol is measured 30**

**minutes later.** The normal response is a stimulated plasma cortisol greater than 20 μg/dl. This test detects primary and secondary adrenal failure, except within a few weeks of onset of pituitary dysfunction (e.g., shortly after pituitary surgery; see Anterior Pituitary Gland Dysfunction, sec. **III.A**).

**B. The distinction between primary and secondary adrenal failure** is usually clear. Hyperkalemia, hyperpigmentation, or other autoimmune endocrine deficits indicate primary adrenal failure, whereas deficits of other pituitary hormones, symptoms of a pituitary mass (e.g., headache, visual field loss), or known pituitary or hypothalamic disease indicate secondary adrenal failure. If the cause is unclear, the **plasma ACTH** level distinguishes primary adrenal failure (in which it is markedly elevated) from secondary adrenal failure. Most cases of primary adrenal failure are due to autoimmune adrenalitis, but other causes should be considered. Radiographic evidence of adrenal enlargement or calcification indicates that the cause is infection or hemorrhage. Patients with secondary adrenal failure should be tested for other pituitary hormone deficiencies and should be evaluated for a pituitary or hypothalamic tumor (see the Anterior Pituitary Gland Dysfunction section).

**IV. Therapy** (*JAMA* 287:236, 2002)

**A. Adrenal crisis** with hypotension must be treated immediately. Patients should be evaluated for an underlying illness that precipitated the crisis.

1. **If the diagnosis of adrenal failure is known, hydrocortisone, 100 mg IV q8h,** should be given, and **0.9% saline with 5% dextrose** should be infused rapidly until hypotension is corrected. The dose of hydrocortisone is decreased gradually over several days as symptoms and any precipitating illness resolve, then changed to oral maintenance therapy. Mineralocorticoid replacement is not needed until the dose of hydrocortisone is less than 100 mg/day.
2. **If the diagnosis of adrenal failure has not been established,** a single dose of **dexamethasone,** 10 mg IV, should be given, and a rapid infusion of 0.9% saline with 5% dextrose should be started. A **Cortrosyn stimulation test** should be performed (see sec. **III.A**). Dexamethasone is used because it does not interfere with measurement of plasma cortisol. After the 30-minute plasma cortisol measurement, hydrocortisone, 100 mg IV q8h, should be given until the test result is known.

**B. Maintenance therapy** in all patients with adrenal failure requires cortisol replacement with prednisone; most patients with primary adrenal failure also require replacement of aldosterone with fludrocortisone.

1. **Prednisone,** 5 mg PO every morning and 2.5 mg PO every evening, should be started. The dose is then adjusted, with the goal being the lowest dose that relieves the patient's symptoms, without causing osteoporosis and other signs of Cushing's syndrome. Most patients require doses between 4 mg PO qd and 5 mg PO bid. Concomitant therapy with rifampin, phenytoin, or phenobarbital accelerates glucocorticoid metabolism and increases the dose requirement (see Appendix C, Drug Interactions).
2. **During illness, injury, or the perioperative period, the dose of prednisone must be increased.** For minor illnesses, the patient should double the dose for 3 days. If the illness resolves, the maintenance dose is resumed. Vomiting requires immediate medical attention, with IV glucocorticoid therapy and IV fluid. Patients can be given a prefilled syringe of dexamethasone, 4 mg, to be self-administered IM for vomiting or severe illness if medical care is not immediately available. **For severe illness or injury,** hydrocortisone, 50 mg IV q8h, should be given, with the dose tapered as severity of illness wanes. The same regimen is used in **patients undergoing surgery,** with the first dose of hydrocortisone given preoperatively. The dose can be tapered to maintenance therapy by 2–3 days after uncomplicated surgery.
3. **In primary adrenal failure, fludrocortisone, 0.1 mg PO qd,** should be given, along with liberal salt intake. The dose is adjusted to maintain

BP (supine and standing) and serum potassium within the normal range; the usual dosage is 0.05–0.2 mg PO qd. **Patients should be educated in management of their disease,** including adjustment of prednisone dose during illness. They should wear a medical identification tag or bracelet.

## Cushing's Syndrome

Cushing's syndrome (the clinical effects of increased glucocorticoid hormone) is most often **iatrogenic,** due to therapy with glucocorticoid drugs. **ACTH-secreting pituitary microadenomas (Cushing's disease)** account for 80% of cases of endogenous Cushing's syndrome. **Adrenal tumors and ectopic ACTH secretion** account for the remainder.

I. **Clinical findings** include truncal obesity, rounded face, fat deposits in the supraclavicular fossae and over the posterior neck, hypertension, hirsutism, amenorrhea, and depression. More specific findings include thin skin, easy bruising, reddish striae, proximal muscle weakness, and osteoporosis. Diabetes mellitus develops in some patients. Hyperpigmentation or hypokalemic alkalosis suggests Cushing's syndrome due to ectopic ACTH secretion.

II. **Diagnosis** is based on increased cortisol excretion and lack of normal feedback inhibition of ACTH and cortisol secretion (*Ann Intern Med* 138:980, 2003).

   A. **The overnight dexamethasone suppression test** (1 mg dexamethasone given PO at 11:00 PM; plasma cortisol measured at 8:00 AM the next day; normal plasma cortisol level <2 μg/dl) or **24-hour urine cortisol** measurement can be done as a screening test. Both tests are very sensitive, and a normal value virtually excludes the diagnosis.

   B. **An abnormal screening test** indicates the need to perform a low-dose dexamethasone suppression test. Dexamethasone, 0.5 mg PO q6h, is given for 48 hours, and urine cortisol is measured during the last 24 hours. Failure to suppress urine cortisol to less than the normal reference range is diagnostic of Cushing's syndrome. Testing should not be done during severe illness or depression, which may cause false-positive results. Phenytoin therapy also causes a false-positive test by accelerating metabolism of dexamethasone. Random plasma cortisol levels are not useful for diagnosis, because the wide range of normal values overlaps those of Cushing's syndrome. After the diagnosis of Cushing's syndrome is made, tests to determine the cause are best done in consultation with an endocrinologist.

## Incidental Adrenal Nodules

Adrenal nodules are a common incidental finding on abdominal imaging studies. Most incidentally discovered nodules are benign adrenocortical tumors that do not secrete excess hormone, but the differential diagnosis includes adrenal adenomas causing Cushing's syndrome or primary hyperaldosteronism, pheochromocytoma, adrenocortical carcinoma, and metastatic cancer.

I. **Evaluation.** The imaging characteristics of the nodule may suggest a diagnosis but are not specific enough to obviate further evaluation (*Endocrinol Metab Clin North Am* 29:27, 2000).

   A. **In patients without a known malignancy elsewhere,** the diagnostic issues are whether a **syndrome of hormone excess** or an **adrenocortical carcinoma** is present. Patients should be evaluated for hypertension, symptoms suggestive of pheochromocytoma (episodic headache, palpitations, and sweating), and signs of Cushing's syndrome (see Cushing's Syndrome, sec. **I**). **Plasma potassium and dehydroepiandrosterone sulfate** should be measured, and an **overnight dexamethasone suppression test** should be performed. Pheochromocytoma should be tested for by either **plasma fractionated metanephrines** or **24-hour urine catecholamines and metanephrines** (*J Clin Endocrinol Metab* 88:553, 2003).

**B. Patients who have potentially resectable cancer elsewhere** and in whom an adrenal metastasis must be excluded may require needle biopsy of the nodule. **Pheochromocytoma should be excluded before biopsy.**

**II. Management** (*Ann Intern Med* 138:424, 2003). Patients with hypertension and hypokalemia should be evaluated for primary hyperaldosteronism in consultation with an endocrinologist. An abnormal overnight dexamethasone suppression test should be evaluated further (see Cushing's Syndrome, sec. **II.B**). If clinical or biochemical evidence of a pheochromocytoma is found, the nodule should be resected after appropriate α-adrenergic blockade with phenoxybenzamine. Elevation of plasma dehydroepiandrosterone sulfate or a large nodule suggests adrenocortical carcinoma. A policy of resecting all nodules greater than 4 cm in diameter appropriately treats the great majority of adrenal carcinomas while minimizing the number of benign nodules that are removed unnecessarily (*Endocrinol Metab Clin North Am* 29:159, 2000). Most incidental nodules are less than 4 cm in diameter, do not produce excess hormone, and do not require therapy. At least one **repeat imaging procedure** 3–6 months later is recommended to ensure that the nodule is not enlarging rapidly (which would suggest an adrenal carcinoma).

## Anterior Pituitary Gland Dysfunction

The anterior pituitary gland secretes **prolactin, growth hormone,** and four **trophic hormones:** corticotropin (ACTH), thyrotropin (TSH), and the gonadotropins, luteinizing hormone and follicle-stimulating hormone. Each trophic hormone stimulates a specific target gland. Anterior pituitary function is regulated by hypothalamic hormones that reach the pituitary via portal veins in the pituitary stalk. **The predominant effect of hypothalamic regulation is to stimulate secretion of pituitary hormones, except for prolactin,** which is inhibited by hypothalamic dopamine production. **Secretion of trophic hormones is also regulated by negative feedback** by their target gland hormone, and the normal pituitary response to target hormone deficiency is increased secretion of the appropriate trophic hormone.

**I. Anterior pituitary dysfunction** can be caused by disorders of either the pituitary or hypothalamus.

**A. Pituitary adenomas** are the most common pituitary disorder. They are classified by size and function. **Microadenomas** are less than 10 mm in diameter and cause clinical manifestations only if they produce excess hormone. They are too small to produce hypopituitarism or mass effects. **Macroadenomas** are greater than 10 mm in diameter and may produce any combination of pituitary hormone excess, hypopituitarism, and mass effects. **Secretory adenomas** produce prolactin, growth hormone, or ACTH. **Nonsecretory macroadenomas** may cause hypopituitarism or mass effects. **Nonsecretory microadenomas** are common incidental radiographic findings, seen in approximately 10% of the normal population, and do not require therapy (*Endocrinol Metab Clin North Am* 29:205, 2000).

**B. Other pituitary or hypothalamic disorders,** such as head trauma, pituitary surgery or radiation, and postpartum pituitary infarction (Sheehan's syndrome) may cause hypopituitarism. Other tumors of the pituitary or hypothalamus (e.g., craniopharyngioma, metastases), inflammatory disorders (e.g., sarcoidosis, histiocytosis X), and infections (e.g., tuberculosis) may cause hypopituitarism or mass effects.

**II. Clinical findings.** Pituitary and hypothalamic disorders may present in several ways.

**A.** In **hypopituitarism** (deficiency of one or more pituitary hormones), gonadotropin deficiency is most common, causing amenorrhea in women and androgen deficiency in men. Secondary hypothyroidism or adrenal failure rarely occurs alone. Secondary adrenal failure causes deficiency of cortisol but not of aldosterone; hyperkalemia and hyperpigmentation do not occur, although life-threatening adrenal crisis may develop.

**B. Hormone excess** is most commonly **hyperprolactinemia,** which can be due to a secretory adenoma or to nonsecretory lesions that damage the hypothalamus or pituitary stalk, resulting in loss of inhibition by hypothalamic dopamine. Growth hormone excess **(acromegaly)** and ACTH and cortisol excess **(Cushing's disease)** are caused by secretory adenomas.

**C. Mass effects** due to pressure on adjacent structures, such as the optic chiasm, include **headaches** and **loss of visual fields or acuity.** Hyperprolactinemia also may be due to mass effect. **Pituitary apoplexy** is sudden enlargement of a pituitary tumor due to hemorrhagic necrosis.

**D. Asymptomatic pituitary adenomas**

**1. If a microadenoma is found** on imaging done for another purpose, the patient should be evaluated for clinical evidence of hyperprolactinemia (see sec. **VI**), Cushing's disease (see the section Cushing's Syndrome), or acromegaly (see sec. **VII**). Plasma prolactin should be measured, and tests for acromegaly and Cushing's syndrome should be performed if symptoms or signs of these disorders are evident. If no pituitary hormone excess exists, therapy is not required. Whether such patients need repeat imaging is not established, but the risk of enlargement is clearly small (*Endocrinol Metab Clin North Am* 29:205, 2000).

**2. Incidental discovery of a macroadenoma** is unusual. Patients should be evaluated for hormone excess (see sec. **II.D.1**) and hypopituitarism (see sec. **III**). Most macroadenomas should be treated because they are likely to grow further.

**III. Diagnosis of hypopituitarism.** Hypopituitarism may be suspected in the presence of clinical signs of target hormone deficiency (e.g., hypothyroidism) or pituitary mass effects.

**A. Laboratory evaluation** for hypopituitarism begins with evaluation of **target hormone function,** including **plasma free $T_4$** and a **Cortrosyn stimulation test** (see Adrenal Failure, sec. **III.A**). If recent onset of secondary adrenal failure is suspected (within a few weeks of evaluation), the patient should be treated empirically with glucocorticoids (see Adrenal Failure, sec. **IV**) and should be tested later, because the Cortrosyn stimulation test cannot detect secondary adrenal failure of recent onset. In men, **plasma testosterone** should be measured. The best evaluation of gonadal function in women is the **menstrual history.**

**B. If a target hormone is deficient,** its trophic hormone is measured to determine whether target gland dysfunction is secondary to hypopituitarism. An elevated trophic hormone level indicates primary target gland dysfunction. In hypopituitarism, trophic hormone levels are not elevated and are usually within (not below) the reference range. Thus, **pituitary trophic hormone levels can be interpreted only with knowledge of target hormone levels,** and **measurement of trophic hormone levels alone is useless in the diagnosis of hypopituitarism.** If pituitary disease is obvious, target hormone deficiencies may be assumed to be secondary and trophic hormones need not be measured.

**IV. Anatomic evaluation of the pituitary gland and hypothalamus is done best by MRI.** However, hyperprolactinemia and Cushing's disease may be caused by

**Table 22-3.** Major causes of hyperprolactinemia

| |
|---|
| Pregnancy and lactation |
| Prolactin-secreting pituitary adenoma (prolactinoma) |
| Idiopathic hyperprolactinemia |
| Drugs |
| Dopamine antagonists (phenothiazines, metoclopramide, risperidone) |
| Others (verapamil, cimetidine, some antidepressants) |
| Interference with synthesis or transport of hypothalamic dopamine |
| Hypothalamic lesions |
| Nonsecretory pituitary macroadenomas |
| Primary hypothyroidism |
| Chronic renal failure |

microadenomas that are too small to be seen with current techniques. The prevalence of incidental microadenomas should be kept in mind when interpreting MRIs (see sec. **I.A**). Visual acuity and **visual fields** should be tested when imaging suggests compression of the optic chiasm.

**V. Treatment of hypopituitarism.** Deficient target hormones should be replaced. Secondary adrenal failure should be treated immediately, especially if patients are to undergo surgery (see Adrenal Failure, sec. **IV.B**). Treatment of secondary hypothyroidism should be monitored by measurement of **plasma free $T_4$** (see Hypothyroidism, sec. **IV.B.2**). Infertility due to gonadotropin deficiency may be correctable, and patients who wish to conceive should be referred to an endocrinologist. Treatment of growth hormone deficiency in adults has been advocated by some, but the benefits and cost-effectiveness of this therapy are not established (*Ann Intern Med* 137:190, 2002). Treatment of pituitary macroadenomas generally requires transsphenoidal surgical resection, except for prolactin-secreting tumors (see sec. **VI.C.2**).

**VI. Hyperprolactinemia** (*Endocrinol Metab Clin North Am* 30:585, 2001). In women, the most common causes of pathologic hyperprolactinemia are prolactin-secreting pituitary **microadenomas** and **idiopathic hyperprolactinemia** (Table 22-3). In men, the most common cause is a prolactin-secreting **macroadenoma.** Hypothalamic or pituitary lesions that cause deficiency of other pituitary hormones often cause hyperprolactinemia. **Medications** are an important cause in men and in women.

**A. Clinical findings.** In women, hyperprolactinemia causes **amenorrhea** or irregular menses and **infertility.** Only approximately one-half of these women have **galactorrhea.** Prolonged estrogen deficiency increases the risk of **osteoporosis.** In men, hyperprolactinemia causes **androgen deficiency** and **infertility** but not gynecomastia; **mass effects and hypopituitarism** are common.

**B. Diagnosis. Hyperprolactinemia is common in young women,** and plasma **prolactin should be measured in women with amenorrhea,** whether or not galactorrhea is present. Mild elevations should be confirmed by repeat measurements. The history should include medications and symptoms of pituitary mass effects (see sec. **II.C**) or hypothyroidism. Laboratory evaluation should include **plasma TSH** and a **pregnancy test** in women. Prolactin levels of greater than 200 ng/ml occur only in prolactinomas, and levels between 100 and 200 ng/ml strongly suggest this diagnosis. Levels lower than 100 ng/ml may be due to any cause except prolactin-secreting macroadenoma, and such levels in a patient with a large pituitary mass suggest that it is not a prolactinoma. Testing for hypopituitarism (see sec. **III**) is needed only in patients with a macroadenoma or hypothalamic lesion. **Pituitary imaging** should be performed in most cases, as large nonfunctional pituitary or hypothalamic tumors may present with hyperprolactinemia.

**C. Therapy**

1. **Microadenomas and idiopathic hyperprolactinemia.** Most patients are treated because of **infertility** or to prevent **estrogen deficiency and osteoporosis.** Some women may be observed without therapy by periodic follow-up of prolactin levels and symptoms. In most patients, hyperprolactinemia does not worsen, and prolactin levels sometimes return to normal. Enlargement of microadenomas is rare.
   a. The **dopamine agonists bromocriptine** and **cabergoline** suppress plasma prolactin and restore normal menses and fertility in most women. Initial dosages are bromocriptine, 1.25–2.5 mg PO qhs with a snack, or cabergoline, 0.25 mg twice a week. Plasma prolactin levels are initially obtained at 2- to 4-week intervals, and doses are adjusted until the lowest dose required to maintain prolactin in the normal range is reached. Maximally effective doses are 2.5 mg bromocriptine tid and 1.5 mg cabergoline twice a week. Initially, patients should use barrier contraception, as fertility may be restored quickly. **Side effects** include **nausea** and **orthostatic hypotension,** which can be minimized by increasing the dose gradually, and usually resolve with continued therapy. Side effects are less severe with cabergoline.
   b. **Women who want to become pregnant** should be managed in consultation with an endocrinologist.
   c. **Women who do not want to become pregnant** should be followed with clinical evaluation and plasma prolactin levels every 6–12 months. Every 2 years, plasma prolactin should be measured after bromocriptine has been withdrawn for several weeks, to determine whether the drug is still needed. Follow-up imaging studies are not warranted unless prolactin levels increase substantially.
   d. Transsphenoidal resection of prolactin-secreting microadenomas is used only in the rare patient who does not respond to or cannot tolerate dopamine agonists. Prolactin levels usually return to normal, but up to one-half of patients experience relapse.
2. **Prolactin-secreting macroadenomas** should be treated with a dopamine agonist (see sec. **VI.C.1.a**), which usually suppresses prolactin levels to normal, reduces tumor size, and improves or corrects abnormal visual fields in 90% of cases. If mass effects are present, the dose should be increased to maximally effective levels over a period of several weeks. Visual field tests, if initially abnormal, should be repeated 4–6 weeks after therapy is started. Pituitary imaging should be repeated 3–6 months after initiation of therapy. If tumor shrinkage and correction of visual abnormalities are satisfactory, therapy can be continued indefinitely, with periodic monitoring of plasma prolactin levels. The full effect on tumor size may take more than 6 months. Further pituitary imaging is probably not warranted unless prolactin levels rise despite therapy.
   a. **Transsphenoidal surgery** is indicated to relieve mass effects and to prevent further tumor growth if the tumor does not shrink or if visual field abnormalities persist during dopamine agonist therapy. However, the likelihood of surgical cure of hyperprolactinemia due to a macroadenoma is low, and most patients require further therapy with a dopamine agonist.
   b. **Women with prolactin-secreting macroadenomas should not become pregnant** unless the tumor has been resected surgically, as the risk of symptomatic enlargement during pregnancy is 15–35%. Barrier contraception is essential during dopamine agonist treatment.

**VII. Acromegaly** (*Endocrinol Metab Clin North Am* 30:565, 2001) is the syndrome caused by growth hormone excess in adults and is due to a growth hormone–secreting pituitary adenoma in the vast majority of cases. Clinical findings include thickened skin and enlargement of hands, feet, jaw, and forehead. Arthritis or carpal tunnel syndrome may develop, and the pituitary adenoma may cause headaches and vision loss. Mortality from cardiovascular disease is increased.

**A. Diagnosis. Plasma insulin-like growth factor I (IGF-1),** which mediates most effects of growth hormone, is the best diagnostic test. Marked elevations establish the diagnosis. If IGF-1 levels are only moderately elevated, the diagnosis can be confirmed by giving 75 mg glucose orally and measuring serum growth hormone q30min for 2 hours. Failure to suppress growth hormone to less than 2 ng/ml confirms the diagnosis of acromegaly. Once the diagnosis is made, the pituitary should be imaged.

**B. Therapy.** The treatment of choice is transsphenoidal resection of the pituitary adenoma. Most patients have macroadenomas, and complete tumor resection with cure of acromegaly often is impossible. If IGF-1 levels remain elevated after surgery, radiotherapy is used to prevent regrowth of the tumor and to control acromegaly.

1. The somatostatin analog **octreotide** in depot form can be used to suppress growth hormone secretion while the effect of radiation is being awaited. A dose of 10–30 mg IM monthly suppresses IGF-1 to normal in most patients (*J Clin Endocrinol Metab* 87:3013, 2002). Side effects include cholelithiasis, diarrhea, and mild abdominal discomfort.
2. **Pegvisomant** is a growth hormone antagonist that lowers IGF-1 to normal in almost all patients (*Lancet* 358:1754, 2001). The dosage is 10–30 mg SC qd. Few side effects have been reported, but patients should be monitored for pituitary adenoma enlargement and transaminase elevation.

## Metabolic Bone Disease

**I. Osteomalacia** is characterized by defective mineralization of osteoid. Bone biopsy reveals increased thickness of osteoid seams and decreased mineralization rate, assessed by tetracycline labeling. **Causes of osteomalacia** include (1) vitamin D deficiency (most common in the house-bound elderly); (2) **malabsorption** of vitamin D and calcium due to intestinal, hepatic, or biliary disease; (3) disorders of vitamin D metabolism (e.g., renal disease, vitamin D–dependent rickets); (4) vitamin D resistance; (5) chronic hypophosphatemia; (6) renal tubular acidosis; (7) hypophosphatasia; and (8) therapy with anticonvulsants, fluoride, etidronate, or aluminum compounds.

**A. Clinical manifestations** include diffuse skeletal pain, proximal muscle weakness, waddling gait, and propensity to fractures. Radiographic findings include osteopenia and radiolucent bands perpendicular to bone surfaces (pseudofractures or Looser's zones). Serum alkaline phosphatase is elevated. Serum phosphorus, calcium, or both may be decreased.

**B. Diagnosis.** Osteomalacia should be suspected in a patient with osteopenia, elevated serum alkaline phosphatase, and either hypophosphatemia or hypocalcemia. **Serum 25-hydroxyvitamin D** [25(OH)D] levels may be low, establishing the diagnosis of vitamin D deficiency or malabsorption. Radiography of the chest, pelvis, and hips may reveal characteristic pseudofractures. If neither serum 25(OH)D nor radiography is diagnostic, a bone biopsy may be required for diagnosis.

**C. Treatment**

1. **Dietary vitamin D deficiency** can initially be treated with vitamin D, 50,000 IU PO weekly for several weeks, to replete body stores, followed

by long-term therapy with 400–1000 IU/day. Preparations include calcium supplements that contain vitamin D (Os-Cal + D, 125 IU/250- or 500-mg tablet), many multivitamins (400 IU/tablet), and vitamin D drops (200 IU/drop or 8000 IU/ml).

2. **Malabsorption of vitamin D** may require therapy with high doses, ranging from 50,000 IU PO/week to 50,000 IU PO qd. The dose should be adjusted to maintain serum 25(OH)D levels within the normal range. Calcitriol, 0.5–2.0 μg PO qd, can also be used. Calcium supplements, 1 g PO qd–tid, may also be required. Serum 25(OH)D, serum calcium, and 24-hour urine calcium should be monitored every 3–6 months to avoid hypercalcemia or hypercalciuria. If the underlying disease responds to therapy, the dose of vitamin D must be reduced accordingly.

II. **Paget's disease** of bone (*J Bone Miner Res* 16:1379, 2001) is a focal skeletal disorder characterized by rapid, disorganized bone remodeling. It usually occurs after age 40 and most often affects the pelvis, femur, spine, and skull. Clinical manifestations include bone pain and deformity, degenerative arthritis, pathologic fractures, neurologic deficits due to nerve root or cranial nerve compression (including deafness), and, rarely, high-output heart failure and osteogenic sarcoma. Most patients are asymptomatic, with disease discovered incidentally because of elevated serum alkaline phosphatase or an x-ray taken for other reasons.

A. **Diagnosis.** The radiographic appearance is usually diagnostic, and biopsy is rarely necessary. Serum alkaline phosphatase is elevated, reflecting the activity and extent of disease. Serum and urine calcium are usually normal but may increase with immobilization, as after a fracture.

B. **Management**

1. **Indications for therapy** include (1) bone pain due to Paget's disease, (2) nerve compression syndromes, (3) pathologic fracture, (4) elective skeletal surgery, (5) progressive skeletal deformity, (6) immobilization hypercalcemia, (7) hypercalciuria with nephrolithiasis, (8) high-output heart failure, and (9) asymptomatic involvement of weight-bearing bones or the skull.

2. **Bisphosphonates** inhibit excessive bone resorption, relieve symptoms, and restore serum alkaline phosphatase and bone deposition to normal in most patients. The effectiveness of therapy is monitored by measuring serum alkaline phosphatase. Patients are treated with a course of therapy with **alendronate,** 40 mg/day for 6 months, or **risedronate,** 30 mg/day for 2–3 months. Serum alkaline phosphatase is monitored every 3 months. Therapy can be repeated when serum alkaline phosphatase rises above normal.

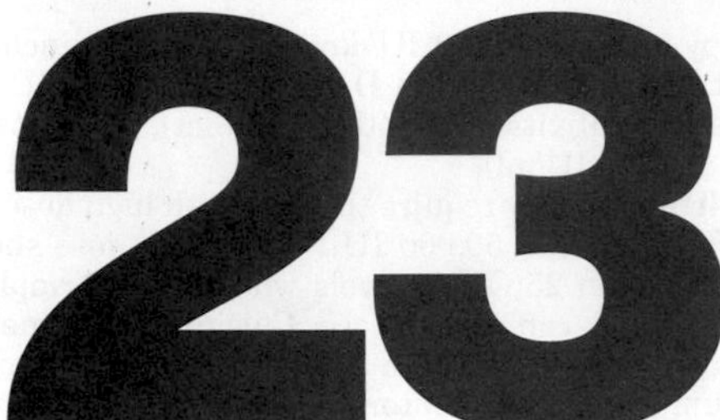

# Arthritis and Rheumatologic Diseases

Leslie E. Kahl

## Therapeutic Approaches to Rheumatic Disease

The etiology of most rheumatologic disorders is unknown. Therapeutic approaches in rheumatology are, therefore, largely palliative. Such approaches involve either local or systemic administration of analgesic, anti-inflammatory, immunomodulatory, or immunosuppressive drugs. Because the same procedures and medications are used for most of the rheumatologic disorders, they are discussed as a group rather than separately under each disorder.

**I. Joint aspiration and injection**

**A. Indications.** Joint aspiration should be performed (1) when an effusion is present in a single joint and its etiology is unclear, (2) for symptomatic relief in a patient with a known arthritis diagnosis, and (3) to monitor the response to therapy in patients with infectious arthritis. Analysis of synovial fluid should include a cell count, microscopic examination for crystals, Gram stain, and culture. Intra-articular glucocorticoid therapy can be used to suppress inflammation when only one or a few peripheral joints are inflamed and infection has been excluded. The joint should be aspirated to remove as much fluid as possible before glucocorticoid injection.

**B. Contraindications. Infection overlying the site to be injected is an absolute contraindication;** significant hemostatic defects and bacteremia are relative contraindications to joint aspiration and injection.

**C. Technique.** The site of aspiration should be cleansed with povidone-iodine solution. Topical ethylchloride spray can be used as a local anesthetic. The site can also be infiltrated with local anesthetic in preparation for the procedure, particularly if there is little or no joint effusion or if there is notable joint space narrowing.

1. **Knee** (Fig. 23-1). The leg should be positioned by gently flexing the knee 10–15 degrees. A rolled towel can be placed in the popliteal fossa to support the knee and allow the quadriceps to relax. The joint is then entered either medially or laterally, immediately beneath the undersurface of the patella.
2. **Ankle** (Fig. 23-2). Aspiration should be performed with the patient supine and the foot perpendicular to the leg. Medial aspiration is performed immediately medial to the extensor hallucis longus tendon, which can be identified by alternately flexing and extending the great toe. A lateral approach can also be used by introducing the needle just distal to the fibula.
3. **Wrist** (Fig. 23-3). Aspiration is performed on the dorsum of the wrist between the distal radius and carpus with the wrist joint flexed slightly. The point of entry for lateral aspiration is just distal to the end of the radius, between the extensor tendons of the thumb. Medial aspiration can also be performed between the distal ulna and the carpus.

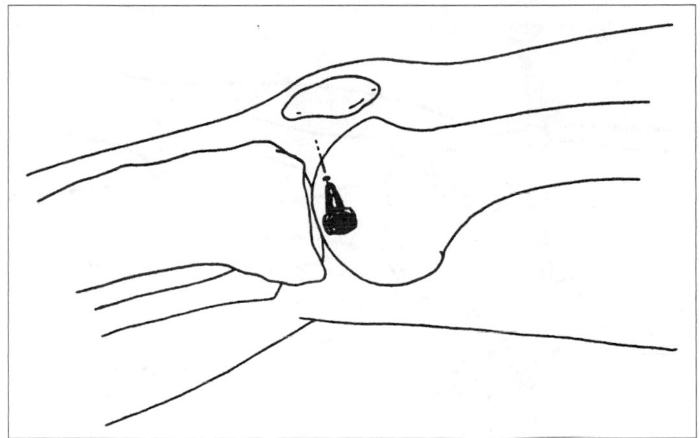

**Fig. 23-1.** Arthrocentesis of the knee: medial approach. [Reproduced with permission from JR Beary III, CL Christian, NA Johanson (eds). *Manual of Rheumatology and Outpatient Orthopedic Disorders* (2nd ed). Boston: Little, Brown, 1987.]

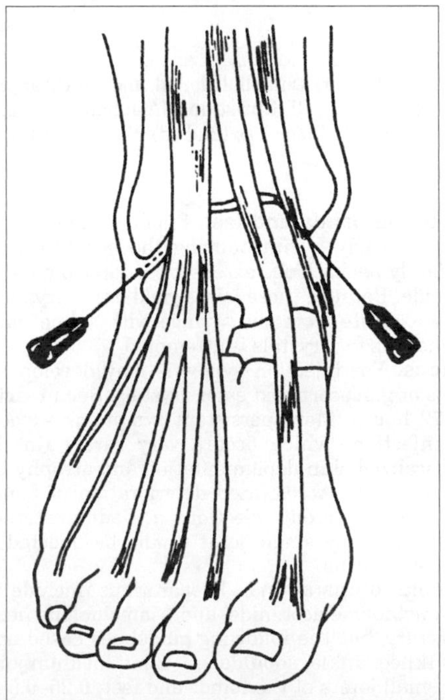

**Fig. 23-2.** Arthrocentesis of the ankle: medial and lateral approaches. [Reproduced with permission from JR Beary III, CL Christian, NA Johanson (eds). *Manual of Rheumatology and Outpatient Orthopedic Disorders* (2nd ed). Boston: Little, Brown, 1987.]

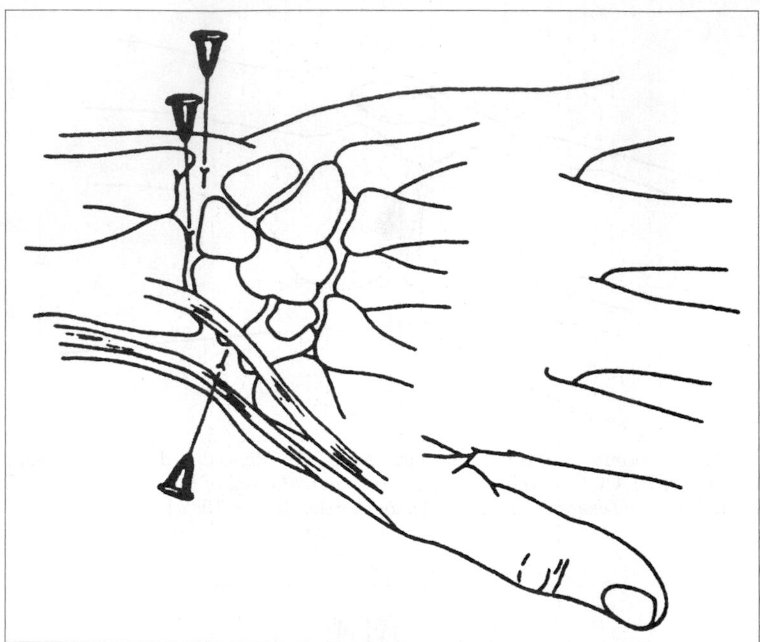

**Fig. 23-3.** Arthrocentesis of the wrist: medial, dorsal, and lateral approaches. [Reproduced with permission from JR Beary III, CL Christian, NA Johanson (eds). *Manual of Rheumatology and Outpatient Orthopedic Disorders* (2nd ed). Boston: Little, Brown, 1987.]

4. **Joints of the hands and feet.** Small joints of the hands and feet are entered similarly by introducing the needle from the dorsal surface immediately beneath the extensor tendon from either the medial or the lateral side. Because these joints yield only very small amounts of fluid, flushing aspirate from the syringe with saline may increase the yield when analysis for crystals is attempted.

D. **Complications.** Postinjection synovitis may develop rarely as a result of phagocytosis of glucocorticoid ester crystals. Such reactions usually resolve within 48–72 hours. More persistent symptoms suggest the possibility of iatrogenic infection, which occurs very rarely (in fewer than 0.1% of patients). Localized skin depigmentation and atrophy may result after glucocorticoid injection. Accelerated deterioration of bone and cartilage also may occur when frequent injections are administered over an extended period. Therefore, any single joint should be injected no more frequently than every 3–6 months.

E. **Glucocorticoid preparations.** Preparations include methylprednisolone acetate, triamcinolone acetonide, and triamcinolone hexacetonide. The dose used is arbitrary, but the following guidelines based on volume are useful: large joints (knee, ankle, shoulder), 1–2 ml; medium joints (wrists, elbows), 0.5–1.0 ml; small joints of the hands and feet, 0.25–0.5 ml. Lidocaine (or its equivalent), up to 1 ml of a 1% solution, can be mixed in a single syringe with the glucocorticoid to promote immediate relief but is not generally used in the digits.

## II. Nonsteroidal anti-inflammatory drugs (NSAIDs)

A. **Therapeutic effects.** These drugs exert their effects principally by inhibiting the constitutive (COX-1) and inducible (COX-2) isoforms of cyclooxygenase. This inhibition produces a mild to moderate anti-inflammatory and analgesic effect via peripheral and central actions. Individual responses to these agents are variable; if one drug is not effective during a 2- to 3-week trial, another should be tried.

**B. Side effects**

1. **GI toxicity** manifests clinically as dyspepsia, nausea, vomiting, or GI bleeding. Nausea and dyspepsia often respond to the addition of an $H_2$-blocking agent or proton pump inhibitor or to a change in NSAID. Direct GI irritation can be minimized by administration after food, by the use of enteric-coated preparations, and by use of the lowest effective dose. However, all NSAIDs have a systemic effect on the GI mucosa, resulting in increased permeability to gastric acid. Most serious GI bleeds during NSAID use occur without prior GI symptoms. **Risk factors for GI bleed** include a history of duodenal-gastric ulceration, age, smoking, ethanol use, and concomitant use of corticosteroids. **Misoprostol,** a synthetic prostaglandin E analog, decreases the risk of NSAID-induced gastric or duodenal ulceration but may cause diarrhea and is an abortifacient. An alternative is high-dose **famotidine,** 40 mg PO bid, or **omeprazole,** 20 mg qd. Diarrhea due to NSAIDs is rare except for the fenamates (e.g., meclofenamic acid, mefenamic acid).
2. **Acute renal failure** is the most common form of renal toxicity, and nephrotic syndrome and acute interstitial nephritis may also occur. **Risk factors** for acute renal failure include preexisting renal dysfunction, CHF, and cirrhosis with ascites. Periodic monitoring of renal function is recommended, particularly in elderly patients. **Sulindac** is relatively less nephrotoxic than other NSAIDs.
3. **Platelet dysfunction** can be caused by all NSAIDs, and particularly aspirin, which is a covalent inhibitor of cyclooxygenase. NSAIDs should be used cautiously or avoided in patients with a bleeding diathesis or those who are taking warfarin and should be discontinued 5–7 days before surgical procedures.
4. **Hypersensitivity reactions** are often seen in patients with a history of asthma, nasal polyps, or atopy. NSAIDs may cause a variety of type I hypersensitivity-like reactions, including urticaria, asthma, and anaphylactoid shock, presumably by increasing leukotriene synthesis. Patients with a hypersensitivity reaction to one NSAID should avoid all NSAIDs and selective COX-2 inhibitors.
5. **Other side effects.** CNS toxicity (headaches, dizziness, dysphoria, confusion, aseptic meningitis) is uncommon. Tinnitus and deafness can complicate NSAID use, particularly with high-dose salicylates. Blood dyscrasias including aplastic anemia have been observed as isolated case reports with ibuprofen, piroxicam, indomethacin, and phenylbutazone. Dermatologic reactions and elevations in transaminases have also been described. Acid-base imbalance is seen with high doses of salicylates. Nonacetylated salicylates have been reported to have less toxicity but also may be less effective.

**III. Selective COX-2 inhibitors**

**A. Therapeutic effects.** These agents exhibit selective inhibition of COX-2, thereby inhibiting inflammation while preserving the homeostatic functions of constitutive COX-1–derived prostaglandins. Their anti-inflammatory and analgesic efficacy is similar to that of traditional NSAIDs.

**B. Side effects. GI symptoms and GI ulcerations** are reduced with these agents in comparison to NSAIDs. **Platelet function** is not impaired, making selective COX-2 inhibitors a good anti-inflammatory option for patients with thrombocytopenia, hemostatic defects, or chronic anticoagulation. In patients who are taking warfarin, however, the INR should be monitored after the addition of a COX-2 inhibitor, as with any medication change. In addition, there has been controversy as to whether the inhibition of prostacyclin but not thromboxane by these agents may promote clotting slightly. **Fluid retention** has been noted with high-dose rofecoxib therapy, and renal function should be monitored in patients at risk of NSAID-induced acute renal failure (see sec. **II.B.2**). **Patients with hypersensitivity reactions to NSAIDs should not use a COX-2 inhibitor, and individuals with a sulfonamide allergy should not use celecoxib.**

**IV. Glucocorticoids** (Table 23-1)

**A. Therapeutic effects.** Glucocorticoids exert a pluripotent anti-inflammatory effect via the inhibition of inflammatory mediator gene transcription.

**B. Preparations, dosages, and routes of administration.** The goal of glucocorticoid therapy is to suppress disease activity with the minimum effective dosage. Prednisone (PO) and methylprednisolone (IV) are generally the preferred drugs because of cost and half-life considerations. IM absorption is variable and therefore is not advised. The dose, route, and frequency of administration are determined by the type of disease and the severity of the disease manifestations. The following are **relative anti-inflammatory potencies** of common glucocorticoid preparations: cortisone, 0.8; hydrocortisone, 1; prednisone, 4; methylprednisolone, 5; dexamethasone, 25.

**C. Side effects.** Adverse effects are related to dosage and duration of administration and, except for cataracts and osteopenia, can be minimized by alternate-day administration once the disease is controlled (twice the daily dose given every other day).

1. **Adrenal suppression.** Glucocorticoids suppress the hypothalamic-pituitary-adrenal axis. Patients who have received more than 10 mg prednisone (or the equivalent) daily for several weeks may have some degree of axis suppression for up to 1 year after cessation of therapy. Adrenal sup-

**Table 23-1.** Corticosteroids and immunomodulatory and immunosuppressive drugs

| Generic name | Tablet size (mg) | Starting dose (mg) | Dose interval | Maximum daily or interval dose (mg) |
|---|---|---|---|---|
| Prednisone | 1, 2.5, 5, 10, 20, 50 | 5–20 (low), 1–2 mg/kg (high) | qd | — |
| Methylprednisolone (IV) | — | 500 | bid for 3–5 d | — |
| Methotrexate | 2.5 | 7.5 | Weekly | 25 |
| Sulfasalazine | 500 | 500 | bid | 3000 |
| Hydroxychloroquine | 200 | 200 | bid | 400 |
| Leflunomide | 10, 20 | 20 | qd | 20[a] |
| Azathioprine | 50 (scored) | 1.5 mg/kg | qd | 2.5–3.0 mg/kg[b] |
| Cyclophosphamide | 25, 50 | 1.0–1.5 mg/kg | qd | 2.5–3.0 mg/kg[a] |
| Cyclophosphamide (IV) | — | 0.5–1.0 g/m$^2$ | Monthly | —[b,c] |
| Cyclosporine | 25, 50, 100 | 2–3 mg/kg | qd | 5 mg/kg |

[a]Treatment can be begun with a loading dose of 20 mg/day for 14 days.
[b]Titrate peripheral WBC count to 3500–4500 cells/μl (with neutrophils >1000).
[c]The addition of 2-mercaptoethanesulfonate (mesna) is recommended.

pression is minimized by dosing in the morning and using a single daily low dose of a short-acting preparation, such as prednisone, for a short period. In patients who are receiving chronic glucocorticoid therapy, hypoadrenalism (anorexia, weight loss, lethargy, fever, and postural hypotension) may occur at times of severe stress (e.g., infection, major surgery) and should be treated with stress doses of glucocorticoids (see Chap. 22, Endocrine Diseases). Mineralocorticoid activity, however, is preserved. These patients should wear a medical-alert bracelet or carry identification.

2. **Immunosuppression.** Glucocorticoid therapy reduces resistance to infections. **Bacterial infections** in particular are related to the dosage of glucocorticoids and are a major cause of morbidity and mortality. Thus, minor infections may become systemic, quiescent infections may be activated, and organisms that usually are nonpathogenic may cause disease. Local and systemic signs of infection may be partially masked, although fever associated with infection generally is not suppressed completely by glucocorticoids. When possible, a skin test for tuberculosis should be placed before glucocorticoid therapy is instituted, and, if it is positive, appropriate prophylaxis is indicated (see Chap. 13, Treatment of Infectious Diseases).
3. **Endocrine abnormalities.** Possible endocrine abnormalities include a **cushingoid habitus** and **hirsutism. Hyperglycemia** may be induced or aggravated by glucocorticoids but usually is not a contraindication to therapy. Insulin therapy may be required, although ketoacidosis is rare. **Fluid and electrolyte abnormalities** include hypokalemia and sodium retention, which may induce or aggravate hypertension.
4. **Musculoskeletal problems. Osteopenia** with vertebral compression fractures is common among patients who are receiving long-term glucocorticoid therapy. Supplemental calcium, 1.0–1.5 g/day PO, should be given along with vitamin D, 800 units, as soon as steroid therapy is begun (*Arthritis Rheum* 44:1496, 2001). A bisphosphonate may be indicated in postmenopausal women or in men or premenopausal women who are at high risk for osteopenia, and calcitonin can be considered for those who cannot tolerate a bisphosphonate. Determination of baseline bone density is appropriate in these patients. A judicious exercise program may be beneficial in stimulating bone formation. **Steroid myopathy** generally involves the hip and shoulder girdle musculature. Muscles are weak but not tender and, in contrast to inflammatory myositis, serum creatine kinase, aldolase, and electromyography are normal. The myopathy usually resolves slowly with a reduction in glucocorticoid dosage and an aggressive exercise program. **Ischemic bone necrosis** (aseptic necrosis, avascular necrosis) caused by glucocorticoid use often is multifocal, most commonly affecting the femoral head, humeral head, and tibial plateau. Early changes can be demonstrated by bone scan or MRI. Early surgical intervention with core decompression remains controversial.
5. **Other adverse effects.** Changes in **mental status** ranging from mild nervousness, euphoria, and insomnia to severe depression or psychosis may occur. **Ocular effects** include increased intraocular pressure (sometimes precipitating glaucoma) and the formation of posterior subcapsular cataracts. **Hyperlipidemia, menstrual irregularities,** increased perspiration with **night sweats,** and **pseudotumor cerebri** also may occur.

V. **Immunomodulatory and immunosuppressive drugs.** These agents can be used to treat rheumatologic disorders (Table 23-1). This group of drugs includes a number of pharmacologically diverse agents that exert anti-inflammatory or immunosuppressive effects. Often, such agents are referred to as *disease-modifying antirheumatic drugs*. They are characterized by a delayed onset of action and the potential for serious toxicity. Consequently, they should be prescribed with the guidance of a rheumatologist or other physician who is experienced in their use and given only to well-informed, cooperative patients who are willing to comply with meticulous follow-up.

**A. Methotrexate,** a purine inhibitor and folic acid antagonist, is used to treat synovitis and myositis and may improve the leukopenia of Felty's syndrome.

1. **Dosage and administration.** Typically, methotrexate is administered as a single PO dose once a week starting with 7.5 mg. Clinical response is usually noted in 4–8 weeks. If no response is attained after 6–8 weeks of therapy, the dosage can be increased by 2.5- to 5.0-mg increments every 2–4 weeks to a maximum of 25 mg/week or until improvement is observed. Dosages above 20 mg/week are generally given by SC injection to promote absorption. Methotrexate in a dosage of 7.5–17.5 mg/week is also used in a treatment regimen for rheumatoid arthritis (RA) in combination with sulfasalazine, 500 mg bid, and hydroxychloroquine, 200 mg bid.
2. **Contraindications and side effects.** Methotrexate is **teratogenic** and should not be used during pregnancy. It should also be avoided in patients with significant hepatic or renal impairment. **Folic acid supplementation** at a dosage of 1–2 mg qd may reduce methotrexate toxicity without impeding its efficacy. Concomitant use of trimethoprim/sulfamethoxazole should be avoided.
   a. **Minor side effects** include GI intolerance, stomatitis, rash, headache, and alopecia.
   b. **Bone marrow suppression** may occur, particularly at higher doses. Blood and platelet counts should be obtained before initiation, monthly during the first 3–4 months and every 6–8 weeks thereafter. Macrocytosis may herald serious hematologic toxicity and is an indication for folate supplementation, dose reduction, or both.
   c. **Cirrhosis** may occur rarely with long-term use. AST, ALT, and serum albumin should be measured every 4–8 weeks. Liver biopsy should be performed if the AST is elevated in five of nine determinations or if the serum albumin level falls below the normal range. Alcohol consumption increases the risk of methotrexate hepatotoxicity.
   d. **Hypersensitivity pneumonitis** may occur but usually is reversible. Patients with preexisting pulmonary parenchymal disease may be at increased risk.
   e. **Rheumatoid nodules** may develop or worsen, paradoxically, in some patients on methotrexate.

**B. Sulfasalazine** is useful for treating synovitis in the setting of RA and the seronegative spondyloarthropathies.

1. The initial **dosage** is 500 mg PO qd, with increases in 500-mg increments weekly until a total daily dose of 2000–3000 mg (given in evenly divided doses) is reached. Clinical response usually occurs in 6–10 weeks.
2. **Contraindications and side effects. Sulfasalazine should not be used in patients with glucose-6-phosphate dehydrogenase deficiency or sulfa allergy.** Nausea is the principal adverse effect and can be minimized by the use of the enteric-coated preparation of the drug. Hematologic toxicity including a reduction in any cell line and aplastic anemia rarely occurs. However, periodic monitoring of blood and platelet counts is warranted.

**C. Hydroxychloroquine** is an antimalarial agent that is used to treat dermatitis, alopecia, and synovitis in systemic lupus erythematosus (SLE) and mild synovitis in RA.

1. **Dosage.** Hydroxychloroquine typically is given at a dosage of 4–6 mg/kg PO qd (200–400 mg) after meals to minimize dyspepsia and nausea.
2. **Contraindications and side effects. Hydroxychloroquine should not be used in patients with porphyria, glucose-6-phosphate dehydro-**

**genase deficiency, or significant hepatic or renal impairment.** It should be avoided during pregnancy. The most common side effects are allergic skin eruptions and nausea. Serious ocular toxicity occurs but is rare with currently recommended dosages. Ophthalmologic evaluation should be performed every 12–18 months.

D. **Leflunomide** is a pyrimidine inhibitor that has been approved for the treatment of RA.
   1. **Dosage and administration.** Treatment is begun with 10 or 20 mg PO qd. If the initial daily dosage is to be 10 mg, a loading dose of 20 mg/day for 14 days can be used. Clinical response is generally seen within 4–8 weeks.
   2. **Contraindications and side effects.** Leflunomide is **teratogenic** and has a very long half-life. Women who plan to become pregnant must discontinue the drug and complete a course of elimination therapy with cholestyramine, 8 g PO tid for 11 days. Plasma levels should then be verified to be less than 0.02 mg/L on two separate tests at least 14 days apart before pregnancy is considered. Leflunomide is **contraindicated** in patients with significant hepatic dysfunction or in those who are receiving rifampin. **GI side effects** are the most common. **Diarrhea** occurs in up to 20% of patients and may require discontinuation of the drug. Dosage reduction to 10 mg/day may provide relief while maintaining efficacy, and loperamide can be used for symptomatic relief. **Elevations in serum transaminase levels** may occur, and transaminase levels should be measured at baseline and then monitored monthly. The dosage should be reduced for confirmed twofold elevations, and greater elevations should be treated with cholestyramine and discontinuation of leflunomide. **Rash** and **alopecia** may occur during therapy.

E. **Azathioprine** is an antimetabolite that is used to treat refractory synovitis or myositis. It can also be used as a steroid-sparing agent.
   1. **Dosage.** Therapy is initiated at 1.5 mg/kg/day PO, given as a single dose or in two divided doses. The dosage can be increased at 8- to 12-week intervals to a maximum of 2.5–3.0 mg/kg/day as long as the WBC count remains at or above 3500–4500 cells/μl with more than 1000 neutrophils. The dosage of azathioprine should be reduced by 60–75% if it is given concomitantly with allopurinol, which blocks its metabolic degradation.
   2. **Side effects.** Adverse effects of azathioprine include an increased incidence of infection, nausea, rare hepatotoxicity, and potential long-term oncogenicity.

F. **Mycophenolate mofetil** is an inhibitor of inosine monophosphate dehydrogenase used to treat lupus nephritis and, occasionally, as a steroid-sparing agent.
   1. **Dosage.** Treatment is initiated at 1 g PO daily and can be increased to 2 g/day if the WBC remains at or above 3500–4500 cells/μl.
   2. **Side effects.** The most common adverse effects with mycophenolate mofetil are nausea, diarrhea, and vomiting. Leukopenia and an increased frequency of opportunistic infections have also been reported.

G. **Cyclophosphamide,** an alkylating agent, is used to treat life-threatening manifestations of SLE and vasculitis.
   1. **Dosage and administration.** Cyclophosphamide can be administered either daily (low-dose PO therapy) or intermittently (high-dose IV bolus therapy). The latter route is probably less toxic but also less immunosuppressive. Oral therapy is initiated at a daily morning dose of 1.0–1.5 mg/kg and can be increased to a maximum of 2.5–3.0 mg/kg/day to obtain a WBC count of 3500–4500 cells/μl, with more than 1000 neutrophils. Peripheral WBC counts should be checked 10–14 days after each dosage change and monthly when on a stable dose. IV therapy is initiated at a dosage of 0.5–1.0 g/m$^2$ every 1–3 months. The goal of therapy is to achieve a nadir WBC count of 3500–4500 cells/μl, with more than 1000 neutrophils, 10–14 days after infusion.

2. **Side effects.** Adverse effects include an increased incidence of infection, hemorrhagic cystitis, GI toxicity (nausea, vomiting), gonadal suppression and sterility, alopecia, pulmonary interstitial fibrosis, and oncogenicity (particularly bladder carcinoma). Patients should be encouraged to take the medication in the morning with a lot of fluid, to void frequently, and to void before going to bed to minimize the risk of hemorrhagic cystitis. With IV therapy, sodium 2-mercaptoethanesulfonate (**mesna**) and large volumes of fluid can be given concomitantly to minimize the risk of hemorrhagic cystitis. Mesna can be administered concomitantly with the cyclophosphamide infusion and repeated 3 and 6 hours later. Each mesna dose should be 20% of the total cyclophosphamide dose. **Antiemetics** may be necessary with high-dose IV therapy. The use of trimethoprim/sulfamethoxazole three times a week for ***Pneumocystis carinii* prophylaxis** should be considered.

H. **Cyclosporine** is occasionally used to treat refractory synovitis. Therapy is initiated at a dose of 2–3 mg/kg/day PO. The dose can be increased to as high as 5 mg/kg/day, but **renal toxicity** is the usual limiting factor. The dosage should be reduced if the serum creatinine level increases more than 30% or if hypertension develops. Other toxicities include hirsutism, anemia, liver dysfunction, and oncogenicity.

VI. **Anticytokine therapies.** New treatments directed at specific cytokines have been developed.

A. **Tumor necrosis factor (TNF) inhibitors** have been approved for treatment of RA and have also been useful in seronegative spondyloarthropathies and some forms of vasculitis. In general, these agents are used in patients with moderate to severe RA who have failed a trial of one or more disease-modifying antirheumatic drugs as listed above. Three preparations are currently available, with similar efficacy and toxicity profiles.

1. **Etanercept** is a fusion protein that consists of the ligand-binding portion of the human TNF receptor linked to the Fc portion of human Ig G. It binds to TNF, blocking its interaction with cell surface receptors, thus inhibiting the inflammatory and immunoregulatory properties of TNF. This preparation is given in a dosage of 25 mg SC twice a week.

2. **Infliximab** is a chimeric monoclonal antibody that binds specifically to human TNF-α, blocking its proinflammatory and immunomodulatory effects. It is given by IV infusion in conjunction with methotrexate, 7.5 mg PO weekly, to reduce production of neutralizing antibodies against infliximab. The recommended treatment regimen includes infliximab infusions of 3 mg/kg at initiation, at 2 and 6 weeks, and every 8 weeks thereafter, along with methotrexate at a dose of at least 7.5 mg/week.

3. **Adalimumab** is a recombinant human IgG–1 monoclonal antibody that is specific to human TNF-α. It can be given in a dosage of 40 mg SC every other week. Some patients form antiadalimumab antibodies, and their regimen may include weekly injections of adalimumab or the addition of low-dose methotrexate. The effect of these agents on RA synovitis can be dramatic, with responsive patients reporting the onset of symptomatic benefit within 1–2 weeks. In addition to their symptomatic benefits, these agents appear to retard joint damage significantly.

4. **Contraindications and side effects**

a. **Serious infections and sepsis,** including fatalities, have been reported during the use of TNF-blocking agents. These drugs are contraindicated in patients with acute or chronic infections, and if serious infection or sepsis occurs, the drug should be stopped. Those with a history of recurrent infections and those with underlying conditions that may predispose to infection should be treated with caution and counseled to be vigilant for signs and symptoms of infection. Upper respiratory and sinus infections are most common.

Tuberculosis has also been noted, and a tuberculin skin test and chest x-ray should be obtained before beginning therapy. Patients who are undergoing elective surgical procedures can omit the last dose of the drug that is scheduled to be given before surgery, as well as the next dose scheduled to follow the surgery. These agents are also contraindicated in patients with congestive heart failure.

b. **Local injection site reactions** are common with etanercept and adalimumab, particularly during the first month of therapy. These reactions are generally self-limited and do not require discontinuation of therapy. Serious systemic allergic reactions are rare but may occur with infliximab infusions.

c. **Other adverse effects** may include induction of antinuclear antibodies and, rarely, a lupus-like illness. A demyelinating disorder has been described, as well as exacerbations of preexisting multiple sclerosis. It is unclear whether the frequency of occurrence of lymphoma may be increased in patients who receive these agents.

B. **Inhibitors of interleukin-1$\alpha$ (IL-1).** Currently, only one inhibitor of interleukin is available for patients with rheumatic diseases, but several more are in development. **Anakinra** is a recombinant form of the naturally occurring IL-1–receptor antagonist that is approved for use in RA. It blocks binding of IL-1 to its receptor, thus inhibiting the proinflammatory and immunomodulatory actions of IL-1. This agent is given in a **dosage** of 100 mg SC qd. Like the TNF blockers, it should not be prescribed to patients with ongoing or recurrent infections. **Adverse effects** include an increased frequency of bacterial infections and injection site reactions. **Anakinra should not be used in conjunction with a TNF blocker because of enhanced risk of serious infection and neutropenia.**

VII. **Plasmapheresis.** Until concomitant therapy with glucocorticoids or immunosuppressives has taken effect, plasmapheresis has been used on an investigational basis in life-threatening situations to control various rheumatic diseases. It is an impractical long-term therapy, and its short-term use remains controversial. A new approach, pheresis across a column bound with staphylococcal protein A, the **Prosorba** column, has been approved for treatment of RA.

## Approach to the Patient with a Single Painful Joint

The first step for diagnosis for a patient with a single painful joint is to **identify the structure involved.** Pain that arises from periarticular (e.g., tendon, bursa), muscular, and neurologic structures may be perceived as joint pain. If the pain arises in the joint itself and a single joint is involved, the major disorders in the differential diagnosis are **trauma, infection,** and **crystalline arthritis.**

I. **Diagnostics studies**

A. **Radiographs** of the joint may be useful in documenting trauma or preexisting joint disease. The presence of chondrocalcinosis on x-ray suggests pseudogout but is not diagnostic (see the section Crystal-Induced Synovitis). Radiographs are usually normal in acute infectious or crystalline arthritis.

B. **Synovial fluid** should be aspirated in all patients with a monarticular arthritis who do not have a preexisting diagnosis that is consistent with the clinical picture. Polyarticular disorders such as RA or lupus (SLE) occasionally present initially as monarthritis, but when a single joint is inflamed out of proportion to other joints in what is typically a polyarticular disorder, infection must be excluded. Synovial fluid cell counts above 5000 nucleated cells/μl suggest an inflammatory etiology. Counts above 50,000 cells/μl may indicate infection, particularly if 75% or more of the cells are polymorphonuclear.

**II. Management** is based on the results of radiographs and synovial fluid analysis. Trauma or internal derangement of the joint can be managed by immobilization of the joint and consultation with an orthopedic surgeon. The treatment of infectious arthritis and crystalline disorders is detailed in the following sections.

## Infectious Arthritis and Bursitis

**Infectious arthritis** is generally categorized into gonococcal and nongonococcal disease. The usual presentation is with fever and an acute monarticular arthritis, although multiple joints may be affected by hematogenous spread of pathogens. **Nongonococcal infectious arthritis** in adults tends to occur in patients with previous joint damage or compromised host defenses. In contrast, **gonococcal arthritis** causes one-half of all septic arthritis in otherwise healthy, sexually active young adults.

**I. General principles of treatment**

**A. Joint fluid examination,** including Gram stain of a centrifuged pellet, and culture are mandatory to make a diagnosis and to guide management. A joint fluid leukocyte count is useful diagnostically and as a baseline for serial studies to evaluate response to treatment. Cultures of blood and other possible extra-articular sites of infection also should be obtained.

**B. Hospitalization** is indicated to ensure drug compliance and careful monitoring of the clinical response.

**C. IV antimicrobials** provide good serum and synovial fluid drug concentrations. Oral or intra-articular antimicrobials are not appropriate as initial therapy.

**D. Repeated arthrocenteses** should be performed daily or as often as necessary to prevent reaccumulation of fluid. Arthrocentesis is indicated to (1) remove destructive inflammatory mediators, (2) reduce intra-articular pressure and promote antimicrobial penetration into the joint, and (3) monitor response to therapy by documenting sterility of synovial fluid cultures and steadily decreasing leukocyte counts.

**E. Surgical drainage** or arthroscopic lavage and drainage are indicated for (1) a septic hip; (2) joints in which either the anatomy, large amounts of tissue debris, or loculation of pus prevent adequate needle drainage (most commonly the shoulder); (3) septic arthritis with coexistent osteomyelitis; (4) joints that do not respond in 3–5 days to appropriate therapy and repeated arthrocenteses; and (5) prosthetic joint infection.

**F. General supportive** measures include splinting of the joint, which may help to relieve pain. However, prolonged immobilization can result in joint stiffness. An NSAID or selective COX-2 inhibitor (see Therapeutic Approaches to Rheumatic Disease, sec. **II**) is often useful to reduce pain and increase joint mobility but should not be used until response to antimicrobial therapy has been demonstrated by symptomatic and laboratory improvement.

**II. Nongonococcal septic arthritis** is caused most often by *Staphylococcus aureus* (60%) and *Streptococcus* species. Gram-negative organisms are less common except with IV drug abuse, neutropenia, concomitant urinary tract infection, and postoperatively. **Initial therapy** is based on the clinical situation and a carefully performed Gram stain, which reveals the organism in approximately 50% of patients. With a positive Gram stain, antibiotic coverage can be focused accordingly. With a nondiagnostic Gram stain, antibiotics should be chosen to cover *S. aureus*, *Streptococcus* species, and *Neisseria gonorrhoeae* in otherwise healthy patients, whereas broad-spectrum antibiotics are appropriate in immunosuppressed patients. IV antimicrobials usually are given for at least 2 weeks, followed by 1–2 weeks of oral antimicrobials, with the course of therapy tailored to the patient's response.

III. **Gonococcal arthritis** is more common than nongonococcal septic arthritis. The clinical spectrum of disease often includes migratory or additive polyarthralgias, followed by tenosynovitis or arthritis of the wrist, ankle, or knee and asymptomatic dermatitis on the extremities or trunk. In contrast to nongonococcal septic arthritis, Gram staining of synovial fluid and cultures of blood or synovial fluid often are negative. Bacteriologic assessment of the throat, cervix, urethra, and rectum may aid in establishing the diagnosis. **Initial treatment is with an IV antibiotic** for the first 1–3 days, generally ceftriaxone, 1 g IV qd, or ceftizoxime, 1 g IV q8h. Response to IV antibiotics is usually noted within the first 24–36 hours of treatment. After clinical improvement is noted, therapy is continued with an oral antibiotic to complete 7–10 days of treatment. Ciprofloxacin, 500 mg PO bid, or amoxicillin/clavulanate, 500–850 mg PO bid, can be used. Treatment of coexisting *Chlamydia* infection should also be considered.

IV. **Nonbacterial infectious arthritis** is common with many viral infections, especially hepatitis B, rubella, mumps, infectious mononucleosis, parvovirus, enterovirus, and adenovirus. It is generally self-limited, lasting for less than 6 weeks, and responds well to a conservative regimen of rest and NSAIDs. Arthralgias (often severe) or a reactive arthritis can also be a manifestation of HIV infection. A variety of fungi and mycobacteria can cause septic arthritis and should be considered in patients with chronic monarticular arthritis.

V. **Septic bursitis,** usually involving the olecranon or prepatellar bursa, can be differentiated from septic arthritis by localized, fluctuant superficial swelling and by relatively painless joint motion (particularly extension). Most patients have a history of previous trauma to the area or an occupational predisposition (e.g., "housemaid's knee," "writer's elbow"). *S. aureus* is the most common pathogen. Septic bursitis should be treated with aspiration, which can be repeated if fluid reaccumulates. Oral antibiotics and outpatient management are usually appropriate, and surgical drainage is rarely indicated. Preventive measures (e.g., knee pads) should be used in patients with occupational predispositions.

VI. **Lyme disease** is caused by the tick-borne spirochete *Borrelia burgdorferi*. Typical manifestations begin with an erythematous annular rash (erythema migrans) and flu-like symptoms. Arthralgias, myalgias, meningitis, neuropathy, and cardiac conduction defects may follow in weeks to a few months. Months later, an intermittent or chronic arthritis in one or a few joints, characteristically including the knee, may develop in untreated patients. The diagnosis is based mainly on the clinical picture and exposure in an endemic area. Unfortunately, serologic studies often give false-negative or false-positive results, and patients may remain seropositive for years following treatment. Antibiotic therapy is required (see Chap. 13, Treatment of Infectious Diseases). NSAIDs are a useful adjunct for arthritis. Vaccination should be considered for people living in high-risk areas who have frequent tick exposures.

## Crystal-Induced Synovitis

Deposition of microcrystals in joints and periarticular tissues results in **gout, pseudogout,** and **apatite disease.** A definitive diagnosis of gout or pseudogout is made by finding intracellular crystals in joint fluid examined with a compensated polarized light microscope. Urate crystals, which are diagnostic of gout, are needle shaped and strongly negatively birefringent. The calcium pyrophosphate dihydrate crystals seen in pseudogout are pleomorphic and weakly positively birefringent. Hydroxyapatite complexes, diagnostic of apatite disease, and basic calcium phosphate complexes can be identified only by electron microscopy and mass spectroscopy. In most cases, the arthritides associated with these compounds are suspected clinically but never confirmed.

I. **Primary gouty arthritis** is characterized by hyperuricemia that is usually due to underexcretion of uric acid (90% of cases) rather than to overproduction. Urate crystals may be deposited in the joints, SC tissues (tophi), and kidneys. Men are much more commonly affected than women; most premenopausal women with gout have a family history of the disease. The clinical phases of gout can be divided into (1) asymptomatic hyperuricemia, (2) acute gouty arthritis, and (3) chronic arthritis.

A. **Asymptomatic hyperuricemia** (uric acid levels >8 mg/dl in men and >7 mg/dl in women) is not routinely treated because of expense, potential drug toxicity, and the low risk for adverse outcome from the hyperuricemia itself.

B. **Acute gouty arthritis** presents as an excruciating attack of pain, usually in a single joint of the foot or ankle. Occasionally, a polyarticular onset can mimic RA. Attacks can be precipitated by surgery, dehydration, fasting, binge eating, or heavy ingestion of alcohol. Although the acute gouty attack will subside spontaneously over several days, prompt treatment can abort the attack within hours. The serum uric acid level is normal in 30% of patients with acute gout and, if elevated, should not be manipulated until an attack has resolved.

1. **NSAIDs** are the treatment of choice for acute gout due to ease of administration and low toxicity. Clinical response may require 12–24 hours, and initial doses should be high, followed by rapid tapering over 2–8 days (see Therapeutic Approaches to Rheumatic Disease, sec. **II**). One approach is to use indomethacin, 50 mg PO q6h for 2 days, followed by 50 mg PO q8h for 3 days and then 25 mg PO q8h for 2–3 days. The long-acting NSAIDs generally are not recommended for acute gout. Selective COX-2 inhibitors have not been critically evaluated for treatment of gout but should also be effective.

2. **Glucocorticoids** are useful when NSAIDs are contraindicated. An intra-articular injection of glucocorticoids produces rapid dramatic relief. Alternatively, prednisone, 40–60 mg PO qd, can be given until a response is obtained and then should be tapered rapidly.

3. **Colchicine** is most effective if given in the first 12–24 hours of an acute attack and usually brings relief in 6–12 hours. In view of the efficacy and tolerability of a short course of NSAIDs, colchicine is not commonly used to treat gout but is useful when NSAIDs or glucocorticoids are contraindicated or not tolerated.

   a. **Oral administration** is often associated with severe GI toxicity. The dosage is 0.5–0.6 mg (1 tablet) q1–2h or 1.0–1.2 mg q2h until symptoms abate, GI toxicity develops, or the maximum dose of 6 mg in a 24-hour period is reached. The dosage should be reduced in elderly patients and in those who have renal or hepatic impairment. No more than 1.2 mg/day should be used after the loading dose.

   b. **IV colchicine** produces faster relief with fewer GI side effects but can cause severe myelosuppression and is rarely used. The drug is diluted in 10–20 ml normal saline and is given slowly over 3–5 minutes through a freely flowing IV to avoid extravasation and tissue necrosis. **Colchicine should not be diluted with or injected into IV tubing that contains 5% dextrose because precipitation will occur.** The initial dose is 2 mg, followed by another 1–2 mg in 6 hours if necessary, to a maximum dose of 4 mg in 24 hours. The dosage should be reduced in the elderly, patients who have been receiving chronic oral colchicine, and those with significant renal or hepatic disease. No further colchicine should be given PO or IV for 7 days.

C. **Chronic gouty arthritis.** With time, acute gouty attacks occur more frequently, asymptomatic periods are shorter, and chronic joint deformity may appear. Colchicine (0.5–0.6 mg PO qd or bid) can be used prophylactically for acute attacks. Aspirin (uricoretentive), diuretics, large alcohol intake, and foods high in purines (sweetbreads, anchovies, sardines, liver, and kidney) should be avoided. The serum uric acid level should be lowered if arthritic attacks are frequent, renal damage is present, or serum or urine uric acid levels are elevated consistently. **Maintenance colchicine, 0.5–0.6 mg PO bid, should be given a few days before manipulation of the uric acid level to prevent precipitation of an acute attack.** If no attacks occur after the uric acid has been maintained in the normal range for 6–8 weeks, colchicine can be discontinued.

1. **Allopurinol,** a xanthine oxidase inhibitor, is effective therapy for hyperuricemia in most patients.
   a. **Dosage and administration.** The initial dosage is usually 300 mg PO qd. Daily doses can be increased by 100 mg every 2–4 weeks to achieve the minimum maintenance dosage that will keep the uric acid level within the normal range. In patients with impaired renal function, the daily dose should be reduced by 50 mg for each 20-ml/minute decrease in the creatinine clearance. For patients with a creatinine clearance below 20 ml/minute, the starting dosage is 100 mg every other or every third day. The daily dose should be decreased also in patients with hepatic impairment. The concomitant use of a uricosuric agent may hasten the mobilization of tophi. If an acute attack occurs during treatment with allopurinol, it should be continued at the same dosage while other agents are used to treat the attack.
   b. **Side effects. Hypersensitivity reactions** from a minor skin rash to a diffuse exfoliative dermatitis associated with fever, eosinophilia, and a combination of renal and hepatic injury occur in up to 5% of patients. Patients who have mild renal insufficiency and are receiving diuretics are at greatest risk. **Severe cases are potentially fatal** and usually require glucocorticoid therapy. Allopurinol may potentiate the effect of oral anticoagulants and blocks metabolism of azathioprine and 6-mercaptopurine, necessitating a 60–75% reduction in dosage of these cytotoxic drugs.
2. **Uricosuric drugs** lower serum uric acid levels by blocking renal tubular reabsorption of uric acid. A 24-hour measurement of creatinine clearance and urine uric acid should be obtained before therapy is started, as these drugs are **ineffective with glomerular filtration rates of less than 50 ml/minute.** They are also not recommended for patients who already have high levels of urine uric acid (800 mg/24 hour) because of the risk of urate stone formation. This risk can be minimized by maintaining a high fluid intake and by alkalinizing the urine. If these drugs are being used when an acute gouty attack begins, they should be continued while other drugs are used to treat the acute attack.
   a. **Probenecid** is given at an initial dosage of 500 mg PO qd, which can be raised in 500-mg increments every week until serum uric acid levels normalize or urine uric acid levels exceed 800 mg/24 hour. The maximum dose is 3000 mg/day. Most patients require a total of 1.0–1.5 g/day in two to three divided doses. Salicylates and probenecid are antagonistic and should not be used together. Probenecid decreases renal excretion of penicillin, indomethacin, and sulfonylureas. Side effects are minimal.
   b. **Sulfinpyrazone** has uricosuric efficacy similar to that of probenecid; however, it also inhibits platelet function. The initial dosage of 50 mg PO bid can be increased in 100-mg increments weekly until serum uric acid levels normalize, to a maximum dose of 800 mg/day. Most patients require 300–400 mg/day in three to four divided doses.

D. **Secondary gout,** like primary gout, can be caused by either defective renal excretion or overproduction of uric acid. Intrinsic renal disease, diuretic therapy, low-dose aspirin, nicotinic acid, cyclosporine, and ethanol all interfere with renal excretion of uric acid. Starvation, lactic acidosis, dehydration, preeclampsia, and diabetic ketoacidosis also can induce hyperuricemia. Overproduction of uric acid occurs in myeloproliferative and lymphoproliferative disorders, hemolytic anemia, polycythemia, and cyanotic congenital heart disease. Management includes treatment of the underlying disorder and allopurinol therapy.

**II. Pseudogout** results when calcium pyrophosphate dihydrate crystals deposited in bone and cartilage are released into synovial fluid and induce acute inflammation. **Risk factors** include older age, advanced osteoarthritis (OA), neuropathic joint, gout, hyperparathyroidism, hemochromatosis, diabetes mellitus, hypothyroidism, and hypomagnesemia. The disease may present as an **acute monarthritis or oligoarthritis** mimicking gout or as a **chronic polyarthritis** resembling RA or OA. Usually the knee or wrist is affected, although any synovial joint can be involved. Dehydration, acute illness, and surgery (especially parathyroidectomy) are common precipitants of an acute attack of pseudogout. As in gout, the therapy of choice for most patients is a brief high-dose course of an **NSAID** (see sec. **I.B.1**). **Oral corticosteroids** can be used (see sec. **I.B.2**), and **colchicine** (PO or IV; see sec. **I.B.3**) also may relieve symptoms promptly, but toxicity limits its use. Maintenance daily PO colchicine may diminish the number of recurrent attacks. Aspiration of the inflammatory joint fluid often results in prompt improvement, and **intra-articular injection of glucocorticoids** may hasten the response. Allopurinol or uricosuric agents have no role in treating pseudogout.

**III. Apatite disease** may present with periarthritis or tendonitis, particularly in patients with chronic renal failure. An episodic oligoarthritis also may occur, and apatite disease should be suspected when no crystals are present in the synovial fluid. Erosive arthritis may be seen, particularly in the shoulder ("Milwaukee shoulder"). The treatment of apatite disease is similar to that for pseudogout.

## Rheumatoid Arthritis

**RA** is a systemic disease of unknown etiology that is characterized by symmetric inflammatory polyarthritis, extra-articular manifestations (rheumatoid nodules, pulmonary fibrosis, serositis, vasculitis), and serum rheumatoid factor in up to 80% of patients. **Sjögren's syndrome,** characterized by failure of exocrine glands, occurs in a subset of patients with RA, producing sicca symptoms (dry eyes and mouth), parotid gland enlargement, dental caries, and recurrent tracheobronchitis. **Felty's syndrome,** the triad of RA, splenomegaly, and granulocytopenia, also occurs in a small subset of patients, and these patients are at risk for recurrent bacterial infections and nonhealing leg ulcers.

The course of RA is variable but tends to be chronic and progressive. Approximately 70% of patients show irreversible joint damage on x-ray within the first 3 years of disease. Work disability is common, and life span is shortened by between 3 and 12 years. Most patients can benefit from an early aggressive treatment program that combines medical, rehabilitative, and surgical services designed with three distinct goals: (1) early suppression of inflammation in the joints and other tissues, (2) maintenance of joint and muscle function and prevention of deformities, and (3) repair of joint damage to relieve pain or improve function (*Arthritis Rheum* 46:328, 2002). **Patients with RA and a single joint inflamed out of proportion to the rest of the joints must be evaluated for coexistent septic arthritis.** This complication occurs with increased frequency in RA and carries a 20–30% mortality.

**I. Medical management**

**A. NSAIDs or selective COX-2 inhibitors** (see Therapeutic Approaches to Rheumatic Disease, secs. **II** and **III**) are used as the initial therapy for RA and as an adjunct to immunomodulatory-immunosuppressive therapy. A longer-acting NSAID may facilitate patient compliance.

**B. Glucocorticoids** are not curative and probably do not alter the natural history of RA; however, they are among the most potent anti-inflammatory drugs available (see Therapeutic Approaches to Rheumatic Disease, sec. **IV**). Unfortunately, once systemic glucocorticoid therapy has been initiated, few RA patients are able to discontinue it completely.

1. **Indications** for glucocorticoids include (1) symptomatic relief while waiting for a response to a slow-acting immunosuppressive or immunomodulatory agent, (2) persistent synovitis despite adequate trials of NSAIDs and immunosuppressive or immunomodulatory agents, and (3) severe constitutional symptoms (e.g., fever and weight loss) or extra-articular disease (vasculitis, episcleritis, or pleurisy).
2. **Oral administration** of 5–20 mg qd usually is sufficient for the treatment of synovitis, whereas severe constitutional symptoms or extra-articular disease may require up to 1 mg/kg PO qd. Although alternate-day glucocorticoid therapy reduces the incidence of undesirable side effects, some patients do not tolerate the increase in symptoms that may occur on the off day. **Intra-articular administration** may provide temporary symptomatic relief when only a few joints are inflamed (see Therapeutic Approaches to Rheumatic Disease, sec. **I**). The beneficial effects of intra-articular steroids may persist for days to months and may delay or negate the need for systemic glucocorticoid therapy.

**C. Immunomodulatory and immunosuppressive agents** appear to alter the natural history of RA by retarding the progression of bony erosions and cartilage loss. Because RA may lead to substantial long-term disability (and is associated with increased mortality), the current trend is to initiate therapy with such agents early in the course of RA (see Therapeutic Approaches to Rheumatic Disease, sec. **V**). Once a clinical response has been achieved, the chosen drug usually is continued indefinitely at the lowest effective dosage to prevent relapse.

1. **Indications** for the use of immunomodulatory or immunosuppressive agents include (1) active synovitis that does not respond to conservative management (e.g., NSAIDs); (2) rapidly progressive, erosive arthritis; and (3) dependence on steroids to control synovitis.
2. **Selection** of an immunomodulatory or immunosuppressive agent is tailored to the character of the patient's disease, taking into account the potential toxicity of these agents (see Therapeutic Approaches to Rheumatic Disease, sec. **V.A.1**) (Table 23-1). **Methotrexate** typically is the initial choice for moderate to severe RA. **Hydroxychloroquine or sulfasalazine** can be used as the initial choice in very mild RA. If response to the initial agent is unsatisfactory after an adequate trial (or if limiting toxicity supervenes), an alternate agent, such as **leflunomide, a TNF or IL-1 blocker, or azathioprine,** can be used.
3. **Combinations of immunomodulatory-immunosuppressive agents** can be used if the patient has a partial response to the initial agent. Common combination therapies include methotrexate with either hydroxychloroquine, sulfasalazine, or both (see Therapeutic Approaches to Rheumatic Disease, sec. **V.A.1**). For severe RA, methotrexate has been combined with leflunomide, azathioprine, or cyclosporin A. Such combinations may lead to synergistic or unexpected toxicities and should be used with appropriate caution.

**II. Corrective surgical procedures,** including synovectomy, total joint replacement, and joint fusion, may be indicated in patients with RA to reduce pain and to improve function. Carpal tunnel syndrome is common, and surgical repair may be curative if local injection therapy is unsuccessful. **Synovectomy** may be helpful if major involvement is limited to one or two joints and if a 6-month trial of medical therapy has failed, but usually it is only of temporary benefit.

Prophylactic synovectomy and débridement of the ulnar styloid should be considered for patients with severe wrist disease to prevent rupture of the extensor tendons. Other procedures that may be beneficial include **total joint replacement** of the hip and knee joints, resection of metatarsal heads in patients with bunion deformities, and subluxation of the toes. Reconstructive hand surgery may be useful in carefully selected patients. **Surgical fusion of joints** usually results in freedom from pain but also in total loss of motion; this is tolerated well in the wrist and thumb. Cervical spine fusion of C1 and C2 is indicated for significant cervical subluxation (>5 mm) with associated neurologic deficits. RA patients undergoing elective surgical procedures should have a lateral cervical spine radiograph in flexion and extensions performed to screen for this subluxation.

**III. Adjunctive measures**

**A. Reactive depression and sleep disorders** are often encountered in patients with rheumatic diseases. Judicious use of antidepressants and sedatives may improve the functional status of selected patients.

**B. Rehabilitative therapy** should be managed by a team of physicians, physical and occupational therapists, nurses, social workers, and psychologists. This approach may benefit patients with any form of arthritis.

1. **Acute care** of inflammatory arthritides involves joint protection and pain relief. Proper joint positioning and splints are important elements in joint protection. Heat is a useful analgesic.
2. **Subacute disease** therapy should include a gradual increase in passive and active joint movement.
3. **Chronic care** encompasses instruction in joint protection, work simplification, and performance of activities of daily living. Adaptive equipment, splints, orthotics, and mobility aids may be useful. Specific exercises designed to promote normal joint mechanics and to strengthen affected muscle groups are useful. Overall cardiac conditioning also improves functional status.

**C. Sicca symptoms** (dry eyes and mouth) can be treated symptomatically with artificial tears and saliva. Assiduous dental and ophthalmologic care is recommended, and drugs that suppress lacrimal-salivary secretion further should be avoided. **Pilocarpine** in a dosage of up to 5 mg PO qid may provide symptomatic relief.

**D. Patient education,** including pamphlets and support groups, is available in many communities through local chapters of the Arthritis Foundation.

## Osteoarthritis

**OA,** or **degenerative joint disease,** is characterized by deterioration of articular cartilage, with subsequent formation of reactive new bone at the articular surface. The disease is more common in the elderly but may occur at any age, especially as a sequel to joint trauma, chronic inflammatory arthritis, or congenital malformation. The joints affected most commonly are the distal and proximal interphalangeal joints of the hands, hips, and knees and the cervical and lumbar spine. OA of the spine may lead to spinal stenosis (neurogenic claudication), with aching or pain in the legs or buttocks on standing or walking.

**I. Medical management.** The objectives of therapy include relief of pain and prevention of disability. **Acetaminophen** in a dosage of up to 1000 mg up to qid is the initial pharmacologic treatment (*Arthritis Rheum* 43:1905, 2000). **Low-dose NSAIDs or selective COX-2 inhibitors** are the next step, followed by full-dose treatment (see Therapeutic Approaches to Rheumatic Disease, secs. **II** and **III**). However, because this patient population is often elderly and may have concomitant renal or cardiopulmonary disease, NSAIDs should be used with caution. NSAID-induced GI bleeding also is increased in the elderly population. **Glucosamine sulfate,** 1500 mg PO qd, may reduce symptoms as well as the rate of cartilage deterioration. **Intra-articular glucocorticoid injections** often are beneficial but probably should not be given more than every 3–6 months (see Therapeutic Approaches to Rheumatic Disease, sec. **I.E**). Systemic steroids and narcotic analgesics should be avoided, although the μ-opioid agonist **tramadol** may be useful as an alternative analgesic agent. **Topical capsaicin** may provide symptomatic relief with minimal toxicity.

**II. Adjunctive measures. Nonpharmacologic approaches** may complement drug treatment of arthritis. Activities that involve excessive use of the joint should be identified and avoided. Brief periods of rest for the involved joint can relieve pain. Poor body mechanics should be corrected and malalignments such as pronated feet may be aided by orthotics. An exercise program to prevent or correct muscle atrophy can also provide pain relief. When weight-bearing joints are affected, support in the form of a cane, crutches, or a walker can be helpful, as well as weight reduction and wearing soft-soled shoes. Consultation with occupational and physical therapists may be helpful. When serious disability results from severe pain or deformity, **surgery** can be considered. Total hip or knee replacement usually relieves pain and increases function in selected patients. OA of the spine may cause radicular symptoms from pressure on nerve roots and often produces pain and spasm in the paraspinal soft tissues. Physical supports (cervical collar, lumbar corset), local heat, and exercises to strengthen cervical, paravertebral, and abdominal muscles may provide relief in some patients. **Epidural steroid injections** may reduce radicular symptoms. **Laminectomy and spinal fusion** should be reserved for patients who have severe disease with intractable pain or neurologic complications. Lumbar spinal stenosis may require extensive decompressive laminectomy for relief of symptoms.

## Spondyloarthropathies

The **spondyloarthropathies** are an interrelated group of disorders characterized by one or more of the following features: (1) spondylitis, (2) sacroiliitis, (3) enthesopathy (inflammation at sites of tendon insertion), and (4) asymmetric oligoarthritis. Extra-articular features of this group of disorders may include inflammatory eye disease, urethritis, and mucocutaneous lesions. The spondyloarthropathies aggregate in families, where they are associated with HLA-B27.

**I. Ankylosing spondylitis (AS)** clinically presents as inflammation and ossification of the joints and ligaments of the spine and of the sacroiliac joints. Hips and shoulders are the peripheral joints that are most commonly involved. Progressive fusion of the apophyseal joints of the spine occurs in many patients and cannot be predicted or prevented. Physical therapy emphasizing extension exercises and posture is recommended to minimize possible late postural defects and respiratory compromise. Patients should be instructed to sleep supine on a firm bed without a pillow and to practice postural and deep-breathing exercises regularly. Cigarette smoking should be discouraged strongly. **Non-salicylate NSAIDs,** such as indomethacin, are used to provide symptomatic relief, and **selective COX-2 inhibitors** should also be effective (see Therapeutic Approaches to Rheumatic Disease, secs. **II** and **III**). **Methotrexate and sulfasalazine** provide benefit in some patients (see Therapeutic Approaches to Rheumatic Disease, sec. **V**) (Table 23-1). **TNF blockade** has been shown to be of benefit even in some patients with apparent fixed deformities. Glucocorticoids and immunosuppressive therapy have been used occasionally in patients who do not respond to other agents. Many patients develop osteoporosis in the fused spondylitic spine and are at risk of spinal fracture. Surgical procedures to correct some spine and hip deformities may result in significant rehabilitation in carefully selected patients. **Acute anterior uveitis** occurs in up to 25% of patients with AS and should be managed by an ophthalmologist. Generally, this problem is self-limited, although glaucoma and blindness are unusual secondary complications.

**II. Arthritis of inflammatory bowel disease** occurs in 10–20% of patients with Crohn's disease or ulcerative colitis and is similar to that of AS. It may also occur in some patients with intestinal bypass and diverticular disease. Clinical features include **spondylitis, sacroiliitis,** and **peripheral arthritis,** particularly in the knee and ankle. Although peripheral joint disease may correlate with the activity of the colitis, spinal disease does not. Joint aspiration may be useful to exclude an associated septic arthritis, but antimicrobials are not effective in the management of sterile synovitis associated with colitis. As in AS, **NSAIDs** (other than salicylates) are the treatment of choice, and **selective COX-2 inhibitors** should also be effective. However, GI intolerance of NSAIDs may be increased among this group of patients, and misoprostol may cause unacceptable diarrhea (see Therapeutic Approaches to Rheumatic Disease, sec. **II**). **Sulfasalazine** also may be beneficial for this form of arthritis (see Therapeutic Approaches to Rheumatic Disease, sec. **V.B**) (Table 23-1). Local **injection of glucocorticoids** and **physical therapy** are useful adjunctive measures.

**III. Reiter's syndrome and reactive arthritis.** Reiter's syndrome is seen predominantly in young men and may occur with increased frequency in patients infected with HIV. *Chlamydia* infection has been implicated in some patients. The clinical syndrome consists of **asymmetric oligoarthritis, urethritis, conjunctivitis,** and characteristic **skin and mucous membrane lesions.** The syndrome is usually transient, lasting from 1 to several months, but recurrences associated with varying degrees of disability are common. A reactive arthritis may follow dysentery caused by *Shigella flexneri*, *Salmonella* species, *Yersinia enterocolitica*, or *Clostridium difficile* infections. Articular manifestations are identical to those of Reiter's syndrome; extra-articular manifestations may occur but tend to be mild. Conservative therapy is indicated for control of pain and inflammation in these diseases. Spontaneous remissions are common, making evaluation of therapy difficult. **NSAIDs** (especially indomethacin) are often useful, and **selective COX-2 inhibitors** should also provide relief (see Therapeutic Approaches to Rheumatic Disease, secs. **II** and **III**). **Sulfasalazine** or **methotrexate** may be of benefit in some patients (see Therapeutic Approaches to Rheumatic Disease, sec. **V**) (Table 23-1). In unusually severe cases, **glucocorticoid therapy** may be required to prevent rapid joint destruction (see Therapeutic Approaches to Rheumatic Disease, sec. **IV**) (Table 23-1). Prolonged antibiotic therapy (such as doxycycline, 100 mg PO bid) may be beneficial in Reiter's syndrome that is related to *Chlamydia*. **Conjunctivitis** usually is transient and benign, but ophthalmologic referral and treatment with topical or systemic glucocorticoids are indicated for **iritis.**

**IV. Psoriatic arthritis.** Seven percent of patients with psoriasis have some form of inflammatory arthritis. Five major patterns of joint disease occur: (1) asymmetric oligoarticular arthritis, (2) distal interphalangeal joint involvement in association with nail disease, (3) symmetric rheumatoid-like polyarthritis, (4) spondylitis and sacroiliitis, and (5) arthritis mutilans. **NSAIDs,** particularly indomethacin, are used to treat the arthritic manifestations of psoriasis, in conjunction with appropriate measures for the skin disease. **Selective COX-2 inhibitors** should also be effective (see Therapeutic Approaches to Rheumatic Disease, secs. **II** and **III**). **Intra-articular glucocorticoids** may be useful in the oligoarticular form of the disease, but injection through a psoriatic plaque should be avoided. Severe skin and joint diseases generally respond well to **methotrexate** (see Therapeutic Approaches to Rheumatic Disease, sec. **V)** (Table 23-1). **Sulfasalazine, leflunomide, TNF-α blockers,** and **hydroxychloroquine** (see Therapeutic Approaches to Rheumatic Disease, sec. **V**) (Table 23-1) may also have disease-modifying effects in polyarthritis. When reconstructive joint surgery is performed, colonization of psoriatic skin with *S. aureus* increases the risk of wound infection.

## Systemic Lupus Erythematosus

**SLE** is a multisystem disease of unknown etiology that primarily affects women of childbearing age. Autoantibodies to nuclear and other autoantigens are the hallmark of disease. The course of this disease is highly variable and unpredictable. Disease manifestations are protean, ranging in severity from fatigue, malaise, weight loss, arthritis or arthralgias, fever, photosensitivity, rashes, and serositis to potentially life-threatening thrombocytopenia, hemolytic anemia, nephritis, cerebritis, vasculitis, pneumonitis, myositis, and myocarditis. Patients with lupus have accelerated coronary and peripheral vascular disease, which should be managed aggressively.

I. **Conservative therapy** is warranted if the patient's manifestations are mild.

A. **General supportive measures** include adequate sleep and avoidance of fatigue, as mild disease exacerbations may subside after a few days of bed rest. For patients with photosensitive rashes, sunscreens with a sun protection factor of 30 or greater, protective clothing, such as a hat and long sleeves, and avoidance of sun exposure are recommended. Isolated skin lesions may respond to topical glucocorticoids.

B. **NSAIDs** usually control SLE-associated arthritis, arthralgias, fever, and serositis but not fatigue, malaise, or major organ system involvement. The response to **selective COX-2 inhibitors** should be similar (see Therapeutic Approaches to Rheumatic Disease, secs. **II** and **III**). Hepatic and renal toxicities of the NSAIDs appear to be increased in SLE. NSAIDs should be avoided in patients with active nephritis.

C. **Hydroxychloroquine** (see Therapeutic Approaches to Rheumatic Disease, sec. **V.C**) (Table 23-1) may be effective in the treatment of rash, photosensitivity, arthralgias, arthritis, alopecia, and malaise associated with SLE and in the treatment of **discoid and subacute cutaneous lupus erythematosus.** Skin lesions may begin to improve within a few days, but joint symptoms may require 6–10 weeks to subside. The drug is not effective for treating fever or renal, CNS, and hematologic problems.

II. **Glucocorticoid therapy** (see Therapeutic Approaches to Rheumatic Disease, sec. **IV**) (Table 23-1)

A. **Indications** for systemic glucocorticoids include (1) life-threatening manifestations of SLE, such as glomerulonephritis, CNS involvement, thrombocytopenia, and hemolytic anemia, and (2) debilitating manifestations of SLE (fatigue, rash) that are unresponsive to conservative therapy.

1. **Dosage.** Patients with severe or potentially life-threatening complications of SLE should be treated with prednisone, 1–2 mg/kg PO qd, which can be given in divided doses. After disease is controlled, prednisone should be tapered slowly, the dosage being reduced by no more than 10% every 7–10 days. More rapid reduction may result in relapse. Alternate-day therapy may reduce many of the adverse effects of long-term glucocorticoid therapy. **IV pulse therapy** in the form of methylprednisolone, 500 mg IV q12h for 3–5 days, has been used in SLE in such life-threatening situations as rapidly progressive renal failure, active CNS disease, and severe thrombocytopenia. Patients who do not show improvement with this regimen probably are unresponsive to steroids, and other therapeutic alternatives must be considered. A course of oral prednisone should follow completion of pulse therapy. Electrolytes should be monitored in patients who receive high-dose steroids.

**III. Immunosuppressive therapy** (see Therapeutic Approaches to Rheumatic Disease, sec. **V**) (Table 23-1)

**A. Indications** for immunosuppressive therapy in SLE include (1) such life-threatening manifestations of SLE as glomerulonephritis, CNS involvement, thrombocytopenia, and hemolytic anemia, and (2) the inability to reduce corticosteroid dosage or severe corticosteroid side effects.

**B. Choice of an immunosuppressive** is individualized to the clinical situation. Often, **cyclophosphamide** is used for life-threatening manifestations of SLE. High-dose IV pulse cyclophosphamide may be less toxic but also less immunosuppressive than is low-dose daily PO cyclophosphamide. **Azathioprine** and **mycophenolate mofetil** are used more often as steroid-sparing agents but may not be as effective as cyclophosphamide in treating nephritis.

**IV. Transplantation and chronic hemodialysis** have been used successfully in SLE patients with renal failure. Clinical and serologic evidence of disease activity often disappears when renal failure ensues. The survival rate in these patients is equivalent to that of patients with other forms of chronic renal disease. Recurrence of nephritis in the allograft rarely occurs.

**V. Pregnancy in SLE.** An increased incidence of second-trimester spontaneous abortion and stillbirth has been reported in some women with antibodies to cardiolipin or the lupus anticoagulant. Neonatal lupus may occur in offspring of SSA/Ro-positive mothers. SLE patients may experience an exacerbation in the activity of their disease in the third trimester or peripartum period. Differentiation between active SLE and preeclampsia often is difficult. Women whose SLE is in good control when they become pregnant are less likely to have a flare of disease during pregnancy.

## Systemic Sclerosis

**Systemic sclerosis (scleroderma)** is a systemic illness of unknown cause that is characterized by thickening and hardening of the skin and visceral organs. Most of the manifestations of scleroderma have a vascular basis (Raynaud's phenomenon, telangiectasias, nail fold capillary changes, early edematous skin changes, nephrosclerosis), but frank vasculitis rarely is seen. The label *scleroderma* includes diffuse scleroderma and limited scleroderma (formerly known as the **CREST syndrome: c**alcinosis, **R**aynaud's phenomenon, **e**sophageal dysmotility, **s**clerodactyly, **t**elangiectasias). **Diffuse scleroderma** is characterized by extensive skin disease, the potential for hypertensive "renal crisis," and shortened survival. **Limited scleroderma,** in contrast, may be associated with primary pulmonary hypertension or biliary cirrhosis and has skin thickening that is limited to the face and the distal forearms and hands. Up to 70% of patients with limited scleroderma have anticentromere antibody, which is not seen in individuals with diffuse scleroderma. No curative therapy for scleroderma exists; instead, treatment focuses on particular organ involvement in a problem-oriented manner.

**I. Raynaud's phenomenon** is a reversible vasospasm of the digital arteries that can result in ischemia of the digits. Patients must be instructed to avoid exposure of the entire body to cold, protect the hands and feet from cold and trauma, and discontinue cigarette smoking. Most pharmacologic approaches have had limited success. **Calcium channel antagonists** (e.g., nifedipine) are the preferred initial agents, although they may exacerbate gastroesophageal reflux and constipation in these patients. Alternative vasodilators, such as prazosin, occasionally are helpful, but significant side effects, especially orthostatic hypotension, may preclude their use. Daily low-dose aspirin therapy is often prescribed for its antiplatelet effects. **Sympathetic ganglion blockade** with a long-acting anesthetic agent may be useful when a patient has progressive digital ulceration that fails to improve with conservative therapy. Surgical digital sympathectomy may also be beneficial.

II. **Skin and periarticular changes.** No therapeutic agent is clearly effective for these cutaneous manifestations, although penicillamine or methotrexate is sometimes used. **Physical therapy** is important to retard and reduce joint contractures.

III. **GI involvement.** Reflux esophagitis generally responds to standard therapy (e.g., **$H_2$-receptor antagonists, proton pump inhibitors,** and **promotility agents;** see Chap. 16, Gastrointestinal Diseases). Occasionally, esophageal strictures require mechanical esophageal dilatation. Decreased motility of bowel segments can occur, leading to bacterial overgrowth, malabsorption, diarrhea, and weight loss. Treatment with broad-spectrum antimicrobials in a rotating sequence including **metronidazole** often improves the malabsorption. Metoclopramide may reduce bloating and distention. Rarely, severe constipation or intestinal pseudo-obstruction may occur.

IV. **Renal involvement.** The appearance of hypertension and renal insufficiency, often associated with a microangiopathic hemolytic anemia, signals a poor prognosis. Aggressive BP control with **angiotensin-converting enzyme inhibitors** may delay or prevent the onset of uremia, particularly in patients with a serum creatinine of less than 3 mg/dl. Angiotensin-receptor blockade does not appear to be as effective.

V. **Cardiopulmonary involvement.** Patchy myocardial fibrosis can result in CHF or arrhythmias. Coronary artery vasospasm can cause angina pectoris and may respond to calcium channel antagonists. Pulmonary involvement includes pleurisy with effusion, interstitial fibrosis, pulmonary hypertension, and cor pulmonale. Standard therapies for these conditions are used (see Chap. 9, Pulmonary Disease). Patients with rapidly progressive pulmonary parenchymal disease may benefit from a course of cyclophosphamide.

## Necrotizing Vasculitis

**Necrotizing vasculitis** is characterized by inflammation and necrosis of blood vessels leading to tissue damage. This diagnosis includes a broad spectrum of disorders that have various causes and involve vessels of different types, sizes, and locations. The immunopathogenic process often involves immune complexes. Although in most cases the inciting antigen has not been identified, vasculitic syndromes have been associated with chronic hepatitis B and C. Table 23-2 summarizes clinical features and diagnostic and treatment approaches to the most common forms of vasculitis.

I. **Clinical features** are diverse and depend in part on the size of the vessel involved. Systemic manifestations including fever and weight loss are also common. The response to therapy and the long-term prognosis of these disorders are highly variable. Vasculitis "mimics" should be considered, including bacterial endocarditis, HIV, atrial myxoma, paraneoplastic syndromes, cholesterol emboli, and cocaine and amphetamine use.

II. **Management** should include consultation with a physician experienced in the treatment of these disorders. Treatment should be tailored to the severity of organ system involvement.

   A. **Glucocorticoids** are the usual initial therapy and are beneficial in most vasculitides (see Therapeutic Approaches to Rheumatic Disease, sec. **IV**) (Table 23-1). Although vasculitis that is limited to the skin may respond to lower doses of corticosteroids, the initial dosage for visceral involvement should be high (prednisone, 1–2 mg/kg/day). **If life-threatening manifestations are present,** a brief course of high-dose pulse therapy with methylprednisolone, 500 mg IV q12h for 3–5 days, should be considered.

**Table 23-2.** Clinical features and diagnostic and treatment approaches to vasculitis

| Vasculitic syndrome | Clinical features | Diagnostic approach | Treatment |
|---|---|---|---|
| Large-vessel involvement | | | |
| Giant-cell arteritis | Headache<br>Jaw claudication | Temporal artery biopsy | Prednisone, 60–80 mg/d |
| Takayasu's arteritis | Finger ischemia<br>Arm claudication | Aortic arch arteriogram | Prednisone, 60–80 mg/d |
| Medium-vessel involvement | | | |
| Polyarteritis nodosa | Skin ulcers<br>Nephritis<br>Mononeuritis multiplex<br>Mesenteric ischemia | Skin biopsy<br>Renal biopsy<br>Sural nerve biopsy<br>Mesenteric angiogram<br>Hepatitis B, C testing | Prednisone, 60–100 mg/d<br>Cyclophosphamide, 1–2 mg/kg/d, can be added |
| Wegener's granulomatosis | Sinusitis<br>Pulmonary infiltrates<br>Nephritis | c-ANCA<br>Lung biopsy | Prednisone, 60–100 mg/d *and* cyclophosphamide, 1–2 mg/kg/d |
| Microscopic polyangiitis | Pulmonary infiltrates<br>Nephritis | p-ANCA<br>Renal biopsy | Prednisone, 60–100 mg/d<br>Cyclophosphamide, 1–2 mg/kg/d, can be added |
| Vasculitis in SLE or RA | Skin ulcers<br>Polyneuropathy | Skin or sural nerve biopsy | Prednisone, 60–80 mg/d<br>Cyclophosphamide, 1–2 mg/kg/d, can be added |
| Small-vessel involvement | | | |
| Hypersensitivity vasculitis | Palpable purpura | Skin biopsy | Prednisone, 20–60 mg/d<br>Discontinue inciting drug |
| Henoch-Schönlein purpura | Palpable purpura<br>Nephritis<br>Mesenteric ischemia | Skin biopsy<br>Renal biopsy | Supportive treatment<br>Prednisone, 20–60 mg/d, may be needed |

c-ANCA, cytoplasmic antineutrophil cytoplasmic antibodies; p-ANCA, perinuclear antineutrophil cytoplasmic antibodies; RA, rheumatoid arthritis; SLE, systemic lupus erythematosus.

B. **Immunosuppressives,** in particular oral cyclophosphamide, often are used in the initial management of necrotizing vasculitis, especially when major organ system involvement (e.g., lung, kidney, or nerve) is present (see Therapeutic Approaches to Rheumatic Disease, sec. **V**) (Table 23-1).

C. **Trimethoprim/sulfamethoxazole** can be used in variants of Wegener's granulomatosis limited to the upper airway and may also be useful in preventing relapse, but is not sufficient treatment for systemic disease. This drug is also used for *P. carinii* prophylaxis in patients who are receiving cyclophosphamide.

## Polymyalgia Rheumatica and Temporal Arteritis

**Polymyalgia rheumatica (PMR)** presents in elderly patients as proximal limb girdle pain, morning stiffness, constitutional symptoms, and an elevated erythrocyte sedimentation rate (ESR). Up to 40% of patients with PMR also have temporal arteritis (TA). TA is a form of vasculitis that presents with headache, scalp tenderness, jaw or tongue claudication, vision disturbances (including blindness), stroke, an elevated ESR (often >100), and, in up to 40% of patients, symptoms of PMR.

I. **Management of PMR.** If PMR is present without evidence of TA, **prednisone,** 10–15 mg PO qd, usually produces dramatic clinical improvement within a few days. The ESR should return to normal during initial treatment, but subsequent therapeutic decisions should be based on ESR and clinical status. Glucocorticoid therapy can be tapered gradually to a maintenance dosage of 5–10 mg PO qd but should be continued for at least 1 year to minimize the risk of relapse. NSAIDs may facilitate reduction in prednisone dosage.

II. **Management of TA.** Patients who are suspected of having TA should be treated promptly with **prednisone,** 1–2 mg/kg/day PO qd, to prevent irreversible blindness. The diagnosis of TA should be confirmed by **temporal artery biopsy,** which is not altered by 3–5 days of prednisone therapy. High-dose steroid therapy should be continued until symptoms have abated and the ESR has returned to normal. The dosage then should be tapered gradually to 10–20 mg, with close monitoring of the ESR and clinical status, and should be maintained for 1–2 years.

## Cryoglobulin Syndromes

**Cryoglobulins** are serum proteins that reversibly precipitate in the cold. Cryoglobulinemia is traditionally categorized as monoclonal (formerly type 1) or polyclonal (mixed; formerly types 2 and 3). Patients with **monoclonal cryoglobulinemia** usually have an underlying lymphoproliferative disorder such as myeloma or lymphoma. Symptoms are related to hyperviscosity (blurring of vision, digital ischemia, headache, lethargy) and respond to treatment of the underlying disorder, although plasmapheresis can be used in the acute setting. The majority of patients with **mixed cryoglobulinemia** have hepatitis C; the remainder of cases are found in association with autoimmune disorders such as SLE or RA, or are idiopathic. Clinical manifestations of mixed cryoglobulinemia are mediated by immune complex deposition (arthralgias, purpura, glomerulonephritis, and neuropathy). **Therapy** for secondary cryoglobulinemic states is directed at the underlying disease. Treatment of hepatitis C with interferon-alpha and ribavirin effectively reduces cryoglobulins, although they may recur when treatment is stopped. Prednisone or immunosuppressive agents can be used to treat cryoglobulinemia due to SLE or RA but may exacerbate hepatitis C (see Chap. 17, Liver Diseases).

## Polymyositis and Dermatomyositis

**Polymyositis (PM)** is an inflammatory myopathy that presents as weakness and occasionally tenderness of the proximal musculature. Diagnosis is corroborated by an abnormal electromyogram, elevated muscle enzyme levels (creatine kinase, aldolase, AST), and muscle biopsy. **Dermatomyositis (DM)** is PM with a concomitant rash. PM-DM can occur in three forms: (1) alone, (2) in association with any of the other autoimmune diseases, or (3) with a variety of neoplasms. Risk factors for malignancy in the setting of myositis include the presence of DM, cutaneous vasculitis, male sex, and advanced age. Screening for common neoplasms, such as colon, lung, breast, and prostate cancer, should be considered in these patients. Certain subsets of disease are associated with myositis-specific antibodies such as Jo-1 and signal recognition particle. These antibodies have therapeutic and prognostic implications, and therefore levels should be measured in all patients. When PM-DM occurs without associated disease, it usually responds well to **prednisone,** 1–2 mg/kg PO qd (see Therapeutic Approaches to Rheumatic Disease, sec. **IV**) (Table 23-1). Systemic complaints, such as fever and malaise, respond to therapy first, followed by muscle enzymes and, finally, muscle strength. Once serum enzyme levels normalize, the prednisone dosage should be reduced slowly to maintenance levels of 10–20 mg PO qd or 20–40 mg PO qod. The appearance of steroid-induced myopathy and hypokalemia may complicate therapeutic assessment. IV infusion of **immunoglobulin** may hasten improvement of severe dysphagia. PM-DM associated with neoplasia tends to be less responsive to glucocorticoid therapy but may improve after removal of an associated malignant tumor. Patients who do not respond or cannot tolerate the side effects of glucocorticoids may respond to methotrexate or azathioprine (see Therapeutic Approaches to Rheumatic Disease, sec. **V**) (Table 23-1). **Physical therapy** is essential in the management of myositis. Bed rest with active assisted range of motion is appropriate during very active disease, with more active exercise prescribed to improve strength once inflammation has been controlled.

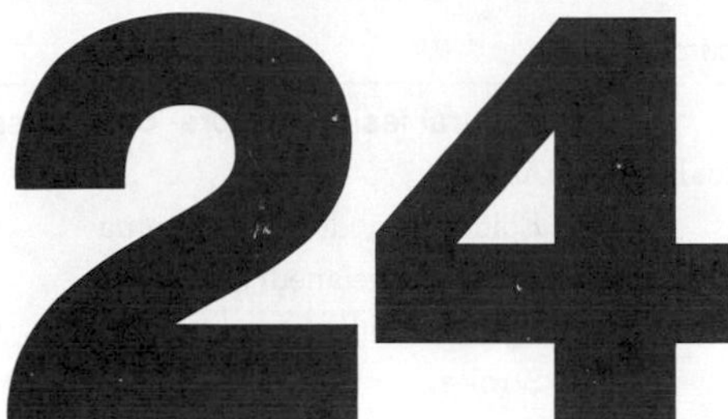

# Neurologic Disorders

Kelvin A. Yamada and
Sylvia Awadalla

## Alterations in Consciousness

**I. Coma** is a state of complete behavioral unresponsiveness to external stimulation in which the patient lies with the eyes closed. Because some causes of coma may lead to irreversible brain damage, expeditious evaluation and treatment must proceed concurrently. The need for neurosurgical intervention must be determined promptly.

**A. Pathophysiology.** Coma results from diffuse or multifocal dysfunction of **both cerebral hemispheres** or of the **reticular activating system** in the brain stem. Unilateral cerebral lesions (e.g., stroke or tumor) rarely impair consciousness unless they produce sufficient mass effect to compress the opposite hemisphere (midline shift or subfalcine herniation) or the brain stem (transtentorial herniation). Mass lesions in the posterior fossa cause coma by compressing the brain stem. Metabolic disorders impair consciousness by diffuse effects on both cerebral hemispheres. See Table 24-1 for a listing of possible etiologies.

**B. Evaluation and management of the comatose patient**

1. The **initial steps** are to control airway and ventilation, administer oxygen, maintain body temperature, and monitor vital signs, including oximetry and continuous ECG.
2. If trauma has or may have occurred, **immobilization of the spine** should be done immediately while arranging radiographs to identify or exclude fracture or instability.
3. An **IV line should be secured,** and adequate circulation should be established. Initial laboratory evaluation should include blood for glucose, electrolytes, BUN, CBC, calcium, ABG, cultures, liver enzymes, ammonia, prothrombin time (PT), activated partial thromboplastin time (aPTT), and blood type and screen. Blood and urine should be sent for toxicologic/drug analysis. A urinalysis should be performed.
4. IV **thiamine** (100 mg), followed by **dextrose** (50 ml 50% dextrose in water = 25 g dextrose), should be administered. Thiamine is administered first because dextrose administration in thiamine-deficient patients may precipitate Wernicke's encephalopathy.
5. IV **naloxone** (opiate antagonist), 0.01 mg/kg, should be administered if opiate intoxication is suspected (coma, respiratory depression, small reactive pupils). Naloxone may provoke opiate withdrawal syndrome in addicted patients. **Flumazenil** (benzodiazepine antagonist), 0.2 mg IV, may reverse benzodiazepine intoxication, but its duration of action is short, and additional doses may be needed. Flumazenil can cause seizures.
6. The **initial assessment** should focus on a **history** of trauma, seizures, medications, alcohol or drug use, and existing medical conditions. The **general physical examination** may reveal a systemic illness associated

**Table 24-1.** Causes of stupor and coma

| Diffuse or metabolic | Structural lesions, supra- or infratentorial |
|---|---|
| CNS infection/inflammation (vasculitis) | Abscess |
| Diabetic ketoacidosis | Epidural/subdural hematoma |
| Drugs and toxins | Hemorrhage/aneurysm |
| Global cerebral ischemia | Hydrocephalus |
| Head trauma | Stroke |
| Hypercalcemia | Tumor |
| Hypernatremia or hyponatremia | Venous occlusion |
| Hypertensive encephalopathy | |
| Hypoglycemia | |
| Hypoxemia or hypercapnia | |
| Liver failure | |
| Renal failure | |
| Sepsis | |
| Subclinical seizures/postictal state | |
| Thiamine deficiency | |

with coma (e.g., cirrhosis, hemodialysis shunt, rash of meningococcemia) or signs of head trauma (e.g., lacerations, periorbital or mastoid ecchymosis, hemotympanum). The **neurologic examination** (see sec. **III**) should localize structural lesions and diagnose brain herniation. Serial examinations are performed to detect and intervene if clinical deterioration occurs.

7. **Herniation** (see sec. **III.F**) must be recognized and treated immediately. Treatment consists of measures to lower intracranial pressure while surgically treatable etiologies are identified or excluded.
   a. Endotracheal intubation is usually performed to enable **hyperventilation** to a carbon dioxide tension ($PCO_2$) of 25–30 mm Hg, which reduces intracranial pressure within minutes by cerebral vasoconstriction. Bag-mask ventilation can be performed if manipulation of the neck is precluded by possible or established spinal instability. Reduction of $PCO_2$ below 25 mm Hg is not recommended because it may reduce cerebral blood flow excessively.
   b. Administration of **mannitol** IV, 1–2 g/kg over 30–60 minutes, osmotically reduces brain free water. The effect peaks at 90 minutes.
   c. **Dexamethasone,** 10 mg IV, followed by 4 mg IV q6h, reduces the edema surrounding a tumor or abscess.
8. As soon as the patient's condition is stable, a **head CT** scan should be obtained to **distinguish operable lesions** (e.g., cerebellar hematoma) from **inoperable lesions** (e.g., pontine hemorrhage). **Coagulopathy** (see Chap. 18, Disorders of Hemostasis) should be corrected if intracranial hemorrhage is diagnosed and before surgical treatment or invasive procedures (e.g., lumbar puncture) are performed. Each patient's circumstance should be carefully assessed before therapeutic anticoagulation is reversed.
9. **Lumbar puncture** is indicated whenever CNS infection is considered and when subarachnoid hemorrhage (SAH) is clinically suspected but not confirmed by neuroimaging. **One should not perform lumbar puncture if a mass lesion or midline shift is present on CT scan. In such**

**cases, if CNS infection is suspected, appropriate broad-spectrum antibiotics and acyclovir should be administered without lumbar puncture** (see Central Nervous System Infections in Chap. 13, Treatment of Infectious Diseases). If cerebrospinal fluid (CSF) is obtained, it should be sent for cell count, protein, glucose, Gram stain, bacterial cultures, and polymerase chain reaction (PCR) for pathogens (particularly herpes simplex). Other potentially helpful studies include detection of bacterial antigens (particularly if antibiotics have been given), acid-fast stain, India ink stain, cryptococcal antigen, and fungal and viral cultures. If possible, extra CSF should be saved and refrigerated.

10. **EEG** is helpful in the diagnosis of subclinical electrical seizures (nonconvulsive status epilepticus). Some conditions have characteristic (not necessarily diagnostic) EEG findings, including hepatic encephalopathy (triphasic waves), herpes simplex virus encephalitis (periodic complexes, PLEDS), and barbiturate or other sedative intoxications (beta activity).
11. If the initial evaluation yields no diagnosis, a metabolic or toxic etiology is most likely. The patient should be admitted to an ICU with continued supportive care while additional diagnostic studies are pursued.

**II. Acute confusional states (delirium)** result from diffuse or multifocal cerebral dysfunction and are characterized by impaired attention, concentration, and memory; fluctuations of consciousness; disorientation and hallucinations; incoherent speech; and agitation.

**A. Etiologies** include those listed in Table 24-1 and also medication effect or withdrawal, drug intoxication or withdrawal (see sec. **II.C** and Drug Overdose in Chap. 25, Medical Emergencies), endocrine disease (i.e., thyroid disorders, diabetes, Cushing's disease), acute intermittent porphyria, confusional migraine, and complex partial seizures. Mild systemic illness commonly produces delirium in an elderly or demented patient, especially in combination with new medications, fever, or sleep deprivation. Structural lesions such as in Table 24-1 can also cause delirium. Acute confusion must be distinguished from **aphasia** [secondary to transient ischemic attack (TIA), stroke, trauma, seizure, abscess, etc.] and transient global amnesia. Acute psychosis can mimic acute delirium, but confusion and depressed consciousness are usually less prominent.

**B.** Guidelines for initial **evaluation and management** are similar to those for the comatose patient (see sec. **I.B**).

1. The **history** may suggest one of the above etiologies. One should carefully review medications and available laboratory results.
2. The **physical and neurologic** examination may reveal systemic illness (e.g., pneumonia) or neurologic signs (meningismus or paralysis) to narrow the differential diagnosis.
3. **Maintenance of adequate airway, circulation (secure IV access), and oxygenation** is an important initial measure. One should obtain a chest radiograph and arterial blood gas and send blood for glucose, electrolytes, BUN, calcium, magnesium, ammonia, thyroid-stimulating hormone, CBC, and cultures. Urine and blood should be sent for urinalysis and drug/toxicologic analysis.
4. **Head CT scan** quickly identifies intracranial hematoma and may demonstrate other structural lesions, such as stroke, SAH, or abscess (see sec. **I.B.8**).
5. **Lumbar puncture** is indicated whenever CNS infection is considered and sometimes to diagnose SAH (see sec. **I.B.9**).
6. Additional measures include administration of IV **thiamine** (100 mg) **followed by** 50 ml 50% **dextrose.** Sedatives are avoided if possible, but, if necessary, low doses of haloperidol (0.5–1 mg), lorazepam (1 mg), or chlordiazepoxide (25 mg) can be used. A quiet well-lit room with close observation is necessary. The use of restraints is discouraged but is sometimes

needed temporarily for patient safety. Restraints should be carefully adjusted and checked periodically to prevent excessive constriction.

C. **Alcohol withdrawal** typically occurs when illness or hospitalization interrupts alcohol intake and deserves emphasis because severe forms carry significant mortality.

1. **Tremulousness, irritability, anorexia, and nausea characterize minor alcohol withdrawal.** Symptoms usually appear within a few hours after reduction or cessation of alcohol consumption and resolve within 48 hours. Treatment includes a well-lit room, reassurance, and the presence of family or friends. Thiamine, 100 mg IM, followed by 100 mg PO qd; multivitamins containing folic acid; and a balanced diet as tolerated should be administered. Chlordiazepoxide (25–100 mg PO q6h) with dosage adjusted until the patient is calm may reduce the incidence of seizures and delirium tremens (*JAMA* 278:144, 1997). Serial evaluation for signs of major alcohol withdrawal is essential; social circumstances often dictate whether this should be done at home or in the hospital.
2. **Alcohol withdrawal seizures,** typically one or a few brief generalized convulsions, occur 12–48 hours after cessation of ethanol intake. Antiepileptic drugs are not indicated for typical alcohol withdrawal seizures. Other causes for seizures (see Seizures, sec. **II**) must be excluded. If hypoglycemia is present, thiamine should be administered before glucose.
3. **Severe withdrawal or delirium tremens** consists of tremulousness, hallucinations, agitation, confusion, disorientation, and autonomic hyperactivity (fever, tachycardia, diaphoresis), typically occurring 72–96 hours after cessation of drinking. Symptoms generally resolve within 3–5 days. Delirium tremens complicates 5–10% of cases of alcohol withdrawal, with mortality up to 15%. Other causes of delirium must be considered in the differential diagnosis (see sec. **II.A**). One should administer supportive management as in sec. **II.C.1.**
   a. **Chlordiazepoxide** is an effective sedative for delirium tremens, 100 mg IV or PO q2–6h as needed (maximum dose, 500 mg in the first 24 hours). One-half the initial 24-hour dose can be administered over the next 24 hours; the dosage can be reduced by 25–50 mg/day each day thereafter. Longer-lasting benzodiazepines (i.e., chloridiazepoxide) facilitate smoother tapering, but shorter-acting agents (i.e., **lorazepam,** 1–2 mg PO or IV q6–8h as needed) may be desirable in older patients and those with reduced drug clearance. In patients with severe hepatic failure, **oxazepam** (15–30 mg PO q6–8h as needed), which is excreted by the kidney, can be used instead of chlordiazepoxide.
   b. **Maintenance of fluid and electrolyte balance** is important. Alcoholic patients are susceptible to hypomagnesemia, hypokalemia, hypoglycemia, and dehydration, which may be severe due to fever, diaphoresis, and vomiting.
   c. Other drugs, including clonidine, atenolol, haloperidol, carbamazepine, and others, have been used to treat alcohol withdrawal. Controlled studies and careful evaluation of the indications for the individual patient must dictate their use for alcohol withdrawal.

**III. Neurologic examination of patients with alteration in consciousness**

A. **Level of consciousness** can be assessed semiquantitatively and followed by all levels of caregivers with the **Glasgow Coma Scale** (Table 24-2). Points are assigned in three categories using the best response and are added together to give scores that range from 3 (unresponsive) to 15 (normal).

B. **Respiratory rate and pattern. Cheyne-Stokes** respirations (rhythmic crescendo-decrescendo hyperpnea alternating with periods of apnea) occur in metabolic coma and supratentorial lesions, as well as in chronic pulmonary disease and CHF. **Hyperventilation** is usually a sign of metabolic acidosis, hypoxemia, pneumonia, or other pulmonary disease but may be caused by upper brain stem injury. **Apneustic breathing** (long pauses after inspira-

**Table 24-2.** Glasgow Coma Scale

| | |
|---|---|
| **Eye opening** | |
| Spontaneous | 4 |
| To voice | 3 |
| To painful stimulation | 2 |
| None | 1 |
| **Best verbal response** | |
| Oriented | 5 |
| Confused | 4 |
| Inappropriate words | 3 |
| Unintelligible sounds | 2 |
| None | 1 |
| **Best motor response** | |
| Follows commands | 6 |
| Localizes pain | 5 |
| Withdraws from pain | 4 |
| Flexor response | 3 |
| Extensor response | 2 |
| None | 1 |

tion), **cluster breathing** (breathing in short bursts), and **ataxic breathing** (irregular breaths without pattern) are signs of brain stem injury and warn of impending respiratory arrest.

C. **Pupil size and light reactivity are extremely valuable neurologic signs.**
   1. **Anisocoria** (asymmetric pupils) in a patient with altered mental status requires diagnosis and treatment, or exclusion, of **uncal herniation.** Anisocoria may be physiologic or produced by mydriatics (e.g., scopolamine, atropine).
   2. **Small but reactive** pupils are seen in narcotic overdose, metabolic encephalopathy, and thalamic or pontine lesions.
   3. **Midposition fixed** pupils imply midbrain lesions and occur in transtentorial herniation.
   4. **Bilaterally fixed and dilated** pupils are seen with severe anoxic encephalopathy or intoxication with drugs such as scopolamine, atropine, glutethimide, or methyl alcohol.

D. **Eye movements.** The **oculocephalic** (doll's eyes) test is performed in a comatose patient (if no cervical injury is present) by quickly turning the head laterally or vertically. With an intact brain stem, the eyes move conjugately opposite the direction of head movement. The **oculovestibular** (cold caloric) test is used if cervical trauma is suspected or if eye movements are absent with the oculocephalic test. To perform the test, the head should be elevated 30 degrees above horizontal and the tympanic membrane visualized to ensure that it is intact and unobstructed. The tympanic membrane should be lavaged with 10–50 ml ice water. In the patient with intact brain stem function, eyes should move conjugately toward the lavaged ear. Vertical gaze can be assessed with simultaneous lavage of both ears.
   1. **Absence of all eye movements** indicates a bilateral pontine lesion or drug-induced ophthalmoplegia (e.g., barbiturates, phenytoin, paralytics).
   2. **Disconjugate gaze** suggests a brain stem lesion.

3. A **gaze preference** conjugately to one side suggests a unilateral pontine or frontal lobe lesion. An associated hemiparesis and oculocephalic and oculovestibular tests help localize the lesion. In **pontine lesions** gaze preference is **toward** the paretic side, and eyes may move toward but do not cross midline. In **frontal lobe lesions** gaze preference is **away** from the paresis, and eyes move conjugately across midline to both sides.
4. **Impaired vertical eye movement** occurs in midbrain lesions, central herniation, and acute hydrocephalus. Conjugate depression and impaired elevation suggest a tectal lesion.

E. **Motor responses** help to assess the level of impaired consciousness (see also Table 24-2). Asymmetric motor responses (spontaneous or stimulus induced) have localizing value.

F. **Herniation** occurs when mass lesions or edema cause shifts in brain tissue. Prompt diagnosis and treatment are necessary to prevent irreversible brain damage and death (see sec. **I.B.7**).

1. **Nonspecific signs and symptoms of increased intracranial pressure** include headache, nausea, vomiting, hypertension, bradycardia, papilledema, sixth nerve palsy, transient visual obscurations, and alterations in consciousness.
2. **Uncal herniation** is caused by unilateral supratentorial lesions and may progress rapidly. The earliest sign is a dilated pupil ipsilateral to the mass, diminished consciousness, and hemiparesis, first contralateral to the mass and later ipsilateral to the mass (Kernohan's notch syndrome).
3. **Central herniation** is caused by medial or bilateral supratentorial lesions. Signs include progressive alteration of consciousness, Cheyne-Stokes or normal respirations followed later by central hyperventilation, midposition and unreactive pupils, loss of upward gaze, and posturing of the extremities.
4. **Tonsillar herniation** occurs when pressure in the posterior fossa forces the cerebellar tonsils through the foramen magnum, compressing the medulla. Signs include altered level of consciousness and respiratory irregularity or apnea.

## IV. Brain death

A. **Brain death** occurs from irreversible brain injury that is sufficient to eliminate all cortical and brain stem function permanently. Because the vital centers in the brain stem sustain cardiovascular and respiratory functions, brain death is incompatible with survival despite mechanical ventilation and cardiovascular and nutritional supportive measures. Brain death is distinguished from persistent vegetative state, in which the absence of higher cortical function is accompanied by intact brain stem function. Although patients in a **persistent vegetative state** are unable to think, speak, understand, or meaningfully respond to visual, verbal, or auditory stimuli, with nutritional and supportive care their cardiovascular and respiratory functions can sustain viability for years. Most hospitals adopt guidelines and criteria for establishing brain death, which should be consulted in each situation. Assessments are usually carried out by attending neurologic or neurosurgical consultants. Summarized below are the major elements of the Barnes-Jewish Hospital and Washington University Medical Center guidelines for establishing brain death.

B. **The first and most critical step in establishing the diagnosis of brain death is to establish an irreversible, untreatable etiology for the brain injury.** Examples include global ischemia (cardiac arrest), asphyxia (near-drowning), intracranial hemorrhage with uncal or central herniation, and severe head trauma with diffuse cerebral edema. Contributing factors that may be reversible, such as hypoxia, hypotension, hypothermia, severe metabolic derangements, and medications that depress consciousness (e.g., barbiturates, benzodiazepines, opiates), should be corrected, but this is not always possible.

**C. The neurologic examination** is a critical element of the diagnosis.
1. The patient is comatose.
2. The patient has no response to visual, auditory, or painful stimulation.
3. The pupils are not reactive.
4. No eye movements occur by oculocephalic or oculovestibular maneuvers (cold calorics, see sec. **III.D**).
5. Corneal, gag, and cough reflexes are absent.
6. Neither spontaneous movement nor motor response to noxious external stimulation occurs. Spinal reflexes do not preclude the diagnosis of brain death.
7. No respiratory effort is seen; the patient requires mechanical ventilation.
   a. The oxygen-apnea test is used to confirm apnea without mechanical ventilation. After ventilation with 100% oxygen to increase oxygen tension, the ventilator is disconnected and a catheter with 6 L/minute oxygen is placed in the endotracheal tube. If there is no respiratory effort when the $PCO_2$ rises above 60 mm Hg, apnea is established.
   b. Arterial or venous blood gas is conveniently obtained if arterial or central IV catheters are in place.
   c. This part of the examination is usually reserved for last because patients are often unstable and the apnea test may produce cardiopulmonary arrest. The possibility that cardiopulmonary arrest may occur must be carefully considered.

**D. Ancillary diagnostic studies** provide supportive data, but brain death is a clinical diagnosis.
1. **EEG** is performed to establish **electrocerebrosilence,** which is the absence of brain-generated electrical activity. Procedures should adhere to guidelines established by the American Electroencephalographic Society (*J Clin Neurophysiol* 11:10, 1994).
2. **Radionuclide** or **conventional four-vessel angiography** demonstrates **absence of cerebral blood flow.**
3. Somatosensory or brain stem auditory **evoked potentials** demonstrate absence of subcortical and cortical responses with intact peripheral responses.

**E.** If brain death is established by the initial evaluation, a repeat evaluation is performed after an interval determined appropriate by the consulting physician to confirm the persistent absence of cortical and brain stem function. If the second examination confirms brain death, the patient is declared dead by the consulting physician and certified in the medical record.

## Seizures

**Generalized convulsive status epilepticus** consists of sustained unconsciousness and continuous or intermittent generalized convulsive seizure activity. Convulsive seizure activity lasting 10 minutes continuously, or intermittently without recovery of consciousness, warrants IV anticonvulsant therapy. Diagnostic evaluation and supportive care must proceed concurrently. Important historical information includes preexisting medical conditions, current medications, drug allergies, and possible precipitating events.

**I. Acute management**

**A.** Acute management includes placement of a soft plastic oral or nasal airway and administration of maximal supplemental oxygen by mask. Bag-mask ventilation and administration of anticonvulsants are usually preferable to attempting endotracheal intubation in a convulsing patient, which often necessitates neuromuscular blockade, although aggressive measures to control the airway may be required. Vital signs, oximetry, and continuous ECG should be monitored. A large-bore IV line (ideally two, one dextrose free) should be placed. **Thiamine** (100 mg) should be given intravenously **followed by** 50 ml 50% **dextrose.** Bed padding reduces traumatic injury. **Laboratory analysis** should include glucose, electrolytes, calcium, magnesium, CBC, BUN, creatinine, ALT, antiepileptic drug levels if indicated, urinalysis, and urine drug screen.

**B. Parenteral anticonvulsants** stop seizures most rapidly but should be reserved for patients with persistent generalized convulsive seizures because of potentially serious adverse effects. If a patient stops convulsing and recovers consciousness, it is safer to administer anticonvulsants orally. The following is one approach to treating persistent convulsive seizures (see also *JAMA* 270:854, 1993; *N Engl J Med* 339:792, 1998). ICU support is typically required; sometimes anesthesiology consultation is needed.

1. **Lorazepam** (0.1 mg/kg at 2 mg/minute up to 4 mg) or **diazepam** (0.2 mg/kg at 5 mg/minute up to 10 mg) stops seizures quickly in most patients. The short duration of action of these drugs requires concomitant administration of maintenance anticonvulsants. Respiratory depression may necessitate intubation and assisted ventilation.
2. **Phenytoin** is the preferred maintenance anticonvulsant (combined with benzodiazepines) for convulsive status epilepticus. The preferred formulation for parenteral administration is **fosphenytoin,** a phosphate ester prodrug of phenytoin. Fosphenytoin is converted in vivo in equimolar concentrations to phenytoin. The loading dose for phenytoin in status epilepticus is 20 mg/kg. **The dose of fosphenytoin is expressed as phenytoin equivalents (PE)** and should be ordered as such (i.e., 20 mg PE/kg). The maximum rate of infusion for fosphenytoin is 150 mg PE/minute; the maximum rate of infusion for phenytoin is 50 mg/minute. Fosphenytoin produces less venous irritation and sclerosis than phenytoin. If phenytoin sodium is administered IV, a large-bore IV infusing dextrose free saline should be used to prevent precipitation in the line. Alternatively, phenytoin can be mixed with normal saline at the bedside and infused immediately. Although fosphenytoin can be administered IM, this route is less desirable in an emergent situation because of delayed time to peak concentrations. BP and cardiac rhythm should be monitored continuously for hypotension and heart block, which often resolve when the administration rate is reduced. Phenytoin and fosphenytoin are contraindicated in heart block.
3. **Phenobarbital** (20 mg/kg at less than 50 mg/minute) should be given if seizures continue after phenytoin loading. Respiratory depression caused by benzodiazepines combined with phenobarbital usually necessitates intubation. When phenobarbital is added to stop recalcitrant seizures, there is no strict dose; it can be administered at 5-mg/kg increments until the seizures are controlled. An IV loading dose of 20 mg/kg generally achieves a serum level of approximately 20 μg/ml within an hour of administration, sufficient to stop most seizures. As with phenytoin, arrhythmias and hypotension may occur during administration, requiring continuous ECG and BP monitoring.
4. A **continuous benzodiazepine infusion** may be a preferable option over phenytoin and barbiturates in some patients. Parenteral valproic acid is another alternative (e.g., in patients with cardiac failure/arrhythmia), with a loading dose of 15 mg/kg.
5. **Barbiturate coma** or **general anesthesia** with neuromuscular blockade may be required to stop seizures that persist despite the previously mentioned measures.

**II. A specific etiology is often associated with status epilepticus,** and its treatment may influence successful management of seizures. Structural abnormalities include primary or metastatic CNS tumors, CNS infections (e.g., bacterial meningitis, herpes encephalitis), CNS inflammatory processes (e.g., CNS lupus), cerebral infarction (more commonly embolic), and acute or preexisting brain injury (e.g., trauma, hemorrhage). Nonstructural precipitants include hypoglycemia, electrolyte abnormalities (e.g., hyponatremia, hypocalcemia), uremia, anoxia, medication effects (e.g., cyclosporine, imipenem, meperidine), drug withdrawal (particularly acute withdrawal of benzodiazepines, barbiturates, antiepileptic drugs), and drug intoxication (e.g., cocaine, methamphetamine). In epileptic patients, subtherapeutic antiepileptic drug levels (noncompliance, drug interaction, etc.) or an acute febrile illness often initiate status epilepticus. Some epileptic patients initially present with status epilepticus. Head CT or MRI and CSF analysis are frequently required to establish a specific diagnosis. **EEG** is useful to diagnose and treat nonconvulsive status epilepticus (see Alterations in Consciousness, sec. **I.B.10**), to guide long-term management and support the clinical diagnosis of epilepsy. Although EEG is not useful during the initial assessment and management of convulsive status epilepticus, it is essential for verifying elimination of electrographic seizures after successful initial treatment of convulsive status epilepticus and for monitoring more aggressive treatments such as barbiturate coma and general anesthesia with neuromuscular blockade.

**III.** The diagnostic approach to a patient with spontaneously terminating seizures with recovery of consciousness is similar to that described in sec. **II.** Depending on the circumstances, outpatient evaluation may be appropriate. If antiepileptic drugs are indicated, oral loading is typically preferred over IV loading.

**IV.** **Maintenance therapy.** After status epilepticus has been successfully treated, and causative factors identified and treated, anticonvulsant drugs are usually maintained, except for benzodiazepines (maintenance phenytoin, 4–7 mg/kg/day; phenobarbital, 1–5 mg/kg/day, IV or PO bid), until the patient can capably manage long-term therapy. Conversion to an oral regimen must be individually tailored. Most patients are adequately treated with a single antiepileptic drug, but others may require adjustment of their previous multiple drug regimen.

## Cerebrovascular Disease

**I.** The hallmark of **stroke** is the abrupt onset of symptoms and neurologic deficits that correspond to interruption of vascular supply to a specific brain region. Although stroke is synonymous with cerebral infarction, fluctuation of functional deficits after stroke onset and reversible deficits known as **TIAs** (deficits resolve within 24 hours) and reversible ischemic neurologic deficits (deficits resolve within a week) suggest that tissue at risk for infarction may be rescued by re-establishing perfusion. **Currently, the most important aspect of stroke management is consideration of stroke as a medical emergency that requires rapid diagnosis and treatment.** Recombinant tissue plasminogen activator **(rt-PA)** is the only proven therapy for acute stroke, but patients must be selected carefully, and administration of rt-PA must commence within 3 hours of stroke onset. Other treatments, including intra-arterial thrombolysis, are available at some centers under research protocols.

**A.** Important **historical information** includes the onset and progression of symptoms and contributory events (e.g., head trauma or seizure). Prior TIA symptoms (e.g., transient monocular loss of vision, aphasia, dysarthria, paresis, or sensory disturbance) are often associated with atherosclerotic vascular disease, the most common cause for stroke. A history of trauma, even minimal, is important, as extracerebral arterial dissections may cause ischemic strokes. Other medical conditions associated with stroke, such as cardiac arrhythmia or valvular disease, connective tissue disease, and sickle cell anemia, should be identified. Classic migraine can mimic stroke and is a risk factor for stroke. In epileptic patients, ictal paralysis is rare, but postictal paralysis (Todd's paralysis) is common after a focal seizure. The diagnosis may be suggested by stroke risk factors such as hypertension, diabetes, smoking, postpartum state, illicit IV drug use, and medications such as oral contraceptives, and management is influenced by these factors.

**B.** **Physical examination** should provide clues that indicate specific diagnostic tests and therapy. **Cardiogenic embolism** accounts for approximately 20% of strokes; physical examination should focus on findings of mitral or aortic stenosis and atrial fibrillation. Embolic disease affects fundi, conjunctivae, nail beds, fingers, and palms. Urinalysis should be performed to evaluate for hematuria. Fever raises concern for infectious etiologies. Meningismus, seizures, or altered mental status suggest meningitis or encephalitis. Septic emboli from bacterial endocarditis can cause meningitis or cerebral or parameningeal abscess. The patient should be examined for evidence of neurocutaneous disease (neurofibromatosis and tuberous sclerosis) and vasculitis (e.g., systemic lupus erythematosus).

**C.** A careful **neurologic examination** reliably establishes the anatomic location of a stroke, which is typically confirmed by neuroimaging. In general, **carotid artery** distribution strokes (anterior circulation) produce combinations of functional deficits (hemiparesis, hemianopsia, cortical sensory loss, often with aphasias or agnosias) contralateral to the affected hemisphere, whereas **vertebral-basilar** strokes (posterior circulation) produce unilateral or bilateral motor/sensory deficits, usually accompanied by cranial nerve and brain stem signs. **Horner's syndrome** (ptosis, miosis, anhidrosis) contralateral to an acute hemiparesis suggests carotid dissection.

**II. Initial assessment and management**

**A.** Vital signs, including oximetry and continuous ECG, should be monitored. Administration of oxygen, placement of IV access, and checking of blood glucose should be done immediately. Laboratory analysis should include CBC with differential and platelet count, PT, activated PTT, and electrolyte panel. ECG (for atrial fibrillation) and a chest radiograph should be obtained.

**B.** Immediately after initial assessment and stabilization, a **noncontrast head CT** scan should be performed to identify various hemorrhagic lesions that influence specific management decisions. The CT scan often confirms a suspected ischemic infarct, unless it is very early after onset (hours) or if the stroke is very small (particularly in the brain stem), in which case MRI is more sensitive. A mass lesion may preclude a diagnostic lumbar puncture for meningitis/encephalitis because it may precipitate brain herniation (see Alterations in Consciousness, sec. **III.F**). Appropriate antimicrobial and antiviral drugs should still be administered.

**C.** **rt-PA** therapy should be considered when a nonhemorrhagic ischemic infarct has been demonstrated and infectious etiologies are excluded, while one continues to pursue a specific diagnosis. Hemorrhagic transformation of infarcts accompanied by higher mortality was observed in some patients treated with rt-PA; therefore, **strict adherence to the American Academy of Neurology/American Heart Association guidelines is recommended** (*Neurology* 47:835, 1996). **Exclusion criteria** include stroke onset longer than 3 hours; extensive infarction evident on CT scan; recent surgery, head trauma, or GI or urinary hemorrhage; seizure at stroke onset; bleeding disorder or anticoagulation with prolonged PT/PTT; and severe uncontrolled hypertension (systolic >185, diastolic >110 mm Hg). The rt-PA dose is 0.9 mg/kg up to a maximum of 90 mg, with the first 10% (maximum, 9 mg) given IV over 1 minute, then the remaining 90% (maximum, 81 mg) given by infusion pump over 1 hour. Aspirin, heparin, and warfarin are not given during the first 24 hours. Systolic BP should be maintained at less than 185 and diastolic BP at less than 110 mm Hg to reduce the patient's risk for hemorrhagic transformation.

**III. Diagnosis and management of specific etiologies**

**A.** Additional diagnostic tests may be required to establish a specific diagnosis.

1. **MRI** scan is more sensitive and accurate than CT in narrowing the differential diagnosis of cerebral lesions, and MR angiography is a useful noninvasive method to evaluate large arteries and veins.
2. **Carotid Doppler** studies enable noninvasive estimation of carotid stenosis. Conventional iodine contrast angiography may be required to diagnose cerebral aneurysm or isolated CNS angiitis and is usually required when carotid endarterectomy is considered (see sec. **III.B.2**).
3. **Transthoracic two-dimensional echocardiography** is helpful to demonstrate intracardiac thrombi, valve vegetations, valvular stenosis or insufficiency, and right-to-left shunting (contrast echocardiogram). In some patients, transesophageal echocardiography is necessary to evaluate the left atrium for thrombi.
4. **CSF** analysis for malignant cells, special cultures, preps (e.g., acid-fast bacilli stain, India ink preparation), or antibody titers (e.g., VDRL) is helpful in the identification of carcinomatous or less common infectious etiologies.
5. **Erythrocyte sedimentation rate, antinuclear antibody, anticardiolipin antibody, hemoglobin electrophoresis, lipid profile,** or other specific tests may be required as indicated to establish a specific diagnosis.

**B. Treatment of atherosclerotic stroke**

1. **Aspirin** reduces stroke morbidity and mortality and is recommended for acute and long-term treatment at doses of 160–325 mg/day (*Lancet* 349:1641 and 1569, 1997). Presently, other antiplatelet aggregating drugs are not recommended for acute stroke treatment (*Stroke* 33:1934, 2002), although they may be alternatives for patients who cannot tolerate or have not responded to aspirin therapy (*Chest* 114:683S, 1998).
2. **Carotid endarterectomy** decreases the risk of stroke and death in patients with recent TIAs or nondisabling strokes and ipsilateral high-grade (70–99%) carotid stenosis (*N Engl J Med* 325:445, 1991). Carotid endarterectomy for asymptomatic high-grade carotid stenosis (≥ 60%) reduces the relative risk of stroke provided that the surgery/angiography complication rate is less than 3% (*JAMA* 273:1421, 1995). Stroke risk factor reduction and antiplatelet therapy are important components of postoperative management (*Stroke* 29:554, 1998).
3. **Heparin, low-molecular-weight heparin, and warfarin** treatment are controversial and not generally recommended for atherosclerotic cerebrovascular disease (*Stroke* 33:1934, 2002); use must be individualized, with potential benefits considered with risks for hemorrhagic complications.

**C. Treatment of cardiogenic embolus.** Anticoagulation is indicated to prevent recurrent embolic strokes. Anticoagulation with heparin should be initiated. **Warfarin** is used for chronic anticoagulation with a target international normalized ratio (INR) of 2–3 for embolic infarcts, the exception being mechanical heart valves, for which an INR of between 2.5 and 3.5 is recommended (see Anticoagulants, sec. **IV**, in Chap. 18, Disorders of Hemostasis). Uncontrolled systemic hypertension is a relative contraindication to long-term anticoagulation because of increased risk for intracranial hemorrhage.

**D. Modification of risk factors,** including systemic hypertension, diabetes, smoking, and possibly elevated lipids and cholesterol, reduces risk for stroke. BP reduction is beneficial even in normotensive stroke patients (*Lancet* 358:1033, 2001). Oral contraceptives may need to be discontinued in women with stroke.

## IV. Intracerebral hemorrhage and SAH

**A.** Intracerebral hemorrhage usually presents with acute onset of focal neurologic deficits that reflect the location and size of the hemorrhage. Headache, vomiting, and altered mental status reflect increased intracranial pressure and often indicate extensive hemorrhage. **Brain herniation and death may**

**occur rapidly.** Head CT scan is necessary to differentiate intracerebral hemorrhage from ischemic stroke.

1. The **etiology** is usually chronic systemic hypertension. The locations of hypertensive intracerebral hemorrhage are putamen/thalamus (70%), pons (10%), cerebellum (10%), and cerebral white matter (10%). Less commonly, intracerebral hemorrhage results from trauma, anticoagulant therapy, saccular aneurysm, arteriovenous malformation, tumor, blood dyscrasia, angiopathy, or vasculitis.
2. **Treatment** consists of supportive care and gradual reduction in BP.
   a. Vascular autoregulation is unpredictably impaired in patients with chronic hypertension and intracerebral hemorrhage. **Higher than normal systemic BP may be required to maintain cerebral perfusion.** Therefore, BP is gradually reduced over days, with careful observation for worsening neurologic deficits, which may reflect cerebral ischemia.
   b. **Surgical consultation is indicated for cerebellar hematomas,** because brain stem compression or obstructive hydrocephalus may develop, and immediate hematoma evacuation or ventricular shunting may be lifesaving. Evacuation of deep cerebral hematomas is rarely beneficial.

B. **SAH** may present with only **sudden onset of severe headache.** Lethargy or coma, fever, vomiting, seizures, and low back pain may also be present. Focal neurologic deficits, nuchal rigidity, and retinal hemorrhages (subhyaloid) suggest SAH. **Complications** of SAH include rebleeding (20% at 2 weeks), vasospasm with ischemic deficits (days 4–14), hydrocephalus, seizures, and hyponatremia.

1. The most common **etiology of SAH** is a ruptured saccular or "berry" aneurysm, which results from defects in the arterial media and internal elastic lamina of large arteries. Other types of aneurysms include fusiform aneurysms (probably secondary to atherosclerosis) and mycotic aneurysms (from septic embolism). Hypertensive intracerebral hemorrhage, arteriovenous malformation, blood dyscrasia, head trauma, cocaine or amphetamine abuse, and tumor are among the other etiologies.
2. **A noncontrast head CT scan is diagnostic** of subarachnoid blood in the sulci and cisternae in 90% of SAH patients in the first 24 hours. In some patients, **lumbar puncture** is necessary to confirm or exclude the diagnosis of SAH. Bloody CSF should be centrifuged immediately and examined for **xanthochromia** (yellow color). Xanthochromia results from RBC lysis and takes several hours to develop, indicating SAH rather than traumatic lumbar puncture. Postcontrast head CT or MRI scan may demonstrate vascular abnormalities, but cerebral angiography is often necessary for definitive diagnosis. Angiography is required for presurgical evaluation of saccular aneurysms.
3. **Treatment** of SAH depends on etiology. Saccular aneurysms are usually treated surgically. The timing of surgery after SAH is controversial and depends on the clinical condition of the patient. Supportive measures while awaiting surgery include bed rest, sedation, analgesia, and laxatives to prevent sudden increases in intracranial pressure or BP. One should **avoid hypotension,** as it may worsen ischemic deficits. Only extreme elevations in BP (diastolic >130 mm Hg) should be treated, and reduction of BP should be gradual, with careful monitoring of BP and the neurologic examination. Nimodipine, a calcium channel blocker, improves outcome in SAH patients and may reduce the incidence of associated cerebral infarction with few side effects. Recommended dosage is 60 mg PO q4h for 21 days, initiated within 4 days of presentation. Volume expansion, induced hypertension, and balloon dilation can occasionally be used to reverse neurologic deterioration due to vasospasm.

# Head Trauma

**I. Initial assessment**

**A. Adequate airway, oxygenation, ventilation, and circulation should be ensured.** The neck should be immobilized in a hard cervical collar to avoid spinal cord injury from manipulating an unstable or fractured cervical spine, and nasal intubation in patients with facial fractures should be avoided. Emergency tracheotomy is sometimes necessary. Hypoventilation and systemic hypotension should also be avoided, as these may reduce cerebral perfusion. Initial supportive measures include obtaining IV access and continuously monitoring vital signs, oximetry, and ECG.

**B. History** focuses on the temporal course of all symptoms, particularly loss of consciousness, occurrence of a lucid interval (which suggests expanding hematoma), and amnesia (which is related to the severity of the blow).

**C.** The **physical examination** should include a careful search for penetrating wounds and other injuries. Hemotympanum, postauricular hematoma (Battle's sign), periorbital hematoma ("raccoon eyes"), and CSF otorrhea/rhinorrhea are indicative of **basilar skull fracture.** The neurologic examination should focus on the level of consciousness (see Alterations in Consciousness, sec. **III,** and Table 24-2), focal deficits, and signs of herniation. Serial examinations must be performed and documented to identify neurologic deterioration early.

**D. Imaging studies.** Head CT is useful for the identification of intracranial hemorrhage; bone window views may be useful for the identification of fractures. Skull and facial radiographs may be necessary to demonstrate some fractures. Cervical radiographs must be performed to exclude fracture or dislocation.

**II. Management**

**A.** Awake, alert patients with **concussion** (posttraumatic confusion, amnesia, with or without transient loss of consciousness, normal neurologic examination and radiographic studies) are observed in the hospital for 24 hours, with hourly neurologic assessment to detect delayed deterioration. Some patients are observed at home by a reliable adult, with instructions for frequent checks and criteria for return. **Neurologic deterioration** after head injury of any severity requires an immediate repeat head CT scan to differentiate between an expanding hematoma that necessitates surgery from diffuse cerebral edema that requires monitoring and reduction of intracranial pressure.

**B. Neurosurgical consultation** is indicated for patients with contusion, intracranial hematoma, cervical fracture, skull fractures, penetrating injuries, or focal neurologic deficits.

1. **If surgery appears imminent** (severe or multiple injuries, intracranial hematoma), restrict oral intake (NPO) and perform preoperative laboratory analysis. In the intubated, comatose patient, modest hyperventilation ($PCO_2 \sim 35$ mm Hg) should be instituted with fluid restriction (avoiding hypotonic fluids). The head should be midline and elevated 30 degrees. Steroids are not indicated. Brain herniation requires immediate countermeasures (see Alterations in Consciousness, sec. **I.B.7**).
2. In **penetrating head trauma,** foreign objects (e.g., knives) should not be moved.
3. **Emergency surgical evacuation** may be lifesaving in acute epidural and subdural hematomas. Epidural hematoma is usually associated with skull fractures across a meningeal artery and may cause precipitous deterioration after a lucid interval. The characteristic noncontrast head CT finding is a lenticular-shaped extra-axial hematoma. Deterioration often follows the classic uncal herniation syndrome (see Alterations in Consciousness, sec. **III.F.2**).

4. **Chronic subdural hematoma** is most common in aged, debilitated, and alcoholic individuals and in anticoagulated patients. Antecedent trauma is often minimal. Symptoms tend to be nonspecific (e.g., headache, confusion, lethargy) and can fluctuate. The need for surgical intervention is determined by the symptoms and degree of mass effect.
5. **Intracerebral hematomas** may be present initially or develop within a contusion. Surgical intervention versus observation depends on the location and size of the hematoma and the patient's neurologic condition.
6. **Skull fractures** increase the risk of epidural hemorrhage and meningitis. Basilar skull fracture is often a clinical diagnosis (see sec. **I.C**).

## Acute Spinal Cord Dysfunction

The hallmark of spinal cord dysfunction is demonstration of a level below which motor, sensory, and autonomic functions are interrupted, due to the spinal cord's segmental functional organization. Rapid diagnosis and treatment may reverse or prevent progression of functional deficits.

I. **Spinal cord compression** typically presents with back pain at the level of compression (some lesions are painless), progressive difficulty in walking, sensory impairment, and urinary retention with overflow incontinence. Rapid deterioration may occur. Etiologies include tumor (primary or metastatic), herniated disk, epidural abscess, hematoma, and vascular malformation. **Transverse myelitis or myelopathy** presents with symptoms and signs similar to cord compression. Transverse myelitis occurs with enteroviruses, herpes zoster, tuberculosis or other granulomatous disease, syphilis, and systemic lupus erythematosus. Transverse myelopathy is caused by infarction (cardiogenic, fibrocartilaginous, or gaseous embolus; hypotension; aortic dissection or surgery) and multiple sclerosis.
   A. **Examination** helps localize the level of dysfunction, but there may be multiple lesions. **Radicular signs** (lancinating pain, paresthesias, and numbness in the dermatomal distribution of a nerve root, with weakness and decreased tone and reflexes in muscles supplied by the root) imply inflammation or compression of the nerve root. Tenderness to spinal percussion over the lesion may be present. **Myelopathic signs** include a band of dysesthesia at the level of a lesion, with bilateral sensory loss and weakness below the level of the lesion. Tone and reflexes are typically diminished below acute lesions (spinal shock); hypertonia, hyperreflexia, and Babinski's signs are present with slowly progressive lesions. Urinary retention commonly accompanies spinal cord compression. Unilateral cord lesions may result in contralateral pain and temperature loss, with ipsilateral weakness and proprioceptive loss **(Brown-Séquard syndrome). Cauda equina syndrome** from compression of the lower lumbar and sacral roots produces sensory loss in a saddle distribution, flaccid leg weakness, decreased reflexes, and urinary/bowel incontinence.
   B. **Imaging studies.** Plain x-rays of the spine may reveal metastatic disease, osteomyelitis, discitis, fractures, or dislocation. MRI scan or myelography with CT scan should be obtained emergently to determine the exact level and extent of the lesion(s). **Imaging should include the entire spine.** Neurosurgical consultation should be obtained before myelography, because occasionally acute postmyelography decompensation occurs with compressive lesions, requiring emergent decompressive laminectomy. For the same reason, lumbar puncture for diagnosis of infection, inflammation, or carcinomatous meningitis should follow exclusion of a compressive lesion.
   C. **Management**
      1. Vital functions should be supported, and preoperative evaluation should be performed.

2. Treatable infections require appropriate antibiotics. Herpes zoster (suggested by a vesicular rash) should be treated with acyclovir (see Antiviral Agents, sec. **II.A**, in Chap. 12, Antimcrobials).
3. **Dexamethasone,** 10 mg IV followed by 4 mg IV q6h, is given for compressive lesions and sometimes for transverse myelitis or spinal cord infarction, although benefit has not been proven for all etiologies.
4. **Neurosurgical consultation should be obtained** because many causes for spinal cord compression are surgically treatable.
5. **Emergent radiation therapy** combined with high-dose steroids is usually indicated for cord compression due to malignancy and generally requires a histologic diagnosis.
6. **Anticipatory acute and long-term supportive care** is important for patients with spinal cord dysfunction. Airway security and adequate ventilation must be confirmed frequently. Pulmonary and urinary infections, skin breakdown at pressure points, joint contractures, and irregular bowel and bladder elimination are common problems. Bladder or rectal distention can cause sympathetic overactivity (headache, tachycardia, diaphoresis, hypertension) as a result of **autonomic dysreflexia.**

**II. Traumatic spinal cord injury** may be obvious from the history or initial examination but must also be excluded in patients who are unconscious, confused, or inebriated when the history regarding trauma is unknown. Penetrating injury, foreign bodies, comminuted fractures, misalignment, and hematoma usually require surgical treatment. **Spinal cord concussion** refers to posttraumatic spinal cord symptoms and signs that resolve rapidly (hours to days).

**A. Immobilization,** especially of the neck, is essential to prevent further injury while the patient's condition is stabilized and radiographic and neurosurgical assessment of the injuries is performed. Vital signs should be continuously monitored, and adequate tissue oxygenation and perfusion should be affirmed. Neurosurgical consultation should be obtained. **Autonomic instability** may lead to fluctuating vital signs and BP. Hypotension may require vasopressors dopamine or dobutamine (see Shock in Chap. 8, Critical Care). α-Adrenergic agonists increase BP but reduce cardiac output and impair spinal cord perfusion. Fluid resuscitation alone usually results in pulmonary edema.

**B. Ventilatory insufficiency** from cervical cord injuries requires immediate airway control and ventilatory assistance, without manipulation of the neck. Bag-mask ventilation, blind nasal intubation, or tracheostomy is typically required.

**C. Examination** may reveal local and radicular pain, local tenderness, weakness in a radicular or myelopathic distribution, sensory loss, absent tone and reflexes, and urinary retention. The presence and extent of injuries should be confirmed with neuroimaging as described previously. Injuries to other systems need to be excluded.

**D. Methylprednisolone,** 30 mg/kg IV bolus, followed by an infusion of 5.4 mg/kg/hour for 24 hours when administered within 3 hours of injury (*N Engl J Med* 322:1405, 1990), and for 48 hours when initiated within 3–8 hours of injury (*JAMA* 277:1597, 1997), may improve neurologic recovery.

## Neuromuscular Disease

**I. Guillain-Barré syndrome** (**GBS,** acute idiopathic demyelinating polyneuropathy)

**A. Presentation** of GBS is typically a rapidly progressive, symmetric ascending paralysis, often after a viral illness (Epstein-Barr virus, cytomegalovirus), gastroenteritis (especially *Campylobacter jejuni*), surgical procedure, or immunization (influenza). Proximal weakness may be pronounced. Cranial nerves, especially the facial nerves, may be involved. Sensory symptoms are usually present and cause discomfort, but objective sensory loss is uncommon. Reflexes are hypoactive or absent, and loss of reflexes on serial examinations is a useful diagnostic feature. CSF protein is usually elevated, without pleocytosis (lymphocytes may be present but are usually <20/μl). **Differential diagnosis** includes arsenic exposure, acute porphyria, tick paralysis, botulism, postdiphtheritic paralysis, and polymyositis. Creatine kinase may be elevated. Nerve conduction studies may assist in the diagnosis (absent H reflexes, prolongation of F-wave latencies, motor conduction block).

**B. Treatment is primarily supportive.** Plasmapheresis and IV immunoglobulin have been shown to be equally effective when carried out early in patients whose conditions are severely compromised or worsening (loss of ambulation, respiratory failure) (*Neurology* 46:100, 1996; *Neurology* 35:1096, 1985). Indications for treatment in mild forms of stable and improving GBS are less clear. Corticosteroids, immunosuppressive drugs, and other agents are not of proven value in GBS. Prevention of exposure keratitis, venous thrombosis, and vigilance for hyponatremia (including SIADH) should be priorities.

1. **Ventilatory function must be closely monitored,** including oximetry, vital capacity, and inspiratory force. Hypoxemia, acidosis, and declining vital capacity (<10–15 cc/kg) and inspiratory force (<25 cm $H_2O$) are indications for ventilatory assistance (see Mechanical Ventilation in Chap. 8, Critical Care).
2. **BP instability.** Paroxysmal hypertension should be managed with short-acting agents that can be titrated against the patient's BP (see Chap. 4, Hypertension). Hypotension is usually caused by decreased venous return and peripheral vasodilatation. Patients on ventilators are particularly prone to hypotension, due to compromised venous return. Treatment consists of intravascular volume expansion with IV fluids. Occasionally, vasopressors are required (see Shock in Chap. 8, Critical Care).
3. **Cardiac arrhythmias** (bradyarrhythmias, including sinus arrest or complete heart block, or tachyarrhythmias) may be a serious complication in GBS; therefore, continuous ECG monitoring is necessary. Hypoxia and electrolyte abnormalities should be excluded as precipitating factors.

**II. Myasthenia gravis (MG)** is an autoimmune disorder that involves antibody-mediated disruption of postsynaptic nicotinic acetylcholine receptors at the neuromuscular junction and is often associated with thymus tumors. Typical symptoms are transient weakness (especially worse after exercise and better after rest), but chronic, persistent weakness may occur. **Presenting signs** include ptosis, diplopia, dysarthria, dysphagia, extremity weakness, and respiratory difficulty. MG is more common in women, and it tends to occur in young women (third decade) and older men (fifth to sixth decade). The clinical course is variable; spontaneous remissions and exacerbations often occur. Progressive deterioration is more likely to occur in the first 3 years. The **differential diagnosis** includes presynaptic neuromuscular junction dysfunction in botulism (see sec. **III**) and the Eaton-Lambert syndrome, a paraneoplastic syndrome associated with carcinoma.

**A.** The **diagnosis** is usually evident from the history and physical examination. Ancillary tests may be useful in confirming the diagnosis.

1. **Edrophonium (Tensilon test)** often produces a marked temporary improvement of strength in myasthenic patients. However, its utility as a diagnostic tool in MG is limited by a high incidence of false positives.
2. Blood **acetylcholine receptor antibody** level remains a highly sensitive and specific assay and is the diagnostic test of choice.
3. **CT of the thorax** is necessary to exclude thymoma.
4. **Repetitive nerve stimulation** (2–3 Hz) typically shows greater than 10% decrement in the amplitude of the compound muscle action potential in MG. In botulism and the Eaton-Lambert syndrome, the response is incremental.

**B. Treatment** of MG follows no specific protocol. The clinician must choose among modalities based on symptoms, lifestyle, and response to treatment. A rapid deterioration in respiratory and swallowing functions necessitates aggressive support, therapy, and correction of precipitating causes (e.g., infection, thyroid dysfunction).

1. **Anticholinesterase** drugs can produce symptomatic improvement in all forms of MG. Pyridostigmine should be started at 30–60 mg PO tid–qid and subsequently titrated to the minimum amount that provides relief of symptoms. Occasional patients require dosing as frequently as q2–3h. Neostigmine methylsulfate, as a continuous IV infusion at one–forty-fifth the total daily dose of pyridostigmine over 24 hours, can be substituted for patients who are not able to take medications orally.
2. **Thymectomy** is an effective treatment for generalized MG and produces complete remission in many patients. However, thymectomy is controversial in children, in adults older than 60 years, and in purely ocular MG. A thymoma is an absolute indication for surgery at any age. In general, thymectomy should be performed electively for moderate to marked generalized MG, early in the course of the disease, and if response to medical treatment is unsatisfactory.
3. **Immunosuppressive drugs** are typically used when additional benefit is needed after cholinesterase inhibitors. High-dose **prednisone** (50 mg qd or higher) is frequently used to achieve rapid improvement, but **hospitalization is advised because an initial exacerbation of weakness often occurs.** Initiating therapy at a lower dose (20 mg qd) followed by dose titration may avoid worsening symptoms. The goal is to identify an effective daily dose, maintain stable improvement, and then taper to an alternate-day regimen. Additional dose reductions can be made gradually. Potential risks of steroid treatment need to be weighed against observed clinical benefit on an individual basis. **Azathioprine,** 1–2 mg/kg PO qd, is an alternative drug for patients who do not respond to steroids or cannot take them. Onset of benefit may require months of treatment. **Side effects** include leukopenia, pancytopenia, infection, GI irritation, and abnormal liver function tests. **Cyclosporine** has been shown to be effective in MG in a double-blind, placebo-controlled clinical trial (*Ann NY Acad Sci* 681:539, 1993). **Cyclophosphamide** and IV **human immunoglobulin** may be beneficial in selected refractory patients.
4. **Plasmapheresis** is used to treat acute exacerbations, impending crisis, and disabling myasthenia that is refractory to other therapies and is used before surgery when postoperative deterioration is possible (e.g., before thymectomy). Benefits are temporary, and no consensus has been reached about exact indications and protocol. Hypotension and thromboembolism are potential complications.
5. **Precipitating factors** include infection, pregnancy, thyroid dysfunction, and drugs. A variety of medications (e.g., aminoglycosides, quinine, beta-blockers, lithium) can worsen or precipitate weakness in myasthenic patients; however, only curariform medications are absolutely contraindicated in MG.

**C. Myasthenic crisis** (the need for assisted ventilation or airway protection, or both) occurs in approximately 10% of patients with MG. Patients with bulbar and respiratory muscle weakness are particularly prone to respiratory failure. Respiratory infection and surgery (e.g., thymectomy) can precipitate crisis. Patients at risk should have pulmonary function monitored closely. Ventilatory support follows the guidelines given in Chap. 8, Critical Care. Anticholinesterases should be temporarily withdrawn from patients who are receiving ventilation support; this avoids uncertainties about overdosage ("cholinergic crisis") and avoids cholinergic stimulation of pulmonary secretions. Steroids, IV immunoglobulins, or plasmapheresis may be helpful. Thymectomy is not part of the emergency treatment of MG.

III. **Botulism** is a disorder of the neuromuscular junction caused by ingestion of an exotoxin produced by *Clostridium botulinum*. The exotoxin interferes with release of acetylcholine from presynaptic terminals at the neuromuscular junction. **Symptoms** begin within 12–36 hours of ingestion and include autonomic dysfunction (xerostomia, blurred vision, bowel and bladder dysfunction) followed by cranial nerve palsies and weakness. **Management** includes removing nonabsorbed toxin with cathartics, neutralizing absorbed toxin with equine trivalent antitoxin (one vial IV with or without one vial IM after normal intradermal horse serum sensitivity test, per the package insert), and providing supportive care (see Bioterrorism, sec. **II.E,** in Chap. 13, Treatment of Infectious Diseases).

IV. **Rhabdomyolysis** secondary to strenuous exercise or metabolic myopathy or from toxic effects (e.g., alcohol) may produce dramatic and painful muscle weakness. Resultant effects include hyperkalemia, myoglobinuria, and renal failure (see Acute Renal Failure, sec. **III.D,** in Chap. 11, Renal Diseases, for management).

V. **Myopathies** (ethanol, steroids, cholesterol-lowering drugs, hypothyroidism) may present with rapidly progressive, proximal muscle weakness. Polymyositis and dermatomyositis should also be considered, particularly if muscle pain is prominent (see Polymyositis and Dermatomyositis in Chap. 23, Arthritis and Rheumatologic Diseases).

VI. **Neuromuscular disorders with rigidity**

A. **Neuroleptic malignant syndrome** is associated with drugs such as haloperidol, phenothiazines, lithium, and reserpine. **Typical features** include fever, obtundation, and muscular rigidity, with elevated creatine kinase and myoglobinuria. **Treatment** includes discontinuing precipitating drug(s), cooling, monitoring and supporting vital functions (arrhythmias, shock, hyperkalemia, acidosis, renal failure), and administering dantrolene (2 mg/kg IV; additional doses q5min up to 10 mg/kg total can be given). Oral bromocriptine can be used in mild cases.

B. High fever, obtundation, and muscular rigidity characterize **malignant hyperthermia syndrome.** Serum creatine kinase is markedly elevated. Renal failure from myoglobinuria and cardiac arrhythmias from electrolyte imbalance can be life-threatening. Multiple genetic mutations are associated with malignant hyperthermia syndrome, with a likely common abnormal elevation in intracellular calcium after triggering factors (e.g., halothane anesthesia). Patients with certain muscle disorders (central core disease, Duchenne muscular dystrophy) are particularly at risk. Successful **management** requires prompt recognition of the syndrome, discontinuation of the offending anesthetic agent, aggressive supportive care that focuses on oxygenation/ventilation, circulation, correction of acid-base and electrolyte derangements, and dantrolene sodium, 1–10 mg/kg/day, to reduce muscular rigidity.

C. **Tetanus** typically presents with generalized muscle spasm (especially trismus) caused by the exotoxin (tetanospasmin) from *Clostridium tetani*. The organism usually enters the body through wounds; onset typically occurs within 14 days of an injury (range, 2–54 days). Mortality may be as high as 50–60%. **Patients who are unvaccinated or have reduced immunity are at risk, underscoring the importance of prevention by tetanus toxoid boosters following wounds.** Tetanus may occur in drug abusers who inject subcutaneously. **Management** consists of supportive care, particularly airway control (laryngospasm) and treatment of muscle spasms (benzodiazepines, barbiturates, analgesics, and sometimes neuromuscular blockade). Cardiac arrhythmias and fluctuations in BP can occur. The patient should be kept in quiet isolation, sedated but arousable. **Specific measures** include wound débridement; metronidazole, 500 mg IV q6h; and human **tetanus immunoglobulin** (3000–5000 U) distributed intramuscularly among several sites proximal to the suspected source of exotoxin. **Active immunization is needed after recovery** (see Appendix F, Immunizations and Post-Exposure Therapies, Tables F-1 and F-3).

## Headache

Headache is a common symptom in hospitalized patients and frequently a presenting symptom in emergency departments. The objective in these settings is to distinguish primary headache syndromes (most commonly migraine), which are treated symptomatically, from secondary headache, which warrants establishment of a specific etiology and treatment. The evaluation and management of primary headache syndromes are typically performed in the outpatient setting; the focus here is on emergent aspects of diagnosis and treatment.

**I. Assessment**

**A. Primary headache syndromes** include **migraines** with (classic) or without (common) aura, **tension** headaches, and **cluster** headaches. Posttraumatic, exertional, cough- and cold-induced, and fleeting ice pick (stabbing) headaches are also considered within the same category after underlying structural lesions have been excluded. The mechanisms of primary headache syndromes are poorly understood but probably include a disturbance in serotonergic neurotransmission. Examination should reveal normal findings during asymptomatic intervals in patients with primary headache syndromes, although transient (usually evolving over several minutes) neurologic deficits including visual field defects, aphasia, and hemiparesis may complicate migraine with aura. The evolution and slower development of neurologic deficits distinguish migraine from the typically abrupt onset of deficits with stroke or TIA.

**B. Secondary headaches** have specific etiologies, and symptomatic features vary depending on the underlying pathology. For example, **SAH** causes abrupt onset of severe pain with neck stiffness (see Cerebrovascular Disease, sec. **IV**). Frontal lobe **tumors** may be asymptomatic until very large, producing headache by compression or traction of pain-sensitive structures such as blood vessels or meninges. In contrast, small tectal tumors cause headache from obstructive hydrocephalus and intracranial hypertension. Headaches from intracranial hypertension may wake the patient from sleep and are worse with postural changes and in the morning on arising from sleep. **Temporal arteritis** (see Polymyalgia Rheumatica and Temporal Arteritis in Chap. 23, Arthritis and Rheumatologic Diseases) typically begins after 50 years of age, which is uncommon for the onset of migraines. Focal neurologic signs suggest an underlying structural lesion, but as mentioned above, transient focal neurologic deficits can occur in migraine. Diplopia from sixth nerve palsy in intracranial hypertension from any cause is considered a false localizing sign (i.e., not necessarily indicating a focal structural lesion).

1. **Intracranial etiologies** include subdural hematoma, intracerebral hematoma, SAH, arteriovenous malformation, brain abscess, meningitis, encephalitis, vasculitis, obstructive hydrocephalus, and cerebral ischemia or infarction. Benign intracranial hypertension (pseudotumor cerebri) presents with headache, papilledema, diplopia, and elevated CSF pressure (>20 cm $H_2O$, relaxed lateral decubitus position).
2. **Extracranial causes** include giant-cell arteritis, sinusitis, glaucoma, optic neuritis, dental disease (including temporomandibular joint syndrome), and disorders of the cervical spine.
3. **Systemic causes** include fever, viremia, hypoxia, carbon monoxide poisoning (measure carboxyhemoglobin), hypercapnia, systemic hypertension, allergy, anemia, caffeine withdrawal, and vasoactive or toxic chemicals (nitrites).
4. **Depression** is a common cause of long-standing, treatment-resistant headaches. Specific inquiry about vegetative signs of depression and exclusion of other causes help to support the diagnosis.

**II. Treatment**

**A. Treatment of secondary headaches is directed at the primary etiology,** such as surgical treatment of cerebral aneurysm causing SAH, evacuation of subdural hematoma, or shunting obstructive hydrocephalus. Diagnostic lumbar puncture for benign intracranial hypertension and meningitis (especially aseptic) often relieves the headache, and the CSF pressure measurement helps guide CSF removal until it is within a normal range (e.g., 10 cm $H_2O$). Alternatively, postural headache after lumbar puncture **("post LP headache")** may occur in some patients.

**B. Acute treatment of migraine,** the most common primary headache syndrome, is directed at aborting the headache. This is easier at onset and often very difficult when the attack is well established. Patients have often used nonprescription analgesics (aspirin, acetaminophen, nonsteroidal anti-inflammatory drugs) and oral prescription medications (isometheptene, butalbital with aspirin or acetaminophen), which are first-line treatments that are most effective early in the course of an attack. Emergent treatments include serotonin agonists and other parenteral medications. Long-term treatment additionally involves prophylactic medications. It is important to review a patient's use of all medications, as they may influence acute management.

1. **Triptans** (serotonin receptor $5HT_{1B}$ and $5HT_{1D}$ agonists) are effective abortive medications that are available in multiple formulations and may be effective even in a protracted attack. **Triptans should not be used in patients with coronary artery disease, cerebrovascular disease, uncontrolled hypertension, migraine accompanied by neurologic deficits, or vertebrobasilar migraine. Sumatriptan**, 6 mg SC, can be repeated in 1 hour (maxiumum, 2 doses/24 hours); 5 or 20 mg nasal (maximum daily dose, 40 mg) or 25–100 mg PO (maximum daily dose, 200 mg) can be repeated in 2 hours. **Zolmitriptan,** 2.5–5.0 mg PO, can be repeated in 2 hours (maximum dose, 10 mg/24 hours). **Rizatriptan,** 5–10 mg PO, can be repeated every 2 hours as needed (maximum dose, 30 mg/24 hours). If the patient is receiving propranolol, the rizatriptan dose is 5 mg and can be repeated every 2 hours to a maximum of 15 mg/24 hours. **Naratriptan,** 1.0–2.5 mg PO, can be repeated in 4 hours (maximum dose, 5 mg/24 hours). **Frovatriptan,** 2.5 mg PO, can be repeated in 2 hours (maximum dose, 7.5 mg/24 hours). **Almotriptan,** 6.25–12.5 mg PO, can be repeated in 2 hours (maximum dose, 25 mg/24 hours). **Eletriptan,** 40 mg PO, can be repeated in 2 hours (maximum dose, 80 mg/24 hours; it cannot be given within 72 hours of ketoconazole, itraconazole, nefazodone, troleandomycin, clarithromycin, ritonavir and nelfinavir). Sometimes headache recurs within 24 hours after complete resolution. Triptans should not be taken within 24 hours of other triptans, isometheptene, or ergot derivatives.
2. **Dihydroergotamine (DHE)** is a potent venoconstrictor with minimal peripheral arterial constriction. Cardiac precautions are indicated in those with a history of angina or peripheral vascular disease or in elderly patients. A dose of 1–2 mg IM or SC can abort a migraine headache before it reaches peak intensity. If an attack has climaxed, 5–10 mg prochlorperazine can be given IV, followed immediately by 0.2 mg DHE IV given over 3 minutes. If tolerated, another 0.8 mg DHE IV is given. This relieves the primary headache in the majority of cases. For intractable migraines (status migrainosus), DHE can be given q8h with IV metoclopramide (*Neurology* 36:995, 1986; *Neurol Clin* 8:587, 1990). DHE 45 NS is administered intranasally, one spray in each nostril. It can be repeated in 15 minutes. The maximum recommended dose is 4 sprays/day.
3. **Ergotamine** is a vasoconstrictive agent that is effective for aborting migraine headaches, particularly if administered during the prodromal phase. Ergotamine should be taken at symptom onset in the maximum dose tolerated by the patient; nausea often limits the dose. Rectal prep-

arations are better absorbed than oral agents. The initial oral dose is 1–2 mg PO. Additional doses of 1–2 mg can be taken every 30 minutes, up to a total dose of 8–10 mg, but these rarely succeed when an initial dose has failed. Rectal (2 mg) administration should be tried in patients who are unresponsive to oral delivery or when emesis prevents oral administration. Dosages that exceed 16 mg/week should be used cautiously to avoid toxicity, which includes angina pectoris, limb claudication, and ergotamine headache and dependency.

4. **Other agents** can be used in the acute treatment of recalcitrant headaches.
   a. Ketorolac, 30–60 mg IM or IV.
   b. Prochlorperazine, 5–10 mg IV, may terminate migraine and helps alleviate nausea. Acute dystonic reactions and hypotension are potential side effects.
   c. Opiate analgesics (see Acute Inpatient Care, sec. **V,** in Chap. 1, Patient Care in Internal Medicine), usually meperidine, 50 mg IM or IV, may be useful for the management of acute headache. Chronic daily headaches should not be treated with narcotic analgesics to prevent addiction and tolerance.

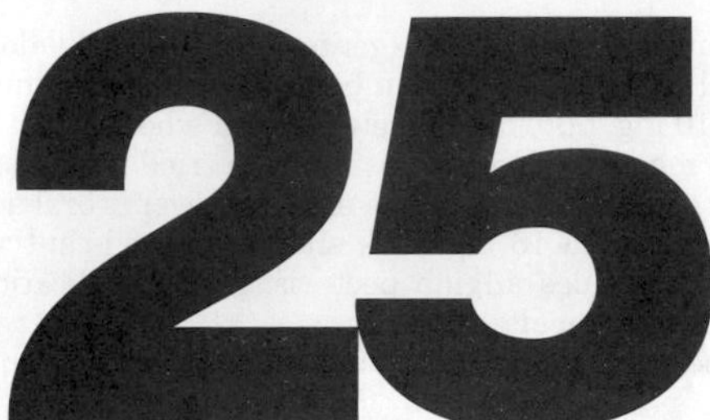

# Medical Emergencies

Daniel Goodenberger

Medical emergencies may not allow time for orderly information gathering and formulation of a narrow differential diagnosis before the initiation of therapy. **The first responsibility** is to provide basic life support (i.e., maintenance of an intact airway, adequate ventilation, and circulation; see Chap. 8, Critical Care).

## Acute Upper Airway Obstruction

In the **conscious patient,** manifestations of airway obstruction may include stridor, impaired or absent phonation, sternal or suprasternal retractions, display of the universal choking sign, and respiratory distress. Look for urticaria, angioedema, fever, or evidence of trauma. The **unconscious patient** may have labored breathing or apnea. Suspect airway obstruction in a nonbreathing patient who is difficult to ventilate. The **differential diagnosis** includes trauma to the face and neck, foreign body, infection (croup, epiglottitis, Ludwig's angina, retropharyngeal abscess, and diphtheria), tumor, angioedema, laryngospasm, anaphylaxis, retained secretions, or blockage of the upper airway by the tongue (in the unconscious patient). **Therapy** is directed at rapid relief of obstruction to prevent cardiopulmonary arrest and anoxic brain damage.

**I. Partial obstruction in the awake patient with adequate ventilation**

**A.** Rapidly take a history, focusing on the causes just listed.

**B.** Perform a directed physical examination, looking for airway swelling, trismus, pharyngeal obstruction, respiratory retractions, angioedema, stridor, wheezing, and grossly swollen lymph nodes and masses in the neck.

If the patient's condition is stable, perform indirect laryngoscopy or fiberoptic nasopharyngolaryngoscopy. A careful examination is unlikely to cause acute airway obstruction in an adult.

**C.** Soft-tissue radiography of the neck (posteroanterior and lateral views) is less sensitive and specific than is direct examination but may be a valuable adjunct. Such radiography should be performed in the emergency department as a portable study, as the patient should not be left unattended. Rapid CT of the airway with constant attendance is an alternative approach where available.

**D.** Treatment is aimed at the underlying disease process; observe the patient carefully and be prepared to intervene to maintain an airway.

**II. Airway obstruction in the awake patient without ventilation.** The most likely causes are a foreign body (usually food) and angioedema. Other causes include infection or posttraumatic hematoma. History is usually unavailable. One should perform the **Heimlich maneuver** (subdiaphragmatic abdominal thrust) repeatedly until the object is expelled from the airway or the patient becomes unconscious (see Chap. 8, Critical Care).

**III. Airway obstruction in an unconscious patient without intact ventilation**

**A.** Such a situation may be due to obstruction by the tongue, or it may be caused by a foreign body, trauma, infection, or angioedema. A history usually is unavailable except from paramedics or relatives. Examination reveals an unresponsive patient with no air movement or paradoxical respiratory efforts.

**B.** The first maneuver should be a head tilt–chin lift if cervical spine trauma is not suspected. Apply a jaw thrust if cervical spine trauma is suspected.

**C.** If these maneuvers are effective, place an oral or nasal airway. If they are ineffective, attempt to ventilate the patient with a bag-valve-mask apparatus. If these attempts are also unsuccessful, rapidly examine the oropharynx and hypopharynx. Avoid a blind finger sweep if it is possible to **examine the airway directly** using a laryngoscope and McGill forceps (if necessary) to remove a foreign body.

**D.** If laryngoscopy cannot be performed immediately and a foreign body is suspected, perform the supine Heimlich maneuver (straddling the supine patient and applying repeated subdiaphragmatic thrusts). Substitute chest thrusts if the patient is very obese or is in late pregnancy.

**E.** Failure of this maneuver should prompt an attempt at direct laryngoscopy and endotracheal intubation. Establish a surgical airway if the patient cannot be intubated. If a surgeon is not immediately available, perform needle cricothyrotomy using a 12- to 14-gauge over-the-needle catheter with high-flow oxygen (15 L/minute from a 50-psi wall source). Cricothyrotomy (see Chap. 8, Critical Care) is a preferred alternative.

## Pneumothorax

Pneumothorax may occur spontaneously or as a result of trauma. Primary spontaneous pneumothorax occurs without obvious underlying lung disease. Secondary spontaneous pneumothorax results from underlying parenchymal lung disease, including chronic obstructive pulmonary disease, interstitial lung disease, necrotizing lung infections, *Pneumocystis carinii* pneumonia, and cystic fibrosis. Traumatic pneumothoraces may occur as a result of penetrating or blunt chest wounds. Iatrogenic pneumothorax occurs after thoracentesis, central line placement, transbronchial biopsy, transthoracic needle biopsy, and barotrauma from mechanical ventilation and resuscitation.

**I.** The **history** reveals that the patient is complaining of ipsilateral chest or shoulder pain, usually of abrupt onset. Dyspnea is usually present, and the patient sometimes has a cough. Symptoms related to an underlying pulmonary disease process may be seen or a history of recent trauma obtained.

**II. Examination** of a patient with a small pneumothorax may be normal. With a larger pneumothorax or with underlying lung disease, there is increased dyspnea and tachypnea. The affected hemithorax may be noticeably larger (due to decreased elastic recoil of the collapsed lung) and relatively immobile during respiration. The patient has decreased breath sounds, decreased vocal fremitus, and a more resonant percussion note. If the pneumothorax is very large, and particularly if it is under tension, the patient may exhibit severe distress, diaphoresis, cyanosis, and hypotension. He or she may have signs of recent procedures or trauma. In addition, one may see such indications of underlying lung disease as clubbing or fever. If the pneumothorax is the result of penetrating trauma or pneumomediastinum, subcutaneous emphysema may be felt.

**III. Diagnosis** is confirmed by a chest radiograph, which reveals a separation of the pleural shadow from the chest wall. A small pneumothorax is more easily seen on a film taken during expiration. Air travels to the highest point in a body cavity; thus, a pneumothorax in a supine patient (who often is receiving positive-pressure ventilation) may be detected as an unusually deep costophrenic sulcus and excessive lucency over the upper abdomen caused by the anterior thoracic air. Tension pneumothorax is a clinical diagnosis; radiographic correlates include mediastinal and tracheal shift away from the pneumothorax and depression of the ipsilateral diaphragm. An ECG may reveal diminished anterior QRS amplitude and an anterior axis shift. In extreme cases, tension pneumothorax may cause electromechanical dissociation.

**IV. Treatment** depends on cause, size, and degree of physiologic derangement.

**A. A small, primary, spontaneous pneumothorax** without a continued pleural air leak may resolve spontaneously. Air is resorbed from the pleural space at roughly 1.5% daily, and therefore a small (~15%) pneumothorax is expected to resolve without intervention in approximately 10 days.

1. Confirm that the pneumothorax is not increasing in size (repeat the chest radiograph in 6 hours if there is no change in symptoms) and send the patient home if he or she is asymptomatic (apart from mild pleurisy). Obtain follow-up radiographs to confirm resolution of the pneumothorax in 7–10 days. Air travel is proscribed during the follow-up period, as a decrease in ambient barometric pressure results in a larger pneumothorax.
2. If the pneumothorax is small but the patient is mildly symptomatic, far from home, or unlikely to cooperate with follow-up, admit the patient and administer high-flow oxygen; the resulting nitrogen gradient will speed resorption.
3. If the pneumothorax is larger than 15–20% or is more than mildly symptomatic, insert a small thoracostomy tube [No. 8 French (Fr.) over a needle] in the second interspace in the midclavicular line; the air can be manually aspirated with a stopcock, attached to a one-way (Heimlich) valve, or, if necessary, connected to suction (*Chest* 119:590, 2001). If the bronchopleural fistula has sealed, cough or Valsalva results in re-expansion with the one-way valve. Most such patients should be hospitalized. If the pneumothorax fails to expand or if there is a continuous large air leak, arrange for insertion of a larger tube with suction (see sec. **IV.B**).
4. Pleural sclerosis to prevent recurrence is recommended by some experts but in most cases is not used after a first episode unless a persistent air leak is present. Doxycycline or a talc slurry can be used via chest tube for patients who wish to avoid surgery or who are at high surgical risk (see Pleural Effusion, sec. **III.C,** in Chap. 9, Pulmonary Disease). Apical bullectomy via thoracoscopy accompanied by pleural sclerosis has a higher success rate (78–91% vs. 95–100%) (*Chest* 119:590, 2001).

**B. Individuals with a secondary spontaneous pneumothorax** usually are symptomatic and require lung re-expansion. Often a bronchopleural fistula persists, and a larger thoracostomy tube and suction are required. If no associated effusion is present, a No. 24–28 Fr. tube is recommended; if fluid is present, choose a larger tube (No. 34–36 Fr.). Attach the thoracostomy tube to a three-bottle suction system or the commercial equivalent (Pleur-evac, Genzyme Biosurgery, Cambridge, MA) and apply 20 cm $H_2O$ suction. Large air leaks may require greater suction. Consult a pulmonologist about pleural sclerosis for persistent air leak and to prevent recurrence. Surgery may be required for persistent air leak and should be considered for high-risk patients for prevention of recurrence.

**C. Iatrogenic pneumothorax** generally is caused either by introducing air into the pleural space through the parietal pleura (e.g., thoracentesis, central line placement) or by allowing intrapulmonary air to escape through breach of the visceral pleura (e.g., transbronchial biopsy). Often no further air leak occurs after the initial event.

1. If the pneumothorax is small and the patient is minimally symptomatic, it can be managed conservatively. If the procedure that caused the

pneumothorax required sedation, admit the patient, administer oxygen, and repeat the chest radiograph in 6 hours to ensure the patient's stability. If the patient is completely alert and the chest x-ray shows no change, the patient can be discharged.

2. If the patient is symptomatic or if the pneumothorax is too large for expectant care, a pneumothorax catheter with aspiration or a one-way valve usually is adequate and can often be removed the following day.
3. Iatrogenic pneumothorax due to barotrauma from mechanical ventilation almost always has a persistent air leak and should be managed with a chest tube and suction.

**D. Tension pneumothorax** results from continued accumulation of air in the chest that is sufficient to shift mediastinal structures and impede venous return to the heart, resulting in hypotension, abnormal gas exchange, and, ultimately, cardiovascular collapse. It can occur as a result of barotrauma due to mechanical ventilation, a chest wound that allows ingress but not egress of air, or a rent in the visceral pleura that behaves in the same way ("ball-valve" effect). Suspect tension pneumothorax when a patient experiences hypotension and respiratory distress on mechanical ventilation or after any procedure in which the thorax is pierced by a needle. When the clinical situation and physical examination strongly suggest this diagnosis, decompress the affected hemithorax immediately with a 14-gauge needle attached to a fluid-filled syringe. Release of air with clinical improvement confirms the diagnosis. Seal any chest wound with an occlusive dressing and arrange for placement of a thoracostomy tube as described in sec. **IV.B.**

## Heat-Induced Illness

Heat illness is due to exposure to increased ambient temperature under conditions in which the body is unable to maintain appropriate homeostasis. Milder syndromes are exertional; the most severe may occur without exercise.

**I. Heat cramps** occur in unacclimatized individuals who engage in vigorous exercise in a hot environment; no published evidence has shown unequivocally that they are a result of salt depletion and hypotonic fluid replacement (*Int J Sports Med* 19:S146, 1998). Cramps typically occur in large muscle groups, most often in the legs. On examination, the patient has moist cool skin, a normal body temperature, and minimal distress. **Treatment** includes rest in a cool environment and salt replacement. Administer 1/2–1 tsp salt or a 650-mg sodium chloride tablet in 500 ml water PO or use a commercially available, oral, balanced electrolyte replacement solution. IV therapy rarely is required, but 2 L normal saline administered over several hours resolves symptoms.

**II. Heat exhaustion** occurs in unacclimatized individuals who exercise in the heat and is partly a result of loss of salt and water. The patient complains of headache, nausea, vomiting, dizziness, weakness, irritability, and cramps. On examination, the patient is diaphoretic, demonstrates piloerection, has postural hypotension, and has normal or minimally increased core temperature. **Therapy** consists of rest in a cool environment, acceleration of heat loss by fan evaporation, and fluid repletion with salt-containing solutions. If the patient is not vomiting and has stable BP, an oral, commercial, balanced salt solution is adequate. If the patient is vomiting or hemodynamically unstable, check electrolytes and give 1–2 L 0.9% saline IV. The patient should avoid exercise in a hot environment for 2–3 additional days.

**III. Heat syncope** affects unacclimatized individuals. Exercise in a hot environment results in peripheral vasodilatation and pooling of blood, with subsequent loss of consciousness. The affected individual regains consciousness promptly when supine, and the body temperature is normal, factors that separate this syndrome from heat stroke. **Treatment** consists of rest in a cool environment, fluid repletion, and a more gradual approach to building exercise endurance.

**IV. Heat stroke** can occur in the face of high core temperature, which causes direct thermal tissue injury. Secondary effects include acute renal failure from rhabdomyolysis. Even with rapid therapy, mortality may reach 76% for body temperatures of 41.1°C (106°F) or higher.

**A. Classic heat stroke** occurs after several days of heat exposure. Individuals at risk include those who are chronically ill, dehydrated, elderly, or obese; who have chronic cardiovascular disease; who abuse alcohol; and who use sedatives, hypnotics, α-adrenergic antagonists, diuretics, anticholinergics, or antipsychotics. Abuse of phencyclidine, cocaine, and amphetamines also may contribute. Risk factors include high humidity and lack of air-conditioning. More than 50% may have infection at presentation (*Ann Intern Med* 129:173, 1998). Typically, these patients have core temperatures higher than 40.5°C (105°F) and are comatose and anhidrotic.

**B. Exertional heat stroke** occurs rapidly in unacclimatized and unfit individuals who exercise in conditions of high ambient temperature and humidity. Those at risk include athletes, soldiers, and laborers, particularly if they lack access to water. Some of the risks associated with classic heat stroke may also be present, and certain congenital diseases that impair sweating may contribute. The core temperature may be lower than 40.5°C; 50% of patients are still sweating at presentation. Individuals with exertional heat stroke are more likely than are those with classic heat stroke to have **disseminated intravascular coagulation (DIC), lactic acidosis, and rhabdomyolysis.**

1. **Diagnosis** is based on the history of exposure or exercise, a core temperature usually of 40.6°C (105°F) or higher, and changes in mental status ranging from confusion to delirium and coma. Differential diagnosis includes malignant hyperthermia after exposure to anesthetic agents, neuroleptic malignant syndrome associated with antipsychotic drugs, anticholinergic poisoning, sympathomimetic toxicity (including cocaine), severe hyperthyroidism, sepsis, meningitis, cerebral malaria, encephalitis, hypothalamic dysfunction due to stroke or hemorrhage, and brain abscess. It is worth noting that neuroleptic malignant syndrome and malignant hyperthermia are both accompanied by severe muscle rigidity.

2. **Therapy**

   a. **Immediate cooling** is necessary. The best method of cooling is controversial. No study has directly compared ice water application with tepid spray. However, ice water lowers body temperature twice as quickly and is the procedure chosen when exertional heat stroke is anticipated (long distance races, military training) (*Int J Sports Med* 19:S150, 1998; *Ann Intern Med* 132:678, 2000). Wrap the patient in sheets that are continuously wetted with ice water. If response is insufficiently rapid, submerge the patient in ice water, recognizing that this may interfere with resuscitative efforts (*Am J Emerg Med* 14:355, 1996). Most emergency facilities that do not care for large numbers of heat illness cases are not equipped for this treatment. In that case, mist the patient continuously with tepid water (20–25°C). Cool the patient with a large electric fan with maximum body surface exposure. Ice packs at points of major heat transfer, such as the groin, axillae, and chest, may further speed cooling. If severely elevated core temperature does not respond to these maneuvers, gastric lavage with ice water may be helpful, although this treatment is controversial (*Crit Care Med* 15:748, 1987). Cold peritoneal lavage is not more effective than evaporative cooling. **Dantrolene sodium** does not appear to be effective for the treatment of heat stroke (*Crit Care Med* 19:176, 1991). However, if malignant hyperthermia due to anesthetic agent is diagnosed, give dantrolene, 2 mg/kg IV repeated q5min as necessary for symptom relief to a total of 10 mg/kg, followed by 1–2 mg/kg qid for 3–4 days. Treat neuroleptic malignant syndrome with dantrolene in the same way, but add bromocriptine, 2.5–5.0 mg PO or per gastrostomy tube q8h. If it is necessary to treat severe hypertension, nitroprusside may be preferable, as it promotes more rapid heat loss via peripheral vasodilation. Shivering and vasoconstriction impair cooling and should be prevented by administration of **chlorpromazine,** 10–25 mg IM, or **diazepam,** 5–10 mg IV. Monitor core temperatures continuously by rectal probe. Tympanic membrane temperature measurement does not correlate well with rectal temperature and may be affected by environmental conditions (*JAMA* 276:194, 1996; *Aviat Space Environ Med* 67:1048, 1996). Oral temperatures are unreliable and are frequently incorrectly low. Discontinue cooling measures when the core temperature reaches 39°C (102.2°F), which should ideally be achieved within 30 minutes. A temperature rebound may occur in 3–6 hours and should be retreated.

b. **Baseline laboratory studies** include CBC; partial thromboplastin time; prothrombin time; fibrin degradation products; electrolytes; BUN; creatinine, glucose, calcium, and creatine kinase levels; liver function tests; arterial blood gases (ABGs); urinalysis; and ECG. Monitor the cardiac rhythm continuously. If an infectious etiology is suspected, obtain appropriate cultures. If a central nervous system etiology is considered likely, CT imaging followed by spinal fluid examination is appropriate.
c. **For hypotension, administer crystalloids;** if refractory, treat with vasopressors and monitor hemodynamics. Avoid pure α-adrenergic agents, as they cause vasoconstriction and impair cooling. Administer crystalloids cautiously to normotensive patients.
d. **Treat rhabdomyolysis** or urine output of less than 30 ml/hour with adequate volume replacement, mannitol (12.5–25 g IV), and bicarbonate (44–100 mEq/L in 0.45% normal saline) to promote osmotic diuresis and urine alkalinization. Despite these measures, **renal failure** may still complicate 5% of cases of classic heat stroke and 25% of cases of exertional heat stroke.
e. **Hypoxemia and acute respiratory distress syndrome (ARDS)** may occur. Treat as described in Chap. 8, Critical Care.
f. **Other complications** include seizures, which should be treated with diazepam and phenytoin. Provide supportive care for hepatic injury, CHF, and coagulopathy.

## Cold-Induced Illness

Exposure to the cold may result in several different forms of injury. An important risk factor is accelerated heat loss, which is promoted by exposure to high wind or by immersion. Extended cold exposure may result from alcohol or drug abuse, injury or immobilization, and mental impairment. **Chilblains** are among the mildest form of cold injury and result from exposure of bare skin to a cold, windy environment (33–60°F). The ears, fingers, and tip of the nose typically are injured, with itchy, painful erythema on rewarming. Treat with rapid rewarming, moisturizing lotions, and analgesics and instruct the patient to avoid re-exposure.

I. **Immersion injury** (trench foot) is caused by prolonged immersion (longer than 10–12 hours) at a temperature <50°F. Treat by rewarming followed by dry dressings. Treat secondary infections with antibiotics.

II. **Frostnip** is the mildest form of frostbite and occurs most frequently on the distal extremities, the nose, or the ear. It is marked by tissue blanching and decreased sensitivity. **Rapid rewarming,** in a water bath at 104–108°F (40–42°C), is the treatment of choice for all forms of frostbite. The water temperature should never be hotter than 112°F.

**III. Superficial frostbite** involves the skin and subcutaneous tissues. Areas with first-degree involvement are white, waxy, and anesthetic; have poor capillary refill; and are painful on thawing. Second-degree involvement is manifested by clear or milky bullae. The treatment of choice is rapid rewarming. Immerse the affected body part for 15–30 minutes; hexachlorophene or povidone-iodine can be added to the water bath. Narcotic analgesics may be necessary for rewarming pain. No deep injury ensues, and healing occurs in 3–4 weeks.

**IV. Deep frostbite** involves death of skin, subcutaneous tissue, and muscle (third degree) or deep tendons and bones (fourth degree).

**A. Diagnosis.** The tissue appears frozen and hard. On rewarming, there is no capillary filling. Hemorrhagic blisters form, followed by eschars. Healing is very slow, and demarcation of tissue with autoamputation may occur. Diabetes mellitus, peripheral vascular disease, an outdoor lifestyle, and high altitude are additional risk factors. More than 90% of deep frostbite occurs at temperatures lower than 6.7°C (44°F) with exposures longer than 7–10 hours.

**B. Treatment.** Treat by rapid rewarming. **Rewarming should not be started until there is no chance of refreezing.** Administer analgesics (IV opioids) as needed. Admit the patient to a surgical service. Elevate the affected extremity, prevent weight bearing, separate the affected digits with cotton wool, prevent tissue maceration by using a blanket cradle, and prohibit smoking. Update tetanus immunization. Intra-arterial vasodilators, heparin, dextran, prostaglandin inhibitors, thrombolytics, and sympathectomy are not routinely justified. Use antibiotics only for documented infection. Amputation is undertaken only after full demarcation has occurred.

**V. Hypothermia** is defined as a core temperature of less than 35°C (95°F). Classification of severity by temperature is not universal. One scheme defines hypothermia as mild at 34–35°C, moderate at 30–34°C, and severe at less than 30°C. The most common cause of hypothermia in the United States is cold exposure due to alcohol intoxication. Another common cause is cold water immersion. Differential diagnosis and other risk factors include extremes of age, cerebrovascular accident, drug overdose, diabetic ketoacidosis, hypoglycemia, uremia, adrenal insufficiency, and myxedema.

**A. Diagnosis** requires accurate monitoring of core temperature. A standard oral thermometer registers only to a lower limit of 35°C. Monitor the patient continuously with a rectal probe with a full range of 20–40°C. Equal efficacy of ear thermistor monitoring has not been demonstrated.

**B. Signs and symptoms** vary with the temperature of the patient at presentation. All organ systems can be involved.

1. **CNS effects.** At temperatures below 32°C, mental processes are slowed and the affect is flattened. At less than 32.2°C (90°F), the ability to shiver is lost, and deep tendon reflexes are diminished. At 28°C, coma often supervenes. Below 18°C, the EEG is flat. On rewarming from severe hypothermia, central pontine myelinolysis may develop.
2. **Cardiovascular effects.** After an initial increased release of catecholamines, there is a decrease in cardiac output and heart rate with relatively preserved mean arterial pressure. ECG changes, manifest initially as sinus bradycardia with T-wave inversion and QT-interval prolongation, may progress to atrial fibrillation at temperatures of less than 32°C. Osborne waves (J-point elevation) may be visible, particularly in leads II and $V_6$. An increased susceptibility to ventricular arrhythmias occurs at temperatures below 32°C. At temperatures of less than 30°C, the susceptibility to ventricular fibrillation is increased significantly, and unnecessary manipulation or jostling of the patient should be avoided. A decrease in mean arterial pressure may also occur, and, at temperatures of less than 28°C, progressive bradycardia supervenes.

3. **Respiratory complications.** After an initial increase in minute ventilation, respiratory rate and tidal volume decrease progressively with decreasing temperature. ABGs measured with the machine set at 37°C should serve as the basis for therapy without correction of pH and carbon dioxide tension ($PCO_2$) (*Arch Intern Med* 148:1643, 1988; *Ann Emerg Med* 18:72, 1989). Supply supplemental oxygen.
4. **Renal manifestations.** Cold-induced diuresis and tubular concentrating defects may be seen.

C. **Laboratory evaluation** includes CBC; coagulation studies; liver function tests; BUN; electrolytes; creatinine, glucose, creatine kinase, calcium, magnesium, and amylase levels; urinalysis; ABGs; and ECG. Obtain toxicology screen if mental status alteration is more profound than expected for temperature decrease. Obtain chest, abdominal, and cervical spine radiographs to evaluate all patients with a history of trauma or immersion injury. Electrolyte abnormalities are common. Serum potassium often is increased. Elevated serum amylase may reflect underlying pancreatitis. Hyperglycemia may be noted but should not be treated, as rebound hypoglycemia may occur with rewarming. DIC may also occur.

D. **Therapeutic measures** include maintenance of the airway and oxygen administration. If intubation is required, the most experienced operator should perform it (see Chap. 8, Critical Care in the section Airway Management and Tracheal Intubation).

1. Conduct CPR in standard fashion. Perform simultaneous vigorous core rewarming; as long as the core temperature is severely decreased, it should not be assumed that the patient cannot be resuscitated. Reliable defibrillation requires a core temperature of 32°C or higher; prolonged efforts (to a core temperature of 35°C) may be justified because of the neuroprotective effects of hypothermia. **Do not begin CPR if an organized ECG rhythm is present,** as inability to detect peripheral pulses may be due to vasoconstriction, and CPR may precipitate ventricular fibrillation. Do not perform Swan-Ganz catheterization, as it may precipitate ventricular fibrillation. If ventricular fibrillation occurs, administer bretylium (5 mg/kg IV) as the agent of choice; lidocaine is an alternative. Avoid procainamide because it may precipitate ventricular fibrillation and increase the temperature that is necessary to defibrillate the patient. Monitor ECG rhythm, urine output, and, possibly, central venous pressure in all patients with an intact circulation.
2. **Rewarming.** The patient should be rewarmed with the goal of increasing the temperature by 0.5–2.0°C/hour, although the rate of rewarming has not been shown to be related to outcome.
   a. **Passive external rewarming** depends on the patient's ability to shiver and thus generate heat. It is effective only at core temperatures of 32°C or higher. Remove wet clothing, cover the patient with blankets in a warm environment, and monitor.
   b. **Active external rewarming** includes application of heating blankets (40–45°C) or warm bath immersion. This type of therapy has been feared to cause paradoxical core acidosis, hyperkalemia, and decreased core temperature, as cold stagnant blood returns to the central vasculature (*J Royal Naval Med Serv* 77:139, 1991), although Danish naval research supports arm and leg rewarming as effective and safe (*Aviat Space Environ Med* 70:1081, 1999). Pending further investigation, limit active rewarming to the trunk of young, previously healthy patients with acute hypothermia and minimal pathophysiologic derangement.
   c. **Active core rewarming is preferred for treatment of severe hypothermia,** although few data are available on outcomes (*Resuscitation* 36:101, 1998).
      (1) **Heated oxygen** is the initial therapy of choice for the patient whose cardiovascular status is stable. This therapeutic maneuver

can be expected to raise core temperatures by 0.5–1.2°C/hour (*Ann Emerg Med* 9:456, 1980). Administration through an endotracheal tube results in more rapid rewarming than delivery via face mask. Administer heated oxygen through a cascade humidifier at a temperature of 45°C or lower.

(2) **IV fluids** can be heated in a microwave oven or delivered through a blood warmer; give fluids only through peripheral IV lines.

(3) **Heated nasogastric or bladder lavage** is of limited efficacy because of low exposed surface area and is reserved for the patient with cardiovascular instability. **Heated peritoneal lavage** with fluid warmed to 40–45°C is more effective than is heated aerosol inhalation, but it should be reserved for patients with cardiovascular instability. Only those who are experienced in its use should perform heated peritoneal lavage, in combination with other modes of rewarming. Closed thoracic lavage with heated fluid by thoracostomy tube has been recommended (*Ann Emerg Med* 19:204, 1990) but is unproved. **Hemodialysis** can be used for the severely hypothermic, particularly when due to an overdose that is amenable to treatment in this way.

(4) **Extracorporeal circulation** (cardiac bypass) is used only in hypothermic individuals who are in cardiac arrest; in these cases, it may be dramatically effective (*N Engl J Med* 337:1500, 1997). Extracorporeal circulation may raise the temperature as rapidly as 10–12°C/hour but must be performed in an ICU or operating room.

3. **Medications.** Give thiamine to most patients with cold exposure, as exposure due to alcohol intoxication is common. Administration of antibiotics is a controversial issue; many authorities recommend antibiotic administration for 72 hours, pending cultures. In general, those patients with hypothermia due to exposure and alcohol intoxication are less likely to have a serious underlying infection than are those who are elderly or who have an underlying medical illness.
4. **Observation.** Admit patients with an underlying disease, physiologic derangement, or core temperature lower than 32°C, preferably to an ICU. Discharge individuals with mild hypothermia (32–35°C) and no predisposing medical conditions or complications when they are normothermic and an adequate home environment can be ensured.

## Near-Drowning

**Predisposing factors** include youth, inability to swim, alcohol and drug use, barotrauma (in scuba diving), head and neck trauma, and loss of consciousness associated with epilepsy, diabetes, syncope, or dysrhythmias. *Near-drowning* is defined as survival for at least 24 hours after submersion in a liquid medium.

I. **Pathophysiology.** Much has been made of the differences in pathophysiology between fresh- and salt-water drownings. However, the **major insults** (i.e., hypoxemia and tissue hypoxia related to $\dot{V}/\dot{Q}$ mismatch, acidosis, and hypoxic brain injury with cerebral edema) are common to both. Hypothermia, pneumonia, and, rarely, DIC, acute renal failure, and hemolysis also may occur.

II. **Treatment.** Begin with resuscitation, focusing on airway management and ventilation with 100% oxygen. Establish an IV line with 0.9% saline or lactated Ringer's solution. The Heimlich maneuver is not indicated unless upper airway obstruction is present (*J Emerg Med* 13:397, 1995).

A. **Immobilize the cervical spine,** as trauma may be present.

B. **Treat hypothermia** vigorously (see the section Cold-Induced Illness).

**C. Obtain** electrocardiogram, serum electrolytes, CBC, ABGs, and chest radiograph. Monitor the cardiac rhythm continuously. Obtain blood alcohol level and drug screen if the mental status is not normal.

**D. Manage pulmonary complications.** Administer 100% oxygen initially, titrating thereafter by ABGs. Intubate the patient endotracheally and begin mechanical ventilation with positive end-expiratory pressure (PEEP) if the patient is apneic, is in severe respiratory distress, or has oxygen-resistant hypoxemia. Administer bronchodilators if bronchospasm is present. Artificial surfactant has not been shown to be useful (*Acad Emerg Med* 2:204, 1995; *Pediatr Emerg Care* 11:153, 1995).

**E. Reserve antibiotics for documented infection.** Pneumonia may be due to water-borne organisms such as *Pseudomonas*, *Aeromonas*, and *Proteus*.

**F. Prophylactic glucocorticoids** have no role (*Heart Lung* 16:474, 1987).

**G. Manage metabolic acidosis** with mechanical ventilation, sodium bicarbonate (if the pH is persistently <7.2), and BP support.

**H. Cerebral edema** may occur suddenly within the first 24 hours and is a major cause of death. Treatment of cerebral edema does not appear to increase survival (*Crit Care Med* 14:529, 1986), and intracranial pressure monitoring does not appear to be effective. Nevertheless, if cerebral edema occurs, hyperventilate the patient to a $PCO_2$ of no less than 25 mm Hg, and administer mannitol (1–2 g/kg q3–4h) or furosemide (1 mg/kg IV q4–6h). Treat seizures aggressively with phenytoin. The routine administration of glucocorticoids is not recommended. Hypothermia or barbiturate "coma" is not indicated (*Pediatrics* 81:630, 1988). It may be necessary to sedate and paralyze the patient to reduce oxygen consumption and facilitate intracranial pressure management.

**III. Observation.** Admit patients who have survived severe episodes of near-drowning to an ICU. Noncardiogenic pulmonary edema may still develop in those individuals with less severe immersions. Admit any patient with pulmonary signs or symptoms, including cough, bronchospasm, abnormal ABGs or oxygen saturation as measured by pulse oximetry ($SpO_2$), or abnormal chest radiograph. Observe the asymptomatic patient with a questionable or brief water immersion for 4–6 hours and discharge the patient if the chest radiograph and ABGs are normal (*Ann Emerg Med* 15:1084, 1986). However, if a documented long submersion, unconsciousness, initial cyanosis or apnea, or even a brief requirement for resuscitation has occurred, the patient **must be admitted for at least 24 hours.**

## Overdosage

**I. Recognition of poisoning and medication overdose** requires a high index of suspicion and careful clinical evaluation. In the most recent year for which information is available, more than 2.2 million toxic exposures occurred in the United States, resulting in more than 1000 deaths (*Am J Emerg Med* 20:391, 2002). Up to 50% of all initial poisoning histories may be incorrect. The ingestion of multiple drugs is common. Seek identification of the drug or drugs ingested and their dosages from the patient's family or friends, private physician, pharmacist, and paramedical personnel. Obtain supporting materials (e.g., pill bottles) and clues regarding the timing of ingestion. Recognition of specific toxic syndromes is often helpful in directing initial management (Table 25-1). Vital signs, neurologic status, pupillary reactions, cardiovascular response, abdominal findings, and unusual odors and excreta, as well as evaluation of ABGs, serum electrolytes, and acid-base abnormalities, may suggest a particular toxin. Order baseline screening of liver and kidney function. Screening of blood, urine, and gastric aspirate for specific toxic agents is important,

**Table 25-1.** Toxic syndromes and possible causes

| Syndrome | Manifestations | Possible causes |
|---|---|---|
| Acquired hemoglobinopathies | Dyspnea, cyanosis, confusion or lethargy, headache | Carbon monoxide<br>Methemoglobinemia (nitrites, phenazopyridine)<br>Sulfhemoglobinemia |
| Anion-gap metabolic acidosis | Variable | Methanol<br>Ethanol<br>Ethylene glycol<br>Paraldehyde<br>Iron<br>Isoniazid<br>Salicylate<br>Vacor<br>Cyanide |
| Anticholinergic | Dry mouth and skin, blurred vision, mydriasis, tachycardia, generalized sunburn-like rash or flushing of skin, hyperthermia, abdominal distention, urinary urgency or retention, confusion, hallucinations, delusions, excitation, or coma | Atropine and other belladonna alkaloids<br>Antihistamines<br>Tricyclics<br>Phenothiazines<br>Jimson seeds |
| Cholinergic | Hypersalivation, bronchorrhea, bronchospasm, urination or defecation, neuromuscular failure, lacrimation | Acetylcholine<br>Organophosphate insecticides<br>Bethanechol<br>Methacholine<br>Wild mushrooms |
| Cyanide | Nausea, vomiting, collapse, coma, bradycardia, no cyanosis, decreased arteriovenous $O_2$ difference with severe metabolic acidosis | Cyanide<br>Amygdalin |
| Extrapyramidal | Dysphoria and dysphagia, trismus, oculogyric crisis, rigidity, torticollis, laryngospasm | Prochlorperazine<br>Haloperidol<br>Chlorpromazine and other antipsychotics<br>Other phenothiazines |
| Narcotic | CNS depression, respiratory depression, miosis, hypotension | Morphine and heroin<br>Codeine<br>Propoxyphene<br>Other synthetic and semisynthetic opiates |
| Salicylism | Fever, hyperpnea, respiratory alkalosis or mixed acid-base disturbance, hypokalemia, tinnitus | Aspirin<br>Other salicylate products |

*(continued)*

**Table 25-1.** Continued

| Syndrome | Manifestations | Possible causes |
|---|---|---|
| Sympathomimetic | Excitation, hypertension, cardiac arrhythmias, seizures | Amphetamines<br>Cocaine<br>Caffeine<br>Aminophylline<br>β Agonists, inhaled or injected |

*Source:* Modified from G Quick, PJ Crocker. Toxic emergency: agent unknown. *Emerg Decisions* 7:44, 1986. Reprinted with permission from Physicians World/Thomson Healthcare, Secaucus, NJ.

but, in most cases, therapy must proceed before such results are available. Abdominal radiography may be useful in detecting retained pills (such as iron). Obtain an ECG and monitor the cardiac rhythm continuously until the ingested agent is identified and thereafter as appropriate. Perform a pregnancy test in women of childbearing years. Although the computerized *Poisindex* (2003; Micromedex, Greenwood Village, CO) system is helpful, seek additional specific advice from the regional poison control center.

**II. Supportive care** is crucial.

**A. Maintain a patent airway** and adequate ventilation. Intubate the trachea if airway protection is required.

**B. Hypotension** usually responds to IV fluids, although vasopressors may be required in refractory cases or in the presence of pulmonary edema. Use dopamine in most situations; choose norepinephrine for overdoses with α antagonists (phenothiazines) and tricyclic antidepressants (due to the proarrhythmic effect of dopamine).

**C. Arrhythmias** may be related to cardiac or autonomic effects; treatment depends on the toxin.

**D. CNS depression** or coma occurs frequently. When present, administer naloxone (2 mg IV) for possible narcotic overdose, give 50% dextrose in water (50 ml IV) or determine finger-stick glucose immediately, administer thiamine (100 mg IV push) for possible Wernicke-Korsakoff syndrome, and give oxygen for possible carbon monoxide intoxication. Give flumazenil for known or suspected benzodiazepine overdose (see sec. **VII.N.2.b**). However, do not give it for unknown overdoses, as this agent may precipitate seizures in cyclic antidepressant overdose. Also, avoid flumazenil administration in patients who have ingested drugs that are known to cause seizures (cocaine, lithium, theophylline, isoniazid, cyclosporine) or who are known to have a preexisting seizure disorder (*Clin Ther* 14:292, 1992).

**III. Prevention of further drug absorption** may be facilitated by gastric emptying (gastric lavage, induced emesis) or by administration of activated charcoal. Gastric emptying procedures, if used, should be initiated within 1 hour of the ingestion. Because most adult overdose patients present several hours after toxic ingestion and because the use of syrup of ipecac may delay subsequent therapy, administration of activated charcoal alone is recommended as the primary GI decontamination procedure for most patients (*Ann Emerg Med* 16:838, 1987). No difference in outcome appears to occur whether gastric emptying plus charcoal or charcoal administration alone is used (*Ann Emerg Med* 14:562, 1985; *Med J Aust* 163:345, 1995). Theoretical exceptions may include phenothiazine overdose (delayed gastric emptying) and drugs that form gastric concretions. Rapidly absorbed agents such as strychnine and cyanide are unlikely to be affected by charcoal administration.

**A. Activated charcoal** adsorbs most drugs, preventing further absorption from the GI tract. Exceptions include alkalis, arsenic and other heavy metals, hydrocarbons, cyanide, ethanol (EtOH) and other alcohols, lithium, ferrous sulfate, carbamate, and mineral acids. It is not indicated for these ingestions. Activated charcoal also promotes efflux of selected drugs (theophylline, phenobarbital, and carbamazepine) from the blood into the bowel lumen. Give 50–100 g activated charcoal, diluted in water, as soon as possible after the toxic ingestion; prehospital administration further enhances recovery. Evidence to support its use more than 1 hour after toxic ingestion is unavailable, and many experts do not recommend its administration after that interval (*J Toxicol Clin Toxicol* 35:721, 1997). Do not use activated charcoal when bowel obstruction or perforation is present or when endoscopy is contemplated. When repeated dosing is used, no more than a single dose of sorbitol or other cathartic should be given. Although **multidose charcoal** has been shown to increase selected drug elimination significantly, it has not yet been demonstrated in a controlled study to reduce mortality in poisoned patients. It is indicated in ingestions of life-threatening amounts of carbamazepine, phenobarbital, theophylline, quinine, dapsone, paraquat, and *Amanita phalloides* (*J Toxicol Clin Toxicol* 37:731, 1999; *BMJ* 319:1414, 1999). It may be of use in overdoses of amitriptyline, cyclosporine, dextropropoxyphene, diazepam, digitoxin, digoxin, disopyramide, methotrexate, nadolol, phencyclidine, phenylbutazone, phenytoin, piroxicam, sotalol, and valproate. Its use in salicylate overdose is controversial. Give an initial dose of 50–100 g and repeat that dose every 4 hours until the patient's condition and laboratory parameters improve. If the patient is obtunded or has an absent gag reflex, the **airway must be protected;** endotracheal intubation may be necessary.

**B.** Because there is no evidence to show that administration of **ipecac** improves outcome and some evidence to suggest an increase in complications (*Ann Emerg Med* 18:56, 1989), and because of its many contraindications, routine use in the emergency center has largely been abandoned (*J Toxicol Clin Toxicol* 35:699, 1997). **Contraindications** to ipecac use include decreased level of consciousness, absent gag reflex, caustic ingestion, convulsions or exposure to a substance that is likely to cause convulsions, and medical conditions that make emesis unsafe. Do not give ipecac for ingestion of unknown toxins, as aspiration may occur if coma or seizures develop.

**C. Gastric lavage** should not be used routinely in the management of the poisoned patient. Exceptions include ingestions of a life-threatening amount of toxin when the patient presents within 60 minutes (*J Toxicol Clin Toxicol* 35:711, 1997) or when concretions are believed to be present. Use a large orogastric tube (No. 28–36 Fr.) for these patients. Contraindications include corrosive ingestion. Lavage should not be performed with an unprotected airway if the patient has lost airway protective reflexes or has ingested hydrocarbons with a high aspiration potential. In these cases, lavage should be performed only **after endotracheal intubation.** Lavage with 200-ml boluses of warm saline, repeated until the effluent is clear, and follow this by instillation of activated charcoal.

**D.** The use of a **cathartic** is not supported by clinical evidence and is therefore not routinely recommended (*J Toxicol Clin Toxicol* 35:743, 1997). If used, give no more than a single dose. Acceptable forms include magnesium citrate, 4 ml/kg (300 ml maximum); sorbitol, 1–2 g/kg (150 g maximum); and magnesium or sodium sulfate, 25–30 g. Do not give magnesium salts to patients with renal failure.

**E. Whole-bowel irrigation** with commercially available polyethylene glycol bowel preparation solution should not be used routinely in the management of the poisoned patient (*J Toxicol Clin Toxicol* 35:753, 1997), as there is no conclusive evidence that it improves outcomes. Exceptions can be considered for toxic ingestions of sustained-release drugs such as β-adrenergic antagonists, calcium channel antagonists, lithium, and theophylline. Evidence is insufficient either to support or exclude its use for iron ingestion with radiographically persistent tablets in the GI tract or body packing with heroin or cocaine. It is contraindicated in the presence of bowel obstruction, ileus, intestinal perforation, and hemodynamic instability and should not be administered to a patient with a compromised unprotected airway. Administer 1–2 L/hour to a total of 10 L; it can be discontinued earlier if the rectal effluent is clear. Obtain an abdominal x-ray to document clearance of iron or drug-containing packets.

F. **Endoscopic or surgical removal, or both,** should be considered only for ingestion of life-threatening agents that have not been or cannot be effectively removed by the above measures, such as button batteries lodged in the esophagus and pharmacobezoars of highly toxic materials and for cocaine body packers with severe toxicity due to rupture of a packet. Endoscopy should not be performed to remove unruptured drug packets, as this intervention may result in rupture and greater toxicity.

IV. **Removal of absorbed drugs** can be achieved by enhancement of renal excretion and extracorporeal methods.

A. **Use forced diuresis only when specifically indicated** because of the risk of causing acid-base disturbances, electrolyte abnormalities, and cerebral or pulmonary edema. Do not attempt forced diuresis in patients with renal insufficiency, cardiac disease, or existing electrolyte abnormalities. Few data support the efficacy of this procedure in improving survival.

1. **Forced alkaline diuresis,** achieving a urinary pH of 7.5–9.0, promotes excretion of drugs that are weak acids, such as salicylates, barbital, and phenobarbital. Administer a solution of sodium bicarbonate, 44–100 mEq, added to 1 L 0.45% saline, at 250–500 ml/hour for the first 1–2 hours. Concomitant administration of potassium chloride may be necessary to treat diuresis-induced hypokalemia and to achieve urinary alkalinization. Exercise great care to avoid excessive volume expansion, especially in the elderly. Administer maintenance alkaline solution and diuretics to maintain a urinary output of 2–3 ml/kg/hour.
2. **Forced acid diuresis** is not recommended for any agent.

V. **Extracorporeal removal of specific toxins by hemodialysis or hemoperfusion** is used when (1) clinical deterioration persists despite intensive supportive therapy, (2) blood levels reach potentially lethal concentrations, (3) a risk of lethal delayed effects exists, and (4) renal or hepatic failure impairs clearance of toxin. Common toxins that can be removed by hemodialysis include toxic alcohols, salicylates, theophylline, and lithium. Generally, compounds with low molecular weight, small volume of distribution, and low degree of protein binding of drug are amenable to removal by hemodialysis. **Specific antidotes** are available that neutralize or prevent the toxic effect of certain drugs (Table 25-2). For information on the pharmacokinetics of the offending agent and specific treatment guidelines, contact the regional poison control center immediately if the drug that was ingested is known.

VI. **Disposition** must be determined. Observe even those patients with apparently trivial overdoses of potentially toxic agents for at least 4 hours before contemplating their discharge. Do not discharge any patient who has taken an intentional overdose without formal psychiatric consultation and assessment of disposition. Refer individuals who experience inadvertent recreational drug overdose for counseling and, possibly, detoxification. Patients who are considered potentially suicidal require constant one-on-one supervision while on the medical service.

VII. **Specific agents**

A. **Acetaminophen** is a common ingredient in many analgesic and antipyretic preparations. Hepatic toxicity is due to depletion of hepatic glutathione and subsequent accumulation of a toxic intermediate metabolite, *N*-acetyl-*p*-benzoquinonimine. Toxicity usually occurs after acute ingestion of more

**Table 25-2.** Antidotes

| Poison or toxic sign | Antidote | Adult dosage |
|---|---|---|
| Acetaminophen | *N*-Acetylcysteine | 140 mg/kg PO, followed by 70 mg/kg q4h for 17 doses |
| Anticholinesterases | Atropine sulfate | 1–5 mg IV (IM, SC) q15min prn to drying of secretions |
| | Pralidoxime (2-PAM) chloride[a] | 1 g IV (PO) over 15–30 min q8–12h × 3 doses prn |
| Benzodiazepines | Flumazenil | 0.2 mg (2 ml) IV over 30 sec, followed by 0.3 mg at 1-min intervals to a total dose of 3 mg |
| Carbon monoxide | Oxygen | 100%, hyperbaric |
| Cyanide | Amyl nitrite[b] *followed by* | Inhalation pearls for 15–30 sec every min |
| | Sodium nitrite[b] *followed by* | 300 mg (10 ml 3% solution) IV over 3 min, repeated in half dosage in 2 hr if persistent or recurrent signs of toxicity |
| | Sodium thiosulfate | 12.5 g (50 ml 25% solution) IV over 10 min, repeated in half dosage in 2 hr if persistent or recurrent signs of toxicity |
| Digoxin | Antidigoxin Fab' fragments | Acute ingestion: Dose (vials) = [ingested digoxin (mg) × 0.8]/0.5<br>Chronic ingestion: Dose (vials) = [serum level (ng/ml) × weight (kg)]/100, infused in 0.9% saline over 15–30 min; repeat if toxicity persists |
| Ethylene glycol (EG) | Fomepizole | 15 mg/kg IV, followed by 10 mg/kg IV q12h for 4 doses, followed by 15 mg/kg IV q12h until the EG level <20 mg/dl |
| | Ethanol[c] | 0.6 g/kg in $D_5W$ IV (PO) over 30–45 min, followed initially by 110 mg/kg/hr to maintain a blood level of 100–150 mg/dl |
| Extrapyramidal signs | Diphenhydramine hydrochloride | 25–50 mg IV (IM, PO) prn |
| | Benztropine mesylate | 1–2 mg IV (IM, PO) prn |
| Heavy metals (e.g., arsenic, copper, gold, lead, mercury) | Chelators[d] | |
| | Calcium disodium edetate (EDTA) | 1 g IV (IM) over 1 hr q12h |
| | Dimercaprol (BAL) | 2.5–5.0 mg/kg IM q4–6h |
| | Penicillamine | 250–500 mg PO q6h |
| | 2,3-Dimercaptosuccinic acid (DMSA, Succimer) | 10 mg/kg PO tid × 5 d, then bid × 14 d |
| Iron | Deferoxamine mesylate | 1 g IM (IV at a rate 15 mg/kg/hr if hypotension) q8h prn |

*(continued)*

**Table 25-2.** Continued

| Poison or toxic sign | Antidote | Adult dosage |
|---|---|---|
| Isoniazid (INH) | Pyridoxine | Amount equal to estimated INH ingestion up to 5 g over 30–60 min; any remainder by IV drip over 12 hr |
| Methanol | Ethanol[c] | See Ethylene glycol |
| Methemoglobinemia | Methylene blue | 1–2 mg/kg (0.1–0.2 ml/kg 1% solution) IV over 5 min, repeated in 1 hr prn |
| Opioids | Naloxone hydrochloride | 0.4–2.0 mg IV (IM, SC, endotracheally) prn |
| Warfarin and related drugs | Vitamin $K_1$ (phytonadione) | 10 mg IM, SC, or IV[e] |
| | Fresh frozen plasma | Variable |

$D_5W$, 5% dextrose in water.
*Note:* This table is only a guide. Antidote usage and dosage depend on the specific clinical situation. The regional poison control center should be contacted for specific therapeutic recommendations.
[a]Pralidoxime is indicated in severe organophosphate poisoning with muscle weakness or fasciculations or respiratory depression.
[b]Nitrites may have an antidotal effect in hydrogen sulfide poisoning.
[c]The requisite ethanol dose depends on prior alcohol use, liver function, and dialysis. Consult the regional poison control center for assistance.
[d]The use of a specific chelating agent or combination of agents depends on the heavy metal involved and on the clinical situation.
[e]Caution should be used when giving vitamin $K_1$ IV. It should be given over 20 min.

than 140 mg/kg, or at least 7.5 g. Precise determination of probable toxicity can be obtained by plotting a plasma acetaminophen level (drawn at least 4 hours after ingestion) on a nomogram in relation to the time since ingestion (Fig. 25-1). However, nearly half of hospitalizations for acetaminophen toxicity are due to toxicity from chronic ingestion, which is increased in those with excess alcohol intake (*Acad Emerg Med* 6:1115, 1999). The nomogram does not provide useful information regarding toxicity of chronic ingestion, however. In this instance, treatment is recommended if there is evidence of liver toxicity and the acetaminophen level is greater than 10 μg/ml. If in doubt, consult with an expert in clinical toxicology or hepatology, or both. The nomogram is also of uncertain usefulness in acute overdose of sustained-release products. In this latter situation, the Rocky Mountain Poison Center recommends that a second drug level be obtained 4–6 hours after the first; if either level falls in the toxic range, antidotal therapy is advised (*Poisindex* 6/2003).

1. **Symptoms** during the first 24 hours include anorexia, vomiting, and diaphoresis. Hepatic enzymes begin to rise 24–36 hours after ingestion and peak (aspartate aminotransferase earliest) 72–96 hours after ingestion. Recovery starts after approximately 4 days unless hepatic failure develops.
2. **Treatment** includes supportive measures and GI decontamination.
   a. Gastric lavage is not indicated. Do not administer ipecac, as its use delays administration of the specific antidote. Administer activated charcoal as soon as possible after the ingestion (see sec. **III.A**). Charcoal appears to provide an additional hepatoprotective effect (*J Toxicol Clin Toxicol* 37:753, 1999).

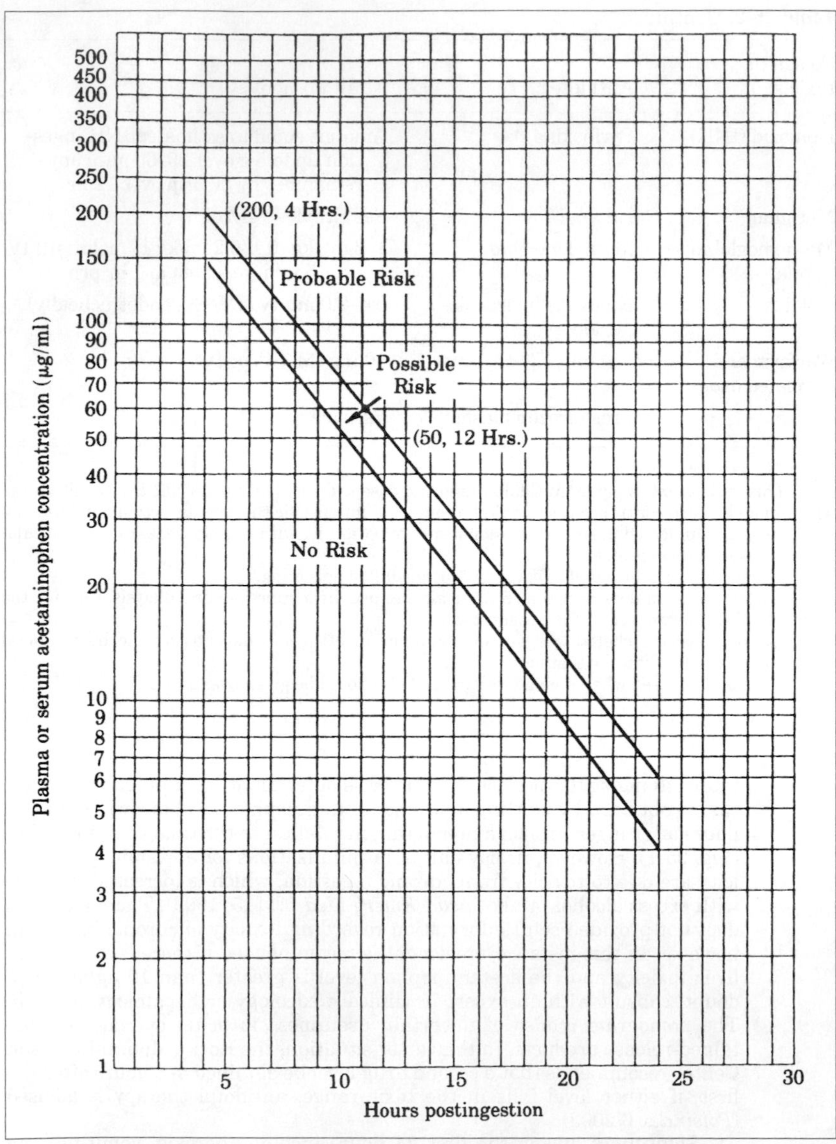


**Fig. 25-1.** Nomogram for acetaminophen hepatotoxicity. (Adapted from BH Rumack, RC Peterson, GG Koch, IA Amara. Acetaminophen overdose: 662 cases with evaluation of oral acetylcysteine treatment. *Arch Intern Med* 141:380, 1981.)

**b.** When the history suggests that a toxic dose has been ingested, do not wait for return of the blood acetaminophen level to administer the first dose of **acetylcysteine (Mucomyst),** a specific antidote that acts as a glutathione substrate. This antidote is most effective in preventing hepatotoxicity if given within 8 hours of ingestion and is recommended up to 24 hours; it may be helpful when administered up to 36 hours after the event if hepatotoxicity is evident (*Lancet* 335:1572, 1990).

**(1) The initial dose** is 140 mg/kg diluted to a 5% solution in a soft drink, juice, or water, given PO or by gastric tube; **it can be given simultaneously with charcoal** without impairment of its efficacy.

**(2)** Subsequent administration (70 mg/kg q4h for a total of 17 doses) is directed by the initial plasma acetaminophen level. **If a toxic level is detected, give the full 17 doses;** if not, no further antidote is indicated. If vomiting occurs less than 1 hour after administration of the antidote, repeat the dose.

**(3)** If vomiting is repetitive and interferes with acetylcysteine administration, use metoclopramide or droperidol, or administer acetylcysteine via a fluoroscopically placed nasoduodenal tube over a period of 30–60 minutes.

**(4) IV acetylcysteine** is not U.S. Food and Drug Administration (FDA) approved but can be considered for those who cannot or will not take oral acetylcysteine. An IV preparation is not available in the United States but can be prepared from the sterile solution for inhalation. Assistance in preparation and a 48-hour protocol can be obtained by contacting the Rocky Mountain Poison Center, 1-800-525-6115. It appears to be more effective than the oral protocol in preventing hepatotoxicity if begun more than 10 hours after ingestion. The initial dose is 140 mg/kg IV over 1 hour, followed by 70 mg/kg q4h for 48 hours. A 20-hour protocol is equally effective if given less than 10 hours after ingestion and is the standard treatment in Great Britain, Canada, and Australia (National Capitol Poison Center, 202-625-3333). The initial dosage is 150 mg/kg IV over 15 minutes in 200 ml 5% dextrose in water ($D_5W$), followed by 50 mg/kg in 500 ml over 4 hours, followed by 100 mg/kg in 500 ml over 16 hours. Side effects include bronchospasm, rash, flushing, and anaphylactoid reaction and are generally dose related. Flushing requires no treatment; treat urticaria with diphenhydramine. Give albuterol and corticosteroids for bronchospasm. Treat angioedema with diphenhydramine, epinephrine, and corticosteroids. Consider administration of IV cimetidine. Administration of acetylcysteine can be safely resumed 1 hour after successful treatment (*Ann Emerg Med* 31:710, 1998).

**c.** Obtain baseline AST, ALT, bilirubin level, BUN, and prothrombin time or international normalized ratio and repeat these readings at least daily for 3 days. Obtain hepatology consultation for consideration of orthotopic liver transplantation if there is biochemical evidence of hepatic failure. Transplantation is considered if the pH is less than 7.3 after 24 hours *or* the prothrombin time is greater than 100 seconds (international normalized ratio >6.5) *and* grade 3–4 coma is present *and* the creatinine is greater than 3.4 mg/dl.

**B. Antidepressants**

**1. Cyclic antidepressants.** Traditional tricyclic antidepressants include amitriptyline, imipramine, desipramine, nortriptyline, doxepin, and protriptyline. Pharmacologic actions include central and peripheral anticholinergic activity, depression of myocardial contractility, slowing of intraventricular and atrioventricular conduction, and CNS effects that are similar to those of phenothiazines. Despite the widespread use of the much safer selective serotonin reuptake inhibitor antidepressants, overdose with cyclic antidepressants is still a leading cause of drug-related death in the United States (*Am J Emerg Med*

20:391, 2002). Overdoses of less than 20 mg/kg cause few fatalities; 35 mg/kg is the approximate median lethal dose, and overdoses in excess of 50 mg/kg are likely to result in death. Next-generation cyclic antidepressants include amoxapine and loxapine (tricyclics with diminished cardiovascular toxicity but increased propensity to severe seizures), maprotiline (a tetracyclic with greater seizure proclivity and cardiovascular toxicity similar to that of older tricyclics), mianserin (a tetracyclic with low propensity for cardiovascular or neurologic toxicity), and trazodone (a noncyclic with minimal cardiovascular and CNS toxicity). Still newer antidepressants include mirtazapine, venlafaxine, bupropion, and nefazadone. Limited data suggest that mirtazapine is relatively nontoxic in overdose (*J Clin Psychiatry* 59:233, 1998). Venlafaxine is also relatively nontoxic in overdose. Symptoms of bupropion overdose include labored breathing, salivation, arched back, ataxia, and convulsions. Symptoms of nefazadone overdose include drowsiness, vomiting, hypotension, tachycardia, incontinence, and coma.

a. **Clinical manifestations** include evidence of cholinergic blockade (mydriasis, ileus, urinary retention, and hyperpyrexia). **Cardiovascular toxicity** occurs as a result of anticholinergic, catecholamine-related, quinidine-like, and α–antagonist effects; these effects result in supraventricular and ventricular arrhythmias, including torsades de pointes, conduction blocks, hypotension, hypoperfusion, and pulmonary edema. **CNS manifestations** range from initial agitation to confusion, stupor, and coma. Seizures may occur, and the resultant metabolic acidosis may worsen cardiac toxicity.

b. **Laboratory evaluation** aids in assessing the severity of the condition and in monitoring progress. Plasma levels correlate poorly with severity of symptoms, although blood levels in excess of 1000 ng/ml have a higher risk of cardiac toxicity. ABGs are useful for ensuring adequate gas exchange and for monitoring alkalinization. ECGs showing limb-lead QRS duration of greater than 100 msec are predictive of seizures; duration greater than 160 msec predicts ventricular dysrhythmias; a terminal 40-msec QRS axis that is more rightward than 120 degrees is even more sensitive (*N Engl J Med* 313:474, 1985; *Ann Emerg Med* 18:348, 1989).

c. **Treatment** includes supportive measures and GI decontamination. Do not administer ipecac syrup, as obtundation may occur rapidly and promote aspiration. Gastric lavage theoretically may be performed regardless of the time of presentation, as cyclic antidepressants delay gastric emptying; however, clinical studies do not show a difference in patients treated in this way versus those given activated charcoal only (*J Emerg Med* 13:203, 1995). Repetitive administration of activated charcoal, 50 g PO or per tube q2–4h, is not routinely recommended. Forced diuresis and hemodialysis are not indicated. Resin or charcoal hemoperfusion removes less than 1–3% of body burden, but this reduction may be associated with improvement of life-threatening cardiac or CNS complications.

   (1) **Cardiac toxicity. Continuous cardiac monitoring is mandatory.** Cyclic antidepressants are protein bound in an alkaline environment and are toxic in an acid environment. Cardiac (and CNS) toxicity therefore is enhanced by metabolic or respiratory acidosis. Initiate treatment prophylactically, as toxic complications often are refractory to therapy once they have developed. Induce **alkalinization** with IV sodium bicarbonate, 1–2 mEq/kg, to maintain an arterial pH of 7.45–7.55. Such an alkaline pH is effective in preventing and treating hypotension, arrhythmias (ventricular and supraventricular), and conduction disturbances. If the

patient is intubated, hyperventilate to a $PCO_2$ of no lower than 25 mm Hg and an arterial pH of 7.45–7.55, as this is an effective means of alkalinization and avoids the administration of large amounts of sodium. Manage refractory ventricular arrhythmias with lidocaine or phenytoin (see Chap. 7, Cardiac Arrhythmias). **Type Ia antiarrhythmics** (procainamide, quinidine, or disopyramide) **are contraindicated** because of additive toxicity. Treat torsades de pointes with magnesium, isoproterenol, and atrial overdrive pacing (see Chap. 7, Cardiac Arrhythmias). Do not use physostigmine unless all other measures for life-threatening arrhythmias have failed. Use temporary ventricular pacing for complete heart block. Treat hypotension that is unresponsive to alkalinization with norepinephrine and fluid administration.

(2) **CNS complications.** Alkalinization does not reverse CNS complications. Physostigmine (2 mg IV over 1 minute) reverses CNS depression rapidly in patients with pure cyclic antidepressant overdose. However, because repeated doses are necessary and physostigmine may cause dysrhythmias and seizures, its use is not recommended for coma. Supportive care of coma usually is adequate. Treat seizures with diazepam and phenytoin (see Chap. 24, Neurologic Disorders). Barbiturates are preferred over phenytoin for drug-induced seizures by some but not all authorities. Status epilepticus should be treated aggressively, including the use of high-dose barbiturates, paralysis, and general anesthesia, to prevent permanent neurologic damage. Treat hyperthermia by cooling.

(3) **Respiratory depression.** Treat this commonly occurring complication with endotracheal intubation and mechanical ventilation. Pulmonary edema and aspiration also are common.

d. **Disposition.** Patients should be admitted to an ICU if they have a depressed level of consciousness, respiratory depression, hypotension, arrhythmia, conduction blocks (including QRS >100 msec), or seizures. Observe any asymptomatic individual with a normal ECG in the emergency department and perform cardiac monitoring of such a patient for 6 hours. If the patient remains asymptomatic, the ECG remains normal, and bowel sounds are normal, the patient may safely undergo assessment for psychiatric disposition. If any signs or symptoms are present, the patient must be admitted. **Caution is imperative:** Twenty-five percent of fatalities occur in patients who are awake and alert at the time of presentation, and three-fourths of these patients are in normal sinus rhythm. After a patient's admission, criteria for discharge from an ICU include normal mental status, absence of all cyclic antidepressant symptoms, and no ECG abnormalities (including sinus tachycardia) for 24 hours. Significant arrhythmias rarely develop in a patient who meets all these criteria.

2. **Selective serotonin reuptake inhibitors** include fluoxetine, sertraline, paroxetine, fluvoxamine, and citalopram.

a. **Symptoms.** Symptoms are usually minimal. Patients may become agitated or drowsy or, occasionally, confused. Ataxia, vertigo, tremor, delusions, or hallucinations may occur, as may nausea and emesis. Seizures are rare, occurring most often after fluoxetine or citalopram overdose (*Am J Emerg Med* 10:115, 1992; *Lancet* 347:1602, 1997). Tachycardia is noted frequently; however, ECG changes and significant cardiovascular toxicity are uncommon, although severe citalopram overdose may have QT prolongation. Fatalities are rare (*J Clin Psychiatry* 59[Suppl]:42, 1998). Simultaneous ingestion of these drugs with tricyclic antidepressants may raise plasma levels of the tricyclic. If they are ingested with other drugs that cause serotonin release, such as clomipramine, monoamine oxidase inhibitors, and L-tryptophan, the serotonin syndrome may result [see sec. **VII.B.2.b.(1)**].

**b. Treatment. Avoid emesis.** Perform GI lavage if the patient presents less than 1 hour after ingestion, and administer charcoal, particularly if he or she is unconscious. Although cardiovascular and CNS toxicity rarely occur, obtain an ECG as a baseline. Admit patients who have taken large overdoses to a medical floor, particularly if they are symptomatic or if there is coingestion. Treat seizures with diazepam and phenytoin. If the patient is asymptomatic and medically stable after 6 hours of observation, psychiatric evaluation and disposition assessment can be made safely.

**(1) Serotonin syndrome** occurs most frequently after ingestion of two or more drugs that increase serotonin levels by different mechanisms. Examples include monoamine oxidase inhibitors, L-tryptophan, amphetamines, cocaine, 3,4-methylenedioxymethamphetamine (MDMA), fenfluramine, serotonin reuptake inhibitors, tricyclic antidepressants, sumatriptan, amantadine, levodopa, and bromocriptine. Symptoms include agitation, confusion, hallucinations, myoclonus, diaphoresis, tremor, shivering, nystagmus, diarrhea, and fever. Drowsiness may progress to coma. Seizures may occur. Autonomic effects include tachycardia, hypertension, tachypnea, mydriasis, flushing, salivation, abdominal pain, and diarrhea. **Hyperthermia** is characteristic. Rigidity, trismus, and opisthotonus may be present. Severe complications include DIC, rhabdomyolysis and renal failure, respiratory failure, and ARDS. **Treatment** is supportive with the administration of activated charcoal. Emesis should not be induced. Consider benzodiazepines for agitation and treat hyperthermia with cooling. Diazepam and phenytoin can be given for seizures. Hypertension can be treated with sedation and, if necessary, nitroprusside. If IV saline is unsuccessful for hypotension, administer norepinephrine. Protect the airway and provide ventilatory support for respiratory failure. Consider the administration of cyproheptadine, 4–8 mg q1–4h, until improvement occurs or a total of 32 mg is given.

### C. Cardiovascular drugs

#### 1. β-Adrenergic antagonists

**a. Symptoms** of β-adrenergic antagonist overdose usually occur within 2 hours of ingestion. Cardiovascular manifestations include bradycardia, atrioventricular block, hypotension, and depression of cardiac function, which results in CHF. Sotalol may cause QT prolongation and torsades de pointes. Bradycardia occurs early but does not predict more serious cardiac disturbances. Although some $\beta_1$-specific agents may have little respiratory effect at the standard dosage in patients with asthma or chronic obstructive pulmonary disease, severe bronchospasm may result from ingestion of any β-adrenergic antagonist, because $\beta_1$ selectivity is lost at high doses. CNS manifestations include drowsiness, coma, hypoventilation, and seizures (caused most frequently by propranolol). Nausea and vomiting may occur, and mesenteric ischemia may be severe, particularly with propranolol ingestion, as a result of decreased cardiac output and unopposed α-agonist activity. β-Adrenergic antagonist overdose may cause hypoglycemia by blockade of counterregulatory mechanisms and may also make the appreciation of hypoglycemic symptoms more difficult. Renal failure may occur as a result of hypotension.

**b. Laboratory studies.** Measurement of serum drug levels is not useful. Obtain serum glucose and electrolyte levels. Record a baseline ECG and monitor cardiac activity continuously.

**c. Therapy**

**(1)** Establish an IV line before any other therapy is undertaken.

**(2)** Consider gastric lavage if the patient is seen within 1 hour of ingestion and administer activated charcoal. A second dose of activated charcoal for sustained-release preparation overdose has been recommended by some because of the theoretical potential for drug desorption, but there is no clinical evidence to support this. **Do not give syrup of ipecac** because of the rapidity with which cardiac compromise may occur. Moreover, the increase in vagal tone associated with emesis may promote cardiovascular collapse. If the patient becomes bradycardic or has other manifestations of a vagal reaction, administer up to 2 mg atropine IV. Consider multidose charcoal for sotalol ingestion.

**(3)** Treat hypotension with IV saline; hemodynamic monitoring may be necessary to gauge optimal fluid resuscitation. **Glucagon** (50–150 μg/kg IV over 1 minute, followed by 1–5 mg/hour in 5% dextrose) increases cardiac contractility and heart rate and is the drug of first choice for β-adrenergic antagonist overdose. Isoproterenol (2–20 μg/minute) may be useful, but high doses (≤200 μg/minute) may be necessary. If the BP does not improve or falls, add norepinephrine. Use epinephrine with caution, particularly with propranolol overdoses, because of the propensity for hypertension and reflex bradycardia. Calcium chloride 10%, 10 ml IV, may also be useful for refractory propranolol overdose. Consider intra-aortic balloon pump for refractory hypotension.

**(4)** For torsades de pointes associated with sotalol overdose, isoproterenol, magnesium, and overdrive pacing may be useful (see Chap. 7, Cardiac Arrhythmias). A pacemaker may be necessary for severe bradycardia or heart block that is unresponsive to medications.

**(5)** Use β-adrenergic agonists and theophylline for bronchospasm.

**(6)** Treat seizures with IV benzodiazepine followed by IV phenytoin.

**(7)** Treat hypoglycemia with IV glucose and, if resistant, IV glucagon.

**(8)** Severe respiratory depression may require mechanical ventilation.

**(9)** Dialysis may be useful in removal of nadolol, sotalol, atenolol, and acebutolol but is ineffective for propranolol, metoprolol, and timolol.

**d. Disposition.** Obtain a baseline ECG and monitor the patient's rhythm for at least 6 hours, even in the absence of symptoms. If any cardiovascular, respiratory, or neurologic symptoms are present, admit the patient to an ICU for therapy and continuous monitoring. If, however, no toxic symptoms have occurred 6 hours after ingestion, disposition guided by psychiatric consultation can be made safely.

**2. Calcium channel antagonists**

**a. Symptoms.** Manifestations of calcium channel antagonist overdose depend on the drug ingested. Hypotension is common, as are nausea and vomiting. Severe bradycardia, atrioventricular block, and asystole are most common after verapamil and diltiazem overdose and less common with the dihydropyridines (e.g., nifedipine, nicardipine, amlodipine), which are more likely to cause reflex tachycardia. Pulmonary edema is most likely to occur after verapamil overdose, as is hypocalcemia. Lethargy, confusion, and coma are common. Seizures are most often due to verapamil, less common with diltiazem, and rare with nifedipine. Hyperglycemia occurs frequently. Cardiovascular manifestations usually are apparent within 1–5 hours after ingestion and may persist for more than 24 hours. Sustained-release preparations, particularly verapamil, may cause rhythm disturbances up to 7 days after ingestion.

b. **Laboratory studies.** These should include serum calcium, magnesium, electrolyte, and glucose levels. Obtain an ECG and monitor the cardiac rhythm. Monitor oxygenation by pulse oximetry, and obtain a chest x-ray.

c. **Therapy**

(1) **Avoid inducing emesis** because of the potential for rapid cardiovascular collapse and aspiration. If the patient presents soon after ingestion, consider gastric lavage followed by administration of charcoal. Consider gastroscopy or whole-bowel irrigation with polyethylene glycol solution for removal of retained sustained-release tablets. A second dose of activated charcoal for sustained-release preparation overdose has been recommended by some because of the theoretical potential for drug desorption, but there is no clinical evidence to support this.

(2) **Treat hypotension** with IV 0.9% saline; if resistant, give IV dopamine. Administer 10% **calcium chloride** (10–20 ml IV) for hypotension, bradycardia, or heart block. Repeat at 10-minute intervals three to four times as necessary. Calcium gluconate (3 g) is preferred when the patient is severely acidotic. A calcium gluconate drip at up to 2 g/hour can be titrated to BP, with monitoring of ECG and serum calcium. **Glucagon** (50–150 $\mu$g/kg IV over 1 minute followed by 1–5 mg/hour) may also be useful for heart block and hypotension. Insulin infusion, 0.1–1.0 U/kg/hour with sufficient dextrose to maintain a normal blood glucose, has also been reported to be successful. If hypotension is resistant to the preceding measures, arrange for placement of an intra-aortic balloon pump.

**(3)** Atropine (up to 2 mg IV) can also be given for bradycardia or atrioventricular block, although it rarely is successful. Isoproterenol is a less desirable alternative. Calcium can be administered as above. Place a transvenous pacemaker for medication-resistant heart block.

**(4)** Treat seizures with an IV benzodiazepine (diazepam or lorazepam; see Chap. 24, Neurologic Disorders) and phenytoin. Hemodialysis and hemoperfusion are not useful to accelerate drug removal.

d. **Disposition.** Admit all patients who have cardiovascular symptoms or seizures or who have ingested a sustained-release preparation to an ICU for continuous cardiovascular monitoring. If the patient has taken a non–sustained-release preparation and is asymptomatic, obtain a baseline ECG and monitor ECG rhythm for at least 8 hours. If, at that point, the patient is completely asymptomatic and has a normal ECG, consider discharge after psychiatric consultation.

3. **Digoxin** (see Chap. 7, Cardiac Arrhythmias for details; for doses of Fab' fragments, see Table 25-2)

D. **Caustic ingestions**

1. **Alkaline ingestions.** These include liquid and crystalline lye, automatic dishwasher detergents, oven cleaners, hair relaxers, and some toilet bowl cleaners. Strong alkali solutions, such as liquid drain cleaner, are the agents most commonly associated with injury.

a. **Symptoms and signs. Deep tissue injury in the aerodigestive tract is common.** Oral burns are common and may cause drooling. A lack of oral burns does not exclude esophageal injury. The overall rate of esophageal injury for alkali ingestions is 30–40%; such injury is suggested by vomiting, drooling, or stridor. Esophageal perforation may occur and result in mediastinitis. Esophageal stricture may develop as a late complication. Gastric injury and perforation also may occur and are much more likely with liquid lye ingestions, as the lye passes rapidly into the stomach. Crystalline lye ingestion may lead to severe upper airway injury with stridor and airway obstruction that necessitate rapid intervention. Other symptoms of alkaline ingestion include oral pain, odynophagia, chest pain, abdominal pain, nausea, and vomiting.

**b. Treatment**

**(1) Immediately rinse the oral cavity** copiously with cold water.

**(2) Do not induce emesis** because it may increase injury. Charcoal administration, cathartic administration, and gastric lavage are not indicated. Administration of charcoal obscures anatomic detail for subsequent endoscopy. Diluents are controversial and may induce emesis. *Poisindex* (6/2003) currently recommends administration of diluents (2–8 oz milk or water), although other experts strongly disagree, and the *Poisindex* consensus was last obtained in 1988. **Do not attempt to neutralize the alkaline agent with a weak acid,** as this results in an exothermic reaction and increases tissue damage.

**(3)** Protect the airway and administer oxygen. Endotracheal intubation or early tracheostomy may be required.

**(4)** Establish an IV line and give fluids guided by vital signs.

**(5)** Obtain chest and abdominal radiographs for evidence of perforation (pneumomediastinum, pleural effusion, and pneumoperitoneum). Obtain CBC, electrolytes, BUN, creatinine, and coagulation parameters; if there are signs suggesting severe burns, type and cross-match blood.

**(6)** If the patient exhibits drooling, stridor, or odynophagia, consult a gastroenterologist to arrange for **immediate endoscopy;** otherwise, it can be deferred 12–24 hours. Avoid use of a nasogastric tube.

**(7)** Obtain surgical consultation.

**(8)** Glucocorticoid treatment of esophageal burns in an attempt to prevent stricture is controversial and generally not recommended. Prophylactic antibiotics are not appropriate.

**(9)** Obtain a barium swallow after 2–4 weeks to assess for esophageal stricture.

**2. Acids.** Common household acids include most toilet bowl cleaners, drain cleaners, metal cleaners, battery acid, and swimming pool cleaners. Tissue injury is generally less deep than that produced by alkaline agents. Gastric and esophageal injury, including perforation, are common. Pyloric stricture may result.

**a. Symptoms and signs** include oral pain, drooling, odynophagia, and abdominal pain. Occasionally, respiratory distress, DIC, hemolysis, and systemic acidosis occur.

**b. Therapy**

**(1)** The mouth should be washed copiously with cold water. Diluent administration often is recommended (with the same caveats as noted above for alkaline ingestions) but has no demonstrated clinical efficacy.

**(2)** Neutralization with a weak base is contraindicated. **Induction of emesis, gastric lavage, and charcoal administration are all contraindicated,** and a nasogastric tube should be avoided. Airway involvement is less likely than with alkaline ingestion.

**(3)** Obtain CBC, prothrombin time, partial thromboplastin time, platelet count, electrolytes, BUN, creatinine, and, in severe burns, type and cross-match.

**(4)** Establish IV access and administer fluids guided by vital signs.

**(5)** Sucralfate (1 g q6h) may decrease symptoms but does not appear to decrease complications or perforation.

**(6)** Unsuspected esophageal and gastric burns and duodenal injury are commonly seen with endoscopy, which should be performed within 24 hours. The likelihood of stricture formation (pyloric or esophageal) and perforation depends on the severity of ingestion.

**(7)** Obtain an upright chest x-ray to detect perforation, and arrange surgical consultation.

**(8)** The administration of glucocorticoids is controversial, but their use probably is of no added benefit. Prophylactic antibiotics are not recommended.

**(9)** Obtain an upper GI radiograph after 2–4 weeks.

**E. EtOH and other alcohols**

**1. EtOH.** The toxicity of EtOH is dose related, but tolerance varies widely, based on prior exposure. Blood levels in excess of 100 mg/dl are associated with ataxia, whereas at 200 mg/dl patients are drowsy and confused. At levels in excess of 400 mg/dl, respiratory depression is common and death is possible.

**a. Laboratory studies.** These should include electrolytes, glucose level, serum osmolality, and blood EtOH level. The blood EtOH level can be rapidly estimated by calculating the osmolal gap (measured osmolality minus calculated osmolality, or measured osmolality minus [2 Na (mEq/L) + (urea [mg/dl])/2.8 + (glucose [mg/dl])/18]. **The standard formula for blood EtOH level in mg/dl equals 4.6 times the osmolal gap** (*Poisindex* 6/2003), in the absence of other low-molecular-weight toxins. However, multipliers ranging from 2.7 (*Schweiz Med Wochenschr* 118:845–848, 1988) to 3.7 (*Ann Emerg Med* 38:653, 2001) have been reported using linear regression from actual in vivo measurements in humans; thus, if the standard multiplier is used, the patient may appear to have a residual osmolal gap, implying the presence of another toxin such as methanol (MeOH) or ethylene glycol (EG) when there is none (see secs. **VII.E.3** and **VII.E.4**).

**b. Treatment.** If the patient's mental status is severely depressed, insert an endotracheal tube before performing gastric lavage if the patient presents less than 1 hour after ingestion. Charcoal is not helpful due to the rapid absorption of EtOH from the stomach. Hemodialysis may be useful for life-threatening overdoses. Administer 100 mg thiamine IV followed by 50 ml 50% dextrose in water IV to any **comatose alcoholic patient.** Admit patients with alcohol intoxication if they have severe underlying illness or significant alcoholic ketoacidosis or if ventilatory support is required. Observe other patients until they are sober (blood alcohol level <100 mg/dl) or can be discharged to the care of a responsible sober adult.

**2. Isopropyl alcohol (IPA).** Most rubbing alcohol is 70% IPA. IPA is more toxic than EtOH at any blood level (50 mg/dl = intoxication, 100–200 mg/dl = stupor and coma). Respiratory depression and hypotension occur at high blood levels. Other symptoms include nausea, vomiting, and abdominal pain.

**a. Laboratory evaluation.** Workup commonly reveals ketosis without acidosis (IPA is metabolized to acetone). Metabolic acidosis usually is related to associated hypotension. IPA concentration in the blood can be measured directly or can be estimated in the same fashion as for EtOH (see sec. **VII.E.1.a**), substituting a multiplier of 6.0 for 4.6. Absence of an osmolal gap does not exclude IPA ingestion. Measure plasma glucose, as hypoglycemia may occur, particularly in children. If diagnosis is in doubt, obtain blood levels of other toxic alcohols and determine acid-base status with ABGs.

**b. Therapy.** Do not induce emesis, as mental status may decline rapidly, with subsequent aspiration. Gastric lavage followed by charcoal administration may be useful if performed within 60 minutes of ingestion. For cutaneous exposures, wash the skin and remove contaminated clothes. Maintain an adequate airway and support BP. Hemodialysis is reserved for patients with persistent hypotension despite supportive therapy.

3. **MeOH.** MeOH is in gas-line antifreeze, carburetor fluid, duplicator fluid, and windshield washer fluid. Sterno Canned Heat fuel contains EtOH and MeOH, and the EtOH that is present may delay manifestations of MeOH toxicity. The toxicity of MeOH is due to its conversion by alcohol dehydrogenase to formaldehyde and then by acetaldehyde dehydrogenase to formic acid. Initial symptoms may include lethargy and confusion, followed by an apparent hangover. Toxic symptoms, which may be delayed 18–24 hours, include headache, visual symptoms (blurring, diminished acuity, and whiteness in the visual field), nausea, vomiting, abdominal pain, tachypnea, and respiratory failure. Coma and convulsions may occur in severe MeOH intoxication.

   a. **Examination.** Typically, examination reveals an uncomfortable patient who may be remarkably tachypneic with decreased visual acuity; optic disk hyperemia may be hard to appreciate. Laboratory studies should include CBC, electrolytes, BUN, creatinine, amylase, urinalysis, EtOH, and MeOH levels, as well as ABGs, which reveal a severe anion-gap metabolic acidosis. Development of the acidosis may be delayed until accumulation of toxic metabolites; coingestion of alcohol may prolong this phase for many hours. The range of toxic ingestion is 15–400 ml. In general, pH and acid-base status are better predictors of toxicity than is the absolute MeOH level. The MeOH level (in mg/dl) can be estimated in the same way as for EtOH (see sec. **VII.E.1**), substituting a multiplier of 3.2 for 4.6. However, the absence of an osmolal gap does not rule out MeOH intoxication, and for the reasons noted in sec. **VII.E.1.a,** EtOH intoxication may result in an apparent osmolal gap that is greater than anticipated, leading to temporary misdiagnosis of intoxication with MeOH or another osmotically active toxin.

   b. **Treatment.** Do not induce emesis. Consider gastric lavage if the patient is seen less than 1 hour after ingestion. Charcoal does not absorb significant amounts of MeOH.

      (1) Give **folinic acid** (leucovorin), 1 mg/kg (maximum, 50 mg) IV, followed by folic acid, 1 mg/kg IV q4h for six doses, to increase the metabolism of formate. IV $NaHCO_3$ for severe acidosis may reduce permanent vision damage.

      (2) **4-Methylpyrazole** (**fomepizole;** an alcohol dehydrogenase antagonist) (*J Emerg Med* 8:455, 1990) is FDA approved for the treatment of MeOH toxicity, although no direct comparison with EtOH has been made. Nevertheless, it is more easily administered than EtOH and does not cause depression of mental status or hypoglycemia. Although much more expensive, it is now the antidote of choice. In the United States, it can be obtained from Orphan Medical, Inc. (1-888-8ORPHAN). Administer fomepizole for the following indications: peak MeOH level in excess of 20 mg/dl, while awaiting levels for an ingestion suspected of being MeOH, or an anion-gap metabolic acidosis after suspicious ingestion. The dosage is 15 mg/kg IV followed by 10 mg/kg IV q12h for four doses. This should be followed by 15 mg/kg IV q12h until the MeOH level is less than 20 mg/dl. During hemodialysis, the dosing interval should be changed to q4h (Table 25-3).

      (3) **EtOH delays metabolism of MeOH to its toxic metabolites** by competing for alcohol dehydrogenase and can be used in situations in which fomepizole is unavailable or contraindicated.

**Table 25-3.** Fomepizole administration during dialysis

| Time from last dose | Dose |
|---|---|
| Beginning of dialysis | |
| <6 hr | None |
| >6 hr | Give next scheduled dose |
| During dialysis | Maintenance dose q4h |
| At conclusion of dialysis | |
| <1 hr | None |
| 1–3 hr | One-half of next scheduled dose |
| >3 hr | Give next scheduled dose |

Administer EtOH for the following indications: peak MeOH level in excess of 20 mg/dl, while awaiting levels for an ingestion suspected of being MeOH, or an anion-gap metabolic acidosis after suspicious ingestion. The **loading dose of EtOH** is 7.6–10 ml/kg of a 10% solution, given IV, or 0.8–1 ml/kg of 95% alcohol, administered PO in orange juice. EtOH for infusion is available as stock 5% or 10% solutions in $D_5W$; the latter is preferred. EtOH (10%) for IV infusion can also be prepared by removing 100 ml $D_5W$ from a 1-L bag and replacing it with 100 ml absolute alcohol. Maintenance dosage varies depending on previous alcohol exposure (Table 25-4). The goal is achievement of a blood alcohol level of 100–130 mg/dl to saturate the available alcohol dehydrogenase and prevent formation of MeOH's toxic metabolites. Check EtOH levels 1 hour after the loading dose and at least two to three times a day during maintenance infusion (some authorities recommend hourly levels). It is ultimately less hazardous to the patient to have blood alcohol levels that are too high than too low. Monitor blood glucose levels, as hypoglycemia may occur. Administer EtOH continuously until the MeOH level is less than 10 mg/dl, the formate level is less than 1.2 mg/dl, there is resolution of

**Table 25-4.** Maintenance ethanol dosage regimens for ethylene glycol and methanol intoxication

| | 10% Ethanol IV (ml/kg/hr) | 40% Ethanol PO (ml/kg/hr) | 95% Ethanol PO (ml/kg/hr) | Hemodialysis with 10% ethanol IV[a] (ml/kg/hr) |
|---|---|---|---|---|
| Moderate drinker | 1.4 | 0.3 | 0.15 | 3.3 |
| Chronic drinker | 2.0 | 0.4 | 0.2 | 3.9 |
| Nondrinker | 0.8 | 0.2 | 0.1 | 2.7 |

[a]Dialysate bath concentration of 100 mg/dl preferable.

*Source:* Modified with permission from E Kuffner, KM Hurlbut. Methanol (management/treatment protocol). In: BH Rumack, DG Spoerke (eds). *Poisindex Information System.* Denver: Micromedex, 2003.

acidosis, CNS symptoms abate, and a normal anion gap is restored. This implies regular monitoring of electrolytes, BUN, creatinine, and ABGs. If MeOH levels cannot be readily measured, administer EtOH for at least 9 days without dialysis (or 1 day with dialysis) and until clinical findings resolve (*Poisindex* 6/2003). Every effort should be made to move the patient to a center where levels and dialysis are available.

(4) **Hemodialysis** generally is indicated for an MeOH level that exceeds 50 mg/dl, severe and resistant acidosis, renal failure, or visual symptoms.

4. **EG and diethylene glycol** are used commonly in antifreeze and windshield deicer. Various metabolites are responsible for toxicity. **Initial symptoms** resemble alcohol intoxication. Vomiting is common. CNS depression, seizures, or coma may occur. CHF and pulmonary edema may occur 12–36 hours after ingestion. Death is most likely in this stage. Oliguric renal failure (from oxalate crystal deposition) may occur 24–72 hours after ingestion. Associated flank pain may be prominent.

a. **Laboratory findings.** Obtain electrolyte, BUN, and creatinine levels; serum osmolality; ABGs; urinalysis; and EtOH and EG levels. Findings include a severe metabolic acidosis with an anion gap (which may be delayed for hours until accumulation of toxic metabolites occurs), an osmolal gap, and oxalate and hippurate crystalluria in addition to hematuria and proteinuria. Serum level can be calculated from the osmolal gap as for EtOH, using a multiplier of 6.2. Fluorescein often is added to antifreeze, and urine fluorescence detected with a Wood's lamp up to 6 hours after ingestion is diagnostic (*Ann Emerg Med* 19:663, 1990), although the accuracy of this has been disputed (*Ann Emerg Med* 38:49, 2001).

b. **Treatment**

(1) Do not induce emesis. Neither gastric lavage nor charcoal administration is likely to be effective but can be considered if the patient presents within 1 hour of ingestion, particularly if the ingestion is mixed with other toxins that are amenable to gastric decontamination. Avoid magnesium salt cathartics because of the likelihood of renal failure.

(2) **Correct life-threatening acidosis** with IV sodium bicarbonate pending dialysis; administration for lesser severity is not justified. Administer 1–3 mEq/kg IV and titrate to achieve a normal pH. Monitor the calcium level, as hypocalcemia may result.

(3) **4-Methylpyrazole (fomepizole)** (*N Engl J Med* 340:879, 1998; *N Engl J Med* 340:832, 1998) is FDA approved for use in EG poisoning. Indications include an EG level in excess of 20 mg/dl, a suspected EG ingestion (while levels are being awaited), or an anion-gap metabolic acidosis with a history of EG ingestion, regardless of level. The dosing is similar to the treatment of MeOH poisoning [see sec. **VII.E.3.b.(2)**]. Treatment with 4-methylpyrazole should continue until the EG level is less than 20 mg/dl (*J Toxicol Clin Toxicol* 37:537, 1999).

(4) **IV EtOH** [although not FDA approved and never studied prospectively; see sec. **VII.E.3.b.(3)**] (Table 25-4) can be used as an alternative when fomepizole is unavailable or contraindicated (hypersensitivity). It should be continued until the EG level is less than 10 mg/dl, with no symptoms and a normal pH. An EtOH level of at least 100 mg/dl should be maintained. If levels are unavailable, infusion should be continued for at least 3 days, or 1 day with dialysis. Every effort should be made to transfer the patient safely to a facility with the capacity to measure EG levels and perform dialysis.

(5) **Administer pyridoxine** (100 mg IV qd) to promote the conversion of glyoxylate to glycine and **thiamine** (100 mg IV qd) to promote the formation of nontoxic alpha-hydroxy-beta-ketoadipic acid.

(6) **Dialysis** is highly effective in severe cases; EtOH infusion should be continued at higher doses (Table 25-4) during dialysis. Indications for dialysis include a glycol level in excess of 50 mg/dl (unless the patient is being given 4-methylpyrazole and the patient is asymptomatic with a normal pH), electrolyte abnormalities that are unresponsive to standard therapy, deteriorating vital signs despite supportive therapy, renal failure, or a pH of less than 7.25–7.30 that is unresponsive to therapy (*J Toxicol Clin Toxicol* 37:537, 1999). Discontinue dialysis when the glycol level is less than 10 mg/dl, the glycolic acid level is undetectable, and the acidosis, clinical status, and anion gap have returned to normal. EG levels can be estimated as for alcohol, using 6.2 as the multiplier of the osmolal gap (see sec. **VII.E.1.a**). When levels cannot be measured easily, continue EtOH administration for at least 3 days without hemodialysis (or for 1 day with hemodialysis) and until clinical findings resolve, whichever is longer (*Poisindex* 6/2003). Measure EtOH levels after the loading dose and two to three times a day during maintenance therapy.

F. **Hydrocarbon ingestions** are characterized by GI upset, pulmonary aspiration, and CNS alterations. Morbidity and mortality usually are attributed to pulmonary aspiration. Low viscosity (e.g., kerosene, gasoline, and liquid furniture polish) is associated with greater aspiration potential. Motor oil, transmission oil, mineral oil, baby oil, and suntan oil usually are nontoxic.

1. **Clinical manifestations** usually are apparent within the first 6 hours and include vomiting, chest or abdominal pain, cough, dyspnea, low-grade fever, arrhythmias, an altered sensorium, seizures, and radiographic evidence of aspiration pneumonitis or pulmonary edema.
2. **Treatment of nontoxic hydrocarbon ingestion** is not required in the absence of symptoms. These agents have high aspiration potential but are associated with little or no GI absorption. Gastric emptying is never necessary. Obtain chest radiographs only if patients have pulmonary symptoms. Such patients can be discharged after 6 hours if they are asymptomatic. Hospitalize patients with an abnormal chest radiograph or ABGs and treat them supportively.
3. **Initiate treatment of toxic hydrocarbon ingestion** by removing contaminated clothing and washing the affected skin to prevent dermatitis and percutaneous absorption.
   a. Provide **supplemental oxygen** to patients with significant aspiration injuries.
   b. **Gastric emptying,** although controversial, is recommended for ingestion of toxic hydrocarbons, particularly halogenated hydrocarbons (trichloroethylene, carbon tetrachloride, methylene chloride) or those that contain toxic additives (e.g., heavy metals, insecticides, nitrobenzene, aniline, or camphor), although some authorities recommend only administration of activated charcoal. Other potentially toxic hydrocarbons (gasoline, benzene, kerosene, lighter fluid, paint thinner, and toluene), except for large suicidal ingestions, do not require gastric emptying. If gastric emptying is performed, this is one of the few potential indications for ipecac, as aspiration appears to be less frequent with the use of ipecac than after gastric lavage. Therefore, in alert patients, induce emesis with ipecac, 30 ml PO. Perform gastric lavage after intubation with a cuffed endotracheal tube in any patient with CNS depression, a depressed gag reflex, or seizures.
   c. **Observe the patient for at least 6 hours** after gastric decontamination. Hospitalize patients who are lethargic or have pulmonary

symptoms or an abnormal pulmonary examination, ABGs, or chest radiograph.

d. **Prophylactic antibiotics or glucocorticoids are not indicated.**

G. **Lithium** is administered as a carbonate or citrate salt for the treatment of psychiatric disease, principally bipolar disorder. Overdose often is suicidal. Excretion is renal. States of dehydration and sodium uptake promote lithium retention and toxicity, as does thiazide diuretic use.

1. **Symptoms** are loosely related to blood level in acute overdose. Therapeutic blood levels range between 0.6 and 1.2 mEq/L. At less than 2.5 mEq/L, symptoms are mild and consist of tremor, ataxia, nystagmus, and lethargy. Between 2.5 and 3.5 mEq/L, the patient may be agitated and confused and have fasciculations, nausea, vomiting, and diarrhea. Levels in excess of 3.5 mEq/L are associated with seizures, coma, cardiac arrhythmias, hypotension, noncardiogenic pulmonary edema, nephrogenic diabetes insipidus, and death. Levels associated with severe symptoms may be lower in those with chronic ingestion.
2. **Laboratory studies** entail checking electrolytes, creatinine, and lithium level. Obtain an ECG and monitor the patient continuously while he or she is being evaluated and treated. Electrolytes may reveal a low anion gap with elevated bicarbonate, and there may be evidence of diabetes insipidus. Lithium levels should be measured repetitively until at least two sequential levels show continued decline.
3. **Treatment**

a. Consider gastric lavage if the patient presents within 1 hour of ingestion. Charcoal does not bind lithium; sodium polystyrene sulfonate (15 g PO qid or 30–50 g per rectum) can decrease absorption (*Ann Emerg Med* 21:1308, 1992). Sustained-release preparations may form concretions. If levels continue to rise despite treatment, perform whole-bowel irrigation with commercial polyethylene glycol solution, 2 L/hour for 5 hours.

b. Establish IV access and hydrate with 0.9% saline to achieve euvolemia. Avoid dehydration, as this promotes renal lithium reabsorption. Treat arrhythmias in standard fashion (see Chap. 7, Cardiac Arrhythmias).

c. Criteria for dialysis are inexact. Consult a nephrologist for consideration of hemodialysis (preferably with a bicarbonate rather than acetate bath) for the following indications: blood level that exceeds 3.5–4.0 mEq/L after an acute ingestion, chronic toxicity with a blood level of more than 2.5 mEq/L, worsening mental status, seizures, dysrhythmias, pulmonary edema, and renal failure. The goal is achievement of a sustained level of 1 mEq/L 8 hours after dialysis, which may necessitate prolonged or repeated dialysis.

H. **Methemoglobinemia** (acquired) can be caused by nitrites, nitroprusside, nitroglycerin, chlorates, sulfonamides, aniline dyes, nitrobenzene, antimalarials, and phenazopyridine. Methemoglobinemia has also been reported after benzocaine topical anesthesia for endoscopy as well as other topical anesthetics (*Am J Med Sci* 318:415, 1999) and after dapsone therapy (*Ann Pharmacother* 32:549, 1998). This discussion does not deal with hereditary methemoglobinemia or hemoglobin M disease. Symptoms include headache, fatigue, lethargy, dyspnea, tachycardia, and dizziness. The patient may be hypotensive due to the vasodilating properties of nitrates as well as tissue hypoxia. Seizures may occur.

1. The **diagnosis** is suggested in patients with a normal oxygen tension (as measured by ABGs) and generalized cyanosis (corresponding to a methemoglobin level of 15% or more) that does not respond to oxygen. Blood with that level of methemoglobin placed on white filter paper appears chocolate-colored when exposed to room air as compared to blood from a normal control. Measured arterial oxygen saturation that is much lower

than that calculated for the alveolar oxygen tension also is suspicious for methemoglobinemia. Final confirmation rests with measurement of a methemoglobin level. Blood levels exceeding 50% indicate severe toxicity, often associated with CNS depression, seizures, coma, and arrhythmias; levels higher than 70% are often fatal. In addition to ABGs and methemoglobin level, obtain CBC, electrolytes, and chest x-ray. Obtain an ECG and monitor the cardiac rhythm continuously.

2. **Treatment** includes supplemental oxygen. **Do not give ipecac** because seizures may occur and promote aspiration. Consider gastric lavage (with airway protection) if the patient presents within 1 hour of ingestion or has coma or seizures. Administer activated charcoal. If signs of hypoxia are present or if the methemoglobin level exceeds 30%, administer **methylene blue,** 1–2 mg/kg in a 1% solution IV over 5 minutes. The dose can be repeated in 1 hour if signs of hypoxia persist and q4h thereafter to a maximum dose of 7 mg/kg. Treat seizures with a benzodiazepine and phenytoin in addition to methylene blue. Treat hypotension with IV fluids and, if resistant, with dopamine. Hospitalize the patient in an ICU if he or she is symptomatic or if the methemoglobin level is greater than 20%. Hyperbaric oxygen and exchange transfusion are extreme measures for severely symptomatic patients.

**I. Opioids**

1. **Symptoms** of opioid overdose are respiratory depression, a depressed level of consciousness, and miosis. However, the pupils may be dilated with acidosis or hypoxia or after overdoses with meperidine or diphenoxylate plus atropine. Overdose with alpha-methylfentanyl ("China white") may result in negative toxicology screens. Heroin may be adulterated with scopolamine, cocaine, or caffeine, complicating the clinical picture. Less common complications include hypotension, bradycardia, and pulmonary edema. Be aware of body packers, who smuggle heroin in their intestinal tracts. Deterioration of latex or plastic containers may result in drug release and death (*Am J Forensic Med Pathol* 18:312, 1997). Drug levels and other standard laboratory tests are of little use. Pulse oximetry and ABGs are useful for monitoring respiratory status.
2. **Treatment** includes airway maintenance, ventilatory and circulatory support, and prevention of further drug absorption. Emesis is contraindicated. Gastric lavage can be considered for oral ingestions that present within 1 hour; administer activated charcoal. Whole-bowel irrigation may be safe and effective for body packers; surgery is not indicated except for obstruction (*Vet Hum Toxicol* 33:353, 1991). Endoscopic removal should not be attempted due to the danger of rupture. **Naloxone hydrochloride** specifically reverses opioid-induced respiratory and CNS depression and hypotension. The initial dose is 2 mg IV; large doses may be required to reverse the effects of propoxyphene, diphenoxylate, buprenorphine, or pentazocine. In the absence of an IV line, naloxone can be administered sublingually (*Ann Emerg Med* 16:572, 1987), via endotracheal tube, or intranasally (*Emerg Med J* 19:375, 2002). Isolated opioid overdose is unlikely if there is no response to a total of 10 mg naloxone. Repetitive doses may be required (duration of action is 45 minutes), and this should prompt hospitalization despite the patient's return to an alert status. If the patient is alert and asymptomatic for 6 hours after an oral ingestion and a single dose of naloxone, or for 4 hours after a single treatment for an IV overdose, he or she can be discharged safely. Methadone overdose may require therapy for 24–48 hours, whereas levo-alpha-acetylmethadol may require therapy for 72 hours. A continuous IV drip that provides two-thirds of the initial dose of naloxone hourly, diluted in $D_5W$, may be necessary to maintain an alert state (*Ann Emerg Med* 15:566, 1986). Body packers should be admitted to an ICU for close monitoring of the respiratory rate and

level of consciousness and remain so until all packets have passed, as documented by CT. Ventilatory support should be provided for the patient who is unresponsive to naloxone and for pulmonary edema.

J. **Organophosphates** are responsible for a number of human poisonings, particularly in developing countries. Parathion and malathion are the most common insecticides involved; they often are contained in hydrocarbon solvent. Suicidal ingestion and agricultural exposure, including dermal absorption, occur. "Nerve gases" used in terrorist biowarfare are anticholinesterases, such as Sarin.

1. **Diagnosis and routine laboratory measurements. Toxic manifestations** are due to inhibition of acetylcholinesterase in the nervous system. **Muscarinic manifestations** include miosis, increased lacrimation, blurred vision, bronchospasm, bronchorrhea, diaphoresis, salivation, bradycardia, urinary incontinence, and increased GI motility, manifested by cramps, nausea, vomiting, and diarrhea. Among the **nicotinic manifestations** are muscle weakness and cramps, muscle fasciculations, hypotension, and respiratory paralysis. CNS toxicity is characterized by anxiety, slurred speech, mental status changes (e.g., delirium, coma, and seizures), and respiratory depression. Complications of ingestion include pulmonary edema, aspiration pneumonia, chemical pneumonitis, delayed polyneuropathy, and ARDS. Nonketotic hyperglycemia and glucosuria are common. Hyperamylasemia may reflect pancreatitis. Red cell cholinesterase and plasma pseudocholinesterase levels are decreased; activities of less than 50% of baseline are associated with poor outcome.

2. **Treatment**

   a. Apply measures to support ventilation and circulation, decontaminate the skin (the medical team should wear rubber gloves, aprons, and shoe covers if there is major skin contamination), and consider gastric lavage for oral poisonings if presentation is within 1 hour of ingestion; **induction of emesis is contraindicated.** Administer activated charcoal. Monitor ABGs and ECG; QTc prolongation is associated with a worse prognosis.

   b. **Atropine** (preservative free, to avoid benzyl alcohol toxicity with large doses) is the drug of choice for organophosphate toxicity. Give an initial dose of 1 mg IV; if the patient experiences no adverse effects, repeat a dose of 2 mg q15min until atropinization (as manifested by drying of secretions, tachycardia, flushing, dry mouth, and dilated pupils) occurs. The average patient requires approximately 40 mg/day, but larger doses (500–1500 mg/day) may be necessary. Intermittent administration may have to be continued for at least 24 hours until the organophosphate is metabolized. Severe cases may require several days or more of therapy, because of slow regeneration of acetylcholinesterase activity. Atropine does not reverse the muscle weakness.

   c. Give **pralidoxime,** 1–2 g IV in 100 ml normal saline over 30 minutes, which reactivates the cholinesterase and counteracts weakness, muscle fasciculations, and respiratory depression. Repeat administration q6–12h to a maximum of 12 g in 24 hours. An alternative is continuous infusion at 500 mg/hour as needed for several days. Unlike organophosphates, carbamate intoxications do not irreversibly inhibit cholinesterase, and thus pralidoxime is not usually required and may worsen symptoms.

   d. Treat **seizures** with a benzodiazepine and phenytoin; if severe seizures require muscle relaxants, **do not use succinylcholine,** which may result in prolonged paralysis.

   e. **Hemoperfusion** should be considered for severe parathion overdoses, although there is little objective evidence to support its use.

f. Support respiratory failure with mechanical ventilation.

K. **Phencyclidine** is a dissociative anesthetic and is available illicitly, mislabeled as LSD, mescaline, psilocybin, and tetrahydrocannabinol. Frequency of use varies widely by geographic region and is frequent in some urban areas but uncommon in many other parts of the United States.

1. **Symptoms** that occur even with small ingestions include agitation, hallucinations, bizarre or violent behavior, hypertension, tachycardia, and horizontal or vertical nystagmus. Patients are relatively impervious to pain and may be catatonic or self-destructive and difficult to subdue. Stupor progressing to coma, hypertension, hyperpyrexia, hypertonicity, and bronchospasm characterizes moderate ingestions. Massive ingestions may lead to hypotension, respiratory failure, rhabdomyolysis, and acute tubular necrosis. Hypoglycemia is common, and death may occur.
2. **Treatment** is primarily supportive. Monitor electrolytes, creatinine, and creatine phosphokinase (CPK). Drug levels are not useful. Minimize sensory input and remove potentially injurious objects from the area. Use diazepam to control agitation; give haloperidol if the agitation is severe. Treat dystonic reactions with diphenhydramine. Control adrenergic manifestations (e.g., hypertension) with β-adrenergic blockade if bronchospasm is not present; sodium nitroprusside may be required in severe cases. Ipecac is contraindicated. Gastric lavage may provoke violent behavior and is recommended only in severe poisonings and only after the airway has been protected. In that case, repeated charcoal administration also may interrupt enterogastric and enterohepatic circulations but has not been demonstrated to have an effect on outcome. Acid diuresis is no longer recommended. Avoid restraints, as they may increase rhabdomyolysis. Treat hyperthermia with cooling and hydration. Seizures are uncommon in adults; treat with benzodiazepines and phenytoin. Consider discharging any patient with low-dose intoxication from the emergency department after his or her symptoms resolve and psychiatric consultation has been obtained. Hospitalize patients with more severe intoxication.

L. **Neuroleptics**

1. **Phenothiazines** that are used commonly include chlorpromazine, thioridazine, prochlorperazine, perphenazine, trifluoperazine, fluphenazine, mesoridazine, haloperidol (a butyrophenone), and thiothixene.
   a. **Overdoses** are characterized by agitation or delirium, which may progress rapidly to coma. Pupils may be mydriatic, and deep tendon reflexes are depressed. Seizures and disorders of thermoregulation, particularly hyperthermia, may occur. Frank neuroleptic malignant syndrome may complicate use of these agents. Hypotension (due to strong α-adrenergic antagonism), tachycardia, arrhythmias (including torsades de pointes), and depressed cardiac conduction occur. Measuring blood levels is not helpful. Radiographs may reveal pill concretions that are present in the stomach despite apparently effective gastric emptying.
   b. **Treatment** includes airway protection, respiratory and hemodynamic support, and administration of activated charcoal. Emesis is contraindicated. Consider gastric lavage, which may be effective hours later due to delayed gastric emptying caused by the phenothiazines. Consider whole-bowel irrigation for ingestion of sustained-release formulations. Monitor the cardiac rhythm and treat ventricular arrhythmias with lidocaine and phenytoin; class Ia agents (e.g., procainamide, quinidine, disopyramide) are contraindicated; avoid sotalol. Treat hypotension with IV fluid administration and α-adrenergic vasopressors (norepinephrine). Dopamine is an acceptable alternative. Paradoxical vasodilation may occur in response to epinephrine administration because of unopposed β-adrenergic response

in the setting of strong α-adrenergic antagonism. Recurrent torsades de pointes may require magnesium, isoproterenol, or overdrive pacing (see Chap. 7, Cardiac Arrhythmias). Treat seizures with diazepam and phenytoin. Treat dystonic reactions with benztropine, 1–4 mg, or diphenhydramine, 25–50 mg, IM or IV. Treat hyperthermia with cooling. Forced diuresis, hemodialysis, and hemoperfusion are not useful. Admit those patients who have ingested a significant overdose for cardiac monitoring for at least 48 hours.

2. **Clozapine** is an atypical neuroleptic.
   a. **Overdose** is characterized by altered mental status, ranging from somnolence to coma (*Pharm Med* 6:169, 1992). Anticholinergic effects occur, including blurred vision, dry mouth (although hypersalivation may occur in overdose), lethargy, delirium, and constipation. Seizures occur in a minority of overdoses. Coma may occur. Physical manifestations include hypotension, tachycardia, fasciculations, tremor, and myoclonus. Agranulocytosis may result. ECG abnormalities are unusual, but atrioventricular block may occur. Serious dysrhythmias rarely occur.
   b. **Treatment.** Monitor BP and respiratory status, including ABGs, if respiratory depression occurs. Obtain an ECG and monitor the cardiac rhythm continuously. Obtain WBC and liver function tests; follow the WBC weekly for 4 weeks. Clozapine levels are not useful. Induction of emesis is contraindicated. Perform gastric lavage if the patient presents within 1 hour of ingestion. Treat hypotension with crystalloids; if resistant, treat with norepinephrine or dopamine. Treat seizures with benzodiazepines and phenytoin. Provide ventilatory support for respiratory failure. No evidence has been shown that forced diuresis, hemodialysis, or hemoperfusion is beneficial. Filgrastim can be given for agranulocytosis. Admit and monitor patients with severely symptomatic overdoses for 24 hours or more.
3. **Olanzapine** is an atypical antipsychotic that is similar to clozapine.
   a. **Overdose** is characterized by somnolence, slurred speech, ataxia, vertigo, nausea, and vomiting (*Ann Emerg Med* 34:279, 1999). Anticholinergic effects occur, including blurred vision, dry mouth, and tachycardia. Seizures are uncommon. Coma may occur. Physical manifestations include hypotension, tachycardia, and pinpoint pupils that are unresponsive to naloxone. Serious dysrhythmias rarely occur.
   b. **Treatment.** Induction of emesis is contraindicated. Consider gastric lavage if presentation is within 1 hour of ingestion. Give activated charcoal. Treat hypotension with fluids and, if ineffective, norepinephrine or dopamine. Give benzodiazepines and phenytoin for seizures. Provide ventilatory support for respiratory failure, which occurs uncommonly.
4. **Risperidone, ziprasidone, and quetiapine** are newer atypical antipsychotics with limited information about overdose. Clinical effects in common include CNS depression, tachycardia, hypotension, and electrolyte abnormalities. QRS and QTc prolongation have occurred with each, but clinically significant ventricular dysrhythmias are uncommon. Do not induce emesis. Consider gastric lavage if presentation is within an hour of ingestion. Administer activated charcoal. Monitor electrolytes, liver function, and electrocardiogram with continuous telemetry. Treat hypotension with fluids, and if severe and persistent, norepinephrine in preference to dopamine. Treat ventricular dysrhythmias with sodium bicarbonate to maintain a pH of 7.45–7.55, and avoid Ia antiarrhythmics (procainamide, quinidine, and disopyramide). Monitor and provide support for respiratory depression. Diuresis, hemodialysis, and hemoperfusion do not appear to be useful.

**M. Salicylate** toxicity may result from acute ingestion or chronic intoxication. Toxicity is usually mild after acute ingestions of less than 150 mg/kg, moderate after ingestions of 150–300 mg/kg, and generally severe with overdoses of 300–500 mg/kg. Toxicity from chronic ingestion typically is due to intake of more than 100 mg/kg/day over a period of several days and usually occurs in elderly patients with chronic underlying illness. Diagnosis often is delayed in this group of patients, and mortality is approximately 25%. Significant toxicity due to chronic ingestion may occur with blood levels lower than those associated with acute ingestions.

1. **Symptoms.** Nausea, vomiting, tinnitus (implying levels >30 mg/dl), hyperpnea, and malaise can occur. Fever suggests a poor prognosis in adults. Severe intoxications are associated with lethargy, convulsions, and coma, which may result from cerebral edema. Noncardiogenic pulmonary edema occurs in up to 30% of adults and is more common with chronic ingestion, cigarette smoking, neurologic symptoms, and older age.
2. **Laboratory data**
   a. Obtain a CBC; electrolyte, BUN, creatinine, and blood glucose levels; and prothrombin and partial thromboplastin times. Prothrombin time prolongation is common.
   b. **ABGs** may reveal an early respiratory alkalosis, followed by metabolic acidosis. Approximately 20% of patients exhibit either respiratory alkalosis or metabolic acidosis alone (*J Crit Illness* 1:77, 1986). Most adults with pure salicylate overdose have a primary metabolic acidosis and a primary respiratory alkalosis. After mixed overdoses, respiratory acidosis may become prominent (*Arch Intern Med* 138:1481, 1978).
   c. **Hypoglycemia,** common in children, is rare in adults.
   d. **Blood levels** must be drawn 6 hours or more after acute ingestion of salicylates to allow prediction of severity of intoxication and patient disposition (Fig. 25-2). Obtaining earlier levels is appropriate in severely intoxicated patients, to guide intervention. Levels in excess of 70 mg/dl at any time represent moderate to severe intoxication; levels of more than 100 mg/dl are very serious and often fatal. This information is useful only for acute overdoses; estimation of severity is invalidated by the use of enteric-coated aspirin or chronic ingestion. Bicarbonate levels and pH are more useful than salicylate levels as prognostic indicators in chronic intoxication.
3. **Treatment**
   a. Consider **gastric lavage** if presentation is within 1 hour of ingestion. Administer activated charcoal. Multidose charcoal may be useful in severe overdose (*Pediatrics* 85:594, 1990) but is not routinely recommended.
   b. **Alkaline diuresis** is indicated for salicylate blood levels that are higher than 40 mg/dl. Administer 88 or 100 mEq (2 ampules) sodium bicarbonate in 1000 ml $D_5W$ at a rate of 10–15 ml/kg/hour if the patient is clinically volume depleted until urine flow is achieved. Maintain alkalinization using the same solution at 2–3 ml/kg/hour, and monitor urine output, urine pH (target pH, 7–8), and serum potassium. Achievement of alkaline diuresis often requires the simultaneous administration of at least 20 mEq/L **potassium chloride.** Because there is little evidence of improved outcome with alkaline diuresis, and because older patients may have cardiac, renal, and pulmonary comorbidity, **avoid vigorous fluid therapy in the elderly,** as pulmonary edema is more likely to occur in this population.
   c. Although acetazolamide causes urine alkalinization, the associated acidemia increases salicylate toxicity, and therefore it must not be used.
   d. **Hemodialysis** is indicated for blood levels in excess of 100–130 mg/dl after acute intoxication but may be useful with chronic toxicity when

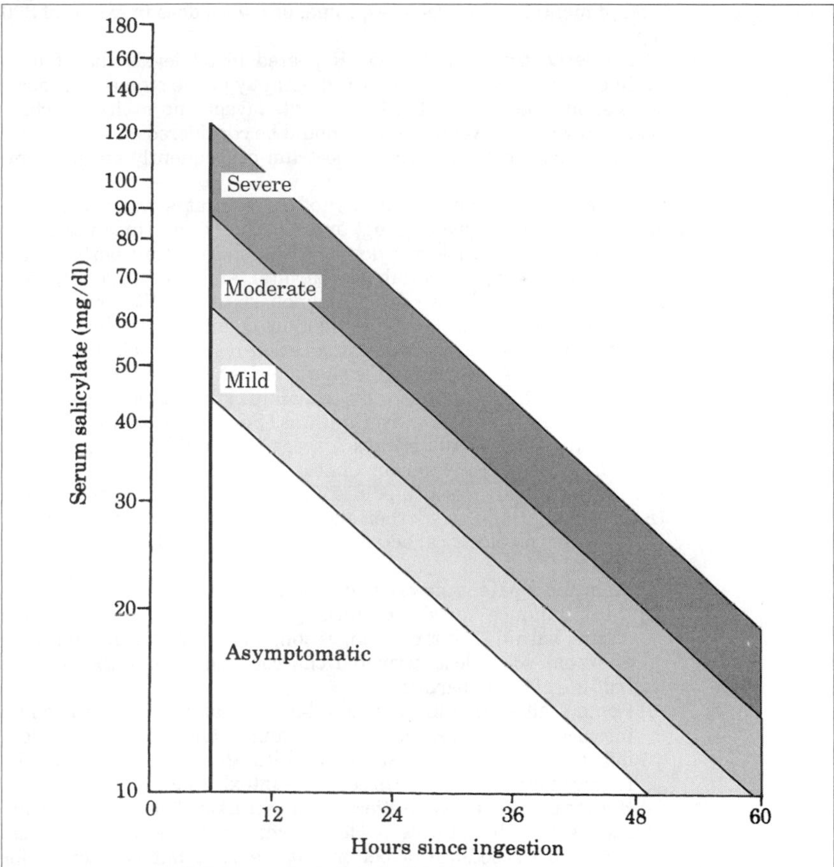


**Fig. 25-2.** Severity of salicylate intoxication. (Adapted from AK Done. Salicylate intoxication. *Pediatrics* 26:800, 1960.)

levels are as low as 40 mg/dl if other indications for dialysis exist. Among these are refractory acidosis, severe CNS symptoms, progressive clinical deterioration, pulmonary edema, and renal failure.

e. **Treatment of pulmonary edema** may also require mechanical ventilation with a high fraction of inspired oxygen concentration and PEEP. Treat **cerebral edema** with hyperventilation and osmotic diuresis. Administer a benzodiazepine (diazepam, 5–10 mg IV q15min up to 50 mg) followed by phenobarbital, 15 mg/kg IV.

f. **Patients with minor symptoms** (nausea, vomiting, tinnitus), an acute ingestion of less than 150 mg/kg, and a first blood level of less than 65 mg/dl can be treated in the emergency department. Blood levels should be repeated q2h until they show a decline. These patients often are medically stable for discharge, and their disposition can be determined based on psychiatric evaluation.

g. **Admit moderately symptomatic patients** for at least 24 hours.

h. **Admit patients with severe overdoses to an ICU.** Severe overdoses are manifested by tachypnea, dehydration, pulmonary edema, altered mental status, seizures, coma, or a total dose in excess of 300 mg/kg.

i. **The elderly are at high risk.** Repeated blood levels that fail to decline should prompt contrast radiography of the stomach; concretions should be subjected to bicarbonate lavage and multidose charcoal, and whole-bowel irrigation should be considered.

N. **Sedative-hypnotics** include a diverse spectrum of frequently abused compounds.

1. **Barbiturates.** Toxic manifestations of barbiturates vary with the amount of ingestion, type of drug, and length of time since ingestion. Toxicity can occur with lower doses of the short-acting barbiturates (e.g., butabarbital, hexobarbital, secobarbital, and pentobarbital) than of the long-acting barbiturates (e.g., phenobarbital, barbital, mephobarbital, and primidone), but fatalities are more common with the latter.

a. **Clinical manifestations.** Mild intoxication resembles alcohol intoxication. Moderate intoxication is characterized by greater depression of mental status, response only to painful stimuli, decreased deep tendon reflexes, and slow respirations. Severe intoxication causes coma and a loss of all reflexes (except the pupillary light reflex). Plantar reflexes are extensor. Characteristic bullae ("barb burns") may be seen over pressure points and on the dorsum of the fingers (*BMJ* 1:835, 1965). Hypothermia and hypotension may occur. In severe cases, no electrical activity is seen on an EEG.

b. **Treatment**

(1) Maintain a patent airway and adequate ventilation.

(2) Do not induce emesis. Perform **gastric lavage** if presentation occurs within 1 hour of ingestion, and **administer activated charcoal.** Multidose activated charcoal markedly decreases the half-life of phenobarbital.

(3) **Forced alkaline diuresis,** similar to that used for salicylate intoxication, is effective in enhancing phenobarbital excretion, but not that of short-acting barbiturates. Its use should be reserved for severe, life-threatening intoxication.

(4) **Hemoperfusion** may be effective for excretion of phenobarbital and short-acting barbiturates. Hemoperfusion is used rather than hemodialysis because of better drug removal but is reserved for patients with stage IV coma with increased blood levels and refractory hemodynamic compromise.

(5) Treat hypotension with crystalloid administration. If this fails, administer norepinephrine or dopamine.

2. **Benzodiazepines.** These agents depress mental and respiratory function when taken in overdose. Fatalities are rare, but mixed overdoses are common. Most overdoses are the result of attempts at self-harm. An exception is flunitrazepam (Rohypnol, "roofies"), which is ten times as potent as diazepam. It is mixed with low-quality heroin and used to soften the effects of cocaine. It is also mixed with alcohol as a "date rape" drug. Effects are similar to those of other benzodiazepines. It may cause hallucinations, and mixing with alcohol increases respiratory depression. It often is not detected on standard toxicology screens.

a. **Symptoms** include drowsiness, dysarthria, ataxia, slurred speech, and confusion.

b. **Treatment.** Do not induce emesis. Consider gastric lavage if presentation is within 1 hour of ingestion. Administer activated charcoal. Provide general supportive measures for hypotension and bradycardia. Rarely, respiratory depression may require intubation. **Flumazenil,** a benzodiazepine antagonist, reverses toxicity without causing respiratory depression. Administer 0.2 mg (2 ml) IV over 30 seconds, followed by 0.3 mg at 1-minute intervals to a total dose of 3 mg. If no response is observed after such treatment, benzodiazepines are unlikely to be the cause of the patient's sedation. If a partial response has occurred, give additional 0.5-mg increments to a total of 5 mg. Rarely, as much as a 10-mg total dose may be necessary for full reversal. If no IV access is available, the drug can be administered by endotracheal tube. Treat recurrence of sedation or respiratory depression by repeating the preceding regimen or by continuous infusion of 0.1–0.5 mg/hour. **If mixed overdose with cyclic antidepressants is suspected or the patient has a known history of seizure disorder, flumazenil should not be used.** Forced diuresis and hemodialysis are ineffective.

3. **Gamma-hydroxybutyrate.** An endogenous short-chain fatty acid that occurs naturally in the body, this illegal substance is not detected by standard toxicology screens. It has emerged as an important intoxicant. It is often sold to participants at large dance parties ("raves") and has been responsible for mass intoxications (*Prehosp Emerg Care* 3:357, 1999). It has also been used as a "date rape" drug. Synonyms include, but are not limited to, "liquid Ecstasy," "liquid E," "grievous bodily harm," "Georgia home boy," "soap," "salty water," and "organic Quaaludes."
   a. **Symptoms** include ataxia, nystagmus, somnolence progressing to coma, vomiting, and random clonic movements of the face and extremities. EEG recording supports the belief that these represent myoclonus and not true seizures. Respiratory depression may progress to apnea.
   b. **Treatment.** Absorption is very rapid, and lavage and activated charcoal administration are of little use. Do not induce emesis. The drug is not antagonized by naloxone or flumazenil. Experimental but no clinical evidence has been found for the use of physostigmine, and its use is not recommended. Administer oxygen and protect the airway; monitor oxygenation. Drug levels are not usually available, and the drug is not detected on routine toxicology screens. Obtain electrolytes and glucose and establish an IV line. Stimulation, including endotracheal intubation, may stimulate violently aggressive behavior. Give atropine for persistent symptomatic bradycardia. Treat hypotension with IV fluids; pressors are rarely necessary. Obtain an ECG and monitor the cardiac rhythm continuously. Intoxication is usually short lived; coma typically lasts for 1–2 hours, and full recovery often occurs within 8 hours. Stable asymptomatic patients can be discharged after 6 hours of observation. Admit any patient who is still clinically intoxicated after 6 hours (*Ann Emerg Med* 31:729, 1998).

O. **Stimulants** include amphetamines and cocaine.

1. **Amphetamines**
   a. **Symptoms.** Toxicity is manifested by hyperactivity, irritability, delirium, hallucinations, psychosis, mydriasis, hyperpyrexia, flushing, diaphoresis, hypertension, arrhythmias, vomiting, and diarrhea. Less common manifestations include acute renal failure secondary to rhabdomyolysis, seizures, CNS hemorrhage, coma, myocardial infarction, aortic dissection, and circulatory collapse.
   b. **Treatment** includes early administration of activated charcoal. **Induction of emesis is contraindicated,** as it may induce seizures. Perform gastric lavage only for recent large ingestions. Establish an IV line and monitor electrolytes, renal function, and CPK. Obtain an ECG and monitor the cardiac rhythm. Treat agitation with diazepam; physical restraints may increase the occurrence of rhabdomyolysis. Treat hallucinations and psychosis with haloperidol. Droperidol, 2.5–5.0 mg IV, may be superior to benzodiazepines for sedation (*Eur J Emerg Med* 4:130, 1997). However, it may cause Q-T prolongation and torsades des pointes; therefore, its use should be reserved for severe agitation that is resistant to benzodiazepines, and continuous cardiac monitoring should be used. Treat severe hypertension with nitroprus-

side or a β-adrenergic antagonist; phentolamine can also be considered (see Chap. 4, Hypertension). Diazepam is the initial drug of choice for seizures, followed by phenytoin or phenobarbital. Arrhythmias usually respond to propranolol or lidocaine. Monitor core temperature. Hyperthermia may require cooling blankets, evaporative cooling, or paralysis; if unsuccessful, dantrolene or bromocriptine may be useful. Hemodialysis is not clearly effective. Treat rhabdomyolysis as outlined in Chap. 11, Renal Diseases. Admit patients with moderate to severe symptoms or with abnormal vital signs.

2. **3-4 Methylenedioxymethamphetamine ("Ecstasy").** This compound is a popular drug of abuse associated with "rave" culture. Surveys have shown that nearly 40% of college students have used it at least once. It is often used in association with prolonged vigorous dancing, causing dehydration and contributing to hyperthermia.
   a. **Symptoms** are due in part to the drug's action as a serotonin releaser. They include hypertension, tachycardia, dilated pupils, diaphoresis, and trismus. Severe intoxications may result in hyperthermia, DIC, muscle rigidity, myoclonus, rhabdomyolysis, acute renal failure, and occasionally the syndrome of inappropriate antidiuretic hormone secretion. Supraventricular and ventricular arrhythmias may occur. Initial confusion and agitation may progress to coma and seizures.
   b. **Treatment.** Toxicology screens are unreliable. Initiation of therapy is based on presumptive diagnosis according to history and presentation. Monitor electrolytes, BUN, creatinine, liver function tests, CBC, coagulation studies, and CPK. Therapy at present is based on case reports and reviews (*Pediatrics* 100:705, 1997). Do not induce emesis, as coma and seizures may occur abruptly. Gastric lavage is useful only if initiated within 1 hour of ingestion. Administer activated charcoal. Establish an IV line and maintain hydration. Treat agitation with benzodiazepines, with preparation to protect the airway and support ventilation. β-Adrenergic antagonists may be useful in treatment of tachycardia and hypertension. Severe hypertension may require nitroprusside. Treat seizures with benzodiazepines followed by phenytoin or phenobarbital. Treat ventricular arrhythmias with lidocaine, phenytoin, or esmolol. Cool the hyperthermic patient with evaporative cooling; consider dantrolene administration. Treat rhabdomyolysis supportively (see Chap. 11, Renal Diseases).
3. **Cocaine**
   a. **Symptoms.** Cocaine causes short-lived CNS and sympathetic stimulation, hypertension, tachypnea, tachycardia, and mydriasis. Depression of the higher nervous centers ensues rapidly and may result in death. Mortality may also result from drug-induced seizures, subarachnoid hemorrhage, stroke, or direct cardiac effects (e.g., coronary artery spasm, myocardial injury, and precipitation of lethal arrhythmias) (*N Engl J Med* 315:1495, 1986). **Myocardial infarction** may be precipitated in individuals without underlying heart disease. Rhabdomyolysis may occur, precipitating renal failure. **Pulmonary edema** may develop abruptly after an individual smokes the free alkaloid form of cocaine ("free base") or its heated bicarbonate precipitant ("crack"). Pneumomediastinum may occur after smoking crack and may progress to pneumothorax. Other pulmonary complications include alveolar hemorrhage, obliterative bronchiolitis, hypersensitivity pneumonitis, and asthma (*Am J Med* 87:664, 1989). Bowel ischemia and necrosis may occur.
   b. **Treatment.** Maintain a patent airway and support respiration and circulation. Obtain CBC, electrolytes, and CPK. Obtain an ECG and monitor the cardiac rhythm continuously. Myocardial ischemia and infarction should be managed as outlined in Chap. 5, Ischemic Heart

Disease. Avoid β-adrenergic antagonists in patients with myocardial ischemia or infarction, as they allow unopposed α-adrenergic vasospasm (*Ann Intern Med* 112:897, 1990). Labetalol may be preferable, and phentolamine may be useful in selected cases. Nitroglycerin can be used for ischemic pain. Treat ventricular arrhythmias with lidocaine; β-adrenergic antagonists may be useful in those without myocardial ischemia. Use benzodiazepines to decrease the stimulatory effect of cocaine and to treat seizures initially. Follow with phenytoin or phenobarbital for longer-term seizure control. Treat noncoronary manifestations of adrenergic stimulation with labetalol; severe or sustained hypertension may require treatment with nitroprusside. Treat rhabdomyolysis and hypotension supportively. Hyperthermia may require a cooling blanket, evaporative cooling, sedation, or paralysis. Diuresis and dialysis are not useful. Admit patients with marked toxicity to an ICU for observation and cardiac monitoring. **Suspected body packers** should undergo abdominal radiography to rule out cocaine-containing packets in the intestinal tract; Gastrografin-enhanced CT may be more sensitive. If such packets are present, perform gentle catharsis with charcoal and psyllium; mineral oil may dissolve latex packets and precipitate toxicity. Admit such patients to an ICU for monitoring, as rupture may be rapidly fatal. Whole-bowel irrigation and surgery probably are rarely necessary, although they have been recommended; surgery is clearly indicated only for bowel obstruction. Attempts at endoscopic removal are contraindicated, as rupture may result. Obtain repeated radiographs until the packets are no longer visible. With appropriate care, mortality is less than 1% (*Am J Med* 88:325, 1990). "Body stuffing" involves smaller amounts of drug. To avoid arrest, body stuffers may ingest crack cocaine that is unwrapped or wrapped only in a layer of cellophane. Abdominal radiography is almost invariably negative. The course is generally benign, presumably due to poor absorption. Nearly three-fourths of patients remain asymptomatic, and most of the rest have only mild to moderate symptoms, including tachycardia and hypertension. Only 4% have severe toxicity, including seizures, dysrhythmias, and death (*Ann Emerg Med* 29:596, 1999; *J Emerg Med* 18:221, 2000). Close observation is nevertheless warranted.

**P. Theophylline**

1. **Symptoms.** Nausea and vomiting are the most common symptoms of theophylline toxicity and are associated with serum levels exceeding 20 mg/ml. Moderate toxicity is largely due to relative epinephrine excess and includes tachycardia, arrhythmias, tremors, and agitation. Severe toxicity results in hallucinations, seizures (which may be refractory to standard therapy), dysrhythmias (including sinus tachycardia, atrial fibrillation, supraventricular tachycardia, and ventricular tachycardia and fibrillation), and hypotension. Rhabdomyolysis occurs occasionally (*Intensive Care Med* 18:129, 1992). Severity of intoxication is modified by chronicity, age of the patient, and the presence of comorbid diseases. Severe toxicity is most common at serum levels in excess of 90 mg/ml in the acutely intoxicated, usually younger individual. Seizures and cardiac toxicity are likely at serum levels of more than 60 mg/ml in the chronically intoxicated and might occur at even lower levels.
2. **Laboratory studies.** Obtain theophylline levels q2h until a plateau is reached. The peak level may be delayed significantly after the ingestion of sustained-release theophylline preparations, with toxic levels persisting 50–60 hours after ingestion. Check potassium, electrolyte, glucose, CPK, calcium, and magnesium levels; BUN; and ABGs. Obtain a baseline ECG and maintain continuous cardiac monitoring. Acid-base abnormalities include respiratory alkalosis and metabolic acidosis. Hypokalemia, hyperglycemia, hypercalcemia, and hypophosphatemia may be present.

**3. Therapy**

**a.** Establish an IV line and perform gastric lavage if the patient has taken a potentially life-threatening acute ingestion. Consider lavage also after a large ingestion of a sustained-release preparation, as a bezoar may form. Avoid the use of ipecac because of the potential for seizures and aspiration. Administer activated charcoal. **Multidose charcoal** decreases the half-life of theophylline by 50%, although it has not been clearly shown to improve outcome. Consider whole-bowel irrigation with polyethylene glycol solution for overdoses with sustained-release preparations and blood levels that continue to rise despite therapy.

**b.** Treat severe nausea with metoclopramide, 10–60 mg IV, or ondansetron, 0.15 mg/kg IV (8–10 mg in the average individual) (*Ann Pharmacother* 27:584, 1993). **Do not use phenothiazines because of their propensity to lower the seizure threshold.**

**c.** Treat hypotension with **IV crystalloids** and, if resistant, with dopamine.

**d.** Phenobarbital is preferred to phenytoin for **seizure prophylaxis** in the severely poisoned patient. The treatment of choice for seizures is a benzodiazepine followed by phenobarbital (10 mg/kg loading dose at 50 mg/minute, followed by up to a total of 30 mg/kg at a rate of 50 mg/minute, followed by 1–5 mg/kg/day to maintain therapeutic plasma levels). Because of the cardiovascular and respiratory depressant activities of barbiturates, careful management of the airway and cardiovascular status are mandatory. For those patients who are refractory to phenobarbital therapy, obtain anesthesiology consultation for administration of pentobarbital; muscle paralysis and general anesthesia can be considered.

**e.** Arrhythmias should be treated as they would be in nonintoxicated patients. β-Adrenergic antagonists may be particularly useful but may precipitate bronchospasm in asthmatics. Because of its short half-life, IV esmolol usually is safer.

**f.** **Hemoperfusion** (charcoal or resin) is preferable to hemodialysis because of faster drug removal and is indicated for (1) intractable seizures or life-threatening cardiovascular complications, regardless of drug level; (2) a theophylline level that approaches or exceeds 100 mg/ml after an acute overdose; (3) a theophylline level of more than 60 mg/ml in acute intoxication, with increasing symptoms, and a patient who is intolerant of oral charcoal administration; (4) a theophylline level in excess of 60 mg/ml in chronic intoxication without life-threatening symptoms; and (5) a theophylline level of more than 40 mg/ml in a patient with chronic intoxication and CHF, respiratory insufficiency, hepatic failure (*J Emerg Med* 11:415, 1993), or age older than 60 years.

**g.** **Disposition.** Admit patients who have chronic intoxication, acute ingestion of sustained-release formulations, acute ingestions with levels that fail to fall or are rising despite therapy, or worsening symptoms. Those with levels that are falling to less than 20 mg/ml and whose symptoms are resolving can be discharged.

## Toxic Inhalants

Toxic inhalants comprise a variety of noxious gases and particulate matter that are capable of producing local irritation, asphyxiation, and systemic toxicity. In the management of exposure victims, identification of the offending agent is critical, and the regional poison control center must be contacted for specific therapeutic guidelines.

**I. Irritant gases** produce cutaneous burns, mucosal irritation, laryngotracheitis, bronchitis, pneumonitis, bronchospasm, and pulmonary edema (which may be delayed up to 24 hours after exposure). The more water-soluble gases (e.g., chlorine, ammonia, formaldehyde, sulfur dioxide, ozone) primarily produce inflammation of the eyes, throat, and upper respiratory tract, whereas the less soluble gases (e.g., phosgene, nitrogen dioxide) tend to cause more damage to the terminal airways and alveoli. Household exposure may result from inadvertent mixture of bleach (sodium hypochlorite) with toilet bowl cleaner (sulfuric acid), which produces chlorine gas, or of bleach with ammonia, which produces chloramine gas.

**A. Treatment.** Maintain a patent airway and adequate oxygenation. Treat bronchospasm with bronchodilators. Severe cough may require narcotic antitussives. Treat noncardiogenic pulmonary edema with oxygen, mechanical ventilation, and PEEP as needed (see Chap. 8, Critical Care). Systemic corticosteroids have no role. Treat skin burns by copious irrigation, removal of contaminated clothing, and tetanus prophylaxis (see Appendix F, Immunizations and Post-Exposure Therapies), if needed. Irrigate the eyes immediately and copiously with water or saline if the patient has had chemical contact. Obtain ophthalmologic consultation for caustic eye burns.

**B. Disposition.** Because the development of pulmonary edema may be delayed, observe asymptomatic patients with normal ABGs and chest radiographs for at least 6 hours. Hospitalize patients with symptoms or signs of upper airway edema or pulmonary involvement.

**II. Simple asphyxiants** (e.g., acetylene, argon, ethane, helium, hydrogen, nitrogen, methane, butane, neon, carbon dioxide, natural gas, and propane) cause hypoxia by displacing oxygen from the inspired air. Morbidity and mortality are related to the extent and duration of the hypoxia. **Treatment** consists of supplemental oxygen and supportive care for symptomatic patients.

**III. Systemic toxic inhalants** are gases that are capable of producing prominent systemic toxicity; they include hydrogen sulfide, methyl bromide, organophosphates (see Overdosage, sec. **VII.J**), carbon monoxide, and hydrogen cyanide. Treatment consists of supportive care and specific therapy directed toward the offending agent.

**A. Carbon monoxide** displaces oxygen from hemoglobin, shifts the oxyhemoglobin dissociation curve to the left, and depresses cellular respiration by inhibiting the cytochrome oxidase system. Direct binding to cardiac myoglobin depresses cardiac function. Toxic manifestations are a consequence of tissue hypoxia. Poisoning usually occurs in poorly ventilated areas in which carbon monoxide is released by fires, combustion engines, or faulty stoves or heating systems. Intoxication is seasonal, with more cases occurring in winter. **Arterial oxygen tension usually is normal; thus, the diagnosis of carbon monoxide poisoning requires a high level of suspicion and direct measurement of arterial oxygen saturation or carbon monoxide (carboxyhemoglobin) levels.** Standard pulse oximetry is not reliable.

**1. Symptoms** correlate imperfectly with the carboxyhemoglobin level. Levels of 20–40% are associated with dizziness, headache, weakness, disturbed judgment, nausea and vomiting, and diminished visual acuity. These symptoms and seasonality frequently lead to a misdiagnosis of influenza. Examination may reveal retinal hemorrhages. Levels of 40–60% are associated with tachypnea, tachycardia, ataxia, syncope, and seizures. The ECG may reveal ST-segment changes, conduction blocks, and atrial or ventricular arrhythmias. Levels in excess of 60% are associated with coma and death. Cherry-red coloration of the lips or skin is a relatively rare, late manifestation. Late complications include basal ganglia infarction and parkinsonism. Less severe, delayed neuropsychiatric symptoms also may occur.

2. **Treatment** begins with administration of **100% oxygen** by tight-fitting mask or endotracheal tube. The latter ensures tissue oxygen delivery and decreases the half-life of carboxyhemoglobin from 4–5 hours to 90 minutes. Measure carboxyhemoglobin levels q2–4h, and continue oxygen administration until blood levels are less than 10%. Obtain electrolytes, CPK, ABGs, and an ECG, and monitor the cardiac rhythm continuously. **Hyperbaric oxygen** (3 atm) has been strongly recommended for patients who have been unconscious at any time and present with neurologic signs or symptoms, ECG changes consistent with ischemia, severe metabolic acidosis, rhabdomyolysis, pulmonary edema, or shock. Hyperbaric treatment of patients who have minor or no symptoms but who have carboxyhemoglobin levels of greater than 25–30% is controversial, as is treatment in pregnancy. A randomized controlled trial showed no acute benefit for hyperbaric oxygen therapy as compared to administration of 100% oxygen (*Med J Aust* 170:203, 1999). However, hyperbaric oxygen appears to improve long-term neurologic outcome (*N Engl J Med* 347:1057, 2002). Consult with an expert in the field when indications are unclear. In no case should patients be transferred to a hyperbaric oxygen facility until their condition is stabilized. Treat seizures with diazepam and phenytoin (see Chap. 24, Neurologic Disorders). Arrhythmias and rhabdomyolysis are treated as described elsewhere.

B. **Hydrogen cyanide** may be present in industrial fumigants, insecticides, and products of combustion of synthetics and plastics. It may be generated as a by-product of phencyclidine manufacture. The gas has a characteristic bitter almond odor. Toxic amounts are absorbed rapidly through the bronchial mucosa and alveoli, and symptoms usually appear seconds after inhalation. Concentrations of 0.2–0.3 mg/L air are almost immediately fatal. Oral exposures to **potassium cyanide** may be due to rodenticides, insecticides, silver polish, artificial fingernail remover (acetonitrile), film developer, laboratory reagents, and amygdalin.

1. **Toxic manifestations** include headache, palpitations, dyspnea, and mental status depression, which may progress quickly to coma, seizures, and death. ECG changes include atrial fibrillation, ventricular ectopy, and abnormal ventricular repolarization. Severe lactic acidosis is present, and venous oxygen content is higher than normal and may approach arterial oxygen content. Do not delay initiation of therapy for measurement of whole-blood cyanide levels.
2. **Therapy** focuses on conversion of hemoglobin to methemoglobin, which binds to the cyanide ion, sparing vital oxidative enzymes.
    a. **Amyl nitrite** (1 broken pearl held under the nostril for 15–30 seconds/minute, repeated every minute, with a new pearl q3min) produces a methemoglobin level of approximately 5%. This should be followed as rapidly as possible with 10 ml 3% **sodium nitrite** IV (0.3 g over 3–5 minutes). If the response is inadequate, one-half of the dose of sodium nitrite should be repeated in 30 minutes. The goal is a measured methemoglobin level of 30%.
    b. Give **sodium thiosulfate** (50 ml of a 25% solution IV) immediately after the sodium nitrite, as it converts the cyanide into thiocyanate, which is excreted in the urine. Repeat one-half the dose in 30 minutes if the response is inadequate.
    c. **Administer 100% oxygen** at all times during treatment to ensure adequate tissue oxygen delivery despite methemoglobinemia. Do not give methylene blue for methemoglobin levels less than 70%, as cyanide may be released. In the event of life-threatening methemoglobinemia, consider exchange transfusion. Monitor the cardiac rhythm continuously.
    d. For severe persistent acidosis (pH <7.2), **administer sodium bicarbonate,** 1 mEq/kg, after the preceding measures have been undertaken.

e. In the event of oral ingestion, empty the stomach by gastric lavage after the preceding measures have been undertaken. Do not induce emesis. Rapid absorption makes administration of activated charcoal of dubious utility.

f. The efficacy of hyperbaric oxygen is controversial but can be considered for those who respond poorly to conventional therapy.

g. In Europe, hydroxocobalamin, 4 g IV (10 ml of a 40% solution administered over 20 minutes), is an effective alternative to the above regimen (*Occup Med* 48:427, 1998). The only preparation available in the United States is a 1% solution, and the requirement for infusion of 4 L makes this impractical. Dicobalt ethylenediaminetetra-acetic acid (dicobalt EDTA) and dimethylaminophenol are antidotes that are not available in the United States. If dicobalt EDTA is available, the dose is 300–600 mg (20–40 ml) IV over 1–5 minutes, followed by a 50-ml flush with $D_5W$. An additional 300 mg can be given in 5 minutes if the clinical response is inadequate.

**C. Hydrogen sulfide** is a colorless gas with a characteristic rotten-egg odor. It is found in mines and sewers as well as petrochemical, agricultural (liquid manure processing), and tanning industries.

1. **Symptoms.** Exposure to low concentrations of hydrogen sulfide causes mucous membrane and eye irritation and vision changes. Higher concentrations cause cyanosis, confusion, pulmonary edema, coma, and convulsions. Rapid death occurs in approximately 6% of cases.

2. **Treatment.** Therapy is similar to that used for hydrogen cyanide. Oxygen 100% and nitrites are used, but thiosulfate is not. The efficacy of nitrites is controversial (*Vet Hum Toxicol* 39:152, 1997). Flush the mucous membranes with saline or water. Consider hyperbaric oxygenation for severe intoxication.

**D. Smoke inhalation** is the cause of death in more than 50% of fire-related fatalities. Thermal injury usually is confined to the upper airway because of the rapid cooling of inhaled gases that occurs proximal to the larynx. Toxic gases released by fire include carbon dioxide, carbon monoxide, hydrogen chloride, phosgene, chlorine, benzene, isocyanate, hydrogen cyanide, aldehydes, oxides of sulfur and nitrogen, ammonia, and numerous organic acids. Carbon monoxide accounts for 80% of mortality in the first 12 hours. The other toxins produce epithelial injury that results in airway edema, increased capillary permeability, and mechanical obstruction from desquamated tissue and secretions. Patients who have lost consciousness, have been exposed to a large quantity of smoke in a closed space, have suffered prolonged inhalation or steam exposure, were involved in an explosion, were with other persons who died or were severely injured, or have sustained facial burns or singed nasal vibrissae are at risk for development of respiratory complications, which may be delayed in onset for up to 3 days. High-risk patients should undergo upper airway endoscopy to rule out any life-threatening airway injury immediately; bronchoscopy rarely provides additional therapeutically useful information. A positive xenon scan predicts increased mortality but is rarely justified. Carboxyhemoglobin levels that exceed 15% are indicative of severe exposure.

1. **Clinical manifestations.** Asphyxiation, expectoration of carbonaceous sputum, hoarseness, dyspnea from upper airway edema, stridor, bronchospasm, and noncardiogenic pulmonary edema are characteristic features of smoke inhalation. Upper airway burns may also be noted. Neurologic manifestations include stupor and coma. Late complications include bacterial pneumonia and pulmonary embolism.

2. **Treatment. Scrupulous airway care is essential,** with frequent suctioning as needed. Endotracheal intubation is required in patients who display evidence of significant upper airway edema or respiratory insufficiency. Bronchoscopy may be necessary to remove endotracheal debris.

Administer **humidified oxygen** to all patients. Give bronchodilators for bronchospasm. Treat ARDS with mechanical ventilation and PEEP. High-frequency flow interruption ventilation has been reported to be effective (*Curr Opin Pulm Med* 3:221, 1997) but is not widely available and requires additional confirmation. Prophylactic antibiotics and glucocorticoids are not indicated. Treat specific intoxications (e.g., cyanide and carbon monoxide poisoning) appropriately. Suspect cyanide intoxication if coma and significant lactic acidosis are present.

3. **Disposition.** Patients who have experienced minor smoke inhalation, who are asymptomatic at 4–6 hours, and who exhibit none of the risk factors just listed can be safely discharged home. Admit asymptomatic patients who have any risk factors for potential respiratory complications for a minimum of 24 hours. Admit patients who have symptoms, significant laboratory abnormalities, or an abnormal alveolar-arterial oxygen gradient to an ICU.

# Appendixes

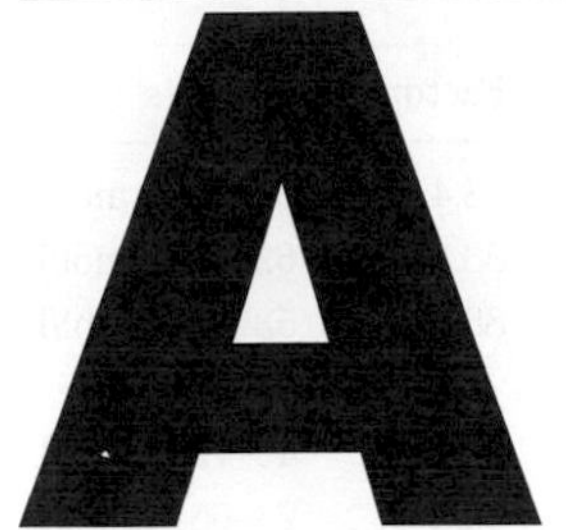

# Barnes-Jewish Hospital Laboratory Reference Values

Ian S. Harris

Reference values for the more commonly used laboratory tests are listed in the following table. These values are given in the units currently used at Barnes-Jewish Hospital and in Systeme International (SI) units, which are used in many areas of the world. Individual reference values can be population and method dependent.

| Test | Current units | Factor[a] | SI units |
|---|---|---|---|
| **Common serum chemistries** | | | |
| Albumin | 3.6–5.0 g/dl | 10 | 36–50 g/L |
| Ammonia (plasma) | 9–33 μmol/L | 1 | 9–33 μmol/L |
| Bilirubin | | | |
| Total[b] | 0.3–1.1 mg/dl | 17.1 | 5.13–18.80 μmol/L |
| Direct | 0–0.3 mg/dl | 17.1 | 0–5.1 μmol/L |
| Blood gases (arterial) | | | |
| pH | 7.35–7.45 | 1 | 7.35–7.45 |
| $PO_2$ | 80–105 mm Hg | 0.133 | 10.6–14.0 kPa |
| $PCO_2$ | 35–45 mm Hg | 0.133 | 4.7–6.0 kPa |
| Calcium | | | |
| Total | 8.6–10.3 mg/dl | 0.25 | 2.15–2.58 mmol/L |
| Ionized | 4.5–5.1 mg/dl | 0.25 | 1.13–1.28 mmol/L |
| $CO_2$ content (plasma) | 22–32 mmol/L | 1 | 22–32 mmol/L |
| Ceruloplasmin | 18–46 mg/dl | 0.063 | 1.5–2.9 μmol/L |
| Chloride | 97–110 mmol/L | 1 | 97–110 mmol/L |
| Cholesterol[c] | | | |
| Desirable | <200 mg/dl | 0.0259 | <5.18 mmol/L |
| Borderline high | 200–239 mg/dl | 0.0259 | 5.18–6.19 mmol/L |
| High | ≥240 mg/dl | 0.0259 | ≥6.22 mmol/L |
| HDL cholesterol[b] | >35 mg/dl | 0.0259 | >0.91 mmol/L |
| Copper (total) | 75–145 mg/dl | 0.157 | 11.8–22.8 mmol/L |
| Creatinine[b] | | | |
| Male age 4–20 yr | 0.2–1.2 mg/dl | 88.4 | 18–106 μmol/L |
| Female age 4–20 yr | 0.2–1.2 mg/dl | 88.4 | 18–106 μmol/L |
| Male age 20–69 yr | 0.7–1.5 mg/dl | 88.4 | 62–133 μmol/L |

| Test | Current units | Factor[a] | SI units |
|---|---|---|---|
| Female age 20–69 yr | 0.6–1.4 mg/dl | 88.4 | 53–124 μmol/L |
| Male age ≥ 70 yr | 0.7–1.7 mg/dl | 88.4 | 62–150 μmol/L |
| Female age ≥ 70 yr | 0.6–1.5 mg/dl | 88.4 | 53–133 μmol/L |
| Ferritin | | | |
| Male adult | 20–323 ng/ml | 2.25 | 45–727 pmol/L |
| Female adult | 10–291 ng/ml | 2.25 | 23–655 pmol/L |
| Folate | | | |
| Plasma | 3.1–12.4 ng/ml | 2.27 | 7.0–28.1 nmol/L |
| Red cell | 186–645 ng/ml | 2.27 | 422–1464 nmol/L |
| Glucose, fasting (plasma) | 65–109 mg/dl | 0.055 | 3.58–6.00 mmol/L |
| Haptoglobin | 30–220 mg/dl | 0.01 | 0.3–2.2 g/L |
| Hemoglobin A1c (estimated) | 4.0–6.0% | 0.01 | 0.04–0.06 |
| Iron (total) (age >13 yr) | | | |
| Male | 45–160 μg/dl | — | 8.1–31.3 μmol/L |
| Female | 30–160 μg/dl | 0.179 | 5.4–31.3 μmol/L |
| Iron-binding capacity | 220–420 μg/dl | 0.179 | 39.4–75.2 μmol/L |
| Transferrin saturation | 20–50% | 0.01 | 0.2–0.5 |
| Lactate (plasma) | 0.7–2.1 mmol/L | 1 | 0.7–2.1 mmol/L |
| Magnesium | 1.3–2.2 mEq/L | 0.5 | 0.65–1.10 mmol/L |
| Osmolality | 275–300 mOsm/kg | 1 | 275–300 mmol/kg |
| Phosphate | 2.5–4.5 mg/dl | 0.323 | 0.81–1.45 mmol/L |
| Potassium (plasma) | 3.3–4.9 mmol/L | 1 | 3.3–4.9 mmol/L |
| Protein, total (plasma) | 6.5–8.5 g/dl | 10 | 65–85 g/L |
| Sodium | 135–145 mmol/L | 1 | 135–145 mmol/L |
| Triglycerides, fasting[c] | <250 mg/dl | 0.0113 | <2.8 mmol/L |
| Troponin I | | | |
| Normal | ≤0.1 ng/ml | 100 | ≤60 ng/L |
| Indeterminant | 0.1–1.4 ng/ml | 100 | 70–140 ng/L |
| Abnormal | ≥1.5 ng/ml | 100 | ≥150 ng/L |
| Urea nitrogen | 8–25 mg/dl | 0.357 | 2.9–8.9 mmol/L |
| Uric acid[b] | 3–8 mg/dl | 59.5 | 179–476 μmol/L |
| Vitamin $B_{12}$ | 180–1000 pg/ml | 0.738 | 133–738 pmol/L |
| **Common serum enzymatic activities** | | | |
| Aminotransferases | | | |
| Alanine (ALT, SGPT) | 7–53 IU/L | 0.01667 | 0.12–0.88 μkat/L |
| Aspartate (AST, SGOT) | 11–47 IU/L | 0.01667 | 0.18–0.78 μkat/L |
| Amylase | 25–115 IU/L | 0.01667 | 0.42–1.92 μkat/L |
| Creatine kinase | | | |
| Male | 30–200 IU/L | 0.01667 | 0.50–3.33 μkat/L |
| Female | 20–170 IU/L | 0.01667 | 0.33–2.83 μkat/L |
| MB fraction | 0–7 IU/L | 0.01667 | 0–0.12 μkat/L |

| Test | Current units | Factor[a] | SI units |
|---|---|---|---|
| Gamma-glutamyl transpeptidase (GGT) | | | |
| Male | 11–50 IU/L | 0.01667 | 0.18–0.83 μkat/L |
| Female | 7–32 IU/L | 0.01667 | 0.12–0.53 μkat/L |
| Lactate dehydrogenase[b] | 100–250 IU/L | 0.01667 | 1.67–4.17 μkat/L |
| Lipase | <100 IU/L | 0.1667 | <1.67 μkat/L |
| 5'-Nucleotidase | 2–16 IU/L | 0.01667 | 0.03–0.27 μkat/L |
| Phosphatase, acid | 0–0.7 IU/L | 16.67 | 0–11.6 nkat/L |
| Phosphatase, alkaline[d] | | | |
| age 10–15 yr | 130–550 IU/L | | 2.17–9.17 μkat/L |
| age 16–20 yr | 70–260 IU/L | | 1.17–4.33 μkat/L |
| age >20 yr | 38–126 IU/L | | 0.13–2.10 μkat/L |
| **Common serum hormone values[e]** | | | |
| ACTH, fasting (8 AM, supine) | <60 pg/ml | 0.22 | <13.2 pmol/L |
| Aldosterone[f] | 10–160 ng/L | 2.77 | 28–443 mmol/L |
| Cortisol (plasma, morning) | 6–30 mg/dl | 0.027 | 0.16–0.81 μmol/L |
| FSH | | | |
| Male | 1–8 IU/L | 1 | 1–8 IU/L |
| Female | | | |
| Follicular | 4–13 IU/L | 1 | 4–13 IU/L |
| Luteal | 2–13 IU/L | 1 | 2–13 IU/L |
| Midcycle | 5–22 IU/L | 1 | 5–22 IU/L |
| Postmenopausal | 20–138 IU/L | 1 | 20–138 IU/L |
| Gastrin, fasting | 0–130 pg/ml | 1 | 0–130 ng/L |
| Growth hormone, fasting | | | |
| Male | <5 ng/ml | 1 | <5 μg/L |
| Female | <10 ng/ml | 1 | <10 μg/L |
| 17-Hydroxyprogesterone | | | |
| Male adult | <200 ng/dl | 0.03 | <6.6 nmol/L |
| Female | | | |
| Follicular | <80 ng/dl | 0.03 | <2.4 nmol/L |
| Luteal | <235 ng/dl | 0.03 | <8.6 nmol/L |
| Postmenopausal | <51 ng/dl | 0.03 | <1.5 nmol/L |
| Insulin, fasting | 3–15 mU/L | 7.18 | ≤144 pmol/L |
| LH | | | |
| Male | 2–12 IU/L | 1 | 2–12 IU/L |
| Female | | | |
| Follicular | 1–18 IU/L | 1 | 1–18 IU/L |
| Luteal | ≤20 IU/L | 1 | ≤20 IU/L |
| Midcycle | 24–105 IU/L | 1 | 24–105 IU/L |
| Postmenopausal | 15–62 IU/L | 1 | 15–62 IU/L |
| Parathyroid hormone | 12–72 pg/ml | — | — |

| Test | Current units | Factor[a] | SI units |
|---|---|---|---|
| Progesterone | | | |
| Male | <0.5 ng/ml | 3.18 | <1.6 nmol/L |
| Female | | | |
| Follicular | 0.1–1.5 ng/ml | 3.18 | 0.32–4.80 nmol/L |
| Luteal | 2.5–28.0 ng/ml | 3.18 | 8–89 nmol/L |
| First trimester | 9–47 ng/ml | 3.18 | 29–149 nmol/L |
| Third trimester | 55–255 ng/ml | 3.18 | 175–811 nmol/L |
| Postmenopausal | <0.5 ng/ml | 3.18 | <1.6 nmol/L |
| Prolactin | | | |
| Male | 1.6–18.8 ng/ml | 1 | 1.6–18.8 μg/L |
| Female | 1.4–24.2 ng/ml | 1 | 1.4–24.2 μg/L |
| Renin activity (plasma)[g] | 0.9–3.3 ng/ml/hr | 0.278 | 0.25–0.91 ng/(L × sec) |
| Testosterone, total | | | |
| Male | 270–1070 ng/dl | 0.0346 | 9.3–37.0 nmol/L |
| Female | 6–86 ng/dl | 0.0346 | 0.21–3.00 nmol/L |
| Testosterone, free | | | |
| Male | 9–30 ng/dl | 0.0346 | 0.31–1.00 pmol/L |
| Female | 0.3–1.9 ng/dl | 0.0346 | 0.0013–0.26 pmol/L |
| Thyroxine, total ($T_4$) | 4.5–12.0 μg/dl | 12.9 | 58–155 nmol/L |
| Thyroxine, free | 0.7–1.8 ng/dl | 12.9 | 10.3–34.8 pmol/L |
| T uptake[h] | 30–46% | 0.01 | 0.3–0.46 |
| Triiodothyronine ($T_3$) | 45–132 ng/dl | 0.0154 | 0.91–2.70 nmol/L |
| $T_4$ index[i] | 1.5–4.5 | 1 | 1.5–4.5 |
| TSH | 0.35–6.20 μU/ml | 1 | 0.35–6.20 mU/L |
| Vitamin D, 1,25-dihydroxy | 15–60 pg/ml | 2.4 | 36–144 pmol/L |
| Vitamin D, 25-hydroxy | 10–55 ng/ml | 2.49 | 25–137 nmol/L |
| **Common urinary chemistries** | | | |
| Delta-aminolevulinic acid | 1.5–7.5 mg/d | 7.6 | 11.4–53.2 μmol/d |
| Amylase | 0.04–0.30 IU/min | 16.67 | 0.67–5.00 nkat/min |
| | 60–450 U/24 hr | — | — |
| Calcium | 50–250 mg/d | 0.250 | 1.25–6.25 mmol/d |
| Catecholamines | <540 μg/d | — | — |
| Dopamine | 65–400 μg/d | — | — |
| Epinephrine | <20 μg/d | 5.5 | <110 nmol/d |
| Norepinephrine | 15–80 μg/d | 5.9 | 88.5–472.0 nmol/d |
| Copper | 15–60 μg/d | 0.0157 | 0.24–0.95 μmol/d |
| Cortisol, free | 9–53 μg/d | 2.76 | 25–146 nmol/d |
| Creatinine | | | |
| Male | 0.8–1.8 g/d | 8.84 | 7.1–15.9 mmol/d |
| Female | 0.6–1.5 g/d | 8.84 | 5.3–13.3 mmol/d |
| 5-Hydroxyindoleacetic acid | <6 mg/d | 5.23 | <47 μmol/d |
| Metanephrine | <1.3 mg/d | 5.46 | <7.1 μmol/d |

| Test | Current units | Factor[a] | SI units |
|---|---|---|---|
| Oxalate | | | |
| Male | 7–44 mg/d | 11.4 | 80–502 μmol/d |
| Female | 4–31 mg/d | 11.4 | 46–353 μmol/d |
| Porphyrins | | | |
| Coproporphyrin | | | |
| Male | ≤96 μg/d | 1.53 | 0–110 nmol/d |
| Female | ≤60 μg/d | 1.54 | 0–92 nmol/d |
| Uroporphyrin | | | |
| Male | ≤46 μg/d | 1.2 | 0–32 nmol/d |
| Female | ≤22 μg/d | 1.2 | 0–26 nmol/d |
| Protein | 0–150 mg/d | 0.001 | 0–0.150 g/d |
| Vanillylmandelic acid (VMA) | <8 mg/d | 5.05 | <40 μmol/d |
| **Common hematologic values** | | | |
| Coagulation | | | |
| Bleeding time[j] | 2.5–9.5 min | 60 | 150–570 sec |
| Fibrin degradation products | <8 μg/ml | — | — |
| Fibrinogen[k] | 150–400 mg/dl | 0.01 | 1.5–4.0 g/L |
| Partial thromboplastin time (activated) | 24–34 sec | 1 | 24–34 sec |
| Prothrombin time | 10.5–14.5[l] sec | 1 | 10.5–14.5 sec[l] |
| INR | 0.78–1.22 | — | — |
| Thrombin time | 11.3–18.5 sec | 1 | 11.3–18.5 sec |
| CBC | | | |
| Hematocrit | | | |
| Male | 40.7–50.3% | 0.01 | 0.407–0.503 |
| Female | 36.1–44.3% | 0.01 | 0.361–0.443 |
| Hemoglobin | | | |
| Male | 13.8–17.2 g/dl | 0.620[m] | 8.56–10.70 mmol/L |
| Female | 12.1–15.1 g/dl | 0.620 | 7.50–9.36 mmol/L |
| Erythrocyte count | | | |
| Male | 4.5–5.7 × $10^6$/μl | 1 | 4.5–5.7 × $10^{12}$/L |
| Female | 3.9–5.0 × $10^6$/μl | 1 | 3.9–5.0 × $10^{12}$/L |
| Mean corpuscular hemoglobin | 26.7–33.7 pg/cell | 0.062 | 1.66–2.09 fmol/cell |
| Mean corpuscular hemoglobin concentration | 32.7–35.5 g/dl | 0.620 | 20.3–22.0 mmol/L |
| Mean corpuscular volume | 80.0–97.6 $\mu m^3$ | 1 | 80.0–97.6 fl |
| Red cell distribution width | 11.8–14.6% | 0.01 | 0.118–0.146 |
| Leukocyte profile | | | |
| Total | 3.8–9.8 × $10^3$/μl | 1 | 3.8–9.8 × $10^9$/L |
| Lymphocytes | 1.2–3.3 × $10^3$/μl | 1 | 1.2–3.3 × $10^9$/L |
| Mononuclear cells | 0.2–0.7 × $10^3$/μl | 1 | 0.2–0.7 × $10^9$/L |
| Granulocytes | 1.8–6.6 × $10^3$/μl | 1 | 1.8–6.6 × $10^9$/L |

| Test | Current units | Factor[a] | SI units |
|---|---|---|---|
| Platelet count | 140–440 × $10^3$/µl | 1 | 140–440 × $10^9$/L |
| Erythrocyte sedimentation rate | | | |
| Male <50 yr | 0–15 sec | — | — |
| >50 yr | 0–20 sec | — | — |
| Female <50 yr | 0–20 sec | — | — |
| >50 yr | 0–30 sec | — | — |
| Reticulocyte count | | | |
| Adults | 0.5–1.5% | 0.01 | 0.005–0.015 |
| Children | 2.5–6.5% | — | — |
| **Immunology testing** | | | |
| Complement (total hemolytic)[n] | 118–226 U/ml | — | — |
| C3 | 75–165 mg/dl | 0.01 | 0.85–1.85 g/L |
| C4 | 12–42 mg/dl | 0.01 | 0.12–0.54 g/L |
| Immunoglobulin | | | |
| IgA | 70–370 mg/dl | 0.01 | 0.70–3.70 g/L |
| IgM | 30–210 mg/dl | 0.01 | 0.30–2.10 g/L |
| IgG | 700–1450 mg/dl | 0.01 | 7.00–14.50 g/L |
| **Therapeutic agents** | | | |
| Amitriptyline (+ nortriptyline) | 150–250 µg/L | — | — |
| Carbamazepine | 4–12 mg/L | 4.23 | 17–51 µmol/L |
| Clonazepam | 10–50 µg/ml | 3.17 | 32–159 nmol/L |
| Cyclosporine (whole blood) | 183–335 ng/ml | | Exact range depends on the type of transplant |
| Digoxin | 0.8–2.0 µg/L | 1.28 | 1.0–2.6 nmol/L |
| Disopyramide | 2–5 mg/L | 2.95 | 6–15 µmol/L |
| Ethosuximide | 40–75 mg/L | 7.08 | 283–531 µmol/L |
| Imipramine | | | |
| Imipramine | 150–300 µg/L | 3.57 | 536–1071 nmol/L |
| Desipramine | 100–300 µg/L | 3.75 | 375–1125 nmol/L |
| Lithium | 0.6–1.3 mmol/L | 1 | 0.6–1.3 mmol/L |
| Nortriptyline | 50–150 µg/L | 3.8 | 190–665 nmol/L |
| Phenobarbital | 10–40 mg/L | 4.3 | 43–172 µmol/L |
| Phenytoin (diphenylhydantoin) | 10–20 mg/L | 3.96 | 40–79 µmol/L |
| Primidone | | | |
| Primidone | 5–15 mg/L | 4.58 | 23–69 µmol/L |
| Phenobarbital | ≤15 µg/L | 4.3 | ≤69 µmol/L |
| Procainamide | | | |
| Procainamide | 4–10 mg/L | 4.23 | 17–42 µmol/L |
| Procainamide + *N*-acetylprocainamide | 6–20 mg/L | — | — |
| Quinidine | 2–5 mg/L | 3.08 | 6.2–15.4 µmol/L |
| Salicylate[o] | 20–290 mg/L | 0.0072 | 0.14–2.10 mmol/L |

| Test | Current units | Factor[a] | SI units |
|---|---|---|---|
| Theophylline | 10–20 mg/L | 5.5 | 55–110 µmol/L |
| Valproic acid | 50–100 mg/L | 6.93 | 346–693 µmol/L |
| **Antimicrobials** | | | |
| Amikacin | | | |
| Trough | 1–8 mg/L | 1.71 | 1.7–13.7 µmol/L |
| Peak | 20–30 mg/L | 1.71 | 34–51 µmol/L |
| 5-Fluorocytosine | | | |
| Trough | 20–60 mg/L | — | — |
| Peak | 50–100 mg/L | — | — |
| Gentamicin | | | |
| Trough | 0.5–2.0 mg/L | 2.09 | 1.0–4.2 µmol/L |
| Peak | 6–10 mg/L | 2.09 | 12.5–20.9 µmol/L |
| Ketoconazole | | | |
| Trough | ≤1 mg/L | — | — |
| Peak | 1–4 mg/L | — | — |
| Sulfamethoxazole | | | |
| Trough | 75–120 mg/L | — | — |
| Peak | 100–150 mg/L | — | — |
| Tobramycin | | | |
| Trough | 0.5–2.0 mg/L | 2.14 | 1.1–4.3 µmol/L |
| Peak | 6–10 mg/L | 2.14 | 12.8–21.4 µmol/L |
| Trimethoprim | | | |
| Trough | 2–8 mg/L | — | — |
| Peak | 5–15 mg/L | — | — |
| Vancomycin | | | |
| Trough | 5–15 mg/L | — | — |
| Peak | 20–40 mg/L | — | — |

ACTH, adrenocorticotropic hormone; fl, femtoliter; fmol, femtomole; FSH, follicle-stimulating hormone; HDL, high-density lipoprotein; INR, international normalized ratio; katal, mole/sec; kPa, kilopascal; LH, luteinizing hormone; µkat, microkatal; nkat, nanokatal; pmol, picomole; TSH, thyroid-stimulating hormone.

[a]A more complete list of multiplication factors for converting conventional units to SI units can be found in *Ann Intern Med* 106:114, 1967, and in *The SI for the Health Professions*. Geneva: World Health Organization, 1977.

[b]Variation occurs with age and gender. This range includes both genders and persons older than 5 yr.

[c]National Institutes of Health Congress Development Panel on Triglycerides, HDL, and Coronary Artery Diseases (*JAMA* 269:505, 1993).

[d]Higher values (up to 350 µU/ml) can be normal in persons younger than 20 yr.

[e]Because most hormones are measured by immunologic techniques and because hormones may vary in molecular weight (e.g., gastrin), most are expressed as mass/L. The reference ranges are method dependent.

[f]Supine, normal unit diet; in the upright position, the reference range is 40–310 ng/L.

[g]High-sodium diet, supplemented with sodium, 3 g/d.

[h]Replaces $T_3$ resin uptake.

[i]$T_4$ × (T uptake).

[j]Template modified after Ivy.

[k]Determined by the Clauss method.

[l]Normal ranges for prothrombin times vary according to the reagent used. Therefore, we report an INR with all prothrombin times ordered.

[m]This factor assumes a unit molecular weight of 16,000; assuming a unit molecular weight of 64,500, the multiplication factor is 0.156.

[n]$CH_{50}$ = reciprocal of dilution of sera required to lyse 50% of sheep erythrocytes.

[o]Therapeutic range for treatment of rheumatoid arthritis (see Chap. 23, Arthritis and Rheumatologic Diseases).

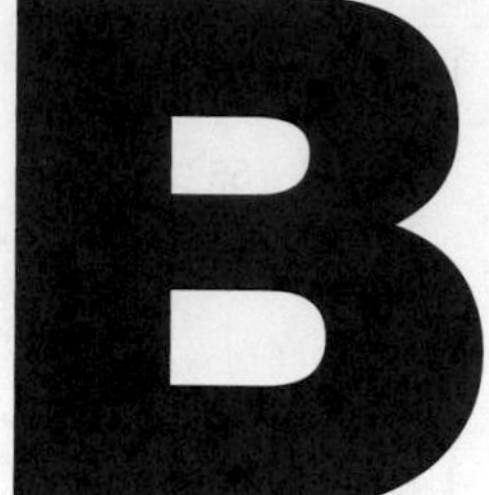

# Pregnancy and Medical Therapeutics

Dorothy (Sara) Hancock

| Class of medication | Relatively safe to use in pregnancy | Limited data or fetal risk appears minimal | Evidence of fetal risk[a] | Significant fetal risk; avoid in pregnancy |
|---|---|---|---|---|
| Analgesics | Acetaminophen | Celecoxib[b] | Aspirin[b] | |
| | | Diclofenac[b] | Codeine[c] | |
| | | Fentanyl[c] | Etodolac[b] | |
| | | Hydrocodone[c] | Indomethacin[b] | |
| | | Hydromorphone[c] | Ketorolac[b] | |
| | | Ibuprofen[b] | Meloxicam[b] | |
| | | Ketoprofen[b] | Nabumetone[b] | |
| | | Meperidine[c] | Oxaprozin[b] | |
| | | Morphine[c] | Propoxyphene[c] | |
| | | Naproxen[b] | Tramadol | |
| | | Oxycodone[c] | | |
| | | Piroxicam[b] | | |
| | | Rofecoxib[b] | | |
| | | Sulindac[b] | | |
| Anticonvulsants[d] | Magnesium sulfate[e] | | Clonazepam | Carbamazepine |
| | | | Ethosuximide | Fosphenytoin |
| | | | Gabapentin | Phenobarbital |
| | | | Lamotrigine | Phenytoin |
| | | | Tiagabine | Primidone |
| | | | Topiramate | Valproic acid |
| Antidepressants/ antipsychotics | | Bupropion | Amitriptyline | Lithium |
| | | Citalopram | Desipramine | Monoamine oxidase inhibitors |
| | | Fluoxetine | Doxepin | |

| Class of medication | Relatively safe to use in pregnancy | Limited data or fetal risk appears minimal | Evidence of fetal risk[a] | Significant fetal risk; avoid in pregnancy |
|---|---|---|---|---|
| | | Paroxetine | Haloperidol | |
| | | Sertraline | Imipramine | |
| | | | Mirtazapine | |
| | | | Nefazodone | |
| | | | Nortriptyline | |
| | | | Olanzapine | |
| | | | Quetiapine | |
| | | | Risperidone | |
| | | | Thioridazine | |
| | | | Trazodone | |
| | | | Venlafaxine | |
| Antidiabetic agents | Insulin | Acarbose | Glimepiride[f] | |
| | | Metformin | Glipizide[f] | |
| | | Miglitol | Glyburide[f] | |
| | | | Pioglitazone | |
| | | | Repaglinide[f] | |
| | | | Rosiglitazone | |
| | | | Troglitazone | |
| Antiemetics | Doxylamine[f] | Chlorpromazine[g] | | |
| | Meclizine[f] | Dimenhydrinate[f] | | |
| | Metoclopramide | Dolasetron | | |
| | Pyridoxine | Granisetron | | |
| | | Ondansetron | | |

| | | | | |
|---|---|---|---|---|
| | | Prochlorperazine[g] | | |
| | | Promethazine[g] | | |
| | | Scopolamine | | |
| | | Trimethobenzamide | | |
| Antihistamines[f] | Chlorpheniramine | Brompheniramine | | |
| | Triprolidine | Cetirizine | | |
| | | Clemastine | | |
| | | Diphenhydramine | | |
| | | Fexofenadine | | |
| | | Hydroxyzine | | |
| | | Loratadine | | |
| Anti-infectants | Amoxicillin | Acyclovir | Amikacin | Fluoroquinolones |
| | Amoxicillin/clavulanic acid | Azithromycin | Ethambutol[l] | Streptomycin[l] |
| | Amphotericin B | Aztreonam | Fluconazole | Tetracyclines |
| | Ampicillin | Chloramphenicol[f] | Gentamicin | |
| | Ampicillin/sulbactam | Clarithromycin | Isoniazid[l] | |
| | Cephalosporins | Clindamycin | Itraconazole | |
| | Clotrimazole (topical)[i] | Famciclovir | Ketoconazole | |
| | Erythromycin[j] | Imipenem/cilastatin | Linezolid | |
| | Miconazole (topical)[i] | Meropenem | Miconazole (systemic) | |
| | Nitrofurantoin | Metronidazole[k] | Pentamidine | |
| | Nystatin | Valacyclovir | Pyrazinamide[l] | |
| | Oxacillin | Valganciclovir | Rifampin[l] | |
| | Penicillin | Vancomycin | Tobramycin | |
| | Piperacillin/tazobactam | | Trimethoprim/sulfamethoxazole[f] | |
| | Ticarcillin/clavulanic acid | | | |

| Class of medication | Relatively safe to use in pregnancy | Limited data or fetal risk appears minimal | Evidence of fetal risk[a] | Significant fetal risk; avoid in pregnancy |
|---|---|---|---|---|
| Antilipemics | | Cholestyramine[h] | Fenofibrate | HMG-CoA reductase inhibitors |
| | | Colesevelam[h] | Gemfibrozil | |
| | | Colestipol[h] | | |
| Antithrombotics | | Clopidogrel | Aspirin[b] | Warfarin |
| | | Dalteparin[m] | | |
| | | Danaparoid[m] | | |
| | | Dipyridamole | | |
| | | Enoxaparin[m] | | |
| | | Heparin[m] | | |
| | | Lepirudin[m] | | |
| | | Ticlopidine | | |
| Cardiovascular drugs | | Atenolol[n] | Amlodipine | Angiotensin-converting enzyme inhibitors |
| | | Clonidine | Diltiazem | Angiotensin II–receptor antagonists |
| | | Digoxin | Felodipine | |
| | | Doxazosin | Nicardipine | |
| | | Hydralazine | Nifedipine | |
| | | Labetalol[n] | Nitrates | |
| | | Lidocaine | Verapamil | |
| | | Methyldopa | | |
| | | Metoprolol[n] | | |
| | | Prazosin | | |
| | | Procainamide | | |
| | | Propranolol[n] | | |

| | | | | |
|---|---|---|---|---|
| | | Quinidine | | |
| | | Terazosin | | |
| | | Timolol[n] | | |
| Cough and cold agents | | Dextromethorphan | Guaifenesin | |
| | | | Pseudoephedrine | |
| Diuretics[o] | | | Amiloride | |
| | | | Bumetanide | |
| | | | Chlorthalidone | |
| | | | Chlorthiazide | |
| | | | Ethacrynic acid | |
| | | | Furosemide | |
| | | | Hydrochlorothiazide | |
| | | | Indapamide | |
| | | | Metolazone | |
| | | | Spironolactone | |
| | | | Torsemide | |
| | | | Triamterene | |
| GI agents | Antacids[p] | Bismuth subsalicylate | | Misoprostol |
| | Attapulgite | Cisapride | | |
| | Kaolin-pectin | Dicyclomine | | |
| | Loperamide | Docusate | | |
| | Metoclopramide | $H_2$-receptor antagonists | | |
| | Psyllium | Lansoprazole | | |
| | | Omeprazole | | |
| | | Pantoprazole | | |
| | | Phenolphthalein | | |

| Class of medication | Relatively safe to use in pregnancy | Limited data or fetal risk appears minimal | Evidence of fetal risk[a] | Significant fetal risk; avoid in pregnancy |
|---|---|---|---|---|
| | | Rabeprazole | | |
| | | Senna | | |
| | | Simethicone | | |
| | | Sucralfate | | |
| Hormonal agents | | | Glucocorticoids[q] (systemic) | Estrogens |
| | | | Progestins[r] | Oral contraceptives |
| Respiratory agents | | Albuterol[s] | Zileuton | |
| | | Beclomethasone (inhalation) | | |
| | | Cromolyn | | |
| | | Flunisolide (inhalation) | | |
| | | Ipratropium | | |
| | | Metaproterenol[s] | | |
| | | Montelukast | | |
| | | Nedocromil | | |
| | | Pirbuterol[s] | | |
| | | Salmeterol[s] | | |
| | | Theophylline | | |
| | | Triamcinolone (inhalation) | | |
| | | Zafirlukast | | |
| Sedatives | | Buspirone | Benzodiazepines[c] | Pentobarbital |
| | | Propofol | | Phenobarbital |
| | | Zolpidem | | |

| | | | | |
|---|---|---|---|---|
| Thyroid agents | Levothyroxine | | | |
| | Thyroid | | | |
| Miscellaneous | Ferrous sulfate | Allopurinol | Azathioprine | Isotretinoin |
| | Potassium chloride | Carisoprodol | Cilostazol | Leflunomide |
| | | Chlorzoxazone | Cyclosporine | Quinine |
| | | Cyclobenzaprine | Modafinil | Tamoxifen |
| | | Etanercept | Naratriptan | Thalidomide |
| | | Flavoxate | Pentoxifylline | |
| | | Oxybutynin | Sumatriptan | |
| | | | Rizatriptan | |
| | | | Zolmitriptan | |

HMG-CoA, 3-hydroxy-3-methylglutaryl coenzyme A.
[a]These medications have some associated risk when used during pregnancy. The potential benefit should be carefully weighed against possible adverse effects.
[b]Use during the third trimester may cause constriction of the ductus arteriosus, which may result in persistent pulmonary hypertension in the newborn. These agents may also inhibit labor and prolong the length of pregnancy.
[c]Regular use during pregnancy may cause physical dependence in the neonate. Avoid use for prolonged periods or in high doses at term.
[d]The risk to the mother may be greater if anticonvulsant therapy is withheld and seizure control is lost. Epilepsy should be treated with the fewest drugs in the lowest doses that are sufficient to prevent convulsions, and pregnant women should be counseled regarding increased risk of malformations.
[e]Drug of choice for convulsions associated with toxemia of pregnancy.
[f]Avoid during the last few weeks of pregnancy.
[g]Generally recognized as safe for mother and fetus if used occasionally in low doses.
[h]These agents are almost totally unabsorbed, but potential adverse effects on the fetus may occur because of impaired maternal absorption of fat-soluble vitamins.
[i]For self-medication, these drugs should not be used in pregnant women unless otherwise instructed by a physician.
[j]Erythromycin estolate has been associated with an increased risk of reversible subclinical hepatotoxicity in approximately 10% of pregnant women; problems with other erythromycins have not been documented.

[k]Avoid use during the first trimester.

[l]Pregnant women with tuberculosis should be managed in concert with an expert in the management of tuberculosis. Untreated tuberculosis represents a far greater hazard to a pregnant woman and her fetus than does treatment of the disease.

[m]Use in the last trimester may increase the risk of maternal bleeding. Maternal osteopenia may be a complication of long-term therapy.

[n]Fetal and neonatal bradycardia, hypotension, hypoglycemia, and respiratory depression have been reported. Whenever possible, avoid therapy during the first trimester and discontinue therapy 2–3 days before delivery.

[o]Routine use of diuretics in pregnancy is not recommended, except for patients with cardiovascular disorders, as these agents do not prevent or alter the course of toxemia and may decrease placental perfusion.

[p]Antacids are generally considered safe as long as chronic high doses are avoided.

[q]Physiologic replacement doses of glucocorticoids administered for treatment of maternal adrenal insufficiency are unlikely to affect the fetus or neonate adversely. Infants born to mothers who received substantial doses of glucocorticoids during pregnancy should be observed carefully for signs of hypoadrenalism.

[r]Progestational agents have been used to prevent habitual or threatened abortion within the first few months of pregnancy and to treat corpus luteum deficiency in early pregnancy.

[s]β-Adrenergic agonists may cause maternal and, to a lesser extent, fetal tachycardia. Maternal hypotension, hyperglycemia, and neonatal hypoglycemia should be expected.

*Source: Drugs in Pregnancy* (2nd ed). New York: Chapman & Hall, 1997; *Drugs in Pregnancy and Lactation* (6th ed). Baltimore: Williams & Wilkins, 2001; *Drug Therapy in Obstetrics and Gynecology* (3rd ed). St. Louis: Mosby–Year Book, 1992; *Drug Information for the Health Care Professional* (USP DI, vol I). Greenwood Village, CO: Micromedex Thomson Healthcare, 2002.

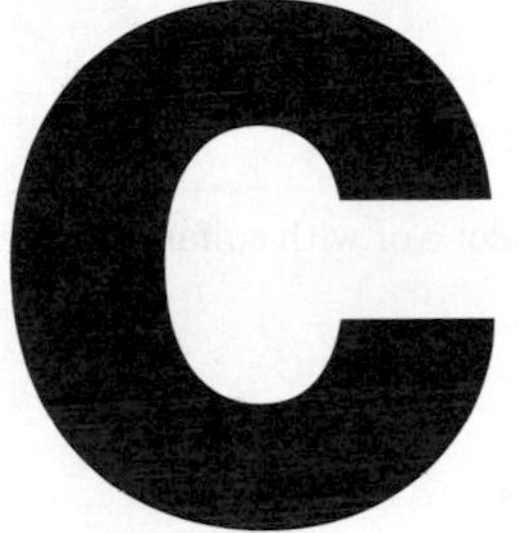

# Drug Interactions

Scott Micek and
Erin Christensen Rachmiel

**Contraindicated drug combinations** are summarized in Table C-1. **Common drug interactions** are summarized in Table C-2. Because new information on drug interactions is continually emerging, it is impossible to include all current drug interactions in a reference text. Information regarding the metabolic pathway of selected medications is included to assist in the prediction of likely drug interactions with new medications. In addition, a list of common substrates, inducers, and inhibitors of the various **cytochrome P-450 isoenzymes** is provided in Table C-3 to allow prediction of likely drug interactions with new medications. For example, if a newly marketed medication is a substrate for CYP2C19, it would be anticipated that coadministration with either omeprazole or fluvoxamine could increase the level and effects of the new medication. A list of drugs associated with **QTc prolongation** is given in Table C-4. The combination of these agents may increase the risk for adverse arrhythmic events.

**Table C-1.** Contraindicated drug combinations

| Medication | Contraindicated drug |
|---|---|
| Alprazolam | Itraconazole |
| | Ketoconazole |
| Bosentan | Cyclosporine |
| | Glyburide |
| Carbamazepine | MAOI |
| Cisapride | See Table C-4 |
| Citalopram | MAOI |
| Clarithromycin | Cisapride |
| | Pimozide |
| | Terfenadine |
| Delavirdine | CYP3A4 substrates (see Table C-3) |
| Dexmethylphenidate | MAOI |
| Dextromethorphan | MAOI |
| Dofetilide | Cimetidine |
| | Hydrochlorothiazide |
| | Ketoconazole |
| | Megestrol |
| | Prochlorperazine |

*(continued)*

**Table C-1.** Continued

| Medication | Contraindicated drug |
| --- | --- |
| | Trimethoprim (alone or with sulfamethoxazole) |
| | Verapamil |
| Efavirenz | Astemizole |
| | Cisapride |
| | Ergot derivatives |
| | Midazolam |
| | Triazolam |
| Eplerenone | CYP3A4 inhibitors (see Table C-3) |
| | Potassium-sparing diuretics |
| | Potassium supplements |
| Erythromycin | Astemizole |
| | Cisapride |
| | Pimozide |
| | Terfenadine |
| Fluconazole | Terfenadine |
| Fluoxetine | MAOI |
| | Thioridazine |
| Fluvoxamine | Astemizole |
| | Cisapride |
| | Pimozide |
| | Terfenadine |
| | Thioridazine |
| Itraconazole | Alprazolam |
| | Astemizole |
| | Cisapride |
| | Dofetilide |
| | Lovastatin |
| | Midazolam |
| | Pimozide |
| | Quinidine |
| | Simvastatin |
| | Triazolam |
| Ketoconazole | Alprazolam |
| | Astemizole |
| | Cisapride |
| | Dofetilide |
| | Terfenadine |
| | Triazolam |
| Methylphenidate | MAOI |
| Nefazodone | Astemizole |
| | Carbamazepine |

(*continued*)

**Table C-1.** Continued

| Medication | Contraindicated drug |
|---|---|
| | Cisapride |
| | Pimozide |
| | Terfenadine |
| | Triazolam |
| Paroxetine | MAOI |
| | Thioridazine |
| Phenelzine (MAOI) | Atomoxetine |
| | Meperidine |
| | Buspirone |
| | Fluoxetine |
| | Guanethidine |
| Proguanil | Aurothioglucose |
| Protease inhibitors | CYP3A4 substrates (see Table C-3) |
| Sertraline | MAOI |
| | Pimozide |
| Sildenafil | Nitrates |
| Tranylcypromine (MAOI) | Atomoxetine |
| | Dibenzazepine derivatives (tricyclic antidepressants) |
| | SSRI |
| | Meperidine |
| | Dextromethorphan |
| | Buspirone |
| | Antihypertensives |
| | Diuretics |
| | Antihistamines |
| | Bupropion |
| | Antiparkinsonism drugs |
| Voriconazole | Astemizole |
| | Barbiturates |
| | Carbamazepine |
| | Cisapride |
| | Ergot alkaloids |
| | Pimozide |
| | Quinidine |
| | Rifabutin |
| | Rifampin |
| | Sirolimus |
| | Terfenadine |

MAOI, monoamine oxidase inhibitor; SSRI, selective serotonin reuptake inhibitor.

**Table C-2.** Common drug interactions

| Medication | Interacting drug | Increases level or effect of: | Decreases level or effect of: |
|---|---|---|---|
| Adenosine | Carbamazepine | Adenosine | |
| | Dipyridamole | Adenosine | |
| | Theophylline | | Adenosine |
| Alendronate | All oral medications | | Alendronate |
| Allopurinol | 6-Mercaptopurine | 6-Mercaptopurine | |
| | Azathioprine | Azathioprine | |
| | Cyclophosphamide | Cyclophosphamide | |
| Almotriptan (3A4, 2D6 substrate) | See Rizatriptan | | |
| Alprazolam (3A4 substrate) | Clarithromycin | Alprazolam | |
| | Diltiazem | Alprazolam | |
| | Erythromycin | Alprazolam | |
| | Fluconazole | Alprazolam | |
| | Fluoxetine | Alprazolam | |
| | Fluvoxamine | Alprazolam | |
| | Grapefruit juice | Alprazolam | |
| | Itraconazole | Alprazolam | |
| | Ketoconazole | Alprazolam | |
| | Nefazodone | Alprazolam | |
| | Quinupristin/dalfopristin | Alprazolam | |
| | Verapamil | Alprazolam | |
| Amiodarone (2C9 inhibitor) | Barbiturates | | Amiodarone |
| | Carbamazepine | | Amiodarone |
| | Cyclosporine | Cyclosporine | |

| | | | |
|---|---|---|---|
| | Digoxin | Digoxin | |
| | Lidocaine | Lidocaine | |
| | Phenytoin | Phenytoin | Amiodarone |
| | Rifampin | | Amiodarone |
| | Warfarin | Warfarin | |
| Amprenavir (3A4 inhibitor) | See Ritonavir | | |
| Antacids | Alendronate | | Alendronate |
| | Isoniazid | | Isoniazid |
| | Itraconazole | | Itraconazole |
| | Ketoconazole | | Ketoconazole |
| | Quinolone antibiotics | | Quinolone antibiotics |
| | Tetracyclines | | Tetracyclines |
| Aripiprazole (2D6 and 3A4 substrate) | Carbamazepine | | Aripiprazole |
| | Ketoconazole | Aripiprazole | |
| | Quinidine | Aripiprazole | |
| Atorvastatin (3A4 substrate) | Bosentan | | Atorvastatin/C/L/S |
| | Clarithromycin | Atorvastatin/C/L/S | |
| | Cyclosporine | Atorvastatin/C/L/S | |
| | Diltiazem | Atorvastatin/C/L/S | |
| | Erythromycin | Atorvastatin/C/L/S | |
| | Fenofibrate | Myopathy or rhabdomyolysis | |
| | Fluconazole | Atorvastatin/C/L/S | |
| | Fluvoxamine | Atorvastatin/C/L/S | |
| | Gemfibrozil | Atorvastatin/C/L/S | |
| | Grapefruit juice | Atorvastatin/C/L/S | |
| | Itraconazole | Atorvastatin/C/L/S | |

(*continued*)

**Table C-2.** Continued

| Medication | Interacting drug | Increases level or effect of: | Decreases level or effect of: |
|---|---|---|---|
| | Ketoconazole | Atorvastatin/C/L/S | |
| | Nefazodone | Atorvastatin/C/L/S | |
| | Niacin | Atorvastatin/C/L/S | |
| | Protease inhibitors | Atorvastatin/C/L/S | |
| | Quinupristin/dalfopristin | Atorvastatin/C/L/S | |
| | Repaglinide | Repaglinide | |
| | Verapamil | Atorvastatin/C/L/S | |
| Atovaquone | Metoclopramide | | Atovaquone |
| | Rifabutin | | Atovaquone |
| | Rifampin | | Atovaquone |
| | Warfarin | Warfarin | |
| Barbiturates (enzyme inducer) | Antiarrhythmics | | Antiarrhythmics |
| | Azole antifungals | | Azole antifungals |
| | Beta-blockers | | Beta-blockers |
| | Chloramphenicol | | Chloramphenicol |
| | Corticosteroids | | Corticosteroids |
| | Cyclosporine | | Cyclosporine |
| | Oral contraceptives | | Oral contraceptives |
| | Protease inhibitors | | Protease inhibitors |
| | Theophylline | | Theophylline |
| | Warfarin | | Warfarin |
| Bosentan (2C9, 3A4, 2C19 inducer) | Atorvastatin | | Atorvastatin |
| | Cyclosporine | | Cyclosporine |

| | | | |
|---|---|---|---|
| | Oral contraceptives | | Oral contraceptives |
| | Glyburide | | Glyburide |
| | Ketoconazole | Bosentan | |
| | Lovastatin | | Lovastatin |
| | Simvastatin | | Simvastatin |
| | Warfarin | | Warfarin |
| Buprenorphine (3A4 substrate) | Erythromycin | Buprenorphine | |
| | Ketoconazole | Buprenorphine | |
| | Protease inhibitors | Buprenorphine | |
| Calcium salts | Alendronate | | Alendronate |
| | Quinolone antibiotics | | Quinolone antibiotics |
| | Tetracyclines | | Tetracyclines |
| Capecitabine | Phenytoin | | Phenytoin |
| | Warfarin | | Warfarin |
| Carbamazepine (enzyme inducer, 3A4 substrate) | Adenosine | Adenosine | |
| | Antiarrhythmics | | Antiarrhythmics |
| | Azole antifungals | | Azole antifungals |
| | Beta-blockers | | Beta-blockers |
| | Chloramphenicol | | Chloramphenicol |
| | Clarithromycin | Carbamazepine | |
| | Corticosteroids | | Corticosteroids |
| | Cyclosporine | | Cyclosporine |
| | Diltiazem | Carbamazepine | |
| | Erythromycin | Carbamazepine | |
| | Fluconazole | Carbamazepine | Fluconazole |
| | Fluvoxamine | Carbamazepine | |

*(continued)*

**Table C-2.** Continued

| Medication | Interacting drug | Increases level or effect of: | Decreases level or effect of: |
|---|---|---|---|
| | Grapefruit juice | Carbamazepine | |
| | Isoniazid | Carbamazepine | |
| | Itraconazole | Carbamazepine | Itraconazole |
| | Ketoconazole | Carbamazepine | Ketoconazole |
| | Nefazodone | Carbamazepine | |
| | Oral contraceptives | | Oral contraceptives |
| | Protease inhibitors | | Protease inhibitors |
| | Quinidine | | Quinidine |
| | Quinupristin/dalfopristin | Carbamazepine | |
| | Theophylline | | Theophylline |
| | Verapamil | Carbamazepine | |
| | Warfarin | | Warfarin |
| | Zonisamide | | Zonisamide |
| Carvedilol (2D6 substrate) | β Agonists | | Carvedilol/L/M/P |
| | Barbiturates | | Carvedilol/L/M/P |
| | Carbamazepine | | Carvedilol/L/M/P |
| | Cimetidine | Carvedilol/L/M/P | |
| | Fluoxetine | Carvedilol/L/M/P | |
| | Paroxetine | Carvedilol/L/M/P | |
| | Phenytoin | | Carvedilol/L/M/P |
| | Quinidine | Carvedilol/L/M/P | |
| | Rifampin | | Carvedilol/L/M/P |
| | Ritonavir | Carvedilol/L/M/P | |

| | | | |
|---|---|---|---|
| Caspofungin | Cyclosporine | Caspofungin | |
| Cefditoren | Antacids | | Cefditoren |
| | $H_2$ antagonists | | Cefditoren |
| Cerivastatin (3A4 substrate) | See Atorvastatin | | |
| Chloramphenicol (2C9 inhibitor) | Barbiturates | | Chloramphenicol |
| | Carbamazepine | | Chloramphenicol |
| | Phenytoin | | Chloramphenicol |
| | Rifampin | | Chloramphenicol |
| | Warfarin | Warfarin | |
| Cilostazol (3A4 substrate) | Clarithromycin | Cilostazol | |
| | Diltiazem | Cilostazol | |
| | Erythromycin | Cilostazol | |
| | Fluconazole | Cilostazol | |
| | Fluvoxamine | Cilostazol | |
| | Grapefruit juice | Cilostazol | |
| | Itraconazole | Cilostazol | |
| | Ketoconazole | Cilostazol | |
| | Nefazodone | Cilostazol | |
| | Omeprazole | Cilostazol | |
| | Protease inhibitors | Cilostazol | |
| | Quinupristin/dalfopristin | Cilostazol | |
| | Verapamil | Cilostazol | |
| Cimetidine (1A2, 2C9, 2D6 inhibitor) | Beta-blockers | Beta-blockers | |
| | Metformin | Metformin | |
| | Phenytoin | Phenytoin | |
| | Procainamide | Procainamide | |

(*continued*)

**Table C-2.** Continued

| Medication | Interacting drug | Increases level or effect of: | Decreases level or effect of: |
|---|---|---|---|
| | Tacrine | Tacrine | |
| | Theophylline | Theophylline | |
| | Tricyclic antidepressants | Tricyclic antidepressants | |
| | Warfarin | Warfarin | |
| Ciprofloxacin (1A2 inhibitor) | Antacids | | Ciprofloxacin |
| | Calcium salts | | Ciprofloxacin |
| | Cyclosporine | Elevated serum creatinine | |
| | Didanosine | | Ciprofloxacin |
| | Glyburide | | Ciprofloxacin |
| | Iron salts | Hypoglycemia | |
| | Probenecid | Ciprofloxacin | |
| | Sucralfate | | Ciprofloxacin |
| | Theophylline | Theophylline | |
| | Warfarin | Warfarin | |
| Cisapride (3A4 substrate) | Clarithromycin | Cisapride | |
| | Erythromycin | Cisapride | |
| | Fluconazole | Cisapride | |
| | Fluvoxamine | Cisapride | |
| | Grapefruit juice | Cisapride | |
| | Itraconazole | Cisapride | |
| | Ketoconazole | Cisapride | |
| | Nefazodone | Cisapride | |
| | Protease inhibitors | Cisapride | |

| | | | |
|---|---|---|---|
| | Quinupristin/dalfopristin | Cisapride | |
| | Zileuton | Cisapride | |
| Citalopram | MAOIs | Serotonin syndrome | |
| | Rizatriptan | Serotonin syndrome | |
| | Sumatriptan | Serotonin syndrome | |
| Clarithromycin (3A4 inhibitor) | Alprazolam | Alprazolam | |
| | Atorvastatin | Atorvastatin | |
| | Carbamazepine | Carbamazepine | |
| | Cerivastatin | Cerivastatin | |
| | Cilostazol | Cilostazol | |
| | Cisapride | Cisapride | |
| | Cyclosporine | Cyclosporine | |
| | Digoxin | Digoxin | |
| | Disopyramide | Disopyramide | |
| | Lovastatin | Lovastatin | |
| | Pimozide | Pimozide | |
| | Simvastatin | Simvastatin | |
| | Theophylline | Theophylline | |
| | Triazolam | Triazolam | |
| Codeine (2D6 substrate) | Fluoxetine | | Codeine |
| | Paroxetine | | Codeine |
| | Quinidine | | Codeine |
| | Ritonavir | | Codeine |
| Corticosteroids | Barbiturates | | Corticosteroids |
| | Carbamazepine | | Corticosteroids |

(continued)

**Table C-2.** Continued

| Medication | Interacting drug | Increases level or effect of: | Decreases level or effect of: |
|---|---|---|---|
| | Phenytoin | | Corticosteroids |
| | Rifampin | | Corticosteroids |
| COX-2 inhibitors (selective) | See NSAIDs | | |
| Cyclosporine (3A4 substrate) | Amiodarone | Cyclosporine | |
| | Barbiturates | | Cyclosporine |
| | Bosentan | | Cyclosporine |
| | Carbamazepine | | Cyclosporine |
| | Caspofungin | Caspofungin | |
| | Clarithromycin | Cyclosporine | |
| | Colchicine | Cyclosporine | |
| | Diltiazem | Cyclosporine | |
| | Erythromycin | Cyclosporine | |
| | Fluconazole | Cyclosporine | |
| | Fluoxetine | Cyclosporine | |
| | Fluvoxamine | Cyclosporine | |
| | Grapefruit juice | Cyclosporine | |
| | Itraconazole | Cyclosporine | |
| | Ketoconazole | Cyclosporine | |
| | Nefazodone | Cyclosporine | |
| | Orlistat | | Cyclosporine |
| | Phenytoin | | Cyclosporine |
| | Protease inhibitors | Cyclosporine | |
| | Quinupristin/dalfopristin | Cyclosporine | |

| | | | |
|---|---|---|---|
| | Rifampin | | Cyclosporine |
| | Simvastatin | Simvastatin | |
| | Sirolimus | Sirolimus | |
| | St. John's wort | | Cyclosporine |
| Dapsone | Didanosine | | Dapsone |
| | $H_2$ antagonists | | Dapsone |
| | Lansoprazole | | Dapsone |
| | Omeprazole | | Dapsone |
| Delavirdine | Alprazolam | Alprazolam | |
| | Cisapride | Cisapride | |
| | Ergot derivatives | Ergot derivatives | |
| | Rifampin | | Delavirdine/efavirenz/nevirapine |
| | Triazolam | Triazolam | |
| Dexmethylphenidate | MAOIs | Hypertensive crisis | |
| | Fosphenytoin | Fosphenytoin | |
| | Phenobarbital | Phenobarbital | |
| | Phenytoin | Phenytoin | |
| | Primidone | Primidone | |
| | Warfarin | Warfarin | |
| Dextromethorphan (2D6 substrate) | Fluoxetine | Serotonin syndrome | |
| | Paroxetine | Serotonin syndrome | |
| Didanosine | Dapsone | | Dapsone |
| | Indinavir | | Indinavir |
| | Itraconazole | | Itraconazole |
| | Ketoconazole | | Ketoconazole |

(continued)

**Table C-2.** Continued

| Medication | Interacting drug | Increases level or effect of: | Decreases level or effect of: |
|---|---|---|---|
| | Quinolone antibiotics | | Quinolone antibiotics |
| | Ribavirin | Didanosine | |
| | Tenofovir | Didanosine | |
| Digoxin | Amiodarone | Digoxin | |
| | Clarithromycin | Digoxin | |
| | Esomeprazole | | Digoxin |
| | Erythromycin | Digoxin | |
| | Quinidine | Digoxin | |
| | Verapamil | Digoxin | |
| Diltiazem (3A4 inhibitor) | Alprazolam | Alprazolam | |
| | Atorvastatin | Atorvastatin | |
| | Carbamazepine | Carbamazepine | |
| | Cerivastatin | Cerivastatin | |
| | Cilostazol | Cilostazol | |
| | Cyclosporine | Cyclosporine | |
| | Lovastatin | Lovastatin | |
| | Simvastatin | Simvastatin | |
| | Sirolimus | Sirolimus | |
| | Triazolam | Triazolam | |
| Disopyramide (3A4 substrate) | Barbiturates | | Disopyramide |
| | Carbamazepine | | Disopyramide |
| | Clarithromycin | Disopyramide | |
| | Erythromycin | Disopyramide | |
| | Fluconazole | Disopyramide | |

| | | | |
|---|---|---|---|
| | Fluvoxamine | Disopyramide | |
| | Grapefruit juice | Disopyramide | |
| | Itraconazole | Disopyramide | |
| | Ketoconazole | Disopyramide | |
| | Phenytoin | | Disopyramide |
| | Quinupristin/dalfopristin | Disopyramide | |
| | Rifampin | | Disopyramide |
| Donepezil | Anticholinergic agents | | Donepezil |
| | Cholinergic agents | Cholinergic effects | |
| Doxercalciferol | Cholestyramine | | Doxercalciferol |
| Efavirenz | See Delavirdine | | |
| Eplerenone (3A4 substrate) | 3A4 inhibitors (Table C-3) | Eplerenone | |
| | Lithium | Lithium | |
| | St. John's wort | | Eplerenone |
| Ertapenem | Probenecid | Ertapenem | |
| Erythromycin (3A4 inhibitor) | Alprazolam | Alprazolam | |
| | Atorvastatin | Atorvastatin | |
| | Carbamazepine | Carbamazepine | |
| | Cerivastatin | Cerivastatin | |
| | Cilostazol | Cilostazol | |
| | Cisapride | Cisapride | |
| | Cyclosporine | Cyclosporine | |
| | Digoxin | Digoxin | |
| | Disopyramide | Disopyramide | |
| | Lovastatin | Lovastatin | |
| | Pimozide | Pimozide | |
| | Simvastatin | Simvastatin | |

(*continued*)

**Table C-2.** Continued

| Medication | Interacting drug | Increases level or effect of: | Decreases level or effect of: |
|---|---|---|---|
| | Theophylline | Theophylline | |
| | Triazolam | Triazolam | |
| Escitalopram | See Citalopram | | |
| Esomeprazole | Digoxin | | Digoxin |
| | Iron salts | | Iron salts |
| | Ketoconazole | | Ketoconazole |
| Fenofibrate | Cyclosporine | Nephrotoxicity | |
| | HMG-CoA reductase inhibitors | Myopathy or rhabdomyolysis | |
| | Warfarin | Bleeding risk | |
| Ferrous sulfate | Alendronate | | Alendronate |
| | Quinolone antibiotics | | Quinolone antibiotics |
| | Tetracyclines | | Tetracyclines |
| Flecainide (2D6 substrate) | Fluoxetine | Flecainide | |
| | Paroxetine | Flecainide | |
| | Protease inhibitors | Flecainide | |
| Fluconazole (2C9, 3A4 inhibitor) | Alprazolam | Alprazolam | |
| | Atorvastatin | Atorvastatin | |
| | Carbamazepine | Carbamazepine | Fluconazole |
| | Cerivastatin | Cerivastatin | |
| | Cilostazol | Cilostazol | |
| | Cisapride | Cisapride | |
| | Cyclosporine | Cyclosporine | |
| | Disopyramide | Disopyramide | |
| | Lovastatin | Lovastatin | |

| | | | |
|---|---|---|---|
| | Phenytoin | Phenytoin | Fluconazole |
| | Simvastatin | Simvastatin | |
| | Triazolam | Triazolam | |
| | Warfarin | Warfarin | |
| Fluoxetine (2D6, 3A4 inhibitor) | Alprazolam | Alprazolam | |
| | Amitriptyline | Amitriptyline | |
| | Benztropine | Benztropine | |
| | Carvedilol | Carvedilol | |
| | Clomipramine | Clomipramine | |
| | Codeine | | Codeine |
| | Cyclosporine | Cyclosporine | |
| | Desipramine | Desipramine | |
| | Dextromethorphan | Serotonin syndrome | |
| | Diazepam | Diazepam | |
| | Flecainide | Flecainide | |
| | Imipramine | Imipramine | |
| | Labetalol | Labetalol | |
| | MAOIs | Serotonin syndrome | |
| | Metoprolol | Metoprolol | |
| | Nortriptyline | Nortriptyline | |
| | Phenytoin | Phenytoin | |
| | Propafenone | Propafenone | |
| | Propranolol | Propranolol | |
| | Rizatriptan | Serotonin syndrome | |
| | Sumatriptan | Serotonin syndrome | |
| | Tramadol | | Tramadol |

(*continued*)

**Table C-2.** Continued

| Medication | Interacting drug | Increases level or effect of: | Decreases level or effect of: |
|---|---|---|---|
| | Triazolam | Triazolam | |
| Fluvastatin | Fenofibrate | Myopathy or rhabdomyolysis | |
| | Gemfibrozil | Myopathy or rhabdomyolysis | |
| | Niacin | Myopathy or rhabdomyolysis | |
| Fluvoxamine (1A2, 2C9, 3A4 inhibitor) | Alprazolam | Alprazolam | |
| | Amitriptyline | Amitriptyline | |
| | Atorvastatin | Atorvastatin | |
| | Carbamazepine | Carbamazepine | |
| | Cerivastatin | Cerivastatin | |
| | Cilostazol | Cilostazol | |
| | Cisapride | Cisapride | |
| | Clomipramine | Clomipramine | |
| | Clozapine | Clozapine | |
| | Cyclosporine | Cyclosporine | |
| | Diazepam | Diazepam | |
| | Disopyramide | Disopyramide | |
| | Imipramine | Imipramine | |
| | Lovastatin | Lovastatin | |
| | MAOIs | Serotonin syndrome | |
| | Phenytoin | Phenytoin | |
| | Pimozide | Pimozide | |
| | Simvastatin | Simvastatin | |
| | Theophylline | Theophylline | |

| | | | |
|---|---|---|---|
| | Triazolam | Triazolam | |
| | Warfarin | Warfarin | |
| Fosphenytoin | See Phenytoin | | |
| Frovatriptan (1A2 substrate) | Ergotamine | | Frovatriptan |
| | Oral contraceptives | Frovatriptan | |
| | Propranolol | Frovatriptan | |
| | Anticholinergic agents | Galantamine | |
| | Cholinergic agents | Cholinergic effects | |
| Galantamine | Cimetidine | Galantamine | |
| | Erythromycin | Galantamine | |
| | Ketoconazole | Galantamine | |
| | Paroxetine | Galantamine | |
| Gemfibrozil | HMG-CoA reductase inhibitors | Myopathy or rhabdomyolysis | |
| Grapefruit juice (3A4 inhibitor) | Alprazolam | Alprazolam | |
| | Atorvastatin | Atorvastatin | |
| | Carbamazepine | Carbamazepine | |
| | Cerivastatin | Cerivastatin | |
| | Cilostazol | Cilostazol | |
| | Cisapride | Cisapride | |
| | Cyclosporine | Cyclosporine | |
| | Disopyramide | Disopyramide | |
| | Lovastatin | Lovastatin | |
| | Pimozide | Pimozide | |
| | Simvastatin | Simvastatin | |
| | Theophylline | Theophylline | |
| | Triazolam | Triazolam | |

(*continued*)

**Table C-2.** Continued

| Medication | Interacting drug | Increases level or effect of: | Decreases level or effect of: |
|---|---|---|---|
| Imatinib (2D6, 3A4 inhibitor and substrate) | Amlodipine | Amlodipine | |
| | Barbiturates | | Imatinib |
| | Carbamazepine | | Imatinib |
| | Clarithromycin | Imatinib | |
| | Dexamethasone | | Imatinib |
| | Erythromycin | Imatinib | |
| | Itraconazole | Imatinib | |
| | Ketoconazole | Imatinib | |
| | Lovastatin | Lovastatin | |
| | Midazolam | Midazolam | |
| | Protease inhibitors | Imatinib | Imatinib |
| | Phenytoin | | Imatinib |
| | Rifampin | | Imatinib |
| | Simvastatin | Simvastatin | |
| | St. John's wort | | Imatinib |
| | Triazolam | Triazolam | |
| | Warfarin | Warfarin | |
| Indinavir | See Ritonavir | | |
| Isoniazid | Carbamazepine | Carbamazepine | |
| | Diazepam | Diazepam | |
| | Phenytoin | Phenytoin | |
| Itraconazole (3A4 inhibitor) | Alprazolam | Alprazolam | |
| | Antacids | | Itraconazole/ketoconazole |
| | Atorvastatin | Atorvastatin | |

| | | | |
|---|---|---|---|
| | Bosentan | Bosentan | |
| | Carbamazepine | Carbamazepine | Itraconazole/ketoconazole |
| | Cerivastatin | Cerivastatin | |
| | Cilostazol | Cilostazol | |
| | Cisapride | Cisapride | |
| | Cyclosporine | Cyclosporine | |
| | Didanosine | | Itraconazole/ketoconazole |
| | Disopyramide | Disopyramide | |
| | Esomeprazole | | Itraconazole/ketoconazole |
| | $H_2$ antagonists | | Itraconazole/ketoconazole |
| | Lansoprazole | | Itraconazole/ketoconazole |
| | Lovastatin | Lovastatin | |
| | Omeprazole | | Itraconazole/ketoconazole |
| | Pantoprazole | | Itraconazole/ketoconazole |
| | Phenytoin | Phenytoin | Itraconazole/ketoconazole |
| | Repaglinide | Repaglinide | |
| | Simvastatin | Simvastatin | |
| | Triazolam | Triazolam | |
| | Warfarin | Warfarin | |
| Ketoconazole (3A4 inhibitor) | See Itraconazole | | |
| Labetalol (2D6 substrate) | See Carvedilol | | |
| Lansoprazole | Dapsone | | Dapsone |
| | Itraconazole | | Itraconazole |
| Letrozole | Tamoxifen | | Letrozole |
| | Ketoconazole | | Ketoconazole |
| Lidocaine | Amiodarone | Lidocaine | |

(continued)

**Table C-2.** Continued

| Medication | Interacting drug | Increases level or effect of: | Decreases level or effect of: |
|---|---|---|---|
| Linezolid | See MAOIs | | |
| Lithium | ACE inhibitors | Lithium | |
| | Acetazolamide | | Lithium |
| | Calcium channel blockers | Increase risk of neurotoxicity | |
| | COX-2 inhibitors (selective) | Lithium | |
| | Diuretics | Lithium | |
| | NSAIDs | Lithium | |
| | Sodium bicarbonate | | Lithium |
| | Theophylline | | Lithium |
| | Urea | | Lithium |
| Lopinavir | See Ritonavir | | |
| Lovastatin (3A4 substrate) | See Atorvastatin | | |
| MAOIs | Amphetamines | Hypertensive crisis | |
| | Meperidine | Hyperpyrexia, agitation, seizures | |
| | Nefazodone | Serotonin syndrome | |
| | Rizatriptan | Rizatriptan | |
| | SSRIs | Serotonin syndrome | |
| | Sumatriptan | Sumatriptan | |
| | Sympathomimetics | Hypertensive crisis | |
| | Tramadol | MAOIs | |
| | Tricyclic antidepressants | MAOIs | |
| | Venlafaxine | Serotonin syndrome | |

| | | | |
|---|---|---|---|
| | Zolmitriptan | Zolmitriptan | |
| Mercaptopurine | Warfarin | | Warfarin |
| | Allopurinol | Mercaptopurine | |
| Metformin | Cimetidine | Metformin | |
| Metoprolol (2D6 substrate) | See Carvedilol | | |
| Metronidazole (2C9 inhibitor) | Disulfiram | Disulfiram | |
| | Warfarin | Warfarin | |
| Moxifloxacin | Antacids | | Moxifloxacin |
| | Calcium salts | Moxifloxacin | |
| | Iron salts | | Moxifloxacin |
| Nefazodone (3A4 inhibitor) | Alprazolam | Alprazolam | |
| | Atorvastatin | Atorvastatin | |
| | Carbamazepine | Carbamazepine | |
| | Cerivastatin | Cerivastatin | |
| | Cilostazol | Cilostazol | |
| | Cisapride | Cisapride | |
| | Cyclosporine | Cyclosporine | |
| | Lovastatin | Lovastatin | |
| | MAOIs | MAOIs | |
| | Simvastatin | Simvastatin | |
| | Triazolam | Triazolam | |
| Nelfinavir | See Ritonavir | | |
| Nevirapine | See Delavirdine | | |
| Niacin | HMG-CoA reductase inhibitors | Myopathy or rhabdomyolysis | |
| NSAIDs | ACE inhibitors | | ACE inhibitors |
| | Diuretics | | Diuretics |
| | Lithium | Lithium | |

*(continued)*

**Table C-2.** Continued

| Medication | Interacting drug | Increases level or effect of: | Decreases level or effect of: |
|---|---|---|---|
| | Methotrexate | Methotrexate | |
| Omeprazole (1A2 inducer, 2C19 inhibitor) | Dapsone | | Dapsone |
| | Diazepam | Diazepam | |
| | Itraconazole | | Itraconazole |
| | Ketoconazole | | Ketoconazole |
| | Phenytoin | Phenytoin | |
| | Theophylline | | Theophylline |
| Oral contraceptives | Antibiotics | | Oral contraceptives |
| | Barbiturates | | Oral contraceptives |
| | Bosentan | | Oral contraceptives |
| | Carbamazepine | | Oral contraceptives |
| | Oxcarbazepine | | Oral contraceptives |
| | Phenytoin | | Oral contraceptives |
| | Rifampin | | Oral contraceptives |
| Oxcarbazepine | Oral contraceptives | | Oral contraceptives |
| | Felodipine | | Felodipine |
| | Fosphenytoin | Fosphenytoin | |
| | Lamotrigine | | Lamotrigine |
| | Phenytoin | Phenytoin | |
| | Verapamil | | Oxcarbazepine |
| Pantoprazole | Ampicillin | | Ampicillin |
| | Iron salts | | Iron salts |
| | Ketoconazole | | Ketoconazole |

| | | | |
|---|---|---|---|
| Paroxetine (2D6 inhibitor) | Benztropine | Benztropine | |
| | Carvedilol | Carvedilol | |
| | Codeine | | Codeine |
| | Desipramine | Desipramine | |
| | Dextromethorphan | Serotonin syndrome | |
| | Flecainide | Flecainide | |
| | Labetalol | Labetalol | |
| | MAOIs | Serotonin syndrome | |
| | Metoprolol | Metoprolol | |
| | Nortriptyline | Nortriptyline | |
| | Propafenone | Propafenone | |
| | Propranolol | Propranolol | |
| | Rizatriptan | Rizatriptan | |
| | Sumatriptan | Sumatriptan | |
| | Tramadol | | Tramadol |
| Phenytoin (enzyme inducer, 2C9 substrate) | Amiodarone | Phenytoin | Amiodarone |
| | Antiarrhythmics | | Antiarrhythmics |
| | Azole antifungals | | Azole antifungals |
| | Beta-blockers | | Beta-blockers |
| | Capecitabine | | Phenytoin |
| | Chloramphenicol | Phenytoin | Chloramphenicol |
| | Cimetidine | Phenytoin | |
| | Corticosteroids | | Corticosteroids |
| | Cyclosporine | | Cyclosporine |
| | Dexmethylphenidate | Phenytoin | |
| | Fluconazole | | Fluconazole |

(*continued*)

**Table C-2.** Continued

| Medication | Interacting drug | Increases level or effect of: | Decreases level or effect of: |
|---|---|---|---|
| | Fluoxetine | Phenytoin | Fluoxetine |
| | Isoniazid | Phenytoin | |
| | Itraconazole | Phenytoin | Itraconazole |
| | Ketoconazole | | Ketoconazole |
| | Omeprazole | Phenytoin | |
| | Oral contraceptives | | Oral contraceptives |
| | Oxcarbazepine | Phenytoin | |
| | Protease inhibitors | | Protease inhibitors |
| | Quinidine | | Quinidine |
| | Theophylline | | Theophylline |
| | Ticlopidine | Phenytoin | |
| | Warfarin | | Warfarin |
| | Zonisamide | | Zonisamide |
| Pimozide (3A4 substrate) | Clarithromycin | Pimozide | |
| | Erythromycin | Pimozide | |
| | Fluconazole | Pimozide | |
| | Fluvoxamine | Pimozide | |
| | Grapefruit juice | Pimozide | |
| | Itraconazole | Pimozide | |
| | Ketoconazole | Pimozide | |
| | Nefazodone | Pimozide | |
| | Protease inhibitors | Pimozide | |
| | Quinupristin/dalfopristin | Pimozide | |

| | | | |
|---|---|---|---|
| | Zileuton | Pimozide | |
| Pravastatin | Fenofibrate | Myopathy or rhabdomyolysis | |
| | Gemfibrozil | Myopathy or rhabdomyolysis | |
| | Niacin | Myopathy or rhabdomyolysis | |
| Procainamide | Cimetidine | Procainamide | |
| Propafenone (2D6 substrate) | Fluoxetine | Propafenone | |
| | Paroxetine | Propafenone | |
| | Protease inhibitors | Propafenone | |
| Propranolol (2D6 substrate) | See Carvedilol | | |
| Quinidine (2D6 inhibitor) | Barbiturates | | Quinidine |
| | Carbamazepine | | Quinidine |
| | Codeine | | Codeine |
| | Desipramine | Desipramine | |
| | Digoxin | Digoxin | |
| | Nortriptyline | Nortriptyline | |
| | Phenytoin | | Quinidine |
| | Rifampin | | Quinidine |
| | Tramadol | | Tramadol |
| Quinupristin/dalfopristin (3A4 inhibitor) | Alprazolam | Alprazolam | |
| | Atorvastatin | Atorvastatin | |
| | Carbamazepine | Carbamazepine | |
| | Cerivastatin | Cerivastatin | |
| | Cilostazol | Cilostazol | |
| | Cisapride | Cisapride | |
| | Cyclosporine | Cyclosporine | |
| | Disopyramide | Disopyramide | |

*(continued)*

**Table C-2.** Continued

| Medication | Interacting drug | Increases level or effect of: | Decreases level or effect of: |
|---|---|---|---|
| | Lovastatin | Lovastatin | |
| | Pimozide | Pimozide | |
| | Simvastatin | Simvastatin | |
| | Triazolam | Triazolam | |
| Repaglinide (3A4 substrate) | Ketoconazole | Repaglinide | |
| | Rifampin | | Repaglinide |
| | Simvastatin | Repaglinide | |
| Rifampin (enzyme inducer) | Antiarrhythmics | | Antiarrhythmics |
| | Atovaquone | | Atovaquone |
| | Azole antifungals | | Azole antifungals |
| | Beta-blockers | | Beta-blockers |
| | Chloramphenicol | | Chloramphenicol |
| | Corticosteroids | | Corticosteroids |
| | Cyclosporine | | Cyclosporine |
| | Oral contraceptives | | Oral contraceptives |
| | Protease inhibitors | | Protease inhibitors |
| | Repaglinide | | Repaglinide |
| | Tamoxifen | Tamoxifen | |
| | Theophylline | | Theophylline |
| | Warfarin | | Warfarin |
| Risedronate | All oral medications | | Risedronate |
| Ritonavir | Atorvastatin | Atorvastatin | |
| | Barbiturates | | Ritonavir/A/I/L/N/S |

| | | | |
|---|---|---|---|
| | Carbamazepine | | Ritonavir/A/I/L/N/S |
| | Cerivastatin | Cerivastatin | |
| | Cilostazol | Cilostazol | |
| | Cisapride | Cisapride | |
| | Cyclosporine | Cyclosporine | |
| | Desipramine | Desipramine | |
| | Flecainide | Flecainide | |
| | Lovastatin | Lovastatin | |
| | Methadone | | Methadone |
| | Phenytoin | | Ritonavir/A/I/L/N/S |
| | Pimozide | Pimozide | |
| | Propafenone | Propafenone | |
| | Rifampin | | Ritonavir/A/I/L/N/S |
| | Simvastatin | Simvastatin | |
| | St. John's wort | | Ritonavir/A/I/L/N/S |
| | Triazolam | Triazolam | |
| Rivastigmine | Anticholinergic agents | | Rivastigmine |
| | Cholinergic agents | Cholinergic effects | |
| Rizatriptan | Ergot derivatives | Rizatriptan | |
| | MAOIs | MAOIs | |
| | SSRIs | Serotonin syndrome | |
| Saquinavir | See Ritonavir | | |
| Sertraline | MAOIs | MAOIs | |
| | Rizatriptan | Serotonin syndrome | |
| | Sumatriptan | Serotonin syndrome | |
| Sildenafil | Indinavir | Sildenafil | |

(*continued*)

**Table C-2.** Continued

| Medication | Interacting drug | Increases level or effect of: | Decreases level or effect of: |
|---|---|---|---|
| | Nitrates | Sildenafil | |
| Simvastatin (3A4 substrate) | See Atorvastatin | | |
| Sirolimus | Cyclosporine | Sirolimus | |
| | Diltiazem | Sirolimus | |
| Sucralfate | Alendronate | | Alendronate |
| | Quinolone antibiotics | | Quinolone antibiotics |
| | Tetracyclines | | Tetracyclines |
| Sulfamethoxazole | Warfarin | Warfarin | |
| Sumatriptan | See Rizatriptan | | |
| Tamoxifen | Aminoglutethimide | Tamoxifen | |
| | Letrozole | | Letrozole |
| | Rifampin | Tamoxifen | |
| Tenofovir | Didanosine | Didanosine | |
| Tetracyclines | Antacids | | Tetracyclines |
| | Calcium | | Tetracyclines |
| | Ferrous sulfate | | Tetracyclines |
| | Sucralfate | | Tetracyclines |
| Theophylline (1A2 substrate) | Adenosine | | Adenosine |
| | Barbiturates | | Theophylline |
| | Carbamazepine | | Theophylline |
| | Cimetidine | Theophylline | |
| | Ciprofloxacin | Theophylline | |
| | Clarithromycin | Theophylline | |

| | | | |
|---|---|---|---|
| | Erythromycin | Theophylline | |
| | Fluvoxamine | Theophylline | |
| | Grapefruit juice | Theophylline | |
| | Omeprazole | | Theophylline |
| | Phenytoin | | Theophylline |
| | Rifampin | | Theophylline |
| | Tacrine | Theophylline | |
| | Ticlopidine | Theophylline | |
| | Zileuton | Theophylline | |
| Ticlopidine | Phenytoin | Phenytoin | |
| | Theophylline | Theophylline | |
| | Warfarin | Warfarin | |
| Tramadol (2D6 substrate) | Cyclobenzaprine | Seizures | |
| | Fluoxetine | Seizures | Tramadol |
| | Meperidine | Seizures | |
| | Paroxetine | Seizures | Tramadol |
| | Quinidine | | Tramadol |
| | SSRIs | Seizures | |
| | Tricyclic antidepressants | Seizures | |
| Triazolam (3A4 substrate) | See Alprazolam | | |
| Valdecoxib (3A4 substrate) | Fluconazole | | Valdecoxib |
| | Ketoconazole | | Valdecoxib |
| | Lithium | Lithium | |
| | Warfarin | Warfarin | |
| Verapamil (3A4 inhibitor) | Atorvastatin | Atorvastatin | |
| | Carbamazepine | Carbamazepine | |

(*continued*)

**Table C-2.** Continued

| Medication | Interacting drug | Increases level or effect of: | Decreases level or effect of: |
|---|---|---|---|
| | Cerivastatin | Cerivastatin | |
| | Cilostazol | Cilostazol | |
| | Cyclosporine | Cyclosporine | |
| | Digoxin | Digoxin | |
| | Lovastatin | Lovastatin | |
| | Oxcarbazepine | | Oxcarbazepine |
| | Simvastatin | Simvastatin | |
| | Triazolam | Triazolam | |
| Voriconazole (2C19, 2C9, 3A4 substrate and inhibitor) | Cyclosporine | Cyclosporine | |
| | Omeprazole | Omeprazole | |
| | Phenytoin | | Voriconazole |
| | Tacrolimus | Tacrolimus | |
| | Warfarin | Warfarin | |
| Warfarin (1A2, 2C9 substrate) | Amiodarone | Warfarin | |
| | Aspirin | Bleeding | |
| | Atovaquone | Warfarin | |
| | Barbiturates | | Warfarin |
| | Bosentan | | Warfarin |
| | Capecitabine | | Warfarin |
| | Carbamazepine | | Warfarin |
| | Cefamandole | Bleeding | |
| | Cefmetazole | Bleeding | |
| | Cefoperazone | Bleeding | |

| | | | |
|---|---|---|---|
| | Cefotetan | Bleeding | |
| | Chloramphenicol | Warfarin | |
| | Cimetidine | Warfarin | |
| | Dexmethylphenidate | Warfarin | |
| | Fluconazole | Warfarin | |
| | Fluvoxamine | Warfarin | |
| | Itraconazole | Warfarin | |
| | Ketoconazole | Warfarin | |
| | Mercaptopurine | | Warfarin |
| | Metronidazole | Warfarin | |
| | NSAIDs | | |
| | Phenytoin | Warfarin (acute) | Warfarin (chronic) |
| | Rifampin | | Warfarin |
| | Salicylates | Bleeding | |
| | Sulfamethoxazole | Warfarin | |
| | Ticlopidine | Warfarin | |
| | Voriconazole | Warfarin | |
| | Zafirlukast | Warfarin | |
| Zafirlukast | Warfarin | Warfarin | |
| Zileuton (1A2, 3A4 inhibitor) | Cisapride | Cisapride | |
| | Theophylline | Theophylline | |
| Ziprasidone (3A4 substrate) | Carbamazepine | | Ziprasidone |
| | Ketoconazole | Ziprasidone | |

(*continued*)

**Table C-2.** Continued

| Medication | Interacting drug | Increases level or effect of: | Decreases level or effect of: |
|---|---|---|---|
| Zonisamide (3A4 substrate) | Carbamazepine | | Zonisamide |
| | Fosphenytoin | | Zonisamide |
| | Phenobarbital | | Zonisamide |
| | Phenytoin | | Zonisamide |

ACE, angiotensin-converting enzyme; C/L/S, cerivastatin/lovastatin/simvastatin; COX, cyclooxygenase; HMG-CoA, 3-hydroxy-3-methylglutaryl coenzyme A; A/I/L/N/S, amprenavir/indinavir/lopinavir/nelfinavir/saquinavir; L/M/P, labetalol/metoprolol/propranolol; MAOIs, monoamine oxidase inhibitors; NSAIDs, nonsteroidal anti-inflammatory drugs; SSRIs, selective serotonin reuptake inhibitors.

**Table C-3.** Substrates, inhibitors, and inducers of hepatic cytochrome P-450 isoenzymes

| CYP1A2 | CYP2C9 | CYP2C19 | CYP2D6 | CYP3A4 |
|---|---|---|---|---|
| **Substrates** | | | | |
| Clozapine | Celecoxib | Amitriptyline | Almotriptan | Almotriptan |
| Cyclobenzaprine | Diclofenac | Clomipramine | Amitriptyline | Alprazolam |
| Imipramine | Fluvastatin | Cyclophosphamide | Cevimeline | Amlodipine |
| Mexiletine | Ibuprofen | Lansoprazole | Clomipramine | Atorvastatin |
| Naproxen | Irbesartan | Omeprazole | Codeine | Buprenorphine |
| Tacrine | Losartan | Pantoprazole | Desipramine | Buspirone |
| Theophylline | Naproxen | Phenytoin | Dextromethorphan | Carbamazepine |
| | Phenytoin | | Flecainide | Cevimeline |
| | Piroxicam | | Haloperidol | Cyclosporine |
| | SMX | | Imipramine | Diazepam |
| | Tamoxifen | | Metoprolol | Diltiazem |
| | Torsemide | | Mexiletine | Disopyramide |
| | Warfarin (S) | | Ondansetron | Ergotamine |
| | | | Paroxetine | Felodipine |
| | | | Propafenone | Fentanyl |
| | | | Risperidone | Indinavir |
| | | | Tamoxifen | Lovastatin |
| | | | Thioridazine | Methadone |
| | | | Timolol | Midazolam |
| | | | Tramadol | Mifepristone |
| | | | Venlafaxine | Nateglinide |
| | | | | Nifedipine |
| | | | | Nisoldipine |
| | | | | Nitrendipine |
| | | | | Pimozide |
| | | | | Quinidine |
| | | | | Repaglinide |
| | | | | Ritonavir |
| | | | | Saquinavir |
| | | | | Sildenafil |
| | | | | Simvastatin |
| | | | | Sirolimus |
| | | | | Tacrolimus |
| | | | | Tamoxifen |
| | | | | Trazodone |

*(continued)*

**Table C-3.** Continued

| CYP1A2 | CYP2C9 | CYP2C19 | CYP2D6 | CYP3A4 |
|---|---|---|---|---|
| | | | | Triazolam<br>Verapamil<br>Zonisamide |
| **Inhibitors** | | | | |
| Cimetidine<br>Ciprofloxacin<br>Clarithromycin<br>Fluvoxamine<br>Ticlopidine | Amiodarone<br>INH<br>Fluconazole<br>Ticlopidine<br>Voriconazole | Fluoxetine<br>Fluvoxamine<br>Ketoconazole<br>Lansoprazole<br>Omeprazole<br>Ticlopidine<br>Voriconazole | Amiodarone<br>Chlorpheniramine<br>Cimetidine<br>Clomipramine<br>Fluoxetine<br>Haloperidol<br>Methadone<br>Paroxetine<br>Quinidine<br>Ritonavir | Amiodarone<br>Cimetidine<br>Clarithromycin<br>Diltiazem<br>Erythromycin<br>Grapefruit juice<br>Itraconazole<br>Ketoconazole<br>Nefazodone<br>Protease inhibitors<br>Quinu-dalfo<br>Verapamil |
| **Inducers** | | | | |
| Carbamazepine<br>Rifampin<br>Tobacco | Bosentan<br>Phenobarbital<br>Rifampin<br>Secobarbital | Bosentan<br>Carbamazepine<br>Rifampin | | Bosentan<br>Carbamazepine<br>Phenobarbital<br>Phenytoin<br>Rifabutin<br>Rifampin<br>St. John's wort |

INH, isoniazid; quinu-dalfo, quinupristin/dalfopristin; SMX, sulfamethoxazole.

**Table C-4.** Drugs associated with QT-interval prolongation[a]

| | | |
|---|---|---|
| Amantadine | Gatifloxacin | Procainamide |
| Amiodarone | Granisetron | Quetiapine |
| Arsenic trioxide | Halofantrine | Quinidine |
| Bepridil | Haloperidol | Risperidone |
| Chloral hydrate | Ibutilide | Salmeterol |
| Chlorpromazine | Indapamide | Sotalol |
| Cisapride | Isradipine | Sparfloxacin |
| Clarithromycin | Levomethadyl | Sumatriptan |
| Disopyramide | Lithium | Tacrolimus |
| Dofetilide | Mesoridazine | Tamoxifen |
| Dolasetron | Methadone | Telithromycin |
| Domperidone | Moxifloxacin | Thioridazine |
| Droperidol | Naratriptan | Tizanidine |
| Erythromycin | Nicardipine | Venlafaxine |
| Felbamate | Octreotide | Ziprasidone |
| Flecainide | Ondansetron | Zolmitriptan |
| Foscarnet | Pentamidine | |
| Fosphenytoin | Pimozide | |

[a]Adapted from http://www.qtdrugs.org.

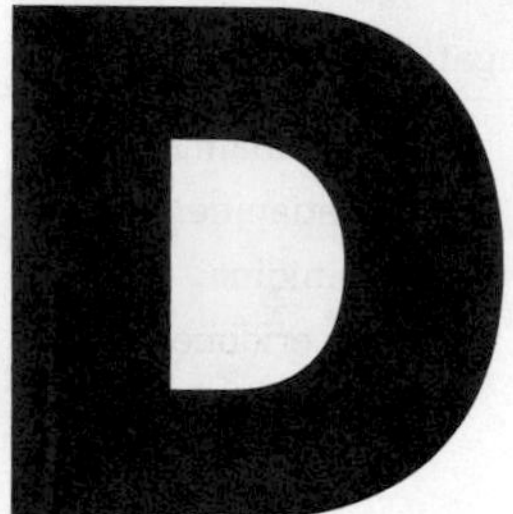

# Intravenous Admixture Preparation and Administration Guide[a]

Robyn A. Schaiff

**Abciximab** (ReoPro)

Diluent: NS

Loading dose: 0.25 mg/kg undiluted over 1 min

Maintenance concentration: 7.5 mg/250 ml NS = 0.03 mg/ml

Infusion rate: 0.125 µg/kg/min (maximum 10 µg/min) for 12 hr

**Aggrastat** (see Tirofiban)

**Aminophylline** (see Theophylline)

**Amiodarone** (Cordarone)

Diluent: $D_5W$ only (glass or polyolefin containers for maintenance infusion)

Loading dosage: 150 mg over 10 min (can repeat), then 1 mg/min for 6 hr

Maintenance concentration: 450 mg/250 ml = 1.8 mg/ml

Infusion rate: 0.5 mg/min (0.5 mg/min = 17 ml/hr)

**Amrinone** [see Inamrinone (Inocor)]

**Angiomax** (see Bivalirudin)

**Argatroban**

Diluent: NS or $D_5W$

Concentration: 250 mg/250 ml = 1 mg/ml

Infusion rate: 2 µg/kg/min—titrate to aPTT 1–3 times control. Dose should be reduced by 50% in moderate hepatic impairment.

**Bivalirudin** (Angiomax)

Diluent: NS or $D_5W$

Concentration: 250 mg/50 ml = 5 mg/ml

Loading dose: 0.75 mg/kg bolus

Infusion rate: 1.75 mg/kg/hr—titrate to ACT goal. Dose should be decreased if $Cl_{Cr}$ <60 ml/min.

**Diltiazem** (Cardizem)

Diluent: NS, $D_5W$

Concentration: 125 mg/125 ml = 1 mg/ml

Initial dosage: 0.25 mg/kg (20 mg) bolus followed by 0.35 mg/kg (25 mg) bolus if necessary

Infusion rate: 5–15 mg/hr; titrate to effect

**Dobutamine** (Dobutrex)

Diluent: NS, $D_5W$

Concentration: 250 mg/250 ml = 1000 µg/ml

Infusion rate: Usually start at 3 μg/kg/min; titrate up to 20 μg/kg/min (Example: For a 70-kg patient to receive 3 μg/kg/min, the drip rate should be 13 ml/hr.)

**Dopamine** (Intropin)

Diluent: NS, $D_5W$

Concentration: 800 mg/500 ml = 1600 μg/ml

Infusion rate: Usually start at 3 μg/kg/min; titrate to effect (Example: For a 70-kg patient to receive 3 μg/kg/min, the drip rate should be 8 ml/hr.)

**Epinephrine**

Diluent: NS or $D_5W$

Concentration: 5 mg/500 ml = 10 μg/ml

Infusion rate: 1–4 μg/min initially; titrate to effect (1 μg/min = 6 ml/hr)

**Eptifibatide** (Integrelin)

Diluent: None—solution is premixed

Loading dose: 180 μg/kg IV bolus. Repeat in 10 min for coronary intervention.

Maintenance concentration: 75 mg/100 ml = 750 μg/ml

Infusion rate: 2 μg/kg/min up to 72 hr. Decrease dose by 50% if serum creatinine = 2–4 mg/dl. Avoid if serum creatinine > 4 mg/dl.

**Esmolol** (Brevibloc)

Diluent: NS, $D_5W$

Concentration: 2.5 g/250 ml = 10 mg/ml

Initial dosage: Loading dosage 500 μg/kg over 1 min

Infusion rate: Usually start at 50 μg/kg/min (21 ml/hr for a 70-kg patient)

**Heparin**

Diluent: NS, $D_5W$, 1/2 NS

Concentration: 25,000 U/250 ml = 100 U/ml

Initial dose: 60–80 U/kg

Infusion rate: Usually start at 14–18 U/kg/hr

**Ibutilide** (Corvert)

Diluent: NS or $D_5W$ or undiluted

Dosage: 1 mg (if weight <60 kg: 0.01 mg/kg) over 10 min; can repeat 10 min after initial infusion

Concentration: Undiluted, 1 mg/10 ml; diluted, 1 mg/50 ml (0.02 mg/ml)

**Inamrinone** (Inocor)

Diluent: NS only (protect from light)

Concentration: 200 mg/100 ml = 2 mg/ml

Initial dosage: Loading dosage 0.75 mg/kg over 2 min

Infusion rate: Usually start at 5 μg/kg/min; titrate up to 15 μg/kg/min[b]

**Integrelin** (see Eptifibatide)

**Lepirudin** (Refludan)

Diluent: NS or $D_5W$

Concentration: 100 mg/250 ml = 0.4 mg/ml

Loading dose: 0.4 mg/kg (0.2 mg/kg if $Cl_{Cr}$ < 60 ml/min)

Maintenance dose: 0.15 mg/kg/hr (decrease dose in renal dysfunction, titrate to prothrombin time 2.0–2.5 times normal)[b]

**Lidocaine**

Diluent: NS, $D_5W$

Concentration: 2 g/500 ml = 4 mg/ml

Infusion rate: 1–4 mg/min (1 mg/min = 15 ml/hr)

**Milrinone** (Primacor)

Diluent: NS or $D_5W$

Loading dosage: 50 μg/kg diluted over 10 min

Concentration: 40 mg/200 ml = 0.2 mg/ml

Infusion rate: 0.375–0.750 μg/kg/min (2 mg/hr = 10 ml/hr)[b]

**Natrecor** (see Nesiritide)

**Nesiritide** (Natrecor)

Diluent: NS or $D_5W$

Concentration: 1.5 mg/255 ml = 6 μg/ml

Loading dose: 2 μg/kg IV bolus

Infusion rate: 0.01 μg/kg/min

**Nicardipine** (Cardene)

Diluent: NS, $D_5W$

Concentration: 25 mg/250 ml = 0.1 mg/ml

Infusion rate: 2–15 mg/hr

**Nitroglycerin**

Diluent: NS, $D_5W$ (glass or polyolefin containers only)

Concentration: 50 mg/250 ml = 200 μg/ml

Infusion rate: Initially 10 μg/min; titrate to effect (10 μg/min = 3 ml/hr)

**Nitroprusside** (Nipride)

Diluent: $D_5W$ only (protect from light)

Concentration: 50 mg/250 ml = 200 μg/ml

Infusion rate: Initially 0.25 μg/kg/min; titrate to effect (10 μg/min = 3 ml/hr)

**Norepinephrine** (Levophed)

Diluent: $D_5W$ only

Concentration: 8 mg/250 ml = 32 μg/ml

Infusion rate: Initially 2 μg/min; titrate (2 μg/min = 4 ml/hr)

**Phenylephrine** (Neo-Synephrine)

Diluent: NS, $D_5W$

Concentration: 10 mg/250 ml = 40 μg/ml

Infusion rate: Initially 10 μg/min; titrate to effect (10 μg/min = 15 ml/hr)

**Procainamide** (Pronestyl)

Diluent: NS, $D_5W$

Concentration: 2 g/500 ml = 4 mg/ml

Loading dose: 17 mg/kg

Infusion rate: 1–4 mg/min (1 mg/min = 15 ml/hr)[b]

**ReoPro** (see Abciximab)

**Theophylline**

Diluent: $D_5W$, NS

Concentration: 800 mg/500 ml =1.6 mg/ml

Initial dosage: Loading dose 5 mg/kg over 20 min

Infusion rate: 0.2–0.6 mg/kg/hr

**Tirofiban** (Aggrastat)

Diluent: NS

Concentration: 12.5 mg/250 ml NS = 0.05 mg/ml

Loading dose: 0.4 μg/kg/min for 30 min

Maintenance infusion: 0.1 μg/kg/min for up to 72 hr. Dose should be 50% lower if $Cl_{Cr}$ <30 ml/hr.

ACT, activated coagulation time; aPTT, activated partial thromboplastin time; $Cl_{Cr}$, creatinine clearance; $D_5W$, 5% dextrose in water; NS, normal saline.

[a]To determine infusion rate:

$$\text{Infusion rate (ml/min)} = \frac{\text{Desired concentration infused } (\mu g/kg/min) \times \text{weight (kg)}}{\text{concentration of solution } (\mu g/ml)}$$

[b]Dependent on renal function.

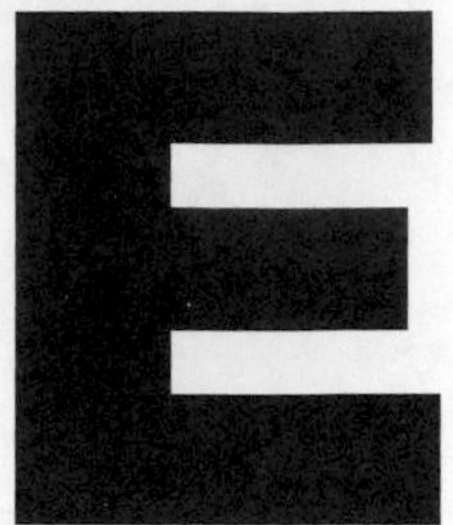

# Dosage Adjustments of Drugs in Renal Failure

Way Y. Huey and
Daniel W. Coyne

| Medication | Route | Adjusted dosing interval (hr) or % normal dose | | | Supplement dose after specific dialysis |
|---|---|---|---|---|---|
| | | >50 ml/min (GFR) | 10–50 ml/min (GFR) | <10 ml/min (GFR) | |
| **Analgesics—nonnarcotic** | | | | | |
| Acetaminophen | H | 4 | 6 | 8 | HD |
| Aspirin | H, R | 4 | 4–6 | A | HD |
| Celecoxib | H | N | N | N | N |
| Diclofenac | H | N | N | N | N |
| Ibuprofen | H | N | N | N | N |
| Indomethacin | H, R | N | N | N | N |
| Ketoprofen | H | N | N | N | N |
| Ketorolac (IM) | H, R | N | N | 50% | N |
| Meloxicam | H | N | — | A | N |
| Nabumetone | H | N | N | N | N |
| Naproxen | H | N | N | N | N |
| Oxaprozin | H | N | N | N | N |
| Piroxicam | H | N | N | N | N |
| Rofecoxib | H | N | N | N | N |
| Sulindac | H, R | N | N | 50% | N |
| Tramadol | H, R | N | 12 | 12 | N |
| **Analgesics—opioid** | | | | | |
| Codeine | H | N | 75% | 50% | N |
| Meperidine | H | N | 75% | 50% | N |
| Morphine | H | N | 75% | 50% | N |
| **Antiarrhythmics** | | | | | |
| Amiodarone | H | N | N | N | N |
| Bretylium | R, H | N | 25–50% | A | ? |
| Digoxin[a] | R | 24 | 36 | 48 | N |
| Disopyramide[a] | R, H | 75% | 15–50% | 10–25% | HD |
| Flecainide[a] | R, H | N | 50% | 50% | N |
| Lidocaine[a] | H, R | N | N | N | N |
| Mexiletine | H, R | N | N | 50–75% | HD |

| Medication | Route | Adjusted dosing interval (hr) or % normal dose | | | Supplement dose after specific dialysis |
|---|---|---|---|---|---|
| | | >50 ml/min (GFR) | 10–50 ml/min (GFR) | <10 ml/min (GFR) | |
| Moricizine | H | N | N | 50–75% | N |
| Procainamide[a] | R, H | 4 | 6–12 | 12–24 | HD |
| Propafenone | H | N | N | 50–75% | N |
| Quinidine[a] | H, R | N | N | N | HD, PD |
| Sotalol | R | N | 30% | 15% | N |
| Tocainide[a] | R, H | N | N | 50% | HD |
| **Antibiotic drugs** | | | | | |
| *Aminoglycosides* | | | | | |
| Amikacin[a] | R | 8–12 | 12 | >24 | HD, PD |
| Gentamicin[a] | R | 8–12 | 12 | >24 | HD, PD |
| Tobramycin[a] | R | 8–12 | 12 | >24 | HD, PD |
| *Antimycobacterial drugs* | | | | | |
| Clofazimine | H | N | N | N | N |
| Cycloserine | R | 12 | 12–24 | 24 | N |
| Ethambutol | R | 24 | 24–36 | 48 | HD, PD |
| Ethionamide | H | N | N | 50% | N |
| Isoniazid | H, R | N | N | N | HD, PD |
| Pyrazinamide | H, R | N | N | 50% | HD, PD |
| Rifabutin | H | N | N | N | N |
| Rifampin | H | N | N | N | ? |
| *Cephalosporins* | | | | | |
| Cefadroxil | R | 12 | 12–24 | 24–48 | HD |
| Cefazolin | R | 8 | 12 | 24–48 | HD |
| Cefdinir | R | 12 | 24 | 48 | HD |
| Cefepime | R | 12 | 16–24 | 24–48 | HD |
| Cefixime | R | 12–24 | 75% | 50% | N |
| Cefonicid | R | N | 50% | 25% | N |
| Cefoperazone | H | N | N | N | N |
| Cefotaxime | R, H | 6–8 | 8–12 | 24 | HD |
| Cefotetan | R | 12 | 24 | 24 | HD, PD |
| Cefoxitin | R | 8 | 8–12 | 24–48 | HD |
| Cefpodoxime | R | 12 | 16 | 24–48 | HD |
| Cefprozil | R | 12 | 16 | 24 | HD |
| Ceftazidime | R | 8–12 | 24–48 | 48 | HD |
| Ceftibuten | R | 24 | 50% | 25% | HD |
| Ceftizoxime | R | 8–12 | 12–24 | 24 | HD |
| Ceftriaxone | R, H | N | N | 24 | N |
| Cefuroxime | R | 8 | 8–12 | 24 | HD |
| Cephalexin | R | 8 | 12 | 12 | HD, PD |

| Medication | Route | Adjusted dosing interval (hr) or % normal dose >50 ml/min (GFR) | 10–50 ml/min (GFR) | <10 ml/min (GFR) | Supplement dose after specific dialysis |
|---|---|---|---|---|---|
| Cephalothin | R | 6 | 6–8 | 12 | HD, PD |
| Cephradine | R | 6 | 50% q6h | 25% q6h | HD, PD |
| Loracarbef | R | 12 | 50% | 3–5 d | HD |
| *Penicillins* | | | | | |
| Amoxicillin/clavulanate | R, H | 8 | 8–12 | 12–24 | HD |
| Ampicillin | R, H | 6 | 6–12 | 12–24 | HD |
| Ampicillin/sulbactam | R, H | 6–8 | 12 | 24 | HD |
| Carbenicillin | R, H | 8–12 | 12–24 | 24–48 | HD, PD |
| Dicloxacillin | R, H | N | N | N | N |
| Mezlocillin | R, H | 4–6 | 6–8 | 8–12 | HD |
| Oxacillin | R, H | N | N | N | N |
| Penicillin G | R, H | N | 75% | 25–50% | HD |
| Piperacillin | R | 4–6 | 6–8 | 12 | HD |
| Piperacillin/tazobactam | R, H | 6 | 8 | 12 | HD |
| Ticarcillin | R | 8 | 8–12 | 24 | HD |
| Ticarcillin/clavulanate | R, H | 3.1 g q4–6h | 2 g q6–8h | 2 g q12h | HD |
| *Quinolones* | | | | | |
| Ciprofloxacin | R | N | 12–24 | 24 | N |
| Enoxacin | R | N | 50% | 50% q24h | N |
| Gatifloxacin | R | N | 50% | 50% | HD, PD |
| Levofloxacin | R | 8–12 | 24 | 48 | N |
| Lomefloxacin | R | N | 75% | 50% | N |
| Moxifloxacin | H | N | N | N | N |
| Norfloxacin | R | N | 12–24 | A | N |
| Ofloxacin | R | N | 12–24 | 24 | N |
| *Other antibacterial drugs* | | | | | |
| Azithromycin | H | N | N | N | N |
| Aztreonam | R | N | 50–75% | 25% | HD, PD |
| Chloramphenicol | R, H | N | N | N | N |
| Clarithromycin | R, H | N | 75% | 50% | N |
| Clindamycin | H | N | N | N | N |
| Dirithromycin | H | N | N | N | N |
| Doxycycline | R, H | N | N | N | N |
| Ertapenem | R, H | N | 50% | ? | HD |
| Erythromycin | H | N | N | N | N |
| Imipenem | R | N | 50% | 25% | HD |
| Linezolid | H, R | N | N | N | HD |

| Medication | Route | Adjusted dosing interval (hr) or % normal dose | | | Supplement dose after specific dialysis |
|---|---|---|---|---|---|
| | | >50 ml/min (GFR) | 10–50 ml/min (GFR) | <10 ml/min (GFR) | |
| Meropenem | R | N | 50% q12h | 50% q24h | HD |
| Metronidazole | R, H | N | N | 50% | HD |
| Pentamidine | ? | N | N | 24–48 | N |
| Quinupristin/dalfopristin | H | N | N | N | N |
| Sulfamethoxazole | R, H | 12 | 18 | 24 | HD |
| Tetracycline | R, H | 12 | 12–18 | 18–24 | N |
| Trimethoprim | R, H | 12 | 18 | 24 | HD |
| Vancomycin[a] (IV) | R | 6–12 | 24–48 | 48–96 | N |
| **Antifungal drugs** | | | | | |
| Amphotericin B | N | 24 | 24 | 24–36 | N |
| Caspofungin | H | 24 | 24 | 24 | N |
| Fluconazole | R, H | N | 50% | 25% | HD |
| Flucytosine | R | 6 | 24 | 24–48 | HD, PD |
| Itraconazole | H, R | N | N | 50% | N |
| Ketoconazole | H | N | N | N | N |
| Miconazole | H | N | N | N | N |
| Terbinafine | R, H | N | ? | ? | ? |
| **Antiviral drugs** | | | | | |
| Abacavir | H | N | N | N | ? |
| Acyclovir (IV) | R | 6 | 24 | 48 | HD |
| Acyclovir (PO) | R | N | 12–24 | 24 | HD |
| Amantadine | R | 12–24 | 24–72 | 72–168 | N |
| Amprenavir | H | N | N | N | ? |
| Cidofovir | R | N | A | A | ? |
| Delavirdine | H | N | ? | ? | ? |
| Didanosine | R | 12 | 24 | 48 | N |
| Efavirenz | H | N | N | N | ? |
| Famciclovir | R | 8 | 12–24 | 48 | HD |
| Foscarnet | R | 25 mg/kg q8h | 15 mg/kg q8h | 6 mg/kg q8h | HD |
| Ganciclovir | R | 12 | 24 | 24 | HD |
| Indinavir | H, R | 8 | ? | ? | ? |
| Lamivudine | R | 12 | 24 | 33% q24h | ? |
| Lopinavir/ritonavir | H | — | — | — | — |
| Nelfinavir | H | N | N | N | ? |
| Nevirapine | H | N | ? | ? | ? |

| Medication | Route | Adjusted dosing interval (hr) or % normal dose >50 ml/min (GFR) | 10–50 ml/min (GFR) | <10 ml/min (GFR) | Supplement dose after specific dialysis |
|---|---|---|---|---|---|
| Rimantadine | H | N | N | 50% | ? |
| Ritonavir | H | N | N | N | ? |
| Saquinavir | H | N | N | N | ? |
| Stavudine | H, R | N | 50% q12–24h | ? | ? |
| Valacyclovir | R | 8 | 12–24 | 50% q24h | HD |
| Zalcitabine | R | 8 | 12 | 24 | ? |
| Zidovudine | H | N | N | N | HD |
| **Anticoagulants** | | | | | |
| *Antithrombin agents* | | | | | |
| Argatroban | H | N | N | N | N |
| Bivalirudin | H, R | — | — | — | ? |
| Dalteparin | R | N | ? | ? | N |
| Enoxaparin | R | N | ? | ? | N |
| Fondaparinux | R | N | | A | — |
| Heparin | H | N | N | N | N |
| Lepirudin | R | N | 15–50% | A | ? |
| Tinzaparin | R | N | ? | A | N |
| Warfarin | H | N | N | N | N |
| *Platelet glycoprotein IIb/IIIa–receptor antagonists* | | | | | |
| Abciximab | — | N | N | N | N |
| Eptifibatide | R | N | 50% | A | A |
| Tirofiban | R | N | 50% if $Cl_{Cr}$ <30 | 50% | N |
| **Cardiovascular agents** | | | | | |
| *Angiotensin-converting enzyme inhibitors* | | | | | |
| Benazepril | H, R | N | 75% | 50% | N |
| Captopril | R, H | N | N | 50% | HD |
| Enalapril | R | N | 75% | 50% | HD |
| Fosinopril | H | N | N | N | N |
| Lisinopril | R | N | 50% | 25% | HD |
| Moexipril | R, H | N | 50% | 50% | ? |
| Perindopril | R, H | N | 50% | 25% | HD |
| Quinapril | H, R | N | 75% | 50% | N |
| Ramipril | R, H | N | 50% | 50% | HD |
| Trandolapril | R, H | N | 50% | A | N |

| Medication | Route | Adjusted dosing interval (hr) or % normal dose >50 ml/min (GFR) | 10–50 ml/min (GFR) | <10 ml/min (GFR) | Supplement dose after specific dialysis |
|---|---|---|---|---|---|
| *Angiotensin II–receptor antagonists* | | | | | |
| Candesartan | GI | M | 50% | 50% | N |
| Eprosartan | H | N | N | N | ? |
| Irbesartan | H | N | N | N | N |
| Losartan | H | N | N | N | N |
| Telmisartan | H | N | N | N | N |
| Valsartan | R | H | N | N | N |
| *β-Adrenergic antagonists* | | | | | |
| Acebutolol | R, H | N | 50% | 25% | N |
| Atenolol | R | N | 50% | 25% | HD |
| Betaxolol | H, R | N | N | 50% | N |
| Bisoprolol | H, R | N | 50% | 25% | N |
| Carteolol | R | 24 | 48 | 72 | ? |
| Carvedilol | H | N | N | N | N |
| Labetalol | H | N | N | N | N |
| Metoprolol | H | N | N | N | HD |
| Nadolol | R | N | 50% | 25% | HD |
| Penbutolol | H | N | N | N | N |
| Pindolol | H, R | N | N | N | ? |
| Propranolol | H | N | N | N | N |
| Sotalol | R | N | 24–48 | ? | ? |
| Timolol | H | N | N | N | N |
| *Calcium channel antagonists* | | | | | |
| Amlodipine | H | N | N | N | N |
| Diltiazem | H | N | N | N | N |
| Felodipine | H | N | N | N | N |
| Isradipine | H | N | N | N | N |
| Nicardipine | H | N | N | N | N |
| Nifedipine | H | N | N | N | N |
| Verapamil | H | N | N | 50–75% | N |
| *Diuretics* | | | | | |
| Acetazolamide | R | 6 | 12 | A | — |
| Bumetanide | R, H | N | N | N | — |
| Furosemide | R | N | N | N | — |
| Indapamide | H | N | N | N | — |
| Metolazone | R | N | N | N | — |
| Spironolactone | R | 6–12 | 12–24 | A | — |
| Thiazide | R | N | N | A | — |

| Medication | Route | Adjusted dosing interval (hr) or % normal dose | | | Supplement dose after specific dialysis |
|---|---|---|---|---|---|
| | | >50 ml/min (GFR) | 10–50 ml/min (GFR) | <10 ml/min (GFR) | |
| Torsemide | H, R | N | N | N | — |
| *Other antihypertensives* | | | | | |
| Clonidine | R | N | N | N | N |
| Doxazosin | H | N | N | N | N |
| Hydralazine (PO) | H | 8 | 8 | 8–16 | N |
| Methyldopa | R, H | 8 | 8–12 | 12–24 | HD, PD |
| Minoxidil | H | N | N | N | HD |
| Nitroprusside | N | N | N | N | N |
| Prazosin | H, R | N | N | N | N |
| Terazosin | R | N | N | N | N |
| **CNS agents** | | | | | |
| *Antidepressants* | | | | | |
| Amitriptyline | H | N | N | N | N |
| Doxepin | H | N | N | N | N |
| Fluoxetine | H | N | N | N | N |
| Imipramine | H | N | N | N | N |
| Nortriptyline | H | N | N | N | N |
| Paroxetine | H | N | N | N | N |
| Sertraline | H | N | N | N | N |
| Trazodone | H | N | N | N | N |
| Venlafaxine | H | N | 75% | 50% | N |
| *Anticonvulsants* | | | | | |
| Carbamazepine[a] | H, R | N | N | 75% | N |
| Ethosuximide[a] | H, R | N | N | 75% | HD |
| Oxcarbazepine | H, R | N | N | N | N |
| Phenobarbital[a] | H, R | N | N | 12–16 | HD, PD |
| Phenytoin[a] | H | N | N | N | N |
| Primidone[a] | H, R | 8 | 8–12 | 12–24 | HD |
| Valproic acid[a] | H | N | N | 75% | N |
| Zonisamide | H,R | N | A | A | ? |
| *Sedatives* | | | | | |
| Alprazolam | H | N | N | N | N |
| Chlordiazepoxide | H | N | N | 50% | N |
| Diazepam | H | N | N | N | N |
| Flurazepam | H | N | N | N | N |
| Lorazepam | H | N | N | N | N |
| Midazolam | H | N | N | 50% | N |
| Temazepam | H | N | N | N | N |
| Zaleplon | H | N | N | ? | N |
| Zolpidem | H | N | N | N | N |

| Medication | Route | Adjusted dosing interval (hr) or % normal dose | | | Supplement dose after specific dialysis |
|---|---|---|---|---|---|
| | | >50 ml/min (GFR) | 10–50 ml/min (GFR) | <10 ml/min (GFR) | |
| *Other psychoactive drugs* | | | | | |
| Aripiprazole | H | N | N | N | N |
| Buspirone | H, R | N | N | 25–50% | HD |
| Chlorpromazine | H | N | N | N | N |
| Citalopram | H | N | N | A | ? |
| Haloperidol | H | N | N | N | N |
| Lithium[a] | R | N | 50–75% | 25–50% | HD, PD |
| Mirtazapine | H | N | ? | ? | ? |
| Ziprasidone | H | N | N | N | N |
| **Others** | | | | | |
| *Antidiabetic drugs* | | | | | |
| Acarbose | GI | N | A | A | N |
| Acetohexamide | H | 12–24 | A | A | N |
| Chlorpropamide | ? | 24–36 | A | A | N |
| Glimepiride | H, R | N | N | N | N |
| Glipizide | H, R | N | N | N | N |
| Glyburide | H, R | N | A | A | N |
| Metformin | R | A | A | A | N |
| Nateglinide | H | N | N | N | — |
| Pioglitazone | H | N | N | N | N |
| Repaglinide | H | N | N | N | N |
| Rosiglitazone | H | N | N | N | N |
| Tolazamide | H | N | N | N | N |
| Tolbutamide | H | N | N | N | N |
| *Antihistamines* | | | | | |
| Azatadine | H | N | N | N | N |
| Cetirizine | H, R | N | 50% | 50% | ? |
| Fexofenadine | H, R | N | 24 | 24 | ? |
| Loratadine | H | N | 48 | 48 | N |
| *Antilipemic drugs* | | | | | |
| Cholestyramine | N | N | N | N | N |
| Clofibrate | H | 6–12 | 12–24 | 24–48 | N |
| Colesevelam | H | N | N | N | N |
| Fluvastatin | H | N | N | ? | N |
| Gemfibrozil | R, H | N | 50% | 25% | N |
| Lovastatin | H | N | N | N | N |
| Pravastatin | R, H | N | N | 50% | N |
| Simvastatin | H | N | N | 50% | N |
| *GI drugs* | | | | | |
| Cimetidine | R | 6 | 8 | 12 | N |

| Medication | Route | Adjusted dosing interval (hr) or % normal dose | | | Supplement dose after specific dialysis |
|---|---|---|---|---|---|
| | | >50 ml/min (GFR) | 10–50 ml/min (GFR) | <10 ml/min (GFR) | |
| Esomeprazole | H | N | N | N | N |
| Famotidine | R, H | N | N | 50% | ? |
| Mesalamine | H | N | N | ? | N |
| Metoclopramide | R, H | N | 75% | 50% | N |
| Misoprostol | R | N | N | N | N |
| Nizatidine | H | N | 24 | 48 | N |
| Omeprazole | H | N | N | N | ? |
| Pantoprazole | H | N | N | N | N |
| Rabeprazole | H | N | N | N | N |
| Ranitidine | R | N | 18–24 | 24 | HD |
| *Other drugs* | | | | | |
| Alendronate | R | N | A | A | ? |
| Allopurinol | R | N | 50% | 10–25% | ? |
| Colchicine (PO) | R, H | N | N | 50% | N |
| Dipyridamole | H | N | N | N | ? |
| Etidronate | R | N | A | A | ? |
| Finasteride | H, R | N | N | N | N |
| Glucocorticoids | H | N | N | N | N |
| Nitrates | H | N | N | N | N |
| Pentoxifylline | H | N | N | N | N |
| Risedronate | R | N | A | A | ? |
| Terbutaline | H, R | N | 50% | A | ? |
| Theophylline | H | N | N | N | HD, PD |
| Ticlopidine | H | N | N | N | ? |
| Tiludronate | R | N | A | A | ? |

A, avoid use; $Cl_{Cr}$, creatinine clearance; GFR, glomerular filtration rate; H, hepatic; HD, hemodialysis; N, none; PD, peritoneal dialysis; R, renal; %, percentage of normal dose; ?, no data.
[a]Serum levels should be used to determine exact dosing.
*Source:* G Aronoff, W Bennett, J Berns, et al. *Drug Prescribing in Renal Failure: Dosing Guidelines for Adults* (4th ed). Philadelphia: American College of Physicians, 1999; CR Gelman, BH Rumack, AJ Hess (eds). *Drugdex System*. Englewood, CO: Micromedex, Inc, 2003; and GK McEvoy (ed). *American Hospital Formulary Service Drug Information*. Bethesda, MD: American Society of Health-System Pharmacists, 2003.

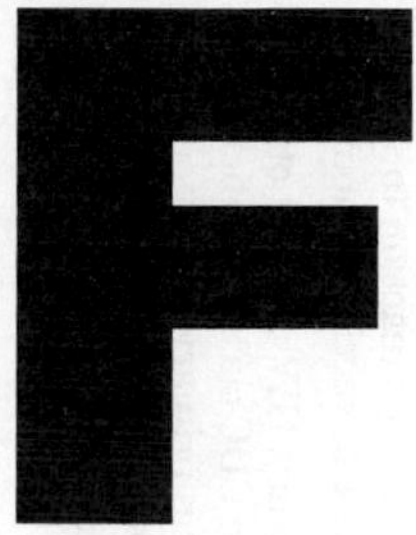

# Immunizations and Post-Exposure Therapies

Alexis M. Elward and
Victoria J. Fraser

**Table F-1.** Routine adult immunizations

| Vaccine | Persons for whom indicated | Dose | Contraindications |
|---|---|---|---|
| Hepatitis A | Travelers to endemic areas, homosexual men, military personnel, illicit drug users, patients with clotting factor disorders, chronic liver disease, occupational risk for infection (i.e., researchers) | 1.0 ml IM (repeated in 6–18 mo for extended immunity)<br>Age ≥ 18 yr<br>HAVRIX: 1440 ELU/dose<br>VAQTA: 50 U/dose | Severe allergic reaction to vaccine or to vaccine component |
| Hepatitis B | Everyone | 1 ml IM (in the deltoid) at 0, 1, and 6 mo (higher dose for immunocompromised and dialysis patients) | Severe allergic reaction to vaccine or to vaccine component |
| Influenza | Everyone ≥ 50 yr, high-risk patients,[a] women who will be in second or third trimester of pregnancy during influenza season, health care workers (consider offering to everyone) | 0.5 ml IM every fall | Severe allergic reaction to vaccine or to vaccine component, including egg protein |
| Pneumococcus | Everyone ≥ 65 yr, high-risk patients[a] ≥ 2 yr old, anatomic or functional asplenia, CSF leak | 0.5 ml IM once (repeated after ≥ 5 yr for highest-risk patients) | Severe allergic reaction to vaccine or to vaccine component |
| Tetanus/diphtheria booster (adult Td) | Everyone | 0.5 ml q10 yr (or a single booster at age 50) | Severe allergic reaction to vaccine or to vaccine component |
| Varicella | All susceptible persons, especially (1) health care workers, (2) persons who live/work in environments where VZV transmission is likely,[b] (3) adolescents and adults living with children, (4) nonpregnant women of childbearing age, (5) international travelers | 0.5 ml SC | Severe allergic reaction to vaccine or to vaccine component<br>Pregnancy, HIV infected other than CDC class N1 deficiency or A1, primary immunodeficiency, neoplasms affecting bone marrow or lymphatic system[c] |

| | | | |
|---|---|---|---|
| Measles | Persons entering college, U.S. travelers to foreign countries, health care workers | 0.5 ml SC | Pregnancy, history of sensitivity to eggs or neomycin; severe immunosuppression |
| Meningococcus | During outbreaks of serogroup C,[d] consider for college freshmen living in dormitories; indicated for patients with terminal complement component deficiencies, functional or anatomic asplenia, travelers to countries where *Neisseria meningitides* is hyperendemic (i.e., sub-Saharan Africa) | 0.5 ml SC | Severe allergic reaction to vaccine or to vaccine component |
| *Haemophilus influenzae* type b (Hib) | All children <5 yr, persons with functional or anatomic asplenia, sickle cell anemia,[e] HIV, Hodgkin's lymphoma[f] | Schedule depends on age; see *MMWR Morb Mortal Wkly Rep* 40(RR-07), 1991 | Severe allergic reaction to vaccine or vaccine component |

CDC, Centers for Disease Control and Prevention; CSF, cerebrospinal fluid; ELU, ELISA units; HAVRIX, hepatitis A vaccine, inactivated; Td, adult tetanus-diphtheria booster; VAQTA, hepatitis A vaccine, inactivated; VZV, varicella-zoster virus.

[a]High-risk patients are those with chronic pulmonary, cardiovascular, metabolic, or renal diseases or hemoglobinopathies, or immunosuppressed or institutionalized persons.

[b]Teachers of young children, day care employees, residents/staff in institutional settings, college students, correctional institution inmates/staff members, military personnel.

[c]Research protocol available through vaccine manufacturer for use in patients with acute lymphocytic leukemia who meet eligibility criteria.

[d]Outbreak is defined as $\geq 3$ probable or confirmed cases within $\leq 3$ months for a primary attack rate of $\geq 10$ cases/100,000 population.

[e]Limited data on antibody response; consider giving $>1$ dose.

[f]Give dose $\geq 2$ weeks before chemotherapy or $\geq 3$ months after the end of chemotherapy [*MMWR Morb Mortal Wkly Rep* 42(RR-04), 1993].

**Table F-2.** Passive immunization

| Disease | Indications and dosage |
|---|---|
| Diphtheria | Suspected respiratory tract diphtheria: diphtheria antitoxin (DAT–equine source), 20,000–120,000 U IM (IV for serious illness) after cultures taken (given in addition to antibiotics). Not routinely recommended for household contacts given significant risk of anaphylaxis (7%) and serum sickness (5%) and equivalent efficacy of antimicrobial prophylaxis (benzathine penicillin, 1.2 million U IM × 1, or erythromycin, 1 g/d in divided doses × 7–10 d). |
| Hepatitis A | **Post-exposure:** within 14 d of known exposure of high-risk persons [unvaccinated household and sexual contacts of infected individual; coworkers of infected food handlers; all staff and children at day care centers where ≥ 1 case has occurred or when cases occur in ≥ 2 households of center attendees; consider for family members of diapered children who attend such a day care center during outbreaks (cases in ≥ 3 families)]: IG, 0.02 ml/kg IM.[a] IG not indicated for casual contacts (e.g., office coworkers). |
| Hepatitis B | **Pre-exposure:** Vaccine prophylaxis preferred (Table F-1).<br>**Post-exposure**: see Table F-5. |
| Measles | For nonimmune contacts within 6 d of exposure: IG, 0.25 ml/kg (maximum 15 ml) for normal host; 0.5 ml/kg (maximum 15 ml) for immunocompromised patients. MMR vaccine may provide some protection if given within 72 hr of initial exposure. |
| Rabies | See Table F-4. |
| Tetanus | See Table F-3. |
| Varicella | Vaccine, 0.5 ml SC within 3 d of exposure (possibly effective up to 5 d post-exposure) or varicella-zoster IG, 1 vial (125 U) IM for each 10 kg body weight (minimum, 125 U; maximum, 625 U) within 96 hr of exposure (optimal if given within 48 hr) [*MMWR Morb Mortal Wkly Rep* 45 (RR-11):1–25, 1996]. |

DAT, direct antiglobulin test; MMR, measles, mumps, rubella.
[a]Anaphylaxis has been reported after injection of IG in IgA-deficient persons. Live attenuated vaccines [MMR, varicella-zoster virus (VZV)] should be delayed after administration of IG (3 mo for MMR, 5 mo for VZV). Patients who received MMR within 2 wk before IG or VZV within 3 wk before IG should be revaccinated.

**Table F-3.** Tetanus prophylaxis

| History of tetanus immunization (doses) | Clean, minor wounds | | Other wounds | |
|---|---|---|---|---|
| | Give Td | Give TIG | Give Td | Give TIG |
| Unknown or <3 doses | Yes | No | Yes | Yes |
| ≥ 3 doses | No if dose within 10 yr; otherwise yes | No | Yes unless last dose within 5 yr | No |

Td, adult tetanus-diphtheria booster; TIG, tetanus immune globulin, 250 U IM, given concurrently with Td at a separate site.

## Management of Rabies

I. **Pre-exposure vaccination** is indicated for persons in high-risk groups, including laboratory workers, veterinarians, animal handlers, and international travelers.[a]

  A. The **dose** is three 1.0-ml injections of human diploid cell vaccine (HDCV),[b] rabies vaccine adsorbed, or purified chick embryo cell vaccine IM (deltoid) on days 0, 7, and 21 or 28.

  B. **Contraindications.** Intradermal HDCV should not be given to travelers taking antimalarial prophylaxis (IM should be used instead).

  C. **Research laboratory and vaccine production workers** should have serum rabies antibody testing every 6 months; spelunkers, veterinarians and staff, animal control and wildlife officers in areas where rabies is enzootic, and laboratory workers who perform rabies diagnostic testing should have serum rabies antibody testing every 2 years.

  D. **Pre-exposure booster vaccination** should be given to people in the above groups to maintain serum titer corresponding to complete neutralization at a 1:5 serum dilution by the rapid fluorescent focus inhibition test.

II. **Post-exposure rabies therapy.** See Table F-4.

  A. For **bats and wild animals,** capturing and sacrificing the animal and performing immunofluorescence on brain tissue provide definitive determination of the animal's rabies status. Except in cases of bites or scratches on the head or neck or bat exposure, it is reasonable to wait for diagnostic testing on the animal before instituting post-exposure therapy. If diagnostic testing on animal brain tissue is negative, no post-exposure therapy is necessary.

  B. **For bites or scratches on the head or neck,** post-exposure therapy should be instituted immediately because of proximity to the central nervous system and potentially shorter incubation period.

  C. **Any bat exposure warrants therapy.** Potential bat exposures also warrant therapy if there is any possibility of an unobserved bite or scratch (i.e., person sleeping in a room, unattended child, demented or obtunded adult).

---

[a]If contact with potentially rabid animals and limited access to medical care are likely.
[b]HDCV can also be given intradermally; the intradermal dose is 0.1 ml on days 0, 7, and 21 or 28.

**Table F-4.** Post-exposure rabies therapy

| Species | Condition of animal at time of attack | Treatment of exposed[a] persons |
|---|---|---|
| Domestic cat, dog, ferret | Healthy and available for 10 d of observation | None unless animal develops rabies |
| | Rabid or suspected rabid | RIG and vaccine[b] |
| | Unknown | Contact public health department |
| Bat[a] | Any | RIG and vaccine[b] |
| Wild skunk, fox, coyote, raccoon, or other carnivore | Unknown; to be regarded as rabid unless proven negative by laboratory testing | RIG and vaccine[b] |
| Wild or domestic rodents (squirrels, rats, mice) and lagomorphs (rabbits, hares) | Unknown: rarely infected with rabies | Contact local health department |

RIG, rabies immunoglobulin.

[a]Exposure: bites or scratches, or animal saliva contaminating abrasions, open wounds, or mucous membranes *except for bats*. **Any bat exposure or potential bat exposures warrants therapy.**

[b]RIG: Administer once to previously unvaccinated persons, 20 IU/kg; best if done immediately (can be given through seventh day after first dose of vaccine administered). Full dose should be infiltrated around wound(s); inject remaining RIG IM at site distant from vaccine administration. **Do not** administer RIG in same syringe or at same anatomic site as vaccine. Previously vaccinated persons (those who received one of the recommended regimens of human diploid cell vaccine, rabies vaccine adsorbed, or purified chick embryo cell vaccine and had a documented rabies antibody titer): two IM 1.0-ml doses of vaccine, days 0 (immediately) and 3.

Vaccine: Five 1-ml doses on days 0, 3, 7, 14, and 28 IM in deltoid (anterolateral aspect of thigh acceptable for children). Gluteal area should not be used, as this results in lower neutralizing antibody titers.

**Table F-5.** Blood-borne pathogen post-exposure guidelines[a]

| Pathogen | Treatment |
|---|---|
| HIV[b] | For percutaneous injury (e.g., bloody needle-stick) or prolonged, excessive exposure of mucous membrane or nonintact skin to blood, blood-contaminated fluids, or potentially infectious material (e.g., cerebrospinal fluid, amniotic fluid), one of the following drug regimens for 4 wk (determine based on resistance in source patient and geographic area): (1) zidovudine, 200 mg PO tid (or 300 mg PO bid), plus lamivudine (3TC), 150 mg PO bid, or (2) 3TC, 150 mg PO bid, plus stavudine (d4T), 40 mg PO bid, or (3) didanosine, 400 mg PO qd, plus d4T, 40 mg PO bid. For highest-risk exposure (e.g., large blood volumes, high HIV viral load, hollow-bore needle), indinavir, 800 mg PO tid, or nelfinavir, 750 mg PO tid, or abacavir, 300 mg PO bid, or efavirenz, 600 mg PO qhs, can be added; consult with experts in occupational health or infectious diseases[c]; occupational health follow-up essential [*MMWR Morb Mortal Wkly Rep* 50(RR-11);1–42, 2001]. |
| | For exposures to other material (e.g., urine), therapy is not recommended. |
| Hepatitis B | For percutaneous injury with blood or blood-contaminated fluids: |
| | Unvaccinated health care worker: Administer hepatitis B immunoglobulin (HBIG), 0.06 ml/kg IM, within 96 hr of exposure; start hepatitis B vaccine series. |
| | Vaccinated health care worker: Check anti-HBs titer. If ≥ 10 IU/ml, no therapy. If <10 IU/ml, give HBIG, 0.06 ml/kg, and booster dose of vaccine or 2 doses of HBIG 1 mo apart (this preferred for health care workers known not to have responded to second vaccine series). |
| Hepatitis C | Immunoglobulin not effective. Ensure occupational health follow-up for baseline and subsequent follow-up testing. |

[a]All blood and body fluid exposures should be reported to the occupational health department. Source patients should be tested for HIV (with consent), hepatitis B surface antigen (HbsAg), and hepatitis C antibody (anti-HCV).

[b]For exposure to patients with known HIV or at high risk for HIV, post-exposure prophylaxis should be started as soon as possible (preferably within 1–2 hr, because there is less evidence for efficacy in preventing transmission after 24–36 hr).

[c]Other antiretrovirals may be indicated if there is a high likelihood that the source patient has drug resistance to components of the standard regimen. If therapy is started for a patient with suspected HIV, it can be stopped if the patient's HIV antibody test is negative, unless there is a high suspicion of acute HIV illness.

## Post-Exposure Prophylaxis Resources

| | |
|---|---|
| National Clinicians Post-exposure Hotline | Telephone: 1-888-448-4911<br>http://www.ucsf.edu/hivcntr |
| CDC (for reporting HIV seroconversions in health care workers with and without post-exposure prophylaxis) | Telephone: 1-800-893-0485 |
| Antiretroviral Pregnancy Registry | Telephone: 1-800-258-4263<br>http://www.apregistry.com |
| U.S. FDA (for reporting unusual or severe toxicity to antiretroviral agents) | Telephone: 1-800-322-1088<br>http://www.fda.gov/medwatch |
| Hepatitis Hotline | Telephone: 1-888-443-7232<br>http://www.cdc.gov/hepatitis |

**Table F-6.** Post-exposure prophylaxis for Centers for Disease Control and Prevention (CDC) class A bioterrorism agents[a]

| Pathogen | Treatment |
|---|---|
| Anthrax | For inhalational exposure, the ACIP recommends that the CDC make vaccination with three doses of AVA available under an investigational drug protocol, to be given 0.5 ml SC at 0, 2, and 4 wk[b]; anthrax vaccine is not currently licensed for use in post-exposure prophylaxis. If vaccine is given, one of the following antibiotic regimens is recommended × 7–14 d after the third dose of vaccine. If antibiotics alone are used, they should be continued for 60 d [*MMWR Morb Mortal Wkly Rep* 51(45):1024–1026, 2002].<br>After exposure to cutaneous or GI anthrax, consider using one of the following antibiotic regimens for 7–14 d:<br>Adults: Ciprofloxacin, 500 mg PO bid *or* doxycycline, 100 mg PO bid<br>Children: Ciprofloxacin, 10–15 mg/kg PO q12h or<br>Doxycycline:<br>>8 yr and >45 kg: 100 mg PO bid<br>>8 yr and ≤ 45 kg: 2.2 mg/kg/dose PO bid<br>≤ 8 yr: 2.2 mg/kg/dose PO bid |
| Botulinum toxin | Close observation of exposed person, treat with equine antitoxin at first sign of illness |
| Pneumonic plague | For close contacts (<2 m), doxycycline, 100 mg PO bid, or ciprofloxacin, 500 mg PO bid for 7 d is preferred (see above for pediatric dosing); chloramphenicol, 25 mg/kg/dose qid is alternative (not used in children <2 yr old); watch closely for fever or cough, promptly initiate parenteral therapy with streptomycin, 1 g IM bid, or gentamicin in symptomatic patients |
| Tularemia | If attacks identified during early incubation period: ciprofloxacin or doxycycline, PO × 14 d (see above for dosing); if attack unrecognized until multiple people ill, observe exposed closely, initiate parenteral therapy at first sign of illness |
| Smallpox | Vaccinate[c] ideally within 3 d of exposure; vaccination 4–7 d after exposure may offer some protection |

ACIP, Advisory Committee on Immunization Practices; AVA, anthrax vaccine adsorbed.
[a]In the event of a bioterrorism attack, the latest recommendations can be accessed via the U.S. Centers for Disease Control and Prevention internet site: http://www.bt.cdc.gov.
[b]The efficacy of alternative dosing schedules is currently under investigation. Contraindications to vaccination are a previous history of anthrax infection or a history of anaphylaxis after AVA or any vaccine components.
[c]An individualized assessment of risks and benefits of vaccination must be made. In general, vaccination for contacts of smallpox cases is recommended even in the presence of usual contraindications (history of or presence of eczema; atopic dermatitis; other acute, chronic, or exfoliative skin conditions; immunosuppression; pregnancy or intent to become pregnant within 4 wk; breastfeeding; age <1 yr). If an exposed person declines vaccination, the alternative strategy is isolation for 19 d.

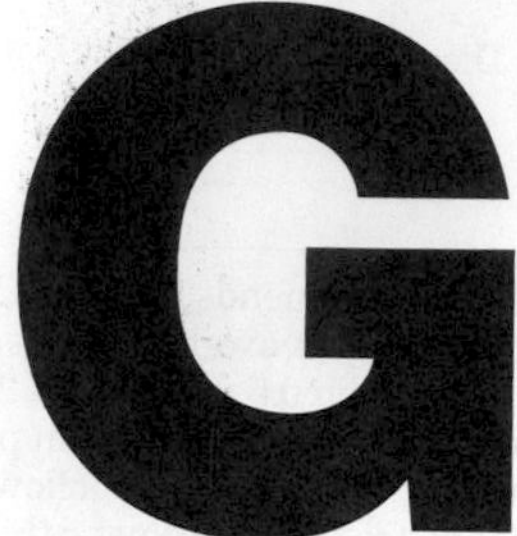

# Infection Control and Isolation Recommendations

Victoria J. Fraser and
Alexis M. Elward

I. **Standard precautions** should be practiced on **all patients at all times** to minimize the risk of nosocomial infection (previously called *body substance isolation* or *universal precautions*).

   A. **Perform hand hygiene,** preferably with an alcohol-based rub or foam, before and after direct patient contact, after contact with the environment, between caring for different patients, and after removing gloves. Soap and water should be used for visibly contaminated hands [*MMWR Morb Mortal Wkly Rep* 51(RR-16):1–45, 2002].

   B. **Wear gloves** when direct contact with moist body substances (e.g., blood, sputum, urine, pus, stool) is anticipated.

   C. **Wear a gown** when clothing is likely to be soiled by a body fluid.

   D. **Wear a mask and goggles or glasses** when splashes of a body fluid are anticipated (e.g., during most invasive procedures).

II. **Specific isolation categories.** In addition to precautions that should be followed for all patients, certain diseases, depending on their mode of spread, **require additional isolation precautions.** Categories and indications for their use may vary slightly among different hospitals. Contact an infection control specialist if there is any uncertainty about what type of isolation a patient might need. The following categories are those suggested by the Centers for Disease Control and Prevention.

   A. **Airborne precautions**

      1. Use a negative-pressure room.
      2. Keep doors closed.
      3. Wear a **respirator, grade N95 or better,** certified by the National Institute for Occupational Safety and Health **(not a surgical mask)** if entering the room of a patient who is suspected of having tuberculosis.
      4. For patients with measles or varicella (e.g., chickenpox) infections, immune persons may enter the room without a mask. Nonimmune persons ideally should not enter the room of such patients, but, if it is absolutely necessary that they enter, they should wear a mask.
      5. If patient transport is absolutely necessary, the patient should wear a **surgical** mask.
      6. Instruct the patient to cover his or her mouth when coughing or sneezing, even if alone.

   B. **Droplet precautions**

      1. Keep doors closed.
      2. Wear a surgical mask if entering the room.
      3. Discard mask **after** leaving the room.
      4. If patient transport is absolutely necessary, the patient should wear a **surgical** mask.

   C. **Contact precautions**

      1. Wear a gown and gloves to enter the room.
      2. Use a dedicated stethoscope and thermometer.
      3. Remove gown and gloves before leaving the room.

4. Perform hand hygiene with an alcohol-based rub or foam or antimicrobial soap before leaving the room.

**III. Isolation for specific infections and duration of isolation** (Tables G-1 and G-2)

**Table G-1.** Isolation for specific infections and duration of isolation

| Isolation type and diseases | Duration of isolation |
|---|---|
| **Airborne** | |
| Tuberculosis (TB) | Until TB is ruled out with three negative acid-fast bacilli smears on consecutive days. (If patient has documented or strongly suspected TB, isolation for hospitalized patients should continue for at least 2 wk of therapy with a good clinical response; however, patients can be discharged during this time if proper follow-up has been arranged with the local health department.) |
| Measles[a] | 4 d after start of rash or for duration of illness if patient is immunocompromised |
| Chickenpox[a]/disseminated zoster[a] | Until all lesions crusted. (Note: Nonimmune persons are potentially contagious days 8–21 after exposure to varicella-zoster virus.) |
| **Droplet** | |
| Adenovirus (pneumonia) | Duration of illness |
| Diphtheria (pharyngeal) | Until cultures are negative (at least 24 hr after stopping antibiotics) |
| Influenza | Duration of illness |
| Meningitis | 24 hr after start of therapy for known or suspected *Neisseria meningitidis* or *Haemophilus influenzae*. This is prudent for all meningitis initially. |
| Mumps[a] | 9 d after onset of swelling |
| Mycoplasma | Duration of illness |
| Parvovirus B19[b] | 7 d for aplastic crisis or for duration of illness if patient is immunosuppressed |
| Pertussis | 5 d after start of therapy |
| Plague (pneumonic) | 72 hr after start of therapy |
| Rubella[b] | 7 d after onset of rash; for congenital rubella place infant on contact precautions during any admission until 1 yr of age unless nasopharyngeal and urine cultures negative after age 3 mo |
| Streptococcal pharyngitis, pneumonia, or scarlet fever in infants and young children | 24 hr after start of therapy |
| **Contact** | |
| Acute infectious diarrhea | Duration of illness |
| Abscess/draining wound | Duration of illness |

(*continued*)

**Table G-1.** Continued

| Isolation type and diseases | Duration of isolation |
|---|---|
| *Clostridium difficile* | Until diarrhea resolves or treatment completed |
| Enterovirus | Duration of illness |
| Herpes simplex (neonatal, primary or disseminated mucocutaneous, severe) | Duration of illness |
| Hepatitis A | Until 1 wk after onset of symptoms |
| Parainfluenza | Duration of illness |
| Respiratory syncytial virus (infants, young children, and immunocompromised adults) | Duration of illness |
| Scabies | 24 hr after start of therapy |
| Viral conjunctivitis ("pink eye") | Duration of illness |
| Oxacillin-resistant *Staphylococcus aureus* | Duration of hospitalization and future hospitalizations[c] |
| Vancomycin-resistant or intermediate-sensitive *S. aureus* | Duration of hospitalization and future hospitalizations[c] |
| Vancomycin-resistant enterococci | Duration of hospitalization and future hospitalizations[c] |
| Multidrug-resistant gram-negative bacteria | Duration of hospitalization and future hospitalizations[c] |

[a]Nonimmune persons should stay out of room if possible.
[b]Nonimmune pregnant women should stay out of room (Barnes-Jewish Hospital policy, not an official Centers for Disease Control and Prevention recommendation).
[c]Unless criteria for discontinuing isolation have been met; consult hospital infection control specialists for specific criteria.

**Table G-2.** Isolation for Centers for Disease Control and Prevention class A[a] agents of bioterrorism

| Isolation type and agent | Duration of isolation |
|---|---|
| **Airborne** | |
| Smallpox[b] | Duration of hospitalization or until scabs fall off |
| Viral hemorrhagic fevers[c] | Duration of hospitalization |
| **Droplet** | |
| Pneumonic plague (*Yersinia pestis*) | Until 72 hr after start of antimicrobial therapy |
| **Contact** | |
| Cutaneous anthrax | Until lesions resolve |
| **Standard precautions** | |
| Inhalational anthrax | Duration of hospitalization |
| Botulism | Duration of hospitalization |
| Tularemia | Duration of hospitalization |

[a]Six class A agents have been identified by the Centers for Disease Control and Prevention. Criteria for inclusion in class A are easily disseminated or transmitted person to person, high mortality, potential for major public health impact, potential for public panic and social disruption, and requirement for special action for public health preparedness.
[b]Contact precautions should be used in handling items potentially contaminated by infectious lesions.
[c]Lassa, Marburg, Ebola, Congo-Crimean. Droplet isolation can be used if the patient does not have prominent coughing, vomiting, diarrhea, or hemorrhaging. Private rooms with potential for conversion of air flow to negative pressure are recommended at admission to avoid later patient transport to negative-pressure isolation.

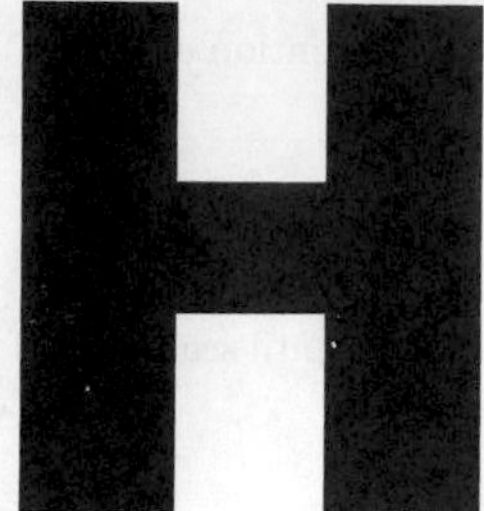

# Clinical Epidemiology

Brian F. Gage and
Bradley Evanoff

## I. Treatment

### A. Clinical trials

1. A **double-blind, randomized controlled trial** is the **gold standard** to evaluate a new treatment. After enrolling consenting patients, such trials typically assign one-half of the participants to receive the experimental therapy and one-half to receive the standard of care (often with a placebo). Participants are then followed prospectively until they experience the end point of interest or until trial termination. **End points** can be a clinical outcome (e.g., an adverse event); a surrogate outcome, such as a significant change in a laboratory value (e.g., cholesterol); or a clinical measurement (e.g., BP).

   When interpreting the results of clinical trials, **clinicians should evaluate validity** by asking the following key questions (*JAMA* 270:2598, 1993):

   **a.** Was the assignment of patients to treatments randomized?
   **b.** Were all patients who entered the trial properly accounted for and attributed at its conclusion?
   **c.** Was follow-up complete?
   **d.** Were patients analyzed in the groups to which they were randomized?
   **e.** Were patients, health workers, and study personnel blind to treatment?
   **f.** Were the groups similar at the start of the trial?
   **g.** Aside from the experimental intervention, were the groups treated equally?

2. **To quantify the risks and benefits of a therapy,** clinicians use standard epidemiologic concepts.

   **a. Patient-years** is the product of the number of patients multiplied by their length of observation in years.
   **b. Incidence rate** can be calculated by dividing the number of adverse events by the number of patient-years.
   **c. Absolute risk reduction (ARR)** is the difference between two incidence rates: $Rate_{therapy} - Rate_{control}$.
   **d. Number needed to treat (NNT)** is the number of patients that have to receive the therapy to prevent one adverse event. NNT can be calculated by taking the reciprocal of ARR (1/ARR).
   **e. Relative risk (RR)** is the ratio of the rate in the experimental group divided by the rate in the control group: $Rate_{therapy}/Rate_{control}$. Studies that compare rates using time-to-event analyses (e.g., Cox proportional hazard regression) often report the **hazard rate,** which is similar to the RR.
   **f. Relative risk reduction (RRR)** is 1 – RR.

### B. Observational studies

Most medical treatments have not been evaluated by double-blinded, randomized, controlled trials. For ethical or logistical reasons, observational stud-

**Table H-1.** 2 × 2 table for an observational study

| Exposure | Disease status | |
|---|---|---|
| | Present | Absent |
| Exposed | a | b |
| Not exposed | c | d |

ies provide the best currently available data for many important questions. Common observational study designs include cohort and case-control studies.

With few exceptions (e.g., nested case-control studies), incidence rates are not available from case-control studies. Thus, the RR and related terms cannot be calculated directly from such trials. However, a similar measure, **the odds ratio (OR),** can be calculated from a case-control study. The OR is calculated from a standard 2 × 2 table (Table H-1) as ad/bc. The results of logistic regression analyses, commonly presented in the medical literature, are also expressed as ORs. For rare events, the OR accurately estimates the RR.

**II. Diagnostic tests**

**A.** Clinicians can use clinical epidemiology to help interpret the results of a physical examination finding or diagnostic test. These tests are described in terms of sensitivity and specificity (Table H-2).

In most cases, clinicians can obtain the sensitivity and specificity from the text of a journal article; however, these values can easily be calculated from raw data using a 2 × 2 table (Table H-3) and the following definitions:

1. **Sensitivity** is the proportion of diseased persons who have a positive test. Sensitivity is also called the **true positive rate** and can be calculated from a/(a + c).
2. **Specificity** is the proportion of nondiseased persons who have a negative test. Specificity is also called the **true negative rate** and can be calculated from d/(b + d).
3. **Positive predictive value** is the proportion of people with a positive test who have the disease, as calculated by a/(a + b).
4. **Negative predictive value** is the proportion of people with a negative test who are free of disease, as calculated by d/(c + d).

**B.** Before applying these results to patient care, clinicians should critically evaluate the studies about the diagnostic test by asking the following key questions (*JAMA* 271:389, 1994):

1. Was there an independent, blind comparison with a reference standard?
2. Did the study include an appropriate spectrum of patients to whom the diagnostic test will be applied?
3. Did the results of the test being evaluated influence the decision to perform the reference standard?
4. Were the methods for performing the test described in sufficient detail to permit replication?
5. Will the reproducibility of the test results and its interpretation be satisfactory in my setting?
6. Will the results change my management?
7. Will patients be better off as a result of the test?

Clinicians can calculate the posttest probability of a disease based on the pretest probability, the results of the test, and sensitivity and specificity of the test.

**C. Likelihood ratios**

The **likelihood ratio (LR)** is the likelihood that a given test result would be expected in a patient with the target disorder compared to the likelihood that a given test result would be expected in a patient without this disorder. The LR can be used to assess the value of a diagnostic test, sign, or symp-

**Table H-2.** Common diagnostic tests at Barnes-Jewish Hospital

| Test | Disease | Threshold | Sensitivity (%) | Specificity (%) |
|---|---|---|---|---|
| B-Natriuretic peptide[a] | Heart failure | >100 pg/ml | 90 | 76 |
| | | >150 pg/ml | 85 | 83 |
| Serial troponin I[b] | Myocardial infarction | >1.0 ng/ml | 90–100 | 83–96 |
| Ferritin[c] | Iron-deficiency anemia | ≤18 ng/mL | 55 | 99 |
| | | ≤45 ng/mL | 82 | 90 |
| D-Dimer, microlatex agglutination assay[d] | DVT or PE | >500 ng/ml | 96 | 39 |
| Helical CT (spiral CT)[e] | PE | 2 mm cuts on CT scan | 70–80 | 91 |
| Prostate-specific antigen[f] | Prostate cancer | ≥4 ng/ml | 18–46 | 91–98 |
| Ventilation-perfusion scan[g] | PE | High probability | 41 | 97 |
| | | High or intermediate probability | 82 | 52 |
| | | Any abnormal result (high, intermediate, or low probability) | 98 | 10 |

DVT, deep venous thrombosis; PE, pulmonary embolism.
[a]*N Engl J Med* 347:161, 2002.
[b]*Ann Emerg Med* 37:478, 2001.
[c]*Am J Med* 88:205, 1990.
[d]*Thromb Haemost* 84:770, 2000.
[e]*Ann Intern Med* 135:88, 2001.
[f]*N Engl J Med* 349:335, 2003.
[g]*JAMA* 263:2753, 1990.

tom. The LR of a positive test (LR+) can be calculated as sensitivity/(1 − specificity). High LRs (>5) make the target disorder substantially more likely in people exhibiting a given result, whereas low LRs (<0.2) make the disease substantially less likely. Likelihood ratios of approximately 1 add no useful clinical information.

**Table H-3.** 2 × 2 table for a diagnostic test

| | Disease status | |
|---|---|---|
| Test status | Present | Absent |
| Test + | a | b |
| Test − | c | d |

The LR is also useful because it allows direct calculation of the posttest odds of disease (posttest odds = pretest odds × LR). In this way, it gives information analogous to the positive or negative predictive values discussed above.

Use of the LR requires the use of **odds of disease** rather than the more familiar probability of disease. Prior probability of disease can be easily converted to pretest odds [pretest odds = prior probability/(1 – prior probability)] and posttest odds can be easily converted to posterior probability [posterior probability = posttest odds/(1 + posttest odds)]. Lists of likelihood ratios for various clinical tests and signs, as well as nomograms and calculators to simplify the use of LR, can be found at www.cebm.utoronto.ca/glossary/lrs.htm.

**D. Receiver operator characteristic (ROC) curve**

The **ROC curve** is a method to plot the discriminatory power of a test using sensitivity and specificity data. The curve plots the sensitivity and specificity of a given test at differing cut points for defining an abnormal test result. The curve thus allows direct visualization of the trade-off between sensitivity and specificity. The upper left-hand corner of the curve represents perfect sensitivity and specificity; the cut points that most closely approach this corner have the greatest discriminant ability. The upper right-hand corner maximizes sensitivity at the expense of poor specificity, whereas the lower left-hand corner maximizes specificity at the expense of sensitivity. Calculation of the area under the ROC curve also allows comparison between two different tests to see which has the greater ability to discriminate between patients with and without a disorder (Fig. H-1).

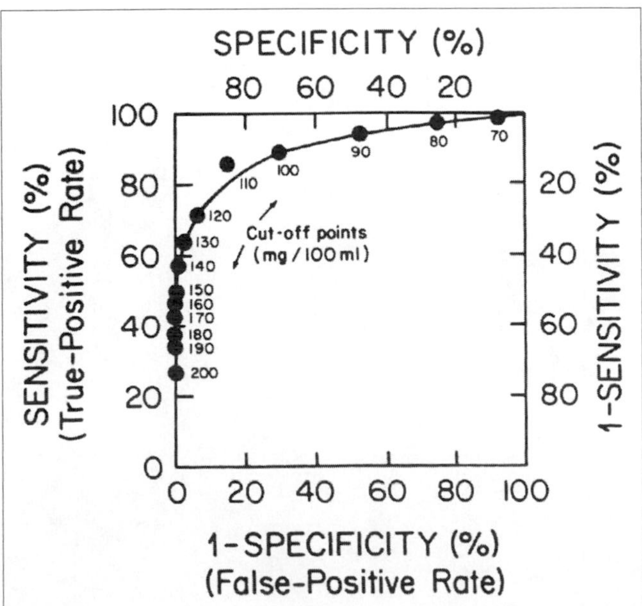


**Fig. H-1.** A receiver operator characteristic curve. The accuracy of 2-hour postprandial blood sugar as a diagnostic test for diabetes mellitus. (Data from *Diabetes Program Guide*, Public Health Service Publication No. 506, 1960.)

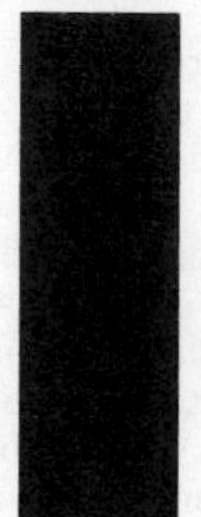

# Advanced Cardiac Life Support Algorithms

Gopa B. Green

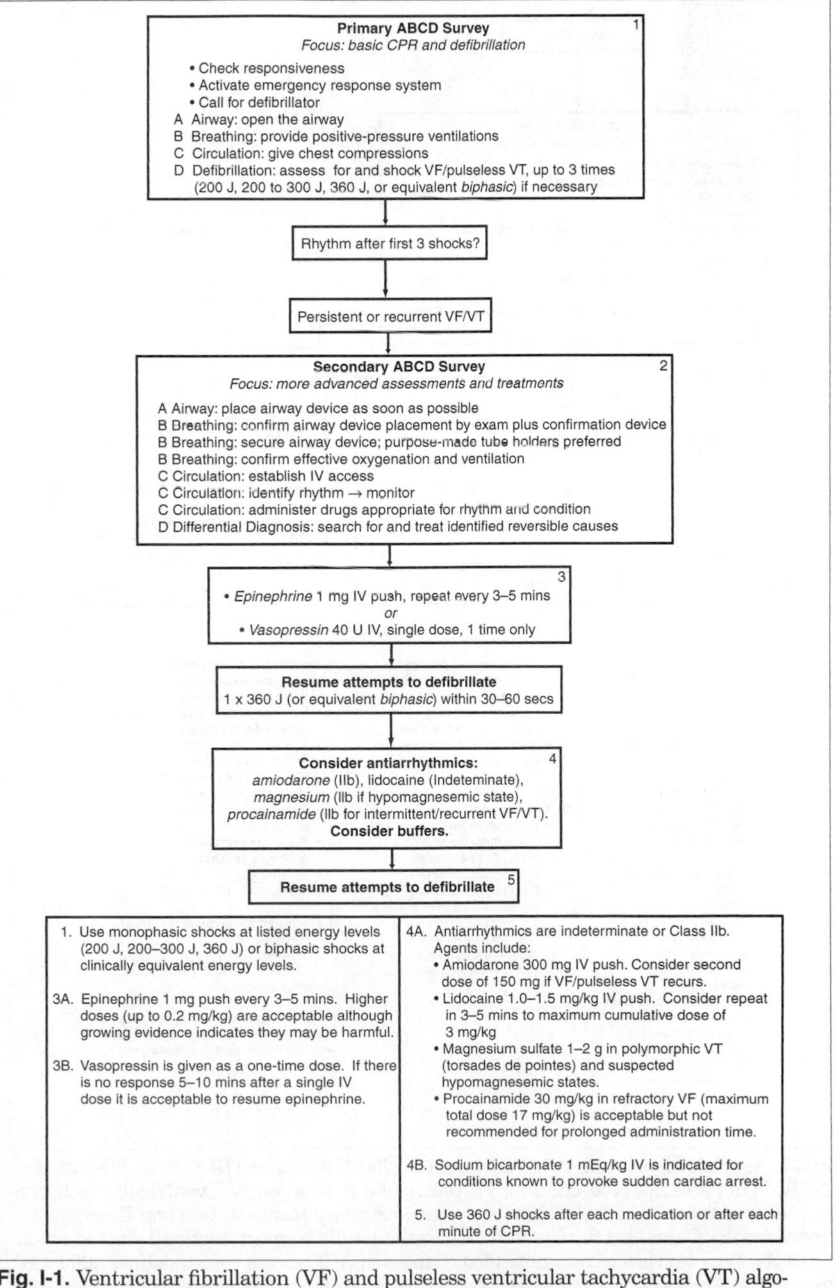


**Fig. I-1.** Ventricular fibrillation (VF) and pulseless ventricular tachycardia (VT) algorithm. [Adapted from Guidelines 2000 for Cardiopulmonary Resuscitation and Emergency Cardiovascular Care. Part 6: advanced cardiovascular life support: section 1: Introduction to ACLS 2000: overview of recommended changes in ACLS from the guidelines 2000 conference. The American Heart Association in collaboration with the International Liaison Committee on Resuscitation. *Circulation* 102(Suppl I):I86, 2000.]

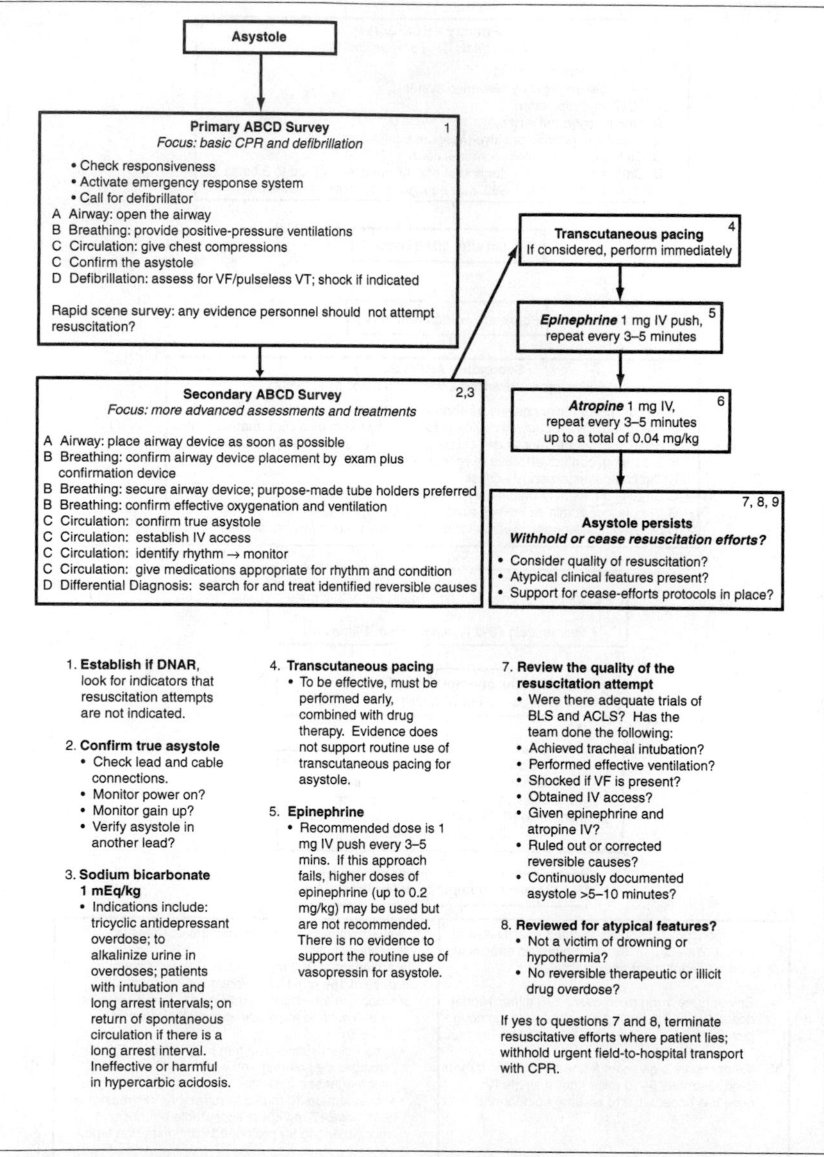

Asystole
Primary ABCD Survey 1
Focus: basic CPR and defibrillation
• Check responsiveness
• Activate emergency response system
• Call for defibrillator
A Airway: open the airway
B Breathing: provide positive-pressure ventilations
C Circulation: give chest compressions
C Confirm the asystole
D Defibrillation: assess for VF/pulseless VT; shock if indicated
Rapid scene survey: any evidence personnel should not attempt resuscitation?
Secondary ABCD Survey 2,3
Focus: more advanced assessments and treatments
A Airway: place airway device as soon as possible
B Breathing: confirm airway device placement by exam plus confirmation device
B Breathing: secure airway device; purpose-made tube holders preferred
B Breathing: confirm effective oxygenation and ventilation
C Circulation: confirm true asystole
C Circulation: establish IV access
C Circulation: identify rhythm → monitor
C Circulation: give medications appropriate for rhythm and condition
D Differential Diagnosis: search for and treat identified reversible causes
Transcutaneous pacing 4
If considered, perform immediately
Epinephrine 1 mg IV push, 5
repeat every 3–5 minutes
Atropine 1 mg IV, 6
repeat every 3–5 minutes
up to a total of 0.04 mg/kg
7, 8, 9
Asystole persists
Withhold or cease resuscitation efforts?
• Consider quality of resuscitation?
• Atypical clinical features present?
• Support for cease-efforts protocols in place?
1. Establish if DNAR, look for indicators that resuscitation attempts are not indicated.
2. Confirm true asystole
• Check lead and cable connections.
• Monitor power on?
• Monitor gain up?
• Verify asystole in another lead?
3. Sodium bicarbonate 1 mEq/kg
• Indications include: tricyclic antidepressant overdose; to alkalinize urine in overdoses; patients with intubation and long arrest intervals; on return of spontaneous circulation if there is a long arrest interval. Ineffective or harmful in hypercarbic acidosis.
4. Transcutaneous pacing
• To be effective, must be performed early, combined with drug therapy. Evidence does not support routine use of transcutaneous pacing for asystole.
5. Epinephrine
• Recommended dose is 1 mg IV push every 3–5 mins. If this approach fails, higher doses of epinephrine (up to 0.2 mg/kg) may be used but are not recommended. There is no evidence to support the routine use of vasopressin for asystole.
7. Review the quality of the resuscitation attempt
• Were there adequate trials of BLS and ACLS? Has the team done the following:
• Achieved tracheal intubation?
• Performed effective ventilation?
• Shocked if VF is present?
• Obtained IV access?
• Given epinephrine and atropine IV?
• Ruled out or corrected reversible causes?
• Continuously documented asystole >5–10 minutes?
8. Reviewed for atypical features?
• Not a victim of drowning or hypothermia?
• No reversible therapeutic or illicit drug overdose?
If yes to questions 7 and 8, terminate resuscitative efforts where patient lies; withhold urgent field-to-hospital transport with CPR.


**Fig. I-2.** Asystole algorithm. ACLS, advanced cardiac life support; BLS, basic life support; DNAR, do not attempt resuscitation; VF, ventricular fibrillation; VT, ventricular tachycardia. [Adapted from Guidelines 2000 for Cardiopulmonary Resuscitation and Emergency Cardiovascular Care. Part 6: advanced cardiovascular life support: section 1: Introduction to ACLS 2000: overview of recommended changes in ACLS from the guidelines 2000 conference. The American Heart Association in collaboration with the International Liaison Committee on Resuscitation. *Circulation* 102(Suppl I):I86, 2000.]

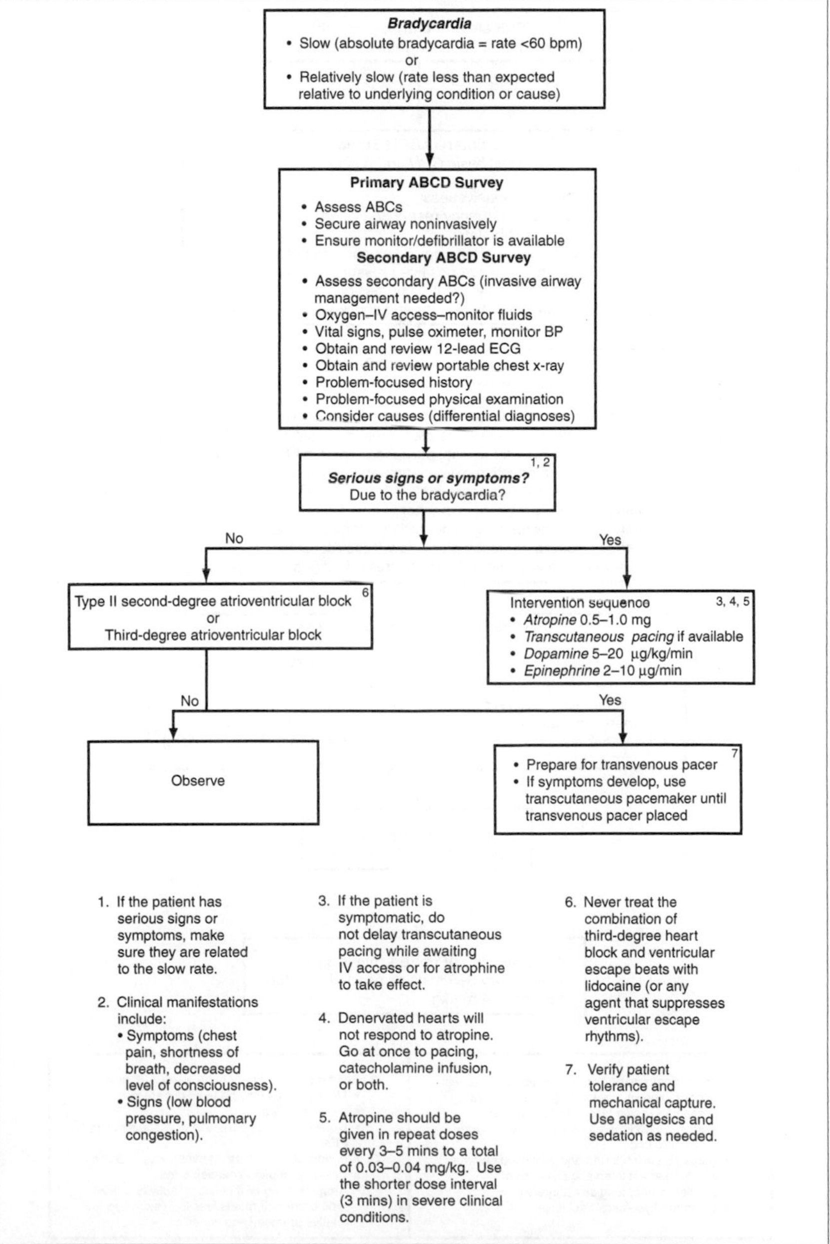


**Fig. I-3.** Bradycardia algorithm. [Adapted from Guidelines 2000 for Cardiopulmonary Resuscitation and Emergency Cardiovascular Care. Part 6: advanced cardiovascular life support: section 1: Introduction to ACLS 2000: overview of recommended changes in ACLS from the guidelines 2000 conference. The American Heart Association in collaboration with the International Liaison Committee on Resuscitation. *Circulation* 102(Suppl I):I86, 2000.]

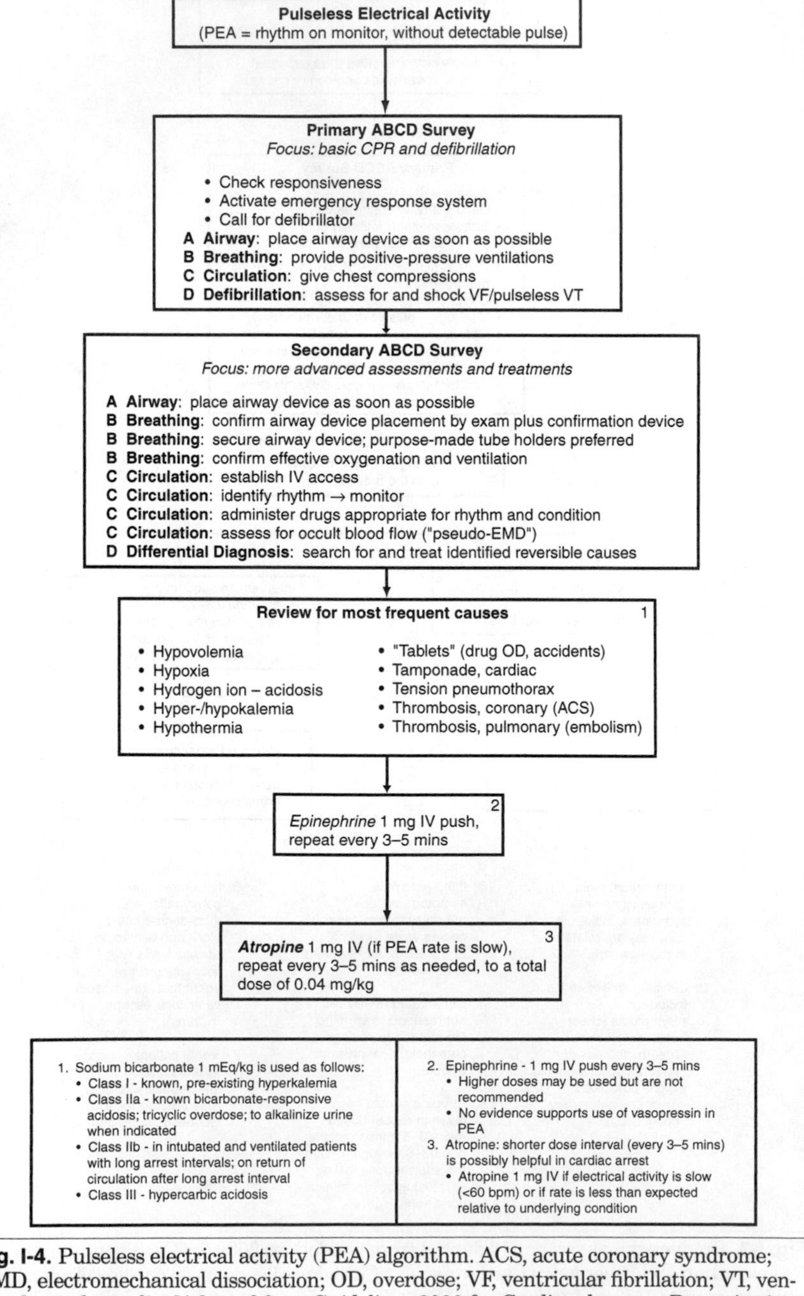


**Fig. I-4.** Pulseless electrical activity (PEA) algorithm. ACS, acute coronary syndrome; EMD, electromechanical dissociation; OD, overdose; VF, ventricular fibrillation; VT, ventricular tachycardia. [Adapted from Guidelines 2000 for Cardiopulmonary Resuscitation and Emergency Cardiovascular Care. Part 6: advanced cardiovascular life support: section 1: Introduction to ACLS 2000: overview of recommended changes in ACLS from the guidelines 2000 conference. The American Heart Association in collaboration with the International Liaison Committee on Resuscitation. *Circulation* 102(Suppl I):I86, 2000.]

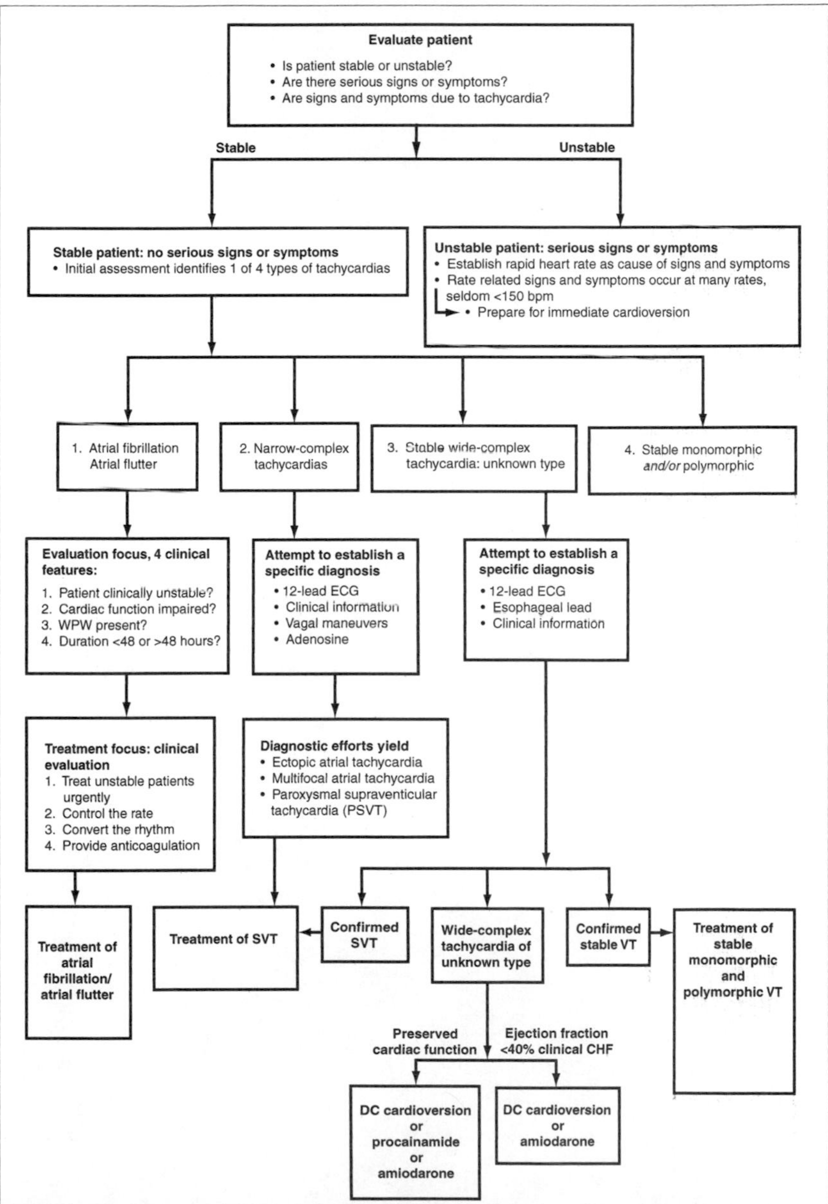


**Fig. I-5.** Tachycardia algorithm. DC, direct current; SVT, supraventricular tachycardia; VT, ventricular tachycardia; WPW, Wolff-Parkinson-White syndrome. [Adapted from Guidelines 2000 for Cardiopulmonary Resuscitation and Emergency Cardiovascular Care. Part 6: advanced cardiovascular life support: section 1: Introduction to ACLS 2000: overview of recommended changes in ACLS from the guidelines 2000 conference. The American Heart Association in collaboration with the International Liaison Committee on Resuscitation. *Circulation* 102(Suppl I):I86, 2000.]

# Index